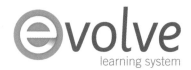
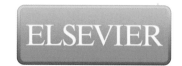
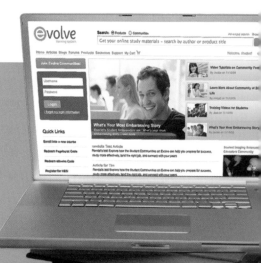
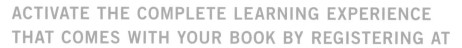
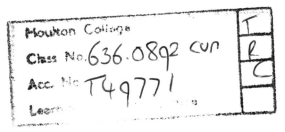

Cunningham's Textbook of

VETERINARY
PHYSIOLOGY

FIFTH EDITION

Cunningham's Textbook of
VETERINARY
PHYSIOLOGY

Bradley G. Klein, PhD

Associate Professor of Neuroscience
Department of Biomedical Sciences and Pathobiology
Virginia-Maryland Regional College of Veterinary Medicine
Virginia Polytechnic Institute and State University
Blacksburg, Virginia

ELSEVIER

3251 Riverport Lane
St. Louis, Missouri 63043

CUNNINGHAM'S TEXTBOOK OF VETERINARY PHYSIOLOGY,   ISBN: 978-1-4377-2361-8
FIFTH EDITION
Copyright © 2013, 2007, 2002, 1997, 1992 by Saunders, an imprint of Elsevier Inc.

ISBN: 978-1-4377-2361-8

Vice President and Publisher: Linda Duncan
Content Strategy Director: Penny Rudolph
Content Manager: Shelly Stringer
Content Development Specialist: Brandi Graham
Publishing Services Manager: Catherine Jackson
Senior Project Manager: Carol O'Connell
Designer: Jessica Williams
Cover Illustration: Lightbox Visual Communications Inc.

Printed in China

Last digit is the print number 9 8 7 6 5 4 3 2 1

This book is dedicated to the veterinary students
throughout the world, because it is these students who give
pleasure, meaning, and value to our teaching

CONTRIBUTORS

S. Ansar Ahmed, DVM, PhD
Department Head
Department of Biomedical Sciences & Pathobiology
Virginia-Maryland Regional College of Veterinary Medicine
Virginia Polytechnic Institute and State University
Blacksburg, Virginia

Steven P. Brinsko, DVM, MS, PhD, DACT
Professor and Chief of Theriogenology
Department of Large Animal Clinical Sciences
College of Veterinary Medicine & Biomedical Sciences
Texas A&M University
College Station, Texas

James G. Cunningham, DVM, PhD
Associate Professor Emeritus
Departments of Physiology and Small Animal Clinical Sciences
College of Veterinary Medicine
Michigan State University
East Lansing, Michigan

Autumn P. Davidson, DVM, MS, DACVIM (Internal Medicine)
Clinical Professor
Veterinary Medicine Teaching Hospital
Department of Medicine and Epidemiology
School of Veterinary Medicine
University of California-Davis
Davis, California

Deborah S. Greco, DVM, PhD, DACVIM
Senior Research Scientist
Nestle Purina Petcare
St. Louis, Missouri

Steven R. Heidemann, PhD
Professor
Department of Physiology
Michigan State University
East Lansing, Michigan

Thomas H. Herdt, DVM, MS, DACVIM, DACVN
Professor and Chief of Nutrition
Department of Large Animal Clinical Sciences and
Diagnostic Center for Population and Animal Health
College of Veterinary Medicine
Michigan State University
East Lansing, Michigan

Bradley G. Klein, PhD
Associate Professor of Neuroscience
Department of Biomedical Sciences and Pathobiology
Virginia-Maryland Regional College of Veterinary Medicine
Virginia Polytechnic Institute and State University
Blacksburg, Virginia

N. Edward Robinson, BVetMed, PhD, MRCVS, DACVIM
Matilda R. Wilson Professor
Departments of Large Animal Clinical Sciences and Physiology
College of Veterinary Medicine
Michigan State University
East Lansing, Michigan

Juan E. Romano, DVM, MS, PhD, DACT
Associate Professor
Department of Large Animal Clinical Sciences
College of Veterinary Medicine and Biomedical Sciences
Texas A&M University
College Station, Texas

Ayman I. Sayegh, DVM, MS, PhD
Professor
Department of Biomedical Sciences
College of Veterinary Medicine
Tuskegee University
Tuskegee, Alabama

Gerhardt G. Schurig, DVM, MS, PhD
Professor and Dean
Department of Biomedical Sciences & Pathobiology
Virginia-Maryland Regional College of Veterinary Medicine
Virginia Polytechnic Institute and State University
Blacksburg, Virginia

†George H. Stabenfeldt, DVM, PhD
Professor
Department of Reproduction
School of Veterinary Medicine
University of California-Davis
Davis, California

---

†Deceased

Robert B. Stephenson, PhD
Associate Professor
Department of Physiology
Michigan State University
East Lansing, Michigan

Jill W. Verlander, DVM
Associate Scientist
Department of Medicine
Division of Nephrology, Hypertension, and Renal
    Transplantation
College of Medicine
University of Florida
Gainesville, Florida

Sharon G. Witonsky, DVM, PhD, DACVIM
Associate Professor
Equine Field Service
Department of Large Animal Clinical Sciences
Virginia-Maryland Regional College of Veterinary Medicine
Virginia Polytechnic Institute and State University
Blacksburg, Virginia

PREFACE

Physiology is the study of the normal functions of the body—the study of the body's molecules, cells, and organ systems and the interrelationships among them. Because the study of medicine is the study of the abnormal functions of the body, it is essential to understand normal physiology if one is to understand the mechanisms of disease. For this reason, physiology and other important sciences basic to medicine are introduced first in the veterinary curriculum.

Physiology is a vast subject, and veterinary students are too busy to learn all that is known about it. Therefore, an effort was made to limit the concepts presented in this book to those germane to the practice of veterinary medicine. Because the scope of physiology encompasses many scientific disciplines and levels of analysis, the authors not only represent the field of physiology, but others such as neuroscience, cell biology, and molecular biology. Some of the authors are also veterinarians, but all have consulted with veterinary clinicians regarding content. Sections on the immune system and cancer underscore the intimate relationship between the understanding of cell and molecular biology, physiological function, and veterinary medicine.

This book is designed for first-year veterinary students. The goal is to introduce the student to the principles and concepts of physiology that are pertinent to the practice of veterinary medicine. Other goals are to introduce the reader to physiopathology and clinical problem-solving techniques and to help the reader understand the relationship between physiology and the practice of veterinary medicine.

This book is designed to be as student friendly as possible. New concepts in the text are introduced by a declarative statement designed to summarize the essential point. This format also helps the reader survey the chapter or review for an examination. These declarative statements are also listed at the beginning of the chapter as an outline of Key Points.

Chapters include one or more Clinical Correlations at the end. These are designed to show the reader how knowledge of physiology is applied to the diagnosis and treatment of veterinary patients. They also provide the student with an additional way to think through the principles and concepts presented, and they can serve as a basis for classroom case discussions.

Several Practice Questions are included in each chapter as another method for students to review the book's content. The brief Bibliography for each chapter is designed to lead the reader to more advanced textbooks, as veterinary students are often too busy to read original literature. However, for those who may find the time, some original literature references are also included in several chapters.

Accompanying resources for the text can be found on Elsevier's Evolve website. These include additional Practice Questions and Clinical Correlations, as well as relevant animations from Elsevier's existing collection. Instructors will appreciate the items in the illustration bank, which can be downloaded into PowerPoint format. A nascent Glossary has been added to the site that will continue to grow in subsequent editions. The terms included represent a subset of the italicized words in the printed text.

In addition to insuring that the information in this latest edition is accurate and up-to-date, some notable improvements include an expansion of the number of figures and in-text Clinical Correlations; reorganization of the introductory chapter of the Gastrointestinal Physiology and Metabolism portion; addition of sections on micturition, visceral afference, and hyperaldosteronism (Conn's Syndrome); expanded information on electrocardiogram and heart sounds, renal system transporters, feline hyperthyroidism, gut peptides, and rumen motility and digesta flow. The expertise of two authors, Drs. Ayman I. Sayegh and Juan E. Romano, has been respectively added to existing expertise in the areas of gastrointestinal physiology and male reproductive physiology. Suggestions of ways to improve this text in subsequent editions are always welcome.

Particular thanks are due to the book's medical illustrator, Mr. George Barile, who drew the new illustrations for this edition and to Ms. Jeanne Robertson who revised much of the existing artwork. Thanks are also in order for the folks at Elsevier who were instrumental in producing the fifth edition, among them Kate Dobson, Carol O'Connell, Heidi Pohlman, Penny Rudolph, Shelly Stringer, and particularly Brandi Graham who always kept a cool head and pleasant demeanor while dealing with innumerable crises and complexities. Drs. Virginia Buechner-Maxwell, Ian Herring, William Huckle, and Bonnie Smith unselfishly provided their valuable opinions on various aspects of the book that resulted in its improvement. Furthermore, this book would not exist without the invaluable expertise of the section authors/editors who worked so hard to make this the best veterinary physiology text possible. A great debt is due to Dr. Jim Cunningham, whose vision, guidance, and expertise made the *Textbook of Veterinary Physiology* a reality and a success. The instructional style he instituted continues in this edition, and will continue in future editions of the text. And last, thanks are due to the many veterinary students whose constructive suggestions for improvements have led to the current edition of the book.

Brad Klein

CONTENTS

Section III: Cardiovascular Physiology

Robert B. Stephenson

Section IV: Physiology of the Gastrointestinal Tract

Thomas H. Herdt and Ayman I. Sayegh

Section V: Endocrinology

Deborah S. Greco and †George H. Stabenfeldt

Section VI: Reproduction and Lactation

Autumn P. Davidson and †George H. Stabenfeldt
Chapter 40 by Juan E. Romano and Steven P. Brinsko

Section VII: Renal Physiology

Jill W. Verlander

†Deceased

Clinical Correlations

Edited by Sharon G. Witonsky

CHAPTER 1

The Molecular and Cellular Bases of Physiological Regulation

KEY POINTS

1. All physiological change is mediated by proteins.
2. Protein function depends on protein shape and shape changes.
3. A series of enzymatic reactions converts tyrosine into the signaling molecules dopamine, norepinephrine, and epinephrine.
4. Muscle contraction and its initiation and cessation depend on the binding specificity and allosteric properties of proteins.
5. Biological membranes are a mosaic of proteins embedded in a phospholipid bilayer.

Transport

1. Only small, uncharged molecules and oily molecules can penetrate biomembranes without the aid of proteins.
2. Molecules move spontaneously from regions of high free energy to regions of lower free energy.
3. Important transport equations summarize the contributions of the various driving forces.
4. Starling's hypothesis relates fluid flow across the capillaries to hydrostatic pressure and osmotic pressure.
5. Membrane proteins that serve the triple functions of selective transport, catalysis, and coupling can pump ions and molecules to regions of higher free energy.
6. Many membrane proteins selectively facilitate the transport of ions/molecules from high to low electrochemical potential.
7. Passive transport of K^+ across the plasma membrane creates an electrical potential.

8. Spatial organization of active and passive transport proteins enables material to pass completely through the cell.
9. Membrane fusion allows for a combination of compartmentalization and transport of material.

Information transmission and transduction

1. Cell signaling often occurs by a lengthy chain of sequential molecular interactions.
2. Signaling pathways begin with the binding of an extracellular molecule to a receptor.
3. Specific physiological information is inherent in the receptor/ligand complex, not in the hormone/neurotransmitter molecule.
4. G-protein–coupled receptors are the largest family (a *superfamily*) of receptors and help regulate almost all physiological processes.
5. Most G-protein–linked information is sent to the cytoplasm by *second messengers*.
6. Ca^{2+} transport across plasma and intracellular membranes is an important second messenger.
7. Cyclic AMP is produced by activation of a membrane-bound enzyme in response to hormone/neurotransmitter binding to receptors.
8. The receptor-mediated hydrolysis of a rare phospholipid of the plasma membrane produces two different second messengers with different actions.
9. Steroid hormones and other lipid signals interact with nuclear receptors, which are transcription factors within the cell.

Physiology is the study of the regulation of change within organisms, in this case higher animals. Our understanding of physiology has changed dramatically in the past 30 years as a result of insight into the molecular basis of biological regulation. This chapter summarizes (and simplifies considerably) our current understanding of the molecular and cellular basis of that regulation. Most of the principles in this chapter apply to all animal cells. The approach taken is one of functional molecular anatomy. That is, the molecular structure of the cell is examined with particular emphasis on the physiological function, in the intact animal, of the molecules and supramolecular structures responsible for the function. Only those aspects of cell function that illuminate the medical physiology of the higher animals are discussed; the reader is referred to the Bibliography for more complete coverage of the cell. Some review of basic concepts and vocabulary is presented. However, the discussion assumes that the reader is familiar with the cell and its constituent molecules,

as presented in courses in general biology and undergraduate courses in biochemistry.

All Physiological Change Is Mediated by Proteins

All physiological change is mediated by a single class of polymeric macromolecules (large molecules), the proteins. Protein function can be subdivided into a number of categories: catalysis, reaction coupling, transport, structure, and signaling.

Catalysis is the ability to increase greatly the rate of a chemical reaction without altering the equilibrium of the reaction. The majority of biochemical reactions occur at a physiologically useful rate only because of protein catalysts, called *enzymes*. Examples of enzymatic catalysis in the synthesis of a class of physiological regulator molecules, catecholamines, are given later in this chapter.

In *reaction coupling*, two reactions are joined together with the transfer of energy. Energy from a spontaneous reaction (similar to water flowing downhill) is funneled to a nonspontaneous reaction (e.g., sawing wood) so that the sum of the two reactions is spontaneous. That is, the energy liberated by the "downhill" reaction is used to drive the "uphill" reaction. This is the basic function of a motor; the "downhill" burning of gasoline is coupled with the "uphill" movement of the car. The ability of proteins to couple spontaneous and nonspontaneous reactions allows cells to be chemical motors, using chemical energy to do various jobs of work. One such job of work, the contraction of striated muscle, is discussed later with particular emphasis on the proteins involved.

Proteins provide a pathway for the *membrane transport* of most molecules and all ions into and out of the cell. Transport and transport proteins are discussed more fully after a discussion of the lipid bilayer membrane, the major obstacle to transport.

Proteins that form filaments and that glue cells to each other and to their environment are responsible for the *structure* and organization of cells and multicellular assemblies (i.e., the tissues and organs of animals). The internal structure of the muscle cell, as well as its ability to do work, is a result of the properties of the muscle proteins discussed later.

At its most basic level, *signaling* requires only a controlled change or difference. Human signaling occurs by way of open and closed electrical circuits (telegraphy), puffs of smoke in the air, and complex black marks on a contrasting background (numbers and letters). As discussed next, a fundamental property of proteins is the ability to change shape. The cell can use changes of protein shape directly to send signals, and the function of some proteins is purely informational. That is, all that some proteins do by changing shape is transmit and transduce information. *Information* can be defined as "any difference that makes a difference," or more simply, any difference that regulates something. Catalysis, coupling, transport, structural, and signaling functions can be combined on individual protein molecules. As will become apparent, such multifunctional proteins carry out many important physiological functions. Also important is that a change in one or more of these protein functions can be used to carry information, to serve as a signal within the cell. Thus, in addition to proteins specialized exclusively to carry information, changes in enzymatic activity or ion transport can also make a difference, transmitting information and triggering an appropriate response.

Protein Function Depends on Protein Shape and Shape Changes

Protein function is founded on two molecular characteristics: (1) proteins can bind to other molecules very specifically; and (2) proteins change shape, which in turn alters their binding properties and their function. The binding specificity of proteins is the result of their complex three-dimensional structure. Grooves or indentations on the surface of protein molecules, called *binding sites,* permit specific interactions with a molecule of a complementary shape, called the *ligand.* This complementary-shape mechanism underlying binding is similar to the shape interaction between a lock and key.

Several aspects of the lock-and-key analogy are worth noting. As with a lock, only a small part of the protein is engaged in binding. The binding is very specific; small changes in the shape of the binding site (keyhole) or the shape of the ligand (key) can cause major changes in protein (lock) behavior. Similar to the lock and key, the complementary-shape interaction serves a recognition function; only those molecules with the right shape affect protein function. This recognition function plays a primary role in information transfer. The protein recognizes a particular

signal by binding to it, thus changing the protein's shape and thus its function. Unlike the majority of locks, however, proteins frequently have multiple binding sites for multiple ligands.

Thus the three-dimensional shape of a protein, its *conformation,* determines protein function. A major force that stabilizes protein conformation is the *hydrophobic interaction.* Oily, *hydrophobic* (water-fearing) amino acids tend to congregate in the middle of a protein away from water, whereas *hydrophilic* (water-loving) amino acids tend to be found on the protein's outer surface interacting with the abundant cellular water. The hydrophobic interaction is also important in stabilizing the interaction of proteins with the lipids of biological membranes, as discussed shortly. Protein shape is also stabilized by *hydrogen bonding* between polar amino acid pairs in the polypeptide (protein) chain.

The same weak forces responsible for protein conformation are also used to hold the ligand in the protein-binding site. The position of the ligand in the binding site is stabilized by hydrogen bonds between the polar groups of the ligand and polar, amino acid side groups lining the binding site, just as hydrogen bonds within the polypeptide chain stabilize the shape of the polypeptide. Precisely because the same forces are responsible for the shape of the protein and for its binding properties, shape influences binding, and in turn, binding can influence protein shape. The ability of proteins to change shape is called *allostery* (Greek, "other shape").

Allosteric changes in protein conformation arise in four general ways. One way, just mentioned, is that most proteins change shape depending on which ligands are bound at particular binding sites (Figure 1-1, *A*). The sequence—specific ligand binding → protein shape change → change in protein-binding properties and protein function → this change regulates something—is a common molecular mechanism underlying physiological control. This method involves no alteration in the covalent structure of the protein.

A second method of producing conformational change, however, occurs as a result of the covalent modification of one or more of the amino acid side groups of the protein (see Figure 1-1, *B*). By far the most common such change is the covalent addition of a phosphate group to the hydroxyl (—OH) group on the side chain of serine, threonine, or tyrosine residues in the protein. This modification is called *phosphorylation.* Because the phosphate group is highly charged, phosphorylation of a protein alters hydrogen bonding and other electrostatic interactions within the protein chain, altering its conformation and functional properties.

In a third method, some physiologically important proteins change shape in response to the electrical field surrounding the protein (see Figure 1-1, *C*). These respond to a voltage change by altering the position of charged amino acids, thus altering protein shape.

The fourth method of protein shape change is the least well understood (not shown). Some proteins change shape in a controlled manner in response to mechanical forces. Although this is not surprising, because all solids and solidlike substances change shape at least slightly in response to force, we know relatively little about mechanosensitive proteins. The best current example is a protein involved in the very early events of hearing that changes its transport of ions in response to the mechanical stimulation by sound (small changes of air pressure in waves).

The significance of binding specificity and allostery can be better appreciated with two examples of their roles in physiological function. The first example is the role of enzymes

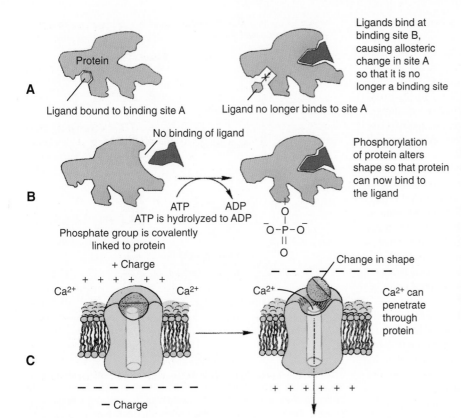

A

Protein

Ligand bound to binding site A

Ligands bind at binding site B, causing allosteric change in site A so that it is no longer a binding site

Ligand no longer binds to site A

B

No binding of ligand

ATP   ADP
ATP is hydrolyzed to ADP

Phosphate group is covalently linked to protein

Phosphorylation of protein alters shape so that protein can now bind to the ligand

C

+ Charge

+ + + + + +

Ca^{2+} Ca^{2+}

− Charge

Ca^{2+} Change in shape

Ca^{2+} can penetrate through protein

+ + + + + +

FIGURE 1-1 Three common mechanisms of allosteric shape change in proteins. **A,** Ligand binding. Ligand binding to an allosteric site (site B) on a protein changes the protein's conformation such that binding site A is altered; ligand no longer binds at site A because of the binding event at site B. **B,** Phosphorylation. Addition of a phosphate group to a serine, threonine, or tyrosine residue of a protein alters the protein's conformation, changing its binding characteristics. In this hypothetical example, phosphorylation activates an otherwise inactive protein. Some proteins inactivate by this mechanism. *ATP,* Adenosine triphosphate; *ADP,* adenosine diphosphate. **C,** Voltage-dependent proteins. The conformation of some proteins, particularly ion channels, is altered by the electrical field surrounding the protein. Shown here is the opening (activation) of a voltage-dependent, gated Ca^{2+} channel when the membrane depolarizes.

in synthesizing three small, structurally similar, nonprotein signaling molecules. This example shows how binding specificity is important in catalytic function and how allostery underlies the regulation of the synthesis. The second example is more complex: the role of proteins in the contraction of muscle. The contraction of muscle shows how proteins can exploit the basic properties of specific binding and allosteric shape change to do more than one job of work at the same time; muscle proteins serve a structural role, serve a catalytic function, and couple the "downhill" hydrolysis of *adenosine triphosphate* (ATP) to do mechanical work, the "uphill" lifting of weight.

A Series of Enzymatic Reactions Converts Tyrosine into the Signaling Molecules Dopamine, Norepinephrine, and Epinephrine

Figure 1-2 is a diagram of the series of reactions by which the amino acid tyrosine is converted into three different signaling molecules: (1) *dopamine,* a brain neurotransmitter; (2) *norepinephrine,* a neurotransmitter of the brain and peripheral autonomic nervous system; and (3) *epinephrine,* an autonomic neurotransmitter and hormone. Dopamine, norepinephrine, and epinephrine share a similar structure. All contain a phenyl (benzene) ring with two hydroxyl groups (i.e., catechol) and an amine group (thus catecholamines). They are among the large number of molecules that function as neurotransmitters. That is, the electrically coded information sent along nerve cells causes the release of a chemical, the neurotransmitter, at the terminal of the neuron, which is next to a target cell, such as another nerve, a muscle, or an endocrine cell. The electrically encoded information of the nerve is transmitted to the target cell by the binding of the neurotransmitter to proteins on the surface of the target

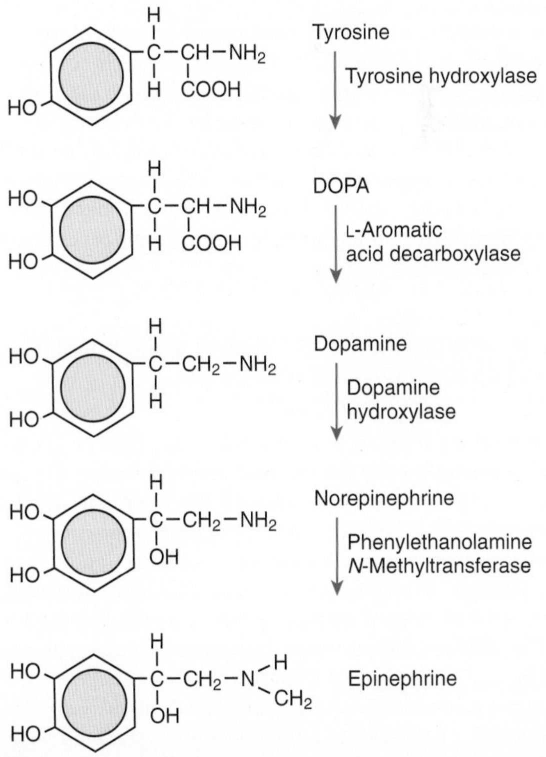

Tyrosine

Tyrosine hydroxylase

DOPA

L-Aromatic acid decarboxylase

Dopamine

Dopamine hydroxylase

Norepinephrine

Phenylethanolamine *N*-Methyltransferase

Epinephrine

FIGURE 1-2 Epinephrine biosynthetic pathway. The amino acid tyrosine is metabolized to the neurotransmitters dopamine, norepinephrine, and epinephrine. The diagram shows the names and structural formulas for each compound in the path and the names of the enzymes that catalyze each reaction. *DOPA,* Dihydroxyphenylalanine.

cell. Proper neurotransmitter synthesis is crucial to nervous function and physiological regulation.

In the first step of catecholamine biosynthesis, tyrosine binds to the enzyme tyrosine hydroxylase, which catalyzes the addition of another hydroxyl group to the phenyl group to form dihydroxyphenylalanine, almost always called *DOPA*. This hydroxyl group alters the enzyme-ligand interaction; the key no longer fits the keyhole. DOPA is released from the tyrosine hydroxylase and is then bound by another enzyme, L-aromatic amino acid decarboxylase. As the name implies, this enzyme catalyzes the removal of the carboxyl group, converting DOPA to dopamine. Dopamine is converted into norepinephrine by the activity of dopamine hydroxylase, which adds yet another hydroxyl group, this time to the two-carbon tail of dopamine. Finally, addition of a methyl group to the amino nitrogen by phenylethanolamine N-methyltransferase gives rise to epinephrine (also called *adrenalin*). Note the binding specificity of the enzymes: whereas the catecholamine structures are all similar to one another, different enzymes bind each one (e.g., epinephrine does not bind to dopamine hydroxylase).

The allosteric properties of one enzyme in this pathway provide an example of physiological regulation. Certain hormones and neurotransmitters cause the *phosphorylation* of tyrosine hydroxylase, the first enzyme in the pathway, increasing its activity. That is, phosphorylation of the enzyme increases the rate at which it catalyzes the conversion of tyrosine to DOPA. Because this step is the slowest in the pathway, an increase in the activity of this protein increases the net rate of synthesis of all the catecholamines. Regulated decreases in the rate of catecholamine synthesis are achieved by a different allosteric mechanism: binding of end products to the enzyme. Dopamine, norepinephrine, and epinephrine can all bind to tyrosine hydroxylase at a site different than the site for tyrosine. These binding events inhibit the enzymatic activity. The inhibition of the pathway by its own end products makes this a classic case of allosteric control called *end-product inhibition*. Many substances regulate their own synthesis by inhibiting an initial enzyme in the pathway. If the cell has enough end products, these products inhibit further synthesis by allosteric changes in the enzyme. This is an example of the following sequence: specific binding → protein shape change → change in protein-binding properties and protein function → this change regulates something.

Muscle Contraction and its Initiation and Cessation Depend on the Binding Specificity and Allosteric Properties of Proteins

There are three types of muscle tissue in vertebrates: (1) *skeletal muscle,* responsible for the animal's ability to move; (2) *cardiac muscle,* a muscle type found only in the heart but structurally similar to skeletal muscle; and (3) *smooth muscle,* which surrounds hollow organs such as blood vessels, gut, and uterus. All three produce tensile force by contracting and shortening the length of the muscle. All muscle contraction occurs by the binding and the allosteric properties of two proteins, actin and myosin. Starting and stopping the contraction process depends on two additional proteins in skeletal and cardiac muscle, troponin and tropomyosin. Contraction initiation and cessation in smooth muscle depend on a different system with different proteins, and are discussed later in this chapter.

Myosin is a large protein whose shape resembles a two-headed golf club. The elongated tail of the myosin molecule corresponds

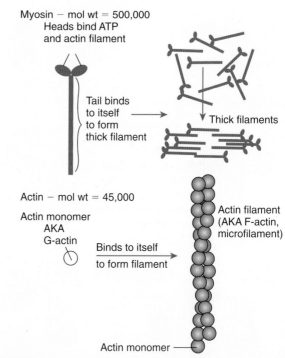

FIGURE 1-3 Assembly of myosin and actin to form filamentous structure. Myosin tails aggregate with one another to form a thick filament, a substructure of striated muscle. Actin monomers (G-actin) are a single polypeptide chain forming a globular protein that can bind to other actin monomers to form actin filament, also called microfilaments. The actin filament is the basic structure of striated muscle thin filaments; thin filaments also have troponin and tropomyosin as part of their structure.

to the shaft of the golf club, and there are two knobs at one end of the tail that, as with golf clubs, are called *heads.* Myosin tails bind specifically to other myosin tails, forming bipolar aggregates called *thick filaments* (Figure 1-3). Myosin heads specifically bind ATP and another muscle protein, actin. Actin binds to itself to form long, thin filaments, called *thin filaments* in muscle and called *F-actin* (filamentous actin) in other cell types. Actin filaments play an important architectural role in all animal cells. Although actin is best understood in muscle cells, all animal cells depend on actin filaments for their shape and for their capacity to migrate in their environment. Actin filaments can be "woven" in various ways to produce different structures, such as ropelike bundles and clothlike networks. These actin bundles and actin networks are used to support the cell in particular shapes, similar to ropes holding up the woven cloth of a tent.

In muscle, the interaction of myosin, ATP, and actin produces contraction and force, as shown in Figure 1-4:

Step A: ATP binds to a myosin head; in this conformation, myosin has little ability to bind to actin.

Step B: Enzymatic activity associated with the myosin head, an *adenosinetriphosphatase* (ATPase), rapidly causes a partial hydrolysis of ATP to *adenosine diphosphate* (ADP) and *inorganic phosphate* (P_i), both of which stay bound to the myosin. With ADP and P_i bound, myosin has a slightly different shape that binds avidly to nearby actin filaments.

Step C: When myosin binds to actin, called *cross-bridging,* the myosin head couples the complete hydrolysis of ATP to a forceful flexing of the myosin head. This allosteric change causes the actin filament to slide past the thick filament. This

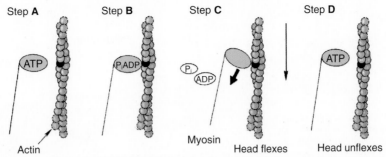

Step **A**   Step **B**   Step **C**   Step **D**

Actin   Myosin   Head flexes   Head unflexes

FIGURE 1-4 Power stroke of actomyosin. **A,** The myosin head has bound to adenosine triphosphate (ATP). In this conformation, myosin has little affinity to bind to actin. **B,** ATP is partially hydrolyzed to adenosine diphosphate (ADP) and inorganic phosphate (P_i); the hydrolysis is partial because the products remain bound to the myosin head. The change in what is bound to the myosin (ADP and P_i, not ATP) has the conformation of myosin so that it binds to actin with high affinity. **C,** Hydrolysis is complete; myosin releases ADP and P_i. This change in what is bound at the myosin head causes an allosteric change in the head; it flexes. Because the myosin head is still bound to the thin filament, the flexion causes the thin filament to slide past the thick filament. **D,** New ATP molecule binds to the myosin head; as for step A, myosin had little affinity for actin in this state, and the head releases from the thin filament and unflexes.

sliding puts the actin filament under tension, which in turn causes the muscle to contract (shorten) against the load of the muscle (i.e., lifting a weight or pumping out blood). All muscle contraction depends on this *sliding filament mechanism* of actin and myosin-based filaments. This same allosteric change of myosin also alters myosin-binding properties so that it releases the ADP and P_i.

Step D: The binding of a new ATP molecule to the myosin head again causes myosin to change shape; the head unflexes and loses its affinity for actin, releasing the cross-bridge, and the cycle can start over. *Rigor mortis* of dead animals is caused by a lack of new ATP to bind to myosin heads. In the absence of ATP, myosin heads remain in Step C (i.e., bound to actin). The muscle is stiff because it is completely cross-bridged together.

This *actomyosin motor* uses the binding and allosteric properties of proteins to (1) create structural filaments capable of withstanding and transmitting mechanical force, (2) catalyze the hydrolysis of ATP, and (3) couple the "downhill" ATP hydrolysis to the "uphill" contraction to produce force. For just the one protein, myosin, there are a number of examples of the characteristic sequence described earlier: specific binding → protein shape change → change in protein-binding properties and protein function → this change makes a difference.

This system of contractile proteins requires some control so that, for example, the heart beats rhythmically and skeletal muscle contraction is coordinated. At the organismal level, skeletal and cardiac muscle contraction is primarily under control by electrical stimulation from nerves or other electrically active cells (see Chapter 6). The transmission of electrical excitation to the actomyosin system is called *excitation-contraction coupling. Excitation-contraction coupling in all types of muscle depends on changes in intracellular calcium ion (Ca^{2+}) concentration.* In skeletal and cardiac muscle, but not smooth muscle, two additional thin-filament proteins, troponin and tropomyosin, are required for this coupling. (Excitation-contraction coupling for smooth muscle is discussed later in this chapter.) In striated muscles, *troponin* binds to tropomyosin and to Ca^{2+}. *Tropomyosin* is a long, thin protein that binds in the groove of the actin filament in such a way that its positions, high in the groove or snuggled down deep in the groove, allow or prevent the myosin head access to the thin

filament (Figure 1-5). Excitation-contraction coupling of striated muscle works as follows:

Step A: Electrical excitation of a striated muscle cell causes an increase in the intracellular concentration of Ca^{2+}.

Step B: The additional Ca^{2+} binds to troponin, causing an allosteric change in troponin.

Step C: Because Ca^{2+} is bound to troponin, which in turn is bound to tropomyosin, the Ca^{2+}-induced change in troponin conformation is transmitted to the tropomyosin molecule. When troponin binds Ca^{2+}, tropomyosin changes its binding to actin in such a way that it exposes the actin site for myosin cross-bridging. (Tropomyosin snuggles down deeper in its actin groove, revealing actin to the myosin head.) As long as troponin binds Ca^{2+}, the muscle contracts by the actomyosin cycle outlined earlier.

Step D: When the Ca^{2+} concentration drops to normal, however, troponin no longer binds Ca^{2+}. This causes tropomyosin to move up in the thin filament groove so that it again blocks the myosin-binding sites on actin. Myosin heads can no longer cross-bridge, and muscle contraction stops.

As with the actomyosin force generation itself, its regulation also shows many examples of the specific binding function. The specific binding of Ca^{2+} to troponin is a purely informational use of protein binding and shape change; that is, troponin has no catalytic, transport, or structural function, but transmits the "on" signal to the next protein. The binding of tropomyosin to actin serves not only a regulatory role but also a structural role; the actin filament is stabilized by tropomyosin, making it less likely to disassemble into actin subunits. The change in the binding geometry of tropomyosin that directly regulates myosin access to actin is a good example of the importance of allosteric change and the following sequence: specific binding (troponin to tropomyosin) → protein (tropomyosin) shape change → change in protein-binding properties (tropomyosin to actin) → a difference in the position of tropomyosin, which in turn regulates the actomyosin motor.

Biological Membranes Are a Mosaic of Proteins Embedded in a Phospholipid Bilayer

Before continuing the discussion of the cellular basis of physiological control, an additional basic structure must be introduced.

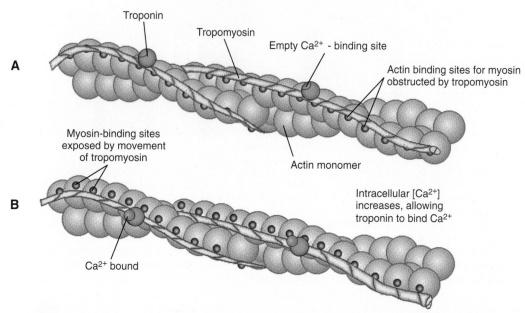

A

B

FIGURE 1-5 Regulation of the actomyosin ATPase and striated muscle contraction by Ca^{2+}. **A,** In the absence of high concentrations of Ca^{2+}, tropomyosin sits in the groove of the actin filament to obstruct the binding sites on actin for myosin. **B,** In the presence of higher Ca^{2+} concentrations, the ion binds to troponin, causing an allosteric change in the interaction of troponin with tropomyosin. This allosteric change in turn changes the interaction of tropomyosin with the actin filament to expose the myosin-binding sites on actin.

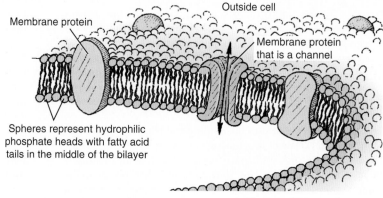

FIGURE 1-6 Fluid mosaic model for biomembranes. Biomembranes consist of a lipid bilayer in which membrane proteins are embedded.

This is the phospholipid bilayer of the biomembranes of cells. *Phospholipids* are molecules that have two long tails of hydrophobic fatty acid and a head containing a charged, hydrophilic phosphate group. Under appropriate aqueous conditions, these molecules spontaneously form an organized membrane structure, similar to the film of a soap bubble. This filmy layer is composed of two layers (a bilayer) of phospholipid molecules. In both layers the hydrophilic heads point outward to hydrogen bond with water, and the oily, fatty-acid tails point inward, toward one another and away from the water. Proteins embedded in this lipid bilayer, called *intrinsic membrane proteins* or just *membrane proteins*, produce the fluid mosaic structure of biomembranes shown in Figure 1-6. All biological membranes share this *fluid mosaic* structure, whether the membrane is the outer plasma membrane separating cytoplasm from extracellular fluid or the membrane surrounding intracellular membranous organelles such as endoplasmic reticulum or lysosomes. It is called a fluid mosaic because of the mosaic of proteins among phospholipids, and because the phospholipid layer is fluid; proteins can move around and diffuse within the plane of the bilayer "like icebergs floating in a phospholipid sea" (the apt phrase of S. J. Singer, one of the originators of the model).

Biological membranes are another crucial molecular structure underlying physiological control. The basic fluid mosaic structure serves four broad functions: (1) compartmentation, (2) selective transport, (3) information processing and transmission, and (4) organizing biochemical reactions in space.

Compartmentation is the ability to separate and segregate different regions by composition and function. For example, the lysosome is a membranous organelle within cells that contains hydrolytic (digestive) enzymes that can potentially digest the cell. The lysosomal membrane compartmentalizes these potentially harmful enzymes, segregating them from the bulk cytoplasm. The rigor mortis, mentioned earlier, that begins shortly after death is transitory because on death the lysosomes begin to break open, releasing their enzymes, and the actomyosin cross-bridges are eventually digested apart.

Clearly, the membrane cannot keep a compartment perfectly sealed; material must enter and leave the cell and its internal compartments. *Selective transport* results partly from the properties of the phospholipid bilayer but mostly from transport proteins embedded in the membrane. These proteins are characteristically selective in their transport functions; for example, the protein that is the specialized ion channel underlying neuronal signaling is 15 times more permeable to sodium ions (Na^+) than to potassium ions (K^+). Transport is a major topic of cell physiology and is discussed in more detail later.

If the cells of an organism are to respond to external changes, they must receive information about the state of the outside world. Just as we higher animals have our sensory organs—eyes, ears, nose, and so forth—arrayed on our outside surface, so too do cells have most of their environmental information processing and transmission apparatus on their external surfaces. These are intrinsic membrane proteins of the plasma membrane, called *membrane receptors*, that serve a purely informational function, as discussed earlier.

At first glance it might seem odd that a fluid membrane could provide spatial organization for biochemical reactions. However, returning to the "icebergs in a phospholipid sea" analogy, random collisions are much more likely for material in the two-dimensional membrane surface than for material moving through the three-dimensional volume of the cytoplasm. (If the Titanic had been able to dive or fly, it would have had additional ways to avoid the iceberg!) This much larger collision probability is exploited by the cell in a number of physiological processes. Membranes can also be fenced off into distinct regions, across which there is limited diffusion of membrane proteins. For example, certain cells in the kidney have two membrane regions that are quite distinct with respect to transport proteins, which is important in the regulation of salt and water balance by the animal.

TRANSPORT

Only Small, Uncharged Molecules and Oily Molecules Can Penetrate Biomembranes Without the Aid of Proteins

Charged particles (i.e., ions) do not pass through a pure phospholipid bilayer because of the inner, hydrophobic region of bilayer. *Polar molecules* (molecules with no net charge but with electrical imbalances) with a molecular weight greater than about 100 daltons are also unable to pass readily through a pure lipid bilayer, thus excluding all sugar molecules (monosaccharides), amino acids, nucleosides, as well as their polymers (polysaccharide, proteins, nucleic acids). On the other hand, some crucially important polar molecules (e.g., water, urea) are small enough to pass through the lipid bilayer. Small, moderate-size, and large molecules that are soluble in oily solvents readily pass through a pure lipid bilayer. Physiologically important molecules in this class include O_2, N_2, and the steroid hormones (see Chapters 33 and 34). However, many toxic, synthetic molecules, such as insecticides, are also in this category.

Molecules Move Spontaneously from Regions of High Free Energy to Regions of Lower Free Energy

The majority of biochemicals do not pass readily through a phospholipid bilayer. Transport of this molecular majority requires a protein pathway across the biomembrane. Also needed is a force causing movement along the pathway. Before elaborating on membrane proteins as pathways through the lipid bilayer, the energy factors that drive the transport are considered.

Objects fall spontaneously because of gravity. This is a manifestation of the principle that movement occurs to minimize the potential energy of the object. Indeed, all change in the universe (at scales greater than the subatomic particles) occurs to minimize the potential energy, also called the *free energy*, of the system. The movement of molecules is strongly affected by forces such as concentration, pressure (both part of chemical potential), and voltage (electrical potential). Molecules move spontaneously from a region of higher concentration to lower concentration, from higher to lower pressure, and from higher to lower electrical potential. Each of these factors—concentration, pressure, and electrical potential—is a source of free energy. The transport of a molecule does not depend necessarily on any one factor; rather, the sum of all the free energy contributions is the determinant of transport. The sum of all the free energy contributions on a substance is usually expressed on a per-mole basis as the electrochemical potential. The *electrochemical potential* is the free energy of the substance, from all sources, per mole of the substance.

For spontaneous transport to occur, there must be a difference in the electrochemical potential of the substance between two regions. The two regions are usually two compartments separated by a membrane. This difference in electrochemical potential is called the *driving force*. Typically, students have little difficulty understanding the direction of spontaneous flow as long as only one factor contributes to the electrochemical potential, pressure, or concentration or the voltage. However, understanding physiological transport, both across cells and across tissues, requires an understanding of the contribution of each factor to the driving force. For example, the flow of fluid from the capillaries of the vascular system depends on the balance between both the hydrostatic pressure difference and the concentration difference of solutes (osmotic pressure) across the capillary. Similarly, movement of Na^+ and K^+ ions across the plasma membrane of nerve cells depends on the driving forces contributed by both voltage differences and ion concentration differences across the membrane.

Material moves spontaneously from regions of high electrochemical potential to low electrochemical potential. Such transport is called *diffusion* or *passive transport*. Net movement of material (i.e., diffusion) stops when the electrochemical difference between regions equals zero. The state at which the free energy or the electrochemical potential difference is zero is called *equilibrium*. Equilibrium means "balance," not equality. Equilibrium is reached when the free energy (electrochemical potential) is balanced; the value on one side is the same as the other. In most cases the source of the free energies on the two sides never becomes equal; the concentrations, the pressure, and the voltages remain different, but their differences "balance out" so that the sum of the free energy differences is zero.

Equilibrium is a particularly important concept because it describes the state toward which change occurs if no work is put into the system. When the system reaches equilibrium, no further net change occurs unless some work is done on the system. The words *net change* are important. Molecules at equilibrium still move and exchange places, but as much goes in one direction as in the other, so there is no net flow of material.

If the cell requires material to move from low to high electrochemical potential (i.e., in the direction away from equilibrium), thus increasing the difference in free energy between two regions, then some driving force, some work, must be provided by some other decrease in free energy. This type of transport is *active transport*. Active transport uses proteins that combine transport and reaction coupling functions; the protein couples the "uphill" movement of material to a "downhill" reaction such as ATP hydrolysis.

Important Transport Equations Summarize the Contributions of the Various Driving Forces

It is worthwhile developing some quantitative aspects of transport, beginning with simple examples and developing equations for the effect of more than one driving force. These equations can be seen as summaries of the physical laws. In most cases the equations describe phenomena with which we have experience by living in a technological society. In these equations, c stands for concentration, V for volume, P for pressure, and so forth; these are common concepts. It is important, however, to think about these equations in real-life terms, not as abstract symbols.

One of these equations relates a hydrostatic (pressure) driving force for water movement that just balances a driving force caused by a chemical potential difference. *Osmosis* is the movement of water across a semipermeable membrane in response to the difference in the electrochemical potential of water on the two sides of the membrane (Figure 1-7). The chemical potential of water is lower in 1 liter (L) of water (H_2O) in which is dissolved 2 millimoles (mmol) of sodium chloride (NaCl) than in 1 L of H_2O in which is dissolved 1 mmol of NaCl. If these two solutions are separated by a pure lipid bilayer, Na^+ and Cl^- ions cannot move to equilibrate the concentration. Rather, the freely permeable water moves from the side with the higher water potential (low concentration of solute) to the side with the lower water potential (higher concentration of solute). Thus, *water follows solute* (a good summary of osmosis), and this water movement dilutes the 2 mmol solution. However, water movement never produces equal concentrations of salt. Rather, another driving force appears as the water moves. The hydrostatic pressure of water increases on the side to which the water moves, increasing the electrochemical potential of the water on that side. Net water movement stops when the increase in water potential from hydrostatic pressure exactly balances the decrease in water potential from the dissolved salt, so that the electrochemical potential becomes equal on both sides of the membrane.

The initial potential difference of water shown in Figure 1-7 is caused by the difference in the concentration of material dissolved in the water. A proper explanation of why the water in a solution has a lower chemical potential than pure water (and why water in a concentrated solution has a lower potential than in a dilute solution) is beyond the scope of this chapter. However, readers familiar with the concept of *entropy* will realize that the disorder of a system increases with the introduction of different particles into a pure substance and with the number of different particles introduced. An analogy would be that a canister with mixed sugar and salt is more disordered, and therefore at higher entropy, than a canister with only pure salt or pure sugar. Also, the disorder of the system increases as more sugar is added to salt (up to 50:50); a pinch of sugar in a canister of salt only increases the disorder slightly. Because an increase in entropy causes a decrease in free energy, the free energy of a solution is decreased as the mole fraction of solute increases.

Osmosis is important to cells and tissues because, generally, water can move freely across them, whereas much of the dissolved material cannot. Given a concentration difference of some nonpermeable substances, the *van't Hoff equation* relates how much water pressure is required to bring the system to equilibrium, that is, the free energy contributed by a pressure difference across the membrane that exactly balances an opposing free energy contribution caused by a concentration difference.

$$\Pi = iRT\Delta c$$

Π = Osmotic pressure, the driving force for water movement expressed as an equivalent hydrostatic pressure in atmospheres (1 atm = 15.2 lb/in^2 = 760 mm Hg). Osmotic pressure is symbolized by Π to distinguish it from other types of pressure terms.

i = Number of ions formed by dissociating solutes (e.g., 2 for NaCl, 3 for $CaCl_2$).

R = Gas constant = 0.082 L atm/mol degree.

T = Temperature on the Kelvin scale; 0° C = 273° K. (RT is a measure of the free energy of 1 mol of material because of its temperature. At 0° C, RT = 22.4 L atm/mol.)

Δc = Difference in the molar concentration of the *impermeable* substance across the membrane.

This equation summarizes a balance of driving forces; P amount of hydrostatic (osmotic) pressure is the same driving force as a particular concentration difference, Δc. The osmotic pressure depends only on the concentration difference of the substance; no other property of the substance need be taken into account. (Those phenomena that depend only on concentration, such as osmotic pressure, freezing-point depression, and boiling-point elevation, are called *colligative properties*.) The van't Hoff equation is strictly true only for ideal solutions that are approximated in our less-than-ideal world only by very dilute solutions. Real solutions require a "fudge factor," called the *osmotic coefficient*,

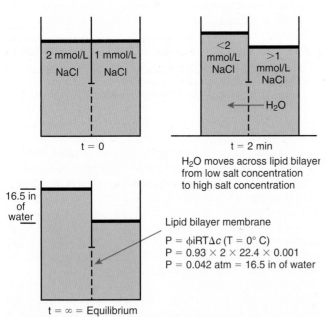

$t = 0$

2 mmol/L NaCl | 1 mmol/L NaCl

$t = 2$ min

<2 mmol/L NaCl | >1 mmol/L NaCl

← H_2O

H_2O moves across lipid bilayer from low salt concentration to high salt concentration

16.5 in of water

$t = \infty$ = Equilibrium

Lipid bilayer membrane

$P = \phi iRT\Delta c$ (T = 0° C)
$P = 0.93 \times 2 \times 22.4 \times 0.001$
$P = 0.042$ atm = 16.5 in of water

FIGURE 1-7 Osmosis. At time *(t)* = 0, two compartments are separated by a lipid bilayer membrane (no transport proteins) that contains salt solutions of differing concentrations. At $t = 2$ minutes, the salt ions cannot move across the membrane to equilibrate their concentration, but water can move. Water moves from the region of higher water potential (low salt) to the region of lower water potential (high salt). Water continues to pass the lipid bilayer until at $t =$ equilibrium; the difference in the height of water between the two sides creates a difference in pressure that is equal but opposite to the difference in the water potential between the two sides. That is, the free energy difference resulting from differing salt concentrations is equilibrated by an equal but opposite free energy difference caused by pressure.

symbolized by Φ (phi). The osmotic coefficient can be looked up in a table, and then plugged into the equation as follows:

$$\Pi = \Phi iRT\Delta c$$

The term Φ*ic* for a given substance represents the osmotically effective concentration of that substance and is often called the *osmolar* or *osmotic concentration,* measured in osmoles per liter (Osm/L). In general, the osmolar concentration of a substance is approximated by the usual concentration times the number of ions formed by the substance; the osmotic coefficient provides a small correction. The osmolarity of a 100 mmol NaCl solution (0.1 mol) is then 0.93 (Φ for NaCl) × 2(NaCl → Na^+ + Cl^-) × 0.1 mol = 0.186 Osm = 186 mOsm.

The previous equation summarizes a phenomenon crucial for physiological function. The greater the concentration difference of an impermeable substance across a membrane, the greater is the tendency for water to move to the side of high concentration. (Water follows solute.) Indeed, if you plug some numbers into this equation, you may be surprised at the large pressures required to balance modest concentration differences. For example, an NaCl concentration difference of 0.1 mol (5.8 g/L) is equilibrated by a pressure (4.2 atm) equal to a column of water 141 ft high (divers must be wary of the bends when ascending from below 70 ft of water). The importance of this is that a small concentration difference can produce a strong force for moving water. The body makes effective use of this to transport water in many tissues: ions/molecules are transported into or out of a compartment → and water follows by osmosis.

Starling's Hypothesis Relates Fluid Flow Across the Capillaries to Hydrostatic Pressure and Osmotic Pressure

An excellent practical example of how a balance of driving forces is responsible for the flow of water and permeable substances across a semipermeable membrane is the movement of water and ions across the single layer of cells (endothelial cells) that compose blood capillaries. The single cell layer composes, in effect, a semipermeable membrane with different transport qualities than that of a simple lipid-bilayer membrane. The junctions between cells are sufficiently permeable to allow small molecules and ions to diffuse between compartments. Only large molecules, most importantly proteins, are unable to move through the holes. The difference in protein concentration between the blood and the water solution surrounding tissue cells, called the *extracellular fluid (ECF)* or *interstitial fluid (ISF),* creates an osmotic pressure for the movement of water with all its dissolved small molecules and ions. This osmotic pressure resulting from dissolved proteins has a special name: *colloid osmotic pressure* or *oncotic pressure.* Protein is more concentrated in the blood than in the interstitial fluid, producing an oncotic pressure of about 0.02 to 0.03 atm = 15 to 25 mm Hg, driving water into the capillary. On the basis of this driving force alone, one would expect the capillaries to fill up with water, thus dehydrating the tissue spaces. However, the heart is a pump that exerts a true hydrostatic pressure on the blood, tending to drive the water (and other permeable molecules) out of the capillaries. The net driving force is the algebraic sum of the oncotic pressure difference and hydrostatic pressure difference between the capillaries and the interstitial fluid, as follows:

$$\text{Net driving force in capillary} = (P_c - P_i) - (\pi_c - \pi_i)$$

P_c = Hydrostatic pressure in the capillary.

P_i = Hydrostatic pressure in the interstitial space (usually near 0).

π_c = Oncotic pressure of blood plasma in capillary (~28 mm Hg).

π_i = Oncotic pressure of interstitial fluid (~5 mm Hg, but depends on the particular tissue).

This equation has enormous relevance to the function of the circulatory system. On the arterial end of capillaries the hydrostatic pressure (P_c) is high, about 35 mm Hg. Plugging this number into the equation along with the others, the net pressure in the capillary is +12 mm Hg; fluid is being driven out of the capillary on the arterial side (*capillary filtration*). The flow of fluid through the resistance of the capillary causes a decline in pressure so that the hydrostatic pressure on the venous side is low, P_c = 15 mm Hg. The oncotic pressures have not changed, so the net driving force on the venous side is –8 mm Hg; there is a net absorption of fluid into the capillary on the venous side (*capillary reabsorption*). This arrangement achieves a major function of the circulatory system; in this way the fluid of the blood circulates among the cells and is then recycled back into the circulatory system.

Pathological alterations in this system emphasize the physiological importance of balance of driving forces for transport. Chronic liver disease occurs with some frequency in horses and dogs, among other mammals. The liver is compromised in its ability to synthesize and secrete a major blood protein, serum albumin. The decline in the concentration of serum albumin lowers the oncotic pressure of the blood. As a result, there is more force to drive fluid out of the capillaries on the arterial side and less driving force for net absorption of fluid on the venous side of capillaries. This causes the tissue spaces of the diseased animals to fill with fluid, a painful and visually obvious symptom called *edema.* The Clinical Correlations section at the end of the chapter provides another example of edema in which increased hydrostatic pressure in the veins and capillaries causes increased capillary filtration and less capillary reabsorption.

Membrane Proteins That Serve the Triple Functions of Selective Transport, Catalysis, and Coupling Can Pump Ions and Molecules to Regions of Higher Free Energy

The van't Hoff equation and Starling's hypothesis deal with passive transport (i.e., movement of material in the direction of lower electrochemical potential). However, the cell moves many ions/molecules against their electrochemical potential. That is, this selective transport requires the expenditure of energy by the cell. Transport in a direction requiring an expenditure of energy (i.e., input of work) is called *active transport.* Active transport depends on intrinsic membrane proteins that use specific binding and allostery to achieve the dual functions of selective transport and reaction coupling. Many (but not all) active transport proteins obtain the energy for transport from ATP hydrolysis; these proteins must function also as enzymes (ATPases).

An important example of active transport is the Na^+,K^+ pump (also known as Na^+,K^+-ATPase). This intrinsic membrane protein consists of four polypeptide chains (2 α + 2 β) and has a mass of approximately 300,000 daltons. This molecule catalyzes the hydrolysis of ATP and couples the hydrolysis energy to the movement of Na^+ out of the cell and K^+ into the cell. This ion pump creates and maintains a considerable concentration gradient across the cell membrane for both ions (Table 1-1).

TABLE 1-1 Concentrations of Various Substances in the Intracellular, Extracellular, and Plasma Fluids

	Concentration (mmol/L)		
	Intracellular	Extracellular	Blood Plasma
Na^+	15	140	142
K^+	150	5	4
Ca^{2+}	0.0001	1	2.5
Mg^{2+}	12	1.5	1.5
Cl^-	10	110	103
HCO_3^-	10	30	27
Phosphate	40	2	1
Glucose	1	5.6	5.6
Protein	4.0	0.2	2.5

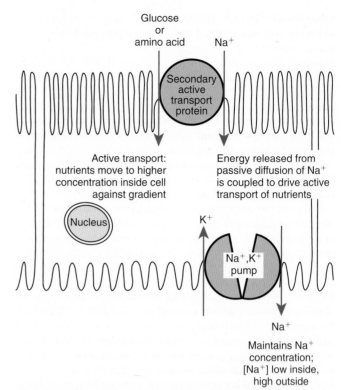

FIGURE 1-9 Secondary active transport as exemplified by uptake of nutrients by gut epithelia. Nutrients such as glucose and amino acids must be actively transported from relatively low concentration in the gut lumen toward higher concentrations within the cells lining the gut. This active transport process uses the concentration gradient of Na^+ ions set up by Na^+, K^+-ATPase (see Figure 1-8) as the source of energy for the active transport process. In other words, the energy released by the passive diffusion of Na^+ into the cell along its concentration gradient is coupled to the energy-requiring transport of glucose or amino acids against their concentration gradients. Thus the secondary active transport protein both serves a transport function and couples the "downhill" transport of Na^+ to the "uphill" transport of nutrients. There are many such secondary active transport processes in the body. For example, the same mechanism shown here is used to reabsorb nutrients from blood filtrate in the kidney.

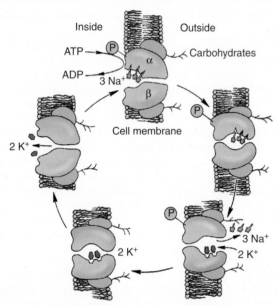

FIGURE 1-8 Hypothetical transport cycle for Na^+, K^+-ATPase. Changes in the conformation of this transport protein driven by ATP hydrolysis and ion-binding events cause three Na^+ ions to be moved out of the cell against a concentration gradient and two K^+ ions to be moved into the cell, also against a concentration gradient, for each ATP hydrolyzed. (Redrawn from a diagram by Dr. Seth Hootman.)

Figure 1-8 shows our current understanding of this protein's structure and outlines the cycle of binding and conformational changes underlying its transport function. The Na^+,K^+-ATPase pumps three Na^+ ions *out* of the cell and two K^+ ions *into* the cell for each ATP molecule hydrolyzed. These directions of ion pumping cause a high Na^+ concentration outside the cell and a low concentration inside, whereas K^+ concentration is high inside and low outside the cell. The different directions of pumping for the two ions depend on differing binding specificity of the pump protein in the two conformational states. The ability of the protein to couple this transport to the enzymatic breakdown of ATP allows the transport to occur against the concentration gradients, from lower to higher electrochemical potentials for both ions. In the particular case of the Na^+, K^+ pump, the number of

transported electrical charges is asymmetrical; three positive charges leave for each two positive charges that enter. This asymmetry of electrical charge transport means that the Na^+, K^+ pump is *electrogenic*, making a minor contribution to the electrical potential (voltage) across cell membranes, as discussed later.

Many different intrinsic membrane proteins actively transport a wide variety of ions and molecules against the transported molecules' electrochemical gradient. Many, such as the Na^+,K^+ pump, couple the energy-requiring "uphill" transport with the "downhill" hydrolysis of ATP. However, any potential source of free energy can be coupled to the energy-requiring transport. Indeed, the gradient of Na^+ set up by the Na^+,K^+ pump is itself used frequently as a source of energy. That is, the "downhill" flow of Na^+ from outside the cell to the inside is a spontaneous reaction whose energy can be coupled to some "uphill" reaction (Figure 1-9). For example, the transport of glucose and many amino acids from the food mass in the small intestine into the cells lining the gut is an active transport process and requires a Na^+ concentration gradient. Transport proteins in the plasma membrane of intestinal epithelial cells couple the spontaneous diffusion of Na^+ into the cell to the inward, energy-requiring transport of the sugar or amino acids. These nutrients are at higher concentration inside the cell than outside, so they must be actively transported into the cell at the expense of the energy stored in the Na^+ electrochemical gradient. That is, the energy from the "downhill" diffusion of Na^+ into the cell is coupled to the "uphill" transport of the nutrient into the cell. Such active transport coupled to Na^+ diffusion across the cell membrane is called *secondary active transport* because of its dependence on the Na^+ concentration gradient established by the primary active transport of the Na^+,K^+ pump.

Examples of transport can be identified in a number of ways. Our examples have been instances in which two ions/molecules must be transported together or not at all, and such transport is called *co-transport*. Co-transport can involve one process of passive transport (diffusion) with an active transport process, as in the two previous examples; it can involve two active transport processes (e.g., Na^+,K^+-ATPase) or two diffusion processes. In the first case, the need for co-transport is energetic; the flow of one ion is needed to drive the other. In the two latter cases, the need for co-transport is a restriction based on the binding properties of the transport protein; it cannot bind one without the other. Co-transport proteins that transport both substances in the same direction are called *symports* or *symporters*. The Na^+/sugar co-transporter in the gut is a symport. Co-transport proteins that transport the two substances in opposite directions (e.g., Na^+,K^+-ATPase) are called *antiports* or *antiporters*. Parenthetically, proteins that transport only a single ion or molecule are called *uniports* or *uniporters*.

Many Membrane Proteins Selectively Facilitate the Transport of Ions/Molecules from High to Low Electrochemical Potential

The movement of ions and of medium and large polar molecules requires a protein molecule to serve as a pathway through the obstruction of the phospholipid bilayer. If the movement of the substance is in the natural direction of its electrochemical gradient (movement from high to low), the transport process is called *facilitated diffusion*. The membrane proteins mediating this transport process through the phospholipid bilayer are *channels* or *carriers* (Figure 1-10). These are distinguished by the extent to which the protein interacts with the transported substance.

Carriers bind the transported substance in the lock-and-key manner, so there is a site-specific binding of the transported substance to the transport protein (see Figure 1-10, *A*). Carrier-mediated transport is typically much slower than channel-mediated diffusion because of the relatively slow binding and unbinding processes. The Na^+,K^+ pump and the Na^+/glucose symport are both examples of carriers.

Channels can be thought of as "protein donuts" embedded in the phospholipid bilayer. The hole in the donut is a pore in the membrane through which small ions such as Na^+, K^+, Ca^+, Cl^-, and H^+ are transported. Although most channels transport ions, a class of channels called *aquaporins* comprises channels for water flow. (Although water can flow through a pure lipid bilayer, this transport is too slow for some functions. Kidney cells, for example, are particularly rich in aquaporins, which are required for the water balance function of the kidney.) For all channels, the pore size and the interaction of the transported material with the amino acid side groups lining the pore allow membrane channels to be selective. Only specific molecules or ions can move through a particular channel. Movement of material through channels is almost as rapid as simple diffusion through a water-filled space of the same area as the channel pore.

The plasma membranes of most cells have passive leaks of ions, particularly K^+. These ionic leaks are typically ascribed to *leak channels,* which are open at all times (see Figure 1-10, *B*). However, most ion channels open or close in response to signals. These latter types are called *gated channels.* The opening and closing of the gates are examples of the allosteric property of proteins. The same signals responsible for allosteric changes in general—ligand binding, phosphorylation, and voltage differences—also control the opening and closing of gated channels, as shown in Figure 1-10. (Because mechanically gated channels are so poorly understood, these are not discussed here.)

Channels that open in response to ligand binding are called *ligand-gated channels* (see Figure 1-10, *C*). The nicotinic acetylcholine receptor is a ligand-gated channel found in skeletal muscle membrane directly beneath incoming neurons (nerve cells). This channel is found also in the membrane of neurons in autonomic ganglia and in the brain. As the name implies, the nicotinic acetylcholine receptor binds to the drug nicotine and the neurotransmitter acetylcholine. In both cases the channel opens in response to ligand binding.

This nicotinic acetylcholine channel plays a key role in transmitting electrical stimulation from neurons to skeletal muscle cells. Briefly, motor neurons release the neurotransmitter acetylcholine in response to the electrical signal coming down the neuron. This acetylcholine binds to and opens the ligand-gated channel on the skeletal muscle. The influx of Na^+ into the muscle cell initiates an electrical response in the muscle, causing the release of Ca^{2+} (through gated channels in the endoplasmic reticulum), in turn causing contraction. (This brief account of neuromuscular transmission, presented only to provide orientation to the function of the acetylcholine channel, is expanded in Chapters 5 and 6.) In the case of the nicotinic acetylcholine receptor/channel, the specific binding and allosteric properties of the protein serve the dual functions of selective transport across the membrane and information reception and transmission to the muscle cell.

Channels that open in response to voltage changes across the membrane are called *voltage-gated* or *voltage-dependent channels* (see Figure 1-10, *D*). This type of channel is largely responsible for the neurons' ability to transmit information along their length and to release neurotransmitter. All voltage-gated channels have a range of membrane potentials that cause them to open; this is the channel's activation range. The minimum membrane potential that causes opening is the channel's *threshold.* The activation range and threshold vary from channel to channel, depending on the conformation of the protein and the electrical properties of the amino acid side groups that form the gate of the channel. In addition to an open and closed configuration, many voltage-dependent channels have a third conformation, called *inactivated.* Like the closed configuration, the inactivated conformation prohibits the diffusion of ions through the channel. Unlike the closed configuration, it does not open immediately in response to changes in membrane potential. Inactivation can be regarded as an enforced rest period for the channel. Voltage-dependent channels that do not inactivate have only open and closed conformations, and they take up one or the other conformation, depending on the membrane potential.

As previously discussed, any of the functions of proteins can be used to transmit information if a difference in the protein function changed the cell. Gated channels, both ligand and

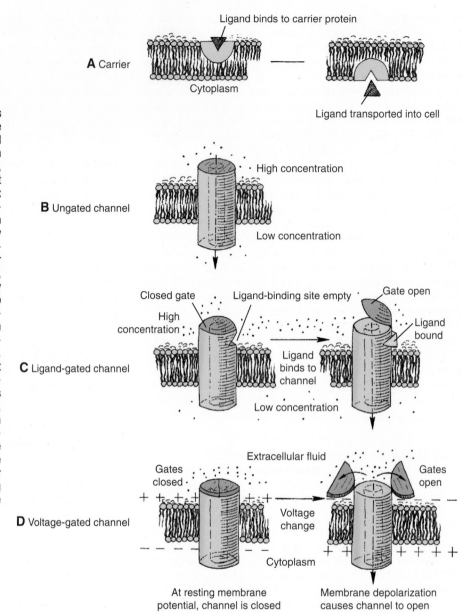

FIGURE 1-10 Types of transport proteins mediating facilitated diffusion. In all cases the ion moves from a region of high potential (shown here as high concentration) to a region of low potential. **A,** Carriers. In a few cases, material is carried by a transport protein that binds tightly to the material, and the complex moves through the lipid bilayer. **B,** Leak channels. These channels are thought not to open and close as do gated channels, and thus they support a small but persistent leak of a particular ion through the pore. Although their existence was long postulated, distinct, ungated leak channels have only recently been identified and isolated, as opposed to leaks through normally gated channels. Selectivity of these and other channels is based on the size of the pore and the weak interactions of ions with the atoms lining the pore. **C,** Ligand-gated channels. The transport protein again forms a pore through the membrane. In the case of gated channels, access of the ion to the pore is controlled by a gate, a substructure of the transport protein that can open and close the pore. In ligand-gated channels the opening and closing of the gate are controlled by the binding of a ligand to the channel. **D,** Voltage-gated channels are similar to ligand-gated channels, except the opening and closing of the gate are controlled by the electrical field around the channel.

voltage gated, are ideal candidates for information transmission because they change their function: opening and closing, permitting or stopping transport. Indeed, the sole physiological function of the nicotinic acetylcholine receptor/channel, as described earlier, is the transmission of information: turning the chemical stimulation by the neuron of the muscle into electrical stimulation (see following discussion) of the muscle membrane, leading to muscle contraction.

Passive Transport of K⁺ Across the Plasma Membrane Creates an Electrical Potential

As just discussed, gated ion channels can convert chemical information into electrical information. Electrical signaling in the animal body is the result of electrical imbalances maintained across the plasma membrane of virtually all cells: cells maintain an electrical potential difference across their plasma membrane. That is, the cell membrane is a battery; if one attaches electrodes to the two ends of a battery, or to the inside and outside of a cell, one finds a voltage difference between the two ends or sides. If

one provides a path for electrical charges to move—a metal wire containing free electrons in the case of a battery, or a membrane channel through which ions can move in the case of the cell—an electrical current flows from higher to lower electrical potential. The diversity of battery-powered devices in our society suggests how many ways this electrical potential can be exploited. The physiology of animals also exploits the baseline electrical potential across the plasma membrane, called the *resting membrane potential.* The word "resting" is added to distinguish the baseline potential from the instantaneous values of membrane potential during the passage of membrane currents.

The resting membrane potential is the indirect result of the concentration gradients of ions across the plasma membrane caused by the activity of the Na⁺,K⁺-ATPase. Partly, this membrane potential is a result of the asymmetry in numbers of ions pumped by the Na⁺,K⁺-ATPase. However, most of the membrane potential is caused by the passive flow of K⁺ through *K⁺ leak channels* in response to the concentration gradient of K⁺ (high inside, low outside). This concentration gradient sets up an electrical driving force (voltage) that exactly balances the concentration driving force. The concentration of K^+ inside a mammalian cell is about 150 mmol; outside in the interstitial fluid, it is about 5 mmol. As a result, K^+ tends to diffuse from the cytoplasm through the leak channel to the interstitial fluid. However, when K^+ alone leaves the cytoplasm without an accompanying negative ion, it causes an electrical imbalance. The exit of K^+ ions leaves the inside of the cell with negative charges not neutralized by positive potassium ions, and the interstitial fluid now has positive K^+ ions not balanced by negative charges. The cell is building an electrical potential difference across the plasma membrane, with the cytoplasm being negative relative to the interstitial fluid.

This electrical potential driving force increases until it balances the concentration driving force for K^+. This situation is analogous to osmosis: the concentration-driven flow of water across a semipermeable membrane creates a different driving force, pressure, that eventually balances the concentration driving force. Similarly, for the resting membrane potential, the concentration-driven flow of K^+ across the semipermeable membrane (semipermeable in the sense that negative ions do not accompany the K^+) creates a different driving force, an electrical voltage, that eventually balances the concentration force. As in the case of osmosis, an equation is used to relate the size of the concentration gradient to the size of the electrical potential that provides an exact balance. This equation is called the *Nernst equation,* as follows:

$$E_X = RT/zF \ln[X_{outside}]/[X_{inside}]$$

E_X = Equilibrium potential for ion X
RT = Gas constant × Absolute temperature
z = Electrical valence for the ion, +1 for Na^+ and K^+, −1 for Cl^-, and so forth
F = Faraday constant = number of coulombs of electrical charge in a mole of ions = 96,500 coulombs/mol
$\ln$ = Natural logarithm (i.e., log to base e)
$[X]$ = Concentration of ion X

A simpler form of this equation can be written by taking advantage of the fact that R and F are constants, T is almost constant under physiological conditions, and the natural log of a number is 2.3 times the common log (log_{10}), as follows (mV, millivolts):

$$E_X = -60 \text{ mV}/z \log[X_{inside}]/[X_{outside}]$$

Because the state of balance between the electrical driving force and the concentration driving force is equilibrium, the value of the electrical potential is called the *equilibrium potential* of the ion. Given the concentrations above for K^+ inside (150 mmol) and outside (5 mmol) the cell, the equilibrium potential for K^+ is:

$$E_{K^+} = -60 \text{ mV}/ + 1 \times \log 150/5$$
$$= -60 \text{ mV} \log 30$$
$$= -60 \text{ mV} \times 1.47$$
$$= -88.2 \text{ mV}$$

Indeed, the measured resting membrane potential across a human muscle cell is −90 mV.

Several aspects of this important equation are worth discussing. If the equilibrium potential for a particular ion is the same as the measured membrane potential, the net driving force for the ion is zero. In this case, there is no net movement, even in the presence of wide-open channels, to provide a path through the membrane. However, for any gradient of a specific ion, if the measured membrane potential is *not* the equilibrium potential of that ion, there is a driving force for the transport of that ion. That is, when the membrane potential is anything other than the equilibrium potential, that ion will flow across the membrane if an appropriate channel is open. Thus the equilibrium potential for an ion provides a "baseline" for comparison with the actual membrane potential to determine whether an ion will tend to move across the plasma membrane. If the measured membrane potential has the same sign but is larger in magnitude than the equilibrium potential, the ion flows in the direction of the electrical potential. If the sign is the same but the magnitude lower, the concentration driving force determines the direction of flow of the ion. If the measured potential has the opposite sign of the equilibrium potential, both electrical and concentration forces are acting on the ion in the same direction. Flow of ions across the plasma membrane (i.e., electrical current) in response to the balance of force between concentration and voltage produces the electrical changes in neurons that underlie the nervous system, as discussed in Chapter 4.

It would be reasonable but incorrect to assume that the transport of ions required to set up the electrical potential measurably alters the concentration gradient. This is untrue because of the large amount of energy required to separate electrical charges. The separation of charge arising from the transport of a few ions balances the energy of quite substantial concentration gradients. Indeed, so few ions move that they cannot be measured by chemical means. Thus, electrical, not chemical, measurements are used routinely to assess transport of ions in cells. The measurable voltage changes caused by immeasurably small concentration changes of ions means also that the electrical phenomena at the membrane persist for many hours, even if the Na^+,K^+-ATPase is inactivated by a toxin. That is, an existing concentration gradient of K^+ would require hours to dissipate at the rate of K^+ leakage characteristic of the plasma membrane. Using the membrane battery analogy, the Na^+,K^+-ATPase is a battery recharger. A portable radio does not require the minute-to-minute services of a battery recharger. Enough energy is stored in the battery to operate the radio for an appreciable period, although the battery recharger is needed eventually. Similarly, enough energy is stored in the K^+ concentration gradient to maintain the membrane potential for a period of time. The Na^+,K^+-ATPase is not required on a minute-to-minute basis, although it is needed ultimately to maintain the concentration gradient on which the resting membrane potential depends.

Spatial Organization of Active and Passive Transport Proteins Enables Material to Pass Completely Through the Cell

Although macromolecules and biomembranes clearly underlie physiological function, many phenomena of the intact animal emerge that are not initially apparent as a simple sum of parts. One interesting example is the spatial organization of plasma membrane transport proteins so that ions move across the cell from one ECF compartment to another. This is called *transcellular transport* or, because it typically occurs across a layer of epithelial cells, *epithelial transport*. This epithelial transport is important in the kidney (see Chapter 42). The plasma membrane of the epithelial cells in the proximal tubules of the kidney contains two distinct regions. The apical membrane regions face the lumen of the tubule and the fluid that will become urine, and the basolateral regions are near the capillaries and the blood. The apical surface contains ungated leak channels for Na^+, whereas the baso-lateral surface contains Na^+,K^+-ATPase molecules. (The membrane proteins in one region are prevented from diffusing into the other by membrane protein "fences" called *tight junctions*.) Na^+ diffuses into the cell on the apical surface from the urinelike fluid driven by both the concentration gradient and the resting membrane potential. When inside the cell, the Na^+ is pumped from the basolateral surface, essentially into the blood, by the Na^+,K^+-ATPase. This allows the kidney to reabsorb and thus conserve Na^+. As long as the Na^+,K^+-ATPase remains restricted to the basolateral surface and the passive channel to the apical membrane, Na^+ can move through the cell from the urinelike fluid in the tubule to the blood in the capillaries. If either protein should lose its spatial restriction, Na^+ would be transported into and out of the cell on the same surface, merely consuming ATP, with no net transport of Na^+ from lumen to capillary.

Membrane Fusion Allows for a Combination of Compartmentalization and Transport of Material

Impermeable molecules can be transported across the cell membrane by means other than membrane proteins. This method involves using membrane itself as a carrier compartment. The lipid bilayer of biological membranes has a structure similar to soap bubbles. As with soap bubbles, small vesicles of biomembrane (essentially "membrane bubbles") can fuse to form larger membrane surfaces. A large membrane surface can also pinch off (requiring fusion of two membrane surfaces) into small vesicles. When these processes occur at the plasma membrane, they are called *exocytosis* and *endocytosis*, respectively (Figure 1-11). More generally, pinching off of membrane or fusion of two membrane vesicles (e.g., for internal membranes) is referred to as *membrane fusion*, whatever the direction. Membrane fusion underlies much of membrane vesicle traffic around the cell. This traffic creates intracellular vesicles, renews plasma membrane by adding newly synthesized membrane, and transports material within the cell and across the plasma membrane. Because the transport is compartmentalized within a membrane bubble, the transported material can be targeted specifically to one or another region of the cell. Also, changes to the "cargo" can occur within a particular membrane compartment, as seen in cholesterol transport.

Exocytosis and endocytosis are crucial in the transport of cholesterol (Figure 1-12). *Cholesterol* is an essential lipid component of many animal biomembranes; the plasma membrane lipids of animals are about 15% cholesterol and 60% phospholipids. Cholesterol is also the starting material for the synthesis of the entire group of hormones called *steroids* (see Chapters 33 and 34). Cholesterol can be synthesized by animals and is also absorbed by meat-eating animals from their diet. Because cholesterol is soluble in oil, it passes from food through the plasma membrane without protein mediation into the cells of the gut lining. However, transport of dietary cholesterol through the circulatory system requires that cholesterol molecules form a complex with a protein molecule to create low-density lipoproteins (LDLs). To take up cholesterol from the circulation, cells bind the LDLs to intrinsic membrane proteins that act as LDL receptors, as shown in Figure 1-12. The receptor/LDL complex then diffuses in the plane of the membrane into specific regions to form coated pits. The coated pit is taken into the cytoplasm by endocytosis. In addition to the transport function, *receptor-mediated endocytosis* functions also to concentrate extracellular material before internalization. The coated pit is not taken into the cell until it has collected the LDLs

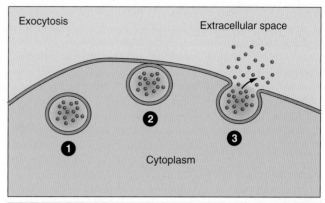

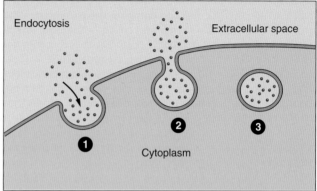

FIGURE 1-11 Two membrane fusion processes: exocytosis and endocytosis. **Top,** In exocytosis, a membrane-bound vesicle from the cytoplasm *(1)* makes contact and fuses with the plasma membrane *(2)*. As the vesicle membrane becomes continuous with the plasma membrane, the contents of the vesicle are released to the extracellular space *(3)*. **Bottom,** In endocytosis, some material from the extracellular space is surrounded by plasma membrane *(1)*, which continues to invaginate until the edges are able to fuse *(2)*, thus pinching off a vesicle from the plasma membrane *(3)*. Membrane fusion can occur between any two compartments within cells separated by lipid bilayer membrane, not only between the cytoplasm and extracellular space, as shown here.

from a much larger volume of ECF than the cell could "drink." The membrane vesicles formed by this endocytosis fuse subsequently to become an *endosome*. The endosome compartment becomes acidic, which causes dissociation of the LDL and the receptor. Through unknown means, the endosome is then able to further separate and compartmentalize the receptor from the LDL. Membrane vesicles containing the now-vacated LDL receptors return to the plasma membrane and fuse by exocytosis. The LDL receptor is recycled to the plasma membrane to pick up more LDL. Experimental evidence suggests that a single LDL receptor molecule can cycle between the plasma membrane and endosomal vesicles more than 100 times before losing its activity. Meanwhile, the LDL moiety is segregated to another endosomal vesicle, which fuses with the lysosome. The lysosome contains hydrolytic enzymes, thus allowing the internalized LDL to be digested. The cholesterol is now available to the cell for steroid synthesis or incorporation into membrane.

Other molecules are also recycled by endocytosis. As with the LDL receptor, for example, many signal receptors, discussed in the next section, are endocytosed back into the cell that released them, saving the cell the effort of synthesizing new receptors. Not all endocytosed molecules are recycled. Many are broken down after their endosome fuses with a lysosome. Indeed, as described

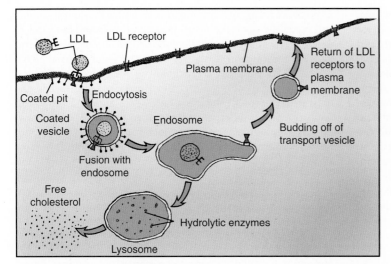

FIGURE 1-12 Processes of membrane fusion involved in cholesterol uptake by cells. Starting at the left, a low-density lipoprotein (LDL)–containing cholesterol binds to an LDL receptor protein of the plasma membrane and undergoes endocytosis, forming an endosome. The receptor is detached from its LDL ligand in the endosome. The LDL portion of the endosome fuses with a lysosome to digest the LDL and produce free cholesterol, while the receptor-containing portion of the endosome pinches off a vesicle to return to the plasma membrane, thus recycling the receptor. (Redrawn from Alberts B, Bray D, Lewis J, et al: *Molecular biology of the cell*, New York, 1983, Garland.)

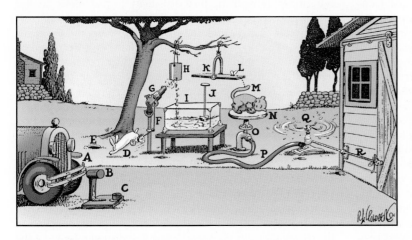

FIGURE 1-13 Rube Goldberg device (garage door opener, circa 1928) as an analogy for the complex cause-and-effect sequence characteristic of cellular chemical signaling. Automobile *(A)* drives into driveway, causing hammer *(B)* to ignite toy cap *(C)*, frightening rabbit *(D)* into its burrow *(E)* and causing pistol *(G)* to fire and so forth, ultimately leading to the opening of the garage door *(R)*. As explained in the text, this whimsical "machine" serves as an analogy for chemical signaling within cells because of the multiple control elements, their connection as a cause-and-effect sequence, and the use of household items, similar to the use of evolutionarily conserved proteins of cells in signaling.

later, this is one method of regulating receptor number on the plasma membrane.

INFORMATION TRANSMISSION AND TRANSDUCTION

Cell Signaling Usually Occurs by a Lengthy Chain of Sequential Molecular Interactions

One of the areas of most rapid progress in cellular physiology has been our understanding of the mechanisms by which extracellular signals, such as hormones, growth factors, and neurotransmitters, alter cellular function, which in turn alters tissue, organ, and animal function. At the molecular level, almost all chemical signaling shares a common "strategy" of mechanism: signals are sent as a long chain of chemical cause-and-effect interactions transmitted between many sequential chemical steps. Indeed, chemical signaling pathways are structured similar to the whimsical "machines" in the cartoons of Rube Goldberg (1883-1970), a famous American newspaper cartoonist. Figure 1-13 shows one of his cartoons from 1928 illustrating an outlandish contraption (a *Rube Goldberg device*) to serve as an automatic garage door opener, realistic versions of which had not yet been invented. The automobile (A) drives in, causing a hammer (B) to ignite a toy cap gun (C), which frightens a rabbit (D) with a string (F) tied to its leg, thus firing a pistol (G), and so forth, until a connection to a rotating water sprinkler causes the carriage-house door to slide open (overhead doors also had not yet been invented). Although

much of the humor of this parody of a machine is lost on us (our attitudes about machines have changed greatly since Goldberg's heyday), Rube Goldberg devices are a surprisingly useful analogy to the overall mechanism of cellular chemical signaling.

Just as the garage door opener of Figure 1-13 depends on a series of sequential cause-and-effect interactions, so chemical signaling occurs by a series of cause-and-effect changes in protein shape and binding. Just as the complex events of Goldberg's device are linked to signal and to actuate garage door opening, so a cascade of changes in protein shape and function are linked to signal and actuate physiological events. Our earlier example of muscle contraction illustrates such a pathway of cause and effect and the analogy to Rube Goldberg devices. Electrical excitation (A) of a muscle cell increases intracellular Ca^{2+} concentration (B), causing Ca^{2+} to bind to troponin (C). This in turn alters the binding of tropomyosin (D) to actin (E) allowing the myosin heads (F) to bind to actin, thus leading to cross-bridging (G) and hydrolysis of ATP and contraction.

As this example indicates, the sequence of cause and effect for both chemical signaling and Rube Goldberg devices is complex. Both involve many different elements, none of which can be identified as **the** controller; all the elements are involved in control. Importantly, this creates multiple sites for regulation and for therapeutic drug action. Just as increasing the caliber of the pistol in the garage door opener would change the response time for opening, so a drug that bound to an element in the middle of a signaling pathway in a cell could increase or decrease the final physiological change in response to a particular hormone, for example. Also related to complexity is that the chain of cause and effect is not obvious; the particular sequence connecting a particular signal (adrenaline binding to a receptor on heart muscle) to a particular outcome (increased cardiac output) must be memorized. However, when the sequence is understood, you can predict from the state of one element in the chain what should happen next. Finally, Rube Goldberg devices were cobbled together from reasonably common household items, such as the bucket, fish tank, sprinkler, and even pistols. Similarly, the elements of chemical-signaling pathways are often highly conserved, and you will see throughout your studies that the same molecules or same basic types of molecules are used in a wide variety of different stimulus-response pathways.

Signaling Pathways Begin with the Binding of an Extracellular Molecule to a Receptor

In addition to the Rube Goldberg–like sequence of signal pathways, another aspect of the overall "strategy" of cellular information transmission is that signaling pathways almost always begin with the environmental signal molecule binding to a protein molecule specialized for information transfer, called a *receptor*. The LDL receptor discussed earlier is involved in the transport of material into cells (see Figure 1-12). However, most other receptors are proteins whose task is to transmit and transduce information to the cell from the extracellular environment. Receptors distinguish among the large number of external signaling molecules (e.g., various hormones, neurotransmitters, growth factors) through the usual protein mechanism of highly specific binding.

Three broad classes of receptors, called *receptor families,* are particularly important in physiological function and are discussed in this chapter and Chapter 2. Two of these families, the *G-protein–coupled receptors* (GPCRs) and the *receptor tyrosine kinases* (RTKs), are intrinsic membrane proteins of the plasma membrane. These membrane receptors bind the signal molecule in the extracellular environment, and the signal is then communicated intracellularly through a Rube Goldberg sequence of "differences that make a difference." The third class of receptors is the *nuclear receptors.* These are not membrane proteins, but rather intracellular proteins that transduce signals from oily, lipidic molecules that can easily enter the cell. Signaling molecules that bind and activate nuclear receptors include steroid and thyroid hormones, fat molecules in the diet, and derivatives of vitamins A and D. The information transduction pathway of nuclear receptors is simpler than that of the membrane receptors in that nuclear receptors are themselves direct regulators of gene transcription; that is, nuclear receptors are transcription factors. Binding of the signal molecule activates the nuclear receptor so that it is then able to bind directly to specific regions of deoxyribonucleic acid (DNA) and stimulate the binding of ribonucleic acid (RNA) polymerase to, and thus production of, messenger RNA from the particular gene or genes in that region of DNA. An example involving the female-specific production of egg protein in hens is discussed later in the chapter.

Specific Physiological Information Is Inherent in the Receptor/Ligand Complex, Not in the Hormone/Neurotransmitter Molecule

Before discussing specific receptors, it is useful to elaborate on some important points about the nature and regulation of the information transfer between the external signal molecule and

receptor. This text provides ample evidence that the same hormone and especially the same neurotransmitter molecule can bind to different receptors. These different receptor-binding events send different information to the cell from the same external signal molecule. For example, acetylcholine is bound by two different receptors, the nicotinic ion channel described earlier and the muscarinic receptor, which is a GPCR, not an ion channel, and sends completely different information to the cell. The hormone/neurotransmitter itself does not contain any specific information; rather, it is a simple signal, such as a phone ringing. One must answer the phone to receive the information. The information content of the hormone/neurotransmitter is really contained in the three-dimensional shape of the receptor molecule. The change in the shape of the receptor on binding the hormone/neurotransmitter is the specific message to the cell.

Cells can make themselves more or less sensitive to the signal of the hormone/neurotransmitter. For example, most cells respond to a prolonged period of exposure to hormone/ neurotransmitter by reducing their sensitivity to that molecule. For membrane receptors, one way is to internalize the receptors by endocytosis, fuse the endosome with a lysosome, and digest the receptor. Typically, membrane receptor number is decreased by endocytosis in response to a sustained high concentration of ligand. This is called *downregulation* of the receptor. This process allows the cell to adapt to high ligand concentrations. Receptor-ligand interaction is a true chemical equilibrium, so the proportion of receptor-ligand complexes, which determines physiological response, depends on the concentration of both receptors and ligands. In the presence of a high ligand concentration, a decrease in receptor number returns the binding equilibrium to the normal proportion of bound/unbound receptors. This allows the cell to respond to increases and decreases in ligand, even at high concentrations of ligand. Another way of regulating the response to a hormone/neurotransmitter is to alter the binding function of the receptor, e.g., by phosphorylating it, so that its affinity for the ligand is reduced (*desensitization*) or increased (*hypersensitization*). Nuclear receptors appear to be less subject to short-term regulation of responsiveness, but at least some nuclear receptors require constant turnover by proteolytic breakdown and new synthesis in order to function.

G-Protein–Coupled Receptors Are the Largest Family (a *Superfamily*) of Receptors and Help Regulate Almost All Physiological Processes

It would be difficult to exaggerate the importance and versatility of information processing that begins with a signal molecule binding to G-protein–coupled receptors. There are approximately 900 GPCRs in humans (Table 1-2). There are an even greater number in animals that depend more on olfaction, with about 1300 in rodents, because smell is mediated by different odorants binding to different GPCRs. An estimated 40% to 50% of all commercial drugs act in a GPCR pathway, exemplifying the importance of GPCRs to medicine. All GPCRs share a similar molecular shape; they are an integral membrane protein composed of a single polypeptide chain that passes in and out of the plasma membrane seven times, resembling a snake (Figure 1-14). As a result, two other names for GPCRs are *seven-transmembrane receptors* and *serpentine receptors*. However, the name GPCRs is more revealing about their mechanism because all also share the same "next step" in their Rube Goldberg signal sequence: they activate a molecular "on-off switch" known

TABLE 1-2 Partial List of G-Protein–Coupled Receptors (GPCRs)

Receptor/Receptor Family*	Example of Function	Drug Ligands
α-Adrenergic	Regulates vasculature	Phenylephrine, oxymetazoline
β-Adrenergic	Regulates heart and vasculature	Atenolol, propranolol
Angiotensin	Principal regulator of blood pressure	Losartan
Calcitonin	Regulates bone resorption	†
Cannabinoid	Unknown but found widely in brain	Marijuana and derivatives
Dopamine	Movement, cognition, and emotions	Chlorpromazine, bromocriptine
Frizzled	Regulates proliferation and differentiation, particularly in stem cells	†
Gastrin	Regulates acid secretion in stomach	Pentagastrin
Glucagon	Regulates "starvation" response	Exendin-4
Histamine	Mediates inflammation and allergy	Diphenhydramine, chlorpheniramine
Muscarinic	Secretion of hormones and neurotransmitters	Atropine, carbachol
Olfactory	Mediates smell	†
Opioid	Mediates analgesia	Morphine, codeine, heroin
Opsins	Mediates light transduction in retina	†
Prostaglandin	Vasodilation	Sulprostone
Serotonin‡	Regulates gut motility, behavioral arousal, feeding, circadian rhythms	Sumatriptan, ketanserin
Vasopressin	Regulates water balance of body	Terlipressin, desmopressin

*In most cases, receptor is named for its ligand.
†None commonly known.
‡One member of the serotonin receptor family is not G-protein–coupled.

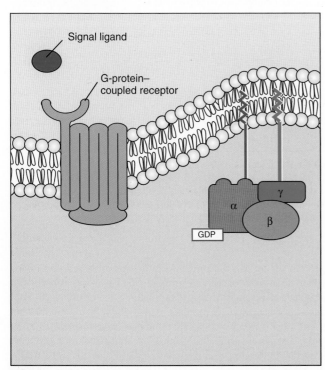

FIGURE 1-14 G-protein–coupled receptor (GPCR) and the heterotrimeric G protein. The hundreds of GPCRs share a similar protein shape, snaking in and out of the membrane seven times. Thus, GPCRs are also called *serpentine receptors* and *heptahelical receptors*. These receptors interact with a membrane-associated guanosinetriphosphatase (GTPase) molecule composed of three different polypeptide subunits *(heterotrimeric)*. The heterotrimeric G protein is not an intrinsic membrane protein, but rather associates with the membrane through lipid tails inserted into the membrane.

as a *G protein,* so called because it is a *guanosinetriphosphatase* (GTPase).

GPCRs bind to a particular type of G protein (another of the many "families" of informational proteins), which is a membrane-associated trimeric protein composed of α, β, and γ subunits. Thus, this type of G protein is called the *heterotrimeric G protein* ("three different subunits"). The heterotrimeric G proteins bind directly to the cytoplasmic domain of a GPCR. Although not intrinsic membrane proteins, heterotrimeric G proteins are closely associated with the plasma membrane through lipid molecules that are posttranslationally added to the subunits and that insert into the lipid bilayer (see Figure 1-14).

As noted, G proteins are molecular "on-off switches" that are also GTPases activated by the binding of a signal molecule to its cognate GPCR. That is, in addition to binding to GPCRs, G proteins also bind *guanosine triphosphate* (GTP) and hydrolyze it to *guanosine diphosphate* (GDP). The binding and hydrolysis of the GTP to GDP underlie the biochemical mechanism of the on-off switch. In Figure 1-15, A, the unstimulated GPCR does not bind to the heterotrimeric G protein, which is in its "off" state by virtue of the α subunit having GDP and the β and γ subunits bound to it. In Figure 1-15, B, a signal ligand binds to its GPCR, activating the receptor and the G protein. The activation of the G protein takes the form of dissociation of the β/γ complex from the α subunit, which allows the α subunit to exchange GDP for GTP. The principal "on" activity of the G protein is represented by the G_α subunit with GTP bound to it. GTP-bound G_α stimulates a variety of enzymes and ion channels that send the signal into the cytoplasm (see Figure 1-15, C), as discussed in the next section. However, the $G_{\beta\gamma}$ complex, once thought to be only an inhibitory factor for the G_α subunit, is now known to activate certain K^+ channels itself and inhibit certain voltage-dependent Ca^{2+}

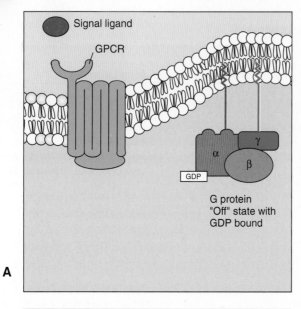

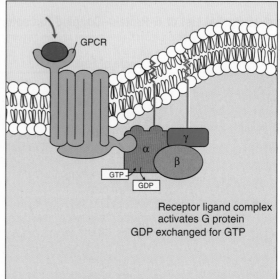

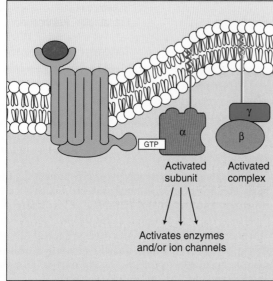

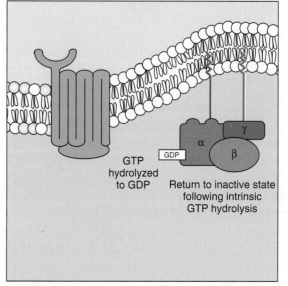

FIGURE 1-15 Duty cycle of heterotrimeric G-protein, a GTPase that acts as a molecular "on-off switch." See text for further details. **A,** Unstimulated GPCR is not bound to the heterotrimeric G protein. **B,** Signal ligand binds to its GPCR, activating receptor and G protein. **C,** GTP-bound Gα subunit stimulates a variety of enzymes and ion channels that send the signal into the cytoplasm. **D,** After stimulating next element in signal pathway, the activated GTP-bound Gα subunit returns to inactive, "off" state because of its intrinsic GTPase activity.

channels. After stimulating the next element in the signal pathway, the activated GTP-bound G$_\alpha$ subunit returns to an inactive, "off" state as a result of its intrinsic GTPase activity (see Figure 1-15, *D*). That is, the bound GTP is hydrolyzed to GDP, and the G$_{\beta\gamma}$ complex rebinds to the G$_\alpha$ subunit, returning it (and the G$_{\beta\gamma}$ complex) to its inactive state, awaiting the next ligand-receptor–binding event.

As noted earlier, one of the aspects of the Rube Goldberg analogy is that the same conserved types of molecules are often used in many different pathways. Among the many protein "differences that make a difference" to transmit information, one of the most widely used is a GTPase that has on-off states based on whether GTP or GDP is bound to it. Thus the heterotrimeric G proteins that couple to GPCRs are only one type of GTPase

protein acting as an on-off switch in signaling pathways. Most other members of the G-protein (GTPase) superfamily are simpler and resemble the G$_\alpha$ subunit alone. For example, one such class of these *small G proteins,* called *Rabs,* helps mediate the membrane fusion processes that underlie exocytosis and endocytosis, discussed earlier. All G proteins share evolutionarily conserved GTP binding and enzymatic hydrolysis sites and a similar on-off mechanism: when GTP is bound, the protein is "on," and when GDP is bound, the protein is "off." Chapter 2 discusses a particular small G protein, Ras, that plays a crucial role in regulating cell division and whose dysfunction plays a major role in cancer. Consequently, G proteins in general are discussed in Chapter 2, and this discussion focuses on signaling mechanisms linked to the heterotrimeric G protein specifically.

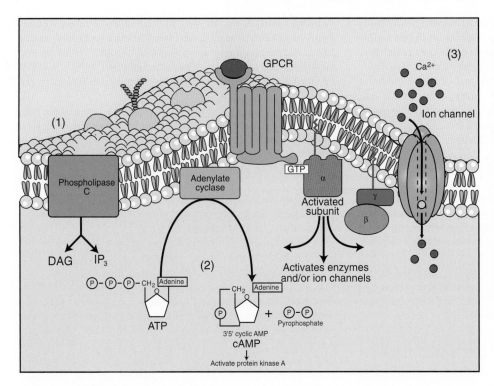

FIGURE 1-16 Activated α subunit of the G protein (Gα) can activate enzymes and ion channels, leading to second-messenger signaling within the cytoplasm. Three principal second messengers send the GPCR information to the cytoplasm. These arise from the activation of ion channels and enzymes stimulated by G$_\alpha$. The second messengers are *(1)* increases in the concentration of inositol 1,4,5-trisphosphate (IP$_3$) in the cytoplasm and increases in the concentration of diacylglycerol (DAG) in the plasma membrane, both as a result of the breakdown of a rare membrane phospholipid, phosphatidylinositol 4,5-bisphosphate (PIP$_2$) by phospholipase C, another G$_\alpha$-stimulated enzyme; *(2)* changes in the concentration of cyclic AMP (cAMP), a special hydrolytic breakdown product of ATP created by the enzyme adenylyl cyclase, which can be activated or inhibited by α subunits; and *(3)* changes in Ca^{2+} concentration within the cytoplasm resulting from transport of Ca^{2+} through gated channels stimulated by G$_\alpha$.

Most G-Protein–Linked Information Is Sent to the Cytoplasm by Second Messengers

As previously noted, the active (heterotrimeric) G protein stimulates an enzyme or ion channel that is associated with the plasma membrane. The ensuing change in ion channel or enzyme function can alter the membrane potential or cause certain molecules/ions to change their concentration in the cytoplasm. Those cytoplasmic ions and molecules that are linked to receptor-ligand binding are called *second messengers*. A second messenger is an ion or molecule that carries the information within the cytoplasm of a cell in response to a signal on the outside surface of a cell (the first message), such as the binding of a hormone or neurotransmitter, or to an electrical event. Most G-protein–linked information is transduced into the cytoplasm in this manner. One of the major advances in our understanding of the molecular basis of physiological signaling is the realization that there are only a few second-messenger systems within animal cells. The most important include the following (Figure 1-16):

1. Two second messengers, inositol 1, 4, 5-trisphosphate (IP$_3$) and diacylglycerol (DAG), are produced by G-protein activation of an enzyme phospholipase C (PLC) (see Figure 1-19 and later discussion).
2. Changes in the concentration of *cyclic adenosine monophosphate* (cAMP).
3. Changes in Ca^{2+} concentration within the cytoplasm.

Clearly, there are many more GPCRs than second messengers. This means that several receptor-mediated events are converted into the same intracellular signal. How does the cell sort out this information? Different cells respond differently to the same second-messenger ion/molecule as a result of the specialized function and makeup of that cell (i.e., the differentiated state it achieved during the development of the animal). For example, smooth muscle cells respond differently to activation of muscarinic acetylcholine receptors (see Table 1-2) than do nerve cells

because the two cells have different proteins that are responsible for their specialized tasks. However, this is only part of the answer, and the specificity of response to the same second messenger and to activation of similar or identical receptors remains an important open question in physiology.

Ca^{2+} Transport Across Plasma and Intracellular Membranes Is an Important Second Messenger

The transport of Ca^{2+} ions through gated channels across the plasma membrane and across intracellular membranes (e.g., endoplasmic reticulum) is a major second messenger system for physiological information transfer. The available evidence suggests that the major role of Ca^{2+} *within* cells is as a physiological signal. In the extracellular compartment, the major physiological function of Ca^{2+} is as the principal mineral of bone. Ca^{2+} is an excellent ion for use as a second messenger because the cytoplasmic concentration of Ca^{2+} is extremely low, about 10^{-7} mol/L in a resting cell. Increases in intracellular Ca^{2+} concentration can be (1) detected easily because the background noise is so low and (2) achieved easily because the Ca^{2+} concentration [Ca^{2+}] in the ECF and in some cellular compartments, such as the endoplasmic reticulum and mitochondria, is 10^4 higher than in the cytoplasm (see Table 1-1). Thus, there is an enormous driving force for Ca^{2+} diffusion into the cytoplasm under most conditions.

Although many GPCRs use Ca^{2+} as one part of their intracellular pathway, the interaction is more complex than usual, as discussed shortly. Thus, we focus here on a simpler and very important example of Ca^{2+} as a second messenger that has already been discussed: the role of Ca^{2+} in regulating the actomyosin ATPase of muscle.

Increased [Ca^{2+}] in the cytoplasm alters cellular function by binding to any of several Ca^{2+}-binding proteins that serve as control proteins. Troponin is one Ca^{2+}-binding protein already mentioned. Reviewing the example of striated muscle contraction from the Ca^{2+} point of view, Ca^{2+} (second messenger) diffuses through gated channels in the endoplasmic reticulum (sarcoplasmic reticulum) of muscle in response to electrical events (first message) on the plasma membrane of the muscle cell. The diffusion of Ca^{2+} from the concentrated storehouse of the sarcoplasmic reticulum increases $[Ca^{2+}]$ in the cytoplasm of the muscle cell, where it binds to troponin. On binding Ca^{2+}, troponin changes its interaction with tropomyosin, which now moves to allow myosin heads access to the actin of the thin filament. The actomyosin ATPase is activated, and muscle contraction ensues.

Calmodulin is a Ca^{2+}-binding protein that plays an important control function in almost all animal cells. As with troponin, calmodulin binds Ca^{2+} when the cytoplasmic $[Ca^{2+}]$ increases. The Ca^{2+}/calmodulin complex activates a large number of different cellular processes. In most such cases, but not all, the Ca^{2+}/calmodulin complex binds to and activates an enzyme. One such enzyme, a protein kinase, is involved in the excitation-contraction coupling in smooth muscle (Figure 1-17), not discussed earlier with the striated muscle types. Protein kinases in general catalyze the hydrolysis of ATP and couple it to the simultaneous phosphorylation of other proteins, as follows:

$$ATP + Protein \xrightarrow[\text{Protein kinase}]{\text{Ca}^{2+}/\text{calmodulin activated}} Protein\ phosphate + ADP$$

In the case of smooth muscle, the particular protein kinase is *myosin kinase,* which, as its name implies, specifically phosphorylates myosin. This phosphorylation increases the affinity of the myosin heads for actin filaments, thus allowing cross-bridging to actin. On formation of the cross-bridge, myosin strokes past the thin filament, producing filament sliding, contraction, and force production by smooth muscle. Cessation of contraction is achieved by cleavage of the phosphate from the myosin by another enzyme, *myosin phosphatase.*

Thus, initiating smooth muscle contraction involves a Rube Goldberg sequence in which environmental stimulation of a smooth muscle cell causes an increase in the intracellular $[Ca^{2+}]$, the second messenger. This in turn leads to a cascade of cause and effect. Increased intracellular $[Ca^{2+}]$ causes calmodulin to bind Ca^{2+}. The Ca^{2+}/calmodulin complex activates the myosin kinase. This enzyme phosphorylates the myosin head, allowing it to cross-bridge to actin. Cross-bridging leads to actomyosin activation, causing filament sliding that is observed as muscle contraction at the tissue level.

This discussion of Ca^{2+} as a second messenger emphasizes one of its major physiological functions: as the second messenger responsible for mediating contraction for all types of muscle (skeletal, cardiac, and striated), although the details of each pathway differ.

Cyclic AMP Is Produced by Activation of a Membrane-Bound Enzyme in Response to Hormone/Neurotransmitter Binding to Receptors

Changes in the activity of membrane-associated enzyme activities are an important mechanism of transmitting information across the cell membrane and are used by most GPCRs. Binding of a signaling molecule to receptors on the extracellular face of the plasma membrane changes the activity of an enzyme located on the cytoplasmic face. The enzyme catalyzes a breakdown reaction; one or more of the breakdown products released into the cytoplasm are second messengers. One important such second-messenger system, and the first to have been discovered, is the

hydrolytic breakdown of ATP to 3′, 5′-adenosine monophosphate, or cAMP, by the enzyme *adenylyl cyclase* (previously called *adenyl cyclase* and *adenylate cyclase*). Cyclic AMP is the second messenger, and adenylyl cyclase is turned on or off as a result of the binding of various hormones and neurotransmitters to cell surface receptors.

As summarized in Figure 1-18, three distinct membrane proteins interact to produce cAMP: (1) any of several receptors, including many GPCRs; (2) the heterotrimeric G protein; and (3) the catalytic protein that actually hydrolyzes ATP to cAMP. Their interaction provides an example of the ability of biomembranes to organize biochemical reactions in space. The likelihood of three proteins colliding and thus being able to interact is much greater in the two-dimensional "phospholipid sea" than in the three-dimensional cytoplasm.

A large number of different hormones/neurotransmitters that bind to different membrane receptors use cAMP to transmit information across the membrane. Among the GPCRs (see Table 1-2) and their hormones/neurotransmitters that use cAMP as their second messenger are *β-adrenergic receptors* that bind epinephrine or norepinephrine, increasing cAMP production and providing important regulation to almost all tissues. The starvation message carried by the binding of glucagon to its receptor (see Chapter 34) is carried to the cytoplasm by an increase in cAMP. *Vasopressin* (also called *antidiuretic hormone,* ADH) binding to its receptors in kidney cells uses cAMP to regulate urine production (see Chapter 33). A number of therapeutic drugs bind to these same receptors and mimic or prevent the physiological action of the hormone/neurotransmitter that normally binds to the receptor.

After ligand binding, the ligand-receptor complex is able to bind to and activate the regulatory G protein (see Figure 1-15, *B*). The G protein in turn changes shape and binds to the catalytic subunit, altering its shape and regulating its ability to bind ATP, and hydrolyzes the catalytic subunit to cAMP (see Figure 1-18). There are two types of G proteins in the adenylyl cyclase system, which differ in their α subunit. The G_s (more specifically, $G_{\alpha s}$, s for stimulatory) activates the catalytic subunit; this is the G protein shown in Figure 1-18. A different G protein, the α subunit of G_i, inhibits adenylyl cyclase when activated. Some diseases are the result of the binding of bacterial toxins to the G proteins. Cholera symptoms result in part from the binding of the toxin of the bacteria *Vibrio cholerae* to the G_s protein, and the irreversible activation of the G_s protein, which in turn irreversibly activates the catalytic subunit. Pertussis (whooping cough) toxin binds irreversibly to and activates G_i, thus inactivating the enzymatic activity.

As suggested by the inhibitory G protein (G_i), regulated decreases in cAMP concentrations are an important part of the cAMP second-messenger system. There are two mechanisms for such decreases: decreasing the rate of cAMP production and eliminating cAMP after formation. The former is achieved by G_i inhibiting the catalytic subunit. Certain inhibitory receptors specifically interact with G_i. Opium and drugs derived from it, such as codeine and morphine, are examples of signaling molecules that bind to inhibitory GPCR (opioid) receptors, activate G_i, and inhibit production of cAMP. Other examples are norepinephrine and epinephrine acting through α_2-adrenergic receptors. Recall that these same neurotransmitters activate adenylyl cyclase when bound to β-adrenergic receptors. This is another example of the principle that the receptor/ligand complex contains the information, not the hormone/neurotransmitter itself.

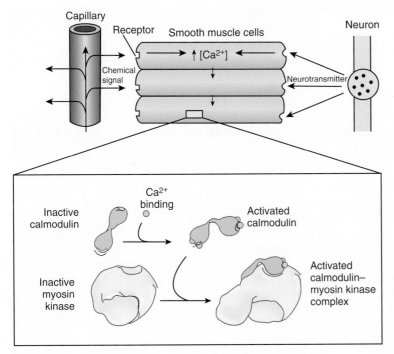

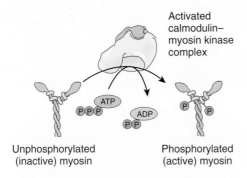

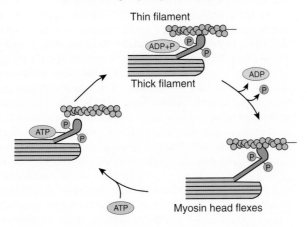

FIGURE 1-17 Role of Ca^{2+} and calmodulin in the regulation of smooth muscle contraction. Smooth muscle regulation is more complex than regulation of striated muscle, and the account here is a simplification. Smooth muscle can be stimulated to contract by a variety of stimuli, including neural signals and soluble chemical signals, as shown here. These external signals all stimulate increased intracellular $[Ca^{2+}]$, which leads to smooth muscle contraction. In the presence of increased intracellular $[Ca^{2+}]$, the Ca^{2+} ions bind to calmodulin, activating it by causing a conformational change. In smooth muscle cytoplasm, the activated Ca^{2+}/calmodulin complex activates myosin kinase, which catalyzes the phosphorylation of myosin. Phosphorylated, activated myosin in turn catalyzes actin-dependent ATP hydrolysis (cross-bridge cycling). Thus, smooth muscle contraction is thick filament regulated, because changes in myosin activate cross-bridging, whereas striated muscle contraction is thin filament controlled, because changes in troponin and tropomyosin of the thin filament activate cross-bridging.

The other control on cAMP levels is elimination of cAMP after formation. This is regulated by the enzyme *cyclic nucleotide phosphodiesteras* (PDE). This enzyme hydrolyzes the 3′ ester bond of the phosphate to the sugar to produce "plain" 5′ AMP (see Figure 1-18). As with myosin kinase discussed earlier, phosphodiesterase is a Ca^{2+}/calmodulin-activated enzyme, so in many cells the activities of the Ca^{2+} and cAMP second-messenger systems antagonize one another.

The increase or decrease in cAMP concentrations most often affects cell function through cAMP's interaction with a particular protein kinase. This protein kinase is called *cAMP-dependent protein kinase*, or *protein kinase A* (PKA). This protein kinase is

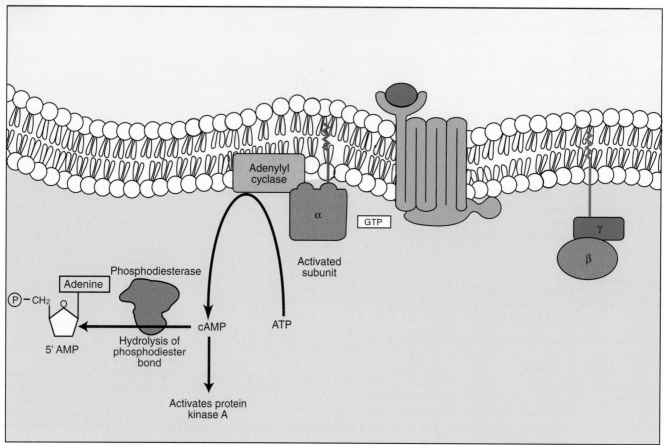

FIGURE 1-18 Activity of cyclic adenosine monophosphate (cAMP) as a second messenger. Cyclic AMP is generated through GPCR-linked activation of adenylyl cyclase, causing hydrolysis of ATP to cAMP. The cAMP thus generated binds to and activates a specific protein kinase, protein kinase A, which in turn can phosphorylate and change the activity of various cellular substrates. When generated, cAMP is broken down by phosphodiesterase (PDE), which hydrolyzes cAMP to "normal" adenosine monophosphate (i.e., 5′ AMP).

distinct from the Ca^{2+}/calmodulin-dependent protein kinase discussed earlier, although the basic outline of action is similar. Protein kinase A is activated by binding cAMP. The higher the concentration of cAMP in a cell, the greater is the number of active protein kinase A molecules. The activated kinase binds to proteins and ATP, hydrolyzing the ATP and phosphorylating the protein. As shown in previous examples, this phosphorylation alters the activity of the target protein, altering its particular characteristic function: catalysis, transport, coupling, and so forth.

Mammals respond to a stressful stimulus by increasing the force and rate of heart contraction, among other physiological effects. This increase in force demonstrates the role of cAMP as a second messenger and the role of Ca^{2+} in GPCR signaling, and it is another example of physiological Rube Goldberg devices based on allosteric changes in proteins. The stressful stimulus causes the adrenal medulla to release epinephrine to the blood, and sympathetic nerves release norepinephrine to the heart. Both catecholamines bind to β-adrenergic GPCRs on the cardiac muscle cells. The receptor-ligand interaction stimulates adenylyl cyclase by way of G_s, increasing intracellular [cAMP], thus increasing protein kinase A activity. Protein kinase A phosphorylates a number of substrates in the cardiac muscle cells, including voltage-dependent Ca^{2+} channels in the plasma membrane. In the phosphorylated state, these channels remain open somewhat longer in response to membrane potentials above threshold.

Consequently, more Ca^{2+} enters the cell for a given electrical stimulation than at lower levels of cAMP. The increase in Ca^{2+} allows more troponin to bind Ca^{2+}; more tropomyosin moves out of the way of myosin heads, causing more cross-bridging and more force production. (Rube Goldberg would have loved modern physiology!)

Another cyclic nucleotide, *cyclic guanosine monophosphate* (cGMP), also serves as a second messenger but is not nearly as widely used as cyclic AMP. Cyclic GMP is the second messenger stimulated by opsins (see Table 1-2) in the rod cells of the retina underlying vision and also causes relaxation of some vascular smooth muscle, including that responsible for penile erection and clitoral engorgement (i.e., blood flow into the corpus cavernosum of both tissues). The role of cGMP in erections is mediated by its activation of cGMP protein kinases, similar to cAMP action via protein kinase A. Activation of cGMP-dependent protein kinase causes relaxation of certain smooth muscles, including those responsible for blood flow to the corpus cavernosum. This has an important clinical correlate: the drug Viagra (sildenafil) inhibits the breakdown of cGMP by a cyclic nucleotide phosphodiesterase, thus increasing blood flow to the penis, and aids erection, but only if neural signals (i.e., sexual stimulation) have stimulated cGMP production initially. This is a good example of how the multistep pathway of cell signaling provides multiple potential sites for appropriate therapeutic intervention; a drug that simply

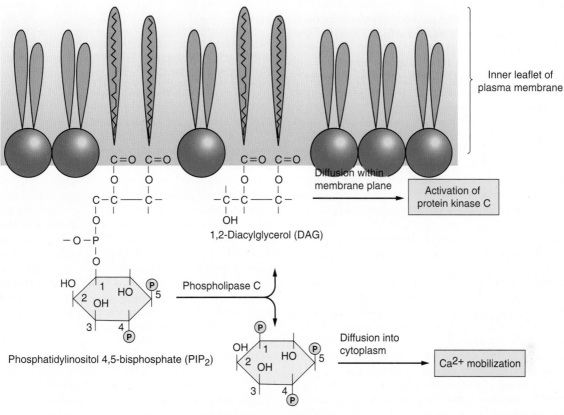

FIGURE 1-19 Hydrolysis of a membrane lipid to produce two second messengers. After appropriate receptor and G-protein activation, the rare membrane phospholipid shown to the left, phosphatidylinositol 4, 5-bisphosphate (PIP_2), is hydrolyzed into two separate second messengers by phospholipase C. The phosphate "head" of the PIP_2 molecule is cleaved to produce the soluble messenger inositol 1, 4, 5-trisphosphate (IP_3), which mobilizes intracellular Ca^{2+}, as well as the lipidic messenger diacylglycerol (DAG), which remains in the membrane and activates protein kinase C.

stimulated cGMP production would cause inappropriate erections, whereas inhibiting its breakdown aids timely erections. Although used mostly by men, sildenafil is also occasionally used for stallions to assist them in "covering" a mare.

In addition to activating protein kinases, cAMP and cGMP can also bind directly to and cause opening of a class of ligand-gated ion channels, cyclic nucleotide–gated ion channels. These ion channels are atypical in that their structure resembles voltage-gated K^+ channels, but they open by directly binding a cyclic nucleotide. These channels play an important role in smell, for which cAMP is the relevant second messenger. In vision, as noted earlier, cGMP is the second messenger, and mutations in the cyclic nucleotide–gated ion channels of cones are responsible for most forms of complete color blindness (but which is rare).

The examples of physiological control by second messengers discussed thus far are short time-scale changes (seconds to hours), which historically have been the purview of "physiologists." It has become increasingly clear, however, that most, if not all, major signals have longer-term (days and weeks) effects based on changes of gene transcription, which in turn mediates changes in growth, differentiation, and long-term behavior. For example, cyclic AMP is now known to be an important regulator of gene transcription controlling learning, production of gametes, and cell division. The effect of cAMP on gene expression is

the result of protein kinase A phosphorylating a specific transcription factor associated with cAMP signaling ("cyclic AMP response element binding protein," or CREB). While space does not allow further discussion of the transcriptional roles of "classic" physiological signal pathways, when dealing with signal pathways it is worthwhile to keep in mind the disclaimer in the first paragraph: only a highly simplified account of cell function is presented here!

The Receptor-Mediated Hydrolysis of a Rare Phospholipid of the Plasma Membrane Produces Two Different Second Messengers with Different Actions

Another second-messenger system differs from both Ca^{2+} and cAMP in that *two* distinct second-messenger molecules are produced as a result of an enzymatic activation by a single receptor/ligand complex. *Phosphatidylinositol* (PI) is a membrane phospholipid that can accept additional phosphate groups by reaction with the —OH groups on the inositol (Figure 1-19). *Phosphatidylinositol 4, 5-bisphosphate* (PIP_2) is the membrane phospholipid that is broken down to produce two important second messengers. PIP_2 is hydrolyzed to *diacylglycerol* (DAG) and *inositol 1, 4, 5-trisphosphate* (IP_3) by a receptor-mediated enzyme called *phospholipase C* (PLC) or phosphoinositidase.

Although many distinct processes are controlled through the PIP$_2$ path, it plays a particularly important role in control of growth and of receptor-mediated secretion. The effect of acetylcholine acting through muscarinic receptors (*not* the nicotinic receptor/ion channel of the nerve-muscle synapse) is often transmitted and transduced through activation of the PIP$_2$ pathway.

The events involved in the receptor-mediated production of IP$_3$ and DAG from PIP$_2$ are similar to those in the production of cAMP. The membrane system appears to consist of three distinct intrinsic membrane proteins: (1) any of several different GPCRs, including the muscarinic acetylcholine receptor and the receptors for some growth factors; (2) a heterotrimeric G protein, similar but not identical to G$_s$ of the cAMP pathway; and (3) the hydrolytic enzyme PLC. A hormone/neurotransmitter or growth factor binds to the receptor, forming a receptor/ligand complex. This complex activates the G protein, which in turn activates the hydrolytic enzyme. At present, only a stimulatory G activity on PLC is known; there is no evidence for an inhibitory G activity in this system.

The activation of the hydrolytic enzyme increases the concentration of IP$_3$, which is water soluble and thus diffuses through the cytoplasm. IP$_3$ binds to and opens ligand-gated Ca^{2+} channels in the endoplasmic reticulum. This releases Ca^{2+} from that high [Ca^{2+}] compartment into the cytoplasm. Ca^{2+} thus becomes the "third messenger" in this system (although this term is not in widespread use) and is another example of a role of Ca^{2+} in GPCR signaling. The ensuing increase in cytoplasmic [Ca^{2+}] affects cellular function by the same mechanisms outlined earlier for Ca^{2+} as a second messenger (e.g., binding to calmodulin), with the Ca^{2+}/calmodulin complex in turn activating various enzyme activities. In receptor-mediated secretion, for example, the binding of acetylcholine to muscarinic receptors in the pancreas (the organ that secretes digestive enzymes) causes an increase in PIP$_2$ breakdown and an increase in cytoplasmic IP$_3$. The IP$_3$ opens ligand-gated Ca^{2+} channels in the endoplasmic reticulum, and intracellular [Ca^{2+}] increases. The process then becomes similar to smooth muscle contraction. Calmodulin binds Ca^{2+}, and the complex activates a protein kinase. However, rather than activating myosin, as for smooth muscle, activation of this protein kinase causes exocytosis of secretory vesicles (membrane bubbles full of secretory product) with the plasma membrane, releasing the enzymes into an extracellular space that is contiguous with the gut.

DAG is also produced on activation of PLC, but it is not at all soluble. DAG diffuses in the plasma membrane, binding to and activating membrane-associated protein kinase, *protein kinase C* (PKC). PKC is not an intrinsic membrane protein and can bind reversibly to the cytoplasmic face of the plasma membrane. PKC phosphorylates other proteins and changes their activity. Because of the membrane-bound character of the enzyme, most evidence indicates that PKC phosphorylates membrane proteins such as receptors and ion channels, regulating their function. In the case of the secretory response to some hormone/neurotransmitter stimulus, PKC generally acts separately but additively with IP$_3$ to produce the response. As with cAMP and protein kinase A, however, much interest focuses on longer-term effects of DAG activation of PKC, particularly its role in growth control and cancer. A class of chemicals long known to promote the onset of cancer, phorbol esters, is a potent substitute for DAG at activating PKC. It is now known that PKC indirectly activates an important transcription factor involved in cell proliferation, nuclear factor kappa B (NF-kB). Thus, as a second messenger and as with cAMP,

DAG has both short-term effects and longer-term transcriptional effects.

Steroid Hormones and Other Lipid Signals Interact with Nuclear Receptors, Which Are Transcription Factors Within the Cell

Nuclear receptors are another large class of protein molecules specialized for information transmission and transduction. Nuclear receptors are sufficiently numerous and diverse that they compose a superfamily of evolutionarily conserved and related receptors, as with the GPCRs. All nuclear receptors are transcription factors that respond to the binding of their cognate lipid signal by regulating which genes are expressed within particular cells under particular conditions. Accordingly, one of the conserved features of nuclear receptors is their DNA-binding domain, which can bind directly to specific sequences of DNA (promoter regions) that control the expression of the neighboring gene(s) (Figure 1-20). As with all other proteins, the DNA-binding function of nuclear receptors is based on their shape. The DNA-binding domain, for example, is a part of the protein shaped into "fingers" by a zinc ion. These *zinc fingers,* also found in many other transcription factors, fit into the grooves of the double helix of DNA at the appropriate base-pair sequence.

Recall that steroid hormones are soluble in oily solvents and are able to diffuse through the lipid bilayer without the mediation of transport proteins. Thyroid hormones are also lipophilic and diffuse through the lipid bilayer. Additionally, several lipid-soluble nutrients are also signaling molecules, including vitamins A and D. Vitamin A is required for vision because it is the covalently bound cofactor for the opsin GPCRs, but it also plays a role in embryonic development. Vitamin D controls Ca^{2+} metabolism. Similarly, saturated and unsaturated fats in the diet are also known to provide signals that control their own breakdown and metabolism and to regulate the differentiation of fat cells (adipose tissue). Consequently, the receptors for these lipid signals are soluble proteins within the target cell. The cellular location of the nuclear receptors varies. Some receptors can be found in the cytoplasm before ligand binding, whereas others are largely restricted to the nucleus (after their initial synthesis in the cytoplasm), but all are functional as transcription factors in the nucleus after activation. The lipid-soluble hormone/nutrient diffuses from the blood into the cell and binds to its receptor, and the hormone/receptor complex is, as in previous examples, the physiologically active entity that ultimately triggers a cellular response. As noted earlier, because the nuclear receptor complex is itself a transcription factor, steroid and thyroid hormones do not require a second messenger; the hormone/receptor complex is itself active within the cell, altering gene expression.

A well-studied example of nuclear receptor action as a regulated transcription factor, with some relevance to veterinary medicine, is the action of estrogen on the reproductive tracts of female chickens (see Figure 1-20). Estrogen is the principal female sex hormone of birds and mammals, and, of course, hens lay eggs in which the embryo and yolk are surrounded by eggwhite. The principal protein of eggwhite is ovalbumin, which is secreted by the epithelial cells of the avian oviduct as the ovum slides by. Thus, one of estrogen's targets in female chickens is oviduct epithelial cells. Estrogen enters the cytoplasm of these cells and binds to its receptor, the *estrogen receptor*. The hormone/receptor complex, but not the ligand-free receptor, is able to mediate estrogen-specific, essentially female-specific, gene transcription. The estrogen receptor complex binds to a sequence of

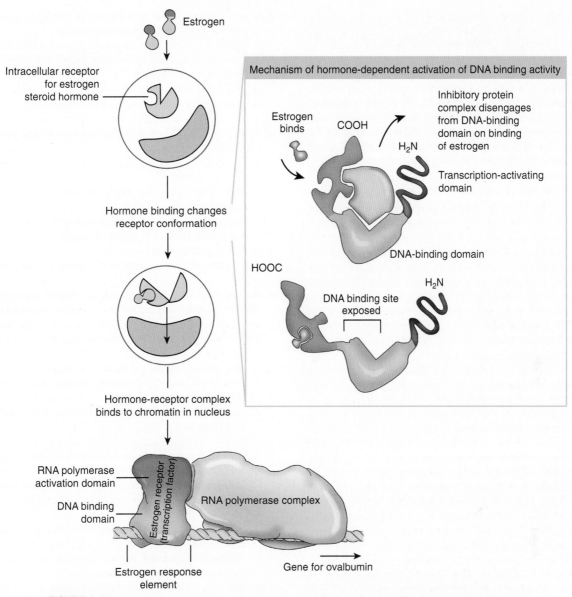

FIGURE 1-20 Steroid hormone action as illustrated by control of ovalbumin expression by estrogen in hens. The steroid hormone estrogen penetrates the lipid bilayer passively because of the oil solubility of the steroid. Inside the cell, the estrogen binds to a cytoplasmic receptor, the estrogen receptor. The binding of estrogen to its receptor causes the receptor protein to change conformation, which in turn changes the DNA-binding activity of the receptor. The hormone/receptor complex enters the nucleus and binds to regulatory sequences of DNA, the estrogen response element. This binding, in turn, activates ribonucleic acid (RNA) polymerase. This initiates transcription of the ovalbumin gene, an estrogen-responsive gene, to produce messenger RNA (mRNA), which is ultimately translated into the ovalbumin protein for secretion.

DNA, called an *estrogen response element,* that controls the transcription of a neighboring gene, for ovalbumin in this case. In other cells of the female, binding of the estrogen receptor to the estrogen response elements of other genes would cause these other female-specific genes to be transcribed and ultimately expressed as a protein (e.g., proteins in yolk of egg). Different steroids bind to different receptors (e.g., male sex hormone testosterone binds to testosterone receptor), which bind to different response elements, leading to different genes expressed (e.g., male-specific gene expression).

Differential gene expression and its regulation were initially pursued primarily by molecular biologists. It rapidly gained importance in physiology, however, and will do so soon in veterinary medicine. Humankind will have fewer scruples about controlling gene expression in animals other than their own species (a fact well illustrated by studies of cancer in mice as discussed in the next chapter). Indeed, understanding control of gene expression may prove more important to veterinary students in the near term than for students of human medicine.

CLINICAL CORRELATIONS

PERIPHERAL EDEMA

History. You examine a 2-year-old cow that has been grazing on poor-quality pasture. The owner states that the cow seems to have a poor appetite, walks slowly, and stands apart from the rest of the herd. The cow has developed swelling beneath the skin of her brisket and ventral thorax.

Clinical Examination. On clinical examination, you find a listless cow standing in a pasture littered with various metal objects. Examination of the cardiovascular system reveals distended jugular veins and abnormal heart sounds characterized by irregular sloshing sounds throughout the cardiac cycle that drastically muffle the first and second heart sounds. Subcutaneous edema (swelling) can be seen throughout the chest and abdomen, but most prominently in the dependent ventral areas of the thorax. Pushing on these swollen areas leaves a dent (pitting edema).

Comment. This is a characteristic history of a cow with hardware disease. The cow, grazing on a pasture littered with metal debris, swallows nails, wire, and so forth. Because these objects are heavier than the feed, they drop into the reticulum, a stomach chamber located just caudal to the diaphragm and heart. With the contractions of the reticulum, a metal object migrates through the reticular wall, diaphragm, and pericardium, leading to an inflammatory response in the pericardium (pericarditis). The resulting process is caused by both inflammation and possible secondary bacterial infections from a contaminated metal object traversing regions of the gastrointestinal tract that contain numerous microorganisms, before the object penetrates the pericardium. An inflammatory exudate fills the pericardial sac; it muffles the heart sounds, and a sloshing sound may be heard on auscultation. As this exudative fluid fills the pericardial sac, it limits the pumping efficiency of the heart by limiting its filling during diastole and by obstructing venous return to the heart (see Chapter 21). The result is left-sided heart failure because the heart cannot circulate (pump) the blood throughout the body. This causes the blood to accumulate initially, leading to an increased hydrostatic pressure in the veins and capillaries. As the capillary hydrostatic pressure rises, capillary filtration is favored over reabsorption, and water leaves the capillary and accumulates in the interstitial space. This accumulated interstitial fluid, primarily as the result of increased capillary filtration, is seen clinically as edema. The other common cause of edema is decreased capillary colloidal osmotic pressure from low serum protein. However, this does not usually play a part in hardware disease.

Treatment. Treatment includes surgical removal of the foreign object or objects, antiinflammatory agents, and antibiotic treatment for the pericarditis. Even though considerable inflammation is present, a secondary bacterial infection often contributes to the response. In such an advanced case, however, treatment often is not completely successful.

PRACTICE QUESTIONS

1. Increasing the extracellular K^+ concentration will:
   a. Have no effect on the resting membrane potential.
   b. Cause the resting membrane potential to decrease (i.e., cause the inside to become less negative with respect to the outside).
   c. Cause the resting membrane potential to increase (i.e., cause the inside to become more negative with respect to the outside).
   d. Increase the concentration potential for K^+ across the plasma membrane.
   e. Require the Na^+,K^+ pump to work harder to pump K^+.

2. G proteins are similar to receptors in that both:
   a. Bind extracellular signaling molecules.
   b. Interact directly with adenylyl cyclase catalytic subunits.
   c. Have activated and inactivated states dependent on ligand binding.
   d. Are extracellular protein molecules.
   e. Directly activate a protein kinase activity.

3. Which of the following statements concerning intracellular Ca^{2+} is false?
   a. It is a second messenger for hormones and neurotransmitters.
   b. It is responsible for excitation-contraction coupling in smooth muscle.
   c. An increase in its concentration in a nerve terminal stimulates the release of a neurotransmitter.
   d. It activates protein kinase A.
   e. Its concentration is increased in the presence of IP_3.

4. If, in a particular capillary bed, the plasma oncotic pressure were to increase and hydrostatic pressure remained constant:
   a. More blood plasma would filter from the capillaries.
   b. The transport effect would be similar to decreasing hydrostatic pressure.
   c. One would suspect a deficiency in blood protein levels.
   d. One would suspect an increase in extracellular fluid protein concentrations.
   e. Fluid reabsorption on the venous side of the capillary bed would decline.

5. Substance X is found to be at a much higher concentration on the outside of a cell than in the cytoplasm, but no transport of X from the extracellular fluid to the cytoplasm occurs. Which of the following statements is inconsistent with this situation?
   a. Substance X has the same electrochemical potential outside and inside the cell.
   b. Substance X is large, is poorly soluble in oil, and has no transport proteins in the membrane.
   c. Substance X is an ion, and the measured membrane potential is the equilibrium potential calculated by the Nernst equation.
   d. Substance X is a steroid molecule.
   e. Substance X is actively transported from the cell to the extracellular fluid.

BIBLIOGRAPHY

Alberts B, Johnson A, Lewis J, et al: *Molecular biology of the cell,* ed 5, New York, 2007, Garland Science.

Lodish H, Berk A, Kaiser CA, et al: *Molecular cell biology,* ed 6, San Francisco, 2007, WH Freeman.

Luttrell LM: Reviews in molecular biology and biotechnology: transmembrane signaling by G protein-coupled receptors, *Mol Biotechnol* 39(3):239–264, 2008.

Novac N, Heinzel T: Nuclear receptors: overview and classification, *Curr Drug Targets Inflamm Allergy* 3(4):335–346, 2004.

Valberg SJ: Diseases of muscles. In Smith BP, editor: *Large animal internal medicine,* ed 4, St Louis, 2008, Mosby.

CHAPTER 2

Cancer: A Disease of Cellular Proliferation, Life Span, and Death

KEY POINTS

1. Cancer arises from genetic dysfunction in the regulation of the cell cycle, cell life span, and cell suicide.

Control of the cell cycle (proliferation)
1. Cell division is the result of a clocklike cell cycle.
2. Cyclin-dependent kinases are the "engines" driving the cell cycle.
3. The CDK "engines" are controlled by both throttle (oncogene) and brake (tumor suppressor) controls.

Growth factor pathway: principal stimulator of cell proliferation
1. The cell cycle is stimulated by growth factors that bind to and activate receptor tyrosine kinases.
2. The Ras oncogene contributes to many cancers and serves as a model for understanding *small G proteins.*
3. The MAP kinase pathway leads to the expression of cyclins and other stimulators of the cell cycle.
4. The MAP kinase pathway also mediates the stimulation of the cell cycle by cell adhesion.

Tumor suppressors: inhibitors of cell cycle
1. Checkpoints in the cell cycle are manned by tumor suppressors.
2. The retinoblastoma and P53 proteins are the main gatekeepers for the cell cycle.

Mechanisms regulating cell suicide and cell life span
1. Apoptosis is the process of cell suicide.
2. Resistance to apoptosis via the intrinsic pathway is a hallmark of cancer.
3. Cellular life span is determined by DNA sequences at the ends of chromosomes.

Tumor origin and the spread of cancer
1. Cancer cells may be related to stem cells.
2. Death by cancer is usually the result of its spread, not the original tumor.
3. Growth of solid tumors depends on development of new blood vessels.

Prospective cancer therapy
1. Cancer therapy has a hopeful but challenging future.

Traditionally, cancer was (and often still is) first detected in humans and domestic animals by clinicians feeling for an unusual mass of cells, tumor cells. Thus, cancer is quite intuitively a disease affecting cellular growth. In the last 25 years, enormous progress has been made in understanding several normal control pathways that regulate cell growth, as well as how these *Rube Goldberg* pathways (see Chapter 1) go wrong in cancer.

The first path to be unraveled, long thought to play a major role in cancer, was the pathway controlling cellular proliferation. Cellular proliferation was known to occur by a regular clocklike cycle of chromosomal doubling followed by mitotic division, called the *cell cycle.* However, almost nothing was known about molecular control of the cell cycle. Progress arose from the study of cancer cells, but importantly also from the study of the proteins synthesized by fertilized sea urchin eggs, how frogs ovulate, and how yeast cells divide. Cell growth depends not only on new cells being formed by cell division, but also on cells dying. As a result of studying in detail the history and fate of every cell that arises during embryonic development to form a soil roundworm (a nematode), it was discovered that cells are programmed to commit "suicide." That is, cells can actively kill themselves using metabolic machinery if the cell has internal damage, such as mutations or oxidative stress. This surprising discovery quickly led to the realization that not only do cancer cells divide inappropriately, but they are also resistant to programmed death and thus continue to divide despite the internal damage. The final general process affecting cellular growth is that normal cells, like the organisms they are part of, have a characteristic life span. However, cancer cells were long known to be "immortal," being able to divide indefinitely. How cells age, or become immortal, was not understood until the process of chromosomal duplication was studied in a ciliated protozoan, similar to the familiar *Paramecium* of college biology laboratories.

As these examples illustrate, our understanding of cellular proliferation, cellular life span, and cell suicide came in large part from the study of problems that first seemed distant from the cancer seen in the clinic. As such, the recent progress on cancer is an unusually dramatic example of the importance of understanding basic biology to understand medicine. The vast majority of cancer studies are conducted on humans and in mice, *the* pre-eminent animal model for cancer, and using cultured cells derived from human and mouse tumors. The much smaller number of studies on domestic animals strongly indicate that the principles derived from humans and mice are generally applicable. However, it is also clear that humans and mice differ in a few aspects of cancer, and thus there are likely to be "special" aspects

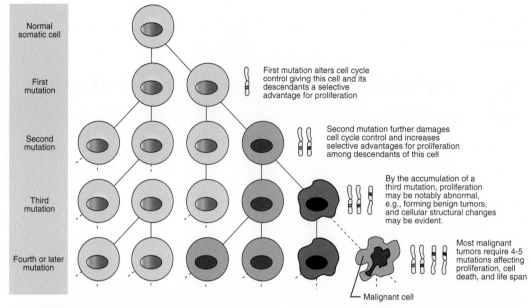

Normal somatic cell

First mutation

First mutation alters cell cycle control giving this cell and its descendants a selective advantage for proliferation

Second mutation

Second mutation further damages cell cycle control and increases selective advantages for proliferation among descendants of this cell

Third mutation

By the accumulation of a third mutation, proliferation may be notably abnormal, e.g., forming benign tumors, and cellular structural changes may be evident.

Fourth or later mutation

Most malignant tumors require 4-5 mutations affecting proliferation, cell death, and life span

Malignant cell

FIGURE 2-1 Clonal basis of cancer. Cancer is the result of the accumulation of mutations in a cell lineage of somatic (nongamete) cells of the body. Beginning with a normal cell, mutations occur by chance or by environmental inputs, such as radiation or cancer-causing chemicals, and accumulate to cause cancer.

of cancer for each species. In the case of domestic animals, different breeds are known to have differing frequencies of various cancers. For example, the reading list at the end of this chapter includes a paper comparing human cancer with the cancer biology of dogs. Veterinary practitioners will need to carefully evaluate the application of knowledge about human and mouse tumors for their patients.

Cancer Arises from Genetic Dysfunction in the Regulation of the Cell Cycle, Cell Life Span, and Cell Suicide

Cancer is a genetic disease (but not usually a hereditary disease) and a uniquely cellular disease. As shown in Figure 2-1, tumors and other cancers arise from the division of a single mutant cell whose descendants accumulate several additional mutations to become increasingly damaged with respect to control of cellular proliferation, life span, and cell death. That is, cancer is a genetic disease caused by the accumulation of mutations in body cells, such as those of the epithelia lining the lungs or the secretory epithelia of the mammary glands.

All the cells of a tumor can trace their ancestry back to a single cell that developed an initial deleterious mutation. This first mutation usually occurs in a gene controlling proliferation, such that the cell produces a mutant protein[1] that is a dysfunctional, more permissive regulator of the cell cycle. This greater "permissiveness" provides the mutant cell with more opportunity to proliferate, and it thus has a selective advantage compared with its normal neighbors. Perhaps because of this selective advantage, or

because of continued exposure to mutagens (e.g., cigarette smoke, agricultural chemicals), a descendant of this cell accumulates another mutation that also affects some aspect of the cell cycle or cell death. This increases the doubly mutant cell's selective advantage further still, and the downward spiral of increasingly abnormal, dividing cells begins to spin out of control. Scientists agree that this accumulation of mutations in individual genes is necessary for cancer to develop, but some think it is not sufficient. Rather, they argue that cancer only results when the accumulation of mutations eventually leads to large-scale genetic instability, such that whole chromosomes are gained and lost. The majority of spontaneous tumors do have cells with abnormal sets of chromosomes, a phenomenon called *aneuploidy*. Whether aneuploidy is necessary for cancer remains to be seen, but there is no disagreement that cancer cells are in some way badly damaged with respect to genes controlling growth.

The mutations leading to cancer are the same type as those that underlie Mendel's familiar laws of heredity. These include base-pair changes, deletions or additions of nucleotides in the gene, and translocation of one piece of a chromosome to another. However, it is important to understand that the *cells* in which the mutations are occurring are different than those underlying Mendel's laws of inheritance. Mendelian inheritance results from mutations occurring in the *germ line* of the organism. These are the cells that will become gametes, either sperm or eggs, and whose deoxyribonucleic acid (DNA) will be passed down to every cell of the offspring. The mutations leading to cancer are occurring in nonreproductive cells throughout the body, called *somatic cells*. These are passed down only to a limited number of other somatic cells by cell division, not to offspring through sexual reproduction. Thus, although cancer is a genetic disease, only about 10% of the time is it a "hereditary disease," that is, the result of mutation inherited from a parent. In general, cancer appears to be the result of the accumulation of mutations leading to genetic instability in a particular lineage of somatic cells.

---

[1]For the many instances when a gene and protein share the same name, this chapter adopts a widely used, but by no means universal, convention for distinguishing genes and their cognate proteins. Gene names are in italics and all lowercase (e.g., *ras*), whereas the protein name has a capitalized first letter and is not italicized (e.g., Ras). This convention is used throughout in preference to the various species-dependent conventions also used in the literature.

Traditionally, cancers are divided into categories based on the cell type involved. Carcinomas are cancers of epithelial cells; sarcomas are derived from connective tissue or muscle; and leukemias are cancers of blood-forming cells. There are many subdivisions based on specific cell types and location of the tumors. However, these names are traditional only; they do not reflect any fundamental differences in the biology of the cancer. Rather, it is now clear that cancers of all types share broadly similar types of dysfunctions controlling cell proliferation, cell suicide, and cell life span.

CONTROL OF THE CELL CYCLE (PROLIFERATION)

Cell Division Is the Result of a Clocklike Cell Cycle

The *Rube Goldberg device* that controls cell growth is particularly complex, with many, many more components than the "garage door opener" of Figure 1-13. To explain these pathways, we begin with the cell cycle that, like the carriage house door, is near the end of the system of control. That is, most of the control elements feed "downstream" to control the cell cycle, or intersect with some aspect of cell cycle control.

Figure 2-2 shows the classic diagram of the cell cycle in which the cell changes its state toward division, progressively going around the diagram, like the hands of a clock. For most mammalian cells, the duration of one cell cycle in culture varies between 18 and 30 hours. Two phases of the cell cycle were identified first and seemed to be where the most important events of the cell cycle occurred. One is *synthesis (S) phase,* during which the DNA is duplicated. The second is *mitosis (M) phase,* during

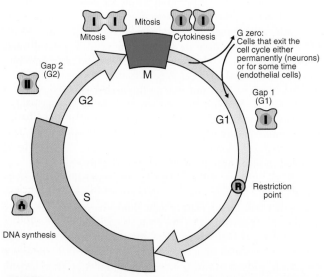

FIGURE 2-2 The mammalian cell cycle. Cell proliferation occurs by a clocklike progression of phases in which characteristic events occur. The most familiar is M phase (mitosis), during which the cytoplasm and replicated chromosomes are distributed to the daughter cells. Cells then enter G1, during which a "decision" is made whether or not to go forward with the cell cycle; this is the R (restriction) point. The events in G1 then allow S (synthesis) phase to proceed, during which the DNA is replicated to produce exactly two copies. After DNA synthesis, the cell prepares for mitosis during G1, and the cycle is complete. Although cells in culture typically go around the cycle continuously, most cells in the body divide only occasionally. These quiescent cells, as well as cells such as neurons that never divide after differentiation, are in G0, a nondividing phase. Under appropriate stimulation, cells can then exit G0 and are said to reenter the cell cycle.

which the duplicated chromosomes are separated to opposite sides of the cell and the cytoplasm divides. In addition to the obvious need for such events if cells are to reproduce, note that both phases must be highly precise. It is crucial for the cell that DNA synthesis produces *exactly* twice the original amount of DNA, no more and no less. Otherwise, there will not be two identical copies of the genetic material to pass on to two identical cells. Similarly, the machinery segregating the duplicated chromosomes during mitosis must partition exactly equal numbers and types of chromosomes to daughter cells, or the cells will be aneuploid. If DNA is not precisely replicated, or if the chromosomes are not properly aligned, the cell cycle is halted, by *checkpoints,* as described later.

However, the events during G1 ("gee-one") and G2 phases remained a mystery. The "G" stands for *gap,* because of the decades-long gap in our understanding of what was happening during this time. Although it was suspected that the cell was preparing itself for DNA synthesis during G1 and preparing for mitosis during G2, the nature of these "preparations" proved difficult to determine. In the mid-1980s, work initially conducted on frog oocytes revealed that specialized protein kinases were activated during G1 and G2 to drive the cell into S phase and M phase, respectively. These special protein kinases are now called *cyclin-dependent kinases* (CDKs).

Cyclin-Dependent Kinases Are the "Engines" Driving the Cell Cycle

Recall from Chapter 1 that protein kinases, which are enzymes that phosphorylate other proteins, are important as elements of signaling pathways. For example, the second messenger cyclic adenosine monophosphate (cAMP) acts by activating protein kinase A (see Figure 1-18), and diacylglycerol as a second messenger activates protein kinase C (see Figure 1-19). Protein kinases play a major role in many aspects of control of the cell cycle; most importantly, CDKs, when activated, can directly cause a cell to enter either S phase or mitosis, whether the cell is ready or not.

Active CDKs are composed of two different types of protein subunits (Figure 2-3). The catalytic subunits (numbered CDK1, CDK2, etc.) are the subunits that have enzymatic activity for hydrolyzing adenosine triphosphate (ATP) and transferring the phosphate group to a protein substrate. The other subunit is an activator of the catalytic subunit and is called a *cyclin;* the abundance of this protein increases and decreases during the cell cycle (i.e., the protein concentration cycles up and down during the cell cycle). Different cyclins are specific for various CDKs and for the different phases of the cell cycle. The various cyclins are identified by letters, such as cyclin A and cyclin B. Cyclins must reach a threshold concentration to activate the catalytic subunit, and the threshold is achieved as a result of protein accumulation from new synthesis during the G phases.

When the cyclins have bound to their appropriate catalytic subunit, the cyclin-CDK complex as a whole is activated by achieving a particular state of *phosphorylation.* There are inhibitory sites of phosphorylation around amino acid 15 of the catalytic subunit, and these must be dephosphorylated. There is also a stimulatory phosphorylation site at amino acid 167, and this must be phosphorylated for cyclin-CDK activity. When activated, the CDK phosphorylates various substrates associated with either S phase or M phase. For example, the cyclin-CDK complex responsible for mitosis directly phosphorylates the protein filaments that strengthen the nuclear membrane (lamins).

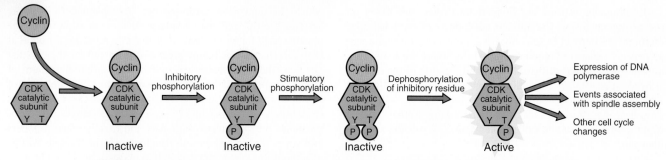

FIGURE 2-3 Activation of the cyclin-CDK "engines" of the cell cycle. Activation of cyclin-dependent kinases depends on the association of a cyclin with a catalytic subunit and then an appropriate pattern of inhibitory and stimulatory phosphorylations on the catalytic subunit.

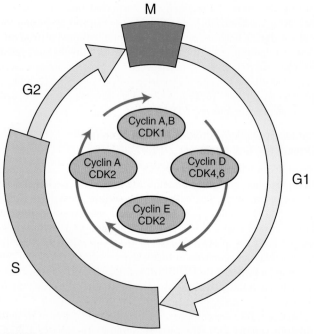

FIGURE 2-4 Cyclins and CDKs around the cell cycle. Different phases of the cell cycle are associated with and driven by different cyclin-CDK pairs, as shown here.

This phosphorylation causes the filaments to disassemble, in turn allowing the nuclear membrane to dissolve, which is an early event of mitosis.

The different phases of the cell cycle are controlled by different cyclin-CDK pairs, as shown in Figure 2-4. Thus the complex of CDK1 with either cyclin B or cyclin A is the particular CDK pair responsible for driving the cell into mitosis. Cyclins E and A interacting with CDK2 play important roles in initiating and maintaining DNA synthesis in S phase. Cyclin D interacting with either CDK4 or CDK6 functions in late G1 in a "decision" by the cell to commit to DNA synthesis. This decision is called the *restriction (R) point* and is discussed in the later section on tumor suppressors.

Given the importance of cyclins and CDKs in driving the cell cycle, one would expect they would have some connection to cancer. Overexpression of cyclin D is associated with human and mouse breast cancer, and ablation of cyclin D provides some protection against breast cancer in mice. Virtually all multiple

myelomas, a type of leukemia, show overexpression of cyclin D. Overexpression of cyclin A is strongly associated with some lung cancers and with testicular cancer of humans, and overexpression of cyclin E is associated with certain human leukemias. Curiously, in contrast to the cyclin subunit, the CDK enzymatic subunit is not known to be mutant in any common cancer.

The CDK "Engines" Are Controlled by Both Throttle (Oncogene) and Brake (Tumor Suppressor) Controls

The CDK-cyclin pairs are controlled by both stimulatory and inhibitory pathways, analogous to an automobile engine controlled by throttle and brake mechanisms. The throttle mechanisms are largely the result of the cell's environmental inputs. That is, various environmental cues, both soluble signal molecules and insoluble molecules found in tissue, are required for cells to divide. However, the pathways sending inhibitory signals to the cell cycle, the "brakes" for cell division, are largely internal and are activated by damage or stress to the cell. In general, these inhibitory signals are like the safety interlocks on an automobile. Just as one cannot start a car in gear, so the cell should not divide if DNA synthesis has not exactly duplicated all the genes and chromosomes, or if something is wrong with the mitotic spindle.

The environmental stimulatory signals for cell division can be as simple and nonspecific as availability of nutrients, to the extent that cells only divide when they have approximately doubled in size through synthetic growth. However, two more specific stimulators of the cell cycle are primarily implicated in cancer. One is the response to soluble growth factors found in the circulation and in the extracellular fluid surrounding cells (see Chapter 1). Growth factors are proteins secreted by a variety of other cell types that are required for the division, and indeed survival, of normal, noncancerous cells. Cancer cells, however, can divide and survive with little or no stimulation from growth factors because of the acquired ability to synthesize growth factors of their own, or the activation of downstream elements in the signaling pathway.

The second stimulatory pathway of general importance in cancer is cell attachment. The cells of multicellular organisms must be tightly attached to one another and to their surrounding matrix, similar to tendon; otherwise we would be jelly, juice, and bubbles on the floor. Also, however, attachment of cells to their surroundings is a source of specific and complex information to the physiology of the cell. One of the most important such messages is a "permissive" signal to divide. Normal cells must be anchored to some substrate in order to respond to other signals to divide. That is, most normal animal cells show *anchorage dependence of growth.* For this reason, vertebrate cells in culture are grown on the surface of a dish or flask, not in suspension the way bacteria are cultured. Again, cancer cells have lost this normal restriction on proliferation, and many cancer cells can divide and survive in suspension. The common test for the absence of anchorage dependence is growth in soft agar: cancer cells will, but normal cells will not, divide and form colonies when suspended in soft agar. Thus, cancer cells can survive unattached while riding the circulation to relocate in a different tissue than that of the original tumor. In this way, cancer is able to spread through the body, a process called *metastasis,* which is ultimately the cause of death in most cases of cancer.

The Rube Goldberg pathways that underlie the proliferative signals of growth factors and adhesion are similar and intersect. These "throttle" contraptions begin with a soluble signal binding to a growth factor receptor and a "solid-state" signal about attachment to the surrounding tissue. However, both pathways quickly converge on the same stimulation pathway for conserved cell division. These stimulatory pathways are driven by proteins that were originally identified as being encoded by genes in viruses that caused cancer in animals. Thus these were named *oncogenes,* literally "cancer genes." A major breakthrough came with the discovery that these oncogenes were actually derived from the host genome, not genes normally encoded in the virus. That is, viruses had stolen cell cycle control genes from their animal host cell. Being viruses, they did not take good care of the animal cell cycle genes they stole. The stolen genes mutated into deranged cell cycle regulators. Subsequently, the same mutant genes that were found in viruses were found to explain many spontaneous cancers in humans and in the long-used experimental tumors of mice. The finding that cancer was caused by abnormal host genes helped confirm that cancer was a somatic genetic disease due to mutations in the tumor cells.

Further analysis revealed that these oncogenes often encode normal stimulators of the cell cycle, and the mutations involved had the effect of permanently activating an element in the cell cycle pathway. You can see how this would work based on the Rube Goldberg cartoon of Figure 1-13. Note that all the elements in the garage door opener are stimulatory; if any one turns "on," a signal is sent "downstream" to cause the garage door to open. If the fish tank of the cartoon were to "mutate" by developing a leak, an "on" signal would be sent downstream of the fish tank, regardless of whether a car had pulled into the driveway. So it is with the oncogene elements controlling the cell cycle. If one of the elements mutates to turn itself "on," that is, acquired a *gain-of-function mutation,* it will stimulate cell division and contribute to cancer. To return to the automobile analogy, oncogenes represent a stuck throttle or accelerator pedal. The normal, well-behaved versions of the oncogene (a watertight fish tank before the bullet, Figure 1-13) are called *proto-oncogenes.* Thus, strictly speaking, oncogenes have their normal equivalent as proto-oncogenes. However, given this awkward usage, increasingly the normal versions are also informally called oncogenes, and it is usually clear from the context whether the mutant or normal version is being discussed. The molecules and molecular events of the oncogene pathway (also called the *growth factor* or *MAP kinase pathway*) are discussed later.

The mechanisms to stop the cell cycle, the "brakes," are called *checkpoints.* Progress through the cell cycle depends on appropriate conditions being reached within the cell before a "decision" is made to go ahead with division. The first such checkpoint occurs before S phase. During G1, the cell checks itself over particularly with respect to DNA damage. The cell has sophisticated pathways to detect and repair DNA damage, such as mismatched bases detected in the double helix. For needed repairs to take place, however, DNA synthesis is delayed; the checkpoint is "engaged." If the DNA is properly repaired, the checkpoint is disengaged, and after the delay, the cell goes ahead into S phase. However, if the DNA damage cannot be repaired, the checkpoint machinery is supposed to signal a more serious consequence. If the checkpoint is not disengaged after about a day, the cell "commits suicide." Thus the checkpoint (or braking machinery) is tied into both the CDK engines and the processes of cell suicide, as described later. Similarly, the second checkpoint is in mitosis and checks for proper mitotic spindle assembly and correct chromosome alignment. Here again, if damage is detected, there are repair mechanisms, and a properly repaired cell will go into M phase after a delay for repair. If no repair can be made, the cell commits suicide.

The molecules and their interactions that underlie both oncogene ("throttle") pathways and checkpoint ("brake") pathways are now covered in greater detail, beginning with the role of growth factors.

GROWTH FACTOR PATHWAY: STIMULATOR OF CELL PROLIFERATION

The Cell Cycle Is Stimulated by Growth Factors that Bind to and Activate Receptor Tyrosine Kinases

The growth factor/oncogene pathway begins with growth factors that function in a familiar way, as discussed in Chapter 1: they bind to and activate an integral membrane protein receptor. Indeed, growth factor receptors belong to the third family of receptors for environmental signals, the *receptor tyrosine kinase* family. This family of signal transducers has some similarities with the G-protein–coupled receptors (GPCRs), but also some important differences. Receptor tyrosine kinases (RTKs) do not require second messengers, but they do function through protein kinase activity (as many GPCRs do). The structure of RTKs is such that binding of ligand (a growth factor) by the extracellular portion of the receptor directly activates protein kinase activity by the cytoplasmic portion of the protein. The receptor itself is an enzyme (Figure 2-5). Thus the RTK carries the message across the plasma membrane, without the need for a second message. RTKs specifically add a phosphate group to a tyrosine residue of the substrate protein. This differs from the protein kinases discussed in Chapter 1 (PKA and PKC), which add the phosphate to serine or threonine residues. Phosphorylation of tyrosine residues within a protein is largely (but not exclusively) specialized to control cell growth pathways, and therefore tyrosine kinase activity generally is associated with stimulation of proliferation.

The growth factors that bind to the RTKs are too diverse to be discussed at length in this chapter. Rather, one important similarity for introductory professional students is that these factors are all poorly named, so do not judge the factor by its name. Sometimes growth factors have "growth factor" in their name; some are referred to as *cytokines;* and some are called *colony-stimulating factors* (for growth of colonies in soft agar, as previously mentioned). Further confusion arises because their names always reflect their history but rarely their broader function. Thus, "epidermal growth factor" stimulates cell division in many more types of cells than only skin cells, but it was discovered using skin cells. The other, more important similarity among growth factors is that whatever their name they share a conserved basic pathway and

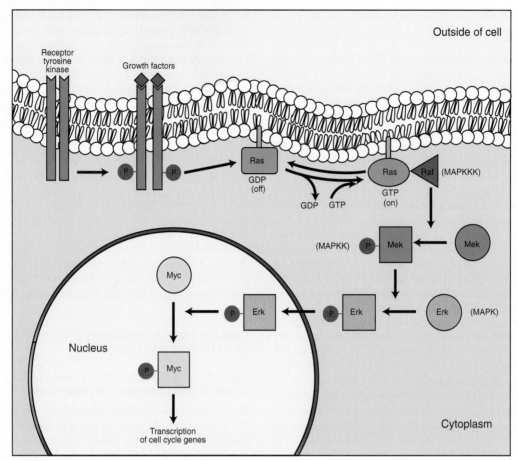

FIGURE 2-5 Growth factor/oncogene pathway. This diagram shows the normal stimulatory pathway by which growth factors lead to cell division. Growth factors bind to membrane receptors (receptor tyrosine kinases, RTKs) that are themselves protein kinases. As shown here, after activation by binding a growth factor, the first protein to be phosphorylated at tyrosine residues is the receptor protein itself. This in turn causes a small G protein, Ras, to exchange GDP for GTP and thus be "turned on." The activated Ras then activates the first protein kinase in a conserved pathway of three kinases, called the MAP kinase pathway. For more detail on Ras and the MAP kinase pathway, see the text. Finally, this series of activating phosphorylations leads to the activation of transcription factors, such as Myc, in turn leading to the expression of genes directly involved in driving the cell cycle (e.g., expression of cyclin D). In this pathway, gain-of-function mutations of the RTKs, Ras, and Myc are particularly important in human cancers.

"strategy" for control, as with the numerous ligands binding GPCRs and nuclear receptors, of their downstream effectors, in this case the CDK engines of the cell cycle. Growth factor activation of RTKs stimulates a pathway involving a G-protein "on-off" molecular switch, the *Ras protein* introduced in Chapter 1, and uses a cascade of protein kinases, both tyrosine and serine-threonine, called the *MAP kinase pathway*. Ultimately, the MAP kinase pathway activates transcription factors, in turn controlling the expression of cyclins, and other direct regulators of CDKs (see Figure 2-5).

The *Ras* Oncogene Contributes to Many Cancers and Serves as a Model for Understanding Small G Proteins

After activation of the RTK, the next major step in the growth factor/oncogene pathway in normal cells is activation of the protein product of the ras proto-oncogene. Investigations of how it worked revealed that the Ras protein was an important member of the small G-protein family of molecular regulators, all of which have intrinsic guanosinetriphosphatase (GTPase) activity and serve as molecular "on-off switches." These proteins control many

basic cellular functions, and the heterotrimeric G protein evolved from Ras-like ancestor proteins (see Chapter 1). Indeed, in yeast it is Ras, not a heterotrimeric G protein, that controls adenyl cyclase and phospholipase C (see Figure 1-18). Figure 2-6 illustrates the duty cycle of this on-off switch and its basic similarity to the alpha subunit (G_α) of the heterotrimeric G proteins. Ras, other small G proteins, and G_α all are in the "on" state when they have guanosine triphosphate (GTP) bound to them (because of receptor activation). All are in the "off" state when the G protein hydrolyzes its GTP so that guanosine diphosphate (GDP) is now bound. You can see how this gene could be discovered as an oncogene, that is, a gene in which a gain-of-function mutation contributes to the development of cancer. If the GTPase activity is lost by mutation, this simple, enzymatic on-off switch remains trapped in the "on" position (the accelerator pedal is stuck). It continues to send an activating signal to the downstream cell cycle machinery without the presence of growth factors or the activation of RTKs. In fact, such mutations in Ras underlie its oncogenic function, and it is estimated that 30% of human cancers have activating mutations in their *ras* gene.

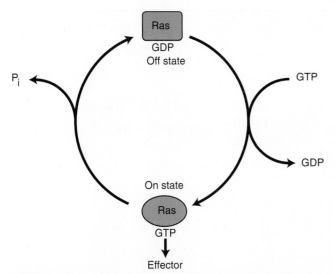

FIGURE 2-6 Duty cycle of the Ras molecular "on-off switch." Ras serves as a model for the activity of small G proteins, of which there are hundreds in the cell. The molecular mechanism of Ras is similar to the alpha subunit of the heterotrimeric G protein, discussed in Chapter 1 and which evolved from Ras-like proteins. As shown here, Ras is in the "off" state when bound to GDP. Activation of RTKs leads to nucleotide exchange: GDP is lost and GTP is bound. In the GTP-bound form, Ras is in the "on" state and sends a stimulatory signal downstream, in this case to Raf in the MAP kinase pathway (see Figure 2-4). Normally, Ras rapidly returns to the off state because an intrinisc GTPase activity of the Ras protein hydrolyzes the GTP to GDP. This nucleotide-dependent on-off cycle is characteristic of all normal small G proteins.

Other small G proteins control a myriad of cellular functions, including others involved in cancer. Thus the Rho subfamily of small G proteins is directly involved in the spread of cancer because it helps regulate actin assembly and activity. As described later, the spread of cancer depends on the ability of cells to migrate through tissues. This "crawling" motility in turn depends on a musclelike mechanism based on actin and myosin (see Figure 1-4). Although the basic, on-off activity of Ras and Rho are the same as that shown in Figure 2-6, Rho is connected to actin, whereas active Ras activates the elements of the MAP kinase pathway.

The MAP Kinase Pathway Leads to the Expression of Cyclins and Other Stimulators of the Cell Cycle

GTP-bound Ras causes the sequential activation of a series of protein kinases, called Raf, Mek, and Erk. Raf phosphorylates and activates Mek, which in turn phosphorylates and activates Erk, as shown in Figure 2-5. This trio of kinases is called *the mitogen-activated protein kinase,* or MAP kinase, pathway (a *mitogen* is a stimulator of mitosis, e.g., a growth factor). If any of these three protein kinases should experience a gain-of-function mutation irreversibly activating the protein kinase, a stimulatory signal is sent down the remainder of the pathway. Thus, as with ras, these three kinase genes act as oncogenes.

One important example of a gain-of-function mutation among the three MAP kinases involves the first of these MAP kinases, Raf. A single–amino-acid mutation in the kinase domain of Raf (a substitution of glutamate for normal valine at amino acid 600) causes permanent activation of Raf in approximately 50% of human melanomas, a very deadly cancer, and is also common in thyroid cancers. As described for mutations in Ras, activation of Raf sends an unregulated stimulatory signal downstream to the other MAP kinases, leading to unregulated proliferation of the cancer cells. Recent clinical progress involving melanoma illustrates the importance of understanding which particular mutations are involved in a given patient's cancer. A newly developed drug, vemurafenib, targets the mutant Raf and significantly prolongs the life span of those melanoma patients harboring this *raf* mutation, but has no effect in cases of melanoma with normal Raf/*raf*.

Raf, Mek, and Erk are a specific example of yet another conserved but diverse general module of information transduction. There are MAP kinase trios other than Raf, Mek, and Erk. Although it is not worthwhile to give names to all the various specific pathways, it should be noted that these trios have a systematic set of names for their elements. Raf is a MAP kinase, kinase, kinase (a MAPKKK). Mek is a MAP kinase, kinase (MAPKK), and Erk protein is the MAP kinase (MAPK) itself. This jargon is awkward, but it is widely used and logical, as Figure 2-5 suggests.

When activated, Erk activates one or more transcription factors that control the transcription and translation of a key regulator of the cyclin-CDK engine. One of these transcription factors, *Myc* ("mick"), is encoded by another important oncogene/proto-oncogene. As with *ras*, the *myc* gene is mutated in a high frequency of human tumors, giving rise to an oncogenic form able to activate the cell cycle. As shown in Figure 2-5, Myc protein is involved in the transcription of a variety of cyclins and of the CDK2 catalytic subunit and plays a significant role in allowing the cell to pass from G1 to S phase. Myc is also involved in many other transcription events related to cell growth, differentiation, and cancer.

This completes the growth stimulatory pathway beginning with a growth factor binding to its RTK receptor that, through Ras, a MAP kinase cascade, and a transcription factor, eventually leads to a direct "throttling up" of a cyclin-CDK engine. This same pathway is used similarly to transduce the information about the other major stimulator of cell division, cell attachment.

The MAP Kinase Pathway also Mediates the Stimulation of the Cell Cycle by Cell Adhesion

As noted earlier, the other major throttle mechanism to regulate the cyclin-CDK engines of the cell cycle is cell adhesion. Cell adhesion, as with growth factor stimulation, ultimately stimulates cyclin-CDK pairs through the MAP kinase pathway. Two types of cell contact are involved in normal growth and proliferation. The most obvious is cell-cell adhesion; most cells are tightly attached to their neighboring cells. The second type is cell adhesion to an extracellular matrix (ECM) of fibrous proteins. Eighty percent of human and mouse cancers arise from epithelial cells (carcinomas), and all epithelial layers are attached to an ECM. The adhesion proteins that bind to other cells or to the ECM are *adhesion receptors*. Adhesion receptors are responsible for the mechanical aspect of attachment, but also act similar to other receptors in transducing information across the plasma membrane. In this case, adhesion receptors communicate the information that the cell is anchored and can divide.

Both cell-cell and cell-ECM adhesion activate the MAP kinase pathway, similar to growth factors, but the Ras intermediate is less important here. Figure 2-7 shows the activation of the MAP kinase pathway as a result of cell-ECM adhesion. The adhesion receptors that bind to ECM are called *integrins* and these activate

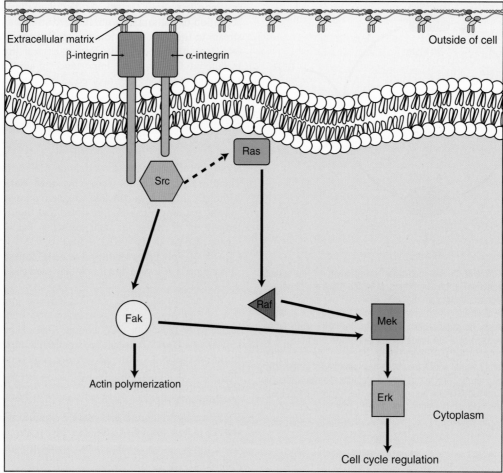

FIGURE 2-7 Cell adhesion functions through the MAP kinase pathway to stimulate cell division. In addition to the growth factor stimulation of proliferation shown in Figure 2-5, normal epithelial cells also require stimulation of the MAP kinase pathway through adhesion to the extracellular matrix. The adhesion receptors are integral membrane proteins called integrins, which are activated by binding proteins of the extracellular matrix. Activation of integrins leads to activation of two protein kinases, Src and focal adhesion kinase (Fak), which in turn activate the MAP kinase pathway.

the MAP kinase pathway via two important intermediates that are oncogenes. One is Src ("sark"), a protein tyrosine kinase and the first oncogene (*src*) to be discovered. Unlike the RTKs previously described, Src is not a receptor. However, Src is located on the inside face of the plasma membrane, where it can interact with adhesion receptors. Another important intermediate is also a protein tyrosine kinase, called Fak (focal adhesion kinase). As before, activation of Src and Fak activate the MAP kinase pathway, leading to increased cell division. Again, mutation or overexpression of *src* and *fak* sends inappropriate stimulation to the cell cycle machinery, which facilitates cancer. As mutant oncogenes, *fak* is associated with aggressive melanomas in humans. The *src* oncogene was named because of its ability to cause sarcomas in chickens.

Several other growth stimulatory pathways work in much the same manner as the growth factor and adhesion pathways. Most stimulatory pathways involve protein kinases and G proteins controlling the transcription of genes encoding proteins that are part of or close to the workings of the cyclin-CDK engines.

Having introduced the fundamentals of stimulatory pathways in the cell cycle, we now change our focus to consider the equally Rube Goldberg–like pathways that provide the brakes to the cell cycle.

TUMOR SUPPRESSORS: INHIBITORS OF CELL CYCLE

Checkpoints in the Cell Cycle Are Manned by Tumor Suppressors

The cell cycle machinery also has crucial "brake" mechanisms that function as checkpoints, as noted earlier. The components of the brake and checkpoint mechanisms were discovered by fusing a normal cell with a cancer cell of the same type, to form a hybrid cell with two nuclei. The resulting hybrid cell invariably showed normal regulation of growth. Apparently, a normal copy of some gene or genes present in the normal cell was able to suppress the altered activity of a mutant gene in the cancer cell. Thus these genes and their encoded proteins were called *tumor suppressors*.

Tumor suppressors play several different functional roles in braking and checking, and they can be divided into two broad types, gatekeepers and caretakers. *Gatekeepers* are genes and proteins that are involved in the actual checkpoint machinery

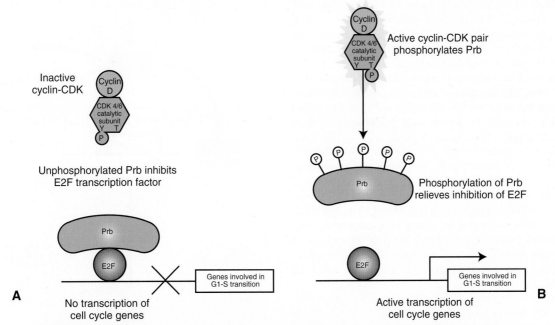

FIGURE 2-8 Retinoblastoma protein and the G1-to-S transition. **A**, In quiescent cells or cells early in G1, retinoblastoma protein (Prb) exists in a nonphosphorylated state that is a direct inhibitor of the E2F transcription factor. The principal CDK pair of G1, cyclin D with CDK4 or CDK6, phosphorylates Prb, releasing its inhibition of E2F. **B**, Activated E2F then participates in the expression of a variety of genes required for S phase, including the cyclins and CDKs of S phase and subunits of DNA polymerase.

connecting cell damage with a halt in the cell cycle. Thus, *P53* (protein of 53-kilodalton mass) is a gatekeeper importantly involved in the pathway that detects DNA damage; it causes a halt in the cell cycle and, if the damage cannot be repaired, signals the cell to undergo programmed death. It is thought that about 50% of human cancers have a mutation in P53. *Caretakers* are usually proteins involved in the repair of damage or the normal maintenance of proteins crucial in the cell cycle. A human example of a caretaker gene and protein is Brca1 (breast cancer 1). This protein is normally involved in the repair of nucleotide mismatches (e.g., G paired with T rather than with C in the complementary DNA strand), and its mutant gene has been found to underlie familial (hereditary) breast cancer in some families.

With these normal functions, one can see how these genes and proteins would suppress tumor activity and cell proliferation. If they are working, DNA is repaired before the cell attempts to divide; this would tend to prevent mutation or other types of genetic instability. However, *loss-of-function mutation* in these genes means the cell now has lost the ability to detect or repair DNA damage. For example, when P53 is nonfunctional, even a badly damaged cell may not receive an adequate signal to commit suicide, and this already-mutant cell can continue to divide. Thus, tumor suppressor genes are associated with loss-of-function mutations in cancer, not gain-of-function mutations as for oncogenes. Returning to the automobile analogy of brakes, mutant tumor suppressor genes resemble dysfunctional braking systems, or no brakes at all.

We focus on two gatekeeper-type tumor suppressors because their role and importance in cancer are clear. The role of caretakers such as Brca1 is both more complex and more uncertain (see suggested reading on *brca* in the Bibliography).

The Retinoblastoma and P53 Proteins Are the Main Gatekeepers for the Cell Cycle

Retinoblastoma is a rare, hereditary, childhood cancer of the retina of the eye. Despite its rarity and that it cannot be induced in mice, retinoblastoma has played an important role in the study of cancer. A statistical study of the disease in the early 1970s provided the best evidence then available that human cancer is a genetic disease. Alfred Knudsen showed that children with retinoblastoma typically inherit one mutant copy from a parent (a *germ line mutation*), but then require a second *somatic mutation* in cells giving rise to the retina. Knudsen's *two-hit hypothesis* was a forerunner to the idea that cancer develops by the accumulation of mutations in a cell lineage. (Retinoblastoma tumors do require the accumulation of additional mutations beyond the two retinoblastoma genes being mutant.) Subsequently, the retinoblastoma gene, *rb*, was the first tumor suppressor gene to be cloned. Study of the encoded protein, Prb, showed that it played a central role in controlling the transition from G1 to S phase of the cell cycle.

The *retinoblastoma protein* is a repressor of a transcription factor whose activity is required for the cell to enter S phase from G1 (Figure 2-8). The transcription factor is E2F, which controls the expression of a wide variety of genes/proteins required for DNA synthesis, including cyclin A, CDK1 (see Figure 2-4), and subunits of DNA polymerase. Prb is a potent inhibitor of E2F only when it is bound to E2F directly, which requires Prb to be in an unphosphorylated state (see Figures 1-1, *B*, and 1-17). The repression of E2F is released by phosphorylation of Prb by cyclin-CDK pairs operating early in G1 in the cell cycle. As discussed, growth factor stimulation of the MAP kinase pathway leads to expression of cyclin D (see Figure 2-5), which in turn makes a pair with either CDK4 or CDK6 to make an active CDK. One of the substrates for cyclin D/CDK4,6 is the retinoblastoma protein. When Prb is phosphorylated by CDK4, 6, it releases from E2F, allowing this transcription factor to promote RNA polymerase activity on genes with E2F promoter regions (see Figure 2-8). It is this release of inhibition by CDK-mediated phosphorylation of Prb that constitutes the molecular mechanism underlying the R-point "decision" to divide late in G1 mentioned earlier and shown in Figure 2-2. If both copies of *rb* are mutant, as in retinoblastoma, there will be no active repressor molecules to bind to E2F, and the decision will always be to divide, regardless of other conditions. E2F then promotes uncontrolled expression of S-phase genes whether or not CDK4, 6 has been activated (in part) by growth factors and adhesion, thus making a contribution to unregulated growth and to cancer. Conversely, in its normal, nonmutant form, Prb tends to suppress tumor formation by acting as a gatekeeper, only allowing the cell "to cross the border" between G1 and into S phase if normal growth factor and adhesion signals are received. Thus, Prb plays a crucial gatekeeper role in healthy, normal cell cycle control.

The other crucial gatekeeper between G1 and S phase is P53. Unlike Prb, P53 does not participate in healthy cell cycles; P53 is only active in response to cell damage, usually DNA damage, or stress, such as low O_2 concentration or oncogene activation (Figure 2-9). The role of P53 is to ensure that stressed/damaged cells are either repaired or, if not, commit suicide before being allowed to replicate their DNA. As a gatekeeper, P53's mechanism is also more direct than Prb; P53 is a transcription factor, and P53 activation stimulates the expression of a protein that is a powerful general inhibitor of all the cyclin/CDK engines. As a transcription factor, P53 also mediates the expression of genes that encode stimulators of cell death, as discussed shortly. Whether the cell responds to P53 by cell cycle arrest to allow repair, or by committing suicide, depends on multiple factors, but presence of an oncogene is among the most important. Normally, the cell cycle arrest activity of P53 is dominant to its death-inducing activity. However, in the presence of oncogenes, including *myc*, suicide is favored. This illustrates clearly the normal tumor suppressor activity of P53: although a cell expressing an oncogene will tend toward increased proliferation, the same oncogene, acting through P53, activates a death pathway to prevent expansion of the mutant cell population.

The activation of P53 occurs in part through mechanisms familiar from previous examples of protein control, including phosphorylation and binding with other proteins. In addition, P53 activity is also regulated simply by an increase in its concentration within the cell. That is, P53 is normally synthesized at a steady but slow rate throughout the cell cycle and is normally degraded at a similar rate. In healthy cells the half-life for a P53 molecule is about 30 minutes, but this increases threefold to sevenfold in response to DNA damage. Even one double-strand break in DNA has been shown to increase P53 concentration rapidly in some cells. Again, it is clear how P53 serves as both a gatekeeper and a tumor suppressor. Activated P53 prevents a cell with DNA damage from crossing the G1-S boundary (its gatekeeper function), which in turn prevents mutant cells from being allowed to accumulate additional mutations (its tumor suppressor function).

However, if the *p53* gene suffers a loss-of-function mutation and the protein cannot act as a transcription factor, a damaged cell will be able to divide, increasing the probability of accumulating further damage and leading to possible cancer. Thus, *p53*/P53 is one of the most important single genes and proteins involved

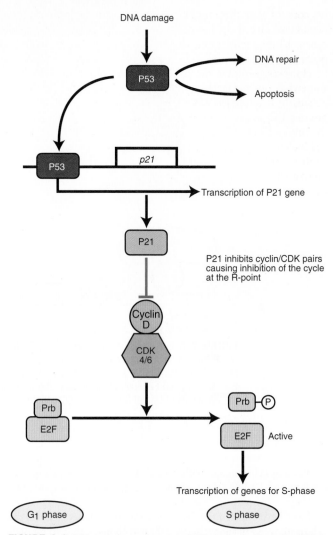

FIGURE 2-9 P53 and the response to DNA damage. Normally, P53 is maintained at low levels in the cell by continuous synthesis and breakdown. DNA damage inhibits breakdown, allowing P53 to build up to functional levels. P53 is itself a transcription factor, and its targets include *p21*, whose protein is a potent inhibitor of all cyclin-CDK pairs. Thus, upregulation of P53 brings the cell cycle to a halt, typically by inhibiting phosphorylation of Prb, as shown here. Subsequently, if the DNA is repaired, P53 returns to low concentration. If the DNA remains damaged, P53 leads to an apoptotic response by mediating expression of pro-apoptotic proteins, as described in the text.

in human cancers; in 1993 the journal *Science* even named it "Molecule of the Year." About 50% of human tumors have a mutation in *p53*, with most of these eliminating DNA binding, disabling its transcription factor activity. When the *p53* gene was "knocked out" in mice, 74% of the animals developed cancers by 6 months of age (young adult). Among experimental mice that had one or two normal copies of the gene, only 1 in 100 animals developed a tumor by 9 months.

In addition to a checkpoint for S phase in which DNA damage provides an important regulatory signal, the other major checkpoint occurs during mitosis. This checkpoint responds to mitotic spindle abnormalities or damage and to abnormalities in the array of chromosomes within the spindle. Again, one can easily see how mutations that disrupted such "safety interlocks" could lead to further damage, by segregating both replicated chromosomes into one daughter cell, for example, with no copy of that chromosome in the other daughter cell. This would lead directly to aneuploidy. Among human cancers, colon cancer is frequently found to have mutations in mitotic checkpoint genes.

However, we leave the topic of mitotic checkpoints at this somewhat intuitive level and do not address the molecular mechanisms in detail. Such an effort would require a lengthy background discussion of the structure, functions, and control of the microtubule-based mitotic spindle, more suitable for a course in cell biology than animal physiology. Instead, we now discuss the controls on cell growth other than proliferation and briefly summarize what is known about programmed cell death and the control of cell life span.

MECHANISMS REGULATING CELL SUICIDE AND CELL LIFE SPAN

Apoptosis Is the Process of Cell Suicide

The process of cell death by external damage, involving cellular swelling, bursting, and engagement of the inflammatory response, has been well described for more than 100 years. This form of cell death is called *necrosis* and is familiar from experiences as common as a cut or abrasion. A rather different process of cell death was described in the 1970s in which cells shrink, the DNA fragments in a systematic way, the plasma membrane bubbles and churns, and the cell breaks up into small pieces that are rapidly engulfed by neighboring cells (Figure 2-10). This neater and

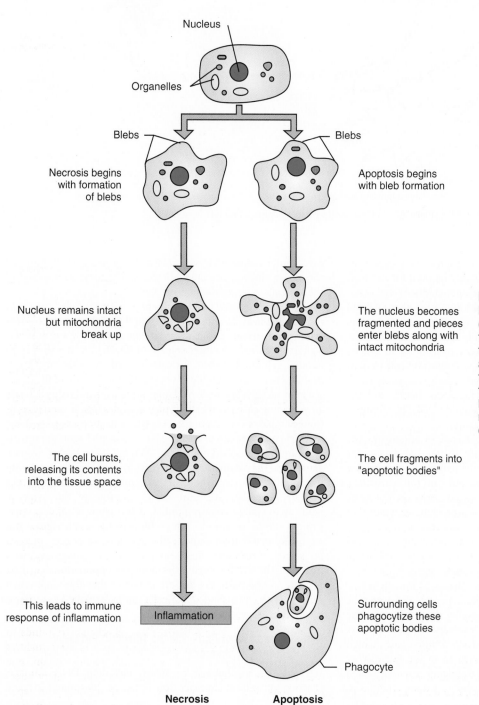

Necrosis   **Apoptosis**

FIGURE 2-10 Necrosis versus apoptosis. Necrosis is cell death as a result of external damage to the cell that leads to bursting of the cell and release of cell contents, leading to inflammation. Apoptosis is cell death as a result of intrinsic mechanisms in which the cell is broken down into cell fragments that then undergo phagocytosis by neighboring cells. This produces no inflammatory reaction and is so "tidy" that apoptosis is difficult to observe.

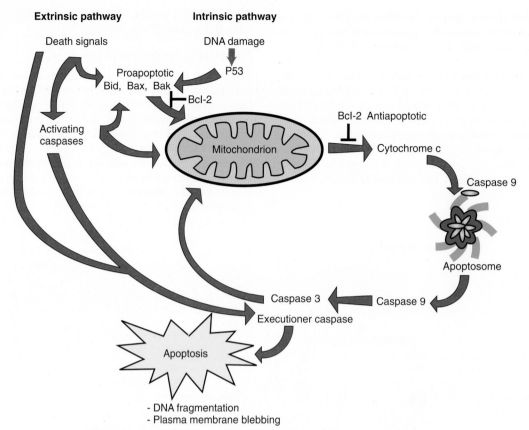

FIGURE 2-11 Extrinsic and intrinsic pathways for apoptosis. See text for details.

cleaner form of cell death was named *apoptosis* (a-pah-toe-sis; Greek, "falling off"). Apoptosis was largely ignored for the next 20 years, until studies of nematode development discovered genes whose only role was to control apoptosis. Further studies revealed the highly conserved mechanisms of apoptosis and its importance in normal development, immune function, and disease. Resistance to apoptosis is clearly a major contributor to cancer. (Conversely, too much apoptosis plays an important role in neurodegenerative diseases and stroke.) Particularly relevant to clinical practice, most cancer drugs and radiation therapy kill the target cells (and unfortunately many bystander cells) by stimulating apoptosis.

There are two broad pathways that lead to apoptosis. The *intrinsic pathway* of apoptosis responds to internal damage or stress from within the cell. The *extrinsic pathway* begins with a signal molecule binding to a "death receptor" on the cell surface (Figure 2-11). However, both pathways converge on the same "executioners." *Caspases* are a family of proteolytic enzymes that have a cysteine amino acid at their active site (the "c" in caspase) and that cleave the substrate proteins at an aspartate amino acid (the "asp" in caspase). Similar to many other proteases, including digestive enzymes and blood-clotting factors, caspases are themselves activated by proteolytic cleavage. That is, as initially translated, the protease contains an inhibitory peptide that must be cleaved away to allow active proteolysis by the enzyme. In the case of the caspases, the activating protease is itself another caspase. Thus, caspases are divided into *activating caspases,* which respond directly to one or another element in the intrinsic or extrinsic pathway, and downstream *executioner caspases,* which lead to specific cleavage of cellular structures. Among other tasks,

executioner caspases cleave cytoskeletal proteins, leading to cell shrinkage, and activate the DNA-degrading enzymes involved in the systematic fragmentation of DNA.

The basic extrinsic pathway of apoptosis, also called the *death receptor pathway,* is unusually short and straightforward considering the extreme and irreversible outcome. An extracellular signal, which can be either soluble or attached to the surface of another cell, binds to and activates a death receptor on the cell destined to commit suicide. The cytoplasmic domain of the death receptor recruits one or two adapter proteins that directly activate an activating caspase, which in turn activates one or more executioner caspases (see Figure 2-11). The activating caspase of the extrinsic pathway can also engage in "cross-talk" with the intrinsic pathway, described shortly, to increase the extent of caspase activation. The extrinsic pathway plays a crucial role in regulating the immune system, where the vast majority of immune cells initially generated are eliminated. The role of the extrinsic pathway in cancer is more limited. A few types of cancers overexpress "decoy receptors," which bind to the death signals but attenuate, rather than activate, the apoptotic response. Interestingly, cancer cells are often responsive to an extrinsic pathway, including the one involved in immune cell elimination, but their normal counterparts are not. It is hoped that this differential sensitivity to extrinsic death signals can be exploited as a therapeutic cancer treatment in the future.

Resistance to Apoptosis Via the Intrinsic Pathway Is a Hallmark of Cancer

Internal cellular damage or stress, including DNA damage, absence of cell anchorage, too little or too much oxygen metabolism, oncogene activation, and radiation damage, can stimulate the intrinsic pathway of apoptosis in normal cells. Most, and perhaps all, cancer cells are more resistant than normal cells to apoptosis through this pathway. Resistance to apoptosis not only increases the probability that the cell will be able to accumulate further genetic damage, but also reduces the likelihood that cancer cells can be eliminated. This is because the antitumor activity of the immune system, as well as most chemotherapy and radiation treatments, depends on apoptosis. Thus, resistance to apoptosis often means resistance to treatment.

The intrinsic pathway is considerably more complex than the extrinsic pathway, and this discussion focuses on three major elements of the pathway involved in activating caspases: P53, the mitochondrion, and the *Bcl family* of proteins (see Figure 2-11). This family of proteins was originally discovered in a cancer ("Bcl" is from B-cell lymphoma, a type of leukemia in which the first such protein was discovered) and includes both pro-apoptotic and anti-apoptotic members. The balance between pro- and anti-apoptotic members determines whether the cell lives or dies. The resistance of cancer cells to apoptosis arises not only from mutations, such as those already described for *p53*, but also from under-expression of pro-apoptotic mediators and overexpression of anti-apoptotic proteins.

We begin with the *mitochondrion,* familiar as the "power-house" of the cell responsible for generating ATP, but also the central control point for the intrinsic pathway of apoptosis. Recall that the mitochondrion has both an inner membrane, responsible for electron transport, and an outer membrane, responsible for compartmentation of this organelle. Pro-apoptotic signals cause the outer membrane of the mitochondria to become leaky, releasing several pro-apoptotic proteins not normally found in the cytoplasm. Among the most important is cytochrome c, an electron transport protein that is only loosely attached to the inner membrane. In the cytoplasm, cytochrome c stimulates the assembly of a multiprotein complex (the apoptosome) that directly stimulates the activity of an activating caspase (caspase-9), ultimately leading to the activation of executioner caspases. What then determines the extent of permeability (leakiness) of the mitochondrial outer membrane?

The Bcl family members are major regulators of mitochondrial outer membrane permeability. The pro-apoptotic members of this family, such as Bax, lead to permeabilization by assembling to form channels in the outer membrane through which cytochrome c can pass. Pro-apoptotic members of the family can also cause the channel through which ATP normally passes into the cytoplasm to open wider than usual. The anti-apoptotic members of the family, such as Bcl-2, seem to function by binding to pro-apoptotic members, inhibiting their activity. In a healthy cell, anti-apoptotic Bcl members are at high enough concentration to neutralize pro-apoptotic activity. Damage increases the amount of pro-apoptotic Bcl molecules and leads to membrane permeabilization. Thus the balance between pro- and anti-apoptotic members of the family controls the permeability state of mitochondria and the survival of the cell.

With about 20 different members of the Bcl family, the balance between pro- and anti-apoptotic Bcl molecules has multiple controls, but P53 activity is certainly a major player. Recall that when activated (e.g., by DNA damage), P53 acts as a transcription factor, and at least three different pro-apoptotic Bcl genes are transcriptionally activated by P53. These include Bax, and also the particularly powerful pro-apoptotic protein, PUMA. Downstream, P53 also activates the transcription of the activating

caspase-9 gene, and the gene of a major cytoplasmic component of the apoptosome. In addition to acting as an activating transcription factor, P53 serves as an inhibitory transcription factor for some genes, including that of the anti-apoptotic Bcl-2 protein. Finally and independent of transcription, activated P53 can directly activate Bax, which is required for its ability to assemble into channel structures. With these multiple effects on apoptotic genes and proteins, P53 is regarded as a central apoptotic control point, in addition to its role in cell cycle regulation.

As noted earlier in the discussion of P53, the importance of apoptosis to tumorigenesis is that with normal apoptosis, almost all damaged cells are eliminated. Without apoptosis, damaged cells live to accumulate additional damage, which illustrates why multiple mutations and dysfunctions are required for tumors to reach a clinically significant stage. The resistance of cancer cells to apoptosis arises from many types of mutations and disruptions of normal gene expression. Perhaps most importantly, mutation of the *p53* gene eliminates its DNA binding and thus transcriptional activity. Related to P53 activity is a protein engaged in P53's normal proteolytic breakdown (see previous discussion). Overexpression of this protein (MDM2) in various cancers of soft tissues inhibits the accumulation of P53 to active levels and therefore inhibits both cell cycle arrest and apoptosis. The anti-apoptotic Bcl-2 protein is overexpressed in a variety of human cancers, including 60% of human follicular lymphomas, but also some lung cancers, melanoma, and prostate cancer. Another common apoptotic lesion seen in cancer cells is overexpression of proteins that bind to and directly inactivate caspases, as well as mutation or loss of expression of the caspases themselves.

Cellular Life Span Is Determined by DNA Sequences at the Ends of Chromosomes

The final major dysfunction of growth control found within cancer cells is the most recently discovered, but also seems to be the most common single molecular lesion in cancers: the expression of a reverse transcriptase called *telomerase.* (A reverse transcriptase is any enzyme that synthesizes DNA from an RNA template.) Telomerase is responsible for replicating *telomeres,* the specialized, noncoding regions of DNA found at the end of chromosomes. However, telomerase is normally expressed only in embryonic cells and in adult *stem cells.* (Stem cells are specialized normal cells that do have limitless replicative potential, such as gamete-generating cells and the blood-forming cells of the bone marrow, as discussed later.) The vast majority of normal somatic cells do not express telomerase, but it is expressed in 85% to 90% of all cancers and is the major determinant of the "immortality" of cancer cells.

Telomeres are segments of highly repetitive DNA, representing hundreds of repeats of the simple nucleotide sequence TTAGGG (in vertebrates), found at the ends of chromosomes. Telomeres serve as caps at chromosomal ends, protecting them against end-to-end joining of chromosomes. Telomeres also prevent the ends of chromosomes from being recognized as sites of DNA damage (double-strand DNA breaks). Most relevant for cancer, telomeres protect against the loss of coding DNA from each chromosomal end with every round of DNA replication; this is needed because normal DNA polymerases have a serious limitation: they cannot fully replicate the end of a double-strand DNA molecule. As a result, the ends of chromosomes become shorter with each round of DNA replication. (Bacteria solve this problem by having circular DNA chromosomes.)

Telomeres are expendable DNA, at the ends of chromosomes, whose progressive shortening does not compromise the coding function of the genome. Although no coding sequence is lost, the shortening of telomeres nevertheless plays an important role in the cell. The shortening of telomeres serves as a kind of clock, measuring the number of times a cell has divided, and the length of the telomere reflects the age of the cell. Through poorly understood mechanisms, cells can detect the length of their telomeres, and when they reach a critically short length, the cell ceases to divide and is said to undergo *senescence* (Latin; "growing old"). As noted earlier, normal cells have a finite life span, such that a cell taken from a middle-aged human will divide 20 to 40 times in culture before senescence. When placed into culture, the number of subsequent cell divisions before senescence reflects the original length of the telomeres. Further, various degenerative diseases, including cirrhosis of the liver, have been shown to accelerate telomere shortening. In principle, senescence is a powerful block to cancer because the original damaged cell (see Figure 2-1) would be unable to divide for a sufficient number of generations to accumulate the necessary multiple mutations required to produce a tumor. Telomerase expression (and other, less common means of elongating telomeres) effectively eliminates this block to cancer development by causing the cells to become immortal.

Telomerase has both protein and RNA components. The protein provides the catalytic reverse transcriptase, allowing the enzyme to elongate the telomere sequence based on the RNA template it carries. That is, the RNA component of telomerase is complementary to the telomere DNA sequence and is used as the template for telomere DNA replication. Telomerase is not expressed in normal adult somatic cells except for stem cells, mentioned earlier. However, immortal tissue culture cells do express telomerase, as do cancer cells. Experimental expression of telomerase in human cells dramatically increases the replicative life span of the cells. Thus the observed expression of telomerase in the vast majority of human cancers permits these cells to divide indefinitely, providing yet another selective advantage for these cells to accumulate other damage over time.

In the last sections of this chapter, we turn our attention to the cancer cell in the context of a *tumor,* which is a population of cancer cells interacting with one another and with surrounding normal tissue. We end our discussion of the intrinsic growth controls of normal and cancer cells with an experimental result that seems to confirm the importance of the types of damage discussed thus far. This experiment showed that four genetic changes were sufficient to transform normal human kidney cells into cancer cells able to form tumors when transplanted into a mouse host (with no immune system). The four genetic changes were to "engineer" into the cells an activating mutation for the *ras* oncogene, inactivation of both the retinoblastoma and P53 proteins, and expression of the catalytic subunit of telomerase. Thus, damage to the genes or expression of these molecules, emphasized here, reflects the minimum requirements for a normal cell to grow as a cancer.

TUMOR ORIGIN AND THE SPREAD OF CANCER

Cancer Cells May Be Related to Stem Cells

As noted in the previous section, some normal adult cells do have unlimited replicative potential. These are *stem cells,* a term that has been much in the news recently. A *stem cell* is a self-renewing cell of high proliferative potential that can also give rise to

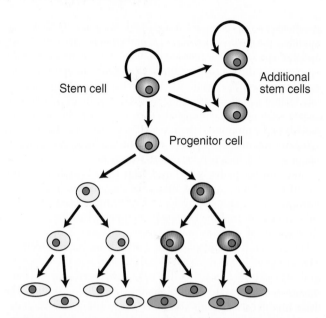

FIGURE 2-12 Stem cells. Stem cells are self-renewing cells of high, sometimes unlimited, replicative potential. Their proliferation forms both additional stem cells and progenitor cells. These progenitor cells divide and eventually differentiate to become one or more types of differentiated somatic cells specialized for certain tasks (e.g., erythrocytes and monocytes of blood).

differentiated cells. Typically, stem cell division produces one cell that remains a stem cell while the other daughter cell differentiates into a specialized cell with the usual limited life span (Figure 2-12). The cell that continues being a stem cell does not lose any developmental capacity and can divide indefinitely, continuing to produce additional stem cells and additional differentiated cells.

Much of the recent attention in the news centers on *embryonic* stem cells. These are embryonic cells that can either continue to form stem cells or differentiate, in principle, to any and every cell type within the body. Even in the adult, however, the maintenance of many normal tissues is critically dependent on stem cells. *Adult* stem cells, however, can only differentiate into a limited array of different cell types, not every cell type in the body. Best understood is that all the various cells of the blood arise from the division of hematopoietic stem cells in the bone marrow; one daughter cell remains a stem cell in the bone marrow while the other differentiates to become one of the several types of blood cells (but the blood stem cell can only form blood cells, not nonblood cells). The cells lining the gut and skin cells also arise from a stable population of adult stem cells, some of whose descendants differentiate into specialized gut and skin cells. For this reason, chemotherapy that is intended to cause apoptosis in cancer cells typically also affects these same populations of normal stem cells; common side effects of chemotherapy include anemia, hair loss, and digestive dysfunction.

Cancer cells resemble stem cells in their immortality, but the relationship of cancer cells to stem cells may go further. Based on the presentation thus far, you may have the mental image of a tumor composed of a uniform population of badly damaged cells, any of which would be capable of forming a new tumor if transplanted. In fact, real tumors are not a homogeneous population of cells, but rather are composed of a variety of cells that differ significantly in their phenotype, despite all being clonal descendants of a single somatic cell, as shown in Figure 2-1. (Keep in mind that all somatic cells of the body are clonal descendants of the fertilized egg, so phenotypic differences arising within clonal lines is not surprising by itself.) Further, experiments with a variety of cancers show that only 1% or less of tumor cells are capable of forming another tumor, even in the same patient (or mouse). Thus, tumors may contain a small subpopulation of *cancer stem cells* that are responsible for producing the heterogeneous cells in the tumor and are uniquely able to continue cancer growth. This would also give tumors the capacity to adapt to their surroundings; because stem cells can differentiate in various ways, differentiated cells that allowed continued growth and survival would be selected.

This hypothesis has been persuasively supported only in leukemias, but it may apply to other cancers as well. Also for leukemias, the cancer stem cells express some marker proteins characteristic of normal hematopoietic stem cells. Further, only those leukemia stem cells expressing certain normal markers are capable of forming new cancers when transplanted. Finally, a possible relationship between cancer and stem cells is that perhaps the genetic changes summarized in this chapter must occur in a normal adult stem cell to produce cancer cells. Here again, the best evidence in favor of such a mechanism comes from leukemias. But the blood is unusual in ways other than just being a fluid rather than a solid tissue, and it is not at all clear that other types of cancers will prove similar.

Indeed, recent results on melanoma, the generally fatal cancer of the skin mentioned earlier in the context of the MAP kinase pathway, challenge some of the concepts of the cancer stem cell hypothesis. For example, a relatively large fraction of melanoma cells, perhaps as much as 25% of the tumor cells, can produce tumors after transplantation. This high frequency is not consistent with scientists' conception of stem cells. More troubling still, some evidence suggests that the ability of melanoma cells to form new tumors is transient. It is as if the "stemness" of melanoma cells is unstable and comes and goes. So the stem cell hypothesis for cancer is a controversial one. On the one hand, those tumors that show stem cell properties raise the possibility that cancer therapy should, perhaps, be directed primarily at cancer stem cells and not the majority of cells in a tumor. And, it might be possible to use stem cell markers for drug targeting, thus sparing the vast majority of cells in the body from side effects of the treatment. On the other hand, we don't know how many cancers or individual tumors will or won't be shown to adhere to the stem cell model. A reading concerning the "premises, promises, and challenges" of cancer stem cells is included in the reading list at the end of this chapter.

Death by Cancer Is Usually the Result of Its Spread, Not the Original Tumor

Death from cancer is often the result of the spread of the cancer from the initial tumor, the *primary tumor,* to various distant sites. This process of cancer cells colonizing other tissues is called *metastasis.* For some cancer types, including leukemias, and those of the brain, the primary tumor itself can be fatal. In contrast, the primary tumor for melanoma is little more than a mole on the skin that does not become life threatening until these cancer cells spread. Although metastasis is the deadliest aspect of cancer, much less is known about it than about the dysfunctions of cell growth leading to the primary tumor.

The best understood aspect of metastasis is that it occurs by a multistep process called the *metastatic cascade.* In this step-by-step process, cells escape from the primary tumor, breaking through tissue barriers to gain access to the circulatory system. The cells are carried until they escape the circulatory system to invade a new tissue (Figure 2-13). The steps of the metastatic cascade suggest that dysfunction of three broad types of cellular function are particularly important: cellular adhesion, cellular motility, and secretion of proteases. How these dysfunctions arise from the genetic damage of growth in the primary tumor is, again, unknown, but mutation resulting from the genetic instability of the primary tumor is typically suggested as a link.

The first step of the metastatic cascade is the loss of cell adhesion by the cancer cell, both to neighboring cells and to the ECM. Accordingly, many types of cancer cells show greatly reduced expression of a cell-cell adhesion receptor, E-cadherin, important for epithelial adhesion. Similarly, primary tumor cells show a wide variety of abnormalities in the number and type of cell-ECM adhesion receptors, integrins, they express. In addition to loosening the bonds to the primary tumor, allowing cells to escape, one hypothesis is that these changes in cell adhesion molecules underlie the curious tendency of various cancers to metastasize preferentially to certain other tissues. Melanoma, for example, has a strong tendency to metastasize to the brain and to bone. Melanoma's particular array of abnormal (for skin) adhesion molecules may represent a "postal code" favoring delivery to a particular distant site.

Having altered its adhesion, enabling escape from the primary tumor, the metastatic cell must make its way toward the circulatory system, enter the circulation (called *intravasation*) to "hitch a ride" around the body. Although "circulation" typically refers to the bloodstream, cancer cells can also be disseminated by traveling within the lymphatic system, which collects extracellular tissue fluid for return to the blood. Indeed, invasion of lymph nodes, which are major collection sites for extracellular fluid and debris, is a common test for initial metastases. For either route, however, the cell's ability to achieve intravasation depends on altering normal motility and expressing proteases. Most animal cell types are capable of "crawling" locomotion using actin and myosin mechanisms similar to muscle contraction (see Figure 1-4). This crawling locomotion is similar to the motility of amebae. Migrating breast cancer cells have been imaged directly and show solitary cells with amoeboid morphology. The entire actin and myosin system of most cancer cells is dysregulated, causing changes in cell shape and the ability and tendency to locomote. For example, normal skin cells are generally quite stationary, but melanoma cells are highly motile. The dysregulation of the actomyosin system results in part from mutations of the Rho family of small, Ras-like G proteins, mentioned briefly earlier. Mutations in *rho* are common among highly metastatic melanoma cells, but such mutations are rare among weakly metastatic melanoma cell lines.

Because cells in solid tissues are crowded together, increased motility appears to be helped by secretion of proteases that digest some of the cell matrix "obstacles" in the cancer cell's path. Epithelial cells give rise to approximately 80% of human cancers. As noted earlier, all epithelial cells are attached to an ECM, which is characterized by a particular type of collagen. Proteases specific for this type of collagen are generally overexpressed by metastatic cells. The number of different proteases and the net amount of protease secreted tend to increase with increasing metastatic potential. In addition, cancer cells appear to have the capacity to

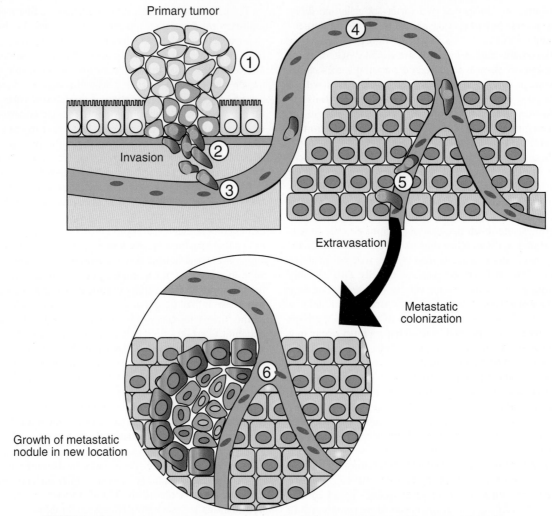

Primary tumor

Invasion

Extravasation

Metastatic
colonization

Growth of metastatic
nodule in new location

FIGURE 2-13 Metastatic cascade, the path from primary tumor to metastatic tumor. Cells of the primary tumor alter their cell adhesion and motility properties to migrate away from the primary tumor site *(1)*. These cells secrete proteases to digest their way through the surrounding tissue *(2)*. They then crawl into the vasculature *(3)*, a process called *intravasation*, where they are then carried passively around the circulation *(4)*. At some point, they adhere to the sides of the blood vessel and crawl out of the vasculature *(5)*, a process called *extravasation*. Some metastatic cells are able to colonize the new location to form a new, deadly metastatic tumor *(6)*.

cause surrounding normal cells to increase their secretion of pro-teases. Proteases not only aid the metastatic cell in intravasation, but also stimulate cell survival and proliferation by largely unknown mechanisms. However, not all ECM represents an obstacle to movement that must be proteolytically degraded. Some types of ECM appear to provide stimulatory pathways for the migrating cells to follow toward the circulation. Migration toward the circulation is also aided by chemoattraction; epidermal growth factor in blood vessels seems to be an attractant for breast cancer cells.

After intravasation, the metastatic cell rides around the circulation until it can attach to the vessel wall. Then, reversing the process of intravasation, the cell "climbs out" of the circulation, which is called *extravasation*. As one might expect, this also depends on changes in adhesion, motility, and protease secretion. After extravasation, the metastatic cell must be able to survive and proliferate in its new environment.

Fewer than 1 in 10,000 cells escaping the primary tumor colonize a new location successfully. It was once assumed that this high rate of failure reflected an "exceedingly rough ride" around the circulatory system. More recent evidence suggests that the limiting factor of metastasis is the survival of the cell in its new location. This represents another example of the natural selection, the "microevolution," occurring in cancer. The foreign environment exerts a strong negative selective pressure on cancer cell arrivals, and the vast majority do not survive. Ironically, our current thinking about metastasis is similar to the "seed and soil hypothesis" first proposed in 1889. Metastasis requires a cancer cell from the primary tumor (the seed) capable of carrying out (selected for) all the steps of the metastatic cascade, and the metastatic cell must colonize a region (the soil) appropriate for its subsequent growth. Normal cells cannot survive in a new location within the same body. Different tissues have different chemical milieus (e.g., different mixes of growth factors), and these are specialized for the survival and growth of the particular cell types found in the region. The process of metastasis necessarily selects for cells capable of growing in a foreign environment. It is thought that most metastatic cells become dormant in their new location and that additional genetic changes are required and must be selected to enable uncontrolled growth. Genes whose products play a role in adapting cells to particular environments have been called *landscaping genes,* another allusion to the current view of metastasis resembling gardening. Mutations in these landscaping genes are postulated to allow growth in the foreign environment, less than 1% of micrometastases grow to a clinically relevant size. A key aspect of this selection process for uncontrolled growth in the foreign location is the secretion by the cancer cells and by surrounding cells of a variety of mediators to stimulate growth of new blood vessels to supply the tumor. Another key feature of selection is remodeling of the local ECM, which normally is required for proliferation. These phenomena of inducing blood supply and remodeling of the ECM are other aspects of metastasis that are poorly understood.

Indeed, it is poorly understood how metastasis actually leads to death except that it often involves a profound and progressive wasting of skeletal muscle and fat in the body called, *cachexia.* This wasting process affects up to 80% of human cancer patients and is responsible for perhaps a third of deaths. Recent experimental results, again with mice, indicate that inhibiting cachexia, even without inhibition of tumor growth, dramatically lengthens the animals' life span. Cachexia is complex, but appears to be due in large part to cancer cells releasing signaling molecules that abnormally stimulate developmental pathways in muscle and fat cells. Activation of these developmental pathways, in turn, leads to abnormally high levels of fat and protein breakdown in the affected cells. Another possible mechanism underlying cachexia involves generalized inflammatory reactions, which attack other aspects of the patient's physiology generally. Possibly the presence of foreign cells, selected for growth in an abnormal location, causes the body's defense mechanisms to be fully mobilized and attack itself, a nightmare of biological "friendly fire" in current military jargon. Presumably, the foreignness of the metastatic tumor explains the highly inappropriate response, which primary tumors typically do not instigate. It is for this reason, in part, that **complete** removal of the primary tumor before metastasis occurs often leads to total recovery. In other cases, death from metastatic disease, like death from some primary tumors, is the result of cancer cells simply overwhelming a vital organ, leading to organ failure.

Growth of Solid Tumors Depends on Development of New Blood Vessels

Tumors, as with normal tissue, require blood vessels to supply them with oxygen and nutrients and to remove waste. Much attention has been focused on the development of tumor capillaries because it is a rate-limiting step in the tumor's growth and progression. Both primary and metastatic tumors require new vessels; without them the tumor remains too small to be visible or palpable, about 1 to 2 mm in diameter. Dormant tumors of this size have been found in autopsies of people who did not die of cancer, so not all tumors develop the blood supply needed for growth. Thus the ability of tumors to stimulate new blood vessel development is a distinct and important step in tumor progression. As this suggests, it is also a relatively early step in tumor progression but is covered here after metastasis because most new vasculature arises from existing capillaries invading new regions of tissue, sharing some features with metastasis.

The discussion of Starling's hypothesis in Chapter 1 notes that blood capillaries are composed primarily of a single layer of a specialized epithelial cell type, the endothelial cell. The first capillaries in the embryo are formed by *vasculogenesis,* the differentiation of precursor cells (angioblasts) to form a basic capillary network. However, most new capillaries are formed by *angiogenesis,* the sprouting and branching of existing capillaries to supply new tissue regions. Larger blood vessels, such as arterioles and veins, all develop from the subsequent growth of capillaries. In the adult, only angiogenesis normally occurs and depends on invasive cellular processes similar to those involved in metastasis: proliferation of existing endothelial cells; migration of the cells into the region to be supplied, involving changes in actin function and adhesion to the surrounding cells; and remodeling the surrounding ECM so the extending cells intercalate among the tissue cells, ultimately to form a hollow tube. Although the cancer cells within a tumor are abnormal, the endothelial cells composing the new capillaries are normal. Thus, tumor capillaries can arise by vasculogenesis (because of the abnormal environment of the tumor) or, and primarily, by angiogenesis. Similarly, the endothelial cells of tumor capillaries respond to the normal stimulatory and inhibitory signals for angiogenesis. Nevertheless, the pathological features of the tumor stimulate abnormal growth of blood vessels, whose pattern, composition, and function differ from normal capillaries.

In normal adult tissue, except for the female reproductive tract, endothelial cells are among the most slowly proliferating cell type. Only 1 in 10,000 adult endothelial cells are in cell division at any one time, compared with about 10% of gut epithelial cells. Normal angiogenesis is under tight regulation by both stimulatory and inhibitory influences. Stimulatory influences include injury and hypoxia which in turn lead to the secretion of angiogenic growth factors such as *vascular endothelial growth factor* (VEGF, "vedge-eff"). This growth factor strongly stimulates endothelial cell proliferation and migration and suppresses apoptosis. VEGF also increases permeability of existing vessels. Inhibitory influences include thrombospondin-1, which is an ECM component that inhibits endothelial cell proliferation and motility. Inhibitory influences also include soluble factors such as angiostatin, which stimulates apoptosis in proliferating endothelial cells, and endostatin, which inhibits the migration of endothelial cells. The growth, stasis, or regression of capillaries depends on the balance between pro- and anti-angiogenic stimuli, much as cellular life and death depend on the balance between pro- and anti-apoptotic signals discussed earlier.

The relative quiescence of normal capillaries is in sharp contrast to capillaries of tumors, which have been compared to wounds that never heal, in that tumor capillaries undergo continuous growth and remodeling. Tumor endothelial cells divide 20 to 40 times more frequently than normal endothelial cells, and tumors typically have a much higher density of vessels than normal tissue. As a result, tumor vasculature is abnormal in structure and function. Tumor vessels can exhibit strange combinations of capillary, venous, and arteriole structures and often incorporate cancer cells as part of the vessel wall. These vessels tend to be convoluted and dilated, follow tortuous paths, and even form dead ends. As a result, blood flow is equally abnormal, with the vessels leakier than normal vessels, and in some cases the blood flows back and forth rather than circulates.

Perhaps the most important factor in this vascular pathology is the high concentration of VEGF in and around tumors. Most human tumors secrete large amounts of VEGF and also cause surrounding tissue to secrete VEGF. Much evidence from experiments on mice supports the crucial role of VEGF in tumor angiogenesis and growth. Antibodies against VEGF suppress growth of existing tumors; cancer cells engineered to be incapable of expressing VEGF were unable to form tumors; and inhibition of the VEGF receptor inhibited the growth of a variety of tumors. In part, the secretion of VEGF by tumor cells seems to be the result of the initial hypoxic conditions of the avascular tumor. Hypoxia is normally a strong inducer of VEGF production, and the centers of many solid tumors show necrotic cells indicative of death from lack of oxygen. In addition, the genetic damage to cells in their progression to a cancer cell also seems to contribute to VEGF overexpression. Mutations of *ras* and overexpression of Bcl-2, the anti-apoptotic factor, have been shown to play important roles in this regard.

Tumor vessels are also substantially more permeable than normal vessels, to the point of being almost hemorrhagic, which is also thought to be caused by overexpression of VEGF (which has an alternative name of *vascular permeability factor*). The leakiness of tumor vessels has several consequences with respect to tumor physiology, spread, and treatment. The high vascular permeability of tumors is believed to aid metastasis in that metastasis requires intravasation of tumor cells into the circulation, and leakier vessels makes this more likely. Leakier vessels also disrupt capillary fluid transport, as discussed in Chapter 1. Recall that capillary filtration and reabsorption depend on the balance between hydrostatic and oncotic forces across the capillary wall. The increased fluid leaking from tumor vessels distends the interstitial space, increasing its hydrostatic pressure and thus reducing the pressure gradient across the capillary wall. The oncotic pressure gradient is also reduced because the leak of proteins into the interstitial space means that the oncotic pressure of the interstitial space approaches that of the blood. The result is uncommonly high net interstitial fluid pressure. This can cause collapse of some vessels, leading to hypoxia of the surrounding tissue and further upregulation of VEGF expression. High interstitial fluid pressure also causes poor fluid transport out of the blood into the tumor. This poor fluid exchange seems to inhibit the delivery of chemotherapeutic agents from the blood to the tumor. Studies on chemotherapy of breast cancer and melanoma show that tumors with high interstitial fluid pressure tended not to respond as well to the therapy.

As with the other insights into tumor biology, the possibility of controlling tumor angiogenesis for therapy is being actively pursued. At this writing, there are more than a dozen anti-angiogenesis compounds being tested. One, bevacizumab (Avastin, an antibody to VEGF), is approved as a first line therapy for metastatic colon cancer, although this same drug has recently been shown to be ineffective for breast cancer. Unlike most cancer therapy that targets the abnormal cancer cell, anti-angiogenic therapy would be targeting normal endothelial cells. These cells are not genetically unstable, and therefore development of drug resistance may be less likely (see following discussion). Also, because normal endothelial cells are unusually quiescent, inhibiting angiogenesis should produce fewer toxic side effects than standard chemotherapies. As with other cell-targeted therapies, however, anti-angiogenesis inhibitors that showed dramatic results in preclinical studies have been much less successful in treating patients.

PROSPECTIVE CANCER THERAPY

Cancer Therapy Has a Hopeful but Challenging Future

Most current cancer therapy makes little or no use of the advances in our understanding of the molecular basis of cancer. Indeed, declines in (human) cancer mortality in the industrialized world are primarily the result of better screening for breast and colon cancer and preventive measures (e.g., discouraging smoking). Both chemotherapy and radiotherapy are typically nonselective (at the cell level) cytotoxic treatments intended to shrink the overall size of tumors, with serious side effects from the general cytotoxicity. Clinical trials to test new cancer drugs nearly always enroll large number of patients with no thought of investigating the particular mutations underlying the patient's tumor. This situation is changing slowly, but perhaps at an accelerated pace, to one of *targeted therapy,* in which the genotype of the tumor is taken into account and, if available, drugs targeting the mutations are used preferentially. An example of targeted therapy, discussed earlier, is the use of vemurafenib to target the Raf mutations occurring in some, but not all, melanomas. A few additional examples of targeted therapy are provided here, but the development of such therapies and of practical molecular diagnosis remains challenging, and often disappointing, with three common themes accounting for treatment failure, reflecting the fundamental properties of cancer. More information about targeted therapy in a paper on "The Evolving War on Cancer," is provided in the reading list for this chapter.

First, despite the success with Raf and melanoma, the accumulation of mutations, along with the differences in this process from individual to individual, means that single molecular markers have not proved very useful in refining diagnosis. For example, assessing the different mutations occurring in such important genes as *ras* or the *p53* gene in breast cancer has had conflicting results in predicting disease outcomes. Presumably this is because these mutations have differing effects, depending on the other mutations involved in the cancer and their interaction with the normal alleles of the individual patient. As a result, it appears that multiprotein/multigene molecular "signatures" will be needed. If such signatures can be developed as body fluid or other relatively noninvasive tests, it could lead to major improvements in treatment, insofar as diagnosing cancer as early as possible is crucial for a favorable prognosis.

The second common theme is that the multiple types of genetic damage and selective processes required for cancer also function to cause resistance to treatment. That is, the unstable and abnormal genetic status of cancer cells that produce the growth abnormalities also lead to abnormal responses to drugs and other interventions. Ironically, a vivid illustration of this is one of the notable successes, one might say the poster child, for targeted therapy in treating cancer. Chronic myeloid leukemia (CML) is known to begin with a specialized mutation (a particular chromosomal translocation) that disrupts the gene for a specific tyrosine kinase, Abl, so that it becomes an activated oncogene. A fairly specific inhibitor of this tyrosine kinase was developed, imatinib (Gleevec), that blocks binding of ATP, disabling kinase activity. This has had marked benefits for patients in the early, chronic stage of CML, which is debilitating but not fatal. In many patients, this drug causes complete remission of CML and has thus far prevented progression to the fatal, acute stage. However, some patients have developed resistance; in most of these cases the *abl* oncogene has mutated yet again such that ATP binding is restored despite Gleevec. More ominously, careful analysis of the blood of CML patients actually in remission indicates a remaining pool of leukemic cells (cancer stem cells apparently), which may subsequently lead to development of resistance in later years. Nevertheless, there are currently more than 20 specific protein kinase inhibitors in clinical trials, and practitioners would welcome additional drugs with the effectiveness of Gleevec, despite its limitations.

In addition to outright mutations leading to cancer, we have mentioned several examples in which changes in gene expression of normal proteins stimulate cancer development. Such a situation underlies another early success of targeted therapy based on a single genetic lesion. Non–small-cell lung cancer is the leading cause of death from cancer in the United States. Some 40% to 80% of these cancers over-express the epidermal growth factor receptor (EGFR), which is an RTK as described earlier. Gefitinib (Iressa) blocks the ATP binding site of EGFR, inhibiting kinase activity similar to Gleevec. As with vemurafenib and *raf* mutations, gefitinib has been shown to be effective among those patients whose non–small-cell lung cancer depends on mutation of the receptor, but not among patients with normal EGFR.

However, changes of gene expression also present a challenge to cancer therapy, particularly with respect to drug resistance, the mechanism of which underlies another, broader example of the obstacle to treatment presented by the genetic status of cancer cells. *Multiple-drug resistance* (MDR) is a phenotype in which cells develop resistance to many current, initially effective, chemotherapeutic agents for a wide variety of cancers. This is the result of the overexpression of a pump protein that causes the efflux of the drug from the cell. As with the selection among cancer cells for continued ability to proliferate, administration of the drug selects for those cancer cell variants that have changes in gene expression, such that the efflux pump reduces the effectiveness of the drug. Thus, new drug development must contend not only with the genetics of cancer, but also the genes and gene expression involved in drug resistance. (An interesting aspect of the drug efflux pump often expressed in cancer cells is that it is also expressed in normal stem cells!)

The third common theme identified as an obstacle to molecular cancer treatments is that, as discussed, cancers reflect physiological dysfunctions at a particularly fundamental level. It is not easy to interfere with these functions without compromising other functions, or interference engages compensatory mechanisms normally serving as "backup" to crucial functions. At the simplest level, interventions that alter these basic mechanisms of cellular life and death often prove to be too disruptive to the physiology of some normal cells to be useful. For example, although vemurafenib, the Raf inhibitor mentioned earlier, and gefitinib, the EGFR inhibitor, have proven effective against some cancers, many other inhibitors in the growth factor/MAP kinase pathway (see Figure 2-5) that showed promise on cultured cells and in mice proved to be too toxic for therapeutic use.

Other results indicate that effective treatments will need to resemble the normal molecular biology of the cell very closely. Experiments attempting to target *p53* are noteworthy in this respect. Because mutation of one *p53* gene will predispose to cancer (if the other copy were lost, an important checkpoint would be lost), activation of the remaining normal copy might protect against cancer. Such enhanced P53 activity did protect against cancer in mice, but the mice also showed notably shortened life span and visible signs of early aging. As shown by this unexpected role of P53 in aging, the central roles played by proto-oncogenes and tumor suppressor genes mean that they often have

multiple roles that complicate development of therapies. In experiments in which expression of activated P53 was limited to mammary tissue, mice were again protected against cancer, but at the cost of inhibiting lactation and mammary development. The best anticancer results obtained from experimentally manipulating P53 expression has come from experiments in which whole artificial chromosomes with the *p53* gene and all its normal control elements were introduced into mice. These mice showed increased resistance to chemically induced cancers with no apparent effects on aging. Introducing genes with all relevant control elements, however, is a rather high hurdle for practical therapies.

Finally, the importance of these normal genes and proteins to cell function means that they often have redundant mechanisms of control. This seems to apply to that other "usual suspect" in cancer, Ras/*ras*. Evidence that association with the plasma membrane via lipid "tails" was required for Ras activity (similar to the alpha subunit of the heterotrimeric G protein, see Figure 1-14) led to the development of drugs, *farnesyl transferase inhibitors* (FTIs), that block addition of the lipid tail. Although FTIs have proved clinically useful against some types of cancer in some patients, their effects are highly variable. One idea is that the FTIs only inhibit one pathway for Ras membrane association. Used alone, these drugs showed only modest effects on tumors, but in combination with standard chemotherapeutic drugs, FTIs worked relatively well on some cancers. However, it was puzzling that some cancers importantly involving *ras* mutations, such as lung cancer, were not affected by the inhibitors. Further, some ras-independent tumors were just as susceptible to FTIs. It now seems that these drugs may not be acting only through Ras membrane association.

As noted earlier, standard chemotherapies and radiation therapies are highly toxic by the usual standards of clinical practice. Cancer therapy is a prime medical example of "drowning men grasping at straws." Thus, the handful of clear successes using targeted therapy based on advances of our molecular understanding of cancer are widely regarded as being hopeful. But the effectiveness of chemical therapies is colored by the enormous success against infectious diseases with antibiotics and vaccines, and of preventing organ-system disease, e.g. cardiovascular disease with GPCR-targeted drugs. These may prove unrealistic models of success for disease at a deeply cellular, genetic level, such as cancer. For veterinary practitioners, a very welcome development would be the use of a domestic animal as a model of cancer, particularly for the development of therapies. The reading list for this chapter includes a paper co-authored by a large group of veterinarians describing the potential advantages of the dog as a cancer model.

CLINICAL CORRELATIONS
DOG THAT COLLAPSED WHILE RUNNING

History. A spayed, 10-year-old female golden retriever collapsed while running outside earlier today. The dog is still very lethargic and does not want to move.

Clinical Examination. The dog has pale mucous membranes with a normal temperature. The capillary refill time is prolonged. Heart rate and respiratory rate are increased. On palpation there appears to be fluid in the abdomen, and the dog is in pain.

Comment. Based on this history and physical examination, there is concern that this dog has hemorrhaged into the abdomen. Hemangiosarcoma is a common tumor of older dogs and originates from a transformed endothelial cell. Dogs often present after having collapsed when the tumor, which is present in the spleen, causes internal bleeding. The dogs must often have emergency surgery to have a splenectomy (spleen removed). In some cases, dogs may show other, nonspecific clinical signs (inappetence, lethargy), so a diagnosis may be made before the dog collapses from acute bleeding. A diagnosis is often made through a combination of modalities, including radiographs, ultrasound, biopsies, histopathology, and immunohistochemistry, to determine the nature of the tumor. In many cases, by the time the diagnosis has been made, the tumor has already metastasized, usually via hematogenous route, to other organs. The lung and liver are more frequently affected, but other sites include kidney, muscle, brain, mesentery, skin, and lymph nodes. Recently it has been demonstrated that canine hemangiosarcomas express platelet-derived growth factor beta (PDGF-β). Suppression of this RTK signaling using imatinib (Gleevec) suppressed the canine cell line in a mouse model.

Treatment. Treatment depends on the stage at which the tumor is diagnosed; in this case, the animal presents with shock and hemorrhage. In these cases the patient is stabilized, surgery is performed, and the spleen (in this patient) is removed. The overall prognosis for these cases is poor because the tumor has usually metastasized by the time the initial diagnosis is made. Radiation therapy is palliative for these cases, and it is sometimes used when there is a large, local unresectable mass. Chemotherapy is usually the treatment of choice, although median survival time for these dogs typically is not long. Medications often include the VAC protocol: doxorubicin, cyclophosphamide, and vincristine. Doxorubicin inhibits DNA synthesis, DNA-dependent RNA synthesis, as well as protein synthesis, and it acts throughout the cell cycle. Cyclophosphamide inhibits DNA replication as well as RNA transcription and replication. Vincristine binds to specific microtubular proteins to inhibit cell division. Complications associated with chemotherapy include myelosuppression and sepsis. Experimental treatments are still being tested and target endothelial cells, blocking adhesion factors and inhibiting growth factors associated with endothelial cell growth.

PRACTICE QUESTIONS

1. Which of the following is associated with normal stimulation of cellular proliferation?
   a. Oncogenes
   b. Tumor suppressor genes
   c. Telomerase
   d. Proto-oncogenes
   e. Caspases

2. In the growth factor pathway, the growth factor first binds to _____ which leads to activation of _____, in turn causing activation of a cascade of _____ enzymes leading to alterations in transcription.
   a. G-protein–coupled receptors; G proteins; adenylyl cyclase
   b. receptor tyrosine kinases; Ras; MAP kinase
   c. receptor tyrosine kinases; Bcl-2; caspase
   d. cyclin-dependent kinases; Prb; telomerase
   e. tumor suppressors; oncogenes; checkpoint

3. Which of the following mediate(s) apoptosis?
   a. Telomerase
   b. Cytochrome c
   c. Receptor tyrosine kinases
   d. Cyclin-dependent kinases
   e. Cyclins

4. The tumor suppressor Prb is a(n) _____ and participates in regulating the cell cycles of _____ cells, whereas P53 is a(n) _____ and participates in regulating the cell cycle of _____ cells.
   a. inhibitor of transcription; healthy; transcription factor; healthy
   b. transcription factor; damaged; inhibitor of apoptosis; healthy
   c. caspase; damaged; inhibitor of transcription; damaged
   d. inhibitor of transcription; healthy; receptor tyrosine kinase; healthy
   e. inhibitor of transcription; healthy; transcription factor; damaged

5. Normal stem cells are similar to cancer cells but differ from normal somatic cells in that normal stem cells and cancer cells both:
   a. Are missing checkpoint controls on the cell cycle.
   b. Have cell cycles that are independent of activation of cyclin-dependent kinases.
   c. Have activated telomerase.
   d. Are resistant to apoptosis in response to DNA damage.
   e. Are able to metastasize to distant, foreign tissues.

VOCABULARY

This chapter is unusual in that it contains a large number of vocabulary words that are specialized for cancer and related topics, words that generally will not be used in later chapters. You should be familiar with these vocabulary words; you should be able to define them and state their role in normal cells, and whether and how they differ in cancer cells.

anchorage dependence of growth
aneuploidy
angiogenesis
apoptosis (intrinsic pathway and extrinsic pathway)
Bcl family
cachexia
caspase(s) (activating and executioner)
cell cycle (G1 phase, S phase, G2 phase, M phase)
checkpoint
cyclin
cyclin-dependent kinase (CDK)
extravasation
gain-of-function mutation
germ line
intravasation
loss-of-function mutation
MAP kinase pathway
MDR phenotype
metastasis
metastatic cascade
oncogenes
P53 primary tumor

Ras
retinoblastoma (Prb)
somatic cells
somatic mutation
stem cells
targeted therapy
telomerase
telomeres
tumor suppressor
vasculogenesis
VEGF

BIBLIOGRAPHY

Chan SR, Blackburn EH: Telomeres and telomerase, *Philos Trans R Soc Lond B Biol Sci* 359(1441):109–121, 2004.

Clevers H: The cancer stem cell: premises, promises and challenges, *Nat Med* 17(3):313–319, 2011.

Goldman JM, Melo JV: Targeting the BCR-ABL tyrosine kinase in chronic myeloid leukemia, *N Engl J Med* 344(14):1084–1086, 2001.

Haber DA, Gray NS, Baselga J: The evolving war on cancer, *Cell* 145(1):19–24, 2011.

Hanahan D, Weinberg RA: Hallmarks of cancer: the next generation, *Cell* 144(5):646–674, 2011.

Harris SL, Levine AJ: The p53 pathway: positive and negative feedback loops, *Oncogene* 24(17):2899–2908, 2005.

Hengartner MO: The biochemistry of apoptosis, *Nature* 407(6805): 770–776, 2000.

Khanna C, Lindblad-Toh K, Vail D, et al: The dog as a cancer model, *Nat Biotechnol* 24(9):1065–1066, 2006.

Khanna C, Paoloni MC: Cancer biology in dogs. In Ostrander EA, Giger U, Lindblad-Toh K, editors: *The dog and its genome*, Cold Spring Harbor, NY, 2005, Cold Spring Harbor Laboratory Press.

Klopfleisch R, von Euler H, Sarli G, et al: Molecular carcinogenesis of canine mammary tumors: news from an old disease, *Vet Pathol* 48(1):98–116, 2011.

Krontiris TG: Oncogenes, *N Engl J Med* 333(5):303–306, 1995.

Langley RR, Fidler I: The seed and soil hypothesis revisited—the role of tumor-stroma interactions in metastasis to different organs, *Int J Cancer* 128(11):2527–2535, 2011.

Tisdale MJ: Molecular pathways leading to cancer cachexia, *Physiology (Bethesda)* 20:340–348, 2005.

Venkitaraman AR: Cancer susceptibility and the functions of BRCA1 and BRCA2, *Cell* 108(2):171–182, 2002.

SECTION II   NEUROPHYSIOLOGY

Bradley G. Klein and James G. Cunningham
Chapter 16 edited by John H. Rossmeisl, Jr.

CHAPTER 3

Introduction to the Nervous System

KEY POINTS

1. The neuron is the major functional unit of the nervous system.
2. The mammalian nervous system has two major subdivisions: the central nervous system and the peripheral nervous system.
3. The central nervous system can be divided into six anatomical regions.

4. The central nervous system is protected by the meninges and cerebrospinal fluid.
5. The nervous system collects and integrates sensory information, formulates a response plan, and produces a motor output.

The nervous system is the first multicellular system described in this book because it is one of the major coordinating systems of the body, and because clarifying many of the concepts that concern the nervous system is important for understanding other systems of the body.

Most clinical signs in veterinary neurology involve abnormal movement (e.g., seizures, paralysis); therefore the physiology of muscle control, posture, and locomotion is emphasized in the following chapters. Because veterinary ophthalmology is an extensive subspecialty, the physiology of vision is also covered. Other sensory systems that can produce easily recognizable clinical signs (e.g., vestibular system, hearing) are discussed in Section II as well. Understanding the autonomic nervous system is essential for understanding pharmacology and the involuntary control of many of the body's most critical functions. Similarly, understanding the blood-brain barrier and the cerebrospinal fluid system is essential to understanding the results of the diagnostic cerebrospinal fluid tap and the homeostasis of the cellular microenvironment of the central nervous system. The electroencephalogram and sensory-evoked potentials are described because of their clinical importance in veterinary medicine. Because of space limitations, only the basic physiological concepts essential to understanding the mechanisms of disease and the practice of veterinary medicine are emphasized. For a more expansive study of neurophysiology, the reader should refer to the texts listed in the chapter bibliographies.

The Neuron Is the Major Functional Unit of the Nervous System

The major functional unit of the nervous system is the *neuron,* a cell type whose shape varies considerably with its location in the nervous system. Almost all neurons have an information-receiving area of the cell membrane, usually called the *dendrite;* a cell body, or *soma,* containing the organelles for most cell metabolic activity; an information-carrying extension of the cell membrane, called an *axon;* and a *presynaptic terminal* at the end of the axon to transmit information to other cells. The axon is often covered with a fatty coating called the *myelin sheath* that enhances the speed of information transfer along the axon's length.

Neurons do not exist in isolation; they are usually interconnected within neural circuits or pathways that serve a specific function (Figure 3-1). Neural circuits/pathways that are related in function are often collectively referred to as *neural systems.* For example, the retinotectal pathway provides information for reflex orientation of the eyes to the position of a light source, whereas the retinohypothalamic pathway carries information affecting the body's physiological rhythms in response to light-dark cycles. These individual neural pathways are both part of the visual system.

The other cell type in the nervous system is the *glial cell.* Glial cells play important roles in producing the myelin sheaths of axons, modulating the growth of developing or damaged neurons, buffering extracellular concentrations of potassium and neurotransmitters, formation of contacts between neurons (synapses), and they participate in certain immune responses of the nervous system. Glial cells do not produce action potentials, but growing evidence indicates that they can indirectly monitor the electrical activity of neurons and use this information to modulate the effectiveness of neural communication. However, not all glial actions are beneficial to the nervous system. Glial-mediated neuroinflammatory responses have been implicated in some neurodegenerative diseases and in the development of chronic pain conditions.

The Mammalian Nervous System Has Two Major Subdivisions: the Central Nervous System and the Peripheral Nervous System

The *central nervous system* (CNS) is divided into the brain and spinal cord (Box 3-1). A series of protective bones surround the entire CNS. The brain is surrounded by the skull, and the spinal cord is surrounded by a series of cervical, thoracic, and lumbar vertebrae and ligaments.

The *peripheral nervous system* (PNS) is composed of the spinal and cranial *nerves* that carry electrical signals, called *action potentials,* away from or toward the CNS. These nerves are bundles of PNS axons. The axons carrying action potentials toward the CNS are called *afferents,* and those carrying such signals away are *efferents.* One way to group the elements of the

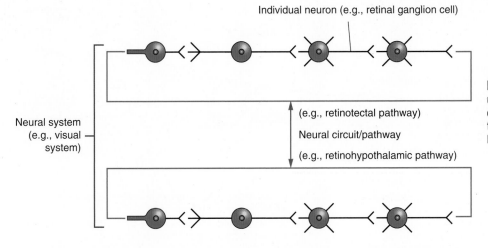

FIGURE 3-1 Individual neurons are usually interconnected within neural circuits or pathways. Neural circuits/pathways that are related in function are often collectively referred to as neural systems.

BOX 3-1 Organization of the Nervous System

Central nervous system (CNS)
  Brain
  Spinal cord

Peripheral nervous system (PNS)
Efferent (motor)
  Somatic—to skeletal muscle
  Visceral—to cardiac muscle
       —to smooth muscle
       —to exocrine glands

Afferent (sensory)
  Somatic—from skin
       —from retina
       —from membranous labyrinth
  Visceral—from thoracic and abdominal organs
       —from olfactory epithelium
       —from taste buds

---

muscle. Action potentials generated by stretch receptors or chemoreceptors (e.g., O_2, CO_2) located within visceral organs of the chest and abdomen are carried to the CNS along *visceral* afferent axons. Visceral efferent and afferent axons are part of the *autonomic nervous system;* the portions of the PNS and CNS responsible for involuntary control of smooth muscle, cardiac muscle, some glands, and many physiological life support functions (e.g., heart rate, blood pressure, digestion).

Peripheral nerve axons converge to form a single spinal nerve at each of the intervertebral foramina. Within the spinal canal, afferent sensory and efferent motor axons are separated; afferent sensory axons enter the spinal cord through the dorsal roots, whereas the efferent motor axons exit the spinal cord through the ventral roots (Figure 3-2).

The PNS and CNS differ in the regenerative ability of their neural axons following physical injury. Peripheral nerve axons can slowly regrow and reconnect to their peripheral targets. Damaged CNS axons do not effectively regenerate due, in large part, to inhibitory features of their local environment. Experimental manipulations of this environment have been shown to improve CNS axonal regrowth.

The Central Nervous System Can Be Divided Into Six Anatomical Regions

The CNS has a longitudinal organization characterized by the phylogenetically oldest parts lying more caudal and the newest portions lying rostral. The CNS can be divided into six major regions (Figure 3-3): the spinal cord and five major brain regions. From caudal to rostral, these brain regions are the medulla, pons, midbrain, diencephalon, and telencephalon. (The cerebellum, a brain structure that lies dorsal to portions of the pons and medulla, is sometimes named as a seventh major region of the CNS.) The medulla, pons, and midbrain form the *brainstem*; the diencephalon and telencephalon form the *forebrain*.

In general, the spinal cord, brainstem, and forebrain represent a hierarchy of functional organization. The spinal cord receives sensory input from and supplies motor output to the trunk and limbs; the brainstem performs these functions for the face and head. Sensory information entering the brainstem is passed to the forebrain, where the most sophisticated forms of information processing take place. Sensory information entering the spinal cord is relayed to the forebrain by way of the brainstem. The forebrain also formulates the most sophisticated forms of motor output. This output is sent to the brainstem for executing

PNS functionally is into sensory and motor subsystems. The elements of spinal and cranial nerves that serve a motor function are (1) axons of somatic efferent neurons, which carry action potential commands from the CNS to junctions, called *synapses,* at skeletal muscles, and (2) axons of visceral efferent neurons, which carry action potentials toward synapses with peripheral neurons that control smooth muscle, cardiac muscle, and some glands. PNS components serving a sensory function are axons of afferent neurons that bring action potential messages to the CNS from peripheral sensory receptors. These receptors are directly or indirectly responsible for transducing energy from the body's external or internal environment into action potentials that travel to the CNS. The intensity of this energy's stimulation of the receptor is encoded by changing the frequency of action potentials as the intensity of stimulation changes.

Spinal and cranial nerve sensory components are axons of (1) somatic afferent neurons and (2) visceral afferent neurons. *Somatic* afferent axons carry action potentials resulting from stimulation of receptors such as the photoreceptors of the eye, auditory receptors of the ear, and stretch receptors of the skeletal

FIGURE 3-2 Spinal cord and the three layers of the meninges within the vertebral canal. Action potentials generated on sensory afferents enter the spinal cord along axons in the dorsal roots. Those generated on motor efferents exit the spinal cord along axons in the ventral roots. (Redrawn from Gardner E: *Fundamentals of neurology,* ed 3, Philadelphia, 1959, Saunders.)

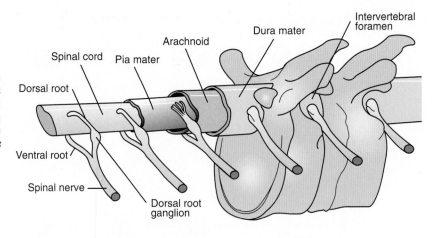

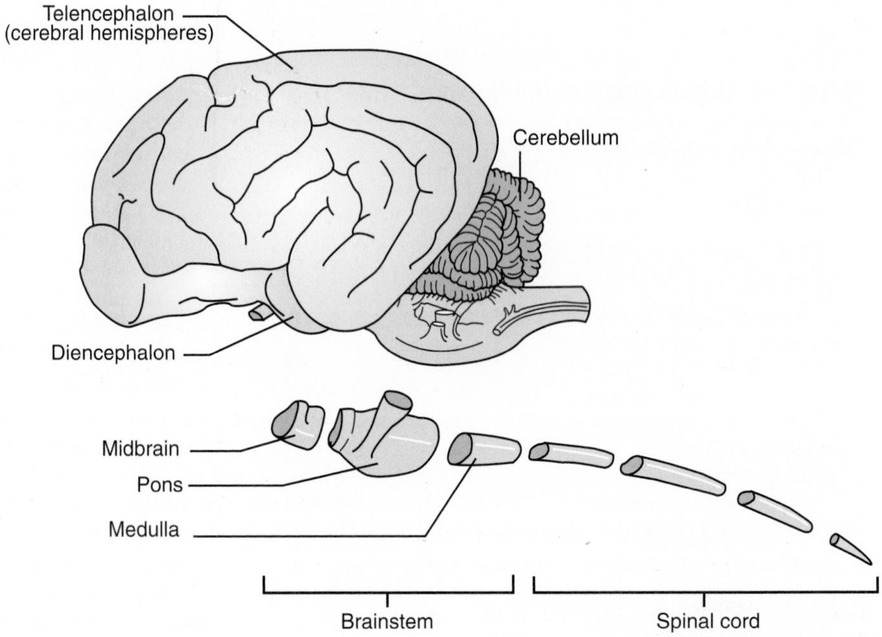

FIGURE 3-3 Central nervous system (CNS) has longitudinal organization in which the phylogenetically oldest parts are caudal and the newest parts are rostral. The CNS can be divided into six major regions: the spinal cord, medulla, pons, midbrain, diencephalon, and telencephalon (cerebral hemispheres).

movement of the face and head or for relay to the spinal cord to execute trunk and limb movement. The forebrain is also capable of sending motor commands directly to the spinal cord. Bundles of axons running from one location to another in the CNS are called *tracts.*

Each of the six CNS regions has distinctive anatomical and functional characteristics. Some of these include the following:

1. The *spinal cord* is the most caudal region in the CNS. Sensory dorsal root axons carry action potentials to the cord that were generated by stimulation of sensory receptors in skin, muscles, tendons, joints, and visceral organs. The spinal cord contains the cell bodies and dendrites of motor neurons whose axons exit through the ventral roots either to reach skeletal muscles or to reach out toward smooth muscle. It also contains tracts of axons carrying sensory information to the brain and motor commands from the brain to the motor neurons. The isolated spinal cord can control simple reflexes, such as muscle stretch reflexes and limb withdrawal from painful stimuli.

2. The *medulla* lies rostral to the spinal cord and resembles it in many ways. By way of cranial nerves, the medulla too receives information from the body's external and internal sensory

receptors and sends motor commands out to skeletal and smooth muscle. Large populations of these receptors and muscles lie in the head and neck region. The cell bodies of medullary neurons that receive the sensory input from cranial nerves or that send the motor output are respectively collected in aggregates called sensory or motor *cranial nerve nuclei.* The cranial nerve nuclei of the medulla play a critical role in life support functions of the respiratory and cardiovascular systems and in aspects of feeding (e.g., taste, tongue movement, swallowing, digestion) and vocalization.

3. The *pons* lies rostral to the medulla and contains the cell bodies of large numbers of neurons in a two-neuron chain that relays information from the cerebral cortex to the cerebellum. The *cerebellum* is not a part of the brainstem but is often described along with the pons because of a similar embryological origin. The cerebellum is important for smooth, accurate, coordinated movement and for motor learning. Cranial nerve nuclei of the pons play important roles in receiving sensory information about facial touch and in the motor control of chewing.

4. The *midbrain,* or *mesencephalon,* lies rostral to the pons and contains the superior and inferior colliculi, which are

important in processing and relaying visual and auditory information that has entered the brain at other levels. The midbrain also contains cranial nerve nuclei that directly control eye movement and that induce pupillary constriction. Some midbrain regions coordinate particular eye movement reflexes.

Each region of the brainstem contains axon tracts carrying action potentials to or from the forebrain, as well as tracts that carry action potentials to or from the spinal cord. Each brainstem region also contains a portion of the *reticular formation*, a netlike complex of many small clusters of cell bodies (nuclei) and loosely organized axonal projections, located near the midline. The reticular formation plays important roles in modulating consciousness and arousal, pain perception, and spinal reflexes, as well as in movement.

5. The *diencephalon* contains the thalamus and the hypothalamus, both of which are large structures consisting of several subnuclei. The *thalamus* is a relay station for and a modulator of information being passed to the cerebral cortex from sensory systems and other brain regions. The *hypothalamus* regulates the autonomic nervous system, controls hormone secretion of the pituitary gland, and plays a major role in physiological and behavioral aspects of homeostasis (e.g., maintenance of temperature and blood pressure; feeding).

6. The *telencephalon,* also commonly referred to as the *cerebral hemispheres,* is made up of the cerebral cortex and a small number of prominent subcortical structures, such as the basal ganglia and hippocampus. The *cerebral cortex* mediates the most complex forms of sensory *integration* and conscious sensory perception. It also formulates and executes sequences of voluntary movement. The *basal ganglia* are a collection of nuclei that modulate the motor functions of cerebral cortex, and the *hippocampus* plays an important role in memory and spatial learning. Considering the function of the hippocampus, it is fascinating that it is one of the very few regions of the adult mammalian brain where new neurons are born.

The Central Nervous System Is Protected By the Meninges and Cerebrospinal Fluid

The entire CNS is surrounded by three protective layers called *meninges*: the pia mater, arachnoid, and dura mater (see Figure 3-2). The innermost layer, lying next to the CNS, is the *pia mater,* which is a single layer of fibroblast cells joined to the outer surface of the brain and spinal cord. The middle layer, the *arachnoid,* so named because of its spiderweb appearance, is a thin layer of fibroblast cells that traps cerebrospinal fluid between it and the pia mater (in the *subarachnoid space*). The outermost meningeal layer, the *dura mater,* is a much thicker layer of fibroblast cells that protects the CNS. Within the brain cavity of the skull, the dura mater is often fused with the inner surface of the bone.

Cerebrospinal fluid (CSF) is a clear, colorless fluid found within the subarachnoid space, the central canal of the spinal cord, and the ventricular system of the brain (see Chapter 15). CSF is produced primarily in the ventricles of the brain, flows down a pressure gradient from the ventricles to the subarachnoid space, where it bathes the surface of the CNS, and from the subarachnoid space eventually passes into the venous system. It is a dynamic fluid, being replaced several times daily. Because CSF can exchange freely with the extracellular fluid of the CNS, it is an important determinant of the neuronal microenvironment, both carrying away metabolic waste and providing certain micronutrients. It can also serve as an important diagnostic tool to indicate CNS infection, inflammation, or tumor activity. CSF also serves as a shock absorber for the CNS during abrupt body movement.

The Nervous System Collects and Integrates Sensory Information, Formulates a Response Plan, and Produces a Motor Output

In simplest terms, the nervous system (1) collects sensory information from its external or internal environment, (2) consciously or unconsciously integrates these various inputs to formulate a response plan, and (3) produces a final motor output that can either change the environment (external or internal) or keep it constant (Figure 3-4). Collecting sensory information and executing the final motor output are the primary responsibilities of the PNS, whereas integration is primarily performed by the CNS. As discussed in Chapter 4, these same functions occur at the level of the individual neuron, which is the principal building block of the nervous system.

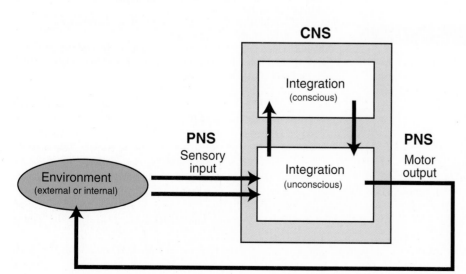

FIGURE 3-4 General functional organization of the nervous system. Sensory input and motor output are primarily mediated by the PNS. Integration is a principal role of the CNS.

CLINICAL CORRELATIONS

NEUROLOGICAL DISEASE IN A HORSE

History. A client calls and asks you to look at a 4-month-old Arabian filly. The owners have had her since birth, and she has always seemed a little clumsy compared with other foals. They think she is getting worse, however, and say she stumbles in the field. She falls over at times when she is playing with the other foals, and she seems very stiff, almost stabbing at the ground when she is walking.

Clinical Examination. The filly is bright and alert. Her temperature, pulse, and respiration are normal. Abnormalities are limited to your neurological examination. She is weak (paresis) in both the hind and the front limbs (grade II), with the hind limbs being worse (grade III). When you assess her conscious proprioception (ataxia), she is also greatly delayed (grade III hind limbs, grade II front limbs). When she walks, the filly seems to slap at the ground (hypermetria), and she drags her toes forward across the ground. You detect no other neurological deficits.

Comment. This filly has *equine degenerative myeloencephalopathy.* An antemortem diagnosis is difficult. Exclusion of other causes is important. Serum vitamin E levels are often, but not exclusively, low. A definitive diagnosis is made at necropsy.

The pathogenesis of the disease is not clear, but risk factors include diets low in vitamin E, use of insecticides, keeping animals on dirt lots, and exposure to wood preservatives. On histopathology, significant changes occur in the medulla and spinal cord. There is diffuse neuronal degeneration of the white matter. Astrocytosis and lipofuscin-like pigment accumulate in affected areas. Demyelination is marked.

Animals with this disease have loss of functional neurons as well as the myelin sheath that surrounds them. As a result, the ability to conduct impulses is greatly affected. Clinically, this affects the animal's ability to respond to external stimuli as well as initiate conscious responses.

Treatment. Supportive treatment is the only therapy that can be given. Keeping horses on green pasture has been shown to be somewhat protective. Supplementing with vitamin E can improve some horses' condition and slow the progression of disease. There are some familial tendencies in Arabian, Appaloosa, Thoroughbred, and Paso Fino horses.

PRACTICE QUESTIONS

1. Which part of a neuron is primarily characterized as the information-receiving component?
   a. Axon
   b. Presynaptic terminal
   c. Cell body
   d. Dendrite
   e. Myelin

2. Which of the following is *not* characteristic of glial cells?
   a. Production of action potentials
   b. Immune responses of the nervous system
   c. Production of the myelin sheaths of axons
   d. Modulating the growth of developing or damaged neurons
   e. Buffering extracellular concentrations of some ions and neurotransmitters

3. The elements of spinal and cranial nerves that carry action potential commands from the CNS to synapses at skeletal muscles are:
   a. Axons of visceral efferent neurons.
   b. Axons of somatic afferent neurons.
   c. Axons of somatic efferent neurons.
   d. The dorsal roots.
   e. Axons of visceral afferent neurons.

4. The thalamus and hypothalamus are components of which major brain division?
   a. Medulla
   b. Pons
   c. Midbrain
   d. Diencephalon
   e. Telencephalon

BIBLIOGRAPHY

Allen NJ, Barres BA: Glia—more than just brain glue, *Nature* 457(7230):675–677, 2009.
Behan M: Organization of the nervous system. In Reece WO, editor: *Duke's physiology of domestic animals,* ed 12, Ithaca, NY, 2004, Comstock Publishing.
Boron WF, Boulpaep EL: *Medical physiology,* ed 2, Philadelphia, 2009, Saunders.
Brodal P: *The central nervous system: structure and function,* ed 4, New York, 2010, Oxford University Press.
Hall JE: *Guyton and Hall textbook of medical physiology,* ed 12, Philadelphia, 2011, Saunders.
Kitchell RL: Introduction to the nervous system. In Evans HE, editor: *Miller's anatomy of the dog,* ed 3, Philadelphia, 1993, Saunders.
Kitchell RL, Evans HE: The spinal nerves. In Evans HE, editor: *Miller's anatomy of the dog,* ed 3, Philadelphia, 1993, Saunders.
Matthews HK: Spinal cord, vertebral and intracranial trauma. In Reed SM, Bayly WM, editors: *Equine internal medicine,* Philadelphia, 1998, Saunders.
Purves D, Augustine GJ, Fitzpatrick D, et al: *Neuroscience,* ed 5, Sunderland, Mass, 2012, Sinauer.
Vallejo R, Tilley DM, Vogel L, et al: The role of glia and the immune system in the development and maintenance of neuropathic pain, *Pain Pract* 10(3):167–184, 2010.

CHAPTER 4

The Neuron

KEY POINTS

1. Neurons have four distinct anatomical regions.
2. Neuronal membranes contain a resting electrical membrane potential.
3. The resting membrane potential is the result of three major determinants.
4. The resting membrane potential can be changed by synaptic signals from a presynaptic cell.
5. Action potentials begin at the axon's initial segment and spread down the entire length of the axon.

There are two major classes of cells in the nervous system: the neuron and the glial cell (see Chapter 3). The neuron is the basic functional unit of the nervous system. The large number of neurons and their interconnections account for the complexity of the nervous system. The number of neurons in the vertebrate nervous system ranges greatly. There are approximately 100 million in a small mammal (e.g., mouse); 100 billion in a human; and more than 200 billion in whales and elephants: far more neurons in a nervous system than people on Earth, and there are 10 to 50 times more glial cells. The structural and functional support provided to neurons by glial cells and their potential to modulate neural communication make an important contribution to the operational integrity of the nervous system. The numbers of cells in the nervous system are huge, but knowing that they have common elements makes it easier to understand them.

Neurons Have Four Distinct Anatomical Regions

A typical neuron has four morphologically defined regions (Figure 4-1): the dendrites, the cell body, the axon, and the presynaptic terminals of the axon. These four anatomical regions are important in the major electrical and chemical responsibilities of neurons: receiving signals from the presynaptic terminals of other neurons (on dendrites), integrating these often-opposing signals (on the initial segment of the axon), transmitting action potential impulses along the axon, and signaling an adjacent cell from the presynaptic terminal. These functions are collectively analogous to the general role of the nervous system: collecting information from the environment, integrating that information, and producing an output that can change the environment.

The *cell body* (also called the *soma* or *perikaryon*) plays a critical role in manufacturing proteins essential for neuronal function. Four organelles are particularly important for this purpose: the nucleus, containing the blueprint for protein assembly; the free ribosomes, which assemble cytosolic proteins; the rough endoplasmic reticulum, in which secretory and membrane proteins are assembled; and the Golgi apparatus, which further processes and sorts secretory and membrane components for transport. The cell body usually gives rise to several branchlike extensions, called *dendrites,* whose surface area and extent greatly exceed those of the cell body. The dendrites serve as the major receptive apparatus of the neuron, receiving signals from other neurons. These signals, usually of a chemical nature, affect specialized receptor proteins *(receptors)* that reside on the dendrites. The cell body also gives rise to the *axon,* a tubular process that is often long (>1 meter in some large animals). The axon is the conducting unit of the neuron, rapidly transmitting an electrical impulse (the action potential) from its initial segment at the cell body to its often distant end at the presynaptic terminal. Intact adult axons lack ribosomes and therefore normally cannot synthesize proteins. Instead, macromolecules are synthesized in the cell body and are carried along the axon to distant axonal regions and to the presynaptic terminals by a process called *axoplasmic transport.* Large axons are surrounded by a fatty, insulating coating called *myelin.* In the peripheral nervous system, myelin is formed by *Schwann cells,* specialized glial cells that wrap around the axon much like toilet paper wrapped around a broomstick. A similar function is performed by glial cells called *oligodendrocytes* in the central nervous system. The myelin sheath is interrupted at regular intervals by spaces called *nodes of Ranvier.* The myelin sheath significantly increases the speed of action potential conduction along the axon.

Axons branch near their ends into several specialized endings called *presynaptic terminals* (or *synaptic boutons*). When the action potential rapidly arrives, these presynaptic terminals transmit a chemical signal to an adjacent cell. The site of contact of the presynaptic terminal with the adjacent cell is called the *synapse,* shown in the inset in Figure 4-1. It is formed by the presynaptic terminal of one cell (presynaptic cell), the receptive surface of the adjacent cell (postsynaptic cell), and the space between these two cells (the *synaptic cleft*). Presynaptic terminals contain chemical transmitter–filled *synaptic vesicles* that can release their contents into the synaptic cleft. The presynaptic terminals of an axon usually contact the receptive surface of an adjacent neuron or muscle cell, usually on the neuron's dendrites, but sometimes this contact is made on the cell body or, occasionally, on the presynaptic terminals of another cell (e.g., for presynaptic inhibition). On many neurons, presynaptic terminals often synapse on

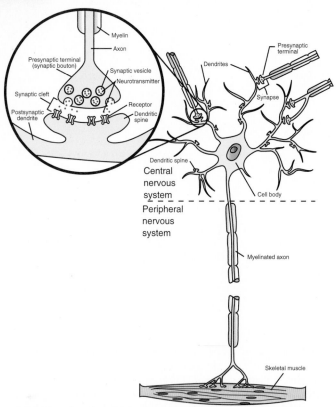

FIGURE 4-1 A typical neuron has four functionally important regions. The cell body manufactures proteins to maintain the neuron; the dendrites receive signals from neighboring neurons; the axon integrates these signals and transmits action potentials some distance along the cell; and the presynaptic terminal signals adjacent cells. The inset shows an enlargement of the circled synapse.

small protrusions of the dendritic membrane called *dendritic spines* (Figure 4-2 and see Chapter 5). The receptive surface of the postsynaptic cell contains specialized receptors for the chemical transmitter released from the presynaptic terminal.

The signaling functions of the morphological components of the neuron can be briefly summarized as follows (Figure 4-3). Receptors, usually dendritic, receive neurochemical signals released from the presynaptic terminals of many other neurons. These neurochemical signals, after being transduced by the receptors into a different form (small voltage changes), are integrated at the initial segment of the axon. Depending on the results of this integration, an action potential (large voltage change) may be generated on the axon. The action potential travels very rapidly to the axon's often distant presynaptic terminals to induce the release of chemical neurotransmitter onto another neuron or muscle cell.

Neuronal Membranes Contain a Resting Electrical Membrane Potential

Neurons, like other cells of the body, have an electrical potential, or voltage, that can be measured across their cell membrane *(resting membrane potential).* However, the electrical membrane potential in neurons and muscle cells is unique in that its magnitude and sign can be changed as the result of synaptic signaling from other cells, or it can change within a sensory organ receptor as a response to transduction of some environmental energy. When the change in membrane potential of a neuron or muscle

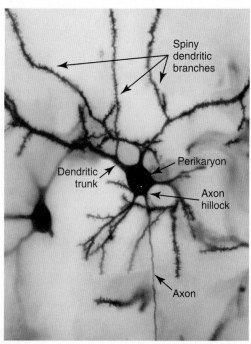

FIGURE 4-2 Morphology of a neuron in mammalian cerebral cortex revealed with the Golgi staining method. The cell body (perikaryon), dendrites, and proximal portions of the axon are visible. Tiny dendritic spines can be seen along the dendrites. The cell body is approximately 20 μm in diameter. (Image courtesy Dr. Ceylan Isgor.)

cell reaches a threshold value, a further and dramatic change in the membrane potential, called an action potential, occurs; this action potential moves along the entire length of the neuronal axon (see later discussion).

The origins of the resting electrical membrane potential are complicated, particularly in a quantitative way. In qualitative terms, however, the resting membrane potential is the result of the differential separation of charged ions, especially sodium (Na^+) and potassium (K^+), across the membrane and the resting membrane's differential permeability to these ions as they attempt to move back down their concentration and electrical gradients (see Chapter 1). Even though the net concentration of positive and negative charges is similar in both the intracellular and extracellular fluids, an excess of positive charges accumulates immediately outside the cell membrane, and an excess of negative charges accumulates immediately inside the cell membrane (Figure 4-4). This makes the inside of the cell negatively charged with respect to the outside of the cell. The magnitude of the resulting electrical difference (or voltage) across the membrane varies from cell to cell, ranging from about 40 to 90 millivolts (mV), and is usually about 70 mV in mammalian neurons. Because the extracellular fluid is arbitrarily considered to be 0 mV, the resting membrane potential is –70 mV, more negative on the inside than on the outside.

The Resting Membrane Potential Is the Result of Three Major Determinants

Three major factors cause the resting membrane potential.
- *The Na^+, K^+ pump.* Cell membranes have an energy-dependent pump that pumps Na^+ ions out of the cell and draws K^+ ions into the cell against their concentration gradients. This maintains the differential distribution of each of these charged ion species across the membrane that underlies their ability to

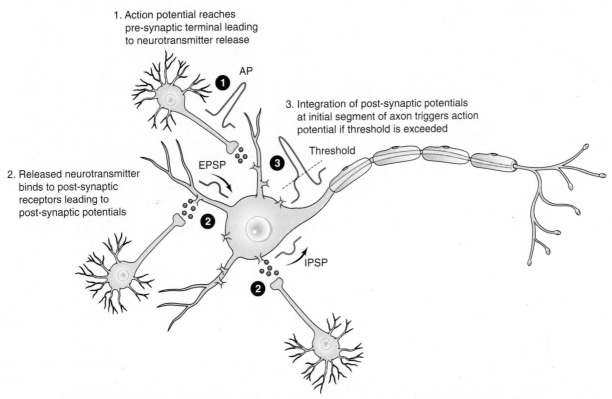

1. Action potential reaches pre-synaptic terminal leading to neurotransmitter release

AP

1

3. Integration of post-synaptic potentials at initial segment of axon triggers action potential if threshold is exceeded

Threshold

3

EPSP

2. Released neurotransmitter binds to post-synaptic receptors leading to post-synaptic potentials

2

IPSP

2

FIGURE 4-3 Overview of neural communication. *AP,* Action potential; *EPSP,* Excitatory post-synaptic potential; *IPSP,* Inhibitory post-synaptic potential. (Portions modified from Klein BG: Membrane potentials: the generation and conduction of electrical signals in neurons. In Reece WO, editor: *Duke's physiology of domestic animals,* ed 12, Ithaca, NY, 2004, Comstock Publishing.)

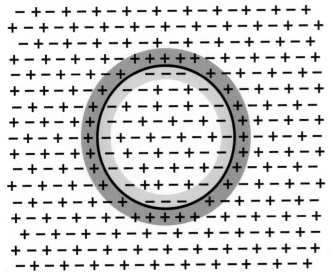

FIGURE 4-4 Net concentrations of positive and negative charges are similar in both the intracellular space and the extracellular space. However, positive charges accumulate immediately outside the cell membrane *(blue),* and negative charges accumulate immediately inside the cell membrane *(lighter blue).*

- An ion species will move toward a dynamic equilibrium if it can flow across the membrane. Using K^+ as an example, the concentration difference across the membrane actively maintained by the Na^+, K^+ pump produces a concentration gradient, or *chemical driving force,* that attempts to push the ion passively across the membrane from high concentration inside the cell toward low concentration outside. If K^+ can flow across ion channels in the membrane, exiting K^+ leaves behind unopposed negative charge (often from negatively charged protein macromolecules trapped inside the cell) that builds an electrical gradient, or *electrical driving force,* pulling K^+ back inside the cell. These opposing gradients eventually produce a dynamic equilibrium, even though there may still be more K^+ inside than outside, as well as a charge imbalance across the membrane. This uneven distribution of charge at dynamic equilibrium produces a voltage across the membrane called the *equilibrium potential* for that ion. When an ion species can flow across a channel in the membrane, it flows toward its equilibrium state, and it drives the voltage across the membrane toward its equilibrium potential.

- *Differential permeability of the membrane to diffusion of ions.* The resting membrane is much more permeable to K^+ than to Na^+ ions because there are vastly more K^+ leak channels than Na^+ leak channels in the membrane. This greater membrane permeability to K^+ means that K^+ ions can more closely approach their dynamic equilibrium state, and equilibrium potential, compared with Na^+ ions, which have difficulty moving across the membrane. Therefore the equilibrium potential for the more permeant K^+ ions (about -90 mV in many mammalian neurons) will have the predominant influence on

produce a voltage across the membrane. The pump itself makes a small, direct contribution to the resting membrane potential because it pushes three molecules of Na^+ out for every two molecules of K^+ drawn into the cell, thus concentrating positive charges outside the cell.

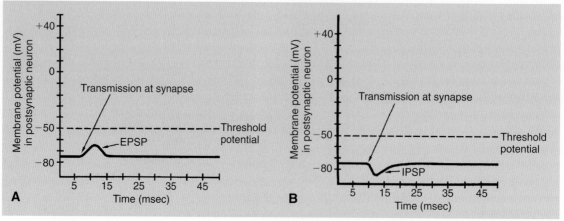

FIGURE 4-5 Postsynaptic potentials. **A**, Excitatory postsynaptic potential *(EPSP)* drives the membrane potential toward threshold. **B**, Inhibitory postsynaptic potential *(IPSP)* drives the membrane potential away from threshold.

the value of the resting membrane potential compared with the equilibrium potential of the vastly less permeant Na⁺ ions (about +70 mV in many mammalian neurons). Therefore, as noted earlier, the resting membrane potential of many mammalian neurons is about –70 mV, close to the equilibrium potential for K⁺.

These three determinants—the Na⁺, K⁺ pump, the movement of a permeant ion toward dynamic equilibrium, and the differentially permeable membrane—are the primary source of the resting membrane potential. The value of this potential can be predicted by the Nernst and Goldman equations; refer to Chapter 1 and the bibliography for a more quantitative understanding of the resting membrane potential.

This discussion of the resting membrane potential has a number of important clinical implications. The Na⁺, K⁺ pump requires energy in the form of adenosine triphosphate (ATP), which is derived from the intracellular metabolism of glucose and oxygen. In fact, it has been estimated that 50% to 70% of the brain's ATP-derived energy is expended on the pump. Because the neuron cannot store either glucose or oxygen, anything that deprives the nervous system of either substrate can lead to impairment of the pump and serious clinical neurological deficits. Fortunately, hormones and other factors normally maintain serum glucose and oxygen levels within narrow limits. Because Na⁺ and K⁺ are important ions involved in establishing the resting membrane potential, it is essential that serum levels of Na⁺ and K⁺ be regulated carefully. The endocrine system (Chapter 33) and kidney (Chapter 41) maintain serum Na⁺ and K⁺ levels within narrow limits. Anything altering serum levels of either ion beyond normal limits also leads to potentially severe neurological deficits.

The Resting Membrane Potential Can Be Changed By Synaptic Signals from a Presynaptic Cell

Although most cells of the body have a resting membrane potential, neurons and muscle cells are unique in that their membrane potential can be altered by a synaptic signal from another cell. Neurotransmitter released from a presynaptic axon terminal binds with receptors on the postsynaptic membrane, resulting in the opening or closing of ion selective channels and changing the membrane potential of the postsynaptic cell. Even though there are trillions of synapses in the nervous system, a presynaptic

signal can alter the postsynaptic membrane potential in basically only two ways: by making it more negative or more positive (less negative). The particular change depends on the nature of the receptor activated by the chemical transmitter that is released from the synaptic vesicles of the presynaptic axon terminal. The change in postsynaptic membrane potential is called a *postsynaptic potential*.

If a chemical synaptic transmission leads to a postsynaptic potential that is more positive in comparison with the resting level (e.g., from –75 to –65 mV), this is said to be an *excitatory postsynaptic potential* (EPSP) (Figure 4-5, *A*). It is called "excitatory" because it increases the chances that the threshold for triggering an action potential will be reached at the initial segment of the postsynaptic cell's axon. When an EPSP changes the postsynaptic membrane potential to a more positive value, the membrane is said to be *depolarized*. Depolarization of the postsynaptic membrane can result if the interaction of the chemical transmitter and its appropriate receptor on the postsynaptic membrane cause (ligand-gated) Na⁺ channels to open. This allows Na⁺ ions to diffuse into the neuron as they begin to flow toward equilibrium across the membrane, moving the membrane potential toward the more positive sodium equilibrium potential. The ion channels that usually change their conductivity as a result of neurotransmitter binding with a receptor are the *ligand-gated* or *chemically gated* ion channels (see Chapter 1).

Because the chemical transmitter is quickly removed from the synapse, the postsynaptic potential change is transient, lasting only a few milliseconds. Furthermore, because the change in ion flow resulting from receptor activation is limited, the magnitude of a postsynaptic potential is often quite small (e.g., 2 to 3 mV). However, it is greatest at the synapse. Although the depolarization spreads over the postsynaptic membrane, it decreases with the distance from the originating synapse, much as the waves created by throwing a stone into a lake decrease in size with the distance from where the stone fell.

If instead the presynaptic neurotransmitter's interaction with the postsynaptic receptor results in opening of the membrane's chemically gated K⁺ channels, then K⁺ ions diffuse out, moving the membrane potential even closer to the equilibrium potential for K⁺ (–90 mV). This change from the resting potential to a more negative membrane potential is called *hyperpolarization*. Such hyperpolarization of the postsynaptic membrane is called an *inhibitory postsynaptic potential* (IPSP) (see Figure 4-5, *B*), because each such transmission makes it less likely that an action potential will result at the axon's initial segment. As with EPSPs, IPSPs spread over the neuron's membrane, and the hyperpolarization decreases with the distance from the originating synapse. It should be noted that only two of the receptor-mediated effects upon chemically gated ion channels, responsible for generating EPSPs or IPSPs, have been discussed earlier.

Action Potentials Begin at the Axon's Initial Segment and Spread Down the Entire Length of the Axon

Both EPSPs and IPSPs on the postsynaptic membrane are the subsequent result of action potentials that occurred on, and synaptic transmission from, many presynaptic cells. The integration of these postsynaptic potentials is important for determining whether neurotransmitter will ultimately be released at the neuron's terminals. However, these postsynaptic potentials decrease in magnitude as they spread along the postsynaptic cell membrane. Because many neurons and muscle cells are long, the cell needs a mechanism for sending an electrical signal from its information-receiving end on the postsynaptic dendritic and soma membrane to the information-transmitting zone at the terminals of the often-lengthy axon. This is accomplished by an explosive event called an *action potential*, a regenerative electrical signal that begins at the axon's initial segment, is triggered by the integration of EPSP and IPSP membrane potential changes, and rapidly spreads down the length of the axon without decreasing in magnitude.

EPSPs and IPSPs can respectively summate on the postsynaptic membrane to produce larger changes in membrane potential than either signal alone. At the axon's initial segment, the arriving EPSPs and IPSPs are integrated. If only a few EPSPs arrive at the axon's initial segment, its membrane potential is not made sufficiently positive to reach its threshold potential (often 10 to 20 mV more positive than the resting potential) for triggering an action potential. However, if many more EPSPs than IPSPs arrive, the initial segment's membrane potential is made positive enough to reach its *threshold potential,* and an action potential is created on the axon. This action potential is the result of the sequential opening of voltage-gated ion channels in the membrane first to sodium and shortly thereafter to potassium.

The explosive changes in membrane potential that characterize the action potential can be described as follows: First, a dramatic and swift depolarization of the axonal membrane potential occurs, in which the inside of the cell actually becomes more positively charged than the outside, followed by a repolarization of the membrane, in which the membrane potential falls back toward the resting potential. The depolarization phase of the action potential is caused by the immediate and extensive opening of voltage-gated Na^+ channels and the consequent influx of Na^+ ions as they attempt to flow toward their equilibrium. As the action potential's depolarization phase continues, the voltage-gated Na^+ channels are spontaneously inactivated, and the voltage-gated K^+ channels, which open with a longer delay than the Na^+ channels, begin to allow even more K^+ ions to exit as they move closer to their equilibrium state. This brings depolarization to a halt and allows repolarization to occur. As repolarization continues, the membrane potential moves temporarily beyond its resting level to a hyperpolarized state. This hyperpolarization is attributable to the flow of K^+ ions out through the voltage-gated K^+ channels, in addition to the flow out through the K^+ leak channels, bringing the membrane potential even closer to the K^+

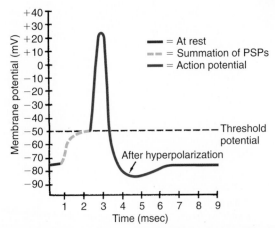

FIGURE 4-6 Axon's membrane potential changes dramatically during an action potential. After threshold is reached by summating postsynaptic potentials (PSPs), the axonal membrane depolarizes, repolarizes, hyperpolarizes, and then returns to its original resting potential. (Modified from Sherwood L: *Human physiology: from cells to systems,* St Paul, 1989, Wadsworth.)

equilibrium potential (–90 mV) than at rest. The membrane potential eventually returns to its resting state as the K^+ voltage-gated channels gradually close. The whole action potential takes about 2 to 3 msec in many neurons but longer in many muscle cells. Figure 4-6 illustrates this sequence of events in a neuron.

An analogy may be helpful for understanding these difficult concepts. Imagine the resting neural membrane as a toilet. The toilet has stored potential energy by filling its water tank. (The neuron has done so by generating the resting membrane potential.) If the handle of the toilet is pushed down only briefly, for a short distance, some water runs into the toilet, but the flush cycle is not initiated. (This is similar to an EPSP without the action potential.) However, if the handle is pushed down far enough and held down long enough, a critical threshold is reached, the flush cycle is triggered, and it must run its course, including the refilling of the tank, before another flush cycle can be started. The action potential is analogous to this flush cycle. It is triggered once a critical depolarization threshold is reached. It usually must run its course, including reestablishing the resting membrane potential, before another action potential can be initiated. Because the flush cycle takes a finite amount of time, only a limited number of flush cycles could be completed in an hour, even if the toilet were flushed again each time the tank refilled. Similarly, because the action potential also has a finite duration, there is a limit to the number of action potentials per second that can be generated on an axon. (However, for both toilets and neurons, strategies can be employed to produce a flush or an action potential before the tank is completely refilled or before the membrane completely returns to the resting potential.)

Certain animal toxins, such as tetrodotoxin from the Japanese puffer fish, can block voltage-gated Na^+ channels and therefore interfere with the generation of action potentials on axons. Many local anesthetics (e.g., lidocaine), which are used in a controlled, clinically efficacious manner, work by a similar mechanism.

The action potential actively propagates from its origin at the initial segment down the axon. The dramatic influx of Na^+ ions that accompanies action potential depolarization of the initial segment's membrane results in the passive spread of these positive charges toward the adjacent resting segment of the membrane. This migration of positive charge on the inner surface of the

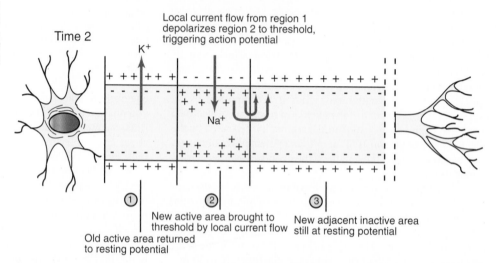

Action potential at region 1 causes
excess of internal positive charge
to passively migrate toward region 2

Time 1

① Active area at peak
of action potential

② Adjacent inactive area
still at resting potential

③ Remainder of axon still at resting potential

Local current flow from region 1
depolarizes region 2 to threshold,
triggering action potential

Time 2

① Old active area returned
to resting potential

② New active area brought to
threshold by local current flow

③ New adjacent inactive area
still at resting potential

FIGURE 4-7 Action potential, first generated in the axon's initial segment *(Time 1, region 1),* moves down the unmyelinated axon as positive charges passively migrate to the immediately adjacent membrane to trigger an action potential there *(Time 2, region 2).* (Redrawn from Sherwood L: *Human physiology: from cells to systems,* St Paul, 1989, Wadsworth.)

membrane, called an *electrotonic current,* depolarizes this adjacent segment to threshold, causing voltage-gated Na$^+$ channels to open. This causes an action potential to develop, which in turn triggers a similar cycle in its adjacent membrane, and so on down the axon. In this way an action potential spreads from the axon's initial segment down to the presynaptic terminal at the axon's far end (Figure 4-7).

The speed with which the action potential is conducted down the axon varies. The internal diameter and the degree of myelination of an axon play a critical role in determining this action-potential conduction velocity. In a small-diameter, unmyelinated axon, the conduction velocity is relatively slow (e.g., 0.5 meters/second [m/sec]); conduction velocities of greater than 90 m/sec (so that a distance as long as a football field is traveled in 1 second), however, are known to occur in large-diameter, heavily myelinated axons. This occurs because the *passive electrotonic current,* responsible for triggering the action potential at the next adjacent patch of axonal membrane, travels faster and farther along wider axons or along myelinated patches of axon. In myelinated axons, exchange of ions across the membrane, and thus generation of the action potential, can only occur at the bare nodes of Ranvier, where a high density of voltage-gated Na$^+$ channels are found. Given the rapid spread of electrotonic current along the myelinated patches *(internodes)* and the comparatively slower process of ion exchange at the nodes, the action potential seems to functionally jump from node to node *(saltatory conduction)* in myelinated axons (Figure 4-8).

The normal facilitation of action-potential conduction velocity by myelin can be appreciated by considering diseases that attack myelin, such as acute idiopathic polyradiculoneuritis ("coonhound paralysis"). Slowing of evoked electrical signals along sensory and motor nerves and depressed spinal reflexes are associated with this condition.

CLINICAL CORRELATIONS

HYPOGLYCEMIA

History. You examine an 8-year-old male boxer dog whose owner complains that the dog experiences seizures, weakness, and confusion around the time he is fed.

Clinical Examination. The findings of the dog's physical examination, including his neurological examination, were within normal limits. His fasting serum glucose level, however, was 29 mg/dL (normal is 70 to 110 mg/dL), and the ratio between serum insulin and serum glucose levels was significantly elevated.

Comment. Neurons depend primarily on oxygen and glucose as metabolites for ATP energy production, and neurons cannot store appreciable quantities of glucose. ATP is needed for maintenance of the normal electrical membrane potential. When deprived of glucose and subsequently ATP, the brain does not function properly; associated clinical signs include seizures, weakness, and confusion. In this animal, these signs were more common at the

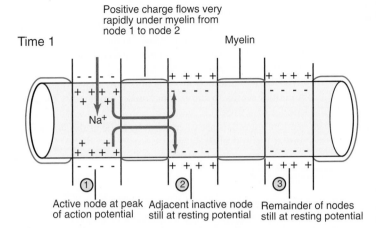

Time 1

Positive charge flows very rapidly under myelin from node 1 to node 2

Myelin

Na+

① Active node at peak of action potential ② Adjacent inactive node still at resting potential ③ Remainder of nodes still at resting potential

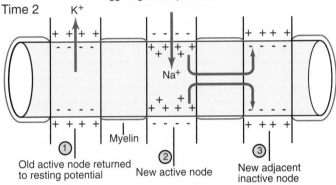

Local current flow from node 1 depolarizes node 2 to threshold, triggering action potential

Time 2

K+

Na+

Myelin

① Old active node returned to resting potential ② New active node ③ New adjacent inactive node

FIGURE 4-8 Saltatory conduction of action potentials in myelinated axons is faster than action-potential conduction in unmyelinated axons because the passive local current flows very rapidly under the myelin to trigger an action potential at the next node. Thus the action potential seems to jump functionally from node to node. (Modified from Sherwood L: *Human physiology: from cells to systems,* St Paul, 1989, Wadsworth.)

time of feeding because as the dog anticipated eating or actually did begin to eat, insulin was released, causing hypoglycemia.

In this case the ratio of insulin to glucose is elevated, probably because of an insulin-secreting tumor of the pancreas. Because insulin facilitates glucose transport through cell membranes, too much insulin results in the transfer of too much serum glucose to the cytoplasm of other cells of the body, thus depriving the brain's neurons of this essential metabolite.

Treatment. Insulinomas can usually be found and removed from the pancreas surgically. After surgical removal of the tumor, additional medical treatment is warranted to maintain normoglycemia. Medications include glucocorticoids, to stimulate gluconeogenesis; diazoxide, to inhibit insulin secretion; streptozocin, which is toxic to the beta cells; and somatostatin, which increases gluconeogenesis. With this tumor type, there is a high rate of metastasis, which means that other tumor sites may remain, in the liver and elsewhere, to overproduce insulin.

SALT TOXICITY IN POT BELLY PIG

History. A client calls you and says that they recently got a young pot belly pig through a friend. The pig was doing well for the first week or so, but now seems to be acting "funny." The pig seems to be depressed, and not as active, walking into things, uncoordinated, and not as responsive when they call her. She also seems like she is not eating or drinking as well, and she may have some loose feces. They have been feeding her dog food, as they have not had a chance to get to the feed store since they got her. They

talked to the owner who they got the pig from, and the owner says that all the other pigs are normal.

Clinical Examination. The pig appears depressed and is not responding normally. Her eyes appear sunken from dehydration, and her gastrointestinal sounds are increased. A brief neurological exam demonstrates depression, ataxia (incoordination) with both her front and hind limbs being equally affected, and blindness. You submit blood for complete blood count and biochemical profile. You also discuss with the owner the possibility to perform a cerebrospinal fluid (CSF) tap to collect a sample of the CSF for analysis to identify the cause of the clinical signs, if it cannot be determined based on the blood work.

Comment. The blood work demonstrates markedly increased levels of sodium and chloride (hypernatremia/hyperchloremia) as well as renal disease (increased blood urea nitrogen [BUN] and creatinine). This pot belly pig has salt toxicity due to the excessive amount of sodium contained in the dog food. The high levels of sodium ingested result in increased levels of sodium in the blood. The sodium in the blood passively diffuses into the CSF and brain. The increased sodium in the brain decreases energy-dependent transport mechanisms and anaerobic glycolysis, which normally function to remove the sodium. Increased sodium levels cause passive movement of fluid to equilibrate the electrolyte and fluid levels, thus causing swelling (edema) as well as inflammation.

Treatment. Animals must be treated with sodium-containing fluids, because decreasing the sodium levels too quickly can exacerbate edema in the brain. Prognosis is guarded.

PRACTICE QUESTIONS

1. When treating critically ill patients with intravenous fluids, which two ions are most important to the neuronal membrane potential?
   a. Na^+ and Cl^-
   b. K^+ and Cl^-
   c. Ca^{2+} and Cl^-
   d. K^+ and Ca^{2+}
   e. Na^+ and K^+

2. The energy required by the Na^+, K^+ neural membrane pump is derived from ATP. In the neuron, this energy results from the nearly exclusive metabolism of oxygen and:
   a. Amino acids.
   b. Fatty acids.
   c. Glucose.
   d. Glycogen.
   e. Proteins.

3. If the number of IPSPs on the dendritic membrane decreases while the number of EPSPs remains the same, what will happen to the action potentials on that neuron?
   a. Probability of triggering action potentials increases.
   b. Probability of triggering action potentials decreases.
   c. Probability of triggering action potentials remains unchanged.
   d. Action potentials would be eliminated.
   e. Action potentials would be conducted with increased velocity.

4. During an excitatory postsynaptic potential in a neural membrane, which of the following is the most important ion flow?
   a. Sodium ions diffuse out of the cell.
   b. Sodium ions diffuse into the cell.
   c. Potassium ions diffuse out of the cell.
   d. Potassium ions pumped in by the Na^+, K^+ pump.
   e. None of the above.

5. Choose the *incorrect* statement below:
   a. Conduction velocity of action potentials is slower in myelinated than in unmyelinated axons.
   b. Conduction velocity of action potentials is faster in myelinated than in unmyelinated axons.
   c. In saltatory conduction of action potentials, the action potential seems to jump functionally from node to node (nodes of Ranvier).
   d. Action potentials are of equal magnitude at the beginning and at the end of an axon.

BIBLIOGRAPHY

Bear MF, Connors BW, Paradiso MA: *Neuroscience: exploring the brain*, ed 3, Philadelphia, 2007, Lippincott, Williams & Wilkins.

Brodal P: *The central nervous system: structure and function*, ed 4, New York, 2010, Oxford University Press.

Garrett LD: Insulinomas: a review and what's new. *Proceedings ACVIM* 2003.

Hall JE: *Guyton and Hall textbook of medical physiology*, ed 12, Philadelphia, 2011, Saunders.

Klein BG: Membrane potentials: the generation and conduction of electrical signals in neurons. In Reece WO, editor: *Duke's physiology of domestic animals*, ed 12, Ithaca, NY, 2004, Comstock Publishing.

Smith MO, George LW: Diseases of the nervous system. In Smith BP, editor: *Large animal internal medicine*, ed 4, St. Louis, 2009, Mosby.

CHAPTER 5
The Synapse

KEY POINTS

1. The anatomy of the neuromuscular junction is specialized for one-way synaptic communication.
2. An action potential on the presynaptic neuron triggers an action potential on the muscle cell through the release of acetylcholine.
3. There is greater variety in the specifics of neuron-to-neuron synaptic transmission than in transmission at the neuromuscular junction.

Neurons communicate with each other and with other cells of the body, such as muscle and secretory cells. In Chapter 4 the generation of the action potential and its rapid conduction down the axon to the presynaptic terminal was discussed. Using these processes, the neuron can rapidly notify its presynaptic terminals, often located far from its cell body, to initiate the transfer of information to other cells. Such communication occurs between cells rapidly, and often focally, at specialized junctions called *synapses* (Greek, "junction" or "to bind tightly"). Synaptic transmission between cells can be either electrical or chemical. At *electrical* synapses, ionic current flows directly between presynaptic and postsynaptic cells as the mediator for signal transmission. Although electrical synapses in the mammalian nervous system appear to be more widespread than originally thought, synaptic transmission is more frequently mediated by a *chemical* messenger. Released from the presynaptic terminals on arrival of the action potential, this chemical messenger rapidly diffuses to the postsynaptic cell membrane, where it binds with receptors. This binding initiates a postsynaptic change in function, often generating a postsynaptic potential.

The best-understood chemical synapse is that between a motor neuron and a skeletal muscle cell (fiber): *the neuromuscular synapse,* also known as the *neuromuscular junction* (Figure 5-1). Given the emphasis in Section II of this text on posture and locomotion, this synapse is the focus of this chapter. Synaptic communication at the neuromuscular junction is fundamentally similar to that between neurons, although there is greater variety in the specifics of neuron-to-neuron synaptic transmission, as also discussed.

The Anatomy of the Neuromuscular Junction Is Specialized for One-Way Synaptic Communication

Motor neurons that synapse on skeletal muscles have their cell bodies located within the central nervous system (CNS), either within the spinal cord or the brainstem. The axons of these motor neurons travel within peripheral nerves, out to the muscle, where each motor neuron synapses on several individual fibers (cells) of the muscle. However, an individual skeletal muscle fiber receives synaptic input from, and therefore its contraction is controlled by, only one motor neuron.

The neuromuscular junction, like most chemical synapses, has (1) a *presynaptic* side; (2) a narrow space between the neuron and muscle fiber, called the *synaptic cleft;* and (3) a *postsynaptic* side (see Figure 5-1). The presynaptic side of the synapse is made up of the terminal (transmitting) portion of the motor neuron. This presynaptic terminal has a swelled, buttonlike appearance and is also called a *synaptic bouton.* The terminal (or synaptic bouton) contains a large number of membranous storage vesicles, called *synaptic vesicles,* which contain the chemical neurotransmitter substance, in this case *acetylcholine.* These synaptic vesicles are lined up in rows along the inner surface of the terminal membrane (Figure 5-2). The presynaptic membrane region associated with each double row of vesicles is called an *active zone* and is the site where the synaptic vesicles will eventually release acetylcholine into the synaptic cleft. The presynaptic terminal also contains mitochondria, an indication of active metabolism in the cytoplasm. Some mitochondrial products (e.g., acetyl-CoA, ATP) play a role in the local synthesis of acetylcholine and in its movement into the synaptic vesicles.

The presynaptic (neural) and postsynaptic (muscle) cell membranes are separated by a narrow space, the synaptic cleft, that is about 50 nm wide (see Figures 5-1 and 5-2). The cleft contains extracellular fluid and a basal lamina, composed of a matrix of molecules, that is a specialized region of the muscle basement membrane. Some of these matrix molecules mediate synaptic adhesion between neuron and muscle.

The postsynaptic muscle cell membrane has several specialized features that facilitate synaptic transmission. Directly opposite the face of the presynaptic terminal, the postsynaptic muscle cell membrane contains receptors for the acetylcholine transmitter (see Figures 5-1 and 5-2). In this focal region the membrane has a series of invaginations, called *junctional folds,* that increase the surface area where acetylcholine receptors can reside. The acetylcholine receptors are most densely packed at the mouth of these junctional folds, and these mouths are closely aligned with the active zones of the presynaptic terminals from which the acetylcholine is released. Thus, there is a good match between the focal region of transmitter release from the neuron and the focal location of the receptors on the muscle fiber. Because the neurotransmitter is found only on the presynaptic neural side

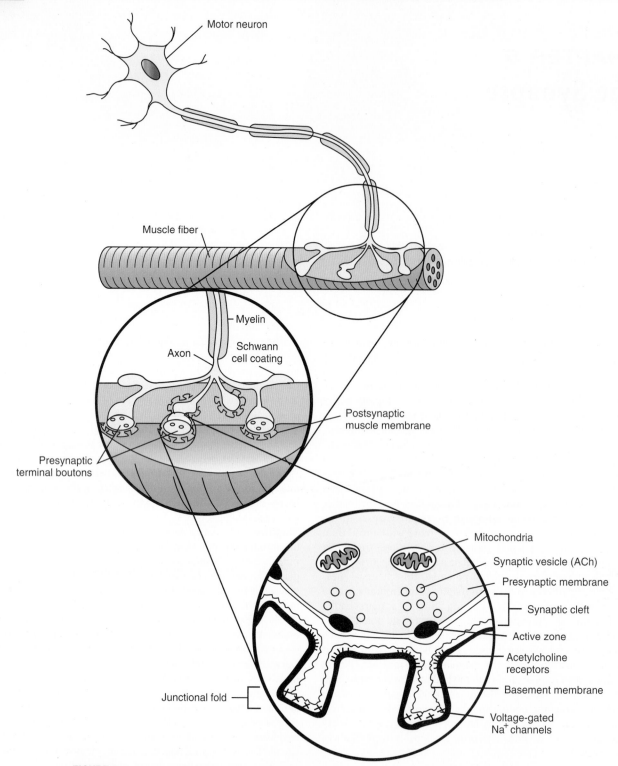

FIGURE 5-1 Synapse between a motor neuron and a skeletal muscle fiber. The neuromuscular junction has a presynaptic (neuronal) side; a narrow space between the neuron and muscle fiber, called the synaptic cleft; and a postsynaptic (muscle) side. *ACh,* Acetylcholine.

of the neuromuscular junction, transmission can go only from neuron to muscle, not in the reverse direction. Also, it should be noted that a motor neuron gives off several presynaptic terminals (synaptic boutons) to an individual muscle fiber. Together, this cluster of terminals is localized to a restricted region of the muscle fiber.

As noted, neurotransmitter signaling across the neuromuscular junction, for purposes of activating muscle fiber contraction, favors the nerve to muscle direction. However, there is some evidence that other types of molecules, in the muscle, may play a role during development in the survival, differentiation, and normal functioning of the presynaptic motor neuron terminals.

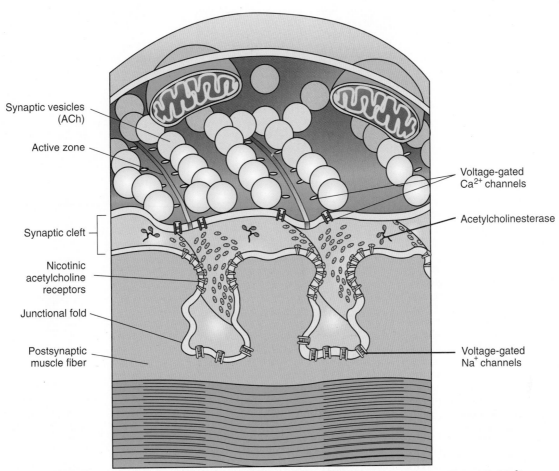

FIGURE 5-2 Presynaptic acetylcholine-filled synaptic vesicles line up at active zones, near voltage-gated Ca²⁺ channels. Released acetylcholine binds with nicotinic acetylcholine receptors at junctional folds on the postsynaptic muscle fiber membrane. (Redrawn and modified from Bear MF, Connors BW, Paradiso MA: *Neuroscience: exploring the brain,* ed 3, Philadelphia, 2007, Lippincott, Williams & Wilkins.)

An Action Potential on the Presynaptic Neuron Triggers an Action Potential on the Muscle Cell Through the Release of Acetylcholine

The function of the neuromuscular junction is to transmit a chemical message unidirectionally between a motor neuron and a skeletal muscle cell (fiber) with a frequency established by the CNS. The arrival of an action potential at the motor neuron terminal triggers the release of the acetylcholine transmitter, which then binds with acetylcholine receptors on the postsynaptic muscle fiber membrane. This leads to the genesis of an action potential along the muscle fiber membrane that ultimately leads to contraction of the fiber.

An action potential on a motor neuron arises at its initial axon segment and then travels along the entire axon, eventually arriving at the presynaptic terminal (see Chapter 4). As previously noted, the exchange of Na⁺ and K⁺ ions, across axonal voltage-gated Na⁺ and K⁺ channels, is responsible for the generation of the action potential and its conduction to the terminal. However, as the action potential arrives at the presynaptic membrane, the wave of depolarization opens voltage-gated Ca²⁺ channels located in this region (see Figure 5-2); as Ca²⁺ flows toward equilibrium across the membrane, the Ca²⁺ enters the presynaptic terminal. This increase in the intracellular Ca²⁺ level is critical for the release of neurotransmitter from the terminal.

Recall that the acetylcholine-containing synaptic vesicles are lined up at the active zones of the presynaptic terminal. They will dock there by the intertwining of binding proteins that respectively reside on the vesicle membrane (synaptobrevin) and on the inner surface of the terminal membrane (syntaxin and SNAP-25) (Figure 5-3). This holds the vesicles near the location of Ca²⁺ entry given that the voltage-gated Ca²⁺ channels are efficiently located in the vicinity of these active zones. When Ca²⁺ flows into the terminal, the ion binds with yet another protein on the synaptic vesicle membrane (synaptotagmin). This triggers fusion of the vesicle with the presynaptic membrane, opening of the vesicle, and release of acetylcholine into the synaptic cleft. After transmitter release, the vesicle membrane is retrieved back into the presynaptic terminal and can be recycled to re-form a vesicle that is then refilled with acetylcholine synthesized in the cytoplasm. Certain bacterial toxins (e.g., botulinum, tetanus) can destroy the binding proteins involved in vesicle docking, ultimately interfering with the ability of the vesicle to release its contents into the synaptic cleft.

After release, acetylcholine then diffuses across the synaptic cleft and binds with transmitter-specific receptors, the *nicotinic acetylcholine receptors,* in the postsynaptic muscle membrane. This specific type of acetylcholine receptor, found at the neuromuscular junction, is so named because it can also bind the

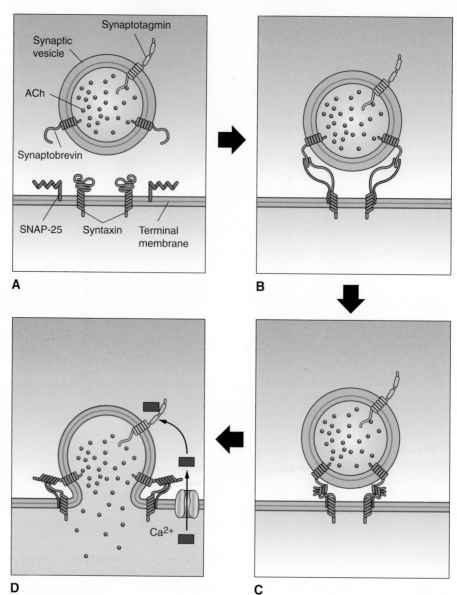

FIGURE 5-3 Release of acetylcholine (ACh) from a synaptic vesicle at the active zone of a motor neuron terminal. **A,** Synaptobrevin is a binding protein on the synaptic vesicle. SNAP-25 and syntaxin are binding proteins at the terminal membrane. Synaptotagmin is a vesicle protein that is a calcium sensor molecule. **B** and **C,** The binding protein on the vesicle intertwines with the binding proteins on the inside of the terminal membrane to dock the vesicle at the terminal membrane. **D,** Depolarization of the terminal membrane, as a result of the action potential, opens voltage-gated Ca^{2+} channels. Ca^{2+} enters the terminal and binds with synaptotagmin. This binding results in fusion of the vesicle and terminal membranes and release of ACh into the synaptic cleft by exocytosis. (Modified from Boron WF, Boulpaep EL: *Medical physiology,* ed 2, Philadelphia, 2009, Saunders.)

alkaloid drug nicotine. There are subtypes of the nicotinic acetylcholine receptor and not all are found on skeletal muscle. Some reside on particular neurons of the central and peripheral nervous systems. The nicotinic acetylcholine receptor is actually a ligand-gated ion channel (see Chapter 1), permeable to small cations, with two binding sites for the acetylcholine molecule. As acetylcholine binds at these two loci, the channel opens and, among other ionic movements, Na^+ ions diffuse into the muscle cell as they attempt to flow toward equilibrium. This contributes to a depolarization of the postsynaptic muscle cell membrane analogous to an excitatory postsynaptic potential (EPSP). However, at the neuromuscular junction, the unitary postsynaptic potential is sufficient to open voltage-gated Na^+ channels deep within the junctional folds and leads to the generation of an action potential on the muscle cell membrane.

Acetylcholine binds with its receptor only briefly (~1 msec). When free, it is destroyed by the enzyme *acetylcholinesterase*. This enzyme, anchored to the basal lamina of the synaptic cleft, inactivates acetylcholine by breaking it down into acetic acid and choline molecules (Figure 5-4). The choline, a precursor of

acetylcholine synthesis, can then be transported back into the presynaptic terminal by a high-affinity transporter protein in the terminal membrane and recycled in acetylcholine synthesis. Chemicals that inhibit acetylcholinesterase, such as some organophosphate insecticides (e.g., malathion, chlorpyrifos) and nerve gases (e.g., sarin), can abnormally prolong the presence of acetylcholine at the synapse, often with disastrous physiological consequences. Because the neurotransmitter is normally destroyed soon after its binding with the muscle membrane receptor, and because more transmitter is not available to attach to the receptors in sufficient quantities until another motor neuron action potential occurs, there is approximately a 1:1 ratio between action potentials on the neuronal and muscle cell membranes.

There Is Greater Variety in the Specifics of Neuron-to-Neuron Synaptic Transmission Than in Transmission at the Neuromuscular Junction

As mentioned earlier, some noteworthy differences exist between synaptic transmission at the neuromuscular junction and neuron-to-neuron synaptic transmission. Although acetylcholine is the

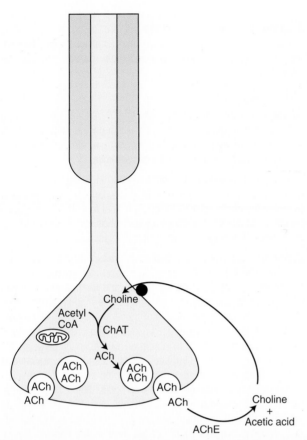

FIGURE 5-4 Synaptic inactivation of acetylcholine *(ACh)*. Released ACh is enzymatically broken down into choline and acetic acid by synaptic acetylcholinesterase. The choline is actively transported back into the terminal and can be reused in ACh synthesis. *ChAT,* Choline acetyltransferase.

BOX 5-1 Members of the Major Neurotransmitter Classes

Amino Acids
Glutamate
Glycine
γ-Aminobutyric acid (GABA)

Amines
Acetylcholine
Serotonin
Histamine

Catecholamines
Dopamine
Norepinephrine
Epinephrine

Peptides*
Substance P
Vasopressin
Somatostatin

Opioids
Leu-enkephalin
Met-enkephalin
β-Endorphin

Purines
Adenosine
Adenosine triphosphate (ATP)

Atypical (Nontraditional)
Gases
Nitric oxide
Carbon monoxide

Endogenous Cannabinoids (Endocannabinoids)
Anandamide
2-Arachidonylglycerol

*Only a partial list of peptide neurotransmitters.

neurotransmitter responsible for the primary postsynaptic effect at the neuromuscular junction, a variety of neurotransmitters, in addition to acetylcholine, can be used to produce the principal postsynaptic effect at neuron-to-neuron synapses (Box 5-1). Furthermore, not all of these transmitters are released from morphologically distinct active zones, although their release from the terminal still appears to depend on Ca^{2+} influx. In such cases, release from the terminal may not always occur directly at the synaptic cleft, resulting in a wider postsynaptic distribution of transmitter. Interestingly, some molecules that are sometimes called *atypical* or *nontraditional neurotransmitters* (e.g., endocannabinoids, nitric oxide) are actually produced in a postsynaptic neuron following traditional synaptic transmission, but then diffuse back across the synaptic cleft to affect the function of the presynaptic terminal. Therefore, neuron-to-neuron communication may not be as specialized for one-way communication as the neuromuscular junction.

The postsynaptic membrane of a neuron-to-neuron synapse can be the soma, dendrites, or even the terminals of the postsynaptic neuron, and junctional folds are not seen at these synapses. However, the dendritic postsynaptic membrane often possesses small protrusions called *dendritic spines* (see Chapter 4). As with the junctional folds on muscle cells, these spines increase the surface area of the postsynaptic membrane and, because of their narrow necks, are thought to provide a means for biochemical isolation between nearby synapses. Further, spines can change size and shape over an animal's lifetime, modulating the functional effectiveness of the synapse. It is therefore thought that spines may play a role in learning and memory. Whereas transmitter release at the neuromuscular junction always produces postsynaptic excitation (membrane depolarization), release at synapses between neurons can produce excitation or inhibition (membrane hyperpolarization). However, synapses on dendritic spines are almost always excitatory.

At the neuromuscular junction, the postsynaptic receptor is almost exclusively the nicotinic acetylcholine receptor, a ligand-gated ion channel. At synapses between neurons, a much greater variety of receptors is available. These may differ from the nicotinic acetylcholine receptor with respect not only to the binding transmitter, but to the receptor mechanism as well (e.g., G-protein coupled; see Chapter 1). Also, several different types of neurotransmitter receptor are often found on a single neuron.

When transmitters other than acetylcholine are employed at neuron-to-neuron synapses, depending on the transmitter, the termination of action of that transmitter may be accomplished by (1) transporter-mediated reuptake of the transmitter itself into the terminal of release or (2) a less specific and somewhat slower form of enzymatic degradation than with acetylcholinesterase. In addition, although simple diffusion of neurotransmitter away from the synapse contributes to the termination of action of most neurotransmitters to some degree, this mode may play a more important role for some neurotransmitters than others. Finally, at neuron-to-neuron synapses, a single action potential on a presynaptic neuron rarely results in a full-blown action potential on the postsynaptic neuron. Some form of summation of presynaptic inputs is required to generate a postsynaptic action potential.

As discussed in Chapter 6, action potentials on the muscle cell membrane lead to contraction, or mechanical shortening, of the muscle cell. When this contraction is combined with the shortening of many muscle cells, movement of the body occurs.

CLINICAL CORRELATIONS

MYASTHENIA GRAVIS

History. You examine a 5-year-old female German shepherd whose owner states that the dog becomes progressively weaker with exercise. The owner also states that recently, just after eating, the dog has begun to vomit food in formed, cylinder-shaped boluses.

Clinical Examination. All abnormalities found on physical examination were referable to the neuromuscular system. After resting, the dog's neurological examination findings were within normal limits. With even moderate exercise, however, the dog became progressively weaker, particularly in the front legs. Intravenous injection of an acetylcholinesterase inhibitor, edrophonium (Tensilon), eliminated all clinical signs of weakness. Radiographs of the chest revealed an enlarged esophagus and thymus.

Comment. The history of an enlarged esophagus (megaesophagus) and the response to an acetylcholinesterase inhibitor confirm the diagnosis of *myasthenia gravis* (grave muscle weakness). This is caused by a failure of transmission of acetylcholine at the neuromuscular synapse. This transmission failure is caused by antibodies produced by the body against its own acetylcholine receptors. The abnormal antibodies bind with the receptors to form complexes, which prevent acetylcholine from binding to the acetylcholine receptors. As a result, no depolarization occurs on the postsynaptic membrane of the cells. Antibodies also alter the junctional folds and number of acetylcholine receptors available to bind with the transmitter. Acetylcholinesterase inhibitors prevent the metabolism of acetylcholine, allowing acetylcholine to remain longer at the synapse, with additional time for binding to the receptors, and thus facilitating normal transmission.

The large amount of skeletal muscle in the dog's esophagus explains its enlargement from paralysis. These patients often regurgitate formed boluses of food shortly after eating.

Myasthenia gravis can be associated with mediastinal masses, usually of the thymus. The autoantibodies that the body makes are often against antigens from the thymus or acetylcholine receptors. In addition to this cause of myasthenia gravis, idiopathic myasthenia gravis is also common.

Treatment. Spontaneous remissions are common, depending on the cause. Until then, oral daily acetylcholinesterase inhibitors are given. Surgical removal of mediastinal masses may also be necessary.

TETANUS

History. A client calls you because their 6-year-old quarter horse gelding stepped on a nail a few days ago on the right front foot. They pulled the nail out, and soaked the foot, but now the horse seems depressed and does not want to move.

Clinical Examination. The horse has an increased temperature (fever) with increased heart rate (tachycardic), and increased pulses of the digital arteries to the right front foot. The leg is warm, swollen, and painful. The horse appears to be very sensitive to any stimulation. The horse is overdue for his vaccinations.

Comment. Exposure to *Clostridium tetani* can occur through cuts/wounds. The bacterium has a neurotoxin, tetanospasmin, that blocks the synaptic release of glycine and gamma-aminobutyric acid (GABA) by cleaving the synaptic vesicle binding protein synaptobrevin. Blocking the release of these transmitters, which normally have an inhibitory effect on motor neurons that innervate skeletal muscles, results in abnormal excitation of these motor neurons. This results in continued muscle stimulation, manifested as hypertonia and muscle spasms. Affected animals can develop a stiff head and neck as well as stiff gait. When they become recumbent, they can develop a sawhorse posture. Muscle spasms are easily elicited, including jaw and lip rigidity, as well as retraction of the eye with presence of the third eyelid. The respiratory muscles are often affected. Because these muscles do not function properly, animals can develop aspiration pneumonia and hypoxia, which are often the cause of death.

Treatment. Treatment is difficult when horses develop clinical signs. They can be given antitoxin to help bind toxin still present. In some situations, horses are also vaccinated against tetanus to help stimulate an antibody response. Horses are placed on antibiotics to kill the *Clostridium*. Additionally, because they are very sensitive to stimulation, horses are placed in a quiet environment and often require sedation. Prognosis is poor in affected animals with approximately 80% mortality.

PRACTICE QUESTIONS

1. At the neuromuscular junction, Ca^{2+} ions are necessary for:
   a. Binding the transmitter with the postsynaptic receptor.
   b. Facilitating diffusion of the transmitter to the postsynaptic membrane.
   c. Splitting the transmitter in the cleft, thus deactivating the transmitter.
   d. Fusing the presynaptic vesicle with the presynaptic membrane, thus releasing the transmitter.
   e. Metabolizing the transmitter within the presynaptic vesicle.

2. A drug that would prevent the release of acetylcholine at the neuromuscular junction would cause what, if any, clinical signs?
   a. Convulsions and excess muscle contractions
   b. Paralysis
   c. No effect on an animal's movement

3. Which one of the following is *true* with regard to the termination of synaptic action at the neuromuscular junction?
   a. The reuptake of intact acetylcholine molecules into the motor neuron terminal is responsible.
   b. Diffusion of acetylcholine away from the synapse is solely responsible.
   c. Acetylcholinesterase rapidly breaks down acetylcholine into choline and acetate.
   d. Dissociation of acetylcholine from the muscarinic receptor, after binding for several seconds, is solely responsible.

4. Several antagonist drugs compete with acetylcholine for the postsynaptic receptor at the neuromuscular junction. If you overdosed your patient with one of these competitive drugs, what would the antidote need to do at the synapse?
   a. Decrease the release of acetylcholine.
   b. Decrease the effectiveness of acetylcholinesterase.
   c. Decrease the influx of Ca^{2+} into the motor neuron terminal.
   d. Decrease the action potential frequency on the motor neuron.
   e. None of the above.

5. Which of the following statements regarding neuron-to-neuron synapses is *false*?
   a. The postsynaptic membrane is always a dendrite.
   b. Dendritic spines increase the surface area of the postsynaptic membrane.
   c. A single action potential on a presynaptic neuron is usually not sufficient to produce an action potential on a postsynaptic neuron.
   d. The neurotransmitter is not always released from a morphologically distinct active zone of the presynaptic terminal.
   e. Depending on the presynaptic neurotransmitter released and the postsynaptic receptor activated, the postsynaptic membrane can be either depolarized or hyperpolarized.

BIBLIOGRAPHY

Bear MF, Connors BW, Paradiso MA: *Neuroscience: exploring the brain*, ed 3, Philadelphia, 2007, Lippincott, Williams & Wilkins.

Boron WF, Boulpaep EL: *Medical physiology*, ed 2, Philadelphia, 2009, Saunders.

Brodal P: *The central nervous system: structure and function*, ed 4, New York, 2010, Oxford University Press.

Hall JE: *Guyton and Hall textbook of medical physiology*, ed 12, Philadelphia, 2011, Saunders.

Hall ZW, Sanes JR: Synaptic structure and development: the neuromuscular junction, *Cell* 72(suppl):99–121, 1993.

Hughes BW, Kusner LL, Kaminski HJ: Molecular architecture of the neuromuscular junction, *Muscle Nerve* 33(4):445–461, 2006.

Klein BG: Synaptic transmission and the neurotransmitter life cycle. In Reece WO, editor: *Duke's physiology of domestic animals*, ed 12, Ithaca, NY, 2004, Comstock Publishing.

Li XM, Dong XP, Luo SW: Retrograde regulation of motoneuron differentiation by muscle beta-catenin, *Nat Neurosci* 11(3):262–268, 2008.

Meyer JS, Quenzer LF: *Psychopharmacology: drugs, the brain, and behavior*, Sunderland, Mass, 2005, Sinauer.

Nestler EJ, Hyman SE, Malenka RC: *Molecular neuropharmacology: a foundation for clinical neuroscience*, ed 2, New York, 2009, McGraw-Hill.

Smith MO, George LW: Diseases of the nervous system. In Smith BP, editor: *Large animal internal medicine*, ed 4, St Louis, 2009, Mosby Elsevier.

CHAPTER 6
The Physiology of Muscle

KEY POINTS

1. Body movement is the result of contraction of skeletal muscle across a movable joint.
2. There are several levels of organization in any skeletal muscle.
3. Action potentials on the sarcolemma spread to the interior of the cell along the transverse tubules.
4. The action potential on the sarcolemma is indirectly coupled to the contraction mechanism through the release of Ca^{2+} from the sarcoplasmic reticulum.
5. The sliding of actin along the myosin molecule results in physical shortening of the sarcomere.

6. Most skeletal muscle fibers can be classified as either fast-contracting or slow-contracting fibers.
7. Muscles change their strength of contraction by varying the number of active motor units or the rate of motor unit activation.
8. The electromyogram is the clinical measurement of the electrical behavior within a skeletal muscle.
9. The structure of cardiac and smooth muscle differs from that of skeletal muscle.
10. The role of Ca^{2+} ions in excitation-contraction coupling in cardiac and smooth muscle is different than in skeletal muscle.

There are three types of muscle in the body: skeletal, cardiac, and smooth muscle. Skeletal muscle makes up about 40% of the body, and smooth muscle and cardiac muscle make up almost 10% more. Because most veterinary patients with disease of the neuromuscular system exhibit abnormalities of movement, it is important to understand how skeletal muscle functions and how it is controlled by the nervous system. Abnormalities of cardiac muscle and smooth muscle feature prominently in many other clinical disorders (e.g., dilated cardiomyopathy, hypertension, detrusor hypertrophy), and such muscle is often the target of pharmacological clinical intervention (e.g., sympathomimetic drugs, adrenergic receptor antagonists).

This chapter explains the physiology of skeletal muscle and includes brief comparisons with cardiac and smooth muscle. Cardiac muscle is discussed more extensively in Section III chapters, and the role of smooth muscle in other body systems is mentioned throughout this book.

Body Movement Is the Result of Contraction of Skeletal Muscle Across a Movable Joint

Skeletal muscle consists of a central, fleshy, contractile muscle "belly" and two tendons, one on each end of the muscle. The muscle and its tendons are arranged in the body so that they originate on one bone and insert on a different bone while spanning a joint. As the muscle contracts, shortening the distance between the origin and insertion tendons, the bones move in relation to each other, bending at the joint (Figure 6-1). When activated by a motor nerve, a skeletal muscle can only shorten. Most joints have one or more muscles on both sides, either to decrease its angle (*flexion*) or to increase its angle (*extension*).

Body movement performed by an animal is the result of contraction of skeletal muscle across a movable joint. It is therefore important to understand the anatomy and physiology of skeletal muscle before discussing how the nervous system choreographs

the contraction of groups of muscle cells to perform an impressive array of body movements.

There Are Several Levels of Organization in Any Skeletal Muscle

Figure 6-2 illustrates the levels of organization in a typical skeletal muscle. Each muscle belly seen during dissection is made up of differing numbers of muscle cells (usually called *muscle fibers*) that span the several inches between the origin and insertion tendons. The fibers range between 5 and 100 µm in diameter and contain multiple nuclei, multiple mitochondria, and other intracellular organelles. The outer limiting membrane of the fiber is called the *sarcolemma*. It consists of a true cell membrane, called the *plasma membrane,* and an outer polysaccharide layer that attaches to the tendons at the cells' extremities. Each muscle fiber is innervated by only one motor neuron, with the neuromuscular junction region located near the middle of the fiber, relative to the ends.

Each muscle fiber is made up of successively smaller subunits (see Figure 6-2). Each fiber contains several hundred to several thousand *myofibrils* arranged in parallel along its length, like a handful of spaghetti. Each myofibril is made up of a linear series of repeating *sarcomeres,* the basic contractile units of the muscle fiber, which can number in the tens of thousands.

The sarcomere has a disk at each end called the *Z disk.* The sarcomere contains several types of large protein molecules responsible for muscular contraction, many of which are polymerized. Numerous thin protein filaments, called *actin,* are attached to the Z disks and extend toward the center of the sarcomere, similar to parallel fingers pointing at each other. Each actin filament consists of two intertwined, helical strands of actin protein and two such strands of *tropomyosin* protein, all wound together as a larger helical complex (see Chapter 1 and Figure 1-5). Also located intermittently along the tropomyosin-actin

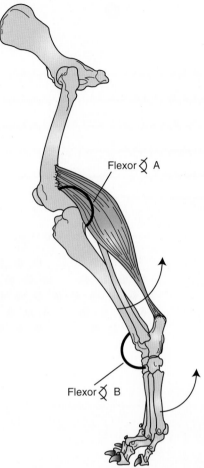

FIGURE 6-1 Body movement is the result of contraction (shortening) of a skeletal muscle attached across a movable joint. Contraction of the muscle will decrease the flexor angle at joint *A* (the stifle joint) and increase the flexor angle at joint *B* (the tarsal joint). This will produce the respective movements about the joints indicated by the *arrows.*

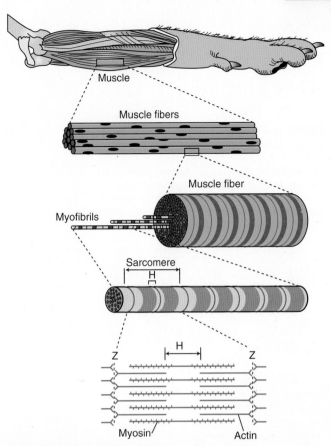

FIGURE 6-2 A typical skeletal muscle has several levels of organization. *H* and *Z* are letters assigned to stripes seen during microscopic examination of skeletal muscle.

strand are complex globular protein molecules called *troponin* that can bind tropomyosin and actin and that have an affinity for calcium (Ca^{2+}) ions. Suspended between and parallel to the actin thin filaments are thicker filaments of *myosin* protein polymers (Figure 6-3). A myosin molecule contains a tail of intertwined helices and two globular heads that can bind both adenosine triphosphate (ATP) and actin (see Figures 1-3 and 1-4). Approximately 500 myosin heads of a thick myosin filament form cross-bridges that interact with actin to shorten the sarcomere as the myosin heads flex and relax. The sarcomere also contains a large protein, *titin*, that helps to maintain the side-by-side relationship of actin and myosin, as well as the resting length during relaxation.

Beneath the plasma membrane of the muscle cell lies the *sarcoplasmic reticulum,* an intracellular storage organelle that forms a reticulated network around the myofibrils (Figure 6-4). This extensive storage sac sequesters Ca^{2+} ions in relaxed muscle and is analogous to the smooth endoplasmic reticulum in other cells.

Located perpendicular to the long axis of the muscle fiber are tubes of plasma membrane formed by periodic invaginations of the sarcolemma (see Figure 6-4). These *transverse tubules,* or *T tubules,* traverse the diameter of the muscle fiber, similar to a flexible drinking straw passing perpendicularly through the

handful of spaghetti (myofibrils) noted earlier. The T tubules snake around the myofibrils, forming junctions with the network of sarcoplasmic reticulum that surrounds the myofibrils (Figure 6-5). These tubules are filled with extracellular fluid and are important because they allow the electrically excitable plasma membrane of the muscle fiber to carry the depolarization of the action potential to the interior of the fiber.

Action Potentials on the Sarcolemma Spread to the Interior of the Cell Along the Transverse Tubules

Skeletal muscle cells have a resting membrane potential, as do neurons, and the muscle cell membrane can be depolarized by synaptic transmission at the neuromuscular junction (see Chapter 5). At this junction, the acetylcholine released by the motor neuron activates nicotinic acetylcholine receptors on the sarcolemma of the muscle cell. The resulting depolarization is sufficient to open enough voltage-gated sodium (Na^+) ion channels, also found at the junctional sarcolemma (see Figure 5-1), to trigger a muscle fiber action potential. Thus, it is at the sarcolemma of the neuromuscular junction that muscle fiber action potentials are generated.

When an action potential is generated near the midpoint of the muscle fiber, it spreads in both directions along the length of the fiber by mechanisms similar to action potential spread in unmyelinated neuronal axons. In contrast to those on axons, however, action potentials on the sarcolemma are also transmitted to the interior of the muscle fiber along the T tubules (see Figure 6-5). This allows the action potential to reach the location

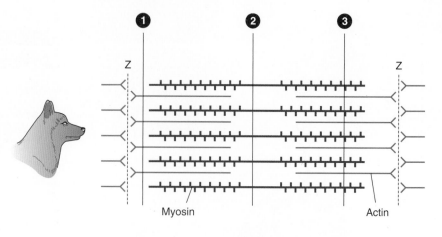

FIGURE 6-3 Parallel arrangement of actin and myosin filaments in a sarcomere. *Top,* The viewer is looking at one end of a sarcomere. *Bottom,* The view of filament organization respectively seen by the observer at each of the three transverse sectioning points indicated in the top part of the figure. (Modified from Boron WF, Boulpaep EL: *Medical physiology,* ed 2, Philadelphia, 2009, Saunders.)

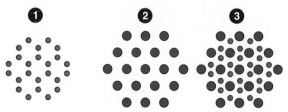

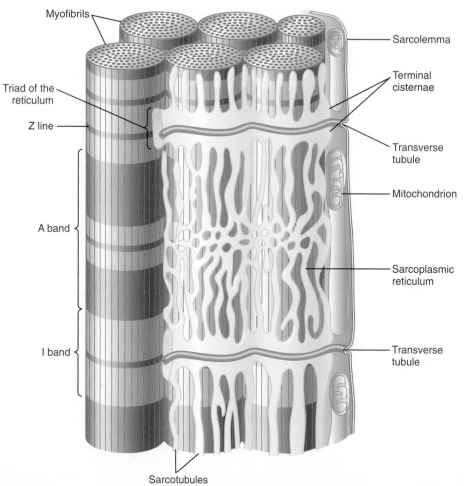

FIGURE 6-4 Diagram of skeletal muscle showing the juxtaposition of myofibrils, transverse (T) tubules, and sarcoplasmic reticula. (Redrawn from Bloom W, Fawcett DW: *A textbook of histology,* Philadelphia, 1986, WB Saunders. Modified after Peachey LD: *J Cell Biol* 25:209, 1965. Drawn by Sylvia Colard Keene. In Guyton AC, Hall JE: *Textbook of medical physiology,* ed 11, Philadelphia, 2006, Saunders.)

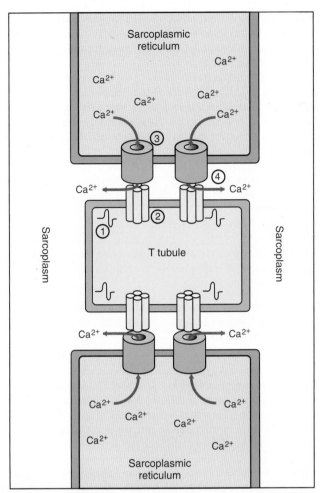

FIGURE 6-5 Relationship between the T tubules (TT) and sarcoplasmic reticulum (SR) during excitation-contraction coupling. *1,* Propagation of action potential produces depolarization of the TT membrane. *2,* Depolarization induces opening of voltage-gated Ca^{2+} channel aggregates in the TT membrane. *3,* Opening of Ca^{2+} release channels on the SR membrane results from mechanical coupling with opening of voltage-gated Ca^{2+} channels on the TT. *4,* Ca^{2+} is released from the SR into the sarcoplasm, where it can bathe the sarcomeres *(not shown)* to induce contraction. (Modified from Boron WF, Boulpaep EL: *Medical physiology: a cellular and molecular approach,* updated edition, Philadelphia, 2005, Saunders.)

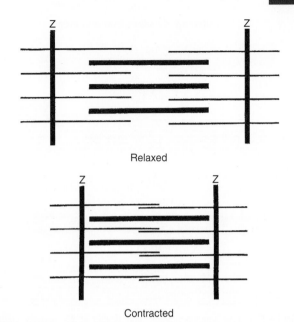

FIGURE 6-6 Sliding of actin along the myosin molecule results in the physical shortening (contraction) of the sarcomere.

of the sarcoplasmic reticulum even in the innermost regions of the muscle fiber. The consequences of the action potential's arrival at the location of the sarcoplasmic reticulum are critical for the coupling of excitation (the action potential) with contraction (shortening) of the sarcomeres of the myofibrils.

The Action Potential on the Sarcolemma Is Indirectly Coupled to the Contraction Mechanism Through the Release of Ca^{2+} from the Sarcoplasmic Reticulum

Whereas in the neuron a rise in cytoplasmic Ca^{2+} at the terminal is critical for initiating the process of transmitter release, a rise in Ca^{2+} in the muscle cell sarcoplasm (cytoplasm of a muscle cell) is critical for initiating *contraction*. At rest, Ca^{2+} ions are pumped out of the sarcoplasm and stored in the sarcoplasmic reticulum using an energy-dependent pump in conjunction with Ca^{2+} binding proteins within the sarcoplasmic reticulum. This leaves too low a concentration of Ca^{2+} in the sarcoplasm to trigger contraction. However, as an action potential spreads along the muscle

fiber surface and into the fiber's core along the T tubules, the depolarization arrives at the junction between the tubules and the sarcoplasmic reticulum (see Figure 6-5). The arrival of the action potential at this junction leads to the release of stored Ca^{2+} ions from the sarcoplasmic reticulum. These Ca^{2+} ions diffuse down their concentration gradient into the sarcoplasm, bathe the sarcomere, then trigger contraction. As the action potential passes, Ca^{2+} is pumped again into the sarcoplasmic reticulum, and relaxation results. This cycle of events is known as *excitation-contraction coupling.*

The link between the action potential on the transverse tubule and Ca^{2+} release from the sarcoplasmic reticulum is mediated by voltage-gated Ca^{2+} channels on the T tubule and Ca^{2+}-induced Ca^{2+} release channels on the sarcoplasmic reticulum (see Figure 6-5). In skeletal muscle a mechanical coupling of these two types of channels is thought to exist; action potential opening of the voltage-gated Ca^{2+} channels of the T tubule produces a direct configurational change in the Ca^{2+}-induced Ca^{2+} release channels on the sarcoplasmic reticulum, allowing the stored Ca^{2+} ions to escape from the sarcoplasmic reticulum into the sarcoplasm. The movement of Ca^{2+} through the opened voltage-gated Ca^{2+} channels on the T tubule, and the Ca^{2+} sensitivity of the Ca^{2+}-induced Ca^{2+} release channels plays a more important role in excitation-contraction coupling in cardiac muscle than in skeletal muscle (see later discussion).

The Sliding of Actin Along the Myosin Molecule Results in Physical Shortening of the Sarcomere

Figure 6-6 illustrates the sarcomere in the relaxed state and in its shorter, contracted state. The sarcomere is changed from its relaxed state to the shorter, contracted state when Ca^{2+} ions become available to the sarcomere. In the presence of Ca^{2+} ions and a sufficient source of ATP, the actin thin filaments are pulled in parallel along the myosin thick filaments by the repetitive movement of the myosin molecule heads, thus shortening the sarcomere. Because each myofibril is made up of a linear series of repeating and connected sarcomeres, the net result is the

Resting, detached conformation

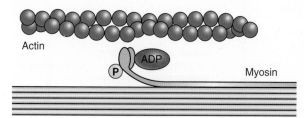

Actin

ADP

P

Myosin

Bound, power-stroke conformation

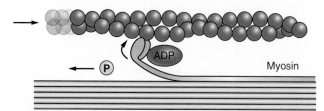

ADP

P

Myosin

FIGURE 6-7 Actin-myosin binding, and flexing of the myosin heads, slides actin along the myosin filaments. *Top,* ATP bound to the myosin head has been hydrolyzed to ADP and inorganic phosphate *(P).* In this state the myosin head is at rest and detached from actin. *Bottom,* The resting myosin head has bound to actin, forming a cross bridge. The dissociation of P from the myosin head induces flexing of the head, pulling the actin filament along the myosin. This has been called the *power-stroke.* (Redrawn from Boron WF, Boulpaep EL: *Medical physiology,* ed 2, Philadelphia, 2009, Saunders.)

physical shortening of the distance between the two ends of the muscle. A more detailed molecular explanation of this sliding filament mechanism of sarcomere shortening is provided in Chapter 1 as an example of the binding specificity and allosteric interactions of proteins. However, the events can be briefly summarized as follows.

At several points along the actin thin filament, there are sites that can bind with the head of the myosin molecule (see Figures 1-4 and 1-5, and accompanying Chapter 1 text). In the absence of Ca^{2+} ions, these sites are either inhibited or covered by the tropomyosin molecules that are normally interwoven within the actin helix. When Ca^{2+} is present and binds with troponin, a regulatory molecule attached to tropomyosin, the troponin molecule undergoes a configurational change. It is thought that this then causes the tropomyosin molecule to move away from and uncover the myosin-binding site on the actin thin filament, permitting actin-myosin binding. Through a cycle that includes binding with and hydrolysis of ATP (to ADP + phosphate), and subsequent dissociation of phosphate, the myosin heads alternately relax and flex while respectively detaching and attaching to the exposed binding sites on the actin thin filament (Figure 6-7). This results in the actin thin filaments sliding in parallel along the myosin thick filaments to shorten the sarcomere (see Figure 6-6). In the absence of Ca^{2+}, the myosin-binding sites on actin again become blocked, and sarcomere relaxation results.

Most Skeletal Muscle Fibers Can Be Classified as Either Fast-Contracting or Slow-Contracting Fibers

Skeletal muscle fibers with short contraction times are sometimes called *fast-twitch fibers.* They tend to be thicker, have extensive sarcoplasmic reticulum for rapid release of Ca^{2+} ions, and have

less extensive blood and mitochondrial supplies because aerobic metabolism is less important. Fast-twitch fibers are fairly rapidly fatigued but are well adapted for jumping, sprinting, and other brief, powerful movements.

In contrast, *slow-twitch fibers* are thinner muscle fibers, have a rich blood and mitochondrial supply, and have a large amount of myoglobin, an iron-containing and oxygen-storing protein similar to hemoglobin. These fibers rely more heavily on oxidative metabolism, are less amenable to fatigue, and are better adapted for the continual contraction of antigravity extensor muscles.

Because slow-twitch fibers have more myoglobin, they are sometimes called *red muscle;* fast-twitch fibers are sometimes called *white muscle.* A third type of fiber, a subclass of fast-twitch fibers, has properties between the two types. Usually, a muscle belly is made up of a blend of these three types, the proportions varying in accordance with the muscle's use. This blend can be changed somewhat with exercise, such as in an athlete training for a different type of sports event.

Muscles Change Their Strength of Contraction by Varying the Number of Active Motor Units or the Rate of Motor Unit Activation

Even though each muscle fiber is innervated by only one neuron, each motor neuron's axon branches as it reaches the muscle and innervates several muscle fibers. A *motor unit* is defined as one alpha (α) motor neuron and all the *extrafusal* (force-generating, striated) muscle fibers that it innervates (Figure 6-8, *A*). All the muscle fibers of each motor unit are of the same functional type (e.g., fast or slow twitch), and an action potential on the motor neuron causes all the muscle fibers to contract simultaneously. In motor units a relationship exists among the functional type of muscle fiber innervated, the number of muscle fibers innervated, and motor neuron size. Small motor units tend to be made up of a motor neuron with a small cell body and a narrow, slower-conducting axon that innervates a small number of slow-twitch fibers. Large motor units have a motor neuron with a large cell body and a faster-conducting, wide axon innervating a large number of fast-twitch fibers. Activation of a small motor unit produces a smaller, slower, less fatiguable increment of contractile force in the muscle compared with a larger motor unit. The neuronal cell bodies of all the motor units from a single muscle form a cluster within the central nervous system (CNS) called the *motor neuron pool* of that muscle (see Figure 6-8, *B*). Within the motor neuron pool for a given muscle, there is a range of motor unit sizes. Muscles with a larger proportion of smaller motor units tend to be amenable to finer control of contractile force.

Although an action potential on a motor neuron produces a simultaneous, brief twitch in all the muscle fibers of the motor unit, the pattern of excitation of the units originating from within the CNS produces the smooth, graded contraction of which most muscles are capable. The CNS can instruct a muscle to contract with greater force primarily by increasing the number of motor units that contract at any one time; this is called *recruitment* or *spatial summation.* The force of contraction can also be increased by increasing the frequency of activation of a motor unit, in which a subsequent twitch begins before relaxation of the previous twitch; this is called *temporal summation.* The recruitment of motor units to increase contractile force occurs in an orderly manner, according to motor unit size, with the smaller units

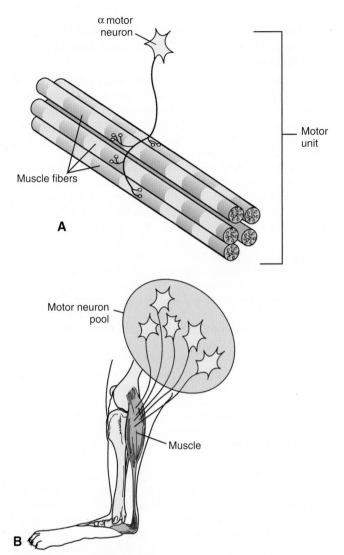

α motor
neuron

Motor
unit

Muscle fibers

A

Motor neuron
pool

Muscle

B

FIGURE 6-8 Innervation of skeletal muscle by α motor neurons of central nervous system (CNS). **A,** A motor unit is an α motor neuron and all the skeletal muscle fibers it innervates. **B,** Neuronal cell bodies of all the motor units from a single muscle form a cluster within the CNS called the *motor neuron pool* of that muscle. (Redrawn from Bear MF, Connors BW, Paradiso MA: *Neuroscience: exploring the brain,* ed 3, Philadelphia, 2007, Lippincott, Williams & Wilkins.)

activated first. This results in force being increased gradually in small, more precise amounts when the muscle force required is low. As the force required increases, faster and larger increases in contractile force are progressively added by orderly activation of the larger motor units. This produces an overall smoothness of contraction, keeping the movement as precise as possible until larger, grosser increments are needed, usually when significant tension has already been generated in the muscle.

In some skeletal muscles the CNS can command some percentage of motor units to be active for extensive periods (various motor units take turns), thus continually shortening the distance between the origin and insertion tendon. When contraction of a whole muscle belly occurs without relaxation, the muscle is said to be in *tetany*. Tetanization of cardiac muscle would be fatal, because heart muscle must relax to allow cardiac filling before it

contracts to pump out the blood. Chapter 19 discusses how cardiac muscle prevents tetany.

The Electromyogram Is the Clinical Measurement of the Electrical Behavior Within a Skeletal Muscle

As an action potential spreads along a muscle fiber, a small portion of the electrical current generated spreads away from the fiber, even to the overlying skin. Electrodes placed on the skin or inserted into the muscle belly can record a summated electrical potential when the muscle contracts. Such a measurement, when visually displayed, is called an *electromyogram* (EMG) and is for skeletal muscle what the electrocardiogram (ECG) is for cardiac muscle. The EMG, often used in conjunction with nerve conduction analysis, helps to determine whether weakness or paralysis is caused by disease in the skeletal muscle, neuromuscular junction, motor neuron, or CNS.

The Structure of Cardiac and Smooth Muscle Differs from That of Skeletal Muscle

As with skeletal muscle, *cardiac muscle* is striated and contains sarcoplasmic reticulum and myofibrils; the fundamental contractile component is formed by actin and myosin subunits (see Figure 19-1). Cardiac muscle also contains transverse tubules, but cardiac muscle differs from skeletal muscle in some important ways. The long skeletal muscle fibers are electrically isolated from each other, whereas the shorter cardiac muscle cells are electrically coupled to each other through end-to-end *intercalated disks* that contain gap junctions. Because gap junctions provide continuity between the cytoplasm of adjacent cells, action potentials can spread from one cardiac muscle cell to another, across these intercalated disks, without the need for chemical neurotransmission to each cell. The cardiac muscle cells can also possess branchlike extensions that form similar connections with some of their parallel neighbors. In fact, as explained in Chapter 19, action potentials arise spontaneously in specialized cardiac muscle cells and then spread throughout a large population of cardiac muscle cells as if they were a functional syncytium. This can result in coordinated contraction of a large region of the heart muscle. The frequency of such action potentials and the force of the resulting contraction are influenced by the autonomic nervous system, but such innervation is not necessary for action potential genesis.

Smooth muscle cells, as with cardiac myocytes, are smaller and shorter than skeletal muscle cells. They do not contain T tubules, and their sarcoplasmic reticulum is poorly developed (Figure 6-9). These cells rely primarily on the transmembrane diffusion of Ca^{2+} ions from the extracellular fluid to induce the actin-myosin interactions responsible for contraction (see following discussion). Although overlapping actin and myosin molecules form the contractile units of smooth muscle cells, the arrangement of these units lacks the structural regularity responsible for the striated appearance of skeletal and cardiac muscle cells. Actin filaments are anchored to *dense bodies* (instead of Z disks), which are found within the cytoplasm as well as in the cell membrane. Therefore, these cells can appear to wrinkle on contraction.

Some smooth muscle cell tissues, usually called *visceral* or *unitary smooth muscle,* have gap junctions between cells and operate similar to a functional syncytium, with cell-to-cell action potential transmission, and coordinated contraction, much as in cardiac muscle. Visceral smooth muscle is abundant in the gastrointestinal tract and other organs of the thoracic and abdominal

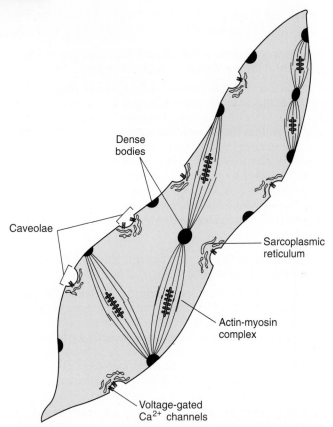

Dense bodies

Caveolae

Sarcoplasmic reticulum

Actin-myosin complex

Voltage-gated Ca²⁺ channels

FIGURE 6-9 General organization of a smooth muscle cell. T tubules are absent, and the sarcoplasmic reticulum is poorly developed. Transmembrane diffusion of extracellular Ca^{2+}, through voltage-gated Ca^{2+} channels in caveolae, plays an important role in initiating contraction. Actin and myosin are present, with actin anchored to dense bodies. Activating the actin-myosin complex can change the cell's shape. (Modified from Guyton AC, Hall JE: *Textbook of medical physiology,* ed 11, Philadelphia, 2006, Saunders.)

cavities. This type of smooth muscle is described more fully in Chapter 28. Another type of smooth muscle cell tissue, usually called *multiunit smooth muscle,* has electrically isolated muscle cells that are capable of contracting independently of each other. Multiunit smooth muscle can be found, for example, in the iris and ciliary body of the eye, where precise control of muscular contraction is needed.

Smooth muscle tissue is innervated by neurons of the autonomic nervous system. In contrast to neuromuscular junctions at skeletal muscle, either acetylcholine or norepinephrine can be released (by different neurons) at junctions with smooth muscle, smooth muscle cells can be either excited or inhibited by their presynaptic input, and a single smooth muscle cell can receive presynaptic input from more than one neuron. Visceral smooth muscle tends to receive a more diffuse innervation from an autonomic neuron, and the neurotransmitter is released at greater distance from the smooth muscle cell, compared with a more focal skeletal neuromuscular junction. In multiunit smooth muscle, it is more common to find synaptic input onto each cell and a synaptic cleft width similar to a skeletal neuromuscular junction. In addition to control by autonomic neurons, various types of smooth muscle tissue can contract in response to self-induced generation of electrical activity, hormonal action, or stretch.

The Role of Ca²⁺ Ions in Excitation-Contraction Coupling in Cardiac and Smooth Muscle Is Different Than in Skeletal Muscle

Contraction of both cardiac and smooth muscle cells results from the sliding together of actin and myosin protein filaments, just as in skeletal muscle. This sliding of actin over myosin requires ATP and does not occur unless Ca^{2+} ions are present, again as in skeletal muscle. However, the origins of the intracytoplasmic Ca^{2+} ions that permit contraction differ.

In skeletal muscle, Ca^{2+} is sequestered in the sarcoplasmic reticulum. With the arrival of the action potential along the sarcolemma and T tubule, Ca^{2+} is released from the sarcoplasmic reticulum and diffuses out into the cytoplasm where it triggers contraction. Here, the mechanical opening of the Ca^{2+}-induced Ca^{2+} release channels of the sarcoplasmic reticulum by the opening of the voltage-gated Ca^{2+} channels of the T tubule is the most significant vehicle for the rise in the cytoplasmic Ca^{2+}. With passage of the action potential, Ca^{2+} is pumped back into the sarcoplasmic reticulum, and the muscle relaxes. In skeletal muscle, little if any influx of extracellular Ca^{2+} (the T tubule lumen is an extension of the extracellular space), through the voltage-gated Ca^{2+} channels of the T tubule, is needed for contraction.

In cardiac muscle the sarcoplasmic reticulum is not as well developed as in skeletal muscle. Therefore the influx of extracellular Ca^{2+}, through the voltage-gated Ca^{2+} channels of the T tubule, and the release of Ca^{2+} from the sarcoplasmic reticulum are both important in triggering contraction. In cardiac muscle the arrival of the action potential along the cell membrane and the T tubules opens voltage-gated Ca^{2+} channels, allowing the influx of extracellular Ca^{2+} ions into the cytoplasm. Some of these Ca^{2+} ions activate the Ca^{2+}-induced Ca^{2+} release channels on the sarcoplasmic reticulum, and these combined sources of increased cytoplasmic Ca^{2+} trigger contraction. If antihypertensive drugs called *calcium channel blockers* are used to block the entry of extracellular Ca^{2+} ions, the force of contraction is reduced. When the action potential has passed, muscle relaxation is accomplished primarily by pumping cytoplasmic Ca^{2+} back into the sarcoplasmic reticulum, although some Ca^{2+} is transported across the sarcolemma into the extracellular space.

In many smooth muscle cells the sarcoplasmic reticulum is poorly developed, and extracellular Ca^{2+} influx plays the principal role in initiating the contractile process. Even though smooth muscle cells have no T tubules, this Ca^{2+} influx is achieved, on membrane depolarization, through activation of voltage-gated Ca^{2+} channels located in shallow depressions of the membrane *(caveolae)* (see Figure 6-9). Calcium channel blockers interfere with this process and can relax smooth muscle in arterial walls, which dilates arteries and lowers blood pressure. Contraction is terminated in many smooth muscle cells primarily by Ca^{2+} transport back into the extracellular space, which is a fairly slow process.

Some receptor-mediated stimulation of smooth muscle cells by neurons or by hormones does not lead to depolarization of the cell membrane, but can lead to contraction of the smooth muscle cell nonetheless. For example, activation of some smooth muscle G protein-coupled membrane receptors (see Figure 1-19), such as those that employ the inositol trisphosphate-diacylglycerol (IP_3-DAG) second messenger pathway, can induce the release of Ca^{2+} stores from the smooth muscle cell sarcoplasmic reticulum, leading to contraction.

The mechanism by which Ca^{2+} induces actin-myosin cross-bridge cycling in smooth muscle differs from that in skeletal and cardiac muscle (see Figure 1-17). In skeletal and cardiac muscle, cross-bridge cycling relies primarily on the Ca^{2+}-induced removal of the tropomyosin block of the actin-binding site. In smooth muscle, cycling relies on a Ca^{2+}-induced increase in the ATPase activity of the myosin head, another slow process. This increase in ATPase activity is brought about when increased intracellular Ca^{2+} initiates a chain of events leading to phosphorylation of the myosin head.

CLINICAL CORRELATIONS

DOWN COW AFTER CALVING

History. A 4-year-old Jersey cow calved earlier this morning; this was her second calf. The producer called you because the cow stood after calving but appeared uncoordinated. Now, a few hours later, the cow is just recumbent and appears dull. She has been offered water and hay but has not accepted either. No other cows are affected. This cow has no history of medical problems.

Clinical Examination. The cow appears dull and does not pay much attention to you or the other activity in the barn. The cow's temperature is slightly low, and her heart rate is slightly increased. Her respirations are normal. She is slightly dehydrated. Her ears are cool to the touch, peripheral pulses are weak, and her rumen contractions are decreased. On examination, she does not appear to have any injuries that would prevent her from standing. Your brief neurological examination is normal, but the cow does have an S-shaped curve to her spine.

Comment. This cow most likely has *hypocalcemia*. Because of the high demands for calcium in the development of the calf in late pregnancy, combined with the production of colostrum and milk, this cow has become hypocalcemic. As reviewed in this chapter, calcium is critical for muscle contractions. Calcium also assists with membrane stabilization of peripheral nerves. Deficits can cause mild tetany, which is sometimes seen in cows with hypocalcemia. Additionally, the release of acetylcholine (ACh) at the neuromuscular junctions is mediated by calcium. Hypocalcemia causes decreased ACh release, which can cause paralysis. All the clinical signs—hypothermia, increased heart rate, weak pulses, paresis, cool extremities, S-shaped curve of the spine, and decreased rumen contractions—can be attributed to hypocalcemia. A definitive diagnosis can be made by measuring ionized calcium. However, most veterinarians and producers will treat based on clinical signs, with the diagnosis confirmed based on response to treatment.

Treatment. Cows are treated with calcium gluconate, which is slowly given intravenously. Most cows will show improvement in clinical signs during the treatment. Cows often become brighter, their rumen contractility and peripheral circulation improve, and their core body temperature normalizes. Most cows attempt to stand after treatment, which is usually about 1 g per 100 pounds. Some cows will relapse and will need to be re-treated.

MALIGNANT HYPERTHERMIA

History. You are called as the attending veterinarian to the veterinary teaching hospital. The large animal clinicians and anesthesiologists have just anesthetized a pig with halothane. The pig is starting to spasm and its temperature is increasing.

Clinical Examination. They have turned off the halothane. The pig is rigid with an increased temperature and increased heart (tachycardic) and respiratory (tachypnic) rates. Laboratory tests demonstrate that the pig has increased muscle enzymes from muscle damage, and is acidotic.

Comment. For most species that develop malignant hyperthermia, there is a defect in the ryanodine receptor (another name for the Ca^{2+}-activated Ca^{2+} release channel on the sarcoplasmic reticulum). This results in increased release of Ca^{2+} into the sarcoplasm, which stimulates the muscles. The uncontrolled muscle activation leads to rigidity, and because of the constant muscle contractions, the pig sustains muscle damage and consumes considerable oxygen. Therefore, the muscle enzymes are increased, and the animal becomes acidotic due to energy and oxygen consumption.

Treatment. Dantrolene can be given to interfere with the release of Ca^{2+} from the sarcoplasmic reticulum. The exact mechanism is unknown; however, because it interferes with Ca^{2+} release, the Ca^{2+} is not available for muscle contractions. As a result, it can cause relaxation of the muscles. In addition, patients should be well ventilated to normalize the blood gas. Fluids are often given to reduce accumulation of creatinine kinase in the muscle, blood, and kidneys. If patients are rehydrated, their acid-base status may normalize due to correction of the lactic acidosis. However, if necessary, bicarbonate can be given to correct acid-base status.

PRACTICE QUESTIONS

1. Troponin and tropomyosin are components of which one of the following structures?
   a. Myosin thick filament
   b. Sarcolemma
   c. T tubule
   d. Actin thin filament
   e. Sarcoplasmic reticulum

2. Action potentials in skeletal muscle cells trigger the release from the sarcoplasmic reticulum of what ion critical to the muscle's contractile process?
   a. Ca^{2+}
   b. Na^+
   c. K^+
   d. Cl^-
   e. HCO_3^-

3. A gross skeletal muscle belly can be instructed (by the central nervous system) to contract more forcefully by:
   a. Causing more of its motor units to contract simultaneously.
   b. Increasing the amount of acetylcholine released during each neuromuscular synaptic transmission.
   c. Increasing the frequency of action potentials in the α motor neuron's axon.
   d. Both a and c.
   e. Both b and c.

4. Which one of the following is *not* found in smooth muscle?
   a. Actin filaments
   b. Myosin filaments
   c. T tubules
   d. Voltage-gated calcium channels
   e. Sarcoplasmic reticulum

5. Choose the *incorrect* statement below:
   a. The muscle fiber and neuronal cell membranes are similar because they both have a resting membrane potential.
   b. A whole muscle, such as the gastrocnemius muscle, can be made to contract more forcefully by increasing the number of motor units contracting.
   c. The muscle membrane's transverse tubular system transmits the action potential to the interior of the muscle cell.
   d. The muscle cell membrane transmits action potentials by saltatory conduction.
   e. The shortening of a skeletal muscle during contraction is caused by the sliding together of actin and myosin filaments.

6. Which one of the following is *least likely* to be significantly associated with a muscle that is primarily involved in brief, powerful movements?
   a. Large α motor neuron cell body
   b. Small motor unit
   c. Fast-twitch fibers
   d. White muscle
   e. Large motor unit

BIBLIOGRAPHY

Bailey JG: Muscle physiology. In Reece WO, editor: *Duke's physiology of domestic animals*, ed 12, Ithaca, NY, 2004, Comstock Publishing.

Bear MF, Connors BW, Paradiso MA: *Neuroscience: exploring the brain*, ed 3, Philadelphia, 2007, Lippincott, Williams & Wilkins.

Boron WF, Boulpaep EL: *Medical physiology*, ed 2, Philadelphia, 2009, Saunders.

Hall JE: *Guyton and Hall textbook of medical physiology*, ed 12, Philadelphia, 2011, Saunders.

Hunt E, Blackwelder JT: Disorders of calcium metabolism. In Smith BP, editor: *Large animal internal medicine*, ed 3, St Louis, 2002, Mosby.

Jiang D, Chen W, Xiao J, et al: Reduced threshold for luminal Ca^{2+} activation of RyR1 underlies a causal mechanism of porcine malignant hyperthermia, *J Biol Chem* 283(30):20813–20820, 2008.

Kandel ER, Schwartz JH, Jessell TM, editors: *Principles of neural science*, ed 4, New York, 2000, McGraw-Hill.

Matthews GG: *Cellular physiology of nerve and muscle*, ed 4, Malden, Mass, 2003, Wiley-Blackwell.

Rosenberg H, Davis M, James D, et al: Malignant hyperthermia, *Orphanet J Rare Dis* 2:21–35, 2007.

CHAPTER 7
The Concept of a Reflex

KEY POINTS

1. A reflex arc contains five fundamental components.
2. Reflex arcs can be segmental or intersegmental.

3. Reflex arcs are widespread in the nervous system, and reflexes underlie a major portion of the neurological examination.

The *reflex arc*, the neural substrate of a reflex, is fundamental to the physiology of posture and locomotion, as well as to the clinical examination of the nervous system. A *reflex* can be defined as an involuntary, qualitatively unvarying response of the nervous system to a stimulus. Reflexes are the simplest behavioral example of the general function of the nervous system: collection of sensory input, integration, and motor output. Reflexes are often both critical for survival and components of more complex behaviors. The anatomy and function of a reflex arc are often fully developed at birth.

A Reflex Arc Contains Five Fundamental Components

All reflex arcs contain five basic components (Figure 7-1). If any one of these five components malfunctions, the reflex response is altered.

1. All reflex arcs begin with a *sensory receptor*. Sensory receptors vary widely within the body but share a common function: they transduce a range of environmental energy, or the presence of an environmental chemical, into a cellular response that directly or indirectly produces action potentials along a sensory neuron. In other words, these receptors collect environmental signals and turn them into a format that can be understood by the nervous system. For example, receptors of the retina transduce light; those in the skin transduce heat, cold, pressure, and other cutaneous stimuli; muscle spindle receptors transduce stretch; and taste receptors transduce chemical stimuli from ingested material. A *primary sensory receptor* is a neuron with a specialized region for stimulus transduction (Figure 7-2; also see Figure 14-6, retinal photoreceptors). A *secondary sensory receptor* is a nonneural cell specialized for stimulus transduction that in turn affects neural activity by releasing neurotransmitter onto a neuron (see Figure 7-2; also see Figure 11-2, vestibular hair cells). Action potentials resulting from stimulus transduction are generated along sensory neurons at a frequency proportional to the intensity of the transduced stimulus. This proportionality between the intensity with which the receptor is stimulated and the frequency of the resulting sensory neuron action potentials is called *frequency coding;* it is one major way the receptor communicates to the central nervous system (CNS) the intensity of light, heat, stretch, and so forth, that it has transduced. Stronger stimuli will also activate a larger number

of sensory receptors, known as the *population code* of stimulus intensity.

2. The next component in a reflex arc, alluded to earlier, is a *sensory neuron* (CNS afferent). These neurons carry action potentials, resulting from receptor activation, to the CNS. Again, in some cases the receptor is just a specialized, usually peripheral, region of the sensory neuron (primary receptors). In other cases the receptor is physically separate from and synapses on the sensory neuron (secondary receptors). Sensory neurons enter the spinal cord by way of the dorsal roots or enter the brain through cranial nerves.

3. The third component of a reflex arc is a *synapse* in the CNS. Actually, for most reflex arcs, more than one synapse occurs in series *(polysynaptic)*. However, some reflex arcs that originate from the muscle spindle are monosynaptic. In polysynaptic reflexes, where one or more neurons lie between the sensory neuron input to the CNS and the motor neuron output, these interposed neurons are called *interneurons* and can be considered part of this third component of the reflex arc.

4. The fourth component is a *motor neuron* (CNS efferent), which carries action potentials from the CNS toward the synapse with the target (effector) organ. Motor neurons leave the spinal cord through the ventral roots, and motor neurons leave the brain through the cranial nerves.

5. The last component is some *target organ* (effector organ) that causes the reflex response. This is usually a muscle, such as the skeletal muscle fibers of the quadriceps muscle of the leg, in the case of the "knee jerk" (muscle stretch) reflex, or the smooth muscle of the iris in the pupillary light reflex. The target could also be a gland, such as a salivary gland in the salivary reflex.

In reality, the final reflex response to a stimulus in mammals is rarely, if ever, the product of a monosynaptic reflex arc acting in isolation. Even if a sensory neuron participates in a monosynaptic reflex arc, it will often give off branches in the CNS that participate in polysynaptic reflex circuits. In addition, even the simplest mammalian reflex responses often involve both the excitation of a given muscle or muscles and the inhibition of another (usually antagonistic) muscle or muscles. The knee jerk reflex is a good illustration of these points (see Figure 8-3). With regard to the individual sensory neurons that underlie this reflex, some

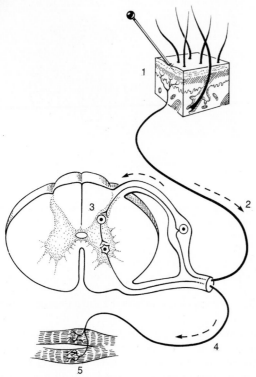

FIGURE 7-1 A reflex arc contains five fundamental components: *1,* a receptor; *2,* a sensory neuron; *3,* one or more synapses in the CNS; *4,* a motor neuron; and *5,* a target organ, usually a muscle. (From De Lahunta A, editor: *Veterinary neuroanatomy and clinical neurology,* ed 2, Philadelphia, 1983, Saunders.)

terminal branches make excitatory monosynaptic connections with motor neurons that activate the quadriceps muscle. Other terminal branches of that same sensory neuron participate in a disynaptic circuit that inhibits motor neurons innervating the antagonistic hamstring muscle.

Also, reflexes do not operate in isolation from the rest of the nervous system. Inputs from other regions of the nervous system, onto the CNS components of a reflex arc, can modulate the sensitivity of the reflex response. For example, if input from the brain to the spinal cord is damaged, reflexes in that region of the cord become exaggerated.

Reflex Arcs Can Be Segmental or Intersegmental

A *segmental reflex* is a reflex in which the reflex arc passes through only a small rostrocaudal portion of the CNS (Figure 7-3, *A*). In such cases the sensory neuron entrance to the CNS, the CNS circuitry, and the motor neuron exit all have a similar rostrocaudal location. The quadriceps stretch reflex (knee jerk reflex) and the pupillary light reflex are examples of segmental reflexes because they use only, respectively, a small number of spinal cord segments (e.g., L4-L6) or a small rostrocaudal region of the brainstem.

In an *intersegmental reflex* the reflex arc traverses many segments of the spinal cord or several major brain divisions (e.g., medulla to midbrain). In one class of intersegmental reflex, the motor neuron exit is located, or extends, a considerable rostral or caudal distance from the location of the sensory neuron entrance to the CNS (see Figure 7-3, *B*). Examples include the vestibulospinal reflexes that produce postural adjustments in response to

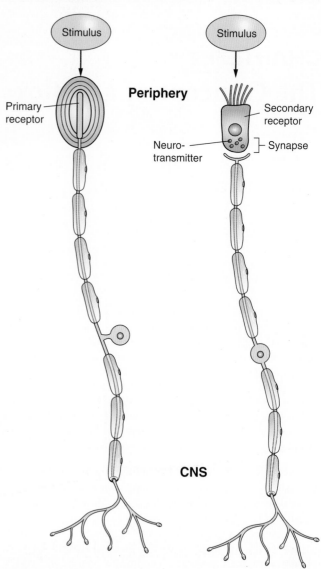

FIGURE 7-2 Primary and secondary sensory receptors. A primary sensory receptor *(left)* is a neuron with a peripheral ending specialized for stimulus transduction. In this particular case, the encapsulated peripheral ending of the neuron transduces the stimulus. The secondary receptor *(right)* is a nonneural cell designed for stimulus transduction, which subsequently releases neurotransmitter onto an adjacent neuron.

acceleration or tilt of the head. The sensory input, originating in the vestibular apparatus of the inner ear, enters the CNS near the pontomedullary border of the brainstem, and the motor neurons exit from the spinal cord, over a large number of spinal cord segments.

For some intersegmental reflexes, the sensory neuron entrance and motor neuron exit are at a similar rostrocaudal location, but the CNS circuitry lying in between travels to and returns from a distant region of the CNS (see Figure 7-3, *C*). These are sometimes referred to as *long-loop* intersegmental reflexes. The proprioceptive positioning reaction is often associated with this category. This reaction involves the animal promptly returning its paw to the normal pad-down position after the clinician flexes it to make the dorsal surface touch the floor or tabletop. The sensorimotor circuitry of this reaction courses from the limb's

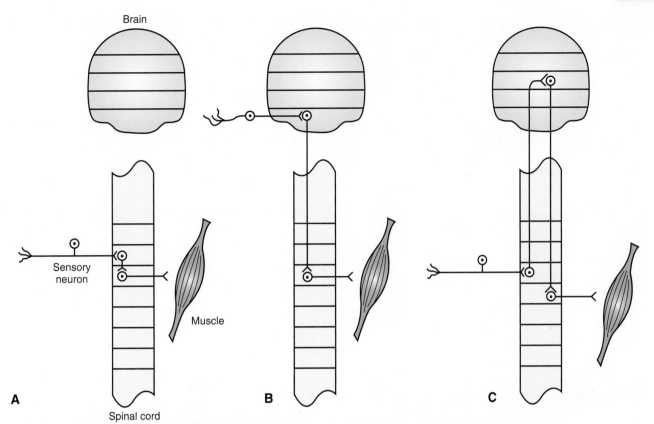

FIGURE 7-3 Segmental and intersegmental reflexes. **A,** In the segmental reflex the sensory neuron input, CNS circuitry, and motor neuron output traverse only a small number of rostrocaudal segments of the CNS. **B,** Intersegmental reflex arcs traverse several CNS segments. In some intersegmental reflexes the sensory neuron input and motor neuron output are separated by several segments. **C,** The long-loop intersegmental reflex arc traverses several CNS segments, even though the sensory input and motor output are located in close rostrocaudal proximity. Horizontal lines delimit either spinal cord segments (e.g., L1, L2) or major brain divisions (e.g., medulla, pons).

peripheral nerves and associated spinal cord segments all the way through the cerebral cortex and back to the limb's spinal cord segments and peripheral nerves.

Reflex Arcs Are Widespread in the Nervous System, and Reflexes Underlie a Major Portion of the Neurological Examination

Reflex arcs are ubiquitous in the nervous system and are the basis of much of an animal's subconscious, involuntary response to its environment. Much of a veterinarian's clinical examination of the nervous system involves evoking reflex responses, such as the pupillary light reflex, muscle stretch (knee jerk) reflex, and flexor reflex.

If any of the five components of the reflex arc malfunctions, the expected reflex response is altered or does not occur. It is important to know the general anatomy, physiology, and expected normal clinical response of the common reflexes in order to perform a neurological examination so that lesions can be localized. For example, loss of pupillary constriction to light in conjunction with normal responses to other visual stimuli, such as avoiding a rapidly oncoming object, suggests that the problem is probably not with the sensory receptor or sensory neuron components of the reflex arc. Several such reflexes are discussed in detail in subsequent chapters.

CLINICAL CORRELATIONS

TRAUMA IN A FOAL

History. Distraught owners call you about their 4-month-old Tennessee Walking Horse colt. He appeared normal this morning when they let him out to pasture with his mother, but later this afternoon, the mare and the foal did not come in to be fed. The owners went out to the pasture and found the mare with the foal, who would not get up. He was lying on his side and seemed unable to position himself sternal. When the owners tried to reposition him, the foal thrashed, trying to get away. You tell the owners not to move the foal and that you will be there soon.

Clinical Examination. The foal appears to be responsive but in great pain and unable to rise. Temperature, pulse, and respirations are all mildly increased. There appears to be a swelling along the cervical (neck) area in the region of C1 to C3. The swelling is hard (bone) and has some fluid (inflammation) as well. There is some crepitus (crackling sound made by bone fragment friction) in the area of the swelling (possible fracture site). The foal displays no other areas of swelling or trauma. Neurological examination reveals normal cranial nerves. In the front limbs the biceps and triceps reflexes seem increased on both sides. Deep pain is present, and cutaneous sensation is increased bilaterally. In the hind limbs the femoral, sciatic, and tibial responses are increased.

Comment. Although it is difficult to localize a fracture definitively, based on history and physical examination a fracture seems likely. The fracture appears to be in the region of C1 to C3. Radiographs would be ideal to make a definitive diagnosis. On neurological testing of the biceps, triceps, sciatic, femoral, and cranial tibial responses, all assess segmental reflex arcs. Because of a high cervical fracture, the descending motor tracts that supply both the thoracic and the pelvic limbs are affected. From point of initiation, the segmental reflexes tested involve the muscle spindles, which detect stretch, followed by sensory fibers in the peripheral nerves, the dorsal root and its ganglion, and the central branches of the sensory fibers projecting onto the ventral horn cell of the same spinal segment. The efferent pathway involves the ventral horn cell (lower motor neuron) followed by the ventral root, motor fibers in the peripheral nerve, neuromuscular junction, and then the myofibers being tested. The presence but exaggeration of the segmental reflexes reflects a change in the modulation of these reflexes by the damaged descending motor tracts that pass through the area of the lesion.

Treatment. The prognosis for this foal is poor. Based on the physical examination and clinical signs, a fracture is likely, and there is little hope for recovery. The complications associated with trying to manage a foal as the fracture heals are enormous. The fracture may not heal, and the foal could have severe residual neurological deficits. In most cases, these foals are euthanized fairly quickly because of the poor prognosis.

PRACTICE QUESTIONS

1. Which of the following is *not* always a component of a reflex arc?
   a. Receptor
   b. Sensory neuron (CNS afferent)
   c. Central nervous system (CNS) interneuron
   d. Motor neuron (CNS efferent)
   e. Target (effector) organ

2. Which of the following regarding sensory receptors is *false*?
   a. They transduce environmental signals, directly or indirectly, into neuronal action potentials.
   b. A primary receptor can be a specialized peripheral region of a sensory neuron.
   c. They directly transduce CNS action potentials into physical activity of a target organ.
   d. They are the initial component of a reflex arc.

3. When the intensity with which a receptor is stimulated is increased, what happens to the *frequency* of action potentials along the sensory neuron from that receptor?
   a. Increases
   b. Decreases
   c. No change

4. Which of the following is *not* an example of a segmental reflex?
   a. Quadriceps stretch reflex
   b. Pupillary light reflex
   c. Vestibulospinal postural reflexes

5. An intersegmental reflex arc is one in which:
   a. The course of the arc is restricted to one or a small number of segments of the CNS.
   b. No target organ is present.
   c. No receptor is present.
   d. The course of the arc traverses several segments of the CNS.
   e. Both b and c.

BIBLIOGRAPHY

Bailey JG: Muscle physiology. In Reece WO, editor: *Duke's physiology of domestic animals*, ed 12, Ithaca, NY, 2004, Comstock Publishing.

Binder MD: Peripheral motor control: spinal reflex actions of muscle, joint and cutaneous receptors. In Patton HD, Fuchs AF, Hille B, et al, editors: *Textbook of physiology*, ed 21, Philadelphia, 1989, Saunders.

Boron WF, Boulpaep EL: *Medical physiology*, ed 2, Philadelphia, 2009, Saunders.

Divers TJ, Smith MO: Spinal fractures and luxations and spinal cord trauma. In Smith BP, editor: *Large animal internal medicine*, ed 3, St Louis, 2002, Mosby.

Hall JE: *Guyton and Hall textbook of medical physiology*, ed 12, Philadelphia, 2011, Saunders.

Kandel ER, Schwartz JH, Jessell TM, editors: *Principles of neural science*, ed 4, New York, 2000, McGraw-Hill.

Lorenz MD, Coates JR, Kent M: Handbook of veterinary neurology, ed 5, Philadelphia, 2010, Saunders.

CHAPTER 8
Skeletal Muscle Receptor Organs

KEY POINT

1. The muscle spindle stretch receptor is an encapsulated organ of specialized muscle fibers with separate motor and sensory innervations.
2. The muscle spindle conveys information about muscle length to the central nervous system.
3. Muscle stretch and action potentials along spindle sensory neurons lead to reflex contraction of the extrafusal muscle fibers.
4. The central nervous system can control spindle sensitivity directly through the gamma (γ) motor neurons.
5. The Golgi tendon organ lies in series between muscle and tendon and detects muscle tension.
6. Free (non-organ) sensory receptors in joints and muscles can provide information about joint position, joint movement, and pain-inducing stimuli of joints and muscles.

Movement, characteristic of all animals, is the end product of skeletal muscle contraction. It is orchestrated by the central nervous system (CNS) through its control of the motor unit (see Chapter 6). To control body movement appropriately, the CNS must (1) assess the effect of gravity on the many muscles of the body, (2) determine the initial position of the body parts to be moved, and (3) detect any discrepancy between the intended movement and the movement that actually occurs. When such discrepancies are detected, appropriate adjustments can be made.

Two important receptor systems have evolved in the skeletal muscles of mammals to provide the CNS with the aforementioned information: the muscle spindle and the Golgi tendon organ (Figure 8-1). The *muscle spindles,* arranged in parallel to the contracting skeletal muscle fibers, provide information about muscle length. The *Golgi tendon organ,* arranged in series with the contracting skeletal muscle fibers, detects muscle tension. This chapter discusses the anatomy and physiology of these two receptor organs; Chapter 10 discusses how the CNS uses the information gathered from these organs to coordinate posture and locomotion. Some of this information is used in reflex arcs of the type described in Chapter 7.

The Muscle Spindle Stretch Receptor Is an Encapsulated Organ of Specialized Muscle Fibers with Separate Motor and Sensory Innervations

The muscle spindle is an encapsulated group of about 3 to 12 small, slender, specialized skeletal muscle fibers (Figure 8-2). Because their capsule is spindle shaped, or *fusiform,* these muscle fibers are called *intrafusal muscle fibers.* The muscle fibers that cause physical shortening of the muscle (the majority of muscle fibers in a muscle belly), located outside the capsule, are called *extrafusal muscle fibers.* Extrafusal muscle fibers often span the length of the gross muscle from origin to insertion tendon; intrafusal muscle fibers and their capsules are much shorter (about 4 to 10 mm long). In addition, the intrafusal muscle fiber endings are attached to the extracellular matrix of, and lie in parallel to,

the extrafusal muscle fibers. Therefore, if the muscle is stretched, lengthening the extrafusal muscle fibers, the intrafusal fibers of the muscle spindle are also stretched.

Unlike extrafusal muscle fibers, the contractile elements of intrafusal muscle fibers are restricted to their polar ends, with none in their middle (equatorial) region. Therefore, their polar ends can contract, but their equatorial region cannot. Such contraction does not directly contribute to the shortening of the gross muscle, but it can tighten the region of the intrafusal fiber that lies between the two poles. As discussed later, this can have a dramatic effect on the muscle spindle's sensitivity for transducing muscle stretch.

Spindle sensory neurons arise from the equatorial region of the intrafusal muscle fibers and carry action potentials from the spindle to the CNS by way of the peripheral nerves. These CNS afferents enter the spinal cord through the dorsal roots (Figure 8-3). The contractile, polar regions of the intrafusal muscle fibers are innervated by motor neurons called *gamma (γ) motor neurons.* Extrafusal muscle fibers—the muscle fibers that cause the physical shortening of the muscle—are supplied by a different population of motor neurons (those that comprise the motor units) called *alpha (α) motor neurons.* Although γ motor neurons go to intrafusal muscle fibers and α motor neurons go to the extrafusal muscle fibers, these CNS efferents both have their cell bodies in the ventral horn of the spinal cord, and their axons leave through the ventral roots.

The Muscle Spindle Conveys Information About Muscle Length to the Central Nervous System

As noted, stretching a muscle can stretch the intrafusal fibers of the muscle spindle that lie parallel to the extrafusal muscle fibers. Stretching (lengthening) the equatorial segment of the intrafusal muscle fiber generates action potentials along the spindle sensory neurons. As the equatorial segment is lengthened, it is believed that stretch-sensitive ion channels open on the sensory neurons, leading to membrane depolarization and action potential generation. Action potentials are generated along the sensory neuron

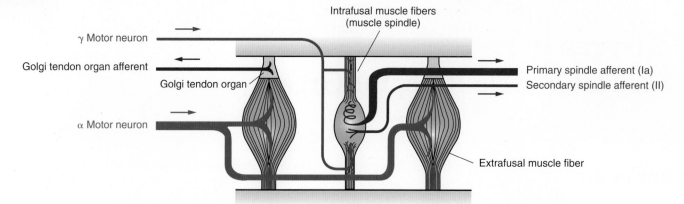

FIGURE 8-1 Skeletal muscles have two important receptors: the muscle spindle and the Golgi tendon organ. The intrafusal muscle fibers (muscle spindle) are arranged in parallel with the extrafusal muscle fibers; the Golgi tendon organ is in series with the extrafusal fibers. *Arrows* indicate direction of action potential flow along respective axons. (Modified from Kandel ER, Schwartz JH: *Principles of neural science,* ed 2, New York, 1985, Elsevier Science.)

output of the muscle spindle in proportion to the amount of lengthening of the middle of the intrafusal muscle fibers. There are actually subclasses of intrafusal fibers (dynamic nuclear bag, static nuclear bag, and nuclear chain) and spindle sensory neurons (Ia, II). This variety allows the sensory neuron output of the spindle to detect not only a change in length during the dynamic phase of muscle lengthening, but also the rate of lengthening, as well as the steady-state length of the muscle as the animal holds the joint still (Figure 8-4).

When a muscle is held at a constant length, such as when a joint is held still, there is usually enough stretch of the muscle's spindles to produce a steady frequency of action potential discharge in the sensory neuron output of the muscle spindle. This steady-state discharge gives the muscle spindle organ the ability to inform the CNS not only about a subsequent lengthening of the muscle, which would produce a proportional increase in action potential discharge, but about a shortening of the muscle as well, which would produce a proportional decrease in action potential discharge from the steady state (see Figure 8-4).

Muscle Stretch and Action Potentials Along Spindle Sensory Neurons Lead to Reflex Contraction of the Extrafusal Muscle Fibers

The sensory output neurons of the muscle spindle enter the CNS, where they make excitatory, monosynaptic connections with α motor neurons that return to the extrafusal fibers of the same muscle (see Figure 8-3). Therefore, stretching a given muscle can lead to a rapid, reflex contraction of that same muscle, bringing it back to its original length. Stretching the muscle lengthens the intrafusal muscle fibers of the spindle, increasing the frequency of action potential discharge along the sensory output neurons of the spindle. This leads to an increase in action potential frequency in the α motor neurons on which the spindle sensory neurons synapse. This produces contraction of the extrafusal fibers innervated by those α motor neurons, which results in contraction (shortening) of the muscle. Contraction of the muscle results in a shortening of the muscle spindle's equatorial region. This eventually reduces the frequency of action potentials occurring on the spindle sensory neurons to the prestretch level, terminating the response. (The cycle is a classic negative-feedback system.)

The reflex just described can be elicited by striking the patellar tendon (insertion tendon of quadriceps muscle) with a blunt object. Because this tendon goes over a *pulley* (the patella), hitting this tendon results in a longitudinal stretch of the whole quadriceps muscle, thus also stretching the muscle spindles. Action potentials from spindle sensory neurons go to the lumbar spinal cord, by way of the dorsal roots, and cause excitatory postsynaptic potentials (EPSPs) on the α motor neurons of the motor units that return to the quadriceps muscle (see Figure 8-3). This causes contraction of the quadriceps muscle and extension of the knee joint, and is an example of the *muscle stretch reflex,* or *myotatic reflex.* When it is applied to the quadriceps muscle, it is called the *knee jerk reflex,* but the mechanisms are present in almost all muscles. However, this is the muscle from which it is easiest to evoke the stretch reflex because it is one of the few whose tendon goes over a sesamoid pulley before inserting on the next bone. Because of the pulley under the tendon, a lateral deflection of the tendon, as from a reflex hammer, results in a longitudinal stretch of the muscle and thus the reflex. Hitting other tendons only moves the muscle belly laterally and does not easily result in the stretch reflex. Therefore, in the clinical neurological examination of most animals, the knee jerk reflex is the most commonly evoked muscle stretch reflex.

The muscle spindle organ and stretch reflex allow the CNS to make automatic, usually unconscious adjustments to muscle stretch imposed by small changes in body position or the weighting of a muscle. Such adjustments can return the muscle to its original length, often returning a joint to its original position. Clinical examination of the stretch reflex provides clues about the peripheral or CNS integrity of its sensory and motor components.

When the stretch reflex acts to return a joint to its original position, the antagonist of the stretched muscle must relax in order for the joint to be able to move. Therefore, in the stretch reflex, some terminal branches of individual spindle sensory neurons do not synapse directly on the α motor neurons of the stretched muscle, but rather synapse on inhibitory spinal interneurons (see Figure 8-3). These neurons, which lie completely within the spinal cord, are also activated by the stretch of the muscle. When they fire action potentials, however, they cause inhibitory postsynaptic potentials (IPSPs) on α motor neurons

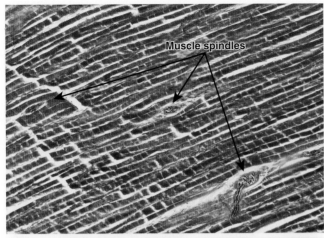

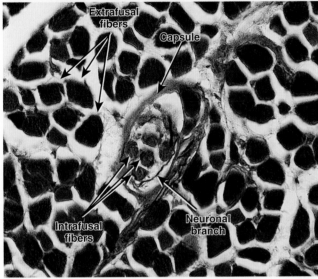

FIGURE 8-2 The muscle spindle receptor is an encapsulated group of specialized (intrafusal) skeletal muscle fibers supplied with both motor and sensory innervation. **A,** Longitudinal section through a skeletal muscle showing that the encapsulated muscle spindles are oriented parallel to the more numerous extrafusal fibers of the muscle. The ends of the muscle spindle are attached to the extracellular matrix of the extrafusal fibers. **B,** Higher-magnification view of a transverse section through a muscle spindle. Intrafusal fibers can be seen within the spindle's tissue capsule. These fibers are fewer, shorter, and more slender than the surrounding extrafusal fibers. A portion of the spindle's innervation can also be seen. (Images courtesy Dr. Tom Caceci, Department of Biomedical Sciences and Pathobiology, College of Veterinary Medicine, Virginia Tech.)

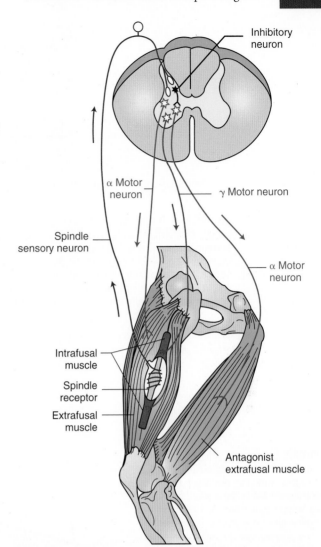

FIGURE 8-3 The muscle spindle stretch reflex (illustrated here as the *knee jerk reflex*) begins when the spindle receptor organ is stretched. This causes action potentials on the receptor's sensory neurons, which in turn cause excitatory postsynaptic potentials on the α motor neurons returning to the extrafusal muscle fibers of that same muscle. Action potentials on the α motor neurons cause extrafusal muscle fibers to contract, and the knee extends ("jerks"). Through an inhibitory interneuron, the α motor neurons to the antagonist muscles are simultaneously inhibited.

that innervate the antagonist of the stretched muscle. This prevents the contraction of the antagonistic muscle.

The Central Nervous System Can Control Spindle Sensitivity Directly Through the Gamma (γ) Motor Neurons

Contraction of the extrafusal muscle fibers is controlled by the larger α motor neurons; intrafusal muscle fibers of the spindle are controlled by the smaller γ motor neurons. The γ motor neurons innervate the intrafusal muscle fibers at their polar ends (see Figures 8-1 and 8-3), the regions containing contractile protein. Action potentials on the γ motor neurons cause shortening of the polar regions of the intrafusal muscle fibers, stretching the equatorial portion.

An important function for this motor innervation of a receptor organ is to regulate the sensitivity of the muscle spindle. Shortening of a gross muscle resulting from initiation of extrafusal muscle fiber contraction has the potential to slacken the intrafusal muscle fibers given their parallel relationship to the extrafusal fibers. This would severely limit the ability of the muscle spindle to transduce stretch. However, this does not normally occur because contraction of the polar regions of intrafusal fibers resulting from γ motor neuron activation is initiated concurrently with shortening of extrafusal fibers caused by α motor neuron activation. This allows the spindle receptor organ to remain taut and sensitive to sudden stretches of the gross muscle over the entire range of its length. This γ motor neuron control mechanism can also function to differentially regulate the sensitivity of the muscle spindle, depending on the type of movement to be made (e.g., novel and unpredictable vs. stereotypical). There

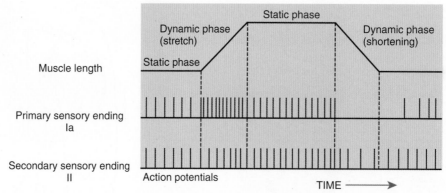

FIGURE 8-4 The muscle spindle can signal the steady-state length of the muscle, as well as the onset and velocity of stretch. When the muscle is stretched, both type Ia and type II spindle sensory neurons have a higher action-potential firing rate at the muscle's new static length. During the dynamic stretching phase, the action-potential firing rate of the type Ia spindle sensory neuron increases rapidly and in proportion to the velocity of stretch. Spindle sensory neurons can also register a decreased steady-state length of the muscle, but type Ia and type II neurons display differential sensitivity to the dynamic phase of shortening. (From Brodal P: *The central nervous system: structure and function,* ed 2, New York, 1998, Oxford University Press.)

FIGURE 8-5 The Golgi tendon organ is located in the tendons of skeletal muscle, in series with the extrafusal fibers. It detects tension in the tendon, produced by muscle contraction, and sends information about this tension to the central nervous system. Sensory neuron branches of the organ are intertwined among braided collagen fibrils *(inset),* which fold up and pinch the neural branches when tension develops in the tendon.

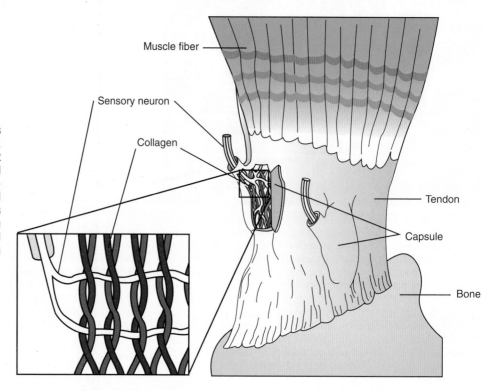

are actually two types of γ motor neurons; one regulates the sensitivity of the muscle spindle to the dynamic phase of stretch (γ_D; gamma dynamic) and one regulates sensitivity to steady-state length (γ_S; gamma static). Chapter 10 describes how co-activation of both the α and γ motor neurons allows the brain to test whether the amount of contraction intended by the brain was what actually occurred.

The Golgi Tendon Organ Lies in Series Between Muscle and Tendon and Detects Muscle Tension

Each Golgi tendon organ is a slender capsule, at the junction between muscle and tendon, in series with 15 to 20 extrafusal skeletal muscle fibers (Figure 8-5). The capsule of each tendon organ contains a complement of braided collagen fascicles, among which the branches of a single sensory neuron are intertwined. This sensory neuron, as with those of the muscle spindle, carries action potentials to the CNS by way of peripheral nerve and dorsal root. The Golgi tendon organ has no motor innervation.

Because the Golgi tendon organ is in series with a group of extrafusal fibers and the tendon, when the extrafusal fibers shorten during contraction, tension is applied to the tendon organ. This causes the braided collagen fibrils of the organ to tighten and squeeze the endings of the sensory neuron. Action potentials are therefore generated and sent to the CNS along the sensory neuron at a frequency proportional to the tension developed by the muscle. In contrast, the muscle spindle is arranged in parallel with the extrafusal muscle fibers, and when they contract, the spindle reduces its action potential frequency.

When action potentials from spindle sensory neurons reach the CNS, as mentioned earlier, they monosynaptically produce EPSPs in the α motor neurons returning to the same muscle. Action potentials along sensory neurons from Golgi tendon organs have the opposite effect: they activate inhibitory interneurons, polysynaptically producing IPSPs on α motor neurons to the same muscle. This leads to a reduced extrafusal muscle fiber contraction.

Free (Non-Organ) Sensory Receptors in Joints and Muscles Can Provide Information About Joint Position, Joint Movement, and Pain-Inducing Stimuli of Joints and Muscles

Input from muscle sensory organs is not the only source of muscle sensory information to the CNS, and is not the only source of sensory information about movement of body parts. Non-organ peripheral endings of sensory neurons, with central projections to the spinal cord, can be found in joint capsules and in ligaments around the joints. Some of these receptors can respond to changes in tension of the joint capsule and can therefore provide information about position of the joint. Some can also respond to the velocity of joint movement. Some joint-associated sensory endings are activated by strong mechanical stimuli, or inflammatory mediators, that are associated with pain sensations (e.g., arthritic pain). Pain-mediating, non-organ sensory endings can also be found in muscle and may contribute to the sensation of muscle soreness. Interestingly, there is a population of non-organ sensory receptors that can be found in both muscles and joints that are thought to trigger circulatory and respiratory reflexes that are associated with onset of body movement.

The two skeletal muscle receptor organs discussed in this chapter provide the CNS with the most important and vital information about muscle length (the spindle) and muscle tension (the Golgi tendon organ), and through their reflex circuitry, they help to keep these parameters within optimal ranges. The information these receptors provide, along with information from receptors of skin and joints, is essential if the CNS is to coordinate posture and locomotion.

CLINICAL CORRELATIONS

FEMORAL NERVE MONONEUROPATHY

History. You examine an 8-year-old male golden retriever. The owner complains that the dog cannot bear weight on the right rear leg.

Clinical Examination. Physical examination deficits are limited to the right rear leg, where you find that the quadriceps femoris muscles are much smaller than those of the left rear leg. The dog cannot bear weight on the right rear leg because the right quadriceps femoris muscles are paralyzed. When you tap on the left patellar tendon with a reflex hammer, the knee briskly extends (the knee jerk or muscle stretch reflex). However, when you tap on the right patellar tendon, no movement occurs.

Comment. The quadriceps femoris muscle group is one of the major antigravity muscle groups of the leg causing the stifle joint (knee joint) to extend. The paralysis in this animal's quadriceps muscle is the reason why he cannot bear weight on the leg. The

small size of the right quadriceps muscle is caused by atrophy, or muscle wasting, which in turn is caused by the loss of α motor neurons to the extrafusal muscle fibers in the quadriceps muscle belly (see Chapter 9). This would also cause a loss of the muscle stretch reflex, because even though the spindle detected the stretch of the muscle belly caused by either gravity or the reflex hammer, the α motor neurons returning to the quadriceps muscle are unable to signal the muscle to contract, thus severing the reflex arc. This syndrome could occur if the femoral nerve is damaged by a tumor or trauma. If the pathological lesion were in the peripheral nerve rather than only in the ventral roots, there would likely be some sensory loss in addition to the motor deficits.

Treatment. This is a *femoral nerve mononeuropathy.* Its treatment depends on the cause of the nerve damage (e.g., trauma, neoplasia, inflammation).

OBTURATOR NERVE PARALYSIS IN A COW POST-CALVING

History. A client calls you about a 2-year-old Holstein cow that calved a few days ago. The calving was difficult (dystocia), and the clients had to pull the calf. Since the calving, the cow has been laying down a lot, and is stiff and uncoordinated when she walks in the barn. She has almost fallen a few times.

Clinical Examination. On examination, she appears to be eating and drinking well. Her temperature, pulse, and respiratory rate are all within normal limits. You watch her get up and lie down and she appears uncoordinated on her right hindlimb. When she is standing, she maintains her leg base wide (abducted). The next time she lies down, you test some of her muscle reflexes, including some of the muscle spindle stretch (myotatic) reflexes. Absence or reduction of such spinal reflexes, and whether the effect is in one muscle group or bilateral, can provide clues to whether there is damage to sensory or motor components of peripheral nerve or whether damage is located in the spinal cord. Exaggeration of reflexes may indicate loss of descending inhibitory control from more rostral parts of the central nervous system. The quadriceps stretch reflex (knee jerk reflex; see this chapter) is tested, although because the animal seems to be able to support its weight on the limb, you do not expect this to be affected. The cranial tibial stretch reflex is also tested by striking the belly of this muscle just below the proximal end of the tibia. The response of this hock flexor is used to assess integrity of the peroneal branch of the sciatic nerve. The pelvic limb flexor reflex is a response to noxious pinching of the skin of the distal limb, involves all the flexor muscles of the limb, and assesses the integrity of the sciatic nerve. All of these reflexes appear normal.

Comment. Based on her history and clinical signs, you suspect obturator nerve paralysis from the trauma during calving. The obturator nerve innervates the adductor, pectineus, and gracilis muscles, which collectively affect hindlimb adduction (drawing nearer to the midline) and hip movements. Thus, the cow can stand and walk, but has problems keeping the limb in a normal position, particularly if the surface is slippery or she is running.

Treatment. Clinical signs are due to inflammation and damage of the obturator nerve. Typically, cows are not treated, and the degree of recovery is based on the extent of inflammation and nerve damage present. More severe cases can be treated with anti-inflammatory drugs or steroids to limit inflammation.

Acknowledgment

The authors thank Dr. Tom Caceci for persevering in the search through his histological specimens to capture the beautiful muscle spindle images of Figure 8-2.

PRACTICE QUESTIONS

1. If the distance between the origin and insertion tendons is increased (the muscle is stretched), what happens to the frequency of action potentials along the sensory axons leaving the muscle spindles in that muscle?
   a. Increases
   b. Decreases
   c. Does not change

2. Activation of the Golgi tendon organ of a given muscle:
   a. Monosynaptically produces EPSPs on the α motor neuron that returns to that muscle.
   b. Is most effectively produced by lengthening of the extrafusal fibers of that muscle.
   c. Polysynaptically produces IPSPs on the α motor neuron that returns to that muscle.
   d. Polysynaptically produces EPSPs on the α motor neuron that returns to that muscle.
   e. Activates motor neurons that return to the Golgi tendon organ itself.

3. Which of the following is *not* characteristic of the muscle spindle?
   a. Encapsulated intrafusal fibers
   b. Sensitivity to muscle tension
   c. Sensitivity to dynamic stretching of the muscle
   d. Lying parallel to the extrafusal muscle fibers
   e. Sensitivity to steady-state length of the muscle

4. Gamma (γ) motor neurons:
   a. Innervate and produce contraction of the equatorial (middle) region of an intrafusal fiber.
   b. Have their cell bodies in the dorsal horn of the spinal cord.
   c. Are never activated at the same time as α motor neurons.
   d. Can regulate the sensitivity of the muscle spindle sensory organ.
   e. Innervate and regulate the sensitivity of the Golgi tendon organ.

BIBLIOGRAPHY

Binder MD: Peripheral motor control: spinal reflex actions of muscle, joint and cutaneous receptors. In Patton HD, Fuchs AF, Hille B, et al, editors: *Textbook of physiology*, ed 21, Philadelphia, 1989, Saunders.

Brodal P: *The central nervous system: structure and function*, ed 4, New York, 2010, Oxford University Press.

Haines DE, editor: *Fundamental neuroscience*, ed 3, New York, 2006, Churchill Livingstone.

Hall JE: *Guyton and Hall textbook of medical physiology*, ed 12, Philadelphia, 2011, Saunders.

Kandel ER, Schwartz JH, Jessell TM, editors: *Principles of neural science*, ed 4, New York, 2000, McGraw-Hill.

Lorenz MD, Coates JR, Kent M: *Handbook of veterinary neurology*, ed 5, Philadelphia, 2010, Saunders.

Purves D, Augustine GJ, Fitzpatrick D, et al: *Neuroscience*, ed 5, Sunderland, Mass, 2012, Sinauer.

Smith MO, George LW: Diseases of the nervous system. In Smith BP, editor: *Large animal internal medicine*, ed 4, St Louis, 2009, Mosby Elsevier.

CHAPTER 9
The Concept of Lower and Upper Motor Neurons and Their Malfunction

KEY POINTS

1. The lower motor neuron is classically defined as the alpha (α) motor neuron.
2. Disease of lower motor neurons causes stereotypical clinical signs.

3. Upper motor neurons lie completely in the central nervous system and control lower motor neurons.
4. Signs of upper motor neuron disease differ from signs of lower motor neuron disease.

The majority of veterinary patients with neurological disease display some abnormality of posture and locomotion. The abnormalities range from weakness or paralysis to spasticity, rigidity, and convulsions. The goal of the diagnostic process for such patients is to determine the location, the extent, and the cause of the lesion. Central to diagnostic logic in neurology is deciding whether the patient's lesion is located in the lower motor neurons or the upper motor neurons. (There are two other possible locations of lesions causing movement disorders: the neuromuscular junction and skeletal muscle.)

This chapter defines lower and upper motor neurons because these concepts are useful in understanding the physiology of posture and locomotion and are essential in locating pathological processes in the nervous system. Malfunctions of these two neuron populations are also described briefly.

The Lower Motor Neuron Is Classically Defined as the Alpha (α) Motor Neuron

The concept of a lower motor neuron is decades old in neurology. The alpha (α) motor neuron is classically defined as a neuron whose cell body and dendrites are located in the central nervous system (CNS) and whose axon extends out through the peripheral nerves to synapse with the extrafusal skeletal muscle fibers (Figure 9-1). The cell bodies of these neurons are located either in the ventral horn of spinal cord gray matter or in cranial nerve nuclei of the brainstem. This is the "final common path" through which CNS commands to a skeletal muscle are channeled to produce movement. This definition predates the discovery of gamma (γ) motor neurons, which innervate muscle spindles. Some authors would include γ motor neurons in the definition of lower motor neurons. Some also consider the pre- and post-ganglionic autonomic neurons to be lower motor neurons (see Chapter 13). The vast majority of clinical signs caused by lower motor neuron disease, however, can currently be explained by the loss or malfunction of the α motor neuron.

Disease of Lower Motor Neurons Causes Stereotypical Clinical Signs

Regardless of the pathological basis for disease of lower motor neurons, a stereotypical set of clinical signs results in the skeletal muscles they innervate.

- *Paralysis* or *paresis*. Disease of the α motor neurons usually prevents the neurons' action potentials from reaching the neuromuscular junction. Therefore, despite the brain's command to the muscle to contract, the message cannot reach the muscle, and paralysis is the result. In fact, such paralysis can be so complete that the adjective *flaccid* is used to describe the paralysis in which no muscle contraction occurs. Because not all the α motor neuron axons of a peripheral nerve may be affected by an insult, and because muscles can be supplied by axons of more than one spinal nerve, paralysis may be incomplete. This symptom is referred to as *paresis*.
- *Atrophy*. Atrophy is the shrinking or wasting of skeletal muscle mass distal to the lower motor neuron lesion (Figure 9-2). This occurs within days of the injury to a nerve. The exact origins of this atrophy are controversial. However, evidence indicates that the reduced frequency of muscle stimulation caused by α motor neuron insult, and the resulting reduced use of the muscle, trigger reductions in muscle protein synthesis and increases in muscle proteolysis. There is evidence that activation of the ubiquitin-proteosome proteolytic pathway underlies this muscle breakdown. The magnitude of this denervation atrophy can be reduced by direct electrical stimulation of the muscle itself. There is also some recent evidence that manually imposed repetitive stretching may reduce denervation atrophy; a molecular signaling pathway suspected to underlie this atrophy reduction has been identified.
- *Loss of segmental and intersegmental reflexes.* Segmental and intersegmental reflexes require a viable α motor neuron in the reflex arc for the reflex response to occur (see Chapter 7). Therefore, such reflexes as the muscle stretch (knee jerk) reflex

Brain

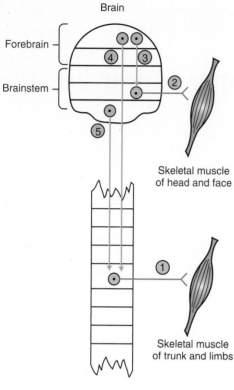

FIGURE 9-1 General organization of lower and upper motor neurons. *Blue,* Lower motor neurons typically originate in the ventral horn of the spinal cord *(neuron 1)* or in cranial nerve nuclei *(neuron 2),* and synapse within skeletal muscle. *Green,* Upper motor neurons typically originate in the brain and project to and control lower motor neurons. Upper motor neurons usually belong to the corticobulbar *(neuron 3),* corticospinal *(neuron 4),* or descending brainstem motor (also called bulbospinal, *neuron 5),* pathways. *Arrowheads* indicate that local synapses may be interposed between the upper and lower motor neurons. *Horizontal lines* delimit either spinal cord segments (e.g., L1, L2) or major brain divisions (e.g., medulla, pons).

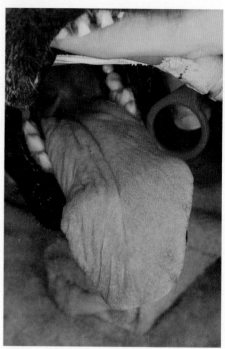

FIGURE 9-2 Atrophy of the right side of the tongue in a golden retriever due to a meningioma that affected the right hypoglossal nerve roots. (From De Lahunta A, Glass E: *Veterinary neuroanatomy and clinical neurology,* ed 3, Philadelphia, 2009, Saunders.)

and the toe-pinch withdrawal (nociceptive) reflex, as well as the proprioceptive positioning reaction, fail to occur because the motor neuron portion of the arc that activates the skeletal muscle is gone.

- *Electromyographic changes.* Within a few days of damage to α motor neurons, abnormal electrical activity of the muscle can be observed on an electromyogram (see Chapter 6).

Damage of α motor neurons occurs often on insult to a peripheral nerve that also contains axons of sensory neurons. Therefore, there may be an accompanying loss of sensory modalities, although this is not a cardinal sign of lower motor neuron damage.

Upper Motor Neurons Lie Completely in the Central Nervous System and Control Lower Motor Neurons

Upper motor neurons are the neurons of the CNS that influence the lower motor neurons. They are typically considered the neurons of origin of the corticospinal (cerebral cortex to spinal cord), corticobulbar (cerebral cortex to brainstem), and descending brainstem motor (brainstem to spinal cord; also called bulbospinal) pathways (see Chapter 10). Upper motor neurons send

axons down to the spinal cord or into the brainstem to control the lower motor neurons (see Figure 9-1).

Signs of Upper Motor Neuron Disease Differ from Signs of Lower Motor Neuron Disease

Lesions of upper motor neurons cause clinical signs that differ significantly from those produced by lower motor neuron disease, although paralysis/paresis may be seen in both scenarios.

- *Inappropriate movement.* Lesions of upper motor neurons can cause a variety of movement disorders, depending on the location of the lesion. Spinal cord disease, affecting portions of upper motor neurons projecting to the cord, often causes various degrees of weakness below the lesion. Disease of the brain that affects upper motor neurons may cause rigidity, seizures, circling gaits, and other inappropriate movements. More specific examples of this general category are presented in Chapters 10, 11, and 12 on the central control of movement, the vestibular system, and the cerebellum, respectively.
- *No atrophy.* Because the lower motor neuron is intact, the muscle does not atrophy. (Modest disuse atrophy may develop much later.)
- *Retained but exaggerated segmental reflexes.* Because the neuronal circuitry of the segmental reflex arc (see Chapter 7) is not interrupted in upper motor neuron disease, reflexes such as the muscle stretch and toe-pinch withdrawal are retained, whereas in lower motor neuron disease, reflexes are depressed or lost. Because upper motor neurons are normally capable of exerting significant inhibitory control over spinal reflexes, however, damage to these neurons can decrease this inhibition, resulting in exaggeration of the reflex response *(hyperreflexia).*

- *Normal electromyogram.* Because the muscle is not atrophied and the lower motor neurons are intact, the electrical activity of the muscle appears normal.

The following clinical correlations illustrate common examples of lower and upper motor neuron disease. Before going to Chapter 10, the reader should understand these concepts and why these dogs have the clinical signs mentioned.

CLINICAL CORRELATIONS

LOWER MOTOR NEURON DISEASE

History. A 2-year-old male German short-haired pointer was admitted to the local veterinary clinic. His vaccinations were current, and the dog had no history of contributing prior illness.

A few days before admission, the dog had a fight with a skunk. For 48 hours before admission, an ascending paralysis developed characterized initially by weakness and then by lack of voluntary movement of first the back legs and then the front legs. No barking was noticed during the illness. The dog was able to control his bladder and bowel and could move his head.

Clinical Examination. On admission, the dog was unable to bear weight on any of his four legs. Other than an elevated respiratory rate, physical examination deficits were limited to the nervous system. The dog was able to eat, drink, and move his head. A severe paralysis was noted in all legs, and no motor response to a toe pinch or tapping of the quadriceps tendon could be elicited. There was widespread atrophy of the muscles of all four legs, as well as those of the thorax and abdomen. The dog did seem to be aware of painful stimuli (deep pain response). There were no cranial nerve deficits. Results of routine blood cell counts and serum chemistry results were within normal limits.

Comment. Generalized atrophy, paralysis, and loss of segmental reflexes indicate widespread, bilateral loss of lower motor neuron function. Fortunately, the disease has spared the muscles of the head and the diaphragm, although the dog's elevated respiratory rate indicates an attempt to compensate for paralysis of some of the respiratory muscles. A clinical diagnosis of *polyradiculoneuritis* (coonhound paralysis) was made. This disease is often preceded by the bite of another animal. Pathological changes are found predominantly in the ventral roots of the spinal cord, where the axons of the lower motor neurons leave the spinal cord. The dorsal roots are usually spared, which explains this dog's apparent ability to feel pain. The clinical signs are those of widespread lower motor neuron disease. The syndrome resembles Guillain-Barré syndrome in humans, and both syndromes have been suggested to be auto-immune in origin.

Treatment. Animals with this form of paralysis usually recover spontaneously. Good nursing care is essential during the illness. A respirator may be necessary temporarily if respiratory paralysis occurs.

UPPER MOTOR NEURON DISEASE

History. A 5-year-old male dachshund is brought to a local veterinary clinic. His vaccination history is current, and the dog has had no contributing past medical or surgical illnesses. Two days before admission, he seemed to be in pain. Throughout the next day the dog became progressively weak in the hind legs.

Clinical Examination. Physical examination abnormalities were limited to the nervous system. The dog was bright, alert, responsive, and able to bear weight normally on the front legs. However, he was weak and unsteady on the hind legs. No atrophy was apparent. All cranial nerve reflexes were normal, as were the spinal segmental reflexes of both front and hind legs. Intersegmental responses, including the proprioceptive positioning reaction, were normal in the front legs but absent in the hind legs (see Chapter 7). Results of a complete blood cell count and serum chemistry analysis were within normal limits.

Comment. Failure to exhibit the normal proprioceptive placing reaction of a paw indicates a lesion somewhere along the sensory or motor routing for this response. This routing includes the peripheral nerves for that limb, the spinal cord rostral to that limb on the same side, and the contralateral side of the brain. However, the absence of atrophy and the retention of segmental reflexes in the affected limbs indicate that the lower motor neurons, neuromuscular junction, and skeletal muscle are normal and that this is an upper motor neuron disease. Because only the hind limbs are affected by weakness and exhibit a deficit in proprioceptive placing, the cervical spinal cord and brain must be normal because motor commands to the front legs are transmitted reliably. Therefore the lesion must be between the front and hind limbs. This is a typical history and a typical clinical presentation for a dog with a *herniated intervertebral disk.*

Treatment. Treatment and prognosis depend on the severity of the spinal cord trauma. Medical management is aimed at reducing edema, vasospasm, inflammation, and other metabolic consequences of the disease that worsen the damage to the spinal cord. When surgery is indicated by the severity of the trauma, the goal is to relieve spinal cord compression. With appropriate medical and surgical management, many dogs recover useful spinal function.

Acknowledgment

The authors thank Dr. Karen Inzana for her thoughtful comments on material in this chapter.

PRACTICE QUESTIONS

1. Which of the following would *not* be considered an upper motor neuron?
   a. Bulbospinal motor neurons
   b. Corticospinal motor neurons
   c. Ventral horn α motor neurons of the spinal cord
   d. Corticobulbar motor neurons

2. You examine a dog that is unable to stand and bear weight on the right rear leg. The right rear leg is much smaller in diameter than the left rear leg. Pinching the toe on the left rear leg results in withdrawal of the left rear leg, but pinching the toe on the right rear leg results in no movement of the right rear leg. The proprioceptive placing response in the left rear leg is normal, but in the right rear leg it is absent. Where is this dog's pathological lesion?
   a. Lower motor neuron to the right rear leg
   b. Lower motor neuron to the left rear leg
   c. Upper motor neuron controlling the right rear leg
   d. Upper motor neuron controlling the left rear leg
   e. Neuromuscular synapse of the left rear leg

3. You examine a dog that is bright, alert, and responsive. She can stand and bear weight on both front legs, but she cannot stand or bear any weight on the back legs. Her knee jerk and toe-pinch withdrawal reflexes are normal in all four legs. There is no atrophy. The proprioceptive positioning response is normal in the front legs but absent in both rear legs. Injecting acetylcholinesterase-inhibiting drugs causes no change in the clinical signs. Where is this dog's pathological lesion most likely located?
   a. Neuromuscular junction
   b. Cervical spinal cord (spinal cord of the neck)
   c. Spinal cord between the front and rear legs (thoracolumbar spinal cord)
   d. Lower motor neurons to the rear legs
   e. Brainstem

4. You examine a dog that is bright, alert, and responsive but unable to stand on any of the four legs. Toe-pinch and knee jerk local (segmental) reflexes are normal in all four legs. There is no atrophy. The proprioceptive positioning response is absent in all four legs. Injecting an acetylcholinesterase-inhibiting drug does not change the clinical signs. Where is this dog's pathological lesion most likely located?
   a. Cervical spinal cord (spinal cord in the neck)
   b. Spinal cord between the front and rear legs (thoracolumbar spinal cord)
   c. Lower motor neurons to all four legs
   d. Neuromuscular junction

5. You are presented with a horse that is unable to stand or support any weight on the hind legs. You electrically stimulate both the sciatic and the femoral nerves with a sufficient stimulus, but neither stimulation results in muscular contraction. However, direct stimulation of both the gastrocnemius and the quadriceps femoris muscles of the rear leg results in muscular contraction. From these observations, what do you logically conclude to be the location of this horse's pathological lesion?
   a. Upper motor neurons controlling the rear legs
   b. Lower motor neurons to the rear legs
   c. Neuromuscular synapses of the rear legs
   d. Muscles of the rear legs
   e. Either b or c

6. You examine a cat that cannot bear weight on the hind legs. The cat is bright, alert, and responsive. Atrophy is present in the back legs. Cranial nerve reflexes are within normal limits, as are segmental reflexes and the proprioceptive positioning responses of the front legs. Knee jerk and toe-pinch withdrawal reflexes are absent in the hind legs. What is the most likely location for this cat's pathological lesion?
   a. Brainstem
   b. Cervical spinal cord (spinal cord in the neck)
   c. Thoracolumbar spinal cord (spinal cord between the front and rear legs)
   d. Lower motor neurons to the front legs
   e. Lower motor neurons to the hind legs

BIBLIOGRAPHY

Agata N, Sasai N, Inoue-Miyazu M, et al: Repetitive stretch suppresses denervation-induced atrophy of soleus muscle in rats, *Muscle Nerve* 39:456–462, 2009.

Brodal P: *The central nervous system: structure and function*, ed 4, New York, 2010, Oxford University Press.

De Lahunta A, Glass E: *Veterinary anatomy and clinical neurology*, ed 3, Philadelphia, 2009, Saunders.

Dow DE, Dennis RG, Faulkner JA: Electrical stimulation attenuates denervation and age-related atrophy in extensor digitorum longus muscles of old rats, *J Gerontol A Biol Sci Med Sci* 60(4):416–424, 2005.

Jackman RW, Kandarian SC: The molecular basis of skeletal muscle atrophy, *Am J Physiol Cell Physiol* 287(4):C834–843, 2004.

Kandel ER, Schwartz JH, Jessell TM, editors: *Principles of neural science*, ed 4, New York, 2000, McGraw-Hill.

Lorenz MD, Coates JR, Kent M: *Handbook of veterinary neurology*, ed 5, Philadelphia, 2010, Saunders.

Purves D, Augustine GJ, Fitzpatrick D, et al: *Neuroscience*, ed 5, Sunderland, Mass, 2012, Sinauer.

Tisdale MJ: Is there a common mechanism linking muscle wasting in various disease types? *Curr Opin Support Palliat Care* 1(4):287–292, 2007.

CHAPTER 10
The Central Control of Movement

KEY POINTS

1. The central nervous system structures that control movement have a hierarchical organization.
2. The spinal cord is the most caudal and simplest level of the movement control hierarchy.
3. Brainstem upper motor neuron pathways are the source of all descending motor system input to the spinal cord, except for one other major pathway.
4. Medial and lateral descending brainstem motor pathways respectively control proximal muscles of posture and more distal muscles of skilled movement.
5. The reticulospinal and vestibulospinal tracts are medial brainstem motor pathways important for keeping the body upright against the pull of gravity.
6. The rubrospinal tract is a lateral brainstem motor pathway that can control distal limb musculature associated with skilled movement.

7. The corticospinal (pyramidal) tract is a direct projection from cerebral cortex to spinal cord responsible for the most skilled voluntary movements of mammals.
8. The corticospinal tract has a massive lateral component controlling the distal musculature and a minor medial component controlling the axial and proximal musculature.
9. The motor cortices of the frontal lobe, the highest level of the motor control hierarchy, consist of three different functional regions.
10. Corticospinal tract co-activation of both alpha (α) and gamma (γ) lower motor neurons may help with small automatic corrections of voluntary movements.
11. The motor system shares some organizational principles with sensory systems.
12. The basal ganglia and cerebellum modulate the activity of motor system components for the respective selection and adjustment of movement.

Unlike the sensory systems, most of which transform physical energy into neural information, the motor system transforms neural information into physical energy. All movement is the result of the contraction of varying numbers of extrafusal skeletal muscle fibers within varying numbers of motor units (see Figure 6-8). These extrafusal muscle fibers do not contract until commanded to do so by the alpha (α) lower motor neuron. The α motor neuron, in turn, does not send such an action potential command until signaled to do so by descending upper motor neurons (see Figure 9-1) or from incoming sensory neurons (or interneurons) in a reflex arc.

Movement can be divided into two general forms. The first is a largely learned, voluntary, conscious, and skilled form, often dominated by flexor muscle activation. The second form is characterized by postural, antigravity muscle activity that is generally subconscious, involuntary, and dominated by extensor muscle contraction. The skilled movement results from fairly discrete contraction of a few muscle groups, many of which are distal to the spinal column. The maintenance of posture often includes longer-term contraction of larger groups of muscles, many of which are located closer (proximal) to the spinal column. Correspondingly, in the spinal cord gray matter, the α motor neurons that control the more distal muscles tend to be located laterally; those controlling the more proximal and axial muscles for posture are located more medially.

Initiating the learned, skilled, voluntary movement of the distal musculature is largely the responsibility of a subgroup of upper motor neuron tracts that project through more lateral regions of the spinal cord white matter and terminate in lateral regions of the spinal cord gray matter. Initiating antigravity and postural muscle activity is the responsibility of upper motor neuron tracts that are associated with more medial regions of the spinal cord white and gray matter, respectively. This lateral-medial distinction is a significant organizational principle in central nervous system (CNS) motor control. Skilled, voluntary movement of the distal musculature is primarily controlled by a lateral system of lower motor neurons and upper motor neuron spinal tracts. More medial systems of such neurons and tracts primarily control postural and antigravity activity of the proximal and axial musculature.

The Central Nervous System Structures That Control Movement Have a Hierarchical Organization

Another organizational principle of the neural control of movement is that it consists of a hierarchy. Generally, simpler movements or movement patterns are organized by more caudal parts of the CNS (Figure 10-1, *bottom portions*), and more complex and skilled patterns are organized by progressively more rostral regions (see Figure 10-1, *top portions*).

The Spinal Cord Is the Most Caudal and Simplest Level of the Movement Control Hierarchy

The spinal cord contains the lower motor neurons that synapse upon the muscles of the trunk and limbs (see Figure 10-1). As noted in Chapter 6, an α lower motor neuron innervates several extrafusal muscle fibers of a single muscle, forming a *motor unit* (see Figure 6-8). The neuronal cell bodies of the motor units of a given muscle are clustered into a *motor neuron pool* located in the ventral horn of spinal cord gray matter. The motor neuron pool of a muscle has a cigar-shaped, longitudinal organization in the cord, often extending rostrocaudally over a few spinal cord segments (e.g., L1-L3; Figure 10-2). These motor neuron pools have a *somatotopic organization* in the ventral horn; that is, their relative position in the CNS corresponds to the relative body position of the muscles that their neurons innervate. In other words, motor neuron pools whose neurons innervate distal muscles of the limbs tend to be located in more lateral parts of the ventral horn, whereas motor neuron pools associated with axial and proximal musculature tend to be located more medially within the ventral horn.

Lower motor neurons projecting out to muscles are often synaptically activated by *premotor neurons* whose cell bodies are usually located in the intermediate zone of spinal cord gray matter (see Figure 10-2). Activating a premotor neuron in the *lateral* part of the intermediate zone on one side of the body will generally activate a modest number of α motor neurons, in the *lateral* part of the ventral horn, on the same side of the body. This

in turn will result in the activation of a modest number of *distal* limb muscles that would generally be used for skilled, voluntary movement. Premotor neuron activation in the *medial* part of the intermediate zone on one side of the body will generally activate a larger number of α motor neurons, in the *medial* part of the ventral horn, often on both sides of the body and often over more than one spinal cord segment. This in turn will result in the extensive activation of *axial* or *proximal* antigravity muscles on both sides of the body. Such a complement of muscles would be required for the involuntary stabilization or adjustment of posture. It can therefore be seen that more lateral parts of the spinal cord gray matter are involved in control of the distal limb musculature of skilled voluntary movement, whereas more medial parts are associated with the axial and proximal musculature of postural control.

The simplest type of motor behavior, the spinal segmental reflex (e.g., the knee jerk reflex; see Chapter 7), can be organized at the level of the spinal cord, without significant control from more rostral divisions of the CNS (e.g., the brain). However, although control from the brain may not be *necessary* for such behaviors, these simple reflexes can often still be influenced by brain input. Furthermore, under different circumstances, the same spinal premotor and α motor neurons that participate in a simple spinal reflex could be activated by the brain to participate in an elegant and skilled sequence of movement.

Brainstem Upper Motor Neuron Pathways Are the Source of All Descending Motor System Input to the Spinal Cord, Except for One Other Major Pathway

Four major axon tracts originate in the brainstem and descend to the spinal cord to influence spinal lower motor neurons: the *vestibulospinal tract,* the *reticulospinal tract,* the *tectospinal tract,* and the *rubrospinal tract* (Figure 10-3). Collectively, the first three are involved in the involuntary maintenance and adjustment of posture and in reflex orientation of the head. Therefore they are principally involved in the control of axial and proximal musculature. The rubrospinal tract is mainly involved in control of distal limb musculature of the type that mediates voluntary skilled movements. These four tracts (often along with components of the basal ganglia and cerebellum) are sometimes referred to as the *extrapyramidal* motor system. This is in contrast to the *pyramidal* motor system that originates in the cerebral cortex, the other major descending motor pathway to the spinal cord, as discussed later. Because the term *extrapyramidal* can encompass

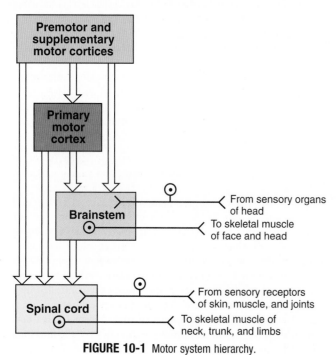

FIGURE 10-1 Motor system hierarchy.

FIGURE 10-2 Somatotopic organization of lower motor neurons in the ventral horn of the spinal cord that respectively supply the distal and axial/proximal musculature. Cell bodies of motor units supplying a given muscle are arranged in longitudinal columns within the ventral horn called *motor neuron pools.* Motor neuron pools to more distal muscles lie laterally to those supplying the axial and proximal musculature. Spinal premotor neurons, which synapse on the motor neurons supplying muscles, are located in the intermediate zone of spinal cord gray matter and also have a somatotopic organization. (Modified from Kandel ER, Schwartz JH, Jessell TM: *Principles of neural science,* ed 3, New York, 1991, Elsevier Science Publishing.)

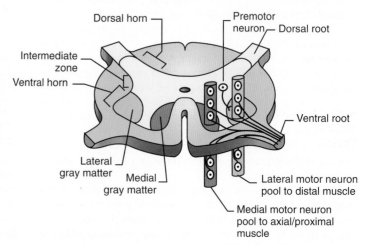

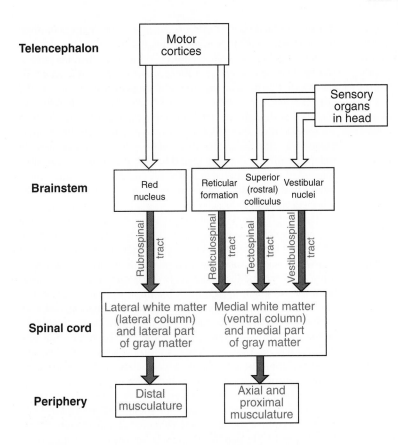

FIGURE 10-3 Organization of the descending brainstem motor pathways to the spinal cord. The medial brainstem motor pathways are the reticulospinal, vestibulospinal, and tectospinal tracts *(labeled red arrows)*. They travel in more medial regions of the spinal cord white matter and synapse within more medial regions of the spinal cord gray matter controlling the axial and proximal musculature. The rubrospinal tract *(labeled green arrow)* is a lateral brainstem motor pathway that travels in more lateral regions of the spinal white matter and synapses within more lateral regions of the spinal gray matter controlling the distal limb musculature. Crossing of some of the pathways is not represented.

such a diverse group of structures, and because it is often applied inconsistently, it is being used less frequently. The four tracts from brainstem to spinal cord are collectively referred to here as the *descending brainstem motor pathways.*

The brainstem, like the spinal cord, contains lower motor neurons that can synaptically activate skeletal muscles, in this case the face and head muscles (see Figure 10-1). The cell bodies of these α motor neurons reside in various cranial nerve nuclei (e.g., facial motor, hypoglossal, oculomotor). The brainstem also receives direct input from sensory organs in the face and head (e.g., eye, vestibular apparatus). Therefore, as in the spinal cord, some fairly simple segmental reflexes can be organized at the brainstem level without the necessity of significant control from other levels of the motor system. Because the brainstem also contains the descending motor pathways to the spinal cord previously noted, however, the brainstem also provides a means by which input from sensory organs in the face and head can reach and control lower motor neurons of the spinal cord that operate muscles of the trunk and limbs (see Figure 10-3). Some of the descending brainstem motor pathways also provide a means by which more rostral regions of the motor system (e.g., motor cortex) can indirectly influence spinal lower motor neurons.

Medial and Lateral Descending Brainstem Motor Pathways Respectively Control Proximal Muscles of Posture and More Distal Muscles of Skilled Movement

The descending brainstem motor pathways to the spinal cord can be divided into a medial group and a lateral pathway. The vestibulospinal, reticulospinal, and tectospinal tracts constitute the *medial brainstem motor pathways,* whereas the rubrospinal tract represents *the lateral brainstem motor pathway* (see Figure 10-3). The groupings are generally based on the relative position of

these tracts within the spinal cord white matter. The axons of the tracts that represent the medial brainstem motor pathways (vestibulospinal, reticulospinal, tectospinal) will mainly travel in more medial regions of the spinal cord white matter (e.g., ventral column) and will synapse within more medial regions of the spinal cord gray matter. Those medial regions of the spinal gray matter contain medial premotor neurons and medial α motor neurons that control the axial and proximal extensor musculature primarily involved in involuntary maintenance and adjustment of posture. Axons of the lateral brainstem motor pathway (rubrospinal) run in a more lateral region of the spinal white matter (lateral column) and synapse in the more lateral spinal gray matter. The premotor and α motor neurons of this region principally control the distal flexor musculature involved in voluntary skilled movement.

Thus, medial brainstem motor pathways project to medial regions of the spinal cord gray matter whose neurons control the more medially located (axial and proximal) extensor muscles of posture, whereas the lateral brainstem motor pathway projects to lateral regions of the spinal gray matter whose neurons control the more laterally located (distal) flexor muscles of skilled movement.

The Reticulospinal and Vestibulospinal Tracts Are Medial Brainstem Motor Pathways Important for Keeping the Body Upright Against the Pull of Gravity

A major responsibility of the medial descending brainstem motor pathways is to maintain the body subconsciously in an upright position against the pull of gravity. The reticulospinal and vestibulospinal tracts play a major role in this involuntary control of the axial and proximal extensor musculature that prevents the animal from falling to the ground. The reticulospinal tract is particularly important in controlling the magnitude of the steady-state contraction level, or *muscle tone,* of these antigravity muscles. The vestibulospinal tract plays an essential role in activating the antigravity muscles in response to destabilization of the body with respect to gravity. Keep in mind that subconscious control of the postural musculature is an integral part of the ability to execute skilled voluntary movement of the distal musculature successfully, because voluntary movement requires a stable platform on which it can proceed.

The reticulospinal tract originates from cell bodies in the *reticular formation* of the brainstem (see Figure 10-3). This is a netlike complex of many small clusters of cell bodies (nuclei) and loosely organized axonal projections, located near the midline. Once thought to be a diffuse and fairly nonspecific system, the reticular formation is now known to contain a number of functionally specific nuclei. In addition to being the origin of a medial descending brainstem motor pathway to the spinal cord, ascending projections of the reticular formation play an important role in modulating consciousness, arousal, and attention. The reticular formation receives a vast array of sensory information and plays an important role in pain perception, respiration, and circulatory function.

Axons of the reticulospinal tract synapse within medial regions of the spinal cord gray matter that primarily control the axial and proximal extensor musculature (see Figure 10-3). Collectively, the tract projects to virtually all rostrocaudal levels of the cord. Portions of the reticulospinal tract that originate from cells in reticular nuclei of the *pons* tend to have an *excitatory* effect on lower motor neurons to the antigravity muscles. Portions of the tract coming from the reticular nuclei of the *medulla* tend to have an *inhibitory* effect on the lower motor neurons to antigravity muscles. These opposing portions of the reticulospinal tract interact to regulate antigravity muscle tone. Influences from other regions of the brainstem, the cerebellum, and the spinal cord endow the pontine reticular nuclei with a high level of spontaneous activity. The effects of such spontaneous excitatory activity on antigravity muscle tone can be tempered by activation of the inhibitory medullary reticular nuclei. Descending projections from the cerebral cortex to the brainstem represent a significant forebrain source of relative control over the two portions of the reticulospinal tract. This cortico-reticulospinal route emphasizes the point that some of the descending brainstem motor pathways provide an indirect way for more rostral levels of the motor system hierarchy to influence spinal lower motor neurons (see Figure 10-3).

The descending cortical projections to the origins of the reticulospinal tract endow that tract with two important motor functions, in addition to its critical role in the subconscious modulation of antigravity muscle tone. The first function is related to skilled voluntary movement requiring a stable postural background, as previously noted. Just *before* the execution of such a voluntary movement, the reticulospinal tract *subconsciously* activates the appropriate axial and proximal musculature that will compensate for the postural destabilization that will be produced by the intended voluntary movement (usually of the distal musculature). The reticulospinal tract also plays a role in the voluntary execution of crude (nonskilled), often stereotypical movements of the proximal limb musculature, such as those involved in simple pointing or locomotion.

As noted in Chapter 8, γ motor neurons are usually activated along with α motor neurons so that muscle spindles maintain their sensitivity to stretch even when the muscle is shortened during contraction. This α-γ *co-activation* is a principle common to the excitation of lower motor neurons by upper motor neurons. Under certain circumstances, however, it appears that this process can be dissociated, such that the γ motor neuron–mediated sensitivity of the muscle spindle, and thus the sensitivity of the stretch reflex, can be adjusted apart from extrafusal muscle contraction. Although the reticulospinal tract participates in α-γ co-activation of lower motor neurons, it appears to be strongly associated with the ability to regulate γ motor neuron activity independently. It is likely that this ability of the reticulospinal tract to modulate independently the sensitivity of the stretch reflex underlies its significant role in adjusting antigravity muscle tone.

The vestibulospinal tract originates from cell bodies in the *vestibular nuclear complex,* which lies primarily in the medulla, just ventral to the fourth ventricle (see Figure 11-8). This complex consists of several subnuclei that receive their principal synaptic input from the eighth cranial nerve fibers carrying sensory input from the vestibular apparatus of the inner ear (see Chapter 11). The vestibular apparatus provides sensory information about the position of the head with respect to gravity and about acceleration of the head through space, thus indicating body position and disturbances of balance. The vestibular nuclear complex also receives significant input from the cerebellum, but not from forebrain levels of the motor system hierarchy.

As in the reticulospinal tract, axons of the vestibulospinal tract synapse within medial regions of the spinal cord gray matter that primarily control the axial and proximal extensor musculature (see Figure 10-3). Also like the reticulospinal tract, vestibulospinal tract axons collectively project to virtually all rostrocaudal levels of the spinal cord. When the vestibular apparatus detects a disturbance of balance, it excites the antigravity musculature in an attempt to counteract the disturbance. Although the vestibulospinal tract principally functions to produce compensatory adjustments to postural disturbances, it seems to make some contribution to antigravity muscle tone as well.

Some aspects of the functions of these two descending brainstem motor pathways can be better understood by considering the clinical state called *decerebrate rigidity.* This condition occasionally results from severe forebrain disease. It also results from surgical transection of the brain at the rostral midbrain level, as discovered by the British neurophysiologist Charles Sherrington. As noted earlier, the portion of the reticulospinal tract originating in the pons, which excites lower motor neurons to antigravity muscles, has a high degree of spontaneous activity. Excitation of the portion of the reticulospinal tract originating in the medulla inhibits the lower motor neurons to antigravity muscles. When the forebrain is disconnected from the brainstem, descending projections from cerebral cortex cannot excite these medullary reticular neurons projecting to the spinal cord, and thus a significant source of inhibition to the lower motor neurons of antigravity muscles is removed. The excitation of the lower motor neurons produced by the spontaneous activity of the pontine reticulospinal neurons has now lost a significant source of opposition, and therefore much greater muscle tone exists in the antigravity muscles. The animal now assumes a hobbyhorse-like posture, often so rigid that the animal stands in a fixed position. Subsequently cutting a portion of the vestibulospinal tract reduces some of this rigidity, so the tract apparently plays some normal role in regulating antigravity muscle tone, in addition to its principal role in responding to postural destabilization with respect to gravity.

As noted, the reticulospinal and vestibulospinal tracts make important contributions to the control of the axial and proximal musculature to keep the body upright. However, the to-and-fro rhythmicity of walking and running is organized by circuits of spinal interneurons that control the lower motor neurons in a repetitive, oscillating manner. Although these spinal neural networks are capable of producing this simple oscillatory behavior without control by more rostral parts of the motor system hierarchy, the reticulospinal tract plays an important role in initiating this locomotor behavior and in controlling its speed.

The *tectospinal tract* is a medial brainstem motor pathway that is principally involved in reflex orientation of the head toward environmental stimuli. The cells of origin of the tectospinal tract are located in the superior colliculus of the midbrain (often called *rostral colliculus* in quadrupeds; see Figure 10-3). Like the other two medial brainstem motor pathways to the spinal cord, the tectospinal tract axons synapse within medial regions of the spinal cord gray matter that primarily control the axial and proximal musculature. However, these axons only project as far as the upper cervical regions of the cord. This is consistent because the tectospinal tract principally controls the musculature that moves the head. The superior colliculus processes visual, auditory, and somatosensory information about the relative position of stimuli in the environment with respect to the organism. The superior colliculus can also control rapid reflex movements (saccades) of the eyes to the stimulus. The tectospinal tract is involved in producing a movement of the head toward the stimulus that corresponds with the rapid eye movement so that the animal's gaze is fixated directly on the stimulus.

The Rubrospinal Tract Is a Lateral Brainstem Motor Pathway That Can Control Distal Limb Musculature Associated with Skilled Movement

As noted, the reticulospinal, vestibulospinal, and tectospinal tracts are medial descending brainstem motor pathways whose axons run rostrocaudally mainly within more medial portions of the spinal white matter and synapse in more medial portions of the spinal gray matter. This region of the spinal gray matter exerts extensive, often bilateral control of the axial and proximal musculature involved in postural control and head orientation. In contrast, the *rubrospinal tract* is a lateral descending brainstem motor pathway whose axons course within more lateral regions of the spinal white matter and synapse in more lateral portions of the spinal gray matter (see Figure 10-3). This region of the spinal gray matter exerts unilateral control over a limited complement of muscles of the distal limbs, often flexors, associated with skilled movements of the extremities.

The rubrospinal tract axons originate in cells of the *red nucleus* (nucleus ruber) of the mesencephalon. The red nucleus receives a very significant descending input from higher levels of the motor system hierarchy in the cerebral cortex. This cortico-rubrospinal route provides a means for the motor cortices to influence indirectly the spinal lower motor neurons that operate the distal limb flexor musculature. Therefore the cortico-rubrospinal route is involved in the voluntary control of musculature that participates in skilled, often manipulative movements of the extremities (although not in the most dexterous movements of the digits). The rubrospinal tract is more important for these types of movements in quadrupeds compared with primates. In primates, direct projections from motor cortices to the spinal cord (the corticospinal tract, described next) are more important than the rubrospinal tract in the control of voluntary

skilled movement of the extremities. As for most nuclei giving rise to tracts that play a direct role in movement, the red nucleus also receives a significant input from the cerebellum. The role of the cerebellum in motor control is briefly described later and in more detail in Chapter 12.

The Corticospinal (Pyramidal) Tract Is a Direct Projection from Cerebral Cortex to Spinal Cord Responsible for the Most Skilled Voluntary Movements of Mammals

The motor cortices of the forebrain constitute the portion of the motor system hierarchy above that of the brainstem and represent the most complex level. As mentioned earlier, these cortical regions are collectively capable of operating spinal lower motor neurons indirectly through some of the descending brainstem motor pathways to the spinal cord (e.g., cortico-reticulospinal route, cortico-rubrospinal route). In mammals a more efficient system exists for the cortical control of spinal lower motor neurons: a direct projection from cells in the motor cortices to the gray matter of the spinal cord. This direct *corticospinal tract,* also referred to as the *pyramidal tract,* is responsible for the most elaborate and dexterous voluntary movement sequences of which mammals are capable, especially movements involving the extremities. However, this tract also participates in less elaborate voluntary movements of the distal musculature and can exert some voluntary control over the postural muscles as well.

The Corticospinal Tract Has a Massive Lateral Component Controlling the Distal Musculature and a Minor Medial Component Controlling the Axial and Proximal Musculature

The corticospinal tract axons primarily originate from cells located in the motor cortices of the frontal lobe of the cerebral hemisphere (Figure 10-4). All cells contributing to the tract are located in layer 5 of the six histological layers of cortical tissue (see Figure 16-1). Along their route from the cerebral cortex, these corticospinal axons pass through the internal capsule of the forebrain, the cerebral peduncles on the ventral surface of the midbrain, and the pontine nuclei within the ventral pons. They emerge on the ventral surface of the medulla, adjacent to the midline, as the pyramids. These appear pyramid-shaped in cross section, partly inspiring the name *pyramidal tract* for axons that pass through them.

As the corticospinal tract axons reach the spinomedullary border, the vast majority (75% in canine to 90% in primates) cross the midline at a structure called the *pyramidal decussation* (see Figure 10-4). The crossing axons then form the *lateral corticospinal tract,* located in the lateral spinal cord white matter, and synapse within lateral regions of the spinal cord gray matter (Figure 10-5). As noted earlier, the lateral regions of the spinal gray matter contain premotor and α motor neurons that primarily control the distal flexor musculature of the extremities that participate in skilled, manipulative, usually voluntary movements. Given this organization, damage to the motor cortices on one side of the body has devastating effects on voluntary skilled movement of the distal flexor musculature on the opposite side of the body. A much smaller percentage of axons traveling in the medullary pyramid do not cross the midline at the pyramidal decussation and remain on the same side of the body to form the much smaller *ventral corticospinal tract* (see Figure 10-4). The axons of this tract are located in more medial regions of the spinal white matter and synapse in more medial regions of the spinal gray matter that control the axial and proximal postural

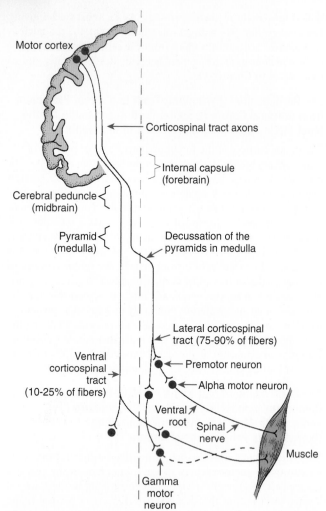

FIGURE 10-4 The corticospinal tract is a direct route primarily from the motor cortices to the contralateral spinal cord gray matter. Most axons of the tract synapse on premotor neurons of the intermediate zone, but some, depending on species phylogeny, synapse directly on α and γ lower motor neurons. About 75% to 90% (again depending upon phylogeny) of the axons of the tract cross the midline at the spinomedullary border to form the lateral corticospinal tract, and about 10% to 25% remain on the same side to form the ventral corticospinal tract. Some prominent anatomical structures formed by corticospinal tract axons within the brain, and their locations, are also indicated.

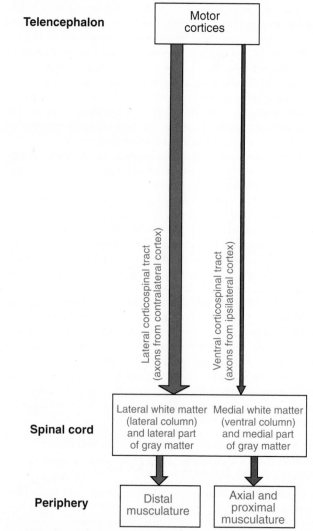

FIGURE 10-5 Somatotopic relationship of corticospinal tract components. Like the descending brainstem motor pathways, the corticospinal tract can be divided into components that respectively travel in more lateral or more medial regions of the spinal cord white matter. The massive and laterally located lateral corticospinal tract synapses in more lateral regions of the spinal cord gray matter that control the distal limb musculature. The axons of this tract originate from the contralateral motor cortices. The much smaller ventral corticospinal tract, whose axons originate from the ipsilateral motor cortices, travels in more medial regions of the spinal white matter and synapses in more medial regions of the spinal gray matter that control the axial and proximal musculature.

musculature (see Figure 10-5). Many axons of the ventral corticospinal tract actually cross the midline, locally, just before synapsing in the spinal gray matter. The ventral corticospinal tract provides a direct means of voluntary control over muscles that are normally involved in a subconscious antigravity function.

The ability of the corticospinal tract to control the most dexterous, skilled movements of the body derives from the synaptic termination pattern of several of its axons. The greater the number of synapses between a neuron in the motor cortices and an α motor neuron in the spinal cord ventral horn, the greater is the number of α motor neurons activated and the less precise the control of the musculature. This is true because each neuron that is excited in the pathway usually activates several postsynaptic neurons. Corticospinal axons bypass synapsing with neurons of the brainstem motor pathways to the cord, but more significantly, some corticospinal axons can bypass synapsing with premotor

neurons of the spinal gray matter, contacting α motor neurons directly. Therefore a given corticospinal neuron can ultimately control smaller numbers of α motor neurons and a smaller complement of the musculature. This permits increased *fractionation* of movement, the increased independence of the actions of different muscles (e.g., the ability to move individual fingers instead of all the fingers together). The proportion of corticospinal neurons making monosynaptic connections with spinal α motor neurons is related to phylogeny. There are no such connections in cats, a small proportion in monkeys, a larger proportion in the anthropoid apes, and a still larger proportion in humans, where the most skilled, fractionated, manipulative movements take place.

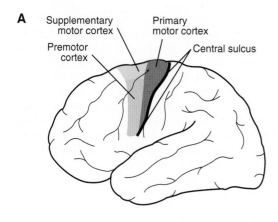

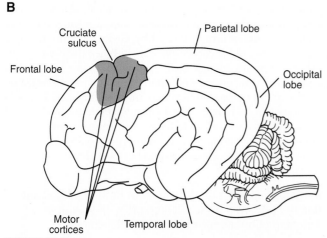

FIGURE 10-6 Motor cortices. **A,** Location of primary motor, supplementary motor, and premotor cortices in the human brain. **B,** Vicinity of the motor cortices in the canine brain.

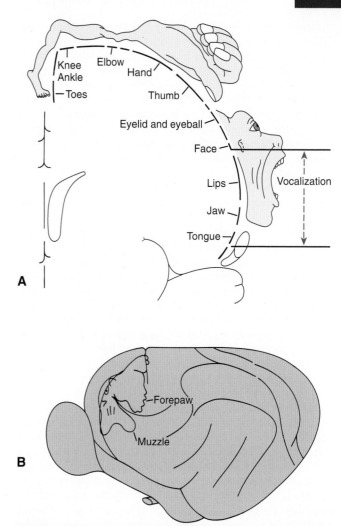

FIGURE 10-7 Somatotopic map of primary motor cortex (MI) showing the origins of axons going to the different skeletal muscles of the body. Body parts represented as proportionally larger have a larger area of MI devoted to their voluntary control, and the movement of that part will generally be that much more precise and fractionated. **A,** In the human, muscles controlling the hand/digits and mouth are disproportionately represented because these muscles are needed for the critical and precise movements of grasping/manipulation and speech. **B,** Primary motor cortex of a cat. (*A* redrawn from Penfield W, Rasmussen T: *The cerebral cortex of man,* New York, 1950, Macmillan; from Berne RM, Levy MN: *Physiology,* ed 2, St Louis, 1988, Mosby; *B* from Prosser CL: *Comparative animal physiology,* ed 3, New York, 1988, Wiley).

As noted, cranial nerve nuclei in the brainstem contain lower motor neurons that travel through cranial nerves to control muscles of the face and head (see Figure 10-1). A significant complement of the axons that leave the motor cortices to form the corticospinal tract will not continue to the spinal cord, but will leave the tract to synapse at the cranial nerve motor nuclei of the brainstem. This complement of axons is referred to as the *corticobulbar tract* ("bulb" being an archaic term for portions of the brainstem). A given cranial nerve nucleus generally receives significant corticobulbar input from both cerebral hemispheres.

The Motor Cortices of the Frontal Lobe, the Highest Level of the Motor Control Hierarchy, Consist of Three Different Functional Regions

The motor cortices of the frontal lobe, the origin of most of the corticospinal tract axons, are composed of the primary motor cortex, the supplementary motor cortex, and the premotor cortex (Figure 10-6; see also Figure 10-1). Although these forebrain regions collectively represent the highest level of the motor control hierarchy, the areas appear to differ with respect to the complexity of motor functions controlled.

In primates the *primary motor cortex* (MI) is located just rostral to the prominent central sulcus and therefore lies along the precentral gyrus (see Figure 10-6, *A*). In many nonprimate mammalian species, a central sulcus is not present and MI appears to lie near the cruciate sulcus (see Figure 10-6, *B*).

Low-level electrical stimulation of a very small region of MI is capable of activating a small number of functionally related muscles. Furthermore, an orderly relationship exists between the region of the body where the muscles are activated and the region of MI stimulated. In this *somatotopic map* of the body musculature in MI, muscles in the caudal part of the body (or the feet in bipeds) can be most easily activated from more dorsomedial parts of MI, whereas muscles in the rostral part of the body (or head in bipeds) can be most easily activated from more ventrolateral parts of MI, with a fairly orderly representation of the other regions of the body between those parts of MI. As shown in Figure 10-7, the musculature of different parts of the body is not equally represented in the somatotopic map. Regions depicted as larger have a larger area of MI devoted to their voluntary muscular control, and thus the movements of that region will generally be that much more precise and fractionated. In the somatotopic map of MI in humans, the hand and the mouth musculatures have a very large proportional representation, reflecting the respective importance of these areas in manipulating objects with the fingers and in articulating speech. The proportional representation of the musculature of the different body parts in MI varies with phylogeny, but the somatotopic maps of the primates tend to be the most detailed, reflecting the most precise control over skilled, voluntary movements.

The *supplementary motor cortex* and the *premotor cortex* are also located in the frontal lobe, just rostral to MI, with supplementary motor cortex positioned dorsomedial to premotor cortex (see Figure 10-6, *A*). Both areas also have a somatotopic map of the body musculature, but it is less precise than in MI. In addition to corticospinal and corticobulbar tract axons, both areas also collectively give rise to axonal projections to nuclei of origin of some descending brainstem motor pathways (see Figure 10-1). Most significantly, however, the supplementary motor and premotor cortices send axons to synapse within MI and thus may represent "supramotor" areas, with an even higher status in the motor control hierarchy than MI; these areas may instruct MI to organize its fairly discrete muscle actions into more elaborate movement patterns. This concept is supported by the fact that, for voluntary movement, neurons in these supramotor areas become active before those of MI.

Evidence indicates that the supplementary motor cortex is particularly important in the *planning and organizing of complex sequences* of the discrete movements normally carried out by MI. For example, supplementary motor cortex appears to be particularly active when an individual mentally rehearses a specific sequence of finger movements. Supplementary motor cortex also appears to be important for instructing the limbs (particularly the forelimbs) on the two sides of the body to work together, simultaneously, to accomplish a task. Premotor cortex appears to play an important role in *preparatory orientation of the body* for the execution of a particular motor task. An example in primates would be rotation of the shoulders and movement of the arms toward a target that is to be manipulated by the hands. Both these areas receive integrated sensory input and visuospatial information (from the posterior parietal cortex), which most likely plays a role in their respective functions.

Using the analogy of playing the piano, we could view MI as being responsible for the simplest muscle activation necessary to press a single piano key, supplementary motor cortex as responsible for planning and organizing the sequence of such finger movements necessary to play a melody, and premotor cortex as responsible for orienting the arms and hands to the correct region of the keyboard to play the various sequences. Of course, the interaction among these areas in determining the appropriate corticospinal (and corticobulbar) tract activity necessary to produce the voluntary movement is certainly more complex than this, and the functional role of these areas in motor control, and how they work together, is still under investigation.

The severity of the deficits resulting from lesions of the corticospinal (pyramidal) system varies with the phylogenetic status of the animal. In primates, such as humans, in whom the pyramidal system is developed extensively, corticospinal tract lesions rostral to the pyramidal decussation cause a dense weakness of the contralateral side of the body. Such one-sided weakness is called *hemiparesis* and is most extensive in the hand and facial muscles (symptoms common in "stroke" in humans). These symptoms are understandable because a huge percentage of the corticospinal tract axons in primates cross the midline at the spinomedullary border (the location of the pyramidal decussation), and the hand and face have the largest proportional representation in primary motor cortex (see Figures 10-4 and 10-7).

In most veterinary species the corticospinal system is not as well developed as in humans, and supraspinal lesions of this system cause much less severe contralateral weakness and little alteration of gait. However, clinical examination can reveal more subtle deficits in voluntary movements of the contralateral limbs. An example is the *proprioceptive positioning reaction*, the ability of an animal to return its paw to a normal, pads-down posture after the clinician flexes it to make the dorsal surface touch the floor or tabletop. This response requires the animal's conscious awareness that the paw is in the flexed position (conscious proprioception) and then requires that the animal be able to respond consciously by returning the paw to its normal posture. This latter motor response in turn is affected by the integrity of the upper motor neurons of the corticospinal tract. When these corticospinal tract neurons are damaged, the animal is slow to return its paw to a normal posture. In addition, toes tend to be dragged on the ground as the leg is drawn forward in normal gait. It should be noted that such deficits could also be produced by damaged corticorubral axons (axons to the red nucleus) originating in the motor cortices. Noting these conscious positioning deficits and other subtle gait changes is important in localizing lesions within the CNS.

Corticospinal Tract Co-Activation of Both Alpha (α) and Gamma (γ) Lower Motor Neurons May Help with Small Automatic Corrections of Voluntary Movements

As noted earlier, α-γ co-activation is a principle common to the excitation of lower motor neurons by upper motor neurons. It has been suggested that such co-activation may permit the muscle spindle to function as an "automatic error correction system" when voluntary movement against a load results in a small deviation from the intended result.

As discussed in Chapter 8, the activation of γ motor neurons along with α motor neurons ensures that the intrafusal muscle fibers remain taut enough to transduce stretch even as the muscle reaches a shorter length on contraction of the extrafusal fibers. The γ motor neuron activation tightens the intrafusal fibers by causing contraction of their polar ends, resulting in adjustment of the muscle spindle sensitivity to the new length of the muscle. It is thought that the α-γ co-activation resulting from a voluntary motor command is meant to produce a contraction of intrafusal fibers that is concordant with extrafusal fiber contraction, such that the muscle spindle is made just sensitive enough to transduce stretch at the new muscle length. Under these circumstances, if the load is more than expected, the α motor neuron activity will not have produced enough extrafusal fiber contraction to shorten the muscle to the new desired length. However, the γ motor neuron activity will have produced the appropriate intrafusal fiber contraction to adjust the muscle spindle sensitivity for the new desired length. This mismatch, where the spindle sensitivity has been adjusted for the new muscle length but the extrafusal fibers have not contracted enough to reach that length, results in a stretching of the muscle spindle and activation of segmental stretch reflex mechanisms. That is, the stretching of the muscle spindle results in more excitatory postsynaptic potentials (EPSPs) on the α motor neurons to the muscle, increasing their action potential firing and increasing the extrafusal fiber contraction to assist with reaching the new desired length.

This type of error correction, in which segmental stretch reflex mechanisms help to accomplish the intended muscle shortening when the corticospinal pathway has not produced the sufficient α motor neuron activity, is called a *servo-assist function*. Thought to result from α-γ co-activation, this servo-assist function is analogous to the power steering in a car, where a compressor in the motor adds power to the driver's turning of the steering wheel when significant resistance is encountered by the tires.

The Motor System Shares Some Organizational Principles with Sensory Systems

With most of the major components and pathways of the motor system now described, it appears that the motor system shares principles of organization common to other brain systems (e.g., sensory systems). One such organizational principle is the existence of topographic maps of the body. As noted, there are organized somatotopic maps of the body's musculature in the motor cortices. Topographic organization also exists in many sensory systems, except it is the peripheral receptor surface that is topographically mapped. For example, CNS components of the somatosensory (touch) system, such as primary somatosensory cortex, contain an organized somatotopic map of the different regions of the skin surface.

Two other principles of organization shared by the motor system and sensory systems are serial and parallel processing of nervous system information. In sensory systems, *serial processing* generally refers to the passage of information from the periphery to successively more rostral regions of the nervous system, in a serial fashion. For example, in the visual system, axons of cells in the retina synapse in the lateral geniculate nucleus of the thalamus, and these thalamic neurons in turn send their axons to synapse in primary visual cortex. Often, in serial processing within the sensory systems, the information collected at successively more rostral levels of the nervous system is organized into

a more sophisticated form. Serial processing can also be observed in the motor system, although in a different direction: from more rostral regions to more caudal regions. The cortico-reticulospinal route is an example of this. However, in motor system serial processing, commands often proceed from areas with more complex organization to those with simpler organization (see Figure 10-1).

Parallel processing refers to the different pathways within a given sensory system operating in parallel, respectively, to carry qualitatively different forms of information. Again, using the somatosensory system as an example, there are separate pathways to cerebral cortex to carry information about gentle touch of the skin and about intense skin contact usually perceived as painful. In the motor system, an example of parallel processing is the respective control of the proximal antigravity musculature by one set of descending brainstem motor pathways (vestibulospinal, reticulospinal) and control of the distal flexor musculature by a different descending brainstem motor pathway (rubrospinal).

Undoubtedly, a combination of both serial and parallel processing is necessary for the integrated function of sensory as well as motor systems.

The Basal Ganglia and Cerebellum Modulate the Activity of Motor System Components for the Respective Selection and Adjustment of Movement

Portions of the motor system are important for proper motor function but do not appear to be directly involved in initiating movement. These structures—the basal ganglia and the cerebellum—serve primarily to modulate the activity of other motor system structures without directly producing movement (Figure 10-8).

The *basal ganglia* are a group of nuclei, the majority of which are deep within the cerebral hemispheres. They include the caudate nucleus and putamen (known collectively as the striatum), the globus pallidus, the substantia nigra, and the subthalamic nucleus. The internal neural circuitry of this multinuclear functional unit is extremely complex and participates in several

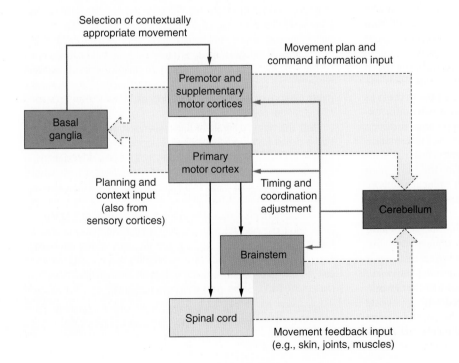

FIGURE 10-8 Modulatory roles of the cerebellum and basal ganglia in relation to the motor system hierarchy. Interposed synaptic relays are not represented.

parallel pathways running through the basal ganglia. The basal ganglia receive input from the motor cortices and many other areas of cerebral cortex and, by way of the thalamus, project output back to the motor cortices, particularly the supplementary motor and premotor cortices (see Figure 10-8). Again, these regions are important in the planning and preparation for movement. Some basal ganglia output projects directly to brainstem nuclei controlling movement.

Generally it is thought that the basal ganglia use the information received from the cortex, including information about the movement plan and the context of the situation, to *help select the appropriate movement pattern while suppressing less appropriate, competing patterns.* Two principal circuits within the basal ganglia play an important role in this process. One circuit acts to facilitate inhibitory output of the basal ganglia, presumably acting to suppress the inappropriate, competing movement pattern. The other circuit acts to reduce inhibitory output of the basal ganglia, presumably "removing the brakes" from the appropriate movement pattern. Dopamine-containing neurons that project from the substantia nigra of the basal ganglia to the striatum of the basal ganglia play an important role in regulating these two circuits. When these dopamine-containing neurons degenerate in humans with Parkinson's disease, severe motor deficits develop, such as difficulty beginning an appropriate movement, slowness of movement, rigidity, and resting tremor. Parkinson's disease does not occur naturally in veterinary species, but some toxins can selectively destroy these dopamine-projecting neurons in nonhuman species, producing some motor deficits seen in the human disease. In horses, ingestion of the yellow star thistle can produce damage of the basal ganglia. Some of the abnormal movements resulting from this damage, involving the lips and tongue of the horse, are reminiscent of such abnormal movements seen in the fingers of human patients with Parkinson's disease. Interestingly, the respective structures in the two species are both used in grasping movements.

The structure and function of the *cerebellum* and its role in motor control are discussed in Chapter 12 and are mentioned only briefly here. The cerebellum's importance in motor control is indicated by the earlier observation that virtually all the nuclei giving rise to the brainstem motor pathways receive output from the cerebellum. Also, the cerebellum indirectly receives input (through pontine nuclei) from the motor cortices (MI, supplementary motor cortex, premotor cortex). As with the basal ganglia, the cerebellum not only receives information from the motor cortices, but indirectly sends information back to them as well. Importantly, the cerebellum receives much sensory information from the skin, joints, muscles, vestibular apparatus, and even the visual system. Therefore the cerebellum receives information about the planning and initiation of movement, as well as continuous sensory feedback about the progress of the movement (see Figure 10-8). The cerebellum in turn can influence activity in the motor cortices and in the brainstem motor pathways to the spinal cord.

Through this organization, it is thought that the cerebellum acts to *compare information about the movement plan with information about how the movement is actually being carried out.* It can then presumably *make adjustments to the ongoing movement itself, or even adjust the movement plan.* Within this framework, the cerebellum appears particularly concerned with gathering sensory feedback about, and with adjusting the control of, the timing of movement. Both experimental and clinical studies have shown that cerebellar damage produces significant deficits in the coordination and smoothness of complex movements. These deficits presumably arise because of problems in the timing of muscle contraction components of the movement. If the muscle contraction components are not properly timed, the movement can appear jerky and uncoordinated, may exhibit improper force, and may not stop at the appropriate time.

CLINICAL CORRELATIONS

FOCAL LESION OF THE MOTOR CORTEX

History. You examine an 11-year-old female boxer dog. Her vaccination history is current. She had an adenocarcinoma of the mammary gland removed 6 months before your examination.

The owner states that over the past few days the dog has become progressively weaker in the left front and left rear legs and occasionally stands with the left front paw flexed such that the dorsal surface touches the ground. On the previous day the dog had a seizure.

Clinical Examination. On physical examination of the patient, you find several routine old-age changes and the results of the mammary surgery. You find also that the dog seems drowsy and is weak on the left front and left rear legs. She has a proprioceptive positioning reaction deficit of both the left front and the left rear leg. Radiographic study of the chest reveals metastatic, neoplastic lesions in the lungs.

Comment. The proprioceptive positioning reaction (or response) is tested by flexing the animal's paw, dorsal side down, while gently supporting her weight. A normal dog senses (conscious proprioception) that the paw is upside down and returns it to the normal pads-down posture (motor response). This is called a response (or reaction), rather than a reflex, because it involves a degree of conscious control. This particular response requires normal function of skin and joint receptors and the peripheral nerve in the tested leg and of the sensory neuron tracts that ascend toward the brain along the ipsilateral (same) side of the spinal cord. Traveling along a multisynaptic pathway, the sensory information crosses to the contralateral (opposite) side of the brain in the brainstem and reaches the contralateral (with respect to the side of the original stimulus) cerebral cortex. As the animal becomes consciously aware that the paw is in an unusual position, action potentials are sent back, down the corticospinal tract, to the lower motor neurons of the muscles of the leg, causing the paw to return to the normal position.

With the wiring diagram of this response in mind, you can see that a deficit in the proprioceptive positioning reaction of the left front and left rear legs could be caused by a lesion of the left cervical spinal cord, the right motor cortex, or supraspinal portions of the right corticospinal tract. This dog's seizure (a manifestation of brain disease) at about the same time suggests that the lesion is in the right cerebral cortex. The brain is a common site for metastasis, and the radiographic lung lesions suggest that the mammary tumor has spread to both the lung and the right side of the brain. The lung contains the first capillary bed that a metastatic cancer cell is likely to encounter when it enters the venous system of the mammary gland. Some cells stop here and grow.

Treatment. Dogs with metastatic mammary carcinomas are usually not treated except to make them more comfortable.

COW WITH HYPOMAGNESEMIA

History. It is May in Southwest Virginia, and a client calls you with a 2-year-old Angus (beef) cow that just calved 2 weeks ago. Early in the morning, they noticed that the cow had been acting a bit abnormal, and then she started to become agitated and hyperexcitable. Within the last 20 to 30 minutes, the cow has gone down, and appears unable to stand. The calf appears to be normal, but appears to be having difficulty nursing due to the cow's agitated state and current recumbency.

Clinical Examination. You rush there immediately, and the cow remains recumbent. She appears unable to stand, and you notice that she has nystagmus, as well as muscle spasms. The temperature, heart rate, and respiratory rate are all increased. You are suspicious that she may progress to convulsions fairly quickly if not treated appropriately.

Comment. You suspect hypomagnesemia based on clinical signs, the recent calving, and that there is lush grass, which is often high in potassium and nitrogen, but low in sodium and magnesium. The lush pasture also increases the pH of the rumen and decreases the transit time in the intestines, both of which cause decreased absorption of magnesium. Magnesium is a cofactor for a vast number of enzymatic reactions and is required for virtually all enzymatic processes involving ATP. It is therefore critical for a huge array of metabolic pathways, including controlling muscle contractions and normal nerve conduction. Thus, deficiency in magnesium limits basic metabolism and activity of the body, and depolarization of nerve and muscle cells is altered. Because both are divalent cations, calcium and magnesium often compete directly in physiological processes. Thus with hypomagnesemia, resulting increased calcium binding alters nerve and muscle activity, including neurotransmitter release and cardiac conduction. Within the central nervous system the decreased magnesium results in decreased impedance to neuronal calcium influx, and this is further exacerbated by receptor-mediated actions of the neurotransmitter glutamate. The excessive influx of calcium leads to abnormally prolonged activation of intraneuronal calcium-mediated signaling, thus causing neurotoxic damage from excessive enzyme activation that can lead to cell death. As a result, signaling from the motor cortex through the ventral and lateral corticospinal tracts, as well as the premotor neurons, α motor neurons, and the muscle, are all affected. This can account for the prominent motor signs in this cow.

Treatment. Immediate treatment with intravenous magnesium is critical. Additional magnesium supplementation is given orally to decrease chances of relapses. Treated animals should not be disturbed for at least 30 minutes. Relapses are common.

PRACTICE QUESTIONS

1. A motor neuron pool located most laterally in the ventral horn of the spinal cord is most likely to operate a muscle controlling movement of the:
   a. Proximal limb.
   b. Neck.
   c. Distal limb.
   d. Abdomen.

2. Which of the following is *true* regarding decerebrate rigidity?
   a. It can result from severe forebrain disease.
   b. Disruption of the cortical control of medullary reticulospinal neurons is a major contributor to the condition.
   c. It can result in a fixed, rigid, hobbyhorse-like posture in the quadruped.
   d. Removal of normal inhibition to some of the antigravity muscles contributes to the condition.
   e. All of the above are true.

3. Which of the following descending brainstem motor pathways controls distal limb musculature associated with skilled movement?
   a. Vestibulospinal tract
   b. Rubrospinal tract
   c. Reticulospinal tract
   d. Tectospinal tract
   e. All of the above play a major role in such control.

4. The corticospinal (pyramidal) tract, in general, initiates what form of movement?
   a. Antigravity movement
   b. Postural adjustment
   c. Skilled, voluntary, mostly flexor movement
   d. Tremulous, jerky movement
   e. None of the above

5. You are presented with a dog with a dense weakness, and proprioceptive placing reaction deficit, of his left front and left back legs. A single pathological site could cause these signs if it were located in the:
   a. Left side of the cervical spinal cord.
   b. Left cerebral cortex.
   c. Right cerebral cortex.
   d. Either a or b
   e. Either a or c

6. The corticospinal tract simultaneously co-activates both the α and the γ lower motor neurons. If the initial co-activation fails to be sufficient to cause the intended shortening of the muscle, sensory neuron activity of the muscle spindle of that muscle will have what influence on the α motor neurons to the same muscle?
   a. Addition of EPSPs
   b. Addition of IPSPs
   c. No influence
   d. Decrease in action potential frequency
   e. Either b or d

BIBLIOGRAPHY

Anderson ME, Binder MD: Spinal and supraspinal control of movement and posture. In Patton HD, Fuchs AF, Hille B, et al, editors: *Textbook of physiology*, ed 21, Philadelphia, 1989, Saunders.

Bear MF, Connors BW, Paradiso MA: *Neuroscience: exploring the brain*, ed 3, Philadelphia, 2007, Lippincott, Williams & Wilkins.

Brodal P: *The central nervous system: structure and function*, ed 4, New York, 2010, Oxford University Press.

De Lahunta A, Glass E: *Veterinary anatomy and clinical neurology*, ed 3, Philadelphia, 2009, Saunders.

Fetz EE: Motor functions of cerebral cortex. In Patton HD, Fuchs AF, Hille B, et al, editors: *Textbook of physiology*, ed 21, Philadelphia, 1989, Saunders.

Fletcher TF: Spinal cord and meninges. In Evans HE, editor: *Miller's anatomy of the dog*, ed 6, Philadelphia, 1993, Saunders.

Haines DE, editor: *Fundamental neuroscience for basic and clinical applications*, ed 3, Philadelphia, 2006, Churchill Livingstone.

Hall JE: *Guyton and Hall textbook of medical physiology*, ed 12, Philadelphia, 2011, Saunders.

Jennings DP: Supraspinal control of posture and movement. In Reece WO, editor: *Duke's physiology of domestic animals*, ed 12, Ithaca, NY, 2004, Comstock Publishing.

Lemon RN: Descending pathways in motor control, *Annu Rev Neurosci* 31:195–218, 2008.

Lorenz MD, Coates JR, Kent M: *Handbook of veterinary neurology*, ed 5, Philadelphia, 2010, Saunders.

McFarlane D: Endocrine and metabolic diseases. In Smith BP, editor: *Large animal internal medicine*, ed 4, St Louis, 2009, Mosby Elsevier.

Nicholls JG, Martin AR, Fuchs PA, et al: *From neuron to brain*, ed 5, Sunderland, Mass, 2012, Sinauer.

Purves D, Augustine GJ, Fitzpatrick D, et al: *Neuroscience*, ed 5, Sunderland, Mass, 2012, Sinauer.

Stewart AJ: Magnesium disorders. In Reed SM, Bayly WM, Sellon DC, editors: *Equine internal medicine*, ed 2, St Louis, 2004, Saunders.

CHAPTER 11

The Vestibular System

KEY POINTS

1. The vestibular system is a bilateral receptor system located in the inner ear.
2. Specialized regions of the vestibular system contain receptors.
3. The semicircular ducts detect rotary acceleration and deceleration of the head.
4. The utricle and saccule detect linear acceleration and deceleration and static tilt of the head.

5. The vestibular system provides sensory information for reflexes involving spinal motor neurons, the cerebellum, and extraocular muscles of the eye.
6. Vestibular reflexes coordinate eye and head movements to maximize visual acuity.

To coordinate posture and locomotion, the brain needs to know not only what movement it intends to command, but also the orientation of the body and what movement the body is actually performing. Chapter 8 describes the muscle spindle, an important source of information for the brain about body position and movement. Another important source of information is the vestibular system. This bilateral receptor system is located in the inner ear and informs the brain about the position and motion of the head.

The vestibular system provides the organism with its sense of equilibrium or balance. It supplies information about the body's orientation or tilt with respect to gravity and about acceleration of the body through space. It does this by detecting (1) static tilt of the head (e.g., the head is held stationary at 5 degrees from vertical), (2) linear acceleration of the head (e.g., the head accelerates in a straight line as an organism begins to run or as your elevator begins to rise), and (3) rotary acceleration of the head (e.g., the head accelerates in a circular fashion as an organism begins to turn its head toward a target or as someone begins to spin you in an office chair). This information is used most often to make automatic, unconscious postural adjustments to keep the organism from falling over as a result of self-imposed or environmentally imposed changes in body orientation. The vestibular system also helps to keep the eyes fixated on a relevant target in the face of such changes in body orientation.

The vestibular system is a common site of pathological lesions. In most veterinary species, lesions of the vestibular system cause a syndrome characterized by head tilt, compulsive rotary movements such as circling or rolling, and spontaneous nystagmus, which is an oscillating movement of the eyes.

To understand how such clinical signs arise and the importance of the vestibular system to the physiology of movement, you need to study its anatomy and function first.

The Vestibular System Is a Bilateral Receptor System Located In the Inner Ear

The inner ear, or *labyrinth,* is made up of two parts: the bony labyrinth and the membranous labyrinth. The bony labyrinth is a system of caverns and tunnels through the petrous temporal bone of the skull. The *bony labyrinth* houses the receptor organs of the vestibular system as well as the receptor organ for hearing, the *cochlea* (Figure 11-1) (see Chapter 17). These receptor organs are part of the *membranous labyrinth,* which consists of thin membranes of epithelium and lies within the bony labyrinth. This epithelial membrane is specialized at some locations to become the sensory receptor cells that form the vestibular and auditory receptor organs. The membranous labyrinth is filled with a fluid called *endolymph* and is separated from the bony labyrinth by a fluid called *perilymph.* The vestibular portion of the membranous labyrinth consists of two major sets of structures: (1) three *semicircular ducts,* located at approximately right angles to each other, and (2) a pair of saclike structures called the *utricle* and *saccule,* sometimes called the *otolith organs.* As discussed later, each major set of structures is respectively involved in transducing a different major class of vestibular stimulus.

Specialized Regions of the Vestibular System Contain Receptors

Each vestibular structure of the membranous labyrinth has a region of epithelial lining that has become specialized into a set of secondary receptor cells (see Chapter 7) called *hair cells* (Figure 11-2). These hair cells form the basis of a sensory receptor organ within each vestibular structure. Each hair cell has several cilia at its apex that are arranged in order according to size. At its base the hair cell synapses with a sensory neuron that carries action potentials to the brainstem. The cell bodies of these sensory neurons are located in Scarpa's ganglia, and their axons collectively form the vestibular portion of the vestibulocochlear nerve (cranial nerve VIII). The cilia from all the hair cells within any one vestibular structure project into a gelatinous mass; displacement of this gelatinous mass in a given direction causes all the hair cell cilia to bend in that direction.

At rest, when the cilia are not deflected, the sensory neurons that synapse with the vestibular hair cells transmit action potentials spontaneously at about 100 per second (Figure 11-3). When the hair cell cilia are bent in a direction toward the largest cilium,

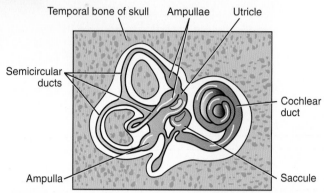

Temporal bone of skull   Ampullae   Utricle

Semicircular
ducts

Cochlear
duct

Ampulla

Saccule

FIGURE 11-1 The bilateral inner ear contains receptor systems for hearing (cochlea) and for detecting the orientation and acceleration/deceleration of the head (vestibular system). The peripheral vestibular apparatus on each side of the head contains a utricle, a saccule, and three semicircular ducts, each with an ampulla at one end.

the hair cells depolarize, the release of transmitter from the hair cells onto the sensory neurons increases, and the action potential frequency of the neurons increases. When the cilia are bent in the opposite direction, toward the smaller cilia, hair cell membranes hyperpolarize, transmitter release decreases, and the action potential frequency of sensory neurons decreases. Therefore, displacement of the hair cell cilia in either of these directions can be detected by the brain as an increase or a decrease from the resting action potential frequency. Deflections in other directions are much less effective. How the brain uses this information to detect the direction of head movement is described later.

The Semicircular Ducts Detect Rotary Acceleration and Deceleration of the Head

Three membranous semicircular ducts are located within corresponding semicircular canals of each bony labyrinth (Figure 11-4). They are positioned at approximately right angles to each other, and both ends of each fluid-filled duct terminate in the utricle. Each semicircular duct has an enlargement at one end, called the *ampulla*, near its junction with the utricle. The ampulla contains a hair cell receptor organ called the *crista ampullaris* (see Figure 11-2). This is a ridge of hair cells that, at their base, synapse on sensory neurons projecting to the central nervous system (CNS) and whose cilia are embedded in an overlying gelatinous mass. This mass, called the *cupula*, attaches to the roof of the ampulla (Figure 11-5). All hair cells of a given crista ampullaris are oriented in the same direction with respect to their cilia. Together, the hair cell ridge and overlying cupula span the diameter of the ampulla.

The semicircular ducts, together with the ampullae and its contents, are involved in transducing rotary acceleration and deceleration of the head. When the head begins to accelerate in a rotary fashion, the semicircular duct and its receptor organ rotate with the head, but the endolymph's acceleration lags behind because of inertia. This relative difference in the rate of acceleration of the semicircular duct and its enclosed endolymph causes the crista ampullaris to "crash into" the slower-moving endolymph. This results in a displacement of the gelatinous cupula in the direction opposite that of head rotation with a corresponding bending of the hair cells. This in turn changes the firing rate of the sensory neurons projecting to the CNS. The opposite happens with deceleration because the semicircular duct and

crista ampullaris slow immediately along with the head while inertia continues to carry the endolymph forward. Stimulation of the crista ampullaris occurs on rotary acceleration or deceleration of the head, not during constant rotational velocity. During the latter, the movement of the endolymph will eventually catch up with the movement of the semicircular ducts and the hair cells will no longer be bent.

Semicircular ducts located on opposite sides of the head, but in approximately the same plane (co-planar), work as a pair to provide the brain with information about the direction and nature of head movement. For instance, a clockwise rotary acceleration of the head would cause bending of the directionally sensitive hair cell cilia in each member of a co-planar pair of semicircular ducts on opposite sides of the head. However, the sensory axons leaving the crista ampullaris from the duct on one side of the head would carry an increased action potential frequency, whereas those from the duct of the other side would carry a decreased action potential frequency. The brain interprets such reciprocal changes in sensory action potential frequency as resulting from clockwise or counterclockwise acceleration or deceleration in a given plane of movement. In reality, rotary acceleration/deceleration in any given plane usually affects all three sets of paired semicircular ducts, but each pair to different degrees. In this way, the bilateral system of six semicircular ducts detects the direction of both rotary acceleration and deceleration of the head and activates or inhibits particular CNS structures to produce the appropriate reflex response.

The Utricle and Saccule Detect Linear Acceleration and Deceleration and Static Tilt of the Head

In the utricle and saccule, the hair cell receptor organ is called the *macula* (see Figure 11-2). It is an oval patch of hair cells with a primarily horizontal orientation on the floor of the utricle and a primarily vertical orientation on the wall of the saccule. The cilia of the macular hair cells extend into a gelatinous layer atop the hair cells. Embedded at the top of this gelatinous mass is a layer of calcium carbonate crystals called *otoliths*. This otolith layer is heavier and denser than the endolymph and other surrounding materials.

Given the organization of the receptor apparatus that lies within the utricle and saccule, these vestibular structures can transduce linear acceleration and deceleration of the head, as well as static head tilt (Figure 11-6). Considering the horizontally oriented macula of the utricle, if the head is accelerated forward in a straight line, movement of the dense otolith layer lags behind that of the macular hair cells. This produces a shearing force that bends the tips of the hair cell cilia, by way of the gelatinous layer, until constant velocity is achieved and the otolith layer catches up with the hair cell layer. In contrast to the crista ampullaris, not all the hair cell clusters of a given macula are oriented in the same direction with respect to their cilia (Figure 11-7). In addition, as previously noted, hair cells of the utricle are oriented in the horizontal plane, whereas those of the saccule are in the vertical plane. Therefore, linear acceleration in a specific direction will bend hair cells of a particular location and orientation in a way that will transiently increase the action potential firing rate of their associated sensory neurons; those of another location and orientation will be bent in a way that transiently decreases the firing rate; and those of yet another location and orientation will be bent in a way that has little or no effect on firing rate. This topographic pattern of hair cell bending and associated transient changes in action potential firing will be different for linear acceleration in a

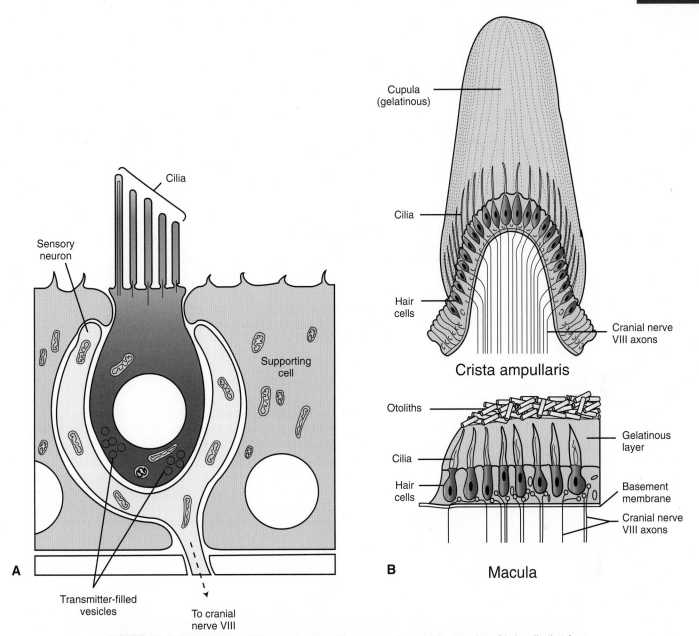

Cupula (gelatinous)

Cilia

Hair cells

Cranial nerve VIII axons

Crista ampullaris

Otoliths

Cilia

Hair cells

Gelatinous layer

Basement membrane

Cranial nerve VIII axons

B Macula

Cilia

Sensory neuron

Supporting cell

Transmitter-filled vesicles

To cranial nerve VIII

A

FIGURE 11-2 Each structure of the peripheral vestibular apparatus contains a region of hair cells that form the basis of a sensory receptor organ. **A,** Each hair cell has several cilia at its apex, arranged in size order, and synapses on a sensory neuron of cranial nerve VIII at its base. **B,** In each ampulla of the semicircular ducts, there is a crest of hair cells whose cilia project into a gelatinous mass called the *cupula,* forming a receptor organ called the *crista ampullaris.* The hair cell receptor organ in the utricle and saccule is the macula, a layer of hair cells whose cilia project up into a gelatinous layer, on top of which lies a layer of calcium carbonate crystals called otoliths.

different direction. The CNS can decipher these various patterns of neural activity to determine the onset and direction of linear acceleration and to initiate an appropriate compensatory response.

Again considering the horizontally oriented macula of the utricle, when the head tilts from the upright position, the heavy and dense otolith layer effectively "falls over" as it is pulled by gravity (see Figure 11-6, *B*). This bends the hair cell cilia, by way of the gelatinous layer, and keeps them bent as long as the head is tilted. This sustained bending (compared with the transient bending during linear acceleration) is translated into sustained changes in action potential firing frequency (compared to transient changes during linear acceleration) in particular populations of associated sensory neurons. In this way the utricle and saccule can inform the brain about a stationary tilt of the head. The direction of the tilt is detected by a similar mechanism as that for detecting the direction of linear acceleration. Astronauts in low gravitational settings receive relatively little information from their utricles and saccules about their stationary head position and must rely more heavily on visual and other sensory cues to detect head position.

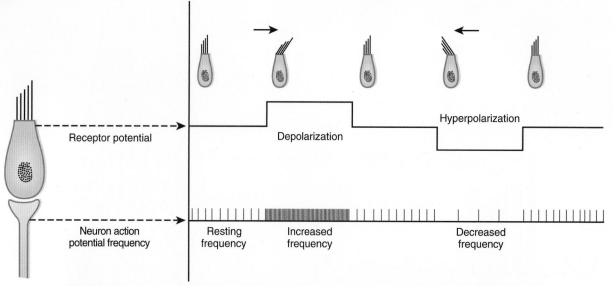

FIGURE 11-3 At rest, sensory neurons on which vestibular hair cells synapse transmit action potentials spontaneously at a rate of about 100 per second. When hair cell cilia are deflected in one direction, the action potential frequency increases; when cilia are deflected in the opposite direction, the frequency decreases.

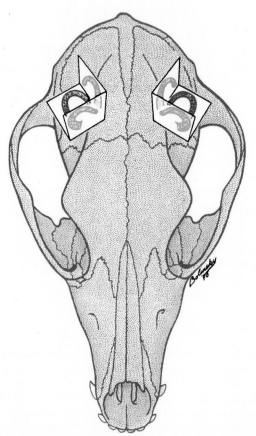

FIGURE 11-4 Three semicircular ducts, each positioned at approximately right angles to the other two, are located on each side of the head and work to detect rotary acceleration and deceleration of the head.

The Vestibular System Provides Sensory Information for Reflexes Involving Spinal Motor Neurons, the Cerebellum, and Extraocular Muscles of the Eye

As noted earlier, vestibular hair cells synapse on sensory neurons whose axons form part of the eighth cranial (vestibulocochlear) nerve and that carry action potentials to the medulla. Almost all these axons synapse in the *vestibular nuclear complex,* a bilateral group of four distinct nuclei occupying a substantial portion of the medulla, and part of the pons, next to the lateral wall of the fourth ventricle (Figure 11-8). From here, second-order neurons (those on which cranial nerve VIII axons synapse) project to three important areas of the nervous system as described below.

Some of the neurons of the vestibular nuclear complex receive significant input from the utricle and saccule (the otolith organs), and their axons in turn form the lateral vestibulospinal tract. This tract provides excitatory facilitation to gamma (γ) and alpha (α) motor neurons of antigravity muscles of the trunk and limbs in response to linear acceleration/deceleration or static tilt of the head (see Chapter 10). Other neurons of the vestibular nuclear complex receive significant sensory input from the crista ampullaris of the semicircular ducts, and their axons in turn form a pathway that projects to cranial nerve nuclei that control eye movements. This pathway, called the *medial longitudinal fasciculus* (MLF), produces compensatory eye movements in response to rotary acceleration/deceleration of the head. The vestibular nuclear complex also sends projections to, and receives projections from, the cerebellum, especially the flocculonodular lobe. Through these reciprocal connections, the cerebellum can fine-tune the coordination of postural and oculomotor reflexes that are controlled by the vestibular system. Finally, some of the projections leaving the vestibular nuclear complex participate in neural circuits leading to cerebral cortex, resulting in conscious vestibular sensations.

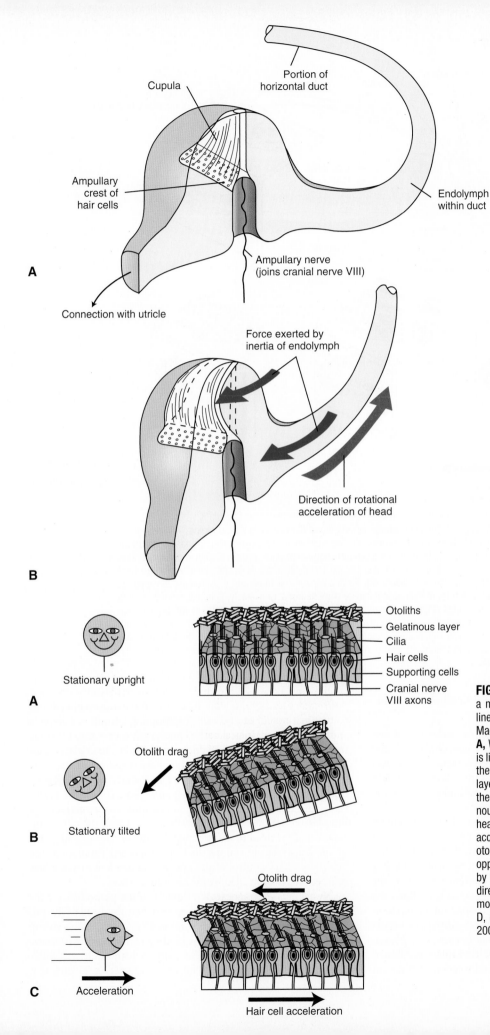

A

Cupula

Portion of horizontal duct

Ampullary crest of hair cells

Endolymph within duct

Ampullary nerve (joins cranial nerve VIII)

Connection with utricle

Force exerted by inertia of endolymph

Direction of rotational acceleration of head

B

FIGURE 11-5 Ampullae of the semicircular ducts contain a crista ampullaris, which transduces rotational acceleration/deceleration of the head. The ducts are filled with endolymph. **A,** Crista ampullaris of the horizontal canal when the head is at rest. **B,** On rotational acceleration of the head in the indicated direction, the relative inertia of the endolymphatic fluid displaces the cupula, and thus the hair cell cilia, in the opposite direction. (Modified from Kandel ER, Schwartz JH, editors: *Principles of neural science,* ed 2, New York, 1985, Elsevier Science Publishing.)

A

Stationary upright

Otoliths
Gelatinous layer
Cilia
Hair cells
Supporting cells
Cranial nerve VIII axons

B

Otolith drag

Stationary tilted

C

Acceleration

Otolith drag

Hair cell acceleration

FIGURE 11-6 Utricle and saccule each contain a macula, which transduces static head tilt and linear acceleration/deceleration of the head. Macula of the utricle is horizontally oriented. **A,** When the head is stationary and upright, there is little or no bending of the hair cell cilia. **B,** When the head tilts and remains tilted, the heavy otolith layer "falls over," producing a drag. This bends the hair cell cilia, by way of the interposed gelatinous layer, in the direction of the tilt. **C,** When the head accelerates in a straight line, the hair cells accelerate in the same direction, but the heavy otolith layer lags behind, producing a drag in the opposite direction. This bends the hair cell cilia, by way of the interposed gelatinous layer, in the direction opposite the acceleration. (Portions modified from Purves D, Augustine GJ, Fitzpatrick D, et al: *Neuroscience,* ed 3, Sunderland, Mass, 2004, Sinauer.)

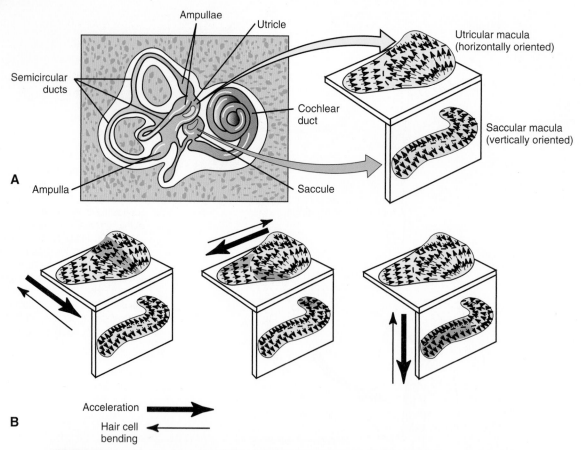

FIGURE 11-7 A, Macula of the utricle is horizontally oriented, and macula of the saccule is vertically oriented. *Small arrows* in a macula represent the approximate orientation of the hair cells in that region, with respect to their cilia. For a given hair cell, the *arrow tip* represents the position of the largest cilium, and the *arrow tail* represents the shortest cilium. **B,** Acceleration in a given direction *(large thick arrows)* results in bending of hair cell cilia in the opposite direction *(large thin arrows)* caused by otolith drag. Hair cells whose cilia are bent directly toward the largest cilium *(green regions)* will be depolarized the most and will produce the greatest increase in action potential frequency in their associated sensory neurons. Conversely, hair cells whose cilia are bent directly away from the largest cilium *(red regions)* will be hyperpolarized the most and will produce the greatest decrease in action potential frequency in their associated sensory neurons. Hair cells whose cilia are bent along other axes will be less significantly affected. (Portions modified from Fuchs AF: Peripheral motor control: the vestibular system. In Patton HD, Fuchs AF, Hille B, et al, editors: *Textbook of physiology,* ed 21, Philadelphia, 1989, Saunders.)

Vestibular Reflexes Coordinate Eye and Head Movements to Maximize Visual Acuity

Vestibular reflex control of the extraocular muscles of the eye, known as the *vestibuloocular reflex* (VOR), coordinates eye and head movements so that as the head turns (rotates), the eyes remain fixed on the original field of vision for as long as possible. Imagine that a dog is seated on a piano stool and you rotate her clockwise to the right. As you rotate her slowly to the right, her eyes rotate in her head slowly to the left so that the eyes remain fixed on the same field of vision as long as possible. As the eyes reach the limit of their leftward excursion, they swiftly move to the right, in the direction of the head movement, until they fix on a new field of vision. If the head continues to rotate, the cycle repeats until constant velocity is achieved. This allows the animal time to interpret a field of vision despite rotary acceleration of the head. When this pattern of eye movement occurs during the VOR, it is referred to as *normal nystagmus* or *physiological nystagmus:* the slow drift opposite head rotation followed by a fast flick back in the direction of head rotation. A transient

postrotatory nystagmus, with the converse eye movement pattern to that just noted, can be seen if a spinning animal or person is suddenly stopped. Inertia of the endolymph causes it to continue rotating in the semicircular duct, pushing on the crista ampullaris, even though the head and duct have stopped moving.

These reflex eye movement patterns require normal sensory input from the semicircular ducts, an intact MLF in the brainstem, and normally functioning motor units of the extraocular muscles (as well as an intact cerebellum). The VOR occurs on rotation of the head in the horizontal plane or the vertical plane, or on clockwise or counterclockwise torsional rotation of the head. Voluntary control of the eyes is independent of vestibular reflexes and is controlled by the cerebral cortex.

Nystagmus may appear occasionally under pathological conditions of the vestibular system, even when the head is at rest. This condition is known as *spontaneous nystagmus.* A persisting head tilt, falling, and compulsive circling or rolling often accompany spontaneous nystagmus in animals with acute vestibular disease. These actions often tend to be oriented in a consistent

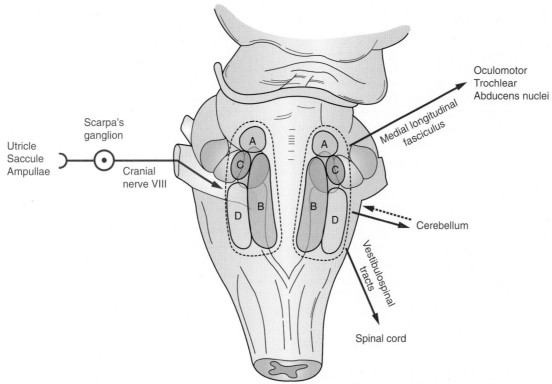

FIGURE 11-8 Dorsal view of the brainstem (with cerebellum removed) and rostral spinal cord showing the vestibular nuclear complex (within *dashed borders*) with its major afferents *(left)* and efferents *(right)*. The vestibular nuclear complex is comprised of the rostral *(A)*, medial *(B)*, lateral *(C)*, and caudal *(D)* vestibular nuclei. The complex spans portions of both the medulla and pons. Different subsets of these nuclei receive afferents from particular portions of the vestibular apparatus, and other subsets give rise to particular efferent pathways, although this characteristic has not been specified in the figure. The *dashed arrow* denotes that the projection to the cerebellum is reciprocal. Note that the afferents and efferents depicted actually exist on both sides of the midline. (Portions from De Lahunta A, Glass E: *Veterinary anatomy and clinical neurology,* ed 3, Philadelphia, 2009, Saunders.)

pattern with respect to the side of a peripheral lesion of the vestibular system. This is presumably a result of abnormal, asymmetric action potential inputs to the brainstem from the vestibular apparatus on the two sides of the head.

Another compensatory reflex that can be elicited by rotational acceleration is the *vestibulocollic reflex* (VCR). This reflex acts to stabilize the head by activating elements of the neck musculature. An extreme example of this reflex is if your dog or cat were in a rowboat with you and the boat suddenly began to roll to one side; the animal's head would move in the direction opposite the roll to try to recapture its original position. Interestingly, the VCR is more effective in species that make minimal eye movements, such as pigeons and owls. In these species the VCR may be serving a significant role in stabilizing gaze.

CLINICAL CORRELATIONS

VESTIBULAR SYNDROME IN A DOG

History. A 3-year-old male cocker spaniel is brought to your clinic. The owner states that for the previous two days, the dog has held his right ear lower than his left ear. He also tends to walk in circles, clockwise to the right. You have treated this dog previously for an infection of the outer right ear.

Clinical Examination. On physical examination of the dog, you find that the outer ear infection persists. You also confirm that the dog persistently tilts his head with the right ear down and circles to the right; you find that he has a spontaneous horizontal nystagmus. Results of the remaining physical and neurological examination are within normal limits.

Comment. Head tilt, circling, and spontaneous nystagmus constitute a common constellation of clinical signs often called the *vestibular syndrome.* It results from abnormality in the vestibular system, usually in the membranous labyrinth. It is frequently caused by the extension of an infection from the outer and middle ear to the labyrinth of the inner ear. This results in an abnormal balance of action potential frequencies between the normal and abnormal sides of the vestibular system, causing asymmetric stimulation of the ocular and postural reflex mechanisms normally controlled by the vestibular nuclei.

Treatment. When such labyrinthitis is caused by bacterial infection, treatment with appropriate antibiotics is often effective in eliminating the clinical signs by returning the peripheral receptor to its normal function. In cases of idiopathic vestibular syndrome in older cats and dogs, spontaneous recovery without treatment is common.

HORSE WITH VESTIBULAR DISEASE

History. A client calls you about a 6-year-old quarter horse mare that has not been eating or drinking well for the last few days. The horse seems depressed, and has been less active than usual in the field. This is the client's favorite mare, and she just returned from training a few months ago. During the spring, she had an episode of *strangles* (also called *distemper*), but she appeared to have recovered uneventfully. Strangles is caused by the bacterium *Streptococcus equi.* She has had no other health issues.

Clinical Examination. The horse appeared to be quieter than expected. She was not very responsive to external stimuli. She had an increased temperature (102.5° F), with normal heart rate and respiratory rate. The mare also had a right-sided head tilt, positional nystagmus (nystagmus that occurs when the head is placed in a particular position) that changes as the head position changes, with the fast phase toward the left, and ventrolateral strabismus (eyes are not focused on the same focal point) on the right side. The mare's strength is normal, but she has conscious proprioceptive deficits (on the right side worse than the left side). Because of this ataxia, she tends to drift to the right when she is standing still and as she walks.

Comment. Based on the deficits, including the head tilt, the mare probably has central vestibular disease. With central vestibular disease, the head tilt is toward the lesion (location of the mass or focus of infection). Additionally, the nystagmus and strabismus are toward the lesion. To determine the cause of the disease, radiographs of the temporomandibular joint (TMJ) should be taken, and a cerebrospinal fluid (CSF) tap with culture should be submitted. Complete white blood cell count and biochemical profile should also be performed to help identify a cause. With the previous history of *Streptococcus equi,* the clinical signs could be caused by either a bacterial otitis or an abscess in the central nervous system/ spinal cord.

Treatment. The horse has an increased white blood cell count, with an increase in neutrophils and fibrinogen. The chemistry panel is normal. Radiographs are normal. The CSF tap shows increased neutrophils and protein present. Culture of the CSF demonstrates *Streptococcus equi.* Bacterial meningitis is the cause of the central vestibular signs. The horse will be treated with intravenous antibiotics, followed by oral antibiotics for an extended period of time. The prognosis is guarded, based on the severity of infection.

PRACTICE QUESTIONS

1. The receptor organ detecting rotary acceleration and deceleration of the head is located in the:
   a. Utricle
   b. Saccule
   c. Ampulla of the semicircular duct
   d. Scala media of the cochlea
   e. Vestibular nuclear complex

2. Which *two* of the following are *not* generally associated with the macula?
   a. Otoliths
   b. Cupula
   c. Detection of linear acceleration of the head
   d. Hair cells
   e. Normal nystagmus

3. You are presented with a dog with a head tilt, compulsive circling, and spontaneous nystagmus. The most likely site of this dog's pathological lesion is the:
   a. Oculomotor nucleus.
   b. Cerebral cortex.
   c. Vestibular system.
   d. Cervical spinal cord.
   e. Spinal accessory (eleventh cranial) nerve.

4. Which one of the following statements is *false?*
   a. All hair cells of a single utricle are oriented in the same direction with respect to their cilia.
   b. In a single vestibular hair cell, displacement of the cilia toward the largest cilium increases the firing rate of the hair cell's associated sensory neuron.
   c. The axons of sensory neurons synaptically associated with vestibular hair cells form the eighth cranial nerve.
   d. A gelatinous layer is associated with the vestibular macula.
   e. The vestibular nuclear complex is located in the brainstem.

5. If a normal dog is sitting on a piano stool and I start to spin (accelerate) the stool to the right, which two of the following will be *false* regarding the observed nystagmus?
   a. The pattern of nystagmus observed at the start of rotation will be seen in reverse briefly after the spinning is abruptly stopped.
   b. An intact medial longitudinal fasciculus (MLF) is important for producing the nystagmus.
   c. The nystagmus will continue long after constant velocity is achieved.
   d. The eyes will drift slowly to the left, as far as they can go, and then flip rapidly back to the right.
   e. Nystagmus will often be observed long after the spinning has stopped, while the dog is stationary.

BIBLIOGRAPHY

Bear MF, Connors BW, Paradiso MA: *Neuroscience: exploring the brain,* ed 3, Philadelphia, 2007, Lippincott, Williams & Wilkins.

Brodal P: *The central nervous system: structure and function,* ed 4, New York, 2010, Oxford University Press.

De Lahunta A, Glass E: *Veterinary anatomy and clinical neurology,* ed 3, Philadelphia, 2009, Saunders.

Fuchs AF: Peripheral motor control: the vestibular system. In Patton HD, Fuchs AF, Hille B, et al, editors: *Textbook of physiology,* ed 21, Philadelphia, 1989, Saunders.

Goldberg JM, Cullen KE: Vestibular control of the head: possible functions of the vestibulocollic reflex, *Exp Brain Res* 210(3–4):331–345, 2011.

Haines DE: *Fundamental neuroscience,* ed 3, New York, 2006, Churchill Livingstone.

Hall JE: *Guyton and Hall textbook of medical physiology,* ed 12, Philadelphia, 2011, Saunders.

Purves D, Augustine GJ, Fitzpatrick D, et al: *Neuroscience,* ed 5, Sunderland, Mass, 2012, Sinauer.

Rush BR: Vestibular disease. In Reed SM, Bayly WM, Sellon DC, editors: *Equine internal medicine,* ed 2, St Louis, 2004, Saunders Elsevier.

Smith MO, George LW: Diseases of the nervous system. In Smith BP, editor: *Large animal internal medicine,* ed 4, St Louis, 2009, Mosby Elsevier.

CHAPTER 12
The Cerebellum

KEY POINTS

1. The cerebellum constantly compares the intended movement with the actual movement and makes appropriate adjustments.
2. Cerebellar histology and phylogeny give clues to cerebellar function.
3. The vestibulocerebellum helps coordinate balance and eye movements.
4. The spinocerebellum helps coordinate muscle tone as well as limb movement.
5. The cerebrocerebellum helps with planning coordinated, properly timed movement sequences.
6. The cerebellum plays a role in motor learning.
7. Cerebellar disease causes abnormalities of movement and further illuminates cerebellar function.

The preceding chapters, which describe the physiology of movement, discuss the function of lower motor neurons through which the central nervous system (CNS) can initiate and control movement by initiating contraction of skeletal muscle. The corticospinal system and the descending brainstem motor system are described in those previous chapters as major subgroups of upper motor neurons that influence the lower motor neurons. More medial portions of those systems coursing through the spinal cord are primarily responsible for the control of axial and proximal antigravity extensor muscles. The more lateral portions primarily control more skilled, learned, voluntary movements caused by contraction of distal flexor muscles. This chapter describes the function of the cerebellum, part of another subgrouping of upper motor neurons critical for proper movement.

The *cerebellum* (Latin, "little brain") is caudal to the cerebral cortex and dorsal to the brainstem (Figure 12-1). Although it constitutes only about 10% of the gross brain volume because of its highly folded structure, the cerebellum contains more than half of all CNS neurons. The outer layer of cerebellar gray matter, the *cerebellar cortex,* has a highly regular, three-layered, histological appearance, which suggests that all cerebellar regions may perform a common underlying task. Like the cerebral cortex, the particular inputs to a given region of cerebellar cortex, and the particular output targets that it influences, in large part account for the functional differences between cerebellar regions. In addition to the cerebellar cortex, and the cerebellar white matter axons entering and leaving the cortex, a group of deep *cerebellar nuclei* is embedded within the cerebellar white matter (Figure 12-2). The cells of these nuclei are a principal origin of the axons leaving the cerebellum. Two large pairs of white matter stalks, the *rostral* and *middle cerebellar peduncles,* respectively carry axons out from and into the cerebellum. A third, smaller pair of cerebellar peduncles, the *caudal cerebellar peduncles,* carry axons both into and out from the cerebellum.

The cerebellum is not necessary for the initiation of movement. Muscle strength remains largely intact with complete destruction of the cerebellum. However, the cerebellum plays a crucial role in the timing and coordination of movement initiated by the parts of the motor system hierarchy discussed in Chapter 10. It does so by adjusting and modulating the output of the motor cortices, corticospinal tract, descending brainstem motor pathways, and spinal cord. Lesions of the cerebellum lead to major clinical deficits in the precision and grace with which movement is accomplished.

The Cerebellum Constantly Compares the Intended Movement with the Actual Movement and Makes Appropriate Adjustments

In performing the essential role of adjusting the timing and coordination of movement, the cerebellum first receives information from components of the motor system hierarchy about the movement it has commanded. It also receives information from muscle spindles, the vestibular and visual systems, and other sensory receptors about the movement the body is actually performing. When the intended movement and the actual movement are not the same, the cerebellum's job is to perform the adjustments necessary to make them the same. For example, if a cat's brain intends that its mouth move to a piece of food in a dish, but sensory receptors inform the cerebellum that the trajectory of the head will cause the mouth to miss the dish, the cerebellum makes appropriate adjustments in the components of the motor system hierarchy to correct the head's trajectory. The correction can be made to the movement in progress and to the plan for subsequent movement.

Cerebellar Histology and Phylogeny Give Clues to Cerebellar Function

The cortex throughout the cerebellum is quite uniform and consists of three layers and only five types of neurons: stellate, basket, Golgi, granule, and Purkinje cells (Figure 12-3). The outermost layer is the *molecular layer* and consists primarily of granule cell axons, known as *parallel fibers* (Figure 12-4); dendrites of neurons located in deeper layers; and scattered inhibitory interneurons, the *stellate* and *basket cells.*

The middle *Purkinje cell layer* of cerebellar cortex consists of the large cell bodies of Purkinje neurons, which have a flat but extremely expansive dendritic field that extends into the molecular layer (see Figures 12-3 and 12-4). This dendritic field is oriented at right angles to the parallel fibers. Therefore, a Purkinje cell is contacted by an expansive array of parallel fiber axons of granule cells, and an individual parallel fiber contacts the dendrites of many Purkinje cells. The stellate and basket cell inhibitory interneurons, noted above, can act to refine, or prune, this extensive spatial pattern of Purkinje cell activation by parallel fibers.

The innermost *granule cell layer* of cerebellar cortex contains the vast number of granule cell somas that give rise to the parallel fibers (see Figures 12-3 and 12-4). This layer also contains occasional Golgi cell bodies. These are inhibitory interneurons that can regulate the overall level of excitation of the Purkinje cells by the granule cell parallel fibers.

Axons of the Purkinje neurons go to the deep cerebellar nuclei, located outside of the cerebellar cortex, embedded in the cerebellar white matter (see Figure 12-2). The Purkinje cells are the only output neurons of the cerebellar cortex and are all inhibitory. They can inhibit the spontaneously active neurons of the deep cerebellar nuclei, whose axons leave the cerebellum. This selective inhibition represents a sensitive temporal refinement of cerebellar processing that supplements the spatial refinement, and the excitation level control, noted above. The cerebellar output neurons participate in regulating the activity of brainstem motor pathways and motor cortices involved in the execution and planning of movement.

The two primary groups of input axons to the cerebellum are the *mossy fiber* and *climbing fiber* axons (see Figure 12-3). Both are excitatory; they cause excitatory postsynaptic potentials (EPSPs) within the cerebellar cortex and, through collateral axons, within the deep cerebellar nuclei (Figure 12-5). The mossy and climbing fibers collectively carry information from components of the motor system hierarchy and from peripheral sensory receptors regarding the planning, initiation, and execution of the movement. The shorter input/output circuit of the cerebellum consists of the climbing and mossy fiber stimulation to the deep cerebellar nuclei, whose output in turn leaves the cerebellum to modify components of the motor system hierarchy. However, the output of the deep cerebellar nuclei is itself modified by inhibition from Purkinje cell axons that originate in cerebellar cortex. The Purkinje cell inhibition of deep cerebellar nuclei is based on the cerebellar cortex's own integration of mossy and climbing fiber inputs. In other words, the same information coming into the cerebellum that drives the cerebellar nuclei is also processed by cerebellar cortex, whose resulting Purkinje cell output refines or "sculpts" the output of the cerebellar nuclei that project to components of the motor system. Within the cerebellar cortex, inhibitory interneurons help to refine or "sculpt" the Purkinje cell output of cerebellar cortex.

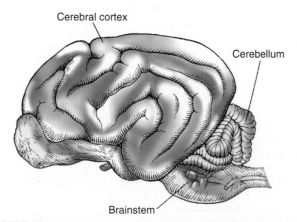

FIGURE 12-1 The cerebellum (Latin, "little brain") is caudal to the cerebral hemispheres and dorsal to the brainstem. (Redrawn from Miller ME, Christiansen GC, Evans HE: *The anatomy of the dog,* Philadelphia, 1964, Saunders.)

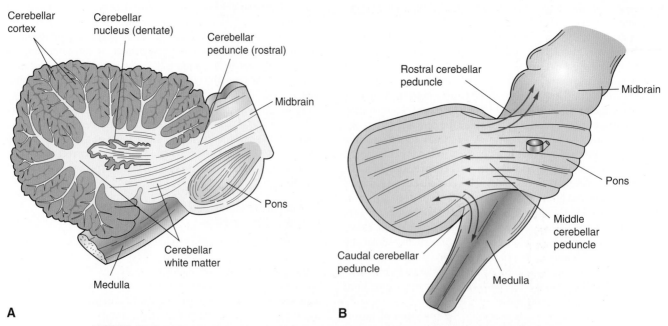

A

B

FIGURE 12-2 A, Mid-sagittal section through the brainstem region showing the internal organization of the cerebellum. **B,** A lateral view of the brainstem region emphasizing the cerebellar peduncles and the principal directions that axons travel within them.

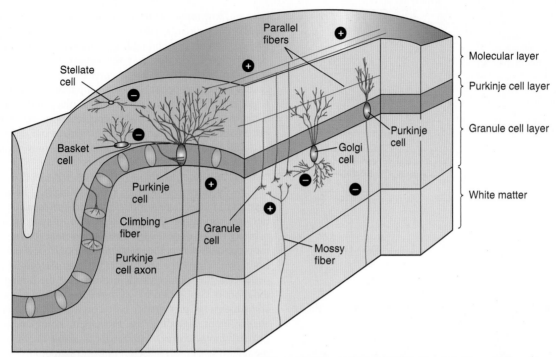

FIGURE 12-3 Five types of neurons are organized into three layers in the cerebellar cortex. A single cerebellar folium is sectioned vertically, in both sagittal and transverse planes, to illustrate the general organization of the cerebellar cortex. A positive sign denotes an excitatory effect of a neural element on its postsynaptic target. A negative sign denotes an inhibitory effect of a neural element on its postsynaptic target. (Modified from Kandel ER, Schwartz JH, editors: *Principles of neural science,* ed 4, New York, 2000, McGraw-Hill.)

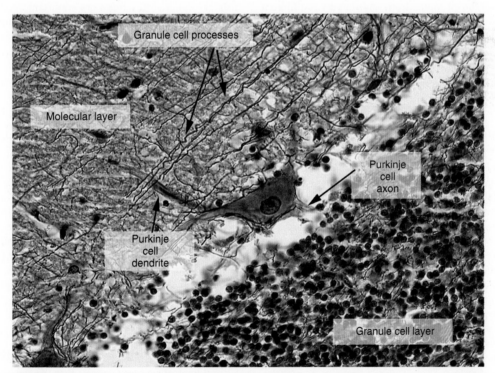

FIGURE 12-4 High-power photomicrograph of the three layers of the cerebellar cortex: granule cell layer, Purkinje cell layer (not labeled), and molecular layer. The image provides a good example of how the parallel fibers, labeled *granule cell processes,* cross the dendritic region of the Purkinje cell in the molecular layer. However, the elaborate branching pattern of the Purkinje cell dendrites is not apparent with this stain. (Image courtesy Dr. Tom Caceci, Department of Biomedical Sciences and Pathobiology, College of Veterinary Medicine, Virginia Tech.)

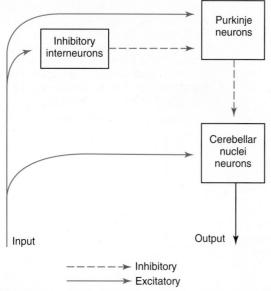

FIGURE 12-5 Input/output organization of the cerebellum. See text for explanation.

Although the cortical synaptology is understood, just how the cerebellum integrates movement feedback with the motor plan and then modifies the output of the deep nuclear neurons is not clear. As noted earlier, because the histological appearance of the cortex is similar throughout the cerebellum, it seems likely that a similar underlying processing mechanism exists in the cortex, regardless of the cerebellar region. However, within the cerebellum, regional variation of inputs from and outputs to different parts of the nervous system renders different motor results from different cerebellar regions. This can be thought of as effectively partitioning the cerebellum into different functional modules. The cerebellum can be divided into three distinct regions from both a functional perspective and a phylogenetic perspective: the *vestibulocerebellum,* the *spinocerebellum,* and the *cerebrocerebellum* (Figure 12-6).

The Vestibulocerebellum Helps Coordinate Balance and Eye Movements

The vestibulocerebellum occupies the flocculonodular lobe and receives most of its afferent input from the vestibular system, by way of the caudal cerebellar peduncles (see Figures 12-2 and 12-6). Its efferent output returns to the vestibular nuclei through these same peduncles either directly from cerebellar cortex or by way of the deep cerebellar nuclei (specifically the fastigial nucleus). The cerebellar output to the vestibular nuclei helps to coordinate the axial and proximal muscles controlling balance, by way of the vestibulospinal tract, and helps to coordinate head and eye movements by way of the medial longitudinal fasciculus (see Chapter 11). In short, the vestibulocerebellum adjusts the coordination of vestibular reflexes. Because this part of the cerebellum was the first to appear in vertebrate evolution, it is sometimes called the *archicerebellum.*

The Spinocerebellum Helps Coordinate Muscle Tone as Well as Limb Movement

The spinocerebellum extends rostrocaudally through the medial portion of the cerebellum (see Figure 12-6). It receives sensory inputs from muscle and cutaneous receptors through the spinal

cord and trigeminal nuclei. It also receives input from neurons in spinal reflex circuits, some of which receive commands from corticospinal or descending brainstem motor pathways. The cerebellar afferents coming from the spinal cord form several spinocerebellar tracts, which mostly enter the cerebellum through the caudal cerebellar peduncle. Some input to the spinocerebellar region also comes directly from the primary motor and primary somatosensory cortices. The spinocerebellum therefore receives information about commands for movement and significant feedback information about the execution of the movement itself. Its outputs travel, through its deep cerebellar nuclei (specifically the fastigial and interpositus), to brainstem nuclei controlling the antigravity musculature (e.g., reticular nuclei), as well as to a brainstem nucleus controlling distal limb musculature (e.g., red nucleus). Some of the spinocerebellar output travels to the primary motor cortex, particularly important for voluntary limb movement, by way of the thalamus. Through these output projections, which leave the cerebellum through the caudal and rostral peduncles, the spinocerebellum can adjust the timing and coordination of "in progress" movement and muscle tone. Such adjustments are presumably based on a comparison of spinocerebellar input regarding the movement command (e.g., from primary motor cortex) with feedback about the ongoing movement itself (e.g., from muscle, joint, and skin inputs). Because this portion of the cerebellum appeared next in evolution, it is sometimes called the *paleocerebellum.*

The Cerebrocerebellum Helps with Planning Coordinated, Properly Timed Movement Sequences

The cerebrocerebellum occupies the lateral cerebellar hemispheres (see Figure 12-6). This region also receives input from the primary motor cortex, but more important, receives a substantial input from premotor and supplementary motor cortices. These cortical inputs reach the cerebellum by way of the corticopontine-cerebellar system, which enters the cerebellum through the massive middle cerebellar peduncles. The cerebrocerebellum does not have direct access to information from peripheral receptors like the spinocerebellum. Its outputs, which travel through the rostral cerebellar peduncles, return to the motor cortices by way of the thalamus. Therefore the cerebrocerebellum is part of a communication loop with regions of motor cortex that are involved in the planning of, and preparation for, movement. Whereas the spinocerebellum helps coordinate the "in progress" execution of movement, the cerebrocerebellum helps the motor cortices with planning ahead for the next appropriate movement so there will be smooth and appropriately timed transitions between components of a movement sequence. The dramatic growth of the cerebrocerebellum and cerebral cortex was the major phylogenetic addition to the brain during primate evolution, and thus it is often called the *neocerebellum.* Presumably this is linked to the primate's ability to perform graceful, intricate, appropriately timed voluntary movements, such as coordinated finger movements as well as mouth and tongue movements necessary for speech.

The Cerebellum Plays a Role in Motor Learning

Several lines of evidence suggest that the cerebellum plays a significant role in motor learning. For example, functional magnetic resonance imaging (fMRI) studies have shown that the cerebellum is very active when learning a new sequence of movements, but it is not as active when the movement becomes relatively automatic. This suggests that the cerebellum is involved in the

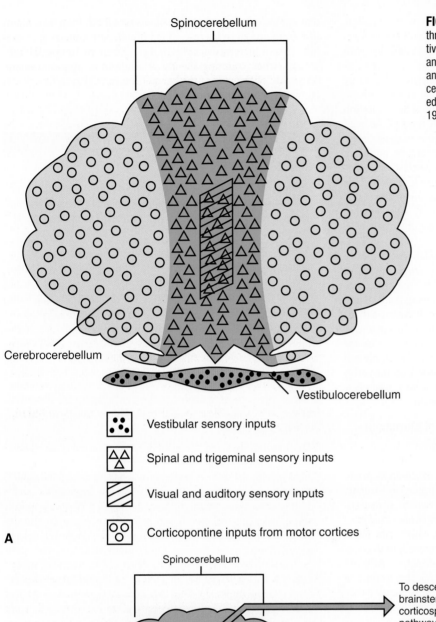

FIGURE 12-6 A, The cerebellum can be divided into three distinct regions, illustrated here with their respective major inputs, from both a functional perspective and a phylogenetic perspective. **B,** Major output targets and general roles of the three functional regions of the cerebellum. (Modified from Kandel ER, Schwartz JH, editors: *Principles of neural science,* ed 2, New York, 1985, Elsevier Science & Technology.)

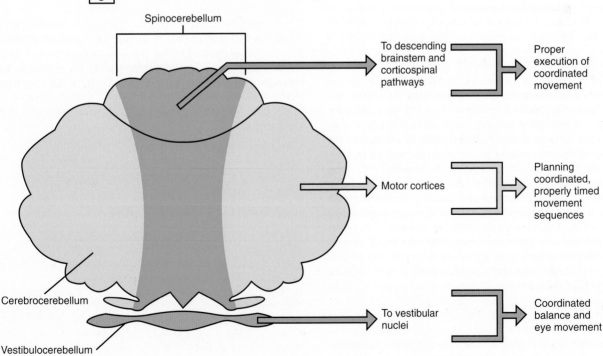

transition from concentrating on learning a new motor skill, such as where to place individual fingers on piano keys to form a chord, to being able to perform that skill automatically, with limited thought. Some reflex behaviors, such as the vestibuloocular reflex (see Chapter 11), although automatic, need to be fine-tuned or adjusted (e.g., with respect to the amount of eye rotation necessary to counteract a given amount of head rotation to keep the gaze fixed on a target) as the proportions of the head change during growth. Damage to certain regions of the cerebellum can prevent this type of adaptive adjustment. In addition, some forms of associative learning, such as some classically conditioned responses, can be abolished after cerebellar lesions. The ability to make motor adaptations after alterations of the visual world, such as learning to throw darts accurately after wearing prism glasses, can also be severely impaired in individuals with cerebellar damage.

Structural and functional changes in cerebellar circuitry have also been observed during motor learning. For example, increases in the number of parallel fiber and climbing fiber synaptic contacts on Purkinje cells have been observed following the learning of complex motor behavior. Furthermore, simultaneous activation of these two types of fibers synapsing on a Purkinje cell, where it is presumed that the climbing fiber is carrying a motor error signal, can produce a long-term depression of Purkinje cell activity. Such depression can have a profound effect on the activity of neurons of the deep cerebellar nuclei that leave the cerebellum to control components of the motor hierarchy.

Cerebellar Disease Causes Abnormalities of Movement and Further Illuminates Cerebellar Function

As discussed, the cerebellum constantly compares the intended movement with the actual movement and makes appropriate adjustments. In cerebellar disease, these appropriate adjustments are not made, resulting in a variety of movement disorders. Affected animals often place their paws far apart *(wide-based gait)* and walk in an uncoordinated manner *(ataxia),* which reflects the inability of the vestibulocerebellum and spinocerebellum to coordinate balance and movement of the axial skeleton. Affected animals also have various degrees of *dysmetria* (inappropriate measure of muscular contraction), in which movements either continue too long or not long enough. This is often manifested as difficulty in bringing the muzzle to a fixed point in space, such as a food dish, and as exaggerated "goose stepping" walking movements. *Asynergia,* a failure of the components of a complex, multiple-joint movement to occur in a coordinated fashion, may also be seen. It is particularly characteristic of damage to the cerebrocerebellum. *Intention tremor* (action tremor), an oscillating movement disorder that is worse when the animal is moving, especially near the end of the movement, is common in cerebellar disease as well. Intention tremors are much less severe when the animal is relaxed and not moving and worsen when a movement is being performed. In animals, intention tremors seem worse in the head and axial (proximal) antigravity muscles. If the vestibulocerebellum is damaged, nystagmus may also be seen (see Chapter 11). These commonly associated clinical signs resulting from cerebellar disease exemplify how the mechanism of disease can be understood through knowledge of normal physiology.

Some clinical studies in humans suggest that the cerebellum may play a role in cognitive functioning as well. Individuals with cerebellar damage have problems making rhythmic movements, which might be expected, but they also appear to have problems judging or perceiving rhythm. Some individuals with cerebellar damage also appear to have problems rapidly shifting their attention from one stimulus to another. Finally, some imaging studies have shown increased activity in the cerebellum, in normal individuals, when counting silently or while imagining movement. The study of the role of the cerebellum in cognitive function is still fairly recent and controversial.

CLINICAL CORRELATIONS

CEREBELLAR HYPOPLASIA

History. An 11-week-old female barn kitten is brought to your clinic for examination. The owner states that this kitten and several others in the litter have been uncoordinated since they began to walk.

Clinical Examination. Physical examination abnormalities are limited to the nervous system. The kitten is bright, alert, and responsive and seems to be of normal size for her age. All cranial nerve and spinal segmental reflexes and intersegmental responses are within normal limits. There is no atrophy. The kitten is uncoordinated (ataxic) when she moves and tends to raise her front paws higher than normal when walking ("goose stepping" hypermetria). She holds her paws far apart when walking. There are coarse, rhythmic movements of her head and proximal antigravity muscles that are absent at rest and severe when she is attempting a precise movement, such as getting her head to a food dish (intention tremor). Her complete blood count and serum chemistry results are within normal limits.

Comment. This kitten demonstrates classic signs of cerebellar disease. The cerebellum constantly compares the intended movement with the actual movement and, when these are not the same, makes the appropriate adjustments. When the cerebellum cannot do this, movement disorders characterized by wide-based gaits, ataxia, dysmetria, asynergia, and intention tremor occur. These movement disorders are worse with precise movement and nearly absent at rest.

This kitten's clinical signs are likely caused by *cerebellar hypoplasia,* in which the cerebellum never developed completely in utero. The in utero infection of *feline panleukopenia virus* results in destruction of the actively dividing granule cells (neurons), with an underdevelopment (hypoplasia) of the granular cell layer of the cerebellum. Purkinje cells may also be affected. Barn cats are often not vaccinated for this disease, and often several kittens in a litter are affected.

Treatment. There is no treatment for cerebellar hypoplasia caused by such in utero viral infection. It is not a progressive disease, and if affected kittens are kept in a fairly safe environment, they can have a normal life span.

NEWBORN CALF UNABLE TO RISE

History. A producer calls to ask about an Angus heifer calf born early today that has not stood. The calf makes efforts but does not seem coordinated enough to stand. The producer has fed the calf with colostrum by tube and wants her examined. This is the second calf this season that has had this problem. They euthanized the other calf after she had not improved over 2 to 3 days. The calves are very valuable, and the producer would like to keep this calf in the herd. Further questioning of the owner reveals an increased percentage of abortions this year. She also bought several new replacement cows last fall that have been introduced to the herd.

Clinical Examination. The calf has a normal temperature, pulse, and respiration. She appears responsive to noise, almost hyper-excitable. There is no evidence of trauma. When the calf is placed in a standing position, she sways back and forth; she tries to maintain a base-wide stance but sometimes falls over or backs up. She appears extremely uncoordinated and hypermetric (movement continuing too long). She scores a 4/5 on ataxia, with 5 being the most severe. Other abnormalities include a greatly delayed menace response and bumping into things when she tries to walk. When she is laid back down and her reflexes are assessed, the calf is hyperreflexic in all her responses.

Comment. Based on this history of the herd and the calf, this herd most likely has a problem with *bovine viral diarrhea virus* (BVDV). This was likely introduced by replacement cows. BVDV would explain the abortions as well as the two affected calves. With BVDV, the virus infects the germinal cells within the cerebellum and kills the Purkinje cells. Infection of these cells results in local inflammation, cell death, hemorrhage, and necrosis. Because of the damage to the Purkinje cells, inhibitory function is disrupted, which affects the vestibulocerebellum, spinocerebellum, and cerebrocerebellum. The deficits in these areas are associated with clinical signs of abnormalities in balance (vestibulocerebellum), eye movement (vestibulocerebellum), ataxia and base-wide stances (vestibulo- and spinocerebellum), and motor coordination and sequencing (spino- and cerebrocerebellum).

Treatment. Because BVDV causes irreversible cell damage, the prognosis for this calf is poor. Even if treatment were available, the calf most likely has BVDV and would shed virus if reintroduced into the herd. Euthanasia is the best option for this calf. The owner should screen the herd and identify infected and persistently infected (PI) animals. Additionally, vaccination with a live versus a killed BVDV vaccine may improve overall outcome.

PRACTICE QUESTIONS

1. Which of the following is principally involved in planning ahead for the next appropriate movement?
   a. Vestibulocerebellum
   b. Spinocerebellum
   c. Cerebrocerebellum
   d. Archicerebellum
   e. Both a and b

2. Loss of the cerebellum causes immediately obvious sensory deficits and prevents the initiation of movement.
   a. True
   b. False

3. Which of the following is *true* regarding cerebellar Purkinje cells?
   a. They are located in the cerebellar cortex.
   b. They have large cell bodies.
   c. They have an extensive dendritic tree.
   d. When active, they inhibit the activity of cells in deep cerebellar nuclei, whose axons leave the cerebellum.
   e. All the above.

4. Loss of the cerebellum causes loss of the muscle stretch reflex.
   a. True
   b. False

5. Cats with congenital malformations of the cerebellum often have ataxia, intention tremor, and wide gait.
   a. True
   b. False

BIBLIOGRAPHY

Brodal P: *The central nervous system: structure and function*, ed 4, New York, 2010, Oxford University Press.

De Lahunta A, Glass E: *Veterinary anatomy and clinical neurology*, ed 3, Philadelphia, 2009, Saunders.

Haines DE, editor: *Fundamental neuroscience for basic and clinical applications*, Philadelphia, 2006, Churchill Livingstone.

Hall JE: *Guyton and Hall textbook of medical physiology*, ed 12, Philadelphia, 2011, Saunders.

Jennings DP: Supraspinal control of posture and movement. In Reece WO, editor: *Duke's physiology of domestic animals*, ed 12, Ithaca, NY, 2004, Comstock Publishing.

Kandel ER, Schwartz JH, Jessell TM, editors: *Principles of neural science*, ed 4, New York, 2000, McGraw-Hill.

Purves D, Augustine GJ, Fitzpatrick D, et al: *Neuroscience*, ed 5, Sunderland, Mass, 2012, Sinauer.

CHAPTER 13

The Autonomic Nervous System

KEY POINTS

1. The peripheral autonomic nervous system differs from the somatic motor system in a number of important ways.
2. The peripheral autonomic nervous system has two subdivisions that originate in the central nervous system and one that does not.
3. The sympathetic nervous system originates from the thoracolumbar spinal cord.
4. The parasympathetic nervous system arises from the brainstem and sacral spinal cord.
5. Most sympathetic and parasympathetic neurons secrete either acetylcholine or norepinephrine as a neurotransmitter.

6. Acetylcholine and norepinephrine have different postsynaptic receptors.
7. Neurotransmitters other than acetylcholine and norepinephrine play some role in peripheral autonomic function.
8. There are general differences in sympathetic and parasympathetic function.
9. Visceral afferent (sensory) neurons play an important role in autonomic nervous system function.
10. The autonomic nervous system participates in many homeostatic reflexes.
11. Preganglionic neurons are influenced by many regions of the brain.

The autonomic nervous system (ANS) is a part of the nervous system that is generally not under conscious, voluntary control, nor is the organism usually conscious of its operation. The ANS is commonly defined as a *peripheral motor system* innervating smooth muscle, cardiac muscle, glandular tissue and the organs of the body cavity, known as *viscera* (e.g., stomach, urinary bladder), that these tissues often comprise. It should be kept in mind, however, that these peripheral targets and their motor innervation are usually part of reflex pathways that also include visceral afferents (see Chapter 3) and central nervous system structures (e.g., hypothalamus), both of which are sometimes included in broader definitions of the ANS.

A principal function of the ANS is maintaining the constancy of the body's internal environment, or *homeostasis*. Toward this end, it regulates such functions as blood pressure, heart rate, intestinal motility, bladder emptying, sweating, and the diameter of the eye's pupil. The ANS has unique anatomy, synaptic transmission, and effect on its various target organs. This chapter describes the general anatomy and function of the ANS. It mainly focuses on its peripheral motor aspects given their relevance to understanding the actions of the large number of drugs that affect the ANS. However, visceral afferents and CNS regulation of autonomic function are touched upon as well. The specific effect of the ANS on particular target organs is described in the chapters for each of the body's systems.

The Peripheral Autonomic Nervous System Differs from the Somatic Motor System in a Number of Important Ways

The ANS differs from the somatic motor system in its target organs, in the number of neurons in its peripheral circuit, and in the nature of the synapse at the target organ. The somatic motor system innervates skeletal muscle, which is the muscle responsible for all movements of the body, as described in Chapters 5 and

6. In contrast, the ANS innervates smooth muscle, cardiac muscle, and glandular tissue (Figure 13-1). Cardiac muscle is the muscle of the heart (see Chapter 19). Smooth muscle is the muscle in blood vessels, in most of the gastrointestinal tract, in the bladder, and in other hollow visceral structures. Gland cells can also be part of visceral organs, as well as comprising nonvisceral glands (e.g., salivary glands, lacrimal gland).

The ANS also differs in the number of neurons it has in the peripheral nervous system (see Figure 13-1). The somatic nervous system has one neuron whose cell body is located in the central nervous system (CNS) and whose axon extends, uninterrupted, to the skeletal muscle, where the peripheral chemical synapse occurs. In contrast, the ANS has two peripheral neurons. The first, called a *preganglionic neuron,* also has its cell body in the CNS, but its axon innervates a second neuron in the chain, called the *postganglionic neuron.* The latter's cell body is in a peripheral structure called a *ganglion,* a collection of neuronal cell bodies outside the CNS. There are chemically mediated synapses both between the preganglionic and postganglionic neurons and between the postganglionic neuron and the cells of its target organ.

The ANS also differs from the somatic motor system in the amount of *myelin* along the peripheral axons; the autonomic postganglionic neurons usually have slowly conducting, unmyelinated axons. In addition, somatic motor neurons always excite their skeletal muscle targets, whereas the autonomic postganglionic neurons can either excite or inhibit their targets. Furthermore, unlike the narrow synaptic cleft at the focal neuromuscular junction of a skeletal muscle cell, ANS target cells are often activated at a greater distance, by a highly branched postganglionic neuron with synaptic boutons (called *varicosities;* see Figure 27-7) distributed all along the length of these branches. This can contribute to a longer latency for, and greater spatial distribution of, postsynaptic cell activation by autonomic postganglionic neurons.

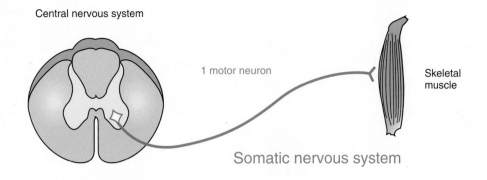

Central nervous system

1 motor neuron

Skeletal muscle

Somatic nervous system

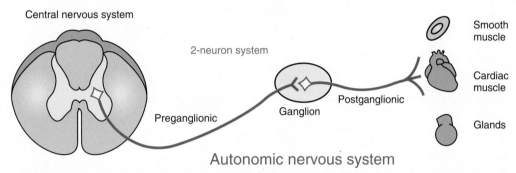

Central nervous system

2-neuron system

Smooth muscle

Cardiac muscle

Glands

Preganglionic

Ganglion

Postganglionic

Autonomic nervous system

FIGURE 13-1 The autonomic nervous system (ANS) differs from the somatic motor system in the number of neurons that it has in the peripheral nervous system. The somatic motor system has one neuron, whose cell body is located in the central nervous system (CNS) and whose axon extends, uninterrupted, to the skeletal muscle, where the peripheral chemical synapse occurs. In contrast, the ANS has two neurons in the path from the CNS to the target. The first, called a *preganglionic neuron,* also has its cell body in the CNS, but its axon innervates a second neuron in the chain, called the *postganglionic neuron.* Its cell body is in a peripheral structure called a *ganglion.*

The Peripheral Autonomic Nervous System Has Two Subdivisions That Originate in the Central Nervous System and One That Does Not

The peripheral ANS is divided into two major subdivisions based on the respective CNS origin of their preganglionic neurons and on their synaptic transmitters at the target organ. These two subdivisions are the *sympathetic nervous system* and the *parasympathetic nervous system.* The *enteric nervous system* can be considered a third subdivision of the peripheral ANS. It is an extensive network of interconnected sensory, motor and interneurons within the gut (gastrointestinal tract) wall that can control gut function independently of the CNS. However, these neurons can also be influenced by the CNS through input from the sympathetic and parasympathetic subdivisions. The enteric nervous system will be discussed in more detail in reference to the regulation of gastrointestinal function in Chapter 27.

The Sympathetic Nervous System Originates from the Thoracolumbar Spinal Cord

The sympathetic nervous system generally has short preganglionic and long postganglionic axons. Preganglionic axons of the sympathetic nervous system leave the spinal cord by way of the ventral roots of the first thoracic through the third or fourth lumbar spinal nerves (Figure 13-2). For this reason, the sympathetic nervous system is often called the *thoracolumbar system.* The preganglionic axons pass through the ventral root and then a communicating branch *(white ramus)* to enter the *paravertebral sympathetic ganglion chain* (also called the *sympathetic trunk),*

where most synapse with a postganglionic neuron (Figure 13-3, *A*). The ganglion chain actually extends from cervical to sacral regions and some of the thoracolumbar preganglionic neurons extend their axons rostrally or caudally within the chain to reach these cervical and sacral ganglia (see Figure 13-3, *A*, asterisk). A large complement of postganglionic axons from each of the chain ganglia enter nearby spinal nerves, through a different communicating ramus *(gray ramus),* and travel to the body wall or extremities to control blood vessels, sweat glands, or hair erector muscles (see Figure 13-3, *A*, #1). Another complement of these postganglionic neurons, mainly from thoracic or cervical chain ganglia, does not enter spinal nerves but forms separate nerves that travel respectively to thoracic viscera (e.g., heart, bronchi) or to organs and glands of the head (e.g., eye, lacrimal gland; see Figure 13-3, *A*, #2).

Some of the thoracolumbar preganglionic axons simply pass through the sympathetic chain ganglia without synapsing there. These axons form *splanchnic nerves* that synapse with postganglionic neurons in *prevertebral ganglia* (see Figure 13-3, *A*, #3), usually named for neighboring blood vessels (e.g., celiac, mesenteric). Postganglionic neurons of the prevertebral ganglia innervate abdominal and pelvic visceral organs. Some of the aforementioned splanchnic nerve fibers bypass the prevertebral ganglia and continue all the way to the *adrenal medulla,* where they synapse with rudimentary postganglionic neurons that make up the adrenal medullary secretory cells (see Figure 13-3, *A*, #4). These vestigial postganglionic neurons secrete their transmitter substance directly into the circulating blood. The transmitter

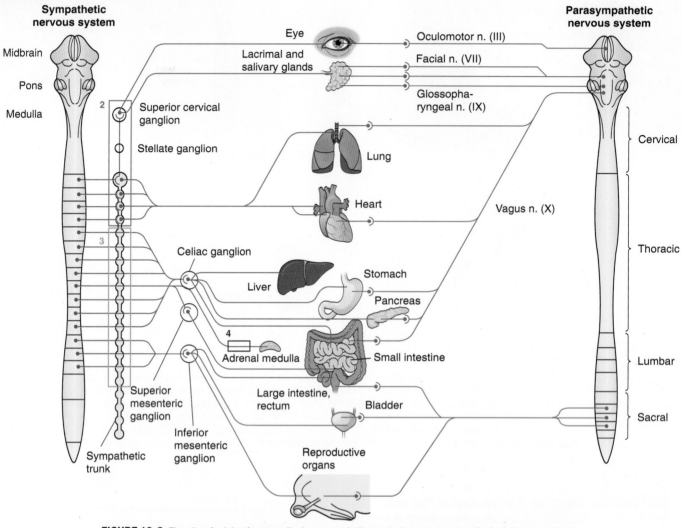

FIGURE 13-2 The site of origin of preganglionic neurons in the central nervous system for both the sympathetic nervous system *(left)* and the parasympathetic nervous system *(right)*. Several sites of projection of postganglionic axons are also shown. The *colored rectangles* highlight different paths that the sympathetic system may take to its targets after leaving the central nervous system. Those paths, with corresponding numbers, are presented in more detail in Figure 13-3. (Modified from Kandel ER, Schwartz JH: *Principles of neural science,* ed 4, New York, 2000, McGraw-Hill.)

substance, acting as a true hormone, is carried by the blood to all tissues of the body.

The Parasympathetic Nervous System Arises from the Brainstem and Sacral Spinal Cord

The parasympathetic nervous system generally has long preganglionic and short postganglionic axons. Preganglionic axons of the parasympathetic system leave the CNS by way of cranial nerves III (oculomotor), VII (facial), IX (glossopharyngeal), and X (vagus) and through several sacral spinal nerves. For this reason, it is called the *craniosacral system* (see Figure 13-2). The parasympathetic preganglionic axons leaving through cranial nerves III, VII, and IX synapse in well defined ganglia outside the skull (e.g., otic, submandibular; see Figure 13-3, *B, top*). The parasympathetic postganglionic neurons project to smooth muscle and glandular targets in the head (e.g., ciliary muscle, parotid gland).

Preganglionic axons leaving through cranial nerve X travel all the way to the body cavity to synapse in more diffuse

parasympathetic ganglia located close to, or within, thoracic and abdominal viscera (see Figure 13-3, *B, bottom*). The short postganglionic neurons control the smooth muscle, cardiac muscle, and glandular cells of these organs.

Parasympathetic preganglionic axons leaving through sacral spinal nerves depart to form pelvic nerves that synapse in diffuse parasympathetic ganglia residing close to, or within, pelvic viscera (e.g. rectum, bladder; see Figure 13-3, *C*). The short postganglionic neurons control these organs, as well as erectile tissue of the genitals.

Most viscera receive both sympathetic and parasympathetic innervation (see Figure 13-2). Although the parasympathetic system originates in brainstem and sacral regions, it can provide parasympathetic innervation to organs in the thoracic and lumbar parts of the body, as just noted, by way of the vagus nerve (cranial nerve X). The sympathetic thoracolumbar system can influence organs in cranial and sacral regions by way of preganglionic sympathetic axons that travel to sympathetic postganglionic neurons in cervical and sacral regions of the sympathetic ganglion chain

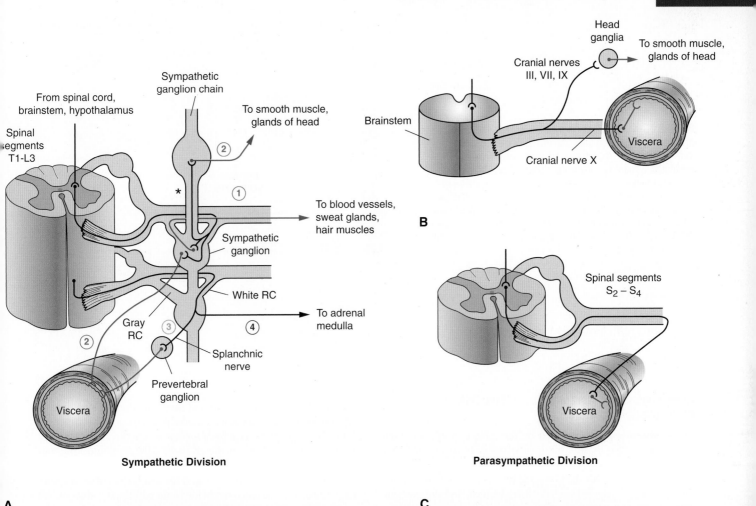

FIGURE 13-3 Synaptic organization of preganglionic and postganglionic neurons of the sympathetic **(A)** and parasympathetic **(B, C)** divisions of the autonomic nervous system. Anatomical locus of each numbered scheme in part **A** can be seen in Figure 13-2, except for #1. See text for further description. *RC,* Ramus communicans (communicating branch). (Modified from Ganong WF: *Review of medical physiology,* ed 13, Norwalk, Conn, 1987, Appleton & Lange.)

(see Figure 13-3, *A*, asterisk). Although blood vessels in all parts of the body receive sympathetic innervation, which most commonly produces vasoconstriction, most do not receive parasympathetic innervation (except those in glands and the external genitals).

Most Sympathetic and Parasympathetic Neurons Secrete Either Acetylcholine or Norepinephrine as a Neurotransmitter

As described in Chapter 5, *acetylcholine* is the neurotransmitter at the somatic neuromuscular synapse. Acetylcholine is also released by the preganglionic neurons at all autonomic ganglia (Figure 13-4). Parasympathetic postganglionic neurons release acetylcholine as well, onto their target organs. Acetylcholine-releasing synapses are often called *cholinergic*. Most anatomically sympathetic postganglionic neurons secrete *norepinephrine* onto their targets. Norepinephrine-releasing synapses are often called *adrenergic*. However, in several species, anatomically sympathetic postganglionic neurons traveling to sweat glands secrete acetylcholine, as do some of the sympathetic postganglionic neurons to blood vessels in skeletal muscle, where they can produce vasodilation.

In the case of the adrenal medulla, incoming preganglionic axons release acetylcholine, but the neuroendocrine-like, postganglionic chromaffin cells release primarily epinephrine and some norepinephrine into the circulating blood. These chromaffin cells can be considered structural and functional analogues of sympathetic postganglionic neurons.

It is important that, when released, the neurotransmitter not linger in the synaptic cleft. The neurotransmitter must be either destroyed in the cleft or dissipated so that the postsynaptic membrane can recover its resting potential and be ready for the next synaptic transmission. Because some synapses can transmit impulses up to several hundred times per second, neurotransmitter destruction must occur quickly. In the case of acetylcholine, acetylcholinesterase destroys the transmitter in the cleft. For norepinephrine, reuptake by the presynaptic neuron is the principal way in which its synaptic effect on the postsynaptic membrane is terminated. The hormonal actions of circulating epinephrine and norepinephrine released by the adrenal medulla, however, are primarily terminated by the enzyme *catechol-O-methyltransferase* (COMT), with a lesser contribution of the enzyme *monoamine oxidase* (MAO). These enzymes are widely distributed in the body, with highest concentrations in the liver and kidney.

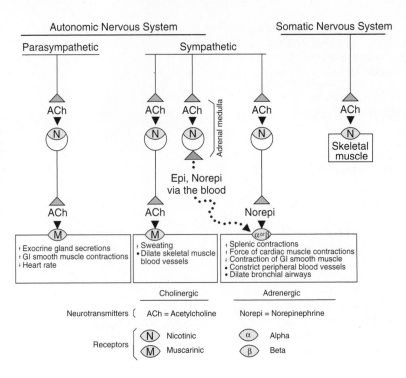

FIGURE 13-4 Classification of autonomic and somatic motor neurons with regard to their transmitter or mediator released, their postsynaptic receptors, and their general influence on the effector organ. Acetylcholine *(ACh)*, released from the pre-synaptic membrane, can stimulate either a muscarinic *(M)* or a nicotinic *(N)* postsynaptic receptor, depending on the particular location of the synapse. Similarly, norepinephrine *(Norepi)* can stimulate either α or β receptors, again depending on the location of the synapse. *Epi,* Epinephrine; *GI,* gastrointestinal.

Acetylcholine and Norepinephrine Have Different Postsynaptic Receptors

The neurotransmitters secreted by the ANS typically stimulate their target organ by first binding with a postsynaptic receptor. These receptors are proteins in the cell membrane. When the transmitter binds with the postsynaptic receptor, the membrane's permeability to selected ions is often changed, and the postsynaptic membrane potential either increases or decreases, with a resulting change in the probability of action potentials in the postsynaptic cell.

Acetylcholine stimulates two different types of receptors (see Figure 13-4). *Muscarinic* acetylcholine receptors are G-protein–coupled receptors (GPCRs; see Chapter 1) found on all the target cells stimulated by postganglionic parasympathetic neurons and by cholinergic postganglionic neurons of the sympathetic nervous system. Faster acting *nicotinic* receptors are ligand-gated ion channels (see Chapter 1) found at all synapses between autonomic preganglionic and postganglionic neurons and at the somatic neuromuscular junction.

The classification of major types and subtypes of neurotransmitter receptors is usually based upon various combinations of the following: responses to agonist or antagonist drugs, distribution among various tissues and organs, signal transduction mechanism (e.g., G protein-coupled, ligand-gated). Muscarinic receptors were named because they are stimulated by *muscarine*, a toadstool poison. Muscarine does not stimulate nicotinic receptors. *Nicotine* stimulates the nicotinic receptors but not muscarinic receptors. Acetylcholine stimulates both, and different drugs block each receptor. For example, atropine blocks muscarinic receptors, whereas curare blocks nicotinic receptors. Although there are respective subtypes of nicotinic (e.g., N_m, N_n) and muscarinic (e.g., M_1-M_5) acetylcholine receptors, there are few therapeutic drugs that can distinguish among subtype members.

Adrenergic receptors are located at synapses between peripheral target tissues and sympathetic postganglionic neurons that release norepinephrine. However, these receptors can also be stimulated by the release of epinephrine and norepinephrine into the bloodstream from the adrenal medulla. There are two major types of adrenergic receptors, called alpha (α) and beta (β) receptors. The β receptors have been further subdivided into $β_1$ and $β_2$ receptors, on the basis of the effect of adrenergic blocking and stimulating drugs. There is now evidence for a third class of β receptor ($β_3$, found in fat cells), and for two classes of α receptors ($α_1$ and $α_2$) that can each be divided into additional subtypes. All adrenergic receptors are GPCRs, and the various subtypes, like the cholinergic receptor subtypes, have differential distributions among various tissues. There are many clinically useful drugs that can distinguish among the members within adrenergic receptor subtype groups.

Neurotransmitters Other Than Acetylcholine and Norepinephrine Play Some Role in Peripheral Autonomic Function

As more of a rule than an exception, individual neurons are capable of releasing more than one neurotransmitter. Multiple release often depends upon how vigorously the neurons are activated by presynaptic stimulation. Therefore, preganglionic and postganglionic sympathetic and parasympathetic neurons that release either acetylcholine or norepinephrine are respectively capable of releasing *co-transmitters* under certain circumstances. Most often these co-transmitters are peptides (e.g., vasoactive intestinal peptide, neuropeptide Y, luteinizing hormone-releasing hormone), but some purine (e.g., ATP) and atypical neurotransmitter (e.g., nitric oxide) co-release has been demonstrated as well. Often the postsynaptic response to release of a neurotransmitter is modified by the release of a co-transmitter from the same neuron. For example, acetylcholine released from parasympathetic postganglionic neurons can activate salivary glands, but co-release of vasoactive intestinal peptide from the same neurons can affect blood vessel diameter in the target region as well.

Acetylcholine and norepinephrine can also be found in the enteric nervous system: acetylcholine is released by excitatory enteric neurons of the gut (see Chapter 27), and postganglionic sympathetic neurons can release norepinephrine into enteric neuronal plexuses to induce inhibition. Like the sympathetic/parasympathetic systems, various enteric neurons also employ vasoactive intestinal peptide, neuropeptide Y, ATP, and nitric oxide. However, the variety of neurotransmitters other than acetylcholine and norepinephrine, employed by neurons of the enteric nervous system, is much more extensive than that found among the sympathetic and parasympathetic systems.

There Are General Differences in Sympathetic and Parasympathetic Function

Although the sympathetic and parasympathetic systems are both important for homeostasis, there are some important general differences in their function.

In physical and some emotional stress, the sympathetic system is capable of a massive, coordinated output with widespread effects on tissues and organs of the body. This causes an increase in heart rate and blood pressure; dilation of the pupil of the eye; an elevation in levels of blood glucose and free fatty acids; and an increased state of arousal. These widespread effects mobilize the body's resources for extra effort in responding to an emergency. Therefore the sympathetic system is sometimes referred to as the *fight or flight* system. The effect of sympathetic discharge not only is widespread but can last longer than effects of parasympathetic discharge because of the prolonged circulation of epinephrine and norepinephrine. Indeed, the adrenal medulla's secretion of epinephrine and norepinephrine into the circulating blood provides prolonged adrenergic stimulation to the entire body, even to some tissues that do not have direct sympathetic postganglionic stimulation.

Under less stressful conditions the sympathetic system plays an important role in homeostasis, but with less universal control within the body. For example, sympathetic control of the skin for thermoregulation, or of the dilator smooth muscle in the iris for enlargement of the pupil in low ambient light, can respectively occur without extensive activation of other organs.

The parasympathetic system is characterized by a greater degree of independent control of tissues and organs, as well as a more precise control within a given tissue or organ, compared with the sympathetic system. In addition, unlike the sympathetic system which innervates virtually all parts of the body, the parasympathetic system does not innervate structures of the body wall and extremities. The parasympathetic system is generally concerned with the restorative aspects of daily living. For example, parasympathetic stimulation assists digestion and absorption of food by increasing gastric secretion, increasing intestinal motility, and relaxing the pyloric sphincter. For this reason, the parasympathetic nervous system is sometimes called the *anabolic* or *restorative* nervous system, as well as the *rest and digest* system.

Many organs of the body have both sympathetic and parasympathetic innervation, each with a reciprocal effect. For example, sympathetic stimulation increases heart rate, whereas parasympathetic stimulation decreases heart rate. Sympathetic stimulation enlarges pupillary diameter, whereas parasympathetic stimulation causes pupillary constriction. These sympathetic and parasympathetic systems work together, along with the enteric system, to exquisitely keep the body's internal environment stable.

Table 13-1 gives a more complete listing of the responses of various organs to adrenergic and cholinergic stimulation by the peripheral autonomic nervous system.

TABLE 13-1 Responses of Effector Organs to Autonomic Nerve Impulses and Circulating Catecholamines

Effector Organ	Cholinergic Impulses: Response	Noradrenergic Impulses Receptor	Noradrenergic Impulses Response
Eye			
Radial muscle of iris	—	α_1	Contraction (mydriasis)
Sphincter muscle of iris	Contraction (miosis)	—	—
Ciliary muscle	Contraction for near vision	β_2	Relaxation for far vision
Heart			
Sinoatrial node	Decrease in heart rate	$\beta_1 > \beta_2$	Increase in heart rate
Atria	Decrease in contractility and shortened AP duration	$\beta_1 > \beta_2$	Increase in contractility and conduction velocity
Atrioventricular (AV) node	Decrease in conduction velocity; AV block	$\beta_1 > \beta_2$	Increase in conduction velocity
His-Purkinje conduction system	Little effect	$\beta_1 > \beta_2$	Increase in conduction velocity
Ventricles	Little effect	$\beta_1 > \beta_2$	Increase in contractility and conduction velocity
Arterioles			
Skeletal muscle, pulmonary, abdominal viscera	Dilation (sometimes skeletal muscle)	α_1 β_2	Constriction Dilation
Coronary, renal	—	α_1, α_2 β_2 (also β_1 renal)	Constriction Dilation
Skin and mucosal, cerebral, salivary gland	—	α_1, α_2 (cerebral α_1 only)	Constriction
Systemic veins	—	α_1, α_2 β_2	Constriction Dilation

Continued

TABLE 13-1 Responses of Effector Organs to Autonomic Nerve Impulses and Circulating Catecholamines—cont'd

Effector Organ	Cholinergic Impulses: Response	Noradrenergic Impulses	
		Receptor	Response
Lung			
Bronchial muscle	Contraction	β_2	Relaxation
Bronchial glands	Stimulation	α_1	Decrease in secretion
		β_2	Increase in secretion
Stomach (Monogastric)			
Motility and tone	Increase	$\alpha_1, \alpha_2, \beta_1, \beta_2$	Decrease (usually)
Sphincters	Relaxation (usually)	α_1	Contraction (usually)
Secretion	Stimulation	α_2	Inhibition
Intestine			
Motility and tone	Increase	$\alpha_1, \alpha_2, \beta_1, \beta_2$	Decrease
Sphincters	Relaxation (usually)	α_1	Contraction
Secretion	Stimulation	α_2	Inhibition
Gallbladder and Ducts			
Gallbladder and ducts	Contraction	β_2	Relaxation
Urinary Bladder			
Detrusor	Contraction	β_2	Relaxation
Trigone and sphincter	Relaxation	α_1	Contraction
Ureter			
Motility and tone	Increase (?)	α_1	Increase
Reproductive System			
Uterus	Variable*	α_1, β_2	Variable
Male sex organs	Erection	α_1	Ejaculation
Skin			
Pilomotor muscles	—	α_1	Contraction
Sweat glands	Generalized secretion	α_1	Localized secretion†
Upper Abdominal Structures			
Spleen capsule	—	α_1	Contraction
		β_2	Relaxation
Adrenal medulla	Secretion of epinephrine and norepinephrine	—	—
Liver	—	α_1, β_2	Glycogenolysis and gluconeogenesis
Kidney	—	α_1	Decreased renin secretion
		β_1	Increased renin secretion
Pancreas			
Acini	Increased secretion	α	Decreased secretion
Islets	—	α_2	Decreased insulin and glucagon secretion
		β_2	Increased insulin and glucagon secretion
Other Glands			
Salivary glands	K^+ and H_2O secretion	α	K^+ and H_2O secretion
Lacrimal glands	Secretion	α	Secretion
Pineal gland	—	β	Increase in melatonin synthesis and secretion

Modified from Westfall TC, Westfall DP: Neurotransmission: the autonomic and somatic motor nervous systems. In Brunton L, Chabner B, Knollman B: *Goodman and Gilman's the pharmacological basis of therapeutics,* ed 12, New York, 2011, McGraw-Hill.
*Depends on stage of estrous cycle, amount of circulating estrogen and progesterone, pregnancy, and other factors.
†On palms of human hands and in some other locations (adrenergic sweating).

Visceral Afferent (Sensory) Neurons Play an Important Role in Autonomic Nervous System Function

Many of the body's visceral functions are regulated by *autonomic reflexes*. As with reflex arcs in the somatic nervous system (see Chapter 7), autonomic reflex arcs also include a sensory side to the arc, including a visceral receptor; a sensory neuron, often called a *visceral afferent* neuron; and one or more synapses in the CNS. The ANS is commonly defined as the peripheral motor preganglionic and postganglionic neurons. Visceral afferent neurons are often not included in this definition, but because they are essential parts of the autonomic reflex arc, they will be described briefly below.

The peripheral portion of a visceral afferent neuron's axon travels toward the CNS along splanchnic, cranial, and pelvic nerves that carry the sympathetic or parasympathetic visceral efferents toward their peripheral targets. Like the somatic afferent neurons carrying touch information from the skin (see Figure 7-2, *left*), the visceral afferent neurons have their cell bodies located in dorsal root or cranial nerve ganglia. The centrally directed portion of the axon synapses in the dorsal horn of the spinal cord or in a cranial nerve nucleus of the brain.

Generally, visceral afferent neurons carrying nociceptive (pain-inducing) information travel in sympathetically characterized nerves (e.g., splanchnic), whereas those carrying non-nociceptive information run within parasympathetically characterized nerves (e.g., vagus, pelvic). Nociceptive stimuli from the viscera can result from strong dilation or contraction of an organ, but are usually chemical in nature, resulting from inflammation or ischemia (restricted blood supply) of an organ. Normal stretch or movement of an organ or blood vessel, or changes in oxygen or carbon dioxide concentration in the blood, are examples of non-nociceptive visceral stimuli.

Non-nociceptive sensory signals from the viscera usually do not reach consciousness, but those that do tend to be diffuse and difficult to localize. Although nociceptive visceral signals often reach consciousness and are initially difficult to localize, the organ source of the pain is often "referred" to (feels like it's coming from) regions of the skin in the general vicinity of the organ. This *referred pain* is thought to result from the convergence of somatic (e.g., skin) afferents and visceral afferents within the dorsal horn of the same spinal cord segment. In human medicine, the locus of the skin pain can be a reliable clue as to the location of the affected organ.

The Autonomic Nervous System Participates in Many Homeostatic Reflexes

Autonomic reflexes are extremely common and are described in detail for each body system in later chapters. A few are described briefly here as examples.

Control of Blood Pressure

Among the body's major priorities is keeping a sufficient blood flow to the brain. Stretch receptors in the internal carotid artery and the aorta detect systemic blood pressure. When these receptors detect a drop in pressure, an increase in activity of sympathetic adrenergic neurons produces peripheral vasoconstriction and increased vascular resistance to increase blood pressure and restore sufficient blood flow to the brain. If blood pressure rises above normal limits in animals, sympathetic adrenergic

vasoconstrictor nerves are inhibited and blood pressure falls back to within normal limits.

Pupillary Light Reflex

When a flashlight is shone into an animal's eye, light stimulates photoreceptors in the retina (see Chapter 14). Sensory action potentials are then transmitted to the brainstem along the optic nerve, where, through several interneurons, parasympathetic cholinergic neurons stimulate the constrictor smooth muscle of the iris. This causes the pupillary diameter to become smaller.

Micturition (Urination)

The normal regulation of *micturition* actually represents a complex interplay of autonomic reflex activity and skeletal muscle control, upon which an element of voluntary regulation is superimposed. Autonomic efferent control of bladder emptying is principally achieved by pelvic parasympathetic output that causes contraction of the bladder wall (detrusor muscle). The ability to store urine is facilitated by sympathetic efferent control originating in the lumbar splanchnic nerves (Figure 13-5, *A*). This sympathetic output will ultimately inhibit contraction of the detrusor muscle directly, as well as indirectly by inhibiting parasympathetic postganglionic neurons that stimulate its contraction. This sympathetic output also facilitates urine storage by contracting the smooth muscle internal sphincter located at the neck of the bladder. Superimposed upon the sympathetic facilitation of urine storage is the contraction of a skeletal muscle external sphincter (urethralis muscle) controlled by somatic motor neurons of the sacral spinal cord, and which is also amenable to conscious voluntary regulation. The sympathetic facilitation of urine storage, together with contraction of the striated external sphincter, can be collectively referred to as the *urine storage reflexes,* which are primarily organized at the level of the spinal cord.

Visceral afferents to the lumbosacral spinal cord from the bladder wall and the urethra provide distention information about the extent of bladder filling. As the bladder begins to fill with urine, this visceral afferent input to the spinal cord activates the urine storage reflexes described previously (see Figure 13-5, *A*).

The distention information regarding bladder filling is also sent from the spinal cord to a region of the midbrain called the *periaqueductal gray* (PAG; see Figure 13-5, *B*). When bladder filling reaches a critical level, the PAG sends a signal to a region of the pons called the *pontine micturition center* (PMC), which, in turn, has projections to the spinal cord that coordinate the components of the *voiding reflexes*. The voiding reflexes include (1) inhibition of the sympathetically mediated storage reflexes, resulting in relaxation of the internal and external sphincters, and (2) excitation of the parasympathetic innervation of the bladder, resulting in bladder contraction.

Of course, animals do not immediately void urine when the bladder is full because survival or social conditions are not always favorable. There is an element of voluntary control over whether the brainstem PMC is activated to trigger the spinal cord voiding reflexes. The distention information sent to the PAG is passed from there to forebrain regions that can consciously perceive bladder fullness and to forebrain regions involved in cognitive (e.g., prefrontal cortex), regulatory (e.g., hypothalamus), and emotional (e.g., amygdala) processes (see Figure 13-5, *B*). These areas will communicate voluntary control–related information back to the PAG regarding the safety and social context of the

URINE STORAGE REFLEXES

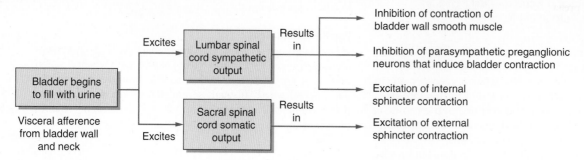

A

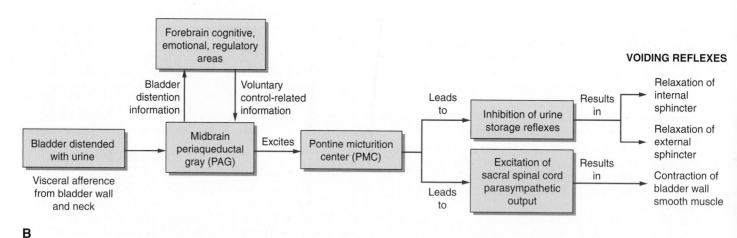

B

FIGURE 13-5 Organization of micturition. **A,** Neural events involved in the urine storage reflexes as the bladder begins to fill with urine. **B,** Neural events involved in the voiding reflexes when the bladder becomes full and distended.

situation. The PAG integrates this information, along with distention signals, to determine whether the PMC should be activated to initiate the voiding reflexes that produce emptying of the bladder.

Gastric secretion of digestive fluids in anticipation of food, and emptying of the rectum in response to filling, are but a few of the many other autonomic reflexes described in more detail throughout this book.

Preganglionic Neurons Are Influenced by Many Regions of the Brain

Much as the lower motor neuron of the somatic system is influenced by the upper motor neuron (see Chapter 9), the preganglionic autonomic neuron is influenced by CNS axons descending from the brainstem and forebrain. However, it should be noted that many of the CNS structures that affect autonomic function cannot be easily assigned a sympathetic or parasympathetic role and many are involved in nonautonomic control in the body, as well.

Many brainstem structures are known to influence autonomic preganglionic neurons in order to control particular visceral functions; we have just seen an example with respect to micturition (e.g., PMC). Another example is the vasopressor center of the medulla that increases peripheral vascular resistance and cardiac output. Often these "centers" are networked clusters

of neurons as opposed to a discrete nucleus. Some brainstem structures are actually comprised of the cell bodies of preganglionic autonomic neurons (e.g., motor nucleus of the vagus).

Most of the brainstem regions that influence autonomic preganglionic neurons receive input from the *hypothalamus* of the diencephalon, a structure that is critical for homeostasis. The hypothalamus coordinates the activity of these brainstem regions as an important means of regulating visceral function for purposes of homeostasis. The hypothalamus exerts its control over these brainstem regions using the guidance of cortical and other telencephalic inputs related to cognitive and emotional processes and with the guidance of both somatic and visceral sensory information. In its critical role in homeostasis, the hypothalamus not only regulates autonomic function, but regulates endocrine function, as well as certain somatic motor actions. By coordinating these three roles, the hypothalamus can produce some complex behaviors related to homeostasis, such as feeding.

Much of the visceral afferent information that will be used by brain structures that influence autonomic preganglionic neurons synapses within the *solitary nucleus* of the medulla. The solitary nucleus then distributes this information, either directly or indirectly, to brainstem or forebrain areas, noted previously, that will influence the autonomic preganglionic neurons. Some of the solitary nucleus output synapses directly on preganglionic neurons of the brainstem, producing some of the simplest autonomic reflexes.

Although the organization of brain structures that affect the function of autonomic preganglionic neurons has been presented in a somewhat straightforward, hierarchal, rostral-to-caudal fashion, the relationship of these brain structures is really more complicated. For example, the hypothalamus can project directly to preganglionic autonomic neurons of the brainstem and spinal cord, there are telencephalic projections to autonomic-related brainstem structures that bypass the hypothalamus, and there are interconnections among different cortical regions that are involved in autonomic function. Therefore, the central control of autonomic function represents more of a complex central autonomic network than a simple hierarchy of control. This complex system of upper motor neurons within the CNS helps coordinate autonomic reflexes and directly influences action potential frequency within preganglionic neurons. As more is learned about these central systems controlling the ANS, their specific role in such conditions as hypertension and various gastrointestinal diseases may become clearer.

CLINICAL CORRELATIONS

HORNER'S SYNDROME

History. A 7-year-old male golden retriever is brought to your clinic for examination. The owner states that during the past 3 weeks, the dog has become progressively weaker in his left front leg and now cannot bear weight on that limb. The owner has also noticed that the dog's left upper eyelid seems to be droopy.

Clinical Examination. Physical examination abnormalities are limited to the nervous system. The dog is bright, alert, and responsive. Cranial nerve reflexes are within normal limits. The dog cannot bear weight on the left front leg, and the leg muscles are atrophied. No segmental reflexes (e.g., toe-pinch withdrawal) or intersegmental responses (e.g., proprioceptive placing) can be elicited in the left front leg. The left upper eyelid droops lower than the right upper lid, and the left pupil is smaller than the right pupil. The left nictitating membrane (third eyelid) is prolapsed (slipped out of place) over part of the cornea, and the left eye seems more sunken into the orbit than the right eye.

Comment. This dog has a lesion of the left brachial plexus, probably a neoplasm. It has caused a lower motor neuron syndrome to the left front leg with atrophy, paralysis, and loss of reflexes. The tumor has damaged the preganglionic neurons of the left sympathetic nervous system as they leave the first two thoracic segments on their way toward the eye. Loss of the sympathetic innervation to the region of the eye causes the small pupil (miosis), drooping of the upper eyelid (ptosis), a sunken appearance in the eye (enophthalmos), and prolapse of the nictitating membrane. This constellation of clinical signs is called *Horner's syndrome.*

Sympathetic preganglionic neurons pass through the brachial plexus (where they were damaged in this dog) and ascend in the vagosympathetic trunk to synapse with the postganglionic neurons in the cranial cervical ganglia. The postganglionic cell axons then go to the region of the eye, where they innervate the dilator smooth muscle cells of the iris. When paralyzed, the constrictor fibers of the iris are unopposed, resulting in miosis. The sympathetic nervous system also innervates several smooth muscle fibers that lift the upper eyelid and help position the nictitating membrane and

the eye within the socket. Because the preganglionic fibers are relatively exposed in the neck, they are usually damaged.

Horner's syndrome can also result from damage to either the postganglionic neurons or the neurons that descend from the hypothalamus to the rostral thoracic cord to control the preganglionic neurons.

Treatment. Treatment involves removing the cause of sympathetic nerve damage, with variable effect upon neural symptoms.

COLIC FROM ADMINISTRATION OF ATROPINE TO TREAT CORNEAL ULCER

History. A client calls you and says that the 14-year-old mare that they are treating for a corneal ulcer is now agitated, looking at her sides, and trying to roll. The mare is not interested in eating or drinking. She was fine this morning when they treated her, but this afternoon, she is looking agitated.

Clinical Examination. The mare has an increased heart rate, respiratory rate, and normal temperature. The eye that has the corneal ulcer is dilated (mydriatic). Her gastrointestinal borborygmi (growling sounds) are decreased in all quadrants. She is given an antiinflammatory medication (banamine, flunixin meglumine). Within a few minutes, she is not as agitated, and she is standing more comfortably. When a nasogastric tube is passed, a moderate amount of gas is present. On palpation per rectum (by way of the rectum), there is some increased gas present in her cecum, but no other abnormal findings. The mare appears to be more comfortable. You ask the client if there have been any changes in treatments, medications, and/or management. When they show you the medications for the corneal ulcer, you realize they had accidentally switched the frequency of administration: they were giving the triple antibiotic 2 times/day and the atropine 4 times/day, instead of the antibiotic 4 times/day and atropine 2 times/day, and they had done this for the last 3 to 4 days.

Comment. Although there are many different causes of colic, it is possible that the colic is due to the inadvertent over-administration of atropine. Atropine can be absorbed systemically from the ophthalmic administration. Atropine blocks the postsynaptic effects of acetylcholine at the level of the muscarinic receptors, and is parasympatholytic (interrupting parasympathetic function), thereby reducing the antagonism of sympathetic effects at the end organs. The resulting relative increase in sympathetic tone can cause an increased heart rate, decreased GI motility, and increased sphincter tone, as well as decreased GI secretions, and urine retention.

Treatment. The horse is treated for colic with banamine, which inhibits cyclo-oxygenase, and is both an antiinflammatory and analgesic. Additionally, the horse is given xyalzine, which is an α_2 adrenergic agonist, with or without butorphanol. Xyalzine will decrease release of neurotransmitters from the neuron by binding to presynaptic α_2 receptors (negative feedback receptors). This decreases sympathetic outflow, including possibly causing bradycardia (decreased heart rate). Butorphanol, which is an opiate that is a κ (kappa) receptor agonist and weak μ (mu) receptor antagonist, is sometimes used as well in combination with xyalzine. In addition to antiinflammatory and possibly analgesics, the horse can also be given mineral oil and/or water via the nasogastric tube to correct possible dehydration. In some cases, if food bolus impaction or ingestion of an excessive or irritating amount of food has occurred, mineral oil may also be given.

PRACTICE QUESTIONS

1. Choose the *incorrect* statement below:
   a. A ganglion is a collection of nerve cell bodies outside the CNS.
   b. Acetylcholine is a chemical transmitter at the parasympathetic postganglionic–to–target organ synapse.
   c. Sympathetic postganglionic neurons are usually longer than those of the parasympathetic system.
   d. The adrenal medulla secretes mostly norepinephrine and relatively little epinephrine.
   e. Muscarinic acetylcholine receptors are found on peripheral targets of parasympathetic postganglionic neurons.

2. A chemical neurotransmitter between preganglionic and postganglionic neurons of the parasympathetic component of the autonomic nervous system is:
   a. Norepinephrine.
   b. Acetylcholine.
   c. Epinephrine.
   d. Serotonin.
   e. γ-Aminobutyric acid.

3. A neurotransmitter most often found at the synapse between sympathetic postganglionic neurons and their targets is:
   a. Norepinephrine.
   b. Epinephrine.
   c. Acetylcholine.
   d. Dopamine.
   e. γ-Aminobutyric acid.

4. Which of the following is *true* regarding sympathetic preganglionic neurons?
   a. Their cell bodies are located in thoracic and lumbar regions of the spinal cord.
   b. Their axons synapse within the sympathetic ganglion chain.
   c. Their axons form splanchnic nerves.
   d. Their axons travel in the ventral root.
   e. All the above are true.

5. Horner's syndrome is caused by the loss of:
   a. Sympathetic innervation to the eye.
   b. Parasympathetic postganglionic innervation to the eye.
   c. Peripheral muscarinic receptors.
   d. Vagus nerve fibers.
   e. Smooth muscle of the iris.

BIBLIOGRAPHY

Benarroch EE: Central autonomic control. In Robertson D, Biaggioni I, Burnstock G, et al, editors: *Primer on the autonomic nervous system*, ed 3, London, UK, 2012, Academic Press.

Boron WF, Boulpaep EL: *Medical physiology*, ed 2, Philadelphia, 2009, Saunders.

Brodal P: *The central nervous system: structure and function*, ed 4, New York, 2010, Oxford University Press.

De Lahunta A, Glass E: *Veterinary anatomy and clinical neurology*, ed 3, Philadelphia, 2009, Saunders.

Fowler CJ, Griffiths D, de Groat WC: The neural control of micturition, *Nat Rev Neurosci* 9(6):453–466, 2008.

Haines DE: *Fundamental neuroscience for basic and clinical applications*, ed 3, Philadelphia, 2006, Churchill Livingstone.

Hall JE: *Guyton and Hall textbook of medical physiology*, ed 12, Philadelphia, 2011, Saunders.

Matsukawa K, Shirai M, Murata J, et al: Sympathetic cholinergic vasodilation of skeletal muscle small arteries, *Jpn J Physiology* 88(1):14–18, 2002.

Nichols JG, Martin AR, Fuchs PA, Brown DA: *From neuron to brain*, ed 5, Sunderland, Mass, 2011, Sinauer.

Papich M: *Saunders handbook of veterinary drugs*, ed 2, St Louis, 2007, Saunders.

Plumb D: *Veterinary drug handbook*, ed 3, Stockholm, Wis, 1999, Pharma Vet Publishing.

Purves D, Augustine GJ, Fitzpatrick D, et al: *Neuroscience*, ed 5, Sunderland, Mass, 2012, Sinauer.

Strain GM: Autonomic nervous system. In Reece WO, editor: *Duke's physiology of domestic animals*, ed 12, Ithaca, NY, 2004, Comstock Publishing.

Stromberg MW: The autonomic nervous system. In Evans HE, editor: *Miller's anatomy of the dog*, ed 3, Philadelphia, 1993, Saunders.

Westfall TC, Westfall DP: Neurotransmission: the autonomic and somatic motor nervous systems. In Brunton L, Chabner B, Knollman B, editors: *Goodman and Gilman's the pharmacological basis of therapeutics*, ed 12, New York, 2011, McGraw-Hill.

CHAPTER 14
The Visual System

KEY POINTS

1. The eye's anatomy is adapted to the eye's role as a visual receptor organ.
2. Through the process of accommodation, the lens changes shape to focus images from various distances onto the retina.
3. The vertebrate retina consists of five major cell types.
4. In some species the fovea minimizes distortion of light compared with other areas of the retina.
5. Tissue layers behind the retina principally absorb light, or can reflect light, depending on the species' habits.
6. Photoreception and transduction of light occur in the rods and cones.

7. Visual image processing in the retina begins as the response of the photoreceptor to light is synaptically transmitted to the ganglion cells by the bipolar cells.
8. The electroretinogram records the electrical response of the retina to a flashing light.
9. Ganglion cell axons transmit action potentials to the visual cortex by way of the lateral geniculate nucleus.
10. The diameter of the pupil is controlled by the autonomic nervous system.
11. The retina, optic nerve, and autonomic nerve supply controlling the pupil can be tested with a flashlight.
12. Aqueous humor determines intraocular pressure.

The eyes are complex sense organs that are basically an extension of the brain. They evolved from primitive light-sensing spots on the surface of invertebrates and in some species have developed many remarkable variations, providing special advantages in various ecological niches. Each eye has a layer of receptors, a lens system for focusing an image on these receptors, and a system of axons for transmitting action potentials to the brain. This chapter describes how these and other components of the eye work.

The Eye's Anatomy Is Adapted to the Eye's Role as a Visual Receptor Organ

Figure 14-1 shows the anatomy of the normal eye in the horizontal plane. The white, outer protective layer encasing most of the eyeball is called the *sclera.* It is modified anteriorly into a clear region called the *cornea* that consists of a specialized arrangement of collagen fibrils with an overlying, stratified, squamous epithelial layer. In the posterior two thirds of the eye the inner surface of the sclera is lined with a vascular and pigmented layer called the *choroid.* Interior to the choroid is the *retina,* the layer containing the photoreceptors.

As light passes through the transparent cornea, it undergoes some bending that will ultimately help to focus it on the retina. After passing through the cornea, the light enters a compartment called the *anterior chamber* (see Figure 14-1). The anterior chamber and the *posterior chamber* are filled with a clear, water-like fluid called *aqueous humor* that supplies important nutrients to the cornea (as well as the lens). Separating the anterior and posterior chambers is a diaphragm of varying size called the *iris.* The iris is a pigmented structure containing dilator and constrictor smooth muscle fibers arranged to vary the diameter of the *pupil,* the hole in the iris through which light passes on its way to the retina. The size of the pupil regulates the amount of light

entering the eye. Behind the iris is the lens. The lens is suspended in the eye by *suspensory ligaments* (known as *zonular fibers*) which attach to the lens and to the *ciliary body,* a muscular structure near the base of the iris. As discussed below, the lens provides variable focusing power, in contrast to the fixed cornea.

Behind the lens is a chamber filled with a gelatinous fluid called the *vitreous humor.* Because of the viscosity of this fluid, the pressure generated by the aqueous humor, and the fairly inelastic nature of the sclera and cornea, the globe of the eye is basically spherical. The vitreous humor also contains phagocytic cells that can clear ocular debris capable of obstructing the light path. Behind the vitreous humor is the neural retinal layer where light is transduced into the electrical activity of neurons. The retina is interrupted at a point where axons of the retina's ganglion cell layer, which travel across the inner surface of the retina, leave the eye on their way to the brain. This point, the *optic disc,* is a recognizable structure when the eye is examined with an ophthalmoscope (Figure 14-2). The interruption of the light-processing retina at the optic disc produces a *blind spot,* another name for the optic disc. The retinal ganglion cell axons leaving the eye at the optic disc give rise to the *optic nerve* (cranial nerve 2), a cranial nerve so rich in axons that there are more axons in both optic nerves than in all the dorsal roots of the spinal cord.

Also visible through the ophthalmoscope, on the surface of the retina, are the *retinal blood vessels* (see Figure 14-2). This network of arteries and veins enters the retina at the optic disc and provides much of the nutrition to the retina. Vessels of the choroid, that enter it after piercing the sclera near the optic disc, provide the remaining nutrition to the retina. Examination of retinal vessels often provides valuable clues to abnormalities elsewhere in the cardiovascular system.

The *lacrimal gland,* located near the lateral canthus (where upper and lower lids meet) of the eye, produces tears in response

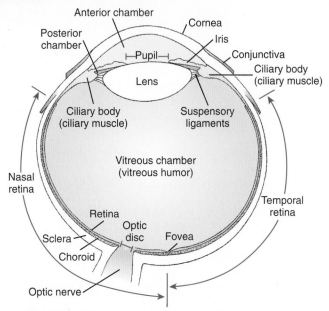

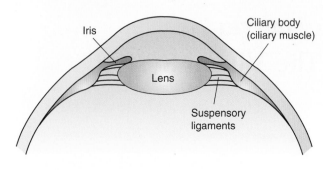

Viewing distant target

FIGURE 14-1 Schematic diagram of a horizontal section through the right eye as viewed from above. (Redrawn from Walls GL: *The vertebrate eye and its adaptive radiation,* Cranbrook Institute of Science, Bulletin 19, 1942.)

Gaze shifts to nearby target

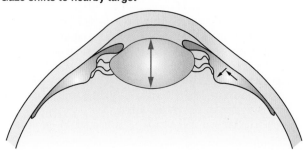

FIGURE 14-3 The process of accommodation as seen in a horizontal section through the eye. As gaze shifts from a distant to a nearby target the ciliary muscle contracts, moving forward and inward *(small black arrows),* releasing tension on the suspensory ligaments. This reduced tension, and the inherent elasticity of the lens, allows the lens to widen antero-posteriorly *(red arrow)* toward its more natural, unstretched, spherical configuration.

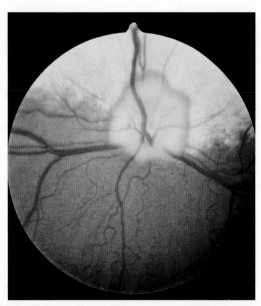

FIGURE 14-2 Ocular fundus (inner posterior surface) of the eye of a medium sized dog, as viewed with an ophthalmoscope, showing the optic disc, retinal blood vessels, and tapetum. The optic disk appears as a light, circular region with a darker border, located just off the center of the image. The reflective tapetum appears as the whiter-colored area surrounding the optic disc and comprising the upper third of the image. (From De Lahunta A, Glass E: *Veterinary anatomy and clinical neurology,* ed 3, Philadelphia, 2009, Saunders.)

to parasympathetic nerve stimulation. Tears then flow over the cornea and are drained into the nose by the nasolacrimal duct. A regular flow of tears across the cornea is essential to the health of the cornea.

The eye is directed toward environmental sources of light by the six striated *extraocular muscles* that originate within the orbit

and attach to the sclera. The muscles can rotate the eye around the dorsoventral, mediolateral, and anteroposterior axes. The third (oculomotor), fourth (trochlear), and sixth (abducens) cranial nerves contribute to this movement.

Through the Process of Accommodation, the Lens Changes Shape to Focus Images from Various Distances onto the Retina

When a camera focuses the images of objects at various distances from the film, the distance between the lens and the film is changed. The eye, however, focuses images by changing the shape of the lens, not by changing the distance between the lens and the retina.

Figure 14-3 shows the process of *accommodation,* whereby the lens adds extra focusing power by changing its shape. The lens of the eye is made up of an elastic *lens capsule* containing laminae of lens fibers that are arranged like the layers of an onion. Given this anatomy, if the eye's lens were taken out of the eye, the lens would assume a spherical shape, principally due to the elasticity of its capsule. When suspended in the relaxed eye, however, the suspensory ligaments pull on the equator of the lens, causing it to flatten in its anterior-posterior dimension. This flattened, less convex lens causes less refraction (bending) of light rays and allows the focus onto the retina of objects more than 20 feet away. To focus the image of objects closer to the eye, however, the lens must assume a more spherical, convex shape. This is accomplished by contraction of the ciliary muscle of the ciliary body. This contraction causes the ciliary muscle to move

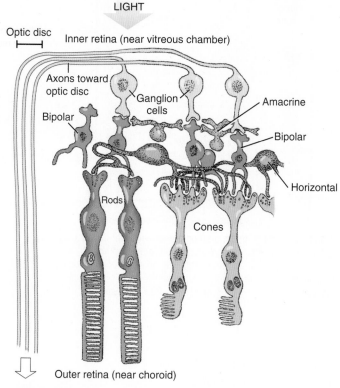

LIGHT

Optic disc

Inner retina (near vitreous chamber)

Axons toward optic disc

Ganglion cells

Amacrine

Bipolar

Bipolar

Horizontal

Rods

Cones

Outer retina (near choroid)

Ganglion cell axons leave eye, forming optic nerve

FIGURE 14-4 Schematic of a patch of vertebrate retina, bordering the optic disc, that shows the five major retinal cell types: photoreceptor cells (either rods or cones), bipolar cells, horizontal cells, amacrine cells, and ganglion cells. The optic disc is formed as retinal ganglion cell axons, which run across the inner surface of the retina, leave the eye to form the optic nerve. (Modified from Kandel ER, Schwartz JH, editors: *Principles of neural science*, ed 2, New York, 1985, Elsevier Science & Technology.)

antero-centripetally (forward and inward), which results in a relaxation of tension on the suspensory ligaments. The result, given the inherent elasticity of the lens capsule, is a more spherical lens with more light refraction that focuses onto the retina the image of nearer objects. The more the ciliary muscle contracts, the more spherical the lens becomes.

In humans, as the lens ages, it becomes less elastic and tends to become less spherical, even when the ciliary muscles contract. This condition is known as *presbyopia.* Many people older than 40 years of age need reading glasses to help their less elastic lens focus on objects nearby. A related condition in dogs and cats, called *nuclear sclerosis,* may begin at around 7 years of age, but it does not appear to produce as significant a visual deficit as in human presbyopia.

The lens should be clear and free of opacities. In *cataracts,* however, the lens becomes more opaque, causing random refraction of light and blurring vision, often leading eventually to blindness.

The Vertebrate Retina Consists of Five Major Cell Types

Given its elegant architecture, the retina, the neural portion of the eye, is capable of considerable processing of the visual image before the information is transmitted toward the brain. The vertebrate retina consists of five major cell types: photoreceptor cells, bipolar cells, horizontal cells, amacrine cells, and ganglion cells (Figure 14-4). As in the cerebral and cerebellar cortices, the arrangement of these component cells is fairly consistent across the retina, suggesting a basic underlying processing mechanism and giving the retina a layered histology. However, local variations in the density of some cell types and in synaptic architecture account for particular functional variations within the retina.

There are two types of retinal photoreceptor cells: *rods* and *cones* (see Figure 14-4). Both rods and cones make direct synaptic connection with the interneurons called *bipolar cells,* which connect the receptors with the ganglion cells. Ganglion cell axons traverse the inner surface of the retina and converge at the optic disc to leave the eye as the optic nerve, sending action potentials to the brain.

Modifying the flow of information at the synapses among the photoreceptors, bipolar cells, and ganglion cells are two interneuron cell types: the horizontal cells and the amacrine cells (see Figure 14-4). The *horizontal cells* mediate lateral interactions among the photoreceptors and bipolar cells. The *amacrine cells* mediate lateral interactions among the bipolar cells and the ganglion cells.

In Some Species the Fovea Minimizes Distortion of Light Compared with Other Areas of the Retina

The retinal ganglion cells are located in the inner retina (closer to the vitreous humor), whereas the photoreceptor cells (rods and cones) are located in the outer retina (closer to the choroid; see Figure 14-4). Therefore, throughout most of the retina, light rays travel through ganglion cells, bipolar cells, amacrine cells, and horizontal cells before reaching the photoreceptors. Although these inner neurons are unmyelinated (the ganglion cell axons become myelinated on leaving the eye) and therefore relatively transparent, they still cause some distortion of light rays.

The *fovea,* an area that demarcates the central retina in many primates, is designed to minimize this distortion. This sloping pit is formed as the neural tissue near the inner surface of the central retina is pushed aside, permitting light rays to have a less obstructed path to the outer retina. Distortion is least in the

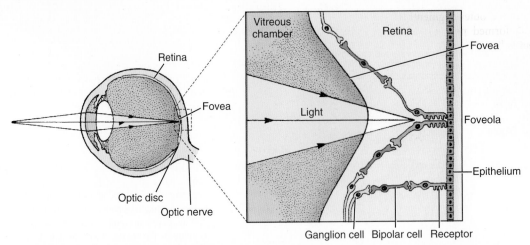

FIGURE 14-5 In most of the retina, light must first pass through inner, and then outer, layers of neurons and their processes before it reaches the photoreceptors. In the center of the fovea (found in many primates), in a region called the *foveola,* these neural elements are shifted aside; therefore, light has an almost unobstructed pathway to the photoreceptors in this region. An enlarged drawing of the foveal region is shown on the *right.* (From Kandel ER, Schwartz JH, editors: *Principles of neural science,* ed 4, New York, 2000, McGraw-Hill.)

center of the fovea, in an area called the *foveola,* where light rays have almost unobstructed access to the photoreceptors (Figure 14-5). This is functionally significant because it allows light to have a less distorted path to the region of the retina associated with the highest visual acuity (ability to discern detail). The optic disc is just nasal to the fovea.

In many mammalian veterinary species, although the central retina is also the area of highest visual acuity, no distinct fovea is formed. However, in these species, as well as primates, major blood vessels that can potentially interfere with the light path avoid passing across the central retina.

Tissue Layers Behind the Retina Principally Absorb Light, or Can Reflect Light, Depending on the Species' Habits

In animals that rely heavily on acute, daylight vision, there is a dark melanin pigment in the epithelial layer between the photoreceptors and the choroid. This pigment absorbs light that has passed by the photoreceptors without stimulating them. If such light were reflected back into the retina, the sharpness of the visual image would be blurred. In nocturnal animals and most domestic mammals, however, there is a patch of reflective material within the choroid called the *tapetum* (see Figure 14-2). When the tapetum is present, the region of the epithelial layer that overlies it does not contain the dark, light-absorbing pigment noted above. This arrangement facilitates the reflection of non-absorbed light back onto the retina allowing it to make optimal use of what light it receives, but at the expense of visual acuity. Reflection of light off the tapetum causes the familiar "night shine" from nocturnal animals' eyes.

Photoreception and Transduction of Light Occur in the Rods and Cones

The anatomical structures of the rod and cone photoreceptors are similar, but there are some important differences. Because they are neurons, the rods and cones are primary receptors. Both cell types are divided into three parts: a synaptic terminal, an inner segment, and an outer segment (Figure 14-6). The photoreceptor synaptic terminal synapses with the bipolar cells. The inner

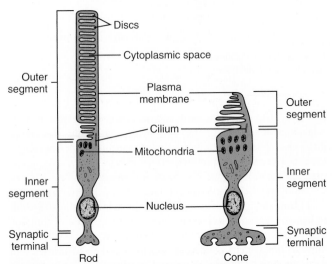

FIGURE 14-6 The two types of photoreceptors, rods and cones, have characteristic structures. Both rod cells and cone cells are differentiated into inner and outer segments connected by a cilium. The inner segments of both cell types contain the nucleus and most of the cell's biosynthetic machinery and are continuous with the synaptic terminals. The membranous discs in the outer segment contain the light-transducing photopigment. The discs in the outer segments of rod cells are separated from the plasma membrane, whereas the discs of cone cells are not. (Modified from O'Brien DF: The chemistry of vision, *Science* 218(4576):961-966, 1982; from Kandel ER, Schwartz JH, editors: *Principles of neural science,* ed 4, New York, 2000, McGraw-Hill.)

segment includes the nucleus, mitochondria, and other cytoplasmic structures. The inner and outer segments are connected by a microtubule-containing cilium. The outer portions are specialized for photoreception. They contain an elaborate array of stacked membranous discs whose membranes contain visual photopigment. *Visual photopigment* is a light-sensitive molecular complex that initiates a biochemical chain of events, transducing light into neural electrical signals.

The discs in the outer segments of the photoreceptors are regularly being formed near the cilium, phagocytized by the pigmented epithelium, and their photopigment cycled back to newly formed discs. Loss of this normal turnover in the outer segment may be important in several retinal diseases (e.g., retinitis pigmentosa). Photopigment of the discs is made up of a protein, called *opsin,* and *retinal,* an aldehyde of vitamin A. The light-sensitive retinal molecule is bound to the opsin, which is a member of the G-protein–coupled membrane receptor family (see Chapter 1). When light is absorbed by a rod or cone, the retinal is transformed in a way that activates the opsin, producing a change in the concentration of an intracellular second messenger, which leads to a change in the membrane potential of the photoreceptor cell. The configurational change in retinal is the only light-sensitive event in vision.

Unlike most sensory receptor cell membranes that depolarize with stimulation, photoreceptors hyperpolarize when struck by light. In rods the visual photopigment is called *rhodopsin.* In the dark, many gated sodium/calcium ion channels remain open, allowing leakage of Na^+ and Ca^{2+} ions into the rod, which keeps the membrane in a depolarized state. When photons of light strike rhodopsin, the resulting change in second-messenger concentration produces a closing of many of the gated Na^+/Ca^{2+} channels. The result is a hyperpolarization of the receptor cell membrane and a decrease in transmitter released at the synapse with the bipolar cell. Photoreception in cones works in a similar manner except that the photopigment opsin is different from that of rhodopsin. Depending on the species, different populations of cones may have different opsins. Because different opsins differ in their ability to absorb particular wavelengths of light, the number of these different cone populations in a species is related to the ability of that species to discriminate different colors.

Differences in the functional properties of rods and cones, differences in their retinal distribution, and differences in the synaptic organization of other retinal neurons to which they pass their information result in a "rod retinal system" and a "cone retinal system" that have different functional attributes (Table 14-1). Because individual rods are more sensitive to light than individual cones, and because several rods feed their synaptic input to a single bipolar cell (convergence), the rod system is the night-vision system concerned with detecting the presence of light. Because of the convergence of many rods on a bipolar cell, however, the rod system is not good for discerning the detail of a visual image (poor visual acuity). Also, because the rods are more highly concentrated in the peripheral retina than the cones, this region is better at detecting the presence of light than discerning its details. Finally, because all rods contain the same

visual photopigment, the rod system cannot discriminate different colors.

As noted, a cone is less sensitive to light than a rod. Also, one or only a few cones feed their synaptic input to a single bipolar cell. Therefore the cone system needs higher levels of illumination to function compared with the rod system. In fact, the cone system actually represents the day-vision system because the rod system does not function well in high levels of illumination. However, due to a lack of convergence onto bipolar cells, the cone system is good at discerning image details. Because the cones have a particularly high density in the region of the fovea, or central retina, this area is the part of the retina with the highest visual acuity. This makes sense considering the fovea, or central retina, is where light falls when an animal looks directly at an object of interest. Again, different populations of cones can contain different photopigments, each differentially sensitive to a range of light frequencies. Thus the cone system is also the color-vision system. Generally, the more cone photopigments present in the retina, each within a different population of cones, the better is the ability of the species to discriminate different wavelengths of light, or to "see" color. In primates there are three different populations of cones, each with a different photopigment. According to the *Young-Helmholtz theory,* the brain assigns color to a given wavelength of light by comparing the relative activation of the different cone populations. Humans who lack one or more of these cone types, as a result of faulty genetic transmission, cannot see colors within particular ranges of the visible spectrum of light. The most common types of such "color blindness" are linked to the X chromosome.

The extent to which various veterinary species perceive color is still controversial. It is believed that mammalian ancestors may have had four different types of cones, whereas early nocturnal mammals may have had only two types of cones, having traded some of their color discrimination ability for rod light sensitivity. Most current mammals, including dogs, have only two types of cones. As noted, primates have three types of cones. It is thought that their successful exploitation of color-rich arboreal environments may have induced selection pressure for additional color discrimination ability, above that imparted by two populations of cones. Modern birds appear to have four populations of cones, one of which is sensitive to light in the ultraviolet (UV) range of the spectrum. Behavioral experiments that show their ability to discriminate UV light suggest that birds have a richer color perception than primates. Lizards, turtles, and some fish also possess UV-sensitive cones. Only primates are known to have the color vision with which humans are familiar.

Visual Image Processing in the Retina Begins as the Response of the Photoreceptor to Light Is Synaptically Transmitted to the Ganglion Cells by the Bipolar Cells

The hyperpolarizing response of the rods and cones to light synaptically influences bipolar cells; in turn, the bipolar cell influences action potential frequencies in the ganglion cell axons on their way to the brain. As alluded to earlier, this transmission of information from the outer to the inner retina can be modulated by the horizontal cells and the amacrine cells (see Figure 14-4). The horizontal cells are in communication with photoreceptor-bipolar cell synapses, and with each other, to allow lateral communication among different photoreceptor-bipolar cell synapses. Amacrine cells can serve a somewhat analogous function with respect to bipolar-ganglion cell synaptic interactions. An interesting consequence of this architecture is that light that hits a specific

TABLE 14-1 Functional Differences Between Rod and Cone Systems

Rod System	Cone System
Most sensitive to light	Less sensitive to light
Night vision (low light)	Day vision (normal indoor and daylight)
Low acuity	High acuity (good at discerning image detail)
Achromatic	Color vision
Peripheral retina	Central retina (fovea)

point on the retina can influence the activity and/or responsiveness to light of cells in an adjacent patch of retina.

Considerable processing of the visual image occurs in the retina, and it is particularly good at detecting luminance changes of small spots of light. The initial stages of color discrimination, contrast detection and enhancement, and directional sensitivity also occur in the retina. The synaptic interactions among photoreceptors, bipolar cells, and horizontal cells play a significant role in contrast enhancement and directional sensitivity. The interactions of amacrine cells with bipolar cells and ganglion cells appear to play a role in processes such as the ability to detect *changes* in the rate of alternation between light and dark. A more detailed description of the synaptic and membrane changes in the chain of transmission within the retina, accounting for these types of retinal image processing, is beyond the scope of this book. To learn more about the many interesting and unusual phenomena occurring in the retina, the reader should refer to the Bibliography.

The Electroretinogram Records the Electrical Response of the Retina to a Flashing Light

The *electroretinogram* (ERG) is a clinical electrophysiological recording from the cornea and skin near the eye. It records the electrical response of the retina to a light flashed into the eye. It has three waves: the *A wave*, corresponding primarily to the activation of visual pigment and photoreceptors; the *B wave*, caused primarily by the response of retinal bipolar cells; and a slower *C wave*, thought to originate in the pigment epithelium. The ERG is a fairly simple, general electrodiagnostic tool for assessing some forms of retinal dysfunction or degeneration.

Ganglion Cell Axons Transmit Action Potentials to the Visual Cortex by Way of the Lateral Geniculate Nucleus

Sets of retinal ganglion cells leaving the eye participate in three important visual pathways: the *retino-geniculo-striate pathway*, the *retino-tectal pathway*, and the *retino-hypothalamic pathway*. The retino-geniculo-striate pathway is principally involved in conscious visual perception of form, color, motion, orientation, and depth. The retino-tectal pathway plays an important role in pupillary reflexes and reflex orientation of the eye to visual targets. The retino-hypothalamic pathway plays a role in the regulation of physiological rhythms by light-dark cycles (e.g., seasonal changes in day length).

For the retinal image, originating from light in the visual field, to reach consciousness, the information must be transferred to the visual cortex. Figure 14-7 shows the retino-geniculo-striate pathway by which the axons of the retinal ganglion cells project to the lateral geniculate nucleus of the thalamus and by which cells in the *lateral geniculate nucleus* project their axons to the primary visual cortex of the occipital lobe. Note that ganglion cell axons from the temporal retina (closest to the ear; see Figure 14-1) travel along the *optic nerve* to the optic chiasm and then project ipsilaterally to the lateral geniculate nucleus on the same side of the brain. Ganglion cell axons from the nasal retina (closest to the nose) come to the *optic chiasm* and cross to the contralateral lateral geniculate nucleus. Retinal ganglion cell axons between the region of the optic chiasm and the lateral geniculate nuclei are referred to as the *optic tracts*. Cells in each lateral geniculate nucleus then send axons to the ipsilateral *primary visual cortex*, in the occipital lobe, by way of the *optic radiations*. This arrangement results in the right half of each

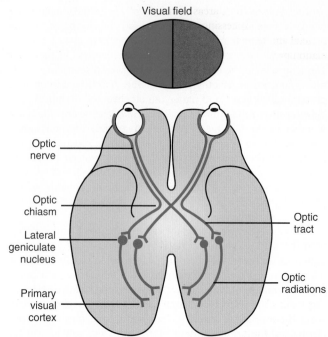

FIGURE 14-7 Retino-geniculo-striate pathway to cerebral cortex. Axons of the retinal ganglion cells project to the lateral geniculate nucleus of the thalamus, and axons from cells of the lateral geniculate nucleus project to the ipsilateral primary visual cortex of the occipital lobe. The right environmental visual field projects to the left half of each retina, and the left environmental visual field projects to the right half of each retina. The right half of each retina sends information to the right lateral geniculate, and from there to the right primary visual cortex. The left half of each retina sends information to the left lateral geniculate, and from there to the left primary visual cortex. Therefore, information from the left visual field arrives in the right primary visual cortex, and information from the right visual field arrives in the left primary visual cortex. The labeled components of each pathway are present on both sides of the brain.

retina sending information to the right primary visual cortex and the left half of each retina sending information to the left primary visual cortex. Light originating in the left half of the environmental visual field generally falls on the right half of the retina of each eye, whereas light originating in the right half of the environmental visual field falls on the left half of the retina of each eye. Given the anatomical map of the retino-geniculo-striate pathway in Figure 14-7, information from an image arising in the left field of vision would be received in the right primary visual cortex, and image information arising from the right field of vision would be received in the left primary visual cortex.

The features of the visual image to which lateral geniculate nucleus cells respond are surprisingly similar to those features processed by the retina (see above). However, more complex feature extraction can begin to be seen in primary visual cortex. For example, while the retina processes information about small spots of light, and the lateral geniculate nucleus processes information about larger spots of light comprised of those smaller spots, primary visual cortex can process information about bars or edges of light that are comprised of those larger spots. In addition, primary visual cortex also processes information about the orientation of those bars or edges and about whether the information comes from one eye or both eyes. Information reaching *primary visual cortex*, or *V1* (also called *striate cortex*), is passed to other occipital lobe areas of visual cortex (e.g., V2, V3) for still more complex processing, then to visual association areas of the parietal and temporal lobes for the highest forms of visual information processing and integration with other sensory modalities. There appears to be parallel processing of retinal information within the retino-geniculo-striate pathway and its higher-order processing regions. One major stream of information in this system apparently is concerned with conscious object identification (e.g., form, color), whereas a parallel stream of information relates to conscious awareness of where an object is located (e.g., motion, position). The three major projection pathways of retinal ganglion cell axons—retino-geniculo-striate, retino-tectal, and retino-hypothalamic—represent another example of the parallel processing of retinal information.

The Diameter of the Pupil Is Controlled by the Autonomic Nervous System

The iris of the eye contains two sets of smooth muscle fibers. One set, arranged in a circular pattern around the pupil, causes the pupil to become smaller *(constrict)* when the fibers contract. These constrictor fibers are innervated by postganglionic parasympathetic neurons whose cell bodies lie in the ciliary ganglion, just behind the eye, and which secrete acetylcholine as the neurotransmitter to the muscle. These parasympathetic postganglionic neurons are activated by parasympathetic preganglionic neurons whose axons travel in the *oculomotor cranial nerve* (cranial nerve 3) and whose cell bodies reside in the *Edinger-Westphal nucleus* of the midbrain.

The other smooth muscle fibers of the iris are arranged radially from the pupil, resembling spokes of a wheel. When these radial smooth muscle fibers contract, they cause the pupil to become larger *(dilate)*. These dilator fibers are innervated by the sympathetic nervous system. The sympathetic preganglionic neurons begin in the first three or four thoracic segments and course cranially in the vagosympathetic trunk to synapse in the superior cervical ganglion of the neck. The sympathetic postganglionic axons originate in cells of this ganglion and course to the region of the eye, where they innervate the dilator fibers of the iris, in addition to a muscle that helps lift the upper eyelid and a muscle that helps keep the "third eyelid" in place at the medial canthus of the eye. The sympathetic postganglionic axons also innervate sweat glands and vascular smooth muscle to the face.

The Retina, Optic Nerve, and Autonomic Nerve Supply Controlling the Pupil Can Be Tested with a Flashlight

When a light is shone into the eye, the pupil of that eye constricts. This action is called the *direct pupillary light reflex* (Figure 14-8). The light triggers the photoreception mechanism, leading to ganglion cell action potentials transmitted along the optic nerve. Some of the ganglion cell axons of the retino-tectal pathway synapse in the pretectal nuclei of the brain (near the diencephalic/mesencephalic border). The pretectal neurons then synapse on the parasympathetic preganglionic neurons of the Edinger-Westphal nucleus (in the mesencephalon), whose axons travel in the oculomotor nerve to synapse on parasympathetic postganglionic neurons in the ciliary ganglion (of the orbit). Stimulation of these postganglionic neurons causes constriction of the pupil by stimulating the constrictor smooth muscle fibers of the iris. A normal direct pupillary light reflex tests the integrity of the retina, the ipsilateral second and third cranial nerves, a limited region of the brainstem, and the iris. Given that a significant proportion of

optic nerve axons cross the midline at the optic chiasm, and that many axons of pretectal neurons also cross the midline (see Figure 14-8, *B*), when a light is shone into one eye, not only does the pupil on the same side constrict (direct pupillary light reflex), but the contralateral pupil also constricts. This action is called the *indirect* or *consensual pupillary light reflex*. It also requires the integrity of the contralateral oculomotor (third) cranial nerve.

Aqueous Humor Determines Intraocular Pressure

Aqueous humor is a clear liquid found in the anterior and posterior chambers of the eye. Its rate of production and absorption is sufficiently high to replace the entire chambers' volume several times a day.

Aqueous humor is produced by the epithelium covering the *ciliary processes,* a system of fingerlike projections on the ciliary body of the posterior chamber. Aqueous humor is thought to be formed by the active transport of sodium, chloride, and bicarbonate ions into the posterior chamber. This establishes an osmotic gradient, causing water to flow passively into the posterior chamber. Aqueous humor flows from the posterior to the anterior chamber through the pupil. Flow is caused by a pressure gradient established by the active process of formation in the posterior chamber.

Aqueous humor is then absorbed into the venous system at the angle between the cornea and the iris. This absorption is driven by a pressure gradient and is assisted, in many species, by a system of trabeculae and canals. If this absorption into the venous system is obstructed, intraocular pressure increases because the production of aqueous humor continues. This pathologic increase in intraocular pressure is called *glaucoma*. As intraocular pressure exceeds intravascular pressure in the blood supply to the retina, blindness results.

CLINICAL CORRELATIONS

HOMONYMOUS HEMIANOPIA

History. You examine a 10-year-old male German shepherd whose owner reports that the dog has recently begun to bump into objects with the left side of his face and has had two seizures. The seizures were characterized by turning of the head to the left and stiffening of the left front leg.

Clinical Examination. Physical examination abnormalities are limited to the nervous system. When presented with a maze of unfamiliar objects in the examination room, the dog collides with objects as if he does not see from the left side. He seems somewhat weak in the left front leg. The dog is otherwise bright, alert, and responsive. Cranial nerve and spinal segmental reflexes are within normal limits, as are intersegmental, proprioceptive placing responses for the right front and right rear legs. However, the proprioceptive placing responses for the left front and left rear legs are quite prolonged.

Comment. This dog's history and neurological examination abnormalities are common in dogs with brain tumors. This dog has a tumor (neoplasm) arising from the meninges over the right posterior cerebral cortex. It is in this posterior (occipital) cortex that the visual image is interpreted from the visual field of the left side (see Figure 14-7). Lesion-induced functional damage to the right

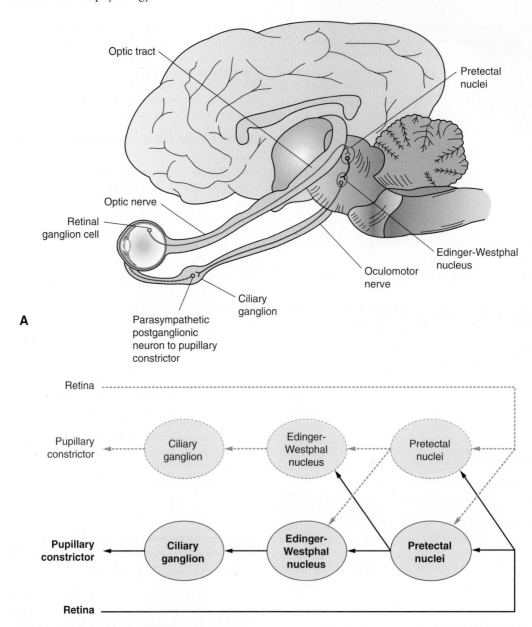

FIGURE 14-8 The pupillary light reflex. **A,** The structures and synapses involved in the direct pupillary light reflex represented on one side of the animal. **B,** Schematic diagram showing connections that cross the midline that are responsible for the consensual (indirect) pupillary light reflex. Retinal axons that cross the midline do so at the optic chiasm (not labeled). Although bilaterally symmetrical, structures and connections originating on one side of the animal have been de-emphasized for ease of interpretation by the reader.

occipital cortex results in loss of vision from the left visual field *(homonymous hemianopia).* Also in the right cerebral cortex, the conscious proprioception response for the left legs is interpreted. This dog's seizures feature turning the head to the left and displaying transient rigidity of the left front leg, because the seizure activity arose from the cerebral cortex at the site of the tumor and spread to the right motor cortex but remained limited to the cerebral cortex on the right side. Because the pyramidal system's corticospinal tract controlling the muscles of the left neck and left front leg arise in the right motor cortex (see Chapter 10), seizure activity causes the transient head turning and left leg stiffness.

Treatment. This dog had a meningioma of the right posterior cerebral cortex. Surgical removal was not attempted in this case.

UVEITIS IN A HORSE

History. A client calls you out to look at their 8-year-old Appaloosa mare's right eye, for squinting, pain, and discharge of a few days duration. The horse does not have any other clinical signs other than the eye.

Clinical Examination. The ophthalmic exam demonstrates a miotic (constricted) pupil, corneal edema (giving it a hazy appearance), and flare (clouding of aqueous humor), of the right eye. You use fluorescein dye to stain the eye, and there is a 3 mm by 4 mm superficial corneal ulcer present. After dilating the eye with tropicamide, you see the optic disc looks edematous (swollen) at the edges. Your exam on the left eye reveals no abnormalities.

Comment. This mare likely has uveitis with an associated corneal ulcer. The uvea is comprised of the choroid, iris, and ciliary body. It is possible that she developed the uveitis, due to a *Leptospira* species (a bacterial spirochete) or another cause, and then because the eye was painful, she scratched the cornea to cause the ulcer. Alternatively, the mare could have developed the ulcer by rubbing her face or from a scratch from a foreign body (i.e., dirt, twigs), and then she developed uveitis secondary to the ulcer.

With uveitis, there is a breakdown of the normal blood-aqueous barrier, allowing protein, cells and fibrin to enter the aqueous humor, clouding it. Corneal endothelial cells are also affected, which can lead to reduced fluid removal from the corneal tissue, resulting in corneal edema. The lacrimal glands, under parasympathetic stimulation, release tears. Because of the inflammation, the ciliary body and pupillary sphincter can constrict or spasm, which can affect the pupil and may be painful.

Treatment. With the corneal ulcer present, steroids are usually not used topically, because there would be a greater chance for infection. The horse is treated with topical atropine, which is an anticholinergic, to help dilate the pupil and relieve ciliary spasm, thus decreasing pain. Horses are also treated with topical antibiotics for possible infection, and also with systemic anti-inflammatory medications, such as flunixin meglumine. In some cases, topical anti-inflammatory medications are also needed. The horse is treated for a few days after the ulcer resolves to maximize the chances of tear production normalizing. If the optic disc is still edematous and the mare is still in pain, based on squinting and/or miotic pupil, she could be switched over to topical steroids to provide better control of inflammation.

PRACTICE QUESTIONS

1. A patient whose left pupil diameter is smaller than normal, whose left upper eyelid droops, and whose left "third eyelid" is abnormally displaced, likely has a lesion of which of the following structures?
   a. Left oculomotor nerve
   b. Left vagosympathetic nerve trunk
   c. Right oculomotor nerve
   d. Right vagosympathetic nerve trunk
   e. Left optic tract

2. Which of the following is *not* characteristic of the cone system?
   a. Many photoreceptors converging on single bipolar cell
   b. Good visual acuity
   c. Multiple photopigments
   d. Day vision
   e. Color vision
   f. All the above are characteristic of the cone system

3. Your friend, a member of the soccer team, is trying without much success to explain the cause for the team's recent losing trend. A variety of implausible explanations are proposed until she mentions that she is progressively losing vision, but only in her left visual field, and has frequent headaches. You recommend that she see a neurologist because she likely has a lesion in her:
   a. Left optic tract
   b. Right optic nerve
   c. Right optic tract
   d. Optic chiasm
   e. Left optic radiations

4. Which of the following regarding the lens is *false*?
   a. It lies behind the iris.
   b. It plays an important role in focusing a visual image on the retina.
   c. It contains layered lens fibers.
   d. Its shape does not normally change.
   e. An increase in its opacity is called a *cataract*.

5. You examine a patient's pupillary light reflexes. Shining a light into the left eye produces both a positive direct and a positive consensual pupillary response. However, shining the light into the right eye produces neither a direct nor an indirect pupillary response. This patient's pathological lesion is located in which of the following structures?
   a. Left optic nerve
   b. Left oculomotor nerve
   c. Right optic nerve
   d. Right oculomotor nerve
   e. Left primary visual cortex

BIBLIOGRAPHY

Bear MF, Connors BW, Paradiso MA: *Neuroscience: exploring the brain*, ed 3, Philadelphia, 2007, Lippincott, Williams & Wilkins.
Brodal P: *The central nervous system: structure and function*, ed 4, New York, 2010, Oxford University Press.
De Lahunta A, Glass E: *Veterinary anatomy and clinical neurology*, ed 3, Philadelphia, 2009, Saunders.
Goldsmith TH: What birds see, *Sci Am* 295(1):68–75, 2006.
Goldstein BE: *Sensation and perception*, ed 8, Pacific Grove, Calif, 2009, Wadsworth.
Haines DE, editor: *Fundamental neuroscience for basic and clinical applications*, ed 3, Philadelphia, 2006, Churchill Livingstone.
Hall JE: *Guyton and Hall textbook of medical physiology*, ed 12, Philadelphia, 2011, Saunders.
Kandel ER, Schwartz JH, Jessell TM, editors: *Principles of neural science*, ed 4, New York, 2000, McGraw-Hill.
Nicholls JG, Martin AR, Fuchs PA, Brown DA: *From neuron to brain*, ed 5, Sunderland, Mass, 2012, Sinauer.
Purves D, Augustine GJ, Fitzpatrick D, et al: *Neuroscience*, ed 5, Sunderland, Mass, 2012, Sinauer.
Sheppard AL, Davies LN: In vivo analysis of ciliary muscle morphologic changes with accommodation and axial ametropia, *Invest Ophthalmol Vis Sci* 51(12):6882–6889, 2010.

CHAPTER 15

Cerebrospinal Fluid and the Blood-Brain Barrier

KEY POINTS

1. Cerebrospinal fluid has many functions.
2. Most cerebrospinal fluid is formed at the choroid plexus of the ventricles.
3. Cerebrospinal fluid flows down a pressure gradient through the ventricular system into the subarachnoid space.
4. Cerebrospinal fluid is absorbed into the venous system.
5. Hydrocephalus is an increased volume of cerebrospinal fluid in the skull.
6. Permeability barriers exist between blood and brain.

Cerebrospinal fluid (CSF) is a clear fluid present in the ventricles (core cavities) of the brain, in the central canal that runs through the core of the spinal cord, and in the subarachnoid space that surrounds the entire outer surface of the brain and spinal cord (Figure 15-1). The CSF contains almost no blood cells, little protein, and differs from plasma with respect to the concentration of various ions. Its rates of formation, flow, and absorption are sufficiently high to cause its replacement several times daily. Sampling its pressure, cell count, and levels of various biochemical constituents is a common diagnostic procedure for central nervous system pathology called a *spinal tap*. Injecting radiopaque dyes into the CSF of the subarachnoid space is the basis of a common neuroradiographic technique called *myelography*, often used in conjunction with computerized tomography (CT scan), which can assess the integrity of the spinal canal. Obstruction of the flow of CSF produces a condition called *hydrocephalus*. An understanding of the formation, flow, and absorption of CSF is essential for understanding these diagnostic procedures and the pathophysiology of hydrocephalus.

The *blood-brain barrier* (BBB) refers to the selective nature of central nervous system (CNS) blood vessels with respect to the materials that can move across their walls, compared with blood vessels in other parts of the body. Understanding the BBB helps clarify how the brain is protected from potentially harmful neuroactive chemicals in the blood, and why it is difficult to deliver certain drugs effectively to the brain.

Cerebrospinal Fluid Has Many Functions

To work properly, the CNS needs protection not only from physical injury but also from significant variation in the local environment of its neurons. A buildup of toxins or a significant change in ionic concentration in this neuronal microenvironment could result in pathological changes in neuronal physiology.

One of the most important functions of CSF is to cushion the brain, protecting it against blows to the head. Because the specific gravities of the brain and CSF are similar, the brain floats in the fluid. Thus the force of a blow to the head is buffered by the CSF instead of being transferred directly to brain tissue.

Because the composition of the CSF is tightly controlled and it is in equilibrium with the extracellular fluid of the brain and spinal cord, the CSF also helps maintain a consistent extracellular microenvironment for the neurons and glia of the CNS. This diffusional equilibrium between the CSF and the extracellular fluid, in conjunction with the flow and multiple daily turnover of the CSF, also makes the CSF an effective waste control system that can remove potentially harmful cellular metabolites. Evidence indicates that these properties may also allow the CSF to function as a brain distribution system for some polypeptide hormones and growth factors that are secreted into the CSF.

Most Cerebrospinal Fluid Is Formed at the Choroid Plexus of the Ventricles

The *ventricles* are a series of interconnected cavities in the core of the brain that have an ependymal cell lining and are filled with CSF (Figure 15-2). The *lateral ventricles* are respectively located in the two cerebral hemispheres, the *third ventricle* is found at the midline of the diencephalon, and the *fourth ventricle* is located between the cerebellum and the dorsal surface of the hindbrain (pons and medulla) (Figure 15-3).

The majority of CSF is formed by a *choroid plexus* located in each of the four ventricles. These are small, cauliflower-like growths of clustered villi that form a portion of the floor or roof of each ventricle (see Figure 15-3). The plexuses consist of tufts of capillaries covered by a layer of ependymal cells. These ependymal cells, unlike the cells lining the rest of the ventricle, form a selective, tight-junction barrier to the secretions of the leaky capillaries and to other surrounding fluids (e.g., CSF, extracellular fluid). Membrane transporters and selective channels regulate the passage of ions and molecules across the ependymal cell barrier, effectively controlling the composition of the CSF being synthesized in the ventricle. The active transport of sodium ions (Na^+) contributes to a net movement of sodium chloride (NaCl) into the ventricles. This osmotic gradient regulates the water content of the CSF as water follows the NaCl passively into the ventricle. There is evidence that some potentially harmful metabolic waste products deposited in the CSF can actually be absorbed and removed by the choroid plexus.

It is important to note that CSF is formed at an almost constant rate, independent of either CSF pressure or blood pressure. Therefore, if CSF pressure or general intracranial pressure were to rise as a result of an obstruction to CSF flow or a space-occupying mass, CSF formation would continue.

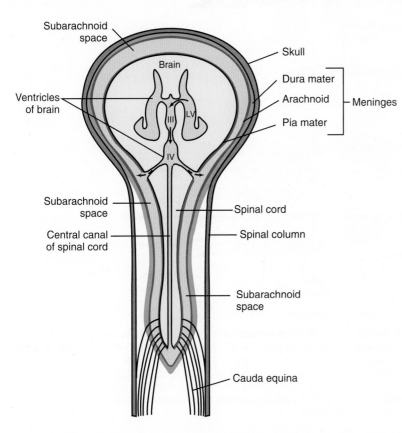

FIGURE 15-1 Schematic diagram of the relationships among the central nervous system, ventricles, cerebrospinal fluid (CSF), and meninges. The CSF is colored pink. *LV,* Lateral ventricle; *III,* third ventricle; *IV,* fourth ventricle; *solid curved arrow,* interventricular foramen; *solid straight arrow,* cerebral aqueduct; *dashed curved arrow,* lateral aperture of the fourth ventricle. (Modified from Behan M: Organization of the nervous system. In Reece WO, editor: *Duke's physiology of domestic animals,* ed 12, Ithaca, NY, 2004, Comstock Publishing.)

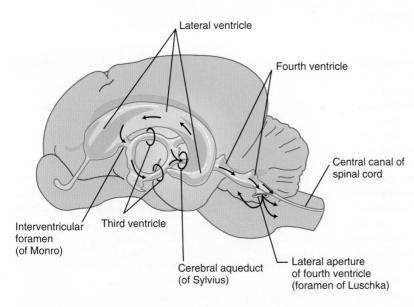

FIGURE 15-2 Lateral view of the ventricular cavities and their approximate spatial position within the brain. *Arrows* represent the flow of cerebrospinal fluid through and ultimately out from the ventricles at the lateral apertures. (From deLahunta A and Glass E: *Veterinary neurology and clinical neurology,* ed 3, St. Louis, 2009, Saunders.)

Cerebrospinal Fluid Flows Down a Pressure Gradient Through the Ventricular System Into the Subarachnoid Space

CSF flows, by bulk, down a pressure gradient from its site of formation at the choroid plexuses through the ventricular system and subarachnoid space into the venous system. Fluid formed in the lateral ventricles passes into the third ventricle through the interventricular foramina (foramina of Monro) (see Figures 15-1, 15-2, and 15-3). The fluid mixes with fluid formed in the third ventricle and from there passes through the *cerebral aqueduct* (aqueduct of Sylvius) of the midbrain into the fourth ventricle.

Fluid in the fourth ventricle passes into the subarachnoid space through two lateral apertures or foramina of Luschka. Some mammals have a third, medially located passageway from fourth ventricle to *subarachnoid space* (foramen of Magendie).

Recall that the brain and spinal cord are encased in bone (the skull and spinal canal, respectively) and are covered by a series of three membranes called the *meninges* (see Chapter 3). From outer to inner, these membranes are the dura, arachnoid, and pia (see Figure 15-1). The subarachnoid space lies between the arachnoid and pia, and when the CSF exits the brain through the apertures (foramina) of the fourth ventricle, the CSF fills the subarachnoid

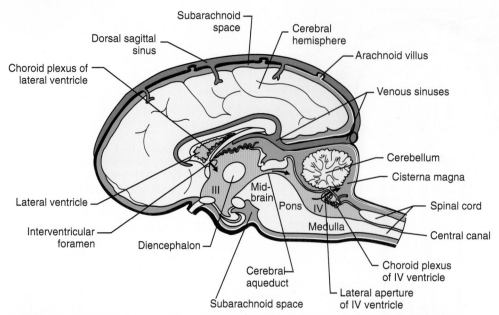

FIGURE 15-3 Midsagittal section of the brain showing portions of the ventricles and subarachnoid space, the choroid plexuses that produce CSF, and the dorsal sagittal sinus into which much of the CSF is absorbed. The cisterna magna is a common location for the sampling of CSF. The CSF within the ventricles is colored *light tan*, and the CSF that has emptied from the ventricles into the subarachnoid space (through the lateral apertures) is colored a *darker tan*. The larger portion of the lateral ventricle lies within the hemisphere, hidden from view. *III*, Third ventricle; *IV*, fourth ventricle. (Modified from Fletcher TF: Spinal cord and meninges. In Evans HE, editor: *Miller's anatomy of the dog*, ed 3, Philadelphia, 1993, Saunders.)

space, spreading out over the entire outer surface of the brain and spinal cord. Thus the entire CNS is essentially floating in a fluid-filled, membranous bag. As the CSF circulates up over the dorsal convexity of the brain, it is absorbed into the venous system near the midline.

The pressure, cell count, and chemical constituents of CSF can be sampled by placing a styletted spinal needle into the subarachnoid space. Anatomically, the most convenient place to perform this varies with species. In humans it is usually performed in the lumbar spinal column because the human spinal cord tapers to a cone (conus medullaris) near the first lumbar vertebra (humans have five lumbar vertebrae) as the dura and arachnoid continue down to around the second sacral vertebra. This provides a relatively large subarachnoid space (lumbar cistern) in the human midlumbar spinal column from which to sample. In most veterinary species, however, the conus medullaris extends to about the sixth or seventh lumbar vertebra, leaving only a small subarachnoid space in the spinal column. Therefore, most veterinary spinal taps are performed by sampling from the subarachnoid space region that is accessed between the skull and the first cervical vertebra (atlas) in anesthetized animals (Figure 15-4). In this location the subarachnoid space, formed as the arachnoid stretches from the caudal cerebellar surface to the dorsal surface of the medulla, is called the *cisterna magna* ("big cistern"; also called cerebellomedullary cistern) and is much deeper than other portions of the subarachnoid space (see Figure 15-3). Spinal taps provide valuable information about such neuropathological lesions as intracranial space-occupying masses and inflammation.

Normal CSF is clear and translucent. Turbidity indicates increased cellularity, and a pink tint suggests the presence of blood. A common cause of increased CSF cell count is inflammation of the CNS. Neutrophils can be indicative of bacterial infec-

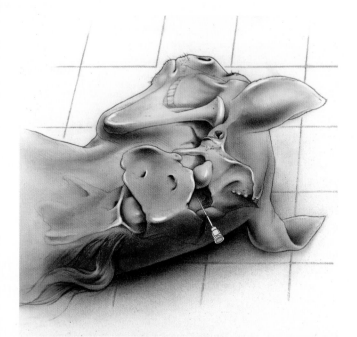

FIGURE 15-4 Region of approach, between the skull and first cervical vertebra (atlas), for collection of a CSF sample from the cisterna magna (cerebellomedullary cistern) in a recumbent horse. (From De Lahunta A, Glass E: *Veterinary anatomy and clinical neurology*, ed 3, Philadelphia, 2008, Saunders.)

tion. Subarachnoid hemorrhage may be responsible for blood in the CSF. Increased CSF protein, in the absence of increased nucleated cell count, can result from conditions such as neurodegeneration or neoplasia. CSF can be cultured if bacterial infection is suspected.

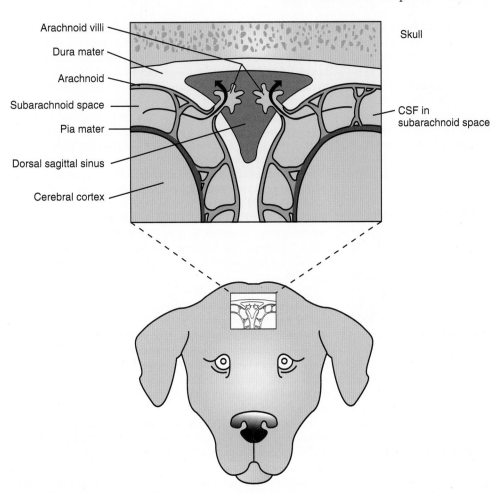

Arachnoid villi

Dura mater

Arachnoid

Subarachnoid space

Pia mater

Dorsal sagittal sinus

Cerebral cortex

Skull

CSF in
subarachnoid space

FIGURE 15-5 Transverse (coronal) section through the dorsal midline of the brain showing the absorption of CSF into the dorsal sagittal sinus through arachnoid villi. The CSF is colored *light blue.* The small window on the dog's head shows the approximate dorsoventral position of the sinus. (Modified from Oliver JE, Lorenz MD: *Handbook of veterinary neurology,* ed 2, Philadelphia, 1993, Saunders.)

Cerebrospinal Fluid Is Absorbed Into the Venous System

CSF is absorbed into the venous system, principally into dura-lined venous sinuses within the skull: the *dorsal sagittal sinus* which lies between the dorsal surfaces of the cerebral hemispheres (see Figure 15-3), and the *transverse sinuses* that lie between the cerebral hemispheres and the cerebellum. In primates, the dorsal sagittal sinus plays the more significant role, while in quadrupeds it is the transverse sinuses. Most of the fluid is absorbed from the subarachnoid space into the dural sinuses through *arachnoid villi* (Figure 15-5, and see Figure 15-3). These are small, fingerlike projections of the arachnoid membrane that poke through the walls of the sinus. Absorption appears to be pressure dependent and is unidirectional; CSF can flow from subarachnoid space to venous sinus, but venous blood cannot normally move from the sinus back into the subarachnoid space. The movement of CSF into the venous sinus is sometimes referred to as a "bulk flow" because all constituents of the fluid, including waste products and other foreign matter (e.g., red blood cells) move into the sinus. Materials cross the cells of the arachnoid villi by both vesicular transport and by the formation and movement of giant, fluid-filled vacuoles. CSF can also cross from subarachoid space to sinus through intercellular spaces between cells of the villi. CSF is produced at a rate of about 1 mL/hr in cats, about 3 mL/hr in dogs and about 20 mL/hr in humans. The entire volume of CSF is replaced several times a day; approximately six times per day in species such as sheep and goat.

In normal animals, CSF pressure is regulated primarily by its absorption at the arachnoid villi because the rate of absorption

can respond to changes in CSF pressure, whereas its formation is fairly constant and independent of changes in pressure. Therefore, any obstruction of CSF absorption into the venous sinus causes CSF pressure to rise almost immediately. In some pathological conditions, such as brain tumors or meningitis, CSF pressure can increase dramatically.

Hydrocephalus Is an Increased Volume of Cerebrospinal Fluid In the Skull

Hydrocephalus is defined as an increased CSF volume in the skull, often associated with an increased ventricular volume and increased intracranial pressure. In theory, hydrocephalus could be caused by too much fluid production at the choroid plexuses, obstruction to its flow through the ventricular system or subarachnoid space, or impaired absorption at the arachnoid villi. In practice, overproduction seems rare, whereas obstruction to flow seems more common, particularly at such vulnerable sites as the narrow cerebral aqueduct (connecting the third and fourth ventricles) and the exits from the fourth ventricle. Such blockages in the ventricular system produce a *noncommunicating hydrocephalus* that results in a buildup of freshly produced CSF in portions of the ventricular system behind the blockage. This causes the ventricular regions inside the brain to expand at the expense of the surrounding brain tissue, and intracranial pressure rises.

Impairment of absorption (a type of *communicating hydrocephalus*) can be secondary to meningitis or hemorrhage, presumably as a result of cellular debris that obstructs the transfer of

CSF from subarachnoid space to venous sinus at the arachnoid villi. This can increase CSF volume in the subarachnoid space, which increases pressure on the outside surface of the brain and increases intracranial pressure.

The pathogenesis of many cases of hydrocephalus is not known. A common form of treatment in humans is surgical implantation of a tube that shunts CSF into the atria of the heart or into the peritoneal cavity, thus relieving episodes of increased CSF pressure and preventing further brain damage. Ventriculo-peritoneal shunts have also been used in veterinary species. The carbonic anhydrase inhibitor acetazolamide or the diuretic furosemide have been used to decrease CSF production.

Permeability Barriers Exist Between Blood and Brain

Many dyes, when injected into the blood, stain other tissues of the body but not the brain. This suggests that the brain's blood vessels have the ability to restrict certain substances from accessing brain tissue. This physiological property of CNS blood vessels is referred to as the *blood-brain barrier* (BBB). The BBB contributes to a stable environment for the neurons and glial cells of the CNS. Such protection from direct exposure to the blood supply is necessary because the composition of blood can significantly vary with factors such as diet, exercise, metabolic activity, illness, age, and exposure to environmental toxins. Many of the varying blood-borne nutrients, metabolites, and toxins are neuroactive and capable of affecting membrane receptors, transporters, or ion channels. In the absence of a BBB, these substances could result in unregulated and undesirable changes in neural activity and behavior.

In most capillaries, water-soluble compounds leave through open clefts between capillary endothelial cells, and exchange is relatively unrestricted. In brain capillaries, however, passage through intercellular clefts is blocked by tight junctions, and exchange of blood solutes is highly selective (Figure 15-6). As a general rule, molecules that are small, uncharged, lipid soluble,

and unbound to plasma proteins (e.g., O_2, CO_2, ethanol, nicotine) can easily pass across the capillary endothelium of the BBB. Some molecules that do not fit this profile (e.g., glucose, some amino acids) are able to pass through the BBB by specific, carrier-mediated transport mechanisms. Brain capillaries have a greater number of mitochondria, which reflects the operation of such transporters. Certain degradative enzymes expressed by brain capillary endothelium (e.g., monoamine oxidase) provide a further restriction on substances that can pass the BBB.

The capillary endothelial cells that characterize the BBB reside within a complex cellular microsystem that also includes surrounding pericytes, glial astrocytic "end-feet," and neurons (see Figure 15-6). This system is called the *neurovascular unit*. The interaction of these elements of the neurovascular unit, although not completely understood, appears important for the development, structural maintenance, and function of the specialized capillary endothelial BBB, which facilitates molecular homeostasis of the brain.

The integrity of the BBB can be compromised by certain pathological states such as ischemic stroke and traumatic brain injury. Reduced integrity of BBB tight junctions are a hallmark of neuroinflammatory disease. Interestingly, even inflammation of peripheral nerves appears to compromise BBB tight junctions. Diseases such as diabetes, as well as multiple sclerosis and Alzheimer's disease in humans, appears to be associated with decreased BBB integrity, although the causative nature is not clear in these cases.

Unfortunately, for many patients, the protection normally afforded to the CNS by the BBB often prevents many antibiotics and other drugs from reaching the brain, particularly drugs with low lipid solubility or drugs bound to plasma proteins. Compounding this problem is the fact that some drugs that do have the properties that would normally permit passive movement through the BBB capillary endothelium are actively moved from the endothelium back out into the blood by carrier-mediated

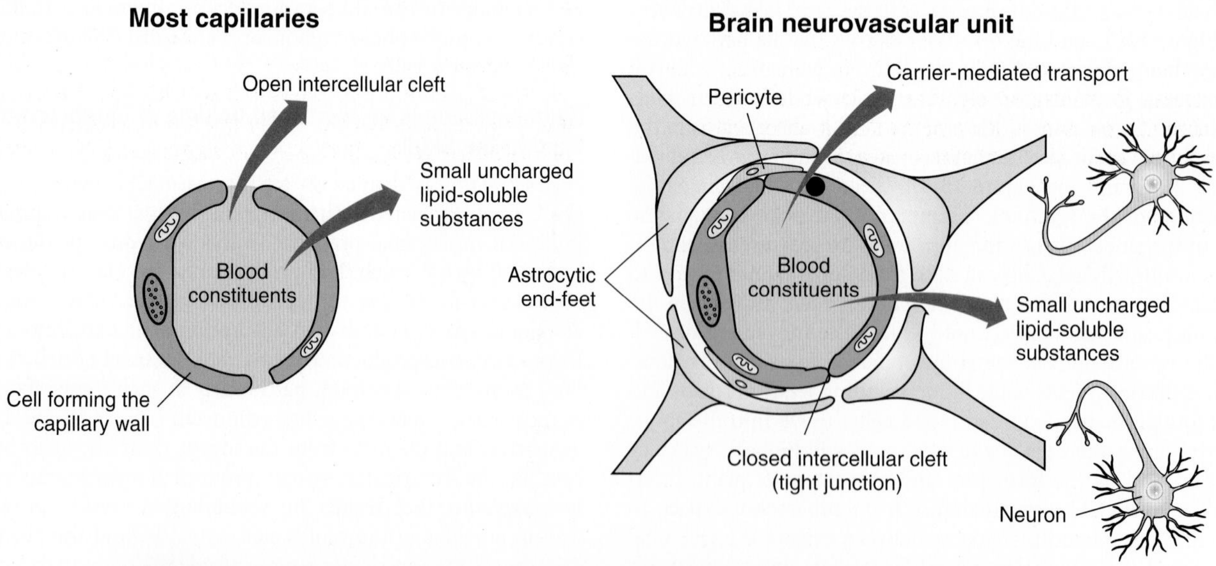

Most capillaries

Open intercellular cleft

Small uncharged lipid-soluble substances

Blood constituents

Cell forming the capillary wall

Brain neurovascular unit

Carrier-mediated transport

Pericyte

Astrocytic end-feet

Blood constituents

Small uncharged lipid-soluble substances

Closed intercellular cleft (tight junction)

Neuron

FIGURE 15-6 Blood-brain barrier (BBB). Unlike most capillaries of the body, cells of brain capillary walls are joined by tight junctions that restrict the passage of material between the cells. These brain capillaries are part of a complex cellular microsystem, called the *neurovascular unit*. The unit also includes surrounding pericytes, glial astrocytic "end-feet," and neurons. Materials leaving brain capillaries must pass through the cells forming the capillary wall. Substances that are not small, uncharged, and lipophilic must be carried across the cells by selective transport mechanisms. Interactions between the elements of the neurovascular unit are thought to contribute to development and maintenance of the tight-junction organization.

transport that seems to have an affinity for some of these drugs. Attempts to circumvent this problem have focused on temporary disruption of the BBB, direct delivery to the brain, "hitching a ride" on particular BBB membrane transporters, and increasing the lipid solubility of drugs.

In some parts of the brain known as the *circumventricular organs,* which include the hypothalamus, the brain capillaries do not form tight junctions, and the BBB is apparently not effective. This is significant because these brain regions are involved in functions such as the control of serum osmolality and glucose levels, hormonal communication, feeding, drinking, and vomiting, and therefore they need to detect the levels of many serum solutes.

CLINICAL CORRELATIONS

INCREASED INTRACRANIAL PRESSURE

History. You examine a 9-year-old female boxer dog. The owner states that recently the dog has seemed drowsier than usual and had what you recognize to be a generalized tonic-clonic seizure the preceding night.

Clinical Examination. Physical examination of the dog reveals a hard, nodular mass of the mammary gland. Other deficits are referable to the nervous system and are characterized by apparent drowsiness and confusion and by a deficit of the proprioceptive positioning reaction of the right front and right rear legs. Lateral radiographs of the chest reveal metastatic, neoplastic lesions in the lungs. The CSF pressure, as measured with a manometer through a needle placed in the cisterna magna, is 310 mm CSF. (The normal CSF pressure in dogs is less than 180 mm CSF.)

Comment. This is a typical case of a dog with a neoplasm of the mammary gland that has spread first to the lungs, which contain the first capillary bed filter encountered by tumor cells as they invade the venous system, and then to the brain. As the tumor mass increases within the fixed encasement of the cranial vault, CSF and other fluid volumes are displaced. Some loss of myelin may compensate temporarily for the expanding intracranial mass, but eventually the expanding tumor, encased in the skull, causes an increase in intracranial pressure, which is reflected in an increased CSF pressure in the cisterna magna. When measuring this pressure, the dog is anesthetized, and a styletted spinal needle is placed in the cisterna magna. The stylet is removed, and a rigid glass or plastic tube (manometer) is attached using a right-angle, three-way valve. CSF rises up the manometer to a height proportional to intracranial pressure. Its height is measured off the millimeter graduations marked on the tube.

The proprioceptive deficits of the right front and right rear legs result from a focal, asymmetric lesion of the left cerebral cortex. The seizure also resulted from this mass. With the mammary mass, metastatic lesions in the lungs, asymmetric neurological signs, seizures, and elevated CSF pressure, it is reasonable to conclude that this dog has an intracranial neoplasm that probably spread from the mammary gland to the lungs and the brain. Computed tomography (CT) or magnetic resonance imaging (MRI) is warranted to further define the tumor in the brain.

Treatment. If this dog had a focal tumor within the CNS, other treatments would be possible. However, extensive treatment in this case would be futile because of the metastatic lesions. Palliative care (affording relief but not cure), steroids, and analgesics will make the animal more comfortable.

SEIZURES IN A FOAL

History. A 2-day-old Arabian colt from an unobserved foaling displays lethargy and inability to rise, and he started to go into seizure in the last hour. The foal stood, but it took longer than normal. The foal has been nursing, but the mare does not appear to have much milk; this is the mare's first foal. The foal seems less active than normal foals and has become more lethargic as the day progressed. Finally, it seemed as though he would not stand, and he had a seizure while traveling to the clinic.

Clinical Examination. The foal has a fever, and pulse and respiration are increased. Mucous membranes are darker red than normal, the membranes are dry (dehydration), and the capillary refill time is prolonged (poor perfusion). Auscultation (listening for sounds within the body) reveals harsh lung sounds and crackles. The umbilicus (navel) is thickened and wet. There is petechiation (petechial hemorrhages) inside the ears and in the sclera. There appears to be signs of uveitis (see Chapter 14) in the eyes. The foal is not responsive to manipulations and thrashes, although not in seizure, while being examined. The foal also lacks a suckle reflex.

Comment. Although many possibilities exist for the cause of seizures in this foal, the two most likely reasons are low glucose level (hypoglycemia) and infection (meningitis). The blood glucose level is high in this foal, so meningitis (inflammation of the meninges) with septicemia is most likely. This foal probably has become septic (blood-borne infection) based on the history and clinical signs, which support that he likely did not receive enough colostrum and may not be receiving enough milk from the mare. Without adequate colostrum and nutrition, the foal's immune system is more susceptible to infection. With the thickened umbilicus, harsh lung sounds, fever, petechiation, uveitis, and seizures, the signs are consistent with septicemia, which is manifesting in different regions of the body. The umbilicus could be infected (omphalophlebitis), the lung sounds are consistent with infection (pneumonia), and seizures are consistent with meningitis.

Complete blood count, chemistry, blood gases, and blood culture are warranted to determine the overall status of the foal. In many cases, these tests will be sufficient to make a diagnosis and determine treatment. In some cases, to make a definitive diagnosis, an atlanto-occipital (A/O) CSF tap (which samples from the cisterna magna) is best because it is closest to the site of the lesion, compared with a lumbosacral tap. The tap also allows a culture to be submitted so that the foal can be treated with the most efficacious antibiotics. When performing the CSF tap, the foal can be sedated with diazepam (Valium). The CSF is submitted for protein, glucose, cytology, and culture. Typically, the protein level is high with meningitis, and cytology shows an increased number of leukocytes (neutrophils). There is always the potential for a false-negative result with the culture.

Treatment. Prognosis for a septic foal with seizures is poor, with many factors to consider. In regard to the meningitis, treatment consists of antibiotics, antiinflammatory agents, and anticonvulsants as needed. Seizures can cause hypoxia to the affected area, which can result in permanent damage. Besides meningitis, other problems include the umbilical infection, respiratory infection, and uveitis. With septicemia, other organs often become infected (joints, gastrointestinal tract, renal system). Additional concerns are potential renal insult caused by dehydration or complications associated with some antibiotics. Supportive care is another consideration. Managing a recumbent foal is challenging, not only for the reasons already listed, but also because of other factors including additional infection, aspiration, and nutritional support.

PRACTICE QUESTIONS

1. Obstruction of cerebrospinal fluid (CSF) flow at the cerebral aqueduct (aqueduct of Sylvius) would lead to dilation (enlargement) of the:
   a. Lateral ventricles.
   b. Fourth ventricle.
   c. Central canal of the spinal cord.
   d. Subarachnoid space.
   e. Conus medullaris.

2. CSF is principally formed at the:
   a. Arachnoid villi.
   b. Aqueduct of Sylvius.
   c. Choroid plexuses.
   d. Subarachnoid space.
   e. Dorsal sagittal sinus.

3. You are performing a spinal tap on an anesthetized horse and measuring CSF pressure. Cellular debris has obstructed the arachnoid villi following meningitis. What would you expect regarding CSF pressure?
   a. Pressure would be higher than normal.
   b. Pressure would be lower than normal.
   c. Pressure would be normal.

4. For many veterinary species, diagnostic sampling of CSF is often performed by placing a sampling needle in the:
   a. Lateral ventricles.
   b. Dorsal sagittal sinus.
   c. Third ventricle.
   d. Cerebral aqueduct of Sylvius.
   e. Cisterna magna.

5. Which *two* of the following are *false* regarding the blood-brain barrier (BBB)?
   a. The BBB is very effective at the circumventricular organs of the brain.
   b. Astrocytic end-feet are thought to be partially responsible for development of the BBB.
   c. Brain capillaries generally have a high number of endothelial tight junctions.
   d. Many dyes injected into the blood can typically penetrate most tissues of the body, but usually not the brain.
   e. Small, uncharged, lipid-soluble molecules do not generally pass through the BBB.

BIBLIOGRAPHY

Abbott NJ, Rönnbäck L, Hansson E: Astrocyte-endothelial interactions at the blood-brain barrier, *Nat Rev Neurosci* 7(1):41–53, 2006.

Boron WF, Boulpaep EL: *Medical physiology*, ed 2, Philadelphia, 2009, Saunders.

Brodal P: *The central nervous system: structure and function*, ed 4, New York, 2010, Oxford University Press.

De Lahunta A, Glass E: *Veterinary anatomy and clinical neurology*, ed 3, Philadelphia, 2009, Saunders.

Di Terlizzi R, Platt SR: The function, composition and analysis of cerebrospinal fluid in companion animals: part I—function and composition, *Vet J* 172(3):422–431, 2006.

Di Terlizzi R, Platt SR: The function, composition and analysis of cerebrospinal fluid in companion animals: part II—analysis, *Vet J* 180(1):15–32, 2009.

Fletcher TF: Spinal cord and meninges. In Evans HE, editor: *Miller's anatomy of the dog*, ed 3, Philadelphia, 1993, Saunders.

Hall JE: *Guyton and Hall textbook of medical physiology*, ed 12, Philadelphia, 2011, Saunders.

Hawkins BT, Davis TP: The blood-brain barrier/neurovascular unit in health and disease, *Pharmacol Rev* 57(2):173–185, 2005.

Mollanji R, Papaiconomou C, Boulton M, et al: Comparison of cerebrospinal fluid transport in fetal and adult sheep, *Am J Physiol Regul Integr Comp Physiol* 281(4):R1215–R1223, 2001.

Paolinelli R, Corada M, Orsenigo F, Dejanaa E: The molecular basis of the blood-brain barrier differentiation and maintenance. Is it still a mystery? *Pharmacol Res* 63(3):165–171, 2011.

Pollay M: The function and structure of the cerebrospinal fluid outflow system, *Cerebrospinal Fluid Res* 7:9, 2010.

Purves D, Augustine GJ, Fitzpatrick D, et al: *Neuroscience*, ed 5, Sunderland, Mass, 2012, Sinauer.

Simard M, Nedergaard M: The neurobiology of glia in the context of water and ion homeostasis, *Neuroscience* 129(4):877–896, 2004.

Thomas WB: Hydrocephalus in dogs and cats, *Vet Clin North Am Small Anim Pract* 40(1):143–159, 2010.

CHAPTER 16
The Electroencephalogram and Sensory-Evoked Potentials

KEY POINTS

1. All areas of the cerebral cortex share common histological features.
2. The electroencephalogram is a common clinical tool.

3. The collective behavior of cortical neurons can be studied noninvasively through the use of macroelectrodes on the scalp.
4. Stimulation of sensory pathways can be recorded as evoked potentials.

When many excitable cells are present in a living tissue, their electrical behavior can be detected by macroelectrodes placed on the body at a distance from these cells. Several clinically important electrophysiological diagnostic procedures are based on this concept.

Underlying these procedures is a theory called *volume conduction*. This theory describes the spread of ionic currents within the extracellular fluid from a group of neurons or muscle cells to more distant points in the body, such as the skin. These ionic currents can be measured from the skin. Their waveforms are characteristic of the tissues from which they arise. The best-known electrophysiological recording is the electrocardiogram from heart muscle (see Chapter 20). The electromyogram from skeletal muscle (see Chapter 6) and electroretinogram (see Chapter 14) are other examples.

This chapter introduces two additional clinical electrophysiological tools: the electroencephalogram and *sensory-evoked potentials*, particularly brainstem auditory-evoked responses. These tools represent two general types of clinical electrophysiological recordings. The first is a record of the spontaneous activity of tissue. The second is a record of potentials that are artificially evoked by electrical or magnetic stimulation of tissue or by activation of sensory receptor organs. Before discussing the electroencephalogram and sensory-evoked potentials, it is necessary to understand more about the histology and electrophysiology of the cerebral cortex.

All Areas of the Cerebral Cortex Share Common Histological Features

Different regions of the cerebral cortex have different functions. For example, the motor cortices (see Chapter 10) project to the brainstem and spinal cord to initiate skilled, learned, conscious movement. The occipital cortex processes visual information received from the retina of the eye (see Chapter 14). The temporal cortex processes similar information from the ear (see Chapter 17). Even though different cortical regions have different functions, they have an underlying histological similarity. Therefore, cortical synaptic processing of information shares common features across regions, but differences in the origin of input signals and the destination of output signals contribute significantly to functional differences among regions. However, cerebral cortical

cells can also work collectively over vast regions of the brain in such normal states as sleep and wakefulness and in such disease states as coma and seizures.

The cerebral cortex contains several different cell types, but most belong to two major classes: pyramidal cells and stellate cells (Figure 16-1). These cells are arranged in six layers (I-VI). The *pyramidal cells,* so named because their cell bodies are pyramid shaped, have dendrites projecting up toward the pial surface of the cortex, usually reaching and branching within layer I. These cells also have basal dendrites that extend horizontally from the cell body. Pyramidal cells are projection neurons, with their axons leaving their cortical region of origin and projecting to other parts of the central nervous system (CNS) or to a different region of cerebral cortex. Pyramidal cells are generally excitatory at their axon's synapse. *Stellate cells,* so named because most have a star-like appearance, are local-circuit interneurons within the cortex and can be either excitatory or inhibitory. The majority of subcortical information arrives at the cortex through a massive input from the thalamic nuclei, most of which is targeted to layer IV. Input from some portions of the thalamus, as well as from other regions of the cerebral cortex, have a more diffuse termination across cortical layers. Information arriving from cortical afferents is processed by local cortical circuitry, and pyramidal cells then carry the processed information to other CNS regions.

As with other regions of the brain, the cerebral cortex contains many more glial cells than neurons. Three types of glial cells are present in the cortex: *astrocytes, oligodendrocytes,* and *microglia.* They do not develop action potentials, but as noted in Chapter 3, they may indirectly monitor neuronal electrical activity and modulate the effectiveness of neural communication. Glia also take up excess potassium ions, neurotransmitter, and toxins from the extracellular space and play a role in immune function. In addition, they help guide the course of developing neurons, play a role in synapse formation, and stabilize the position of neurons, thus the origin of the term glia ("glue").

The Electroencephalogram Is a Common Clinical Tool

It has been known since the 1930s that a fluctuating electrical voltage reflecting brain activity could be recorded from macroelectrodes on the scalp (Figure 16-2). Such a recording is known

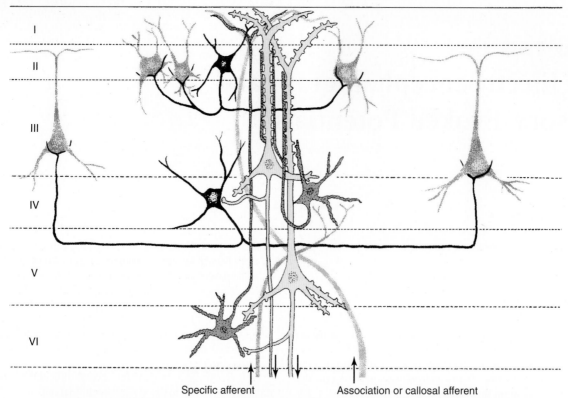

FIGURE 16-1 The principal neuron types and their interconnections have a basic similarity in the various regions of the cerebral cortex. Note that the two large pyramidal cells *(yellow)* in layers III and V receive multiple synaptic contacts from the star-shaped interneuron (stellate cell, *violet*) in layer IV. Basket cell *(black)* inhibition is directed to the somata of cortical neurons. Major input to the cortex derives from specific thalamic nuclei (*specific afferent*) and is directed mostly to layer IV; association and callosal inputs (*association or callosal afferent*) have a more widespread termination pattern among the cortical layers. (From Kandel ER, Schwartz JH, editors: *Principles of neural science,* ed 2, New York, 1985, Elsevier Science & Technology.)

as an *electroencephalogram* (EEG). The frequency of the waveform recorded varies inversely with its amplitude. Both frequency and amplitude change with changes in levels of arousal (Figure 16-3). An alert animal has a fairly high-frequency, fairly low-amplitude EEG, whereas a more relaxed animal has a slower-frequency, higher-amplitude EEG. A sleeping animal usually begins sleep by exhibiting a slow-wave, high-amplitude EEG. Paradoxically, there are periods of high-frequency, low-amplitude EEG during the sleep cycle. Four frequency ranges have been given names: *alpha* (8-13 Hz), *beta* (13-30 Hz), *delta* (0.5-4 Hz), and *theta* (4-7 Hz).

This technique has been applied clinically since the early 1960s. Abnormal EEG activity has been associated empirically with several brain diseases. In human neurology, EEGs have been used to classify the epilepsies, to localize lesions, and to help define "brain death." EEGs have not been as widely used in veterinary medicine but still have clinical utility in veterinary neurology.

We now discuss where these scalp recordings originate and how they relate to brain function.

The Collective Behavior of Cortical Neurons Can Be Studied Noninvasively Through the Use of Macroelectrodes on the Scalp

The scalp EEG records a fluctuating voltage resulting from changes in postsynaptic potentials in thousands of neurons below the electrode. Each change in voltage has a polarity.

By convention, changes in voltage measured by extracellular electrodes, such as those on the scalp, have a standard direction of deflection when observed on the recorder device. When the voltage change is in a positive direction, the recorded deflection is "down"; when in a negative direction, the deflection is "up" (Figure 16-4). The polarity of the voltage change at the scalp depends on the nature and location of the postsynaptic potential change. If an *excitatory postsynaptic potential* (EPSP) occurs in a deep cortical layer, positive ions (e.g., Na^+) enter the cell there, leaving the extracellular fluid at that location relatively negative. Through principles of volume conduction, this leaves the extracellular fluid near the cortical surface positive with respect to the deeper, negatively charged region of extracellular fluid (see Figure 16-4; for simplicity, only one cell is indicated). This results in a positive voltage change being recorded at the scalp macroelectrode near the cortical surface. Based on the same principles, if the EPSP occurs near the cortical surface (see Figure 16-4), the voltage recorded from the scalp is negative. The polarity of these changes would be reversed for *inhibitory postsynaptic potentials* (IPSPs).

Voltage changes recorded from the scalp are the result of the summated extracellular voltage changes caused by the postsynaptic potentials of a large number of active cortical neurons, primarily pyramidal cells, because the voltage change from any one neuron is too small to record. Action potentials contribute little to the EEG with scalp electrodes.

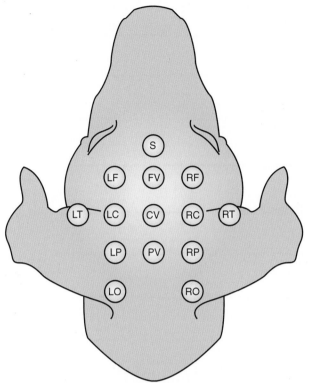

FIGURE 16-2 Commonly used points of scalp electrode attachment (electrode montage) for recording the electroencephalogram (EEG). Recordings are typically made from multiple paired combinations of electrodes.

The *amplitude* (height) of voltage fluctuations in the scalp-recorded EEG is a function of how many cortical cells are changing their postsynaptic potentials in the same direction at the same time. Because a high-amplitude voltage change would result from a large number of neurons firing synchronously, a high-amplitude, slow-frequency EEG is said to be a *synchronized EEG*. When neurons are firing more or less at random, a low-amplitude, high-frequency EEG results, said to be a *desynchronized EEG*.

The *frequency* with which EEG voltage changes occur is largely determined by the *reticular activating system*. As noted in Chapter 10, ascending projections of the reticular formation play an important role in modulating consciousness, arousal, and attention. Many of these projections synapse primarily in the thalamus, hypothalamus, or directly in the cerebral cortex in a diffuse fashion. Diffuse cortical projections from portions of the thalamus (intralaminar nuclei) and hypothalamus (lateral hypothalamus), along with diffuse, direct cortical projections from the reticular formation, likely regulate consciousness and arousal. Neurons that project to cortex from specific sensory relay nuclei of the thalamus and receive reticular formation input probably influence attention. The term reticular activating system collectively refers to these ascending reticular formation neurons and the neurons that relay their activity to the cortex, both of which affect consciousness, arousal, and attention.

Stimulation of Sensory Pathways Can Be Recorded as Evoked Potentials

Large areas of the brain and the spinal cord are not reflected in the EEG. Other clinical electrophysiological recordings can help examine the function of these areas.

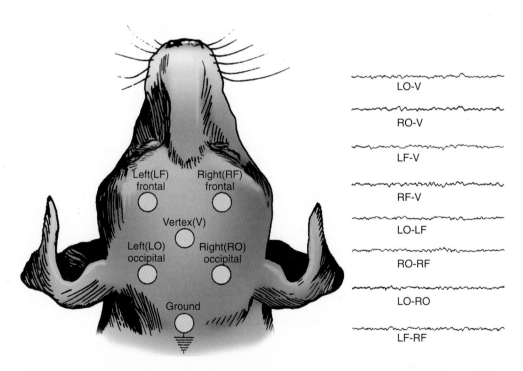

FIGURE 16-3 EEG recorded from various combinations of lead points using an older, simpler electrode configuration (the Redding configuration). It shows the difference in frequency and amplitude between an alert animal *(44),* a relaxed animal *(45),* and an animal in light sleep *(80).* Note the decrease in frequency and increase in amplitude in the progression from alert to relaxed to light sleep. (From Oliver JE, Hoerlein BF, Mayhew IG, editors: *Veterinary neurology,* Philadelphia, 1987, Saunders.)

Continued

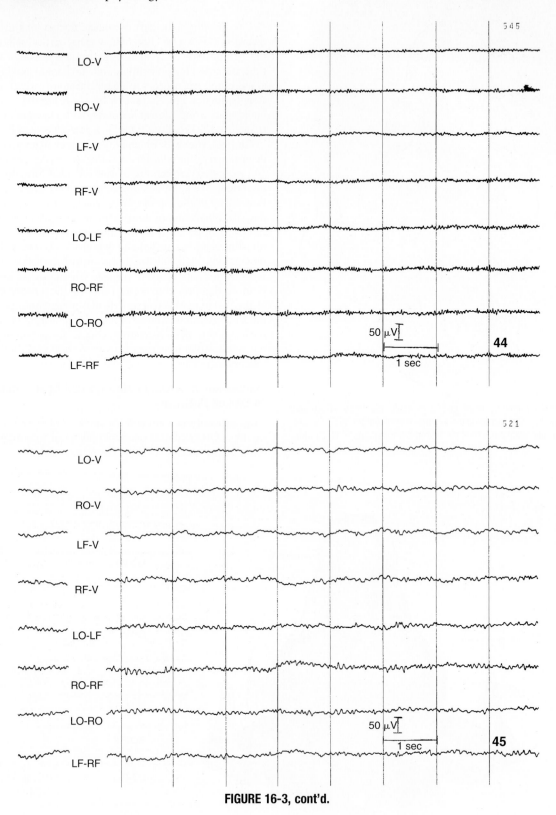

FIGURE 16-3, cont'd.

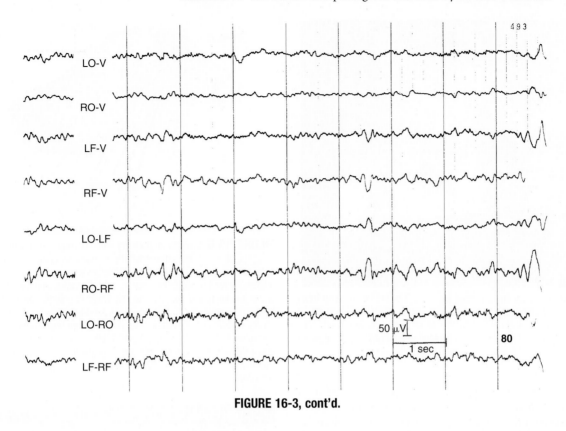

LO-V

RO-V

LF-V

RF-V

LO-LF

RO-RF

LO-RO

LF-RF

50 μV

1 sec

80

493

FIGURE 16-3, cont'd.

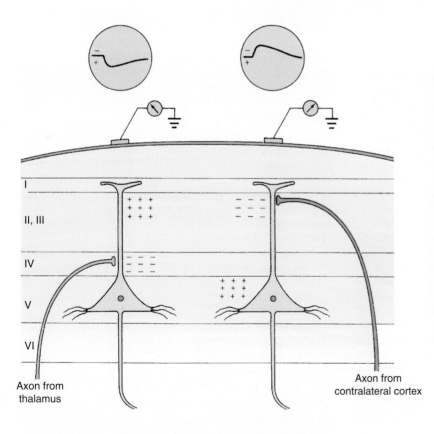

I

II, III

IV

V

VI

Axon from
thalamus

+ + +
+ + +
+ + +

− − −
− − −

− − −
− − −

+ + +
+ + +
+ + +

Axon from
contralateral cortex

FIGURE 16-4 Scalp recordings and underlying synaptic mechanisms. **Left,** Potential recorded from a scalp electrode after activation of thalamic inputs. The terminals of thalamocortical neurons make excitatory connections on cortical neurons predominantly in layer IV. Thus the site of inward current flow (sink) in layer IV leaves the extracellular fluid at that location relatively negative and the extracellular fluid near the cortical surface relatively positive. Because the recording electrode is located on the scalp, near the cortical surface, it records a positive potential. By convention, a positive extracellularly recorded potential is, unlike intracellular recordings, a downward deflection. **Right,** Potential recorded from an excitatory callosal afferent originating in the contralateral cortex. The axon of this callosal neuron terminates in a superficial cortical layer. A negative potential (upward deflection) is recorded because the electrode is closer to the site of inward current flow, which leaves the extracellular fluid near the cortical surface relatively negative. (From Kandel ER, Schwartz JH, editors: *Principles of neural science,* ed 2, New York, 1985, Elsevier Science & Technology.)

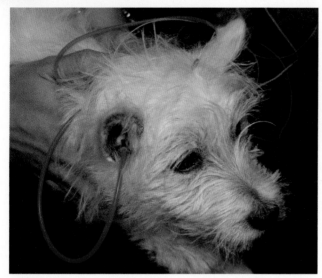

FIGURE 16-5 Canine instrumented for a BAER examination using tubal ear inserts *(thick red and blue tubes)* and a vertex-mastoid skin electrode montage *(thin wires)*. (Image courtesy of Dr. John H. Rossmeisl, Jr., Department of Small Animal Clinical Sciences, Virginia-Maryland Regional College of Veterinary Medicine, Virginia Tech.)

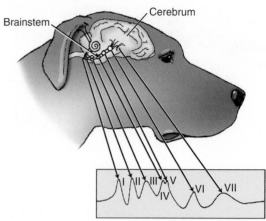

FIGURE 16-6 Brainstem auditory-evoked response (BAER): idealized diagram of waveforms recorded by signal averaging. Neural elements believed to generate sequentially the auditory waves are grouped as follows. Wave I reflects the cochlea, spiral ganglia, and cranial nerve VIII. Wave II reflects the cochlear nuclei. Wave III reflects the nucleus of the trapezoid body. Waves IV and V reflect the lateral lemniscus and lemniscal nuclei, and caudal colliculus, respectively (these two waves are frequently combined to form one wave). Wave VI reflects the medial geniculate body. Wave VII reflects auditory radiations. Positive is upward. (From Oliver JE, Hoerlein BF, Mayhew IG, editors: *Veterinary neurology,* Philadelphia, 1987, Saunders.)

Synaptic activity in a sensory pathway can be recorded from the scalp by a computerized technique that averages out the more random background EEG activity and averages in the electrical response to multiple stimulations of a sensory system. Such signals are called *sensory-evoked potentials.*

Because scalp macroelectrodes can more easily record the EEG electrical signals generated from the closer cerebral cortical cells, these higher-voltage signals must be eliminated; otherwise, they would mask the sensory-evoked potentials. Because the background EEG signals are relatively random, a computer can average them together and functionally erase them from the recording while at the same time averaging the nonrandom sensory-evoked potential signals recorded from multiple stimulations of a sensory pathway. In this way, scalp macroelectrodes can be used to record electrical events generated in brain locations distant from the recording electrode. For this reason, these sensory-evoked potentials are often called *far-field potentials.*

One such sensory-evoked potential is the *brainstem auditory-evoked response* (BAER). This clinical electrophysiological procedure, in which the electrode placement is configured to include early activity from the caudal brainstem, records the electrical events for 10 msec after a click stimulus to the ear (Figure 16-5). Usually, seven waves are recorded, thought to be generated by neural activity in components of the auditory pathway from the auditory nerve through the auditory radiations leaving the medial geniculate nucleus of the thalamus (Figure 16-6). Recordings longer than 10 msec are sometimes taken, and these are referred to as *middle latency recordings.* These later waves reflect cortical response to auditory stimulation. BAER is used in animals and humans to assess brainstem function in general, and auditory function in particular. Other sensory-evoked potentials can be recorded from the visual system, the somatosensory system, and other sensory modalities.

BAER is also often used with simultaneous EEG recording in the confirmation of brain death. A flat EEG, a very crude indicator of brain death, combined with a viable BAER can suggest that the functional deficit may not be irreversible.

CLINICAL CORRELATIONS

BRAIN TUMOR

History. You examine a 13-year-old Boston terrier. The owner states that during the past 3 weeks the dog has had seizures of increasing frequency, characterized by turning the head to the right, rigidity of the right front and right hind legs, collapsing to the ground, and urination. More recently, the dog has seemed weak, drowsy, and confused. He tends to walk in circles and seems weak on the right front leg.

Clinical Examination. Important physical examination deficits are referable to the nervous system. The dog seems weak, drowsy, confused, and unsteady in gait. He tends to walk in counterclockwise circles. Cranial and spinal segmental reflexes are within normal limits. Proprioceptive positioning reaction is abnormal in the right front leg and normal in the other three legs (see Chapters 7 and 10). An EEG reveals that the dominant frequency is slower and the amplitude higher over the left parietal cortex than over the rest of the brain. Occasional bursts of electrical spiking activity can also be seen from the area of the left parietal cortex. A computed tomography (CT) or magnetic resonance imaging (MRI) scan is warranted to determine the presence and nature of a tumor suspected from the EEG patterns. MRI provides the best imaging of intracranial lesions to determine whether this is a primary tumor (originating from the brain tissue) or a secondary tumor (originating from other tissue; e.g., osteosarcoma, lymphosarcoma).

Comment. This is an old dog, with a recent history of progressive, asymmetric brain disease. The history suggests a focal intracranial lesion, perhaps a brain tumor. A focal lesion is further confirmed by the EEG and brain imaging. Brain tumors within the cerebral hemispheres often cause focal slowing of the EEG frequency with increased amplitude. This is called a *slow-wave focus.* The tumor itself is electrically silent, but its effects on the surrounding cerebral cortex are slowing, and the intermittent bursts of electrical spikes represent seizure activity within the cortex. Between clinical seizures, these spikes can still be seen with the EEG, but they do not spread widely enough within the cortex to cause a clinical seizure. During a clinical seizure, this abnormal electrical activity spreads more widely to otherwise normal brain tissue, causing the various motor and other events of the seizure. Why such spikes only occasionally spread to incorporate more distant parts of the brain to cause seizures, and why seizures stop, is still unknown.

Treatment. Many forms of seizure disorders can be managed successfully by removing the underlying cause, or the frequency of the seizures can be reduced with antiepileptic medication. In this dog the cause is likely a brain tumor. Depending on the nature of the tumor, surgery and radiation therapy may be possible and may extend the dog's life. However, the prognosis is likely poor. Antiepileptic and steroid medication may improve the quality of the dog's remaining life.

PRACTICE QUESTIONS

1. Which of the following regarding EEG is *false*?
   a. Its measurement relies on volume conduction.
   b. It predominantly measures postsynaptic potentials in the cerebral cortex.
   c. It is commonly used to measure the activity of a small number of neurons.
   d. It is a measure of the spontaneous activity of brain tissue.
   e. Both a and d.

2. A lesion in which of the following brain structures would be least likely to have a significant effect on the EEG?
   a. Cerebral cortex
   b. Thalamus
   c. Hypothalamus
   d. Cerebellum
   e. Reticular activating system

3. Which of the following statements is *true*?
   a. A slow-frequency, high-amplitude EEG is said to be "desynchronized."
   b. The EEG alone is used to confirm brain death.
   c. There are some periods of high-frequency, low-amplitude EEG during sleep.
   d. The EEG is usually measured in response to the stimulation of a sensory receptor organ.

4. The BAER requires averaging out the random background EEG activity before it can be observed.
   a. True
   b. False

5. A brain tumor may cause focal slowing of the EEG from the brain tissue immediately surrounding the tumor.
   a. True
   b. False

BIBLIOGRAPHY

Bagley RS: *Fundamentals of veterinary clinical neurology*, Ames, Iowa, 2005, Blackwell Publishing.

Bear MF, Connors BW, Paradiso MA: *Neuroscience: exploring the brain*, ed 3, Philadelphia, 2007, Lippincott, Williams & Wilkins.

Bergman RL: Intracranial neoplasia in dogs. *Proceedings, ACVIM,* 2005.

Ducote JM, Dewey CW: Neurodiagnostics. In Dewey CW, editor: *A practical guide to canine and feline neurology*, Ames, Iowa, 2003, Iowa State Press.

Haines DE, editor: *Fundamental neuroscience for basic and clinical applications*, ed 3, Philadelphia, 2006, Churchill Livingstone.

Hall JE: *Guyton and Hall textbook of medical physiology*, ed 12, Philadelphia, 2011, Saunders.

Kandel ER, Schwartz JH, Jessell TM, editors: *Principles of neural science*, ed 4, New York, 2000, McGraw-Hill.

Lorenz MD, Kornegay JN: *Oliver and Lorenz's handbook of veterinary neurology*, ed 4, Philadelphia, 2004, Saunders.

Poma R, Chambers H, da Costa RC, et al: MRI measurement of the canine auditory pathways and relationship with brainstem auditory evoked responses, *Vet Comp Orthop Traumatol* 21(3):238–242, 2008.

Strain GM: Consciousness and higher cortical function. In Reece WO, editor: *Duke's physiology of domestic animals*, ed 12, Ithaca, NY, 2004, Comstock Publishing.

Williams DC, Aleman T, Holliday TA, et al: Qualitative and quantitative characteristics of the electroencephalogram in normal horses during spontaneous drowsiness and sleep, *J Vet Intern Med* 22(3):630–638, 2008.

CHAPTER 17

Hearing

KEY POINTS

1. Sound waves are alternating phases of condensation and rarefaction (pressure waves) of molecules in the external environment.
2. Outer and middle ears funnel sound waves to the cochlea.
3. The cochlea is located in the inner ear.
4. The cochlea transduces sound waves to action potentials of the eighth cranial nerve.

5. Deciphering of sound wave frequency begins in the cochlea.
6. Action potentials from the cochlea are transmitted up through the brainstem to the cerebral cortex.
7. Deafness results from an interruption in the hearing process.

Our lives are enriched by music and conversation, and altered by the sounds of danger. Many mammalian species have a particularly acute sense of hearing. Hearing depends on the remarkable properties of hair cell receptors in the cochlea that mediate transduction of sound into action potentials that are then sent to the brain. Fortunately, the auditory system is not usually a site of pathological lesions in veterinary medicine, except for occasional congenital defects and exposure to ototoxic drugs. Nevertheless, hearing is sufficiently important to warrant a brief discussion of its physiology.

Sound Waves Are Alternating Phases of Condensation and Rarefaction (Pressure Waves) of Molecules in the External Environment

Sound waves are longitudinal vibrations of molecules in the external environment characterized by alternating phases of condensation and rarefaction (increases and decreases in pressure). These alternating changes in pressure produce the sensation of sound after they strike the tympanic membrane and are subsequently transduced into neural signals that ultimately reach the cerebral cortex. Sound waves reaching the tympanic membrane can be expressed as changes in sound pressure as a function of time (Figure 17-1).

In general, the subjective *loudness* of the sound is correlated with the *amplitude* of a sound wave; the subjective *pitch* is correlated with the *frequency* of the wave. The amplitude of a sound is usually quantified according to the logarithmic *decibel scale,* which expresses the energy of the sound relative to the energy of a standard reference sound. This standard sound, representing 0 decibels (dB), is the threshold for human hearing where the sound of the background movement of air molecules can almost be heard. Normal conversation is about 60 dB, and the loudest tolerable sound for humans is about 120 dB, about 1 million times the threshold amplitude. The loudest reported dog barking has been recorded as 108 dB. Sound frequency, the number of pressure oscillation cycles per unit time, is usually expressed in units called hertz (Hz), where 1 Hz equals 1 cycle per second.

Outer and Middle Ears Funnel Sound Waves to the Cochlea

The outer ear, composed of the fleshy part (pinna) and the ear canal, funnels sound waves to the *tympanic membrane,* or eardrum (Figure 17-2). Some animals can move the pinna to more effectively collect sound waves, and the natural shape of the pinna can act to selectively filter certain sound frequencies. The eardrum is a membrane between the outer and the middle ear. The middle ear is an air-filled cavity in the temporal bone and is connected to the nasopharynx by the auditory (eustachian) tube. Three tiny bones—the malleus, incus, and stapes—collectively called the *ossicles,* are connected to each other and are located in the middle ear. The malleus is connected to the eardrum, and the stapes is connected to the oval window, a membranous separation between the middle and the inner ear. The ossicles transfer vibration of the eardrum to the oval window in a manner that avoids a significant loss of energy as the sound wave is transferred from the air-filled outer ear to the fluid-filled inner ear. Two small skeletal muscles are also located in the middle ear, with one attached to the malleus and one attached to the stapes. Their contraction reduces the transfer of vibration between the eardrum and the oval window. This can function to protect the inner ear from very loud sounds.

The Cochlea Is Located in the Inner Ear

The inner ear (labyrinth) contains the receptor organs of two sensory systems: (1) the vestibular system, which detects acceleration and static tilt of the head (see Chapter 11), and (2) the auditory system, which detects and analyzes sound. The inner ear consists of the *bony labyrinth* and, within the bony labyrinth, the *membranous labyrinth.* The bony labyrinth is a series of tunnels within the petrous temporal bone. Inside these tunnels, surrounded by a fluid called *perilymph,* is the membranous labyrinth. The membranous labyrinth follows the contour of the bony labyrinth and contains *endolymph.* The vestibular and auditory portions of the inner ear are contiguous, and the "membranous tunnel within a bony tunnel" design is an anatomical feature of both parts. The auditory portion of this inner ear complex is called the *cochlea* (see Figure 11-1).

The cochlear portion of the labyrinth is coiled like a snail shell. If we could mentally uncoil this arrangement to a linear form and then take a transverse section through it, perpendicular to the long axis (like cutting a salami and then looking at the cut end), we would see two membranes, the basilar and Reissner's, dividing the cochlea into three chambers, or *scalae* (Figure 17-3). The dorsally located *scala vestibuli* and ventrally located *scala tympani* contain perilymph. The flexible middle scala, or *scala media* (cochlear duct), is formed by the membranous portion of the labyrinth and contains endolymph. The *basilar membrane* is the floor of the scala media, and atop this membrane lies the hair cell receptor organ for hearing called the *organ of Corti*. An anchored, gel-coated ridge, called the *tectorial membrane,* lies just atop the

hair cells of the organ of Corti. The morphological organization just described is virtually the same all along the length of the cochlea, except that the scala vestibuli and scala tympani connect with each other at the distal end (farthest from the oval window).

The Cochlea Transduces Sound Waves to Action Potentials of the Eighth Cranial Nerve

The organ of Corti mediates the transduction of sound waves into action potentials. The hair cell receptors of the organ of Corti are similar in structure and function to the hair cells that form the vestibular sensory organs. The hair cells synapse on sensory neurons that form the cochlear portion of the eighth cranial (vestibulocochlear) nerve, which projects to the brainstem's *cochlear nuclei.* The cell bodies of these sensory neurons reside in the *spiral ganglion* (see Figure 17-3). Sound-induced bending of the hair cell cilia changes the frequency of action potentials on the eighth nerve fibers.

Sound waves in the external environment are collected by the outer ear and cause vibrations of the tympanic membrane. These vibrations are transmitted through the middle ear by movement of the ossicles and result in similar vibrations of the oval window of the cochlea. As the oval window vibrates, sound energy is transferred down through the perilymph of the scala vestibuli and down through the endolymph of the scala media to the basilar membrane. This energy produces a series of traveling waves that begin near the base of the basilar membrane (closest to the oval window) and move along its length. The situation is analogous to whipping the free end of a rope that is stationary at the opposite end. A diagram of this transmission is shown in Figure 17-4. The movement of the traveling wave causes portions of the flexible basilar membrane to move up and down. Because the organ of Corti sits atop the basilar membrane, this up-and-down motion causes the hair cell cilia to be sheared back and forth against the anchored, overlying tectorial membrane (Figure 17-5). This, in turn, changes the release of transmitter from the hair cells onto the eighth nerve neurons, which in turn alters the action potential firing rate of these neurons. It is at this point that the organ of Corti has transduced the sound wave energy into neural activity. As the amplitude of an environmental sound wave increases (normally perceived as a louder sound), a longer area

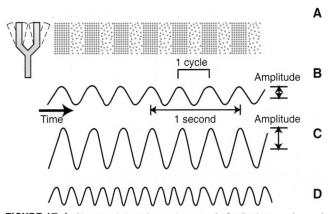

FIGURE 17-1 Characteristics of sound waves. **A,** Cyclical expansion and contraction of the tuning fork produce a cyclical compression and rarefaction of air molecules and a cyclical change in air pressure. **B,** Cyclical change in air pressure corresponding to a pure tone. The number of cycles per second is the frequency of the tone and is expressed in hertz (Hz). The frequency of the tone in *B* is 3 Hz. The amplitude of the wave reflects the magnitude of the pressure increase and is usually expressed in decibels (dB). **C,** Tone with a greater amplitude is perceived as louder than *B*. **D,** Tone with a greater frequency is perceived as having a higher pitch than *B* and *C*.

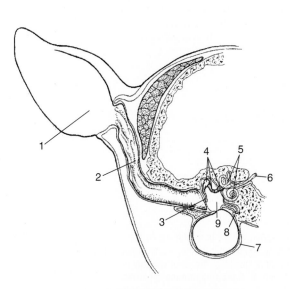

Schematic section through the left ear

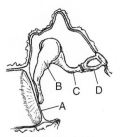

The auditory ossicles

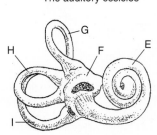

The bony labyrinth

FIGURE 17-2 Schematic diagrams of a section through the left ear, the auditory ossicles, and the bony labyrinth. *1,* Pinna; *2,* ear canal; *3,* tympanic membrane; *4,* auditory ossicles; *5,* bony labyrinth; *6,* eighth cranial nerve; *7,* tympanic bulla; *8,* eustachian tube; *9,* middle ear; *A,* tympanic membrane; *B,* malleus; *C,* incus; *D,* stapes; *E,* cochlea; *F,* utricle; *G, H,* and *I,* semicircular canals. (From Getty R: *Atlas for applied veterinary anatomy,* ed 2, Ames, Iowa, 1964, Iowa State University Press.)

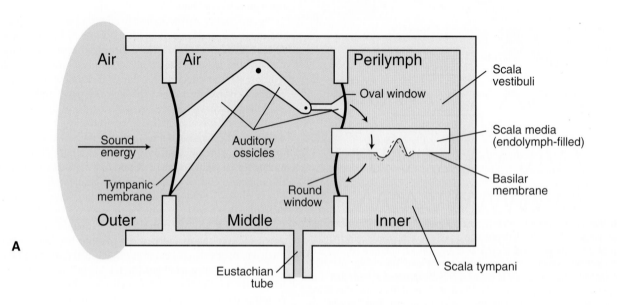

FIGURE 17-3 Schematic representation of a section through one of the turns of the cochlea. (From Hall JE: *Guyton and Hall textbook of medical physiology,* ed 12, Philadelphia, 2011, Saunders.)

Reissner's membrane
Tectorial membrane
Stria vascularis
Scala vestibuli
Spiral limbus
Scala media
Spiral prominence
Spiral ganglion
Organ of Corti
Basilar membrane
Scala tympani
© 2004 Schenk

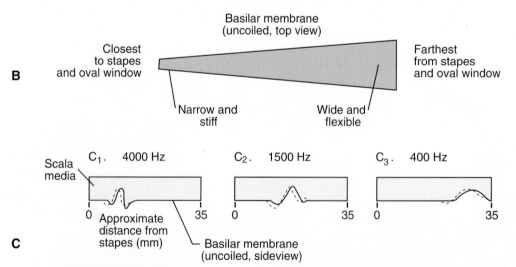

Air
Air
Perilymph
Scala vestibuli
Oval window
Sound energy
Auditory ossicles
Scala media (endolymph-filled)
Basilar membrane
Tympanic membrane
Round window
Scala tympani
Outer
Middle
Inner
Eustachian tube

A

Basilar membrane (uncoiled, top view)

Closest to stapes and oval window

Farthest from stapes and oval window

Narrow and stiff

Wide and flexible

B

Scala media

C_1. 4000 Hz

C_2. 1500 Hz

C_3. 400 Hz

0   Approximate distance from stapes (mm)   35

0   35

0   35

Basilar membrane (uncoiled, sideview)

C

FIGURE 17-4 Schematic representation of the transmission of sound energy from the outer ear to the inner ear. **A,** Sound energy enters the air-filled outer ear and vibrates the tympanic membrane, which produces movement of the ossicles in the air-filled middle ear. Ossicular movement displaces the oval window of the fluid-filled inner ear, resulting in a traveling wave on the basilar membrane. **B,** Basilar membrane is narrow and stiff at the base and wider and more flexible farther from the base. **C,** As the frequency of a sound decreases, the region of maximum displacement of the basilar membrane, produced by the traveling wave, is located progressively farther from the base. (Redrawn from Lippold OCJ, Winton FR: *Human physiology,* ed 6, New York, 1972, Churchill Livingstone.)

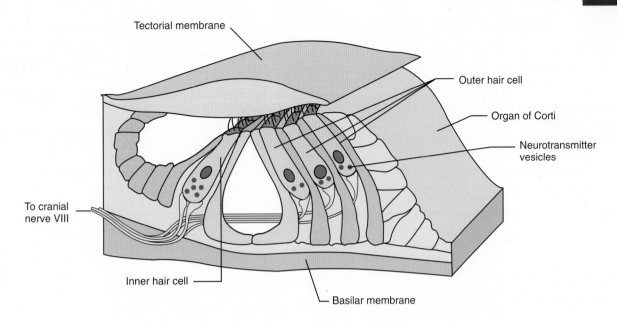

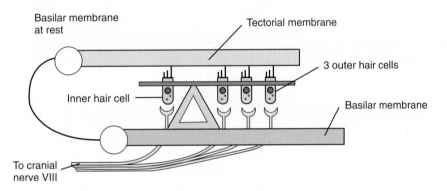

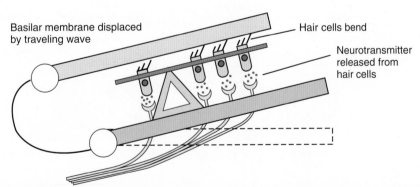

FIGURE 17-5 Transduction of sound into neural activity occurs at the organ of Corti. **A,** Structural organization of the organ of Corti and its hair cell receptors, sitting atop the basilar membrane. **B,** Traveling waves along the basilar membrane displace the membrane and organ of Corti upward, shearing hair cell cilia against the overlying tectorial membrane. This bending of the cilia induces the release of neurotransmitter from the hair cells onto sensory neurons of the eighth cranial nerve. (Modified from Goldstein EB: *Sensation and perception,* ed 6, Pacific Grove, Calif, 2002, Wadsworth.)

of the basilar membrane is displaced. This results in a larger number of hair cells shearing against the tectorial membrane, which in turn affects the activity of a larger number of eighth nerve neurons. This is one way that sound intensity is coded by the nervous system.

Deciphering of Sound Wave Frequency Begins in the Cochlea

The physical properties of the basilar membrane are not uniform along its length. It is narrower and relatively stiffer at its base (near the oval window), and it becomes progressively wider and more flexible toward its apex (see Figure 17-4, *B*). Thus the resonant properties of the membrane are not uniform. A region near the base is significantly displaced by a high-frequency sound, and as the sound frequency decreases, the region of significant displacement is located progressively closer to the apex (see Figure 17-4, *C*). Because the organ of Corti sits atop the basilar membrane, high-frequency sounds are most likely to affect hair cells and their associated eighth nerve neurons near the base of the membrane. As frequency decreases, the hair cells and neurons that are activated are located progressively closer to the apex. Given this orderly relationship between the frequency of a sound wave and the region of the cochlea that is activated by that frequency, the cochlea is said to have a *tonotopic organization*. Therefore a principal means by which the nervous system begins to decipher the frequency of a sound is through the location of the hair cells and neurons that are most affected by that sound.

Among species, there is a rough positive correlation between the number of coils or turns in the cochlea and the size of the frequency range for hearing, although there are exceptions for some species with specialized cochleas (e.g., horseshoe bat, kangaroo rat). The upper frequency range of hearing appears to be negatively correlated with the distance between the two ears.

Action Potentials from the Cochlea Are Transmitted Up Through the Brainstem to the Cerebral Cortex

Action potentials arising in the cochlea travel along the cochlear portion of the eighth cranial nerve to the cochlear nuclei in the medulla oblongata. From there, neural activity is synaptically relayed, in a sequential manner, to the *superior olivary complex* (a group of nuclei spanning the pontomedullary border region), the *inferior colliculus* of the midbrain, the *medial geniculate nucleus* of the thalamus, and finally to the *auditory cortex* of the temporal lobe (Figure 17-6). Conscious perception of sound occurs in the cerebral cortex. Because of extensive connections of central auditory neurons across the midline, information originating in the cochlear nuclei on one side can reach other auditory nuclei on both sides of the brain. However, information originating from a given cochlea is predominantly conducted to the contralateral auditory cortex. Each nucleus in the auditory pathway has a tonotopic representation of sound frequency but is specialized to process particular features of sound. For example, the superior olivary complex plays a major role in determining which side of the head an environmental sound source is coming from. Important environmental cues for this directional localization are differences in the intensity, and in the time of arrival, of a sound at the two different ears. On the other hand, the medial geniculate nucleus is specialized to detect certain combinations of frequencies, as well as timing patterns among sounds.

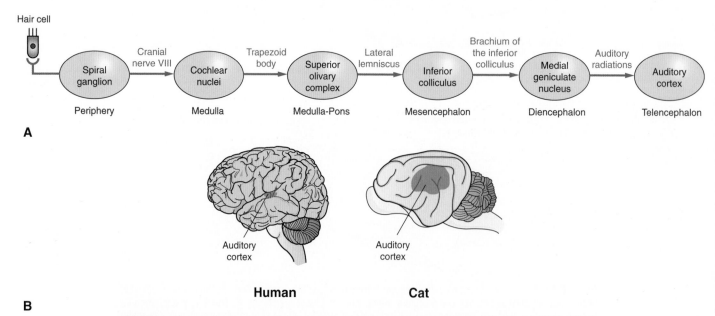

FIGURE 17-6 Principal components of the auditory pathway from hair cell to cerebral cortex. **A,** *Ovals* represent ganglia (peripheral nervous system) or nuclei (central nervous system) and *arrows* represent named axonal connections between them. Major brain divisions (e.g., medulla, pons, etc.) where the structures reside are also noted. **B,** The temporal lobe location of auditory cortex in the human and cat brains. (Modified from Bear MF, Connors BW, Paradiso MA: *Neuroscience: exploring the brain,* ed 3, Philadelphia, 2007, Lippincott, Williams & Wilkins.)

Deafness Results From an Interruption in the Hearing Process

Clinical deafness may result from a loss of sound transmission in the outer or middle ear, called *conduction deafness,* or from malfunction of the cochlear hair cells or eighth nerve fibers, called *nerve deafness* or *sensorineural deafness.* Given that auditory information from one ear is significantly distributed to both sides of the central nervous system, unilateral damage to the auditory system in the brain is often difficult to detect or to localize with a traditional hearing test. In veterinary medicine, inflammatory lesions and neoplasms of the outer or middle ears are frequently the cause of conduction deafness. Sometimes the inflammation can secondarily spread to the inner ear to also cause sensorineural deafness. Deafness in young animals is usually caused by a congenital defect in the cochlea (inherited sensorineural deafness), frequently associated with white coat coloration. Certain antibiotics, diuretics, and antineoplastic agents have ototoxic properties capable of damaging cochlear structures (acquired sensorineural deafness). Like humans, dogs and cats are also susceptible to age-related hearing loss (*presbycusis*).

CLINICAL CORRELATIONS

CONGENITAL DEAFNESS

History. An owner brings you an 8-week-old, almost completely white, male Dalmatian and reports that the pup does not appear to hear anything.

Clinical Examination. Your physical examination reveals a seemingly normal, healthy Dalmatian pup except for his apparent deafness. He does not seem to respond to voice commands or loud noises. Vestibular and all other neurological reflexes are within normal limits. A brainstem auditory-evoked response (see Chapter 16) is flat, which suggests that the brain has not received any signal from the cochlea.

Comment. Congenital deafness is fairly common in dogs and other animals with white coat color. It is usually caused by the partial or complete absence of the cochlea and occasionally by the absence of other neural elements in the auditory pathway. This is known as *nerve deafness* or *sensorineural deafness* and is usually present at birth (congenital). Why it is linked to white coat coloration is under investigation, but the pattern suggests that this is a genetically determined failure, usually bilateral, of the cochlea to develop. This dog can have a relatively normal life as long as the owners are attentive.

PRACTICE QUESTIONS

1. Which one of the following is the *first* to be displaced by sound energy entering the ear?
   a. Oval window
   b. Tectorial membrane
   c. Basilar membrane
   d. Tympanic membrane
   e. Stapes

2. Hair cells similar to those of the organ of Corti are important for the function of which *two* of the following sensory organs?
   a. Muscle spindle
   b. Retina
   c. Crista ampullaris
   d. Golgi tendon organ
   e. Utricular macula

3. Which one of the following statements is *false?*
   a. An increase in sound wave frequency is perceived as an increase in pitch.
   b. The area of greatest displacement of the basilar membrane moves closer to its base (toward the oval window) as the sound wave frequency decreases.
   c. A decrease in sound wave amplitude is perceived as decreased loudness.
   d. An increase in sound wave amplitude displaces a longer region of the basilar membrane.
   e. Contraction of muscles attached to the ossicles reduces the sound energy reaching the inner ear.

4. Which one of the following cranial nerves transmits sound to the brain?
   a. Second
   b. Seventh
   c. Eighth
   d. Tenth

5. Of the following brain nuclei, which one receives auditory information *last?*
   a. Medial geniculate nucleus
   b. Cochlear nuclei
   c. Superior olivary complex
   d. Inferior colliculus

BIBLIOGRAPHY

Bear MF, Connors BW, Paradiso MA: *Neuroscience: exploring the brain,* ed 3, Philadelphia, 2007, Lippincott, Williams & Wilkins.

Brodal P: *The central nervous system: structure and function,* ed 4, New York, 2010, Oxford University Press.

De Lahunta A, Glass E: *Veterinary anatomy and clinical neurology,* ed 3, Philadelphia, 2009, Saunders.

Goldstein EB: *Sensation and perception,* ed 8, Pacific Grove, Calif, 2009, Wadsworth.

Haines DE, editor: *Fundamental neuroscience,* ed 3, New York, 2006, Churchill Livingstone.

Hall JE: *Guyton and Hall textbook of medical physiology,* ed 12, Philadelphia, 2011, Saunders.

Purves D, Augustine GJ, Fitzpatrick D, et al: *Neuroscience,* ed 5, Sunderland, Mass, 2012, Sinauer.

Strain GM: Deafness prevalence and pigmentation and gender associations in dog breeds at risk, *Vet J* 167(1):23–32, 2004.

Strain GM, Myers LJ: Hearing and equilibrium. In Reece WO, editor: *Duke's physiology of domestic animals,* ed 12, Ithaca, NY, 2004, Comstock Publishing.

CHAPTER 18

Overview of Cardiovascular Function

KEY POINTS

1. Because normal cardiovascular function is essential for life and health, a practical understanding of cardiovascular function and dysfunction is vital to the veterinary clinician.
2. Cardiovascular dysfunctions sometimes reflect primary cardiovascular disturbances or diseases, but more often they are secondary consequences of noncardiovascular disturbances or diseases.
3. Substances transported by the cardiovascular system include nutrients, waste products, hormones, electrolytes, and water.
4. Two modes of transport are used in the cardiovascular system: bulk flow and diffusion.
5. Because diffusion is very slow, every metabolically active cell in the body must be close to a capillary carrying blood by bulk flow.
6. The pulmonary and systemic circulations are arranged in series, but the various organs within the systemic circulation are arranged in parallel.
7. Cardiac output is the volume of blood pumped each minute by one ventricle.
8. The perfusion pressure for the systemic circulation is much greater than the perfusion pressure for the pulmonary circulation.
9. Each type of blood vessel has physical properties suited to its particular function.
10. Blood is a suspension of cells in extracellular fluid (plasma).
11. The cellular component of blood includes red blood cells, white blood cells, and platelets.
12. Most of the oxygen in blood is carried in chemical combination with the protein hemoglobin within red blood cells.

Because Normal Cardiovascular Function Is Essential for Life and Health, a Practical Understanding of Cardiovascular Function and Dysfunction Is Vital to the Veterinary Clinician

Cardiovascular physiology is the study of the function of the heart, the blood vessels, and the blood. The primary function of the cardiovascular system can be summarized in one word: *transport*. The bloodstream transports numerous substances that are essential for life and health, including the oxygen and nutrients required by every cell in the body. Blood also carries carbon dioxide and other metabolic waste products away from metabolically active cells and delivers them to the lungs, kidneys, or liver, where they are excreted.

To appreciate the importance of cardiovascular transport, consider what happens if the heart stops contracting and circulation ceases: unconsciousness results within about 30 seconds, and irreversible damage to the brain and other sensitive body tissues occurs within a few minutes. However, circulation does not have to stop completely for significant dysfunction to occur. For example, the loss of as little as 10% of the normal blood volume can impair exercise performance.

In each tissue of the body, normal function depends on the delivery of adequate blood flow. The higher the rate of metabolism in a tissue, the greater is the requirement for blood flow. The condition of inadequate blood flow to any tissue is called *ischemia*. Even transient ischemia leads to *dysfunction*. Persistent ischemia leads to permanent tissue damage (*infarction*) and eventually to cell death (*necrosis*).

Many veterinary students have difficulty understanding cardiovascular physiology. They tend to agree with William Harvey, the father of cardiovascular physiology, whose initial impression was that the motions of the heart and the blood were so complicated that they could be comprehended only by God. Harvey persisted, however, in a careful, deliberate study of cardiovascular function and in 1628 set forth the first proof that the heart propels blood through the blood vessels in a circulatory pattern. Before Harvey's time, it was thought that blood flowed out of the heart into the blood vessels and then returned to the heart by backward flow in the same vessels. In other words, blood was thought to flow in a tidal manner, in much the same way that air flows through a single set of airways: first into the lungs and then back out.

We now take for granted that the cardiovascular system is a *circulatory system*, not a tidal system. However, the circularity of the cardiovascular system is precisely what makes it difficult to understand. It has no clear beginning or ending, and disturbances in one part of the cardiovascular system end up affecting all other parts as well. In recognition of this complexity, Chapters 18 to 26 are written with the goal of identifying the most basic and important concepts of *normal cardiovascular function* and explaining them in a way that best prepares the reader to understand, diagnose, and treat *cardiovascular dysfunction* (cardiovascular disease). The remainder of this chapter reviews the general features of the cardiovascular system. Chapters 19 to 25 discuss the various elements of the cardiovascular system in detail. Chapter 26 summarizes cardiovascular function and dysfunction by describing the overall effects of heart failure, hemorrhage, and exercise.

Cardiovascular Dysfunctions Sometimes Reflect Primary Cardiovascular Disturbances or Diseases, But More Often They Are Secondary Consequences of Noncardiovascular Disturbances or Diseases

Impairment in the transport functions of the cardiovascular system is encountered frequently in veterinary medicine. Some of these cardiovascular dysfunctions are *primary,* in that the fundamental disturbance or disease process affects the cardiovascular system directly. One example of primary cardiovascular dysfunction is *hemorrhage* (loss of blood from blood vessels). Another is *myocarditis* (literally, muscle-heart-inflammation), which can be caused by a toxic chemical or by a viral or bacterial infection that inflames the heart muscle and impairs the ability of the heart to pump blood.

Cardiovascular dysfunction and disease can be either *congenital* (present at birth) or *acquired* (developing after birth). Congenital cardiovascular diseases frequently involve defective heart valves, which either cannot open fully or cannot close completely. Congenital cardiac defects are common in certain breeds of dogs and horses. Although a heart that has a congenital defect or an acquired disease may be able to pump an adequate amount of blood when the animal is at rest, it usually cannot deliver the increased blood flow required by the body during exercise. When a dysfunction in the heart impairs its ability to pump the amount of blood flow normally needed by the body, the condition is called *heart failure* (or pump failure). The patient with heart failure classically exhibits a limited ability or willingness to exercise (*exercise intolerance*).

Parasites are a common cause of acquired cardiovascular dysfunction. In dogs, for example, adult heartworms (*Dirofilaria immitis*) lodge in the right ventricle and pulmonary artery, where they impede the flow of blood. These worms also release substances into the circulation that disrupt the body's ability to control blood pressure and blood flow. In horses, bloodworms (*Strongylus vulgaris*) lodge in the mesenteric arteries and decrease the blood flow to the intestine. The resulting intestinal ischemia depresses digestive functions (motility, secretion, and absorption), and the horse exhibits signs of gastrointestinal distress (*colic*).

In many other disease states, cardiovascular complications develop even though the cardiovascular system is not the primary target of the disease. These *secondary cardiovascular dysfunctions* often become the most serious and life-threatening aspects of the disease. For example, severe burns or persistent vomiting or diarrhea leads to substantial losses of water and *electrolytes* (small, soluble ions in the body fluids; e.g., Na^+, Cl^-, K^+, Ca^{2+}). Even if the blood volume is not depleted to dangerously low levels in these conditions, the alteration in electrolyte concentrations can lead to abnormal heart rhythms (*cardiac arrhythmias)* and ineffective pumping of blood by the heart (heart failure). The electrolyte abnormalities in such a patient can be made even worse if incorrect fluid therapy is given. Incorrect fluid therapy can also lead to an accumulation of excess fluid in the tissues of the body; this "waterlogging" of tissues is called *edema*. If the excess fluid gathers in the lung tissue, the condition is called *pulmonary edema.* Pulmonary edema is life threatening because it slows the flow of oxygen from the pulmonary air sacs (*alveoli*) into the bloodstream.

Pulmonary edema is a secondary complication in many disease states. A further example is *shock-lung syndrome,* which results when toxic substances in the body trigger an increase in the permeability of the lung blood vessels. These "leaky" vessels allow water, electrolytes, plasma proteins, and white blood cells to leave the bloodstream and accumulate in the lung tissue and airways. The resulting pulmonary edema can lead to death.

Whereas the effects of shock-lung syndrome are most serious in the pulmonary circulation, other types of shock depress the cardiovascular system in general. *Hemorrhagic shock* is a generalized cardiovascular failure caused by severe blood loss. *Cardiogenic shock* is a cardiovascular collapse caused by heart failure. *Septic shock* is caused by bacterial infections in the bloodstream (*bacteremia*). *Endotoxic shock* occurs when endotoxins (fragments of bacterial cell walls) enter the bloodstream; this often occurs when the epithelial lining of the intestines becomes damaged. Epithelial damage can result from bacterial infections in the intestines or from ischemia in the intestinal walls (as with bloodworms in horses). When the intestinal epithelium breaks down, endotoxins from the intestine can enter the bloodstream. These endotoxins then cause the body to produce substances that depress the pumping ability of the heart. The resulting heart failure leads to low blood flow and ischemia in all the vital body organs. Kidney (or renal) failure, respiratory failure, central nervous system (CNS) depression, and death follow.

Anesthetic overdose is another clinical problem in which the most serious and life-threatening symptoms are the secondary cardiovascular complications. Most anesthetics depress the CNS, and the resulting abnormal neural signals to the heart and the blood vessels can depress cardiac output and lower blood pressure. Some anesthetics, particularly the barbiturates, also depress the pumping ability of the heart directly.

There are many other examples of primary and secondary cardiovascular dysfunction, but those just mentioned illustrate the importance and variety of cardiovascular dysfunctions encountered in veterinary medicine. The distinction between primary and secondary cardiovascular dysfunction is sometimes unclear, but this difficulty simply emphasizes how intimately the cardiovascular system is interconnected with all the other body systems and how dependent all the other systems are on the normal functioning of the cardiovascular system.

Substances Transported by the Cardiovascular System Include Nutrients, Waste Products, Hormones, Electrolytes, and Water

The blood transports the metabolic substrates needed by every cell of the body, including oxygen, glucose, amino acids, fatty acids, and various lipids. The blood also carries away from each cell in the body various metabolic waste products, including carbon dioxide, lactic acid, the nitrogenous wastes of protein metabolism, and heat. Although the heat produced by metabolic processes within cells is not a material waste product, its transport by the cardiovascular system to the body surface is essential, because tissues deep within the body would otherwise become overheated and dysfunctional.

Blood also transports vital chemical messengers: the hormones. Hormones are synthesized and released by cells in one organ and are carried by the bloodstream to cells in other organs, where they alter organ function. For example, insulin, which is produced by cells of the pancreas, is carried by the blood to cells throughout the body, where it promotes the cellular uptake of glucose. Inadequate insulin production (as in type 1 diabetes) results in inadequate entry of glucose into cells, whereas glucose concentrations in the blood rise to very high levels. The low intracellular glucose concentration is particularly disruptive to neural function, and the consequences can be serious (diabetic coma) or lethal. Another hormone, *adrenaline* (a mixture of *epinephrine* and *norepinephrine*), is released into the bloodstream by cells in the adrenal medulla during periods of stress. The epinephrine and norepinephrine circulate to various body organs, where they have effects that prepare a threatened animal for the "fight or flight" response. These effects include an increase in heart rate and cardiac contractility, dilation of skeletal muscle blood vessels, an increase in blood pressure, increased glycogenolysis, dilation of the pupils and airways, and piloerection (hair standing on end).

Finally, the blood transports water and essential electrolytes, including Na^+, Cl^-, K^+, Ca^{2+}, H^+, and HCO_3^-. The kidneys are the organs primarily responsible for maintaining normal water and electrolyte composition in the body. The kidneys accomplish this by altering the electrolyte concentrations in blood as it flows through the kidneys. The altered blood then circulates to all other organs in the body, where it normalizes the water and electrolyte content in the extracellular fluids of each tissue.

Two Modes of Transport Are Used in the Cardiovascular System: Bulk Flow and Diffusion

Blood moves through the heart and blood vessels by bulk flow. The most important feature of bulk flow is that it is rapid over long distances. Blood that is pumped out of the heart travels quickly through the aorta and its various branches; within 10 seconds it reaches distant parts of the body, including the head and limbs. Transport requires energy, and the source of energy for bulk flow is a hydrostatic pressure difference; unless the pressure at one end of a blood vessel is higher than the pressure at the other end, flow will not occur. The difference in pressure between two points in a blood vessel is called the *perfusion pressure difference* or, more often, simply *perfusion pressure*. Perfusion literally means "through-flow," and the perfusion pressure is the pressure difference that causes blood to flow through blood vessels. The muscular pumping action of the heart creates the perfusion pressure that constitutes the driving force for bulk blood flow through the circulation.

It is important to distinguish between perfusion pressure difference and *transmural pressure difference* (usually shortened to *transmural pressure*). Transmural means "across the wall," and transmural pressure is the difference between the blood pressure inside a blood vessel and the fluid pressure in the tissue immediately outside the vessel (transmural pressure equals inside pressure minus outside pressure). Transmural pressure is the pressure difference that would cause blood to flow out of a vessel if a hole were poked in the vessel wall. Transmural pressure is also called *distending pressure*, because it corresponds to the net outward "push" on the wall of a blood vessel. Figure 18-1 emphasizes the distinction between perfusion pressure and transmural pressure.

Diffusion is the second mode of transport in the cardiovascular system. Diffusion is the primary mechanism by which dissolved substances move across the walls of blood vessels, from the bloodstream into the interstitial fluid, or vice versa. *Interstitial fluid* is the extracellular fluid outside capillaries. It is the fluid that bathes each cell of a tissue. Most of the movement of substances between the blood and the interstitial fluid takes place across the walls of the *capillaries,* the smallest blood vessels. For a substance (e.g., oxygen) to move from the bloodstream to a tissue cell, it diffuses across the wall of a capillary and into the tissue interstitial fluid, and then diffuses from the interstitial fluid into the tissue cell.

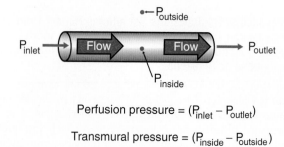

Perfusion pressure = $(P_{inlet} - P_{outlet})$

Transmural pressure = $(P_{inside} - P_{outside})$

FIGURE 18-1 Fluid pressures associated with a blood vessel. P_{inlet}, P_{outlet}, and P_{inside} refer to blood pressure within the vessel. $P_{outside}$ refers to the pressure in the tissue fluid (interstitial fluid) immediately outside the blood vessel. Perfusion pressure is the pressure difference *along the length* of a blood vessel. Transmural pressure (distending pressure) is the pressure difference *across the wall* of the vessel, indicated here at the midpoint of the vessel. Perfusion pressure is the driving force for blood flow through the vessel, whereas transmural pressure is the driving force that would cause blood to flow out of the vessel if there were a hole in it.

The source of energy for diffusion is a *concentration difference.* A substance diffuses from the bloodstream, across the wall of a capillary, and into the interstitial fluid only if the concentration of the substance is higher in the blood than in the interstitial fluid (and if the capillary wall is permeable to the substance). If the concentration of a substance is higher in the interstitial fluid than in the blood, the substance will diffuse from the interstitial fluid into the capillary blood. It is important to distinguish *diffusion,* in which a substance moves passively from an area of high concentration toward an area of low concentration, from *active transport,* in which substances are forced to move in a direction opposite to their concentration gradient. In general, substances are not transported actively across the walls of capillaries. The movement of substances between the bloodstream and the interstitial fluid occurs by passive diffusion.

Because Diffusion Is Very Slow, Every Metabolically Active Cell in the Body Must Be Close to a Capillary Carrying Blood by Bulk Flow

To understand more fully how the two types of transport (bulk flow and diffusion) are used in the cardiovascular system, consider the transport of oxygen from the outside air to a neuron in the brain. With each inspiration, fresh air containing oxygen (O_2) moves by bulk flow through progressively smaller airways (trachea, bronchi, and bronchioles) and finally enters the alveolar air sacs (Figure 18-2, *A*). The thin walls separating alveoli contain a meshwork of capillaries (see Figure 18-2, *B*). Blood flowing through these *alveolar capillaries* passes extremely close (within 1 μm) to the air in the alveoli (see Figure 18-2, *C*). The blood in an alveolar capillary has just returned from the body tissues, where it gave up some of its oxygen. Therefore the concentration of oxygen in alveolar capillary blood is lower than the concentration of oxygen in alveolar air. This concentration difference causes some oxygen to diffuse from the alveolar air into the capillary blood.

A large dog has about 300 million alveoli, with a total surface area of about 130 m² (equal to half the surface area of a tennis court). This huge surface area is laced with pulmonary capillaries. Thus, even though only a tiny amount of oxygen diffuses into each pulmonary capillary, the aggregate uptake of oxygen into the pulmonary bloodstream is substantial (typically, 125 mL

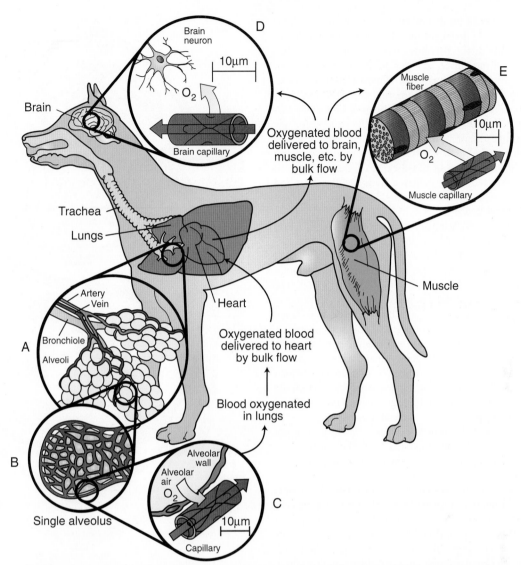

FIGURE 18-2 Oxygen (O_2) is transported from the atmosphere to cells throughout the body by a combination of bulk flow and diffusion. First, O_2 moves by bulk flow through the airways, from the atmosphere to the alveoli (tiny air sacs) of the lungs *(inset A)*. The wall of each alveolus contains a meshwork of alveolar (pulmonary) capillaries *(inset B)*. O_2 readily diffuses from the alveolar air into the blood that is flowing through the alveolar capillaries *(inset C)*. Bulk flow of blood next carries this O_2 to the heart; from there it is delivered by bulk flow into the capillaries of all the body organs (except the lungs). In the brain *(inset D)*, skeletal muscle *(inset E)*, and other tissues, O_2 moves by diffusion from the capillary blood into the interstitial fluid and then into the tissue cells, where it is utilized to support oxidative metabolism. Bulk flow is rapid; it can transport O_2 to all parts of the body within a few seconds. Diffusion is slow; it can transport O_2 efficiently only over distances less than 100 µm (note distance scales in insets C, D, and E). Oxygenated blood has a bright-red color; deoxygenated blood is darker and bluish red.

O_2/minute in a large, resting dog, increasing by a factor of 10 or more during strenuous exercise). In summary, both the large alveolar surface area and the proximity of alveolar air to the blood in alveolar capillaries promote efficient diffusion of oxygen; it takes less than 1 second for the blood in an alveolar capillary to become oxygenated.

As it leaves the lungs, each 100 mL of oxygenated blood normally carries 20 mL of oxygen. About 1.5% of this oxygen is carried in solution; the other 98.5% is bound to the protein *hemoglobin* within the *erythrocytes* (red blood cells). The oxygenated blood moves by bulk flow from the lungs to the heart. The heart pumps this oxygenated blood out into the aorta, and from there

it is distributed via a complex system of branching arteries to all parts of the body (including the brain and skeletal muscles, as illustrated in Figure 18-2). Capillaries in the brain bring a bulk flow of oxygenated blood very close to each brain neuron (see Figure 18-2, *D*). Metabolic processes within the neurons consume oxygen, so the oxygen concentration inside neurons is low. The gradient of oxygen concentration between the capillary blood (high) and the neurons (low) provides the driving force for oxygen to diffuse first from the blood into the interstitial fluid and then into the neurons.

Each brain neuron must be within about 100 µm of a capillary carrying blood by bulk flow if diffusion is to deliver oxygen rapidly enough to sustain normal metabolism in the neuron. Diffusional exchange over distances up to 100 μm typically takes only 1 to 5 seconds. If the distance involved were a few millimeters, diffusion would take minutes to occur. Diffusion of oxygen a few centimeters through body fluid would take hours. Therefore, normal life processes require that every metabolically active cell of the body be within about 100 μm of a capillary carrying blood by bulk flow. If this bulk flow is interrupted for any reason, perhaps because of a *thrombus* (blood clot) in the artery that delivers blood to a particular region of a tissue, that region of tissue becomes ischemic. As stated earlier, ischemia leads to dysfunction; persistent, severe ischemia leads to infarction and eventually to necrosis. *Cerebral infarction* causes the condition commonly known as *stroke.*

Figure 18-2, *E*, shows a capillary carrying bulk flow of blood past a skeletal muscle cell (muscle fiber). Oxygen moves by diffusion from the capillary blood into the muscle interstitial fluid and then into the muscle cell, where it is consumed in the metabolic reactions that provide energy for muscle contraction. The oxygen consumption of a skeletal muscle depends on the severity of its exercise; at a maximum, oxygen consumption may reach levels 40 times greater than the resting level. Because of its tremendous metabolic capacity, muscle tissue has an especially high density of capillaries. In fact, several capillaries are typically arrayed around each skeletal muscle fiber. This arrangement provides more surface area for diffusional exchange than would be possible with a single capillary and brings the bulk flow of blood extremely close to all parts of each skeletal muscle cell.

Heart muscle, like skeletal muscle, consumes a large amount of oxygen. Oxygenated blood is carried from the aorta to the heart muscle by a network of branching *coronary arteries.* This blood next moves by bulk flow into *coronary capillaries,* which pass close by each cardiac muscle cell. If a thrombus interrupts the bulk flow of blood in a coronary artery, the heart muscle cells supplied by that artery become ischemic. Ischemia develops even if the cardiac muscle deprived of blood flow lies within a few millimeters of the left ventricular chamber, which is filled with oxygen-rich blood. Oxygen simply cannot diffuse rapidly enough from the ventricular chamber to the ischemic cells to sustain their metabolism. Ischemic cardiac muscle loses its ability to contract forcefully; also, cardiac arrhythmias may develop. Severe myocardial ischemia causes a *myocardial infarction,* or heart attack.

Coronary artery disease and *cerebrovascular disease* are encountered more often in human medicine than in veterinary medicine. In contrast, *cardiac disease* (dysfunction of the heart muscle or valves, as distinguished from disease of the coronary arteries) is encountered more often in veterinary medicine than in human medicine. Therefore, Chapters 19 to 26 place more emphasis on cardiac physiology than on vascular physiology.

The Pulmonary and Systemic Circulations Are Arranged In Series, But the Various Organs Within the Systemic Circulation Are Arranged in Parallel

As shown in Figure 18-3, blood is pumped from the left ventricle into the aorta. The aorta divides and subdivides to form many arteries, which deliver fresh, oxygenated blood to each organ of the body, except the lungs. The pattern of arterial branching that delivers blood of the same composition to each organ is called *parallel.* After blood passes through the capillaries within individual organs, it enters veins. Small veins combine to form progressively larger veins, until the entire blood flow is delivered to the right atrium by way of the *venae cavae* (pleural of vena cava,

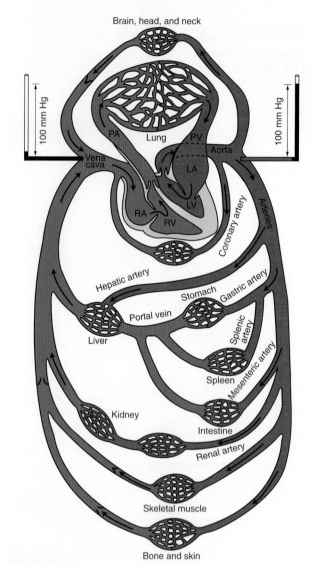

FIGURE 18-3 General layout of the cardiovascular system, showing that the systemic and pulmonary circulations are arranged in series and that the organs within the systemic circulation are arranged in parallel. *LA,* Left atrium; *LV,* left ventricle; *PA,* pulmonary artery; *PV,* pulmonary vein; *RA,* right atrium; *RV,* right ventricle. Oxygenated blood has a bright-red color; deoxygenated blood is darker and bluish red. The drawing also shows that, if an open tube containing mercury *(black)* were stuck into the aorta, the normal blood pressure within the aorta would push mercury nearly 100 mm upward into the tube, at which point the upward force of the blood pressure would be equalized by the downward force of gravity acting on the mercury. In contrast, the blood pressure in the *venae cavae* is much lower (typically about 3 mm Hg), as illustrated on the left side of the drawing. (Modified from Milnor WR: *Cardiovascular physiology,* New York, 1990, Oxford University Press.)

includes both superior vena cava and inferior vena cava). The blood vessels between the aorta and the *venae cavae* (including the blood vessels in all organs of the body except the lungs) are collectively called the *systemic circulation.* From the right atrium, blood passes into the right ventricle, which pumps it into the pulmonary artery. The pulmonary artery branches into progressively smaller arteries, which deliver blood to each alveolar (pulmonary) capillary. Blood from pulmonary capillaries is collected in pulmonary veins and brought to the left atrium. Blood then passes into the left ventricle, completing the circuit. The blood vessels of the lungs, including the pulmonary arteries and veins, constitute the *pulmonary circulation.* The pulmonary circulation and the heart are collectively termed the *central circulation.* The pulmonary circulation and the systemic circulation are arranged in *series;* that is, blood must pass through the pulmonary vessels between each passage through the systemic circuit.

In one pass through the systemic circulation, blood generally encounters only one capillary bed before being collected in veins and returned to the heart, although a few exceptions to this rule exist. One exception occurs in the *splanchnic circulation,* which supplies blood to the digestive organs. As shown in Figure 18-3, blood that leaves the gastric, splenic, or mesenteric capillaries enters the *portal vein.* The portal vein carries splanchnic venous blood to the liver, where the blood passes through another set of capillaries before it returns to the heart. This arrangement of two systemic capillary beds in series is called a *portal system.* The splanchnic portal system allows nutrients that have been absorbed from the gastrointestinal tract to be delivered directly to the liver. There the nutrients are transformed for storage or allowed to pass into the general circulation. The liver also receives some blood directly from the aorta through the hepatic artery.

The kidneys also contain a portal system. As shown in Figure 18-3, blood enters a kidney by way of a renal artery and passes through two sets of capillaries (called *glomerular* and *tubular*) before returning to the venous side of the systemic circulation. Large amounts of water, electrolytes, and other solutes are filtered out of the blood as it passes through the glomerular capillaries. Most of this filtered material is subsequently reabsorbed into the bloodstream as it flows through the peritubular capillaries. The remainder becomes urine. The kidneys use the *renal portal system* to adjust the amounts of water, electrolytes, and other critical solutes in the blood.

A third portal system is found in the brain and is important in the control of hormone secretion by the pituitary gland. After traversing capillaries in the hypothalamus, blood enters portal vessels that carry it to the anterior pituitary gland *(adenohypophysis)* and to another set of capillaries (see Figures 33-16 and 33-17). As blood traverses the hypothalamic capillaries, it picks up several signaling chemicals that control the release of pituitary hormones. When this blood reaches capillaries in the anterior pituitary gland, these substances diffuse out of the bloodstream and into the pituitary interstitial fluid, where they act on pituitary cells to increase or decrease their secretion of specific pituitary hormones. This system is called the *hypothalamic-hypophyseal portal system.*

To summarize, except for a few specialized portal systems, blood encounters only one capillary bed in a single pass through the systemic circulation.

Cardiac Output Is the Volume of Blood Pumped Each Minute by One Ventricle

In a resting dog, it takes about 1 minute for blood to traverse the entire circulation (from the left ventricle back to the left ventricle). Because the pulmonary and systemic circulations are in series, the volume of blood pumped by the right side of the heart each minute must equal the volume of blood pumped by the left side of the heart each minute. The volume of blood pumped per minute by either the left ventricle or the right ventricle is called *cardiac output.* Among the mammalian species typically encountered in veterinary medicine, cardiac output at rest is approximately 3 liters per minute per square meter (L/min/m²) of body

surface area. A large dog (e.g., German shepherd) typically has a body surface area a little less than 1 m² and a cardiac output at rest of about 2.5 L/min.

In an animal at rest, blood entering the aorta is divided so that approximately 20% of it flows through the splanchnic circulation and 20% through the kidneys. Another 20% goes to the skeletal muscles. The brain receives about 15% of the cardiac output, and the coronary arteries carry about 3% of the cardiac output. The remainder goes to skin and bone.

The Perfusion Pressure for the Systemic Circulation Is Much Greater Than the Perfusion Pressure for the Pulmonary Circulation

When the left ventricle contracts and ejects blood into the aorta, the aorta becomes distended with blood, and aortic blood pressure rises to a peak value called *systolic pressure* (typically 120 mm Hg). Between ejections, blood continues to flow out of the aorta into the downstream arteries. This outflow of blood from the aorta causes aortic pressure to decrease. The minimal value of aortic blood pressure, just before the next cardiac ejection, is called *diastolic pressure* (typically 80 mm Hg). A typical appearance of the pressure pulsations in the aorta is shown in the middle panel of Figure 22-7. The *mean aortic pressure* (average value of the pulsatile blood pressure in the aorta) is about 98 mm Hg. This means that, if an open tube containing mercury were stuck into the aorta, the blood pressure within the aorta would push mercury 98 mm upward into the tube; at which point the upward force of the blood pressure would be equalized by the downward force of gravity acting on the mercury.

The mean aortic pressure represents a potential energy for driving blood through the systemic circulation. As blood flows through the systemic blood vessels, this pressure energy is dissipated through friction. The potential energy (blood pressure) remaining by the time the blood reaches the *venae cavae* is only 3 mm Hg. Therefore the perfusion pressure for the systemic circuit is typically 98 mm Hg minus 3 mm Hg, or 95 mm Hg.

Right ventricular contractions cause pulsatile ejections of blood into the pulmonary artery. The resulting, pulsatile variations in pulmonary arterial blood pressure typically have a peak (systolic) value of 20 mm Hg and a minimum (diastolic) value of 8 mm Hg. The typical value for mean pulmonary artery blood pressure is 13 mm Hg. The blood pressure in pulmonary veins (at the point where they enter the left atrium) is typically 5 mm Hg. Under these conditions the perfusion pressure for blood flow through the lungs is 8 mm Hg (i.e., 13 mm Hg minus 5 mm Hg).

The same volume of blood (the cardiac output) flows each minute through the systemic circulation and through the lungs; however, as is evident from the typical values just given, the perfusion pressure for the systemic circuit is much greater than the perfusion pressure for the lungs. The reason for this difference in perfusion pressure is that the systemic vessels offer more friction against blood flow (i.e., have a higher *resistance*) than do the pulmonary vessels. Therefore the systemic circulation is referred to as the *high-pressure, high-resistance side of the circulation.* The pulmonary circuit is called the *low-pressure, low-resistance side.*

By convention, blood pressures are always measured with reference to atmospheric pressure. Thus an aortic pressure of 98 mm Hg means that the blood pressure in the aorta is 98 mm Hg higher than the atmospheric pressure outside the body. Also, by convention, blood pressure is measured at heart level. This is why, in human medicine, blood pressure cuffs are typically applied over the brachial artery (in the upper arm); the brachial artery is at the same level as the heart. If blood pressure is measured in an artery or vein at a level different from heart level, an arithmetic correction should be made so that the pressure is reported as if it had been measured at heart level. This correction is necessary because gravity pulls downward on blood and therefore affects the actual pressure of blood within vessels. Gravity increases the actual blood pressure in vessels lying below heart level and decreases the actual pressure in vessels above heart level. The gravitational effect is significant in an animal the size of a dog and substantial in an animal the size of a horse. The correction factor for the effect of gravity is 1 mm Hg for each 1.36 cm above or below heart level.

Each Type of Blood Vessel Has Physical Properties Suited to Its Particular Function

In a resting animal, at any one moment, about 25% of the blood volume is in the central circulation and about 75% is in the systemic circulation (Table 18-1). Most of the blood in the systemic circulation is found in the veins. Only 20% of the systemic blood is found in the arteries, arterioles, and capillaries. Therefore, systemic veins are known as the *blood reservoirs* of the circulation. Arteries function as *high-pressure conduits* for rapid distribution of blood to the various organs. Arterioles are the "gates" of the systemic circulation; they *constrict* or *dilate* to control the blood flow to each capillary bed. Although only a small fraction of the systemic blood is found in capillaries at any one time, it is within these *exchange vessels* that the important diffusional transport takes place between the bloodstream and the interstitial fluid.

Table 18-2 compares the various types of vessels in the systemic circulation of a dog. As the aorta branches into progressively smaller vessels, the diameters of the vessels become smaller, but the number of vessels increases. One aorta supplies blood to 45,000 terminal arteries, each of which gives rise to more than 400 arterioles. Each arteriole typically branches into about 80 capillaries. The capillaries are so small in diameter that red blood cells must pass through in single file. However, because of the sheer number of capillaries, the total cross-sectional area of the capillaries is much greater than the cross-sectional area of the preceding arteries and arterioles. Because capillary blood flow is spread out over such a large cross-sectional area, the flow velocity within capillaries is low. Blood moves rapidly (about 13 cm/sec) through the aorta and large arteries. At this speed, blood is delivered from the heart to all parts of the body in less than 10 seconds. The velocity of blood flow decreases as the blood leaves arteries and enters arterioles and capillaries in each tissue. The velocity of blood flow in capillaries is so slow that blood typically takes about 1 second to travel the 0.5 mm length of a capillary. During this time, diffusional exchange takes place between the capillary blood and the interstitial fluid. Blood from the capillaries is collected by venules and veins and is carried quite rapidly back to the heart.

An understanding of the normal dynamics of blood flow provides a basis for interpretation of *capillary refill time,* which is measured during a typical clinical physical examination. The examiner locates an area of non-pigmented epithelial membrane (most commonly a non-pigmented area of the gums). Such tissue is normally pink, due to an adequate flow of well-oxygenated blood through the small vessels (arterioles, capillaries, and venules). The examiner applies firm finger pressure to the area for 1 or 2 seconds, which compresses all the small blood vessels and squeezes the blood out of them. Immediately upon release of the finger pressure, the tissue appears very pale, due to the absence of blood in the small vessels. A normal circulation will restore blood flow through the small vessels and the pink color will return within 1 to 2 seconds (the normal capillary refill time). A prolonged capillary refill time is indicative of poor perfusion of the tissue and, by inference, a sluggish circulation.

Figure 18-4 depicts the branching pattern of the systemic vessels and graphs the velocity of blood flow within the different

TABLE 18-1 Distribution of Blood Volume in the Cardiovascular System of a Normal Dog

Distribution	Percent
Between Central and Systemic Circulations	
Central circulation	25
Systemic circulation	75
TOTAL	100
Within the Various Vessels of the Systemic Circulation	
Arteries and arterioles	15
Capillaries	5
Venules and veins	80
TOTAL	100

TABLE 18-2 Geometry of Systemic Circulation of a 30-kg Resting Dog

Vessel	Number	Inside Diameter (mm)	Total Cross Sectional Area (cm^2)	Length (cm)	Velocity of Blood Flow (cm/sec)	Mean Blood Pressure (mm Hg)
Aorta	1	20.0	3.1	40.0	13.0	98
Small arteries	45,000	0.14	6.9	1.5	6.0	90
Arterioles	20,000,000	0.030	140.0	0.2	0.3	60
Capillaries	1,700,000,000	0.008	830.0	0.05	0.05	18
Venules	130,000,000	0.020	420.0	0.1	0.1	12
Small veins	73,000	0.27	42.0	1.5	1.0	6
Venae cavae	2	24.0	9.0	34.0	4.5	3

Modified from Minor WR: *Cardiovascular physiology,* New York, 1990, Oxford University Press.

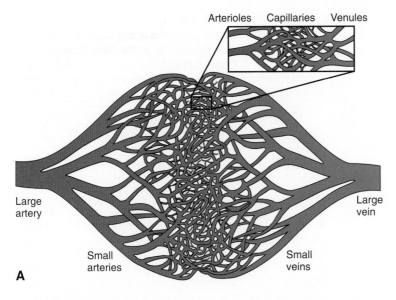

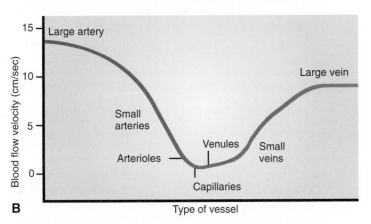

FIGURE 18-4 As the systemic arteries branch to form small arteries, arterioles, and capillaries **(A),** the total cross-sectional area of the vessels increases, so the forward velocity of blood flow decreases **(B).** As blood from the capillaries is collected into venules and veins, the total cross-sectional area is reduced, so the velocity of blood flow increases again. Therefore, blood moves quickly from the heart to the microvessels, where it stays for a few seconds before moving rapidly back to the heart.

types of vessels. This figure emphasizes the rapidity of bulk flow through large vessels and the relatively slow flow through the capillaries. Note that the *velocity* of blood flow is lowest in the capillaries; however, the same *volume* of blood necessarily flows each minute through an artery, the capillaries that it feeds, and the veins draining the capillaries.

In addition to having a large cross-sectional area (and therefore slow velocity of blood flow), capillaries have a large surface area. The total surface area of the walls of all the capillaries in the systemic circulation of a large dog is about 20 m², which is nearly 30 times greater than the dog's body surface area. The large surface area of capillaries helps promote efficient diffusional exchange between the capillary blood and the interstitial fluid.

Blood Is a Suspension of Cells in Extracellular Fluid (Plasma)

As shown in Figure 18-5, blood can be separated into its cellular and liquid components by centrifugation. The liquid phase of blood is lighter in weight than the cells and therefore ends up on the top of the centrifuge tube. This acellular or extracellular liquid in blood is called *plasma*. Water constitutes 93% of the plasma volume. About 5% to 7% of the plasma volume is made up of protein molecules. The presence of proteins gives plasma its typical pale-yellow color. The *plasma proteins* are synthesized in the liver and are added to the bloodstream as it passes through

the liver capillaries. Globulin, albumin, and fibrinogen are the primary plasma proteins. Globulin and albumin are important in the immune responses of the body. Fibrinogen is important in the process of blood clotting. If blood is removed from the body and allowed to stand for a few moments, the soluble fibrinogen molecules polymerize to form an insoluble matrix of fibrin. This causes the blood to congeal, or *coagulate*. Coagulation can be prevented by adding an anticoagulant to the blood; the most common anticoagulants are heparin and citrate. An anticoagulant must be added in preparation for separating blood into its cellular and plasma fractions by centrifugation.

Many important substances, in addition to plasma proteins, are dissolved in plasma. Plasma contains several ions *(electrolytes)* in solution. The dominant cation is sodium (Na^+). The predominant anions are chloride (Cl^-) and bicarbonate (HCO_3^-). Other ions are present in lesser amounts, as indicated in Table 18-3. The concentration of each plasma electrolyte must be kept within narrow limits for body function to be normal, and numerous control systems accomplish this regulation. In general, the plasma electrolytes can diffuse readily across capillary walls; therefore, interstitial fluid and plasma typically have similar electrolyte concentrations.

Plasma contains small amounts of gases (O_2, CO_2, and N_2) in solution. In the lungs, O_2 enters the blood as dissolved O_2, but most of this O_2 quickly combines with hemoglobin (in the red

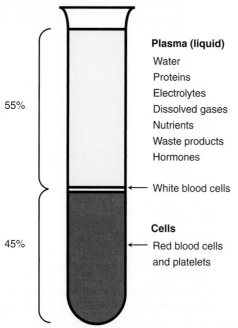

Plasma (liquid)
Water
Proteins
Electrolytes
Dissolved gases
Nutrients
Waste products
Hormones

55%

← White blood cells

Cells

45%

← Red blood cells and platelets

FIGURE 18-5 Anticoagulated blood can be separated into an extracellular fluid component (plasma) and a cellular component (cells) by centrifugation. Plasma is a solution of many important substances in water. The presence of proteins gives plasma its typical pale-yellow color. The cells are heavier than the plasma, and they settle to the bottom. Most of the cells are red blood cells. The white blood cells are slightly lighter in weight than the red blood cells, and they form a thin buffy coat on the top of the red cell layer. Most of the platelets end up in the buffy coat, although at slow centrifuge speeds ("soft spin"), platelets tend to remain suspended in the plasma. The fraction of cells in blood is called the hematocrit. In this example the hematocrit is 45%.

TABLE 18-3 Some Constituents of Canine Plasma (in Addition to Water, the Main Constituent)

Component	Normal Range	Units
Plasma Proteins (Carried in Colloidal Suspension)		
Globulin (total)	2.7-4.4	g/dL
Albumin	2.3-3.1	g/dL
Fibrinogen	0.15-0.30	g/dL
Electrolytes (Dissolved)		
Na^+	140-150	mmol/L
K^+	3.9-5.1	mmol/L
Ca^{2+} (ionized)	1.2-1.5	mmol/L
Mg^{2+} (ionized)	0.5-0.9	mmol/L
Cl^-	110-124	mmol/L
HCO_3^-	17-24	mmol/L
HPO_4^{2-} and $H_2PO_4^-$	1-1.4	mmol/L
H^+	38-49	nmol/L*
(H^+ expressed as pH)[†]	(7.31-7.42)	
Dissolved Gases (Values for Arterial Plasma)		
O_2	0.26-0.30	mL/dL
CO_2	2-2.5	mL/dL
Examples of Nutrients, Waste Products, Hormones		
Cholesterol	140-280	mg/dL
Glucose	76-120	mg/dL
Triglycerides	40-170	mg/dL
Urea nitrogen	8-28	mg/dL
Creatinine	0.5-1.7	mg/dL
Bile acids (fasting)	0-8	μmol/L
Thyroxine (T_4)	1.5-4	nmol/L*

Modified from Latimer KS, Mahaffey EA, Prasse KW: *Duncan & Prasse's veterinary laboratory medicine: clinical pathology,* ed 4, Ames, Iowa, 2003, Wiley-Blackwell.
*Note that [H^+] and [Thyroxine] are in nanomolar units; 10^3 nmol = 1 μmol, and 10^3 μmol = 1 mmol.
[†]pH = −log [H^+], where [H^+] is expressed in molar units; pH is dimensionless.

blood cells). As a consequence, about 98.5% of the total O_2 in blood is carried as *oxyhemoglobin* and only about 1.5% as dissolved O_2. Likewise, only a small portion of the carbon dioxide (CO_2) in blood is carried in the dissolved form. Most of the CO_2 becomes hydrated to form HCO_3^- or combines with hemoglobin or plasma proteins to form *carbamino compounds.*

Nutrient substances dissolved in plasma include glucose, amino acids, lipids, and some vitamins. Dissolved metabolic waste products (in addition to CO_2) include urea, creatinine, uric acid, and bilirubin. Plasma also contains many hormones (e.g., insulin, epinephrine, thyroxine), which are present in exceedingly tiny, but critically important amounts. Table 18-3 lists some of the normal constituents of plasma.

The Cellular Component of Blood Includes Red Blood Cells, White Blood Cells, and Platelets

Cells normally constitute 30% to 60% of the blood volume (depending on the species). The fraction of cells in blood is called the *hematocrit* (see Figure 18-5). The hematocrit is determined by adding an anticoagulant to some blood and then centrifuging it in a tube. The cells are somewhat heavier than plasma and settle to the bottom of the tube during centrifugation. Because centrifugation results in a packing of the blood cells in the bottom of the tube, the hematocrit is sometimes called the *packed cell volume.* Most of the cell component looks red because most of the blood cells are *erythrocytes* (red blood cells, RBCs). Erythrocytes acquire their red color from hemoglobin.

The *leukocytes* (white blood cells, WBCs) are slightly lighter in weight than the RBCs; in a centrifuge tube the WBCs gather in a white *buffy coat* on top of the RBCs. The buffy coat is normally very thin because there are about 1000 times more RBCs than WBCs. Leukocytes are critical in immune and allergic responses of the body. The subtypes of leukocytes include neutrophils, lymphocytes, monocytes, eosinophils, and basophils. A laboratory analysis of the total number and relative distribution of the various WBC subtypes *(differential WBC count)* provides important clues in the diagnosis of disease. Both erythrocytes and leukocytes are made in the bone marrow. They develop, by mitosis and differentiation, from a common line of progenitor cells, the *pluripotent* (uncommitted) *stem cells.*

The cellular component in a centrifuge tube also contains *platelets,* or *thrombocytes,* which are cellular fragments from their precursor cells, the *megakaryocytes.* The megakaryocytes reside in the bone marrow, and they shed bits of their cytoplasm, bounded by cell membrane, into the bloodstream. Platelets participate in *hemostasis* (the control of blood loss from injured or severed blood vessels). In this process a clumping together of platelets (*platelet aggregation*) begins to create a physical barrier across openings in blood vessels. The platelets also release the substance *serotonin*, which causes the blood vessels to constrict, thereby reducing blood pressure and blood flow at the site of injury. Additional substances released from the platelets, along with fibrinogen and several clotting factors in the plasma, lead to the coagulation of blood and the formation of a stable, fibrin-based blood clot.

Coagulation and clotting involve complex, interconnected sequences of chemical reactions (*the coagulation cascade*). A key step in the coagulation cascade is the formation in the plasma of *thrombin,* an enzyme that catalyzes the transformation of fibrinogen to fibrin. Several laboratory tests are used to assess the status of an animal's coagulation system. Two common tests involve determination of the *prothrombin time* (PT) and the *partial thromboplastin time* (PTT).

If blood is allowed to coagulate and then is centrifuged, the fibrin and other plasma clotting factors settle to the bottom along with the RBCs, WBCs, and platelets. The liquid portion remaining above (essentially plasma without fibrinogen and other clotting factors) is called *serum.* Most of the common clinical blood chemistry analyses are performed on serum. Examples include the determination of concentrations of electrolytes and cholesterol.

If blood is treated with an anticoagulant and then allowed simply to sit in a tube (without centrifugation), the erythrocytes slowly begin to settle. For reasons that are not completely understood, the rate of their settling tends to be increased to above normal in certain disease states and decreased to below normal in others. Therefore the *erythrocyte sedimentation rate* (ESR) is a clinically useful diagnostic measurement. An important caveat is that the normal ESR varies substantially between species; for example, it is much more rapid in equine blood than in canine blood.

Blood cell counts are performed by manual or automated scanning of a very small volume (e.g., 1 μL) of anticoagulated whole blood. Table 18-4 presents a summary of normal hematologic values for the dog.

TABLE 18-4 Canine Hematology

Test	Normal Range	Units
Hematocrit	35-57	%
Blood Cell Counts		
Red blood cells	5000-7900	$\times 10^3/\mu L$
White blood cells	5-14	$\times 10^3/\mu L$
Platelets	210-620	$\times 10^3/\mu L$
Hemoglobin Measures		
Blood hemoglobin	12-19	g/dL
MCH (mean corpuscular hemoglobin)	21-26	pg
MCHC (mean corpuscular hemoglobin concentration)	32-36	g/dL

Modified from Latimer KS, Mahaffey EA, Prasse KW: *Duncan & Prasse's veterinary laboratory medicine: clinical pathology,* ed 4, Ames, 2003, Wiley-Blackwell.

Most of the Oxygen in Blood Is Carried in Chemical Combination with the Protein Hemoglobin Within Red Blood Cells

Of the 20 mL of O_2 normally carried in each 100 mL of oxygenated blood, only 1.5% (0.3 mL) is carried in dissolved form. The remaining 98.5% is carried in chemical combination with hemoglobin (in RBCs). *Oxygenated hemoglobin* (oxyhemoglobin, HbO_2) is bright red. When O_2 is released, HbO_2 becomes *reduced hemoglobin* (Hb), which is dark bluish red. The adequacy of oxygenation of an animal's blood can be judged somewhat by looking at the color of its nonpigmented epithelial membranes (e.g., gums, nostrils, or inside surfaces of eyelids). Well-oxygenated tissues appear pink. Poorly oxygenated tissues appear bluish (*cyanotic*) because of the prevalence of reduced Hb.

The ability of blood to carry oxygen is determined by the amount of hemoglobin in the blood and by the chemical characteristics of that Hb. For example, each deciliter (dL) of normal dog blood contains about 15 g of Hb. Each gram of Hb can combine with 1.34 mL of O_2, when fully saturated. Thus, each deciliter of fully oxygenated, normal blood carries 20 mL of O_2. Several disease states (*hemoglobinopathies*) result in the synthesis of chemically abnormal Hb, with a diminished capacity to bind O_2. Also, several common toxins, including carbon monoxide (CO) and nitrates, cause life-threatening alterations in the ability of Hb to bind O_2.

Because hemoglobin is localized inside RBCs, it is possible to derive several clinically useful relationships among the blood Hb content, RBC count, Hb content of each RBC, and hematocrit. For example, if a normal dog has 15 g of Hb in each deciliter of blood and an RBC count of 6 million cells per microliter (μL) blood, it follows that each RBC (on average) contains 25 picograms (pg) of Hb:

$$\frac{15 \text{ g of hemoglobin/dL of blood}}{6 \times 10^6 \text{ red blood cells/}\mu L \text{ of blood}} = 25 \times 10^{-12} \text{ g of Hb/RBC}$$

The value calculated in this way is called the *mean corpuscular hemoglobin* (MCH).

An easier calculation, which serves the same purpose, is to determine how much hemoglobin is contained in each deciliter of packed RBCs. For example, if a dog has 15 g Hb/dL of blood and has a hematocrit of 50%, the Hb concentration in the RBC portion of the blood must be 30 g of Hb/dL of packed RBCs:

$$\frac{15 \text{ g of hemoglobin/dL of blood}}{0.5 \text{ dL of red blood cells/dL of blood}} = 30 \text{ g of Hb/dL of RBCs}$$

The value calculated in this way is called the *mean corpuscular hemoglobin concentration* (MCHC). For simplicity, the calculation is often summarized as follows:

$$MCHC = [\text{hemoglobin}]/\text{hematocrit}$$

The brackets around "hemoglobin" denote concentration.

An abnormally low value of MCH or MCHC is clinically important because it points to a deficit in hemoglobin synthesis (i.e., not enough Hb being made to load up each RBC). In contrast, an abnormally low value for Hb by itself is less informative; hemoglobin concentration in the blood could fall below normal for several reasons, including a deficit in Hb synthesis, a deficit in RBC synthesis, or a "watering down" of the blood either by addition of excess plasma fluid or by loss of RBCs.

Deviations from a normal hematocrit (Hct) can have important consequences in terms of the ability of blood to carry oxygen. Hematocrit also affects the viscosity of blood, as shown in Figure 18-6. *Viscosity* is a measure of resistance to flow. For example, honey is more viscous (more resistant to flow) than water. Plasma, by itself, is about 1.5 times more viscous than water because of the presence of plasma protein molecules (albumin, globulin, fibrinogen). The presence of cells in blood has an even greater effect on viscosity. Blood with an Hct of 40% has twice the viscosity of plasma. For Hct exceeding 50%, viscosity increases rapidly. An abnormally high hematocrit is called *polycythemia,* which literally means "many cells in the blood." The blood of a patient with polycythemia can carry more than the normal 20 mL of O_2/dL of blood (provided that the MCHC is normal), and this may be viewed as beneficial. However, the increased viscosity makes it difficult for the heart to pump the blood. Therefore, polycythemia creates a heavy workload for the heart and can lead to heart failure, particularly if the cardiac muscle is not healthy.

The opposite problem, in which the hematocrit is too low, is called *anemia.* Anemia literally means "no blood," but the word is used to refer to any condition in which there are abnormally few RBCs in each dL or a condition in which there is an abnormally low hemoglobin concentration in each RBC (i.e., MCH and/or MCHC is low). Each deciliter of blood of an anemic patient carries less than the normal 20 mL of O_2. Therefore, cardiac output must be increased above normal to deliver the normal amount of O_2 to the tissues each minute. The necessity to increase cardiac output also imposes an increased workload on the heart and can lead to the failure of a diseased heart. Thus, Hct within the normal range provides the blood with enough Hb to carry an adequate amount of O_2 without putting an undue workload on the heart. For additional information about the transport of O_2 and CO_2 in blood, see Chapter 48.

Figure 18-7 provides an idea of the relative sizes and shapes of the major constituents of blood. The plasma proteins are much, much larger than the ions and nutrient molecules that are dissolved in plasma. RBCs and WBCs are many, many times larger than the plasma proteins. In fact, as mentioned earlier, blood cells are so large that they can barely squeeze through a typical capillary.

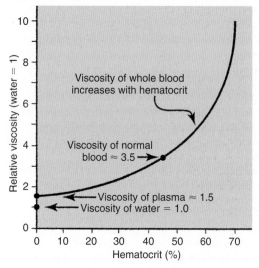

FIGURE 18-6 Plasma is more viscous than water because of the presence of plasma proteins. Blood is more viscous than plasma because of the presence of blood cells. Blood viscosity increases sharply when the fraction of cells (hematocrit) increases above 50%.

CLINICAL CORRELATIONS

LETHARGIC KID GOAT

History. A 6-month-old female kid goat is presented for lethargy and difficulty breathing. Two months ago, in April, the owners bought this goat and another at a sale as pets for their children. The goats have been provided with a small amount of goat feed daily, along with access to a pasture. The owners noticed that both goats were initially very playful, but both have seemed progressively lethargic during the last month. Also, they seem to have more difficulty breathing, even at rest. No vaccinations, deworming, or other treatments have been given.

Clinical Examination. The goat is somewhat thin and is reluctant to stand. There is a swelling (likely edema fluid) under the jaw. The goat's temperature is slightly elevated. The pulse and respiratory rates are moderately increased. The mucous membranes

FIGURE 18-7 Relative size and shape of the major constituents of blood. The figure emphasizes two points: first, that the plasma protein molecules are huge compared with the other plasma solutes, such as glucose, Na^+, and Cl^-; and second, that the blood cells (red and white) are huge compared with plasma protein molecules. Numbers under constituents are their molecular weights (in daltons). The scale *(upper left)* indicates a length of 10 nm. In comparison, the diameter of the red blood cell is 7.5 μm, which is 750 times larger than the scale marker.

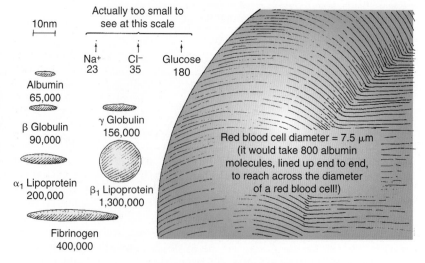

are very pale, which makes the capillary refill time difficult to assess. Respiratory sounds are increased (suggesting possible pulmonary edema). There are no other abnormal findings on physical examination.

Comment. The very pale mucous membranes suggest marked anemia. Indeed, centrifugation of a blood sample reveals that the goat's packed cell volume (Hct) is only 12%. Plasma protein concentration is also below normal, at 4.5 g/dL. Given the lack of deworming, you suspect parasitic infection associated with *Hemonchus contortus, Ostertagia,* or *Trichostrongylus.* A fecal analysis is positive for *Hemonchus* and *Ostertagia.*

Parasitism is a common problem in sheep and goats. The parasites mentioned damage the abomasum, which results in blood loss. The consequent anemia would explain the goat's lethargy, because anemia limits O_2 delivery to the organs, especially during exercise. The elevated respiratory rate and heart rate reflect the animal's attempts to compensate for low O_2 delivery to the tissues by increasing air flow into the lungs and blood flow through the circulation. Plasma protein is lost along with RBCs. This *hypoproteinemia* could account for the edema, because the proteins in plasma exert an important osmotic effect to oppose the tendency for plasma water to leak out of capillaries and into the tissue (interstitial) fluid (see Chapter 23).

Treatment. Ideally, a transfusion of whole blood would be given to help restore both RBCs and plasma proteins; the kid would then be dewormed. However, even if appropriate whole blood were available, transfusion in such an animal is risky. This goat's ability to deal with stress has been severely compromised, and even the physical restraint needed to administer a transfusion might trigger physical collapse or even death. On the other hand, without the transfusion, the animal has little chance of recovery if only treated for the parasites.

COLIC AND ENDOTOXIC SHOCK IN HORSE SECONDARY TO STRONGYLUS PARASITISM

History. A 1-year-old Standardbred filly is brought to your clinic by its new owner because the horse has been restless, rolling, kicking at its belly, and pawing the ground. The owner reports that the horse has had a poor appetite for several days and now refuses both hay and grain. The owner says he has dewormed the filly recently, but her previous deworming history is unknown.

Clinical Examination. The horse is underweight and has a dull hair coat. It is obvious that she is in pain. Physical examination reveals an abnormally high temperature (103.5° F), rapid labored breathing (40 breaths/min), and an elevated heart rate (80 beats/min). All limbs feel cool to the touch. The mucous membranes are abnormally dark, and the capillary refill time is prolonged (both these observations indicate sluggish circulation). Gastrointestinal auscultation of all four quadrants yields abnormal findings; no gastrointestinal *borborygmus* is heard on either the left or the right side, dorsally or ventrally. A rectal examination reveals several distended loops of bowel.

You perform *abdominocentesis* and withdraw some peritoneal fluid. Normally, peritoneal fluid is clear and straw colored; the fluid from this horse is darker yellow than normal and has a turbid appearance. Measurements with a refractometer indicate that the peritoneal fluid contains five times more protein than normal. Microscopic examination of the fluid reveals the presence of four

times the normal number of WBCs, specifically neutrophils, and the cells contain bacteria.

Outcome. You tell the owner that the filly appears to have a badly damaged bowel and that the prognosis is poor. You inform him that surgical treatment is possible, but expensive postoperative complications are likely because infection appears to have spread into the peritoneum. After considering the options, the owner decides against surgery. You institute supportive therapy with intravenous (IV) fluids, analgesics, and antibiotics. Depending on the extent of compromise to the bowel, horses can respond to medical management. However, based on the signs that this filly is showing, including that the filly already has signs of peritonitis, the prognosis is grave.

The horse's condition deteriorates over the next 12 hours. The heart rate increases progressively to 100 beats/min. The mucous membranes show evidence of declining blood flow (darker color and longer capillary refill time). The horse begins to wheeze and becomes lethargic. Bowel sounds continue to be absent. Despite the delivery of IV fluids, there is no output of urine. With the owner's consent, you euthanize the horse.

Necropsy examination indicates that this horse had thrombi (vascular obstructions) in several major branches of her mesenteric arteries, probably secondary to a severe infestation of bloodworms *(Strongylus vulgaris).* Several areas of the intestine were necrotic. Gram-negative bacteria were cultured from both the peritoneal fluid and the blood. The lungs were edematous, and excessive fluid was found in the airways and intrapleural space.

Comment. In horses, *S. vulgaris* lodges in mesenteric arteries and decreases the blood flow to the intestine. Deworming a severely infested horse can precipitate acute intestinal ischemia, because the dead/dying worms break away from the walls of major mesenteric arteries and drift into smaller arteries, which they occlude. Also, the dying worms release substances that trigger the formation of blood clots in the arteries. Digestive processes become disrupted and may cease entirely. Intestinal ischemia and gaseous distention of the bowel cause severe pain. With persistent ischemia, segments of the bowel become permanently damaged (infarcted). Ischemic damage to the intestinal epithelium allows intestinal bacteria and bacterial products (endotoxins) to enter the peritoneum and the blood. WBCs move from the bloodstream into the peritoneal fluid, where they combat the bacteria by engulfing them (phagocytosis). However, the infection overwhelms the immune system. Bacteria and endotoxins (from gram-negative bacteria) cause the body to produce substances that depress the heart and disrupt the capillary endothelium, especially in the lungs. The resultant combination of heart failure and pulmonary edema leads to respiratory failure and subsequent renal failure. The progression of dysfunction becomes irreversible.

PRACTICE QUESTIONS

1. According to Table 18-2, how long does it take for blood to travel the length of a canine capillary?
   a. 0.05 second
   b. 0.1 second
   c. 1 second
   d. 10 seconds
   e. 20 seconds

2. The amount of blood pumped by the left ventricle in 1 minute would equal:
   a. The amount of blood that flowed through the coronary circulation (in the same minute).
   b. One half of the cardiac output.
   c. Two times the cardiac output.
   d. The amount of blood that flowed through all organs of the systemic circulation, except for coronary blood flow.
   e. The amount of blood that flowed through the lungs.

3. A transfusion of normal plasma into a normal dog would:
   a. Decrease the hematocrit of the recipient's blood.
   b. Increase the viscosity of the recipient's blood.
   c. Decrease the mean corpuscular hemoglobin concentration (MCHC) in the recipient's plasma.
   d. Increase the number of cells in the recipient's blood.
   e. Decrease the concentration of proteins in the recipient's plasma.

4. Which of the following sequences of capillary beds might a red blood cell encounter in a normal circulation?
   a. Lungs, skin, lungs, brain
   b. Spleen, liver, mesentery, lungs
   c. Coronary, kidney (glomerular), kidney (tubular), lungs
   d. Lungs, coronary, stomach, liver
   e. Brain, lungs, liver, coronary

5. The walls of most capillaries have pores or clefts in them, which are approximately 4 nm in diameter (4×10^{-9} m). According to Figure 18-7:
   a. A capillary pore is many times larger in diameter than a sodium ion.
   b. An albumin molecule is approximately 2.5 times longer than the diameter of a capillary pore.
   c. The diameter of a red blood cell is many times greater than the diameter of a capillary pore.
   d. A molecule of β globulin or γ globulin could just about squeeze through a capillary pore if it were lined up exactly right.
   e. All of the above are correct.

6. Suppose that the following conditions exist in a particular blood vessel: blood pressure (BP) inside vessel at inlet = 60 mm Hg, BP inside vessel at midpoint = 45 mm Hg, BP inside vessel at outlet = 30 mm Hg, BP outside vessel at midpoint = 5 mm Hg. Under these conditions:
   a. Perfusion pressure for blood flow through this vessel = 30 mm Hg.
   b. Perfusion pressure for blood flow through this vessel = 15 mm Hg.
   c. Distending pressure at the vessel midpoint = 45 mm Hg.
   d. Distending pressure at the vessel midpoint = 40 mm Hg.
   e. Both a and d are correct.

7. Compared with the systemic circulation, the pulmonary circulation:
   a. Carries more blood flow per minute.
   b. Has a lower perfusion pressure.
   c. Has a higher resistance to blood flow.
   d. Carries blood that has a lower hematocrit.
   e. Contains a higher blood volume.

BIBLIOGRAPHY

Bowman DD: *Georgis' parasitology for veterinarians*, ed 9, Philadelphia, 2009, Saunders.

Ettinger SJ, Feldman EC: *Textbook of veterinary internal medicine: diseases of the dog and cat*, ed 7, St Louis, 2010, Elsevier/Saunders.

Hill RW, Wyse GA, Anderson M: *Animal physiology*, Sunderland, Mass, 2008, Sinauer.

Jain NC: *Essentials of veterinary hematology*, Philadelphia, 1993, Lea & Febiger.

Kaneko JJ, Harvey JW, Bruss ML: *Clinical biochemistry of domestic animals*, ed 6, Oxford, UK, 2008, Elsevier.

Kumar V, Abbas AK, Fausto N, Aster J: *Robbins and Cotran pathologic basis of disease*, ed 8, Philadelphia, 2010, Saunders.

Latimer KS: *Duncan & Prasse's veterinary laboratory medicine: clinical pathology*, ed 5, Ames, Iowa, 2011, Wiley-Blackwell.

Milnor WR: *Cardiovascular physiology*, New York, 1990, Oxford University Press.

Mohrman DE, Heller LJ: *Cardiovascular physiology*, ed 7, New York, 2010, McGraw-Hill.

Patteson MW: *Equine cardiology*, Oxford, UK, 1996, Blackwell Science.

Physick-Sheard PW: Parasitic arteritis. In Colahan PT, Merritt AM, Moore JN, et al: *Equine medicine and surgery*, ed 5, vol 1, St Louis, 1999, Mosby–Year Book.

Reagan WJ, Irizarry Rovira AR, DeNicola DB: *Veterinary hematology: atlas of common domestic and non-domestic species*, ed 2, Ames, Iowa, 2008, Wiley-Blackwell.

Reece WO: *Dukes' physiology of domestic animals*, ed 12, Ithaca, NY, 2004, Comstock Publishing.

Reed SM, Bayly WM, Sellon DC, editors: *Equine internal medicine*, ed 3, St Louis, 2009, Elsevier/Saunders.

Schmidt-Nielsen K: *Animal physiology: adaptation and environment*, Cambridge, UK, 1997, Cambridge University Press.

Thrall MA, Baker DC, Campbell TW, et al, editors: *Veterinary hematology and clinical chemistry: text and case presentations (set)*, Philadelphia, 2004, Lippincott, Williams & Wilkins.

Weiss DJ, Wardrop KJ: *Schalm's veterinary hematology*, ed 6, Ames, Iowa, 2010, Wiley-Blackwell.

CHAPTER 19
Electrical Activity of the Heart

KEY POINTS

1. Contraction of cardiac muscle cells is triggered by an electrical action potential.
2. The contractile machinery in cardiac muscle is similar to that in skeletal muscle.
3. Cardiac muscle forms a functional syncytium.
4. Cardiac contractions are initiated by action potentials that arise spontaneously in specialized pacemaker cells.
5. A system of specialized cardiac muscle cells initiates and organizes each heartbeat.
6. Cardiac action potentials are extremely long.
7. Membrane calcium channels play a special role in cardiac muscle.
8. The long duration of the cardiac action potential guarantees a period of relaxation (and refilling) between heartbeats.
9. Atrial cells have shorter action potentials than ventricular cells.
10. Specialized ion channels cause cardiac pacemaker cells to depolarize to threshold and form action potentials.
11. Sympathetic and parasympathetic nerves act on cardiac pacemaker cells to increase or decrease the heart rate.
12. Cells of the atrioventricular node act as auxiliary pacemakers and protect the ventricles from beating too fast.
13. Sympathetic nerves act on all cardiac muscle cells to cause quicker, more forceful contractions.
14. Parasympathetic effects are opposite to those of sympathetic activation but are generally restricted to the sinoatrial node, atrioventricular node, and atria.
15. Dysfunction in the specialized conducting system leads to abnormalities in cardiac rhythm (arrhythmias).
16. Atrioventricular node block is a common cause of cardiac arrhythmias.
17. Cardiac tachyarrhythmias result either from abnormal action potential formation (by the sinoatrial node or ectopic pacemakers) or from abnormal action potential conduction ("reentry").
18. Common antiarrhythmic drugs affect the ion channels responsible for the cardiac action potential.

Contraction of Cardiac Muscle Cells Is Triggered by an Electrical Action Potential

The heart is a muscular pump that propels blood through the blood vessels by alternately relaxing and contracting. As the heart muscle relaxes, the atria and ventricles fill with venous blood. During cardiac contraction, some of this blood is ejected into the arteries. Cardiac contraction takes place in two stages: (1) the right and left atria begin to contract, and (2) after a delay of 50 to 150 milliseconds (msec), the right and left ventricles begin to contract. Atrial contraction helps to finish filling the ventricles with blood. The delay allows time for this "topping up" of ventricular volume. Ventricular contraction ejects blood out of the left ventricle into the aorta and out of the right ventricle into the pulmonary artery. After the atria and ventricles contract, they relax and begin to refill. The entire contractile sequence is initiated and organized by an electrical signal, an *action potential,* which propagates from muscle cell to muscle cell, through the heart.

This chapter begins with a brief description of how cardiac muscle contracts, followed by a detailed description of the action potentials that initiate and organize the heart's contractions. Several common electrical dysfunctions of the heart are then discussed.

Throughout this chapter, comparisons are made between cardiac and skeletal muscle (Table 19-1). In both cardiac and skeletal muscle, an electrical action potential in each muscle cell is necessary to trigger a contraction. The molecular mechanisms that carry out the contraction are also similar in both types of muscle. However, important differences exist between cardiac and skeletal muscle in the characteristics of the action potentials that initiate contractions.

The Contractile Machinery in Cardiac Muscle Is Similar to That in Skeletal Muscle

Cardiac muscle, like skeletal muscle, has a *striated* appearance under the light microscope (Figure 19-1). These cross-striations have the same structural basis in cardiac muscle as in skeletal muscle (see Figure 6-2). Each striated cardiac muscle cell *(muscle fiber)* is made up of a few hundred myofibrils. Each *myofibril* has a repetitive pattern of light and dark bands. The various bands within a myofibril are given letter designations (A band, I band, Z disk). The alignment of these bands in adjacent myofibrils accounts for the striated appearance of the whole muscle fiber. Each repeating unit of myofibrillar bands is called a *sarcomere.* This name, which means "little muscle," is apt because a single sarcomere constitutes the contractile subunit of the cardiac muscle. By definition, a sarcomere extends from one Z disk to the next, a distance of approximately 0.1 mm, or 100 μm.

As in skeletal muscle, each cardiac muscle sarcomere is composed of an array of thick and thin filaments. The *thin filaments* are attached to the Z disks; they interdigitate with the thick filaments. The thin filaments are composed of *actin* molecules. The

TABLE 19-1 Sequence of Events in Contraction of Skeletal Muscle and Cardiac Muscle

Skeletal Muscle	Cardiac Muscle
Action potential is generated in somatic motor neuron	*Note:* Action potentials in autonomic motor neurons are not needed to initiate heartbeats
Acetylcholine is released	*Note:* Neurotransmitters are *not* needed to make the heart beat
Nicotinic cholinergic receptors on muscle cell membrane are activated	*Note:* Activation of receptors is *not* needed—a completely isolated or denervated heart still beats
Ligand-gated Na^+ channels in muscle membrane open	Pacemaker Na^+ channels spontaneously open (and K^+ channels close) in membranes of pacemaker cells
Muscle membrane depolarizes to threshold level for formation of action potential	Pacemaker cell membranes depolarize to threshold for formation of action potential
Action potential forms in muscle cell but does not enter other cells	Action potential forms in a pacemaker cell and then propagates from cell to cell throughout the whole heart
Note: Skeletal muscle cells *do not* have slow Ca^{2+} channels	During action potential, extracellular Ca^{2+} ("trigger" Ca^{2+}) enters cell through "slow" Ca^{2+} channels
Action potential causes Ca^{2+} release from sarcoplasmic reticulum; Ca^{2+} binds to troponin	Entry of extracellular trigger Ca^{2+} causes release of more Ca^{2+} from sarcoplasmic reticulum; Ca^{2+} binds to troponin
Actin's binding sites are made available for actin-myosin cross-bridge formation	Actin's binding sites are made available for actin-myosin cross-bridge formation
Cross-bridge cycling generates contractile force between actin and myosin filaments	Cross-bridge cycling generates contractile force between actin and myosin filaments
Muscle contracts (brief "twitch"); Ca^{2+} is taken up by sarcoplasmic reticulum	Heart contracts (complete "beat" or "systole"); Ca^{2+} is taken up by sarcoplasmic reticulum or pumped back out of cell into extracellular fluid
Muscle relaxes	Heart relaxes

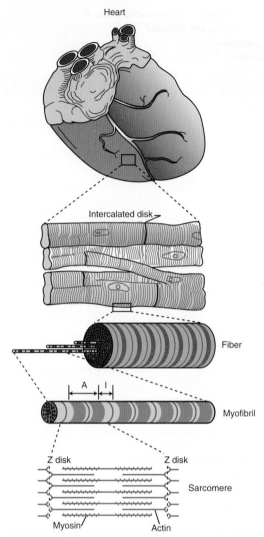

FIGURE 19-1 Under the light microscope, cardiac muscle fibers (muscle cells) are seen to be striated, similar to skeletal muscle. Electron microscopy reveals that the striations result from an orderly arrangement of actin (thin) filaments and myosin (thick) filaments into muscular subunits called sarcomeres (as shown in *bottom drawing*). Like skeletal muscle, a sarcomere is the structural and functional subunit of cardiac muscle. Unlike skeletal muscle fibers, however, cardiac muscle fibers often branch, and they link end to end with neighboring fibers at structures called intercalated disks. Unseen within the intercalated disks are nexi, or gap junctions, which are minute cytoplasmic channels that allow action potentials to propagate from cell to cell.

thick filaments are composed of *myosin* molecules. In the presence of adenosine triphosphate (ATP) and calcium ions (Ca^{2+}), myosin and actin interact in a series of steps called the *cross-bridge cycle*, which results in contraction and force generation in each sarcomere and therefore in the whole muscle cell (for details, see Figures 1-3, 1-4, 1-5, and 6-6).

Cardiac Muscle Forms a Functional Syncytium

Although the molecular basis of contraction is the same for cardiac and skeletal muscle, the two muscle types differ in regard to electrical linkages between neighboring cells, and this difference has important consequences. Individual skeletal muscle cells are electrically isolated (insulated) from one another, so action potentials cannot "jump" from one skeletal muscle cell to another. As described in Chapter 5, an action potential in a skeletal muscle cell is initiated only in response to an action potential in the somatic motor neuron that innervates the skeletal muscle cell. Each neural action potential causes release of the neurotransmitter acetylcholine, which activates nicotinic cholinergic receptors on the skeletal muscle cell, which in turn depolarizes the muscle cell to threshold for the formation of an action potential. When formed, the action potential propagates along the length of that particular muscle cell and then stops. The muscle action potential causes the cell to contract. Neighboring cells may or may not contract at the same time, depending on whether action potentials are initiated in the neighboring cells by their motor neurons.

In contrast, cardiac muscle cells are electrically linked to one another. When an action potential is started in a single cardiac muscle cell, it propagates along the length of that cell. At specialized points of contact with neighboring cells, ionic currents created by the action potential flow into the neighboring cells and initiate action potentials in those cells, too. Because cardiac action potentials propagate from cell to cell through cardiac tissue, neighboring cardiac muscle cells all contract in synchrony, as a unit, and then they all relax. In this regard, cardiac muscle tissue behaves as if it were a single cell. Cardiac muscle is therefore said to form a *functional syncytium* (literally, "acts like same cell").

The specialized cellular structures that allow cardiac action potentials to propagate from cell to cell are evident under the light microscope (see Figure 19-1). Cardiac muscle appears as an array of fibers (individual cardiac muscle cells) that are arranged approximately in parallel but with some branching. Adjacent cells are joined together by dark-appearing structures called *intercalated disks*. Electron microscopy has revealed that within these disks are tiny open channels between neighboring cells. These *nexi*, or *gap junctions*, provide points of contact between the intracellular fluid of adjacent cells. When an action potential depolarizes the cell on one side of an intercalated disk, positive ions flow through the gap junctions and into the neighboring cell. This local, ionic current depolarizes the neighboring cell to threshold for the formation of an action potential. In effect, an action potential propagates from cell to cell through the gap junctions that are located within the intercalated disks. Skeletal muscle does not have intercalated disks or nexi (gap junctions).

Cardiac Contractions Are Initiated by Action Potentials That Arise Spontaneously in Specialized Pacemaker Cells

Because cardiac muscle tissue forms a functional syncytium, and because a cardiac action potential leads to contraction, any one cardiac muscle cell can initiate a heartbeat. In other words, if a single cardiac muscle cell depolarizes to threshold and forms an action potential, that action potential will propagate from cell to cell, throughout the heart, and cause the whole heart to contract. Most cardiac muscle cells have the property of remaining stable at a resting membrane potential; they never form action potentials by themselves. However, a few specialized cardiac muscle cells have the property of depolarizing spontaneously toward the threshold for the formation of action potentials. When any one of these specialized cells reaches threshold and forms an action potential, a heartbeat results. Cardiac cells that depolarize spontaneously toward threshold are called *pacemaker cells* because they initiate heartbeats and therefore determine the rate, or pace, of the heart.

Although all spontaneously depolarizing cells in the heart are called pacemaker cells, only one pacemaker cell, the one that reaches threshold first, actually triggers a particular heartbeat. In the normal heart, the pacemaker cells that depolarize most quickly to threshold are located in the *sinoatrial* (SA) *node*. The SA node is in the right atrial wall, at the point where the *venae cavae* enter the right atrium.

Because it has spontaneously depolarizing pacemaker cells, the heart initiates its own muscle action potentials and contractions. Motor neurons are not necessary for initiating cardiac contractions, whereas they are needed for initiating skeletal muscle contractions. Motor neurons (sympathetic and parasympathetic)

do affect the heart rate, by influencing the rapidity with which the pacemaker cells depolarize to threshold, but the pacemaker cells initiate action potentials, and therefore heartbeats, even without any sympathetic or parasympathetic influences. Thus a denervated heart still beats, whereas a denervated skeletal muscle remains relaxed (in fact, paralyzed). The ability of the heart to beat without neural input enables surgically transplanted hearts to function. When a donor's heart is connected to a recipient's circulation during cardiac transplantation, no nerves are attached to the transplanted heart. The pacemaker cells in the transplanted heart initiate its action potentials and contractions. The only factor missing is control of the heart rate through cardiac sympathetic and parasympathetic nerves.

A System of Specialized Cardiac Muscle Cells Initiates and Organizes Each Heartbeat

Each normal heartbeat is initiated by an action potential that arises spontaneously in one of the pacemaker cells in the SA node (Figure 19-2). When formed, the action potential propagates rapidly, from cell to cell, across the right and left atria, causing both atria to contract. Next, the action potential propagates *slowly*, from cell to cell, through a special pathway of cardiac muscle cells that lies between the atria and the ventricles. This pathway consists of the *atrioventricular* (AV) *node* and the first part of the *AV bundle*, also called the *bundle of His*. The AV node and AV bundle provide the only route for the propagation of action potentials from the atria to the ventricles. Elsewhere, the atria and ventricles are separated by a layer of connective tissue, which can neither form nor propagate action potentials. In addition to providing the only conductive pathway between the atria and the ventricles, the AV node and the first part of the AV bundle have the special property of very slow conduction of action potentials. It takes 50 to 150 msec for an atrial action potential to travel through the AV node and the first part of the AV bundle; that is, it takes 50 to 150 msec for an atrial action potential to propagate into the ventricles. Slow conduction through the *AV junction* creates the delay between atrial and ventricular contractions.

When past the slowly conducting cells of the AV junction, the cardiac action potential enters a branching network of specialized cardiac cells that have the property of extremely rapid propagation of action potentials. The transition zone from slowly conducting to rapidly conducting cells is located within the AV bundle, which has slowly conducting cells in its first portion

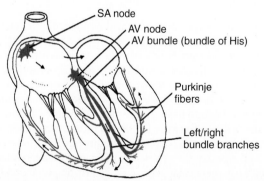

FIGURE 19-2 Specialized conduction system of the heart is responsible for the initiation and organization of cardiac contractions. The system is composed of specialized cardiac muscle fibers, not nerves. *AV,* Atrioventricular; *SA,* sinoatrial.

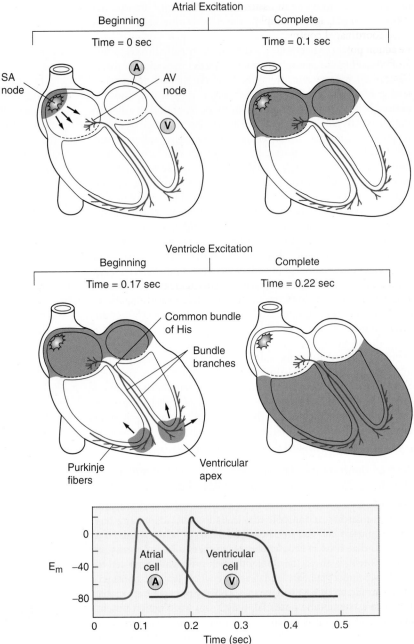

FIGURE 19-3 Heart is pictured at four instants during initiation of a normal contraction. *Shading* indicates areas of heart where an action potential is underway. *Top left* (time = 0 sec), Pacemaker cell in the sinoatrial *(SA)* node has just reached threshold, and an action potential has begun to propagate outward across the atria. *Top right* (time = 0.1 sec), Action potential has reached all parts of both atria (action potential underway in all atrial cells). *Middle left* (time = 0.17 sec), Action potential has passed through the atrioventricular *(AV)* node and down the bundle branches and has just reached the ventricular apex. *Middle right* (time = 0.22 sec), Action potential has just finished propagating outward through the walls of both ventricles (action potential is underway in all ventricular cells, but all atrial cells have finished their action potential). *Bottom,* Graph shows the timing of action potentials in a left atrial cell (at location labeled *A, top left*) and in a left ventricular cell (labeled *V, top left*). Their locations make these among the last atrial and ventricular cells to be depolarized as an action potential propagates across the atria and ventricles, respectively. *E$_m$,* Membrane potential in millivolts.

(connected to the AV node) and rapidly conducting cells beyond that. The rapidly conducting portion of the AV bundle splits to form the *left* and *right bundle branches.* At the ventricular apex, the bundle branches break up into a dispersed network of *Purkinje fibers,* which carry the action potential rapidly along the inner walls of both ventricles. The Purkinje fibers propagate action potentials into the normal ventricular muscle fibers within the inner walls *(subendocardial layers)* of both ventricles. From there, the action potentials propagate quite rapidly outward, from cell to cell, through the ventricular walls. As the action potential reaches each ventricular muscle fiber, that fiber contracts. The extremely rapid conduction of the cardiac action potential, from cell to cell, through the latter portion of the AV bundle, the bundle branches, and the Purkinje system results in a nearly synchronous contraction of all the fibers in both ventricles.

The SA and AV nodes, AV bundle, bundle branches, and Purkinje fibers are collectively called the *specialized conduction system of the heart.* This system is composed of specialized cardiac muscle cells, not nerves. The particular characteristics of the components in the specialized conduction system cause each heartbeat to follow a specific, patterned sequence. In a normal beat, both atria contract, almost simultaneously. Next, there is a brief pause (caused by slow propagation of the action potential through the AV node). The two ventricles then contract, almost simultaneously. Finally, the entire heart relaxes and refills.

Figure 19-3 reemphasizes the role of the specialized conduction system in initiating and organizing a normal cardiac contraction. In this "time lapse" illustration, atrial excitation begins at time t = 0, when one SA node cell has reached threshold and an action potential is just beginning to propagate out of the SA node and into regular atrial tissue. Within 0.1 second, the action potential has propagated completely across the right and left atria, and a coordinated contraction of both atria is just beginning. As the action potential propagates across the atria, it also depolarizes the first cells in the AV node, beginning at time t = 0.04 second. While the atria are in a depolarized (excited) state, the action potential is propagating slowly from cell to cell through the AV node and first part of the AV bundle. After traversing this slowly conducting region, the action potential propagates rapidly through the remainder of the bundle of His and its branches. The action potential arrives at the ventricular apex at time t = 0.17 second. Note that it takes about 0.13 second [(0.17 − 0.04) second] for the action potential to travel through the AV node and bundles; that is, 0.13 second represents a typical delay between atrial depolarization and ventricular depolarization. From the ventricular apex, the Purkinje fibers propagate the action potential rapidly throughout both ventricles. Ventricular excitation (depolarization) is complete by time t = 0.22 second, and both ventricles contract. By this time the atria have repolarized to a resting state and are relaxing. After ventricular excitation and contraction, the ventricles relax, and the whole heart remains in a resting state until the next beat is originated by an SA node pacemaker cell.

Cardiac Action Potentials Are Extremely Long

Two major differences between action potentials in skeletal muscle and cardiac muscle have already been mentioned: First, action potentials propagate from cell to cell in cardiac muscle, whereas skeletal muscle cells are electrically isolated from one another. Second, the heart has pacemaker cells, which form spontaneous action potentials, whereas a skeletal muscle cell only depolarizes and forms action potentials when "commanded" to do so by its motor neuron.

A third important difference between skeletal and cardiac action potentials is their duration (Figure 19-4). The entire action potential in a skeletal muscle lasts only 1 to 2 msec. A cardiac action potential lasts about 100 times longer (100-250 msec). Prolongation of the cardiac action potential is brought about by prolonged changes in the permeability of the cardiac muscle membrane to sodium, potassium, and calcium ions (Na^+, K^+, and Ca^{2+}). Cardiac muscle cell membranes have Na^+ and K^+ channels similar to those found in skeletal muscle, but the timing of their opening and closing is different in cardiac muscle. In addition, cardiac cell membranes also have special Ca^{2+} channels that are not present in skeletal muscle. The movement of extracellular Ca^{2+} through cardiac Ca^{2+} channels has an especially important role in prolonging the cardiac action potential. The presence of Ca^{2+} channels and the important role of extracellular Ca^{2+} in the action potential is the fourth major difference between cardiac and skeletal muscle.

In addition to learning about the special significance of the membrane Ca^{2+} channels in cardiac muscle, it is useful to review the roles of K^+ and Na^+ channels in skeletal muscle and to emphasize some ways in which cardiac K^+ and Na^+ channels are similar to those in skeletal muscle. As explained in Chapter 4, many of the K^+ channels in a neuron or skeletal muscle cell membrane are open when the cell is at rest, and most of the Na^+ channels are closed. As a result, the resting cell is much more permeable to K^+ than to Na^+. As a result, there is a greater tendency for positive K^+ to exit from the cell than for positive Na^+ to enter. This imbalance is the main factor responsible for a resting membrane potential (polarization) in which the inside of the cell membrane is

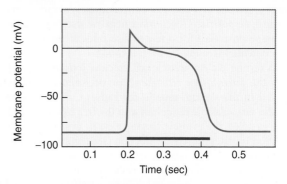

Cardiac muscle cell

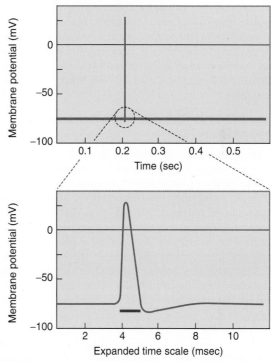

Nerve or skeletal muscle cell

FIGURE 19-4 Action potentials in cardiac muscle cells *(top)* last 100 times longer than action potentials in nerve or skeletal muscle cells *(middle)*. *Bottom,* The nerve or skeletal muscle action potential is shown on a greatly expanded time scale to illustrate that an action potential in a nerve or skeletal muscle cell has a different shape than a cardiac action potential, as well as a much shorter duration. The prolonged phase of depolarization in cardiac muscle cells is called the *plateau* of the action potential. The *dark bars* under each action potential indicate the length of the absolute refractory period.

negative in comparison with the outside. The resting membrane potential in skeletal muscle cells is typically between −70 and −80 mV (see Figure 19-4, *bottom*). An action potential is created when something *depolarizes* the cell (makes it less negative inside). Specifically, depolarization to the *threshold voltage* for opening the voltage-gated Na^+ channels allows an influx of extracellular Na^+ into the cell. This rapid entry of positive ions causes the cell membrane to become positively charged on its inside surface. This positive membrane potential persists for only a moment, however, because the Na^+ channels become *inactivated* very quickly. Na^+ entry ceases, and the cell rapidly repolarizes toward its resting membrane potential. Repolarization is also promoted by the opening of additional K⁺ channels. In fact, this opening of extra K⁺ channels may cause neurons and skeletal muscle cells to become *hyperpolarized* (even more negative than normal resting membrane potential) for a few milliseconds at the end of each action potential (see Figure 19-4, *bottom*).

In a resting skeletal muscle cell, calcium ions are sequestered within the *sarcoplasmic reticulum*. The occurrence of an action potential in the skeletal muscle cell causes Ca^{2+} to be released from the sarcoplasmic reticulum into the free intracellular fluid, which is called the *cytosol*. The increase in cytosolic Ca^{2+} concentration initiates muscle contraction (see Figure 1-5). The contraction initiated by a single action potential is very brief in skeletal muscle, because the cytosolic Ca^{2+} is rapidly pumped back into the sarcoplasmic reticulum by active transport, and the muscle relaxes. Note that the Ca^{2+} responsible for initiating skeletal muscle contraction comes entirely from the intracellular storage site, the sarcoplasmic reticulum. No extracellular Ca^{2+} enters the cell during the action potential, because skeletal muscle cells do not have membrane Ca^{2+} channels. In cardiac muscle, in contrast, membrane Ca^{2+} channels and the entry of extracellular Ca^{2+} into the cells play key roles in both action potentials and contractions.

Membrane Calcium Channels Play a Special Role in Cardiac Muscle

Figure 19-5 depicts a cardiac muscle cell action potential and the sequence of changes in K⁺, Na⁺, and Ca^{2+} permeability that are responsible for the action potential. As the time line begins (on the left side of each graph), the cardiac cell is at a normal, negative resting membrane potential of about –80 mV. The cardiac membrane potential is negative at rest for the same reason that skeletal muscle cells have negative resting membrane potentials: many K⁺ channels are open at rest, and most of the Na⁺ channels are closed. As a result, membrane permeability to K⁺ is much higher than membrane permeability to Na⁺ (see Figure 19-5, *middle two graphs*). In resting cardiac cells, the membrane Ca^{2+} channels are closed, so Ca^{2+} permeability is very low (see Figure 19-5, *bottom*); extracellular Ca^{2+} ions are prevented from entering the cardiac cells.

As in skeletal muscle, a cardiac action potential is created when the cell is depolarized to the threshold voltage for opening the voltage-gated Na⁺ channels. The rapid influx of extracellular Na⁺ into the cell causes the cell membrane to become positively charged on its inside surface (*Phase 0* in Figure 19-5, *top*). The Na⁺ channels inactivate very quickly, which causes the Na⁺ permeability to decrease quickly; the membrane begins to repolarize (*Phase 1*). However, in cardiac muscle, repolarization is interrupted, and there is a prolonged plateau of depolarization, which lasts about 200 msec (*Phase 2*). The plateau of the cardiac action potential is brought about by two conditions that do not occur in nerves or skeletal muscle fibers: (1) some K⁺ channels close, so K⁺ permeability decreases; and (2) many of the Ca^{2+} channels open, so Ca^{2+} permeability increases. Because the Ca^{2+} concentration is higher in the extracellular fluid than in the intracellular fluid, Ca^{2+} flows through the open Ca^{2+} channels and into the cytosol. The combination of reducing the exit of K⁺ from the cell and allowing the entrance of Ca^{2+} into the cell keeps the cell membrane in a depolarized state. After about 200 msec, the K⁺ channels reopen, and the Ca^{2+} channels close; K⁺ permeability increases, and Ca^{2+} permeability decreases. The combination of increasing the exit of K⁺ from the cell and shutting off the entrance of Ca^{2+} into the cell causes the cell to repolarize (*Phase 3*) and

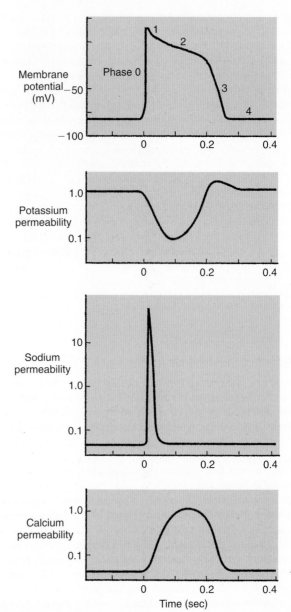

FIGURE 19-5 Membrane potential of a cardiac muscle cell *(top)* is determined by the relative permeabilities of the cell membrane to K⁺ *(second from top)*, Na⁺ *(second from bottom)*, and Ca^{2+} *(bottom)*. At rest *(left side of graphs)*, the cell is much more permeable to K⁺ than to Na⁺ or Ca^{2+}. (That is, the number of open K⁺ channels greatly exceeds the number of open Na⁺ or Ca^{2+} channels.) A cardiac action potential *(middle of graphs)* is produced by a characteristic sequence of permeability changes to K⁺, Na⁺, and Ca^{2+} (i.e., changes in the number of open K⁺, Na⁺, and Ca^{2+} channels). The action potential ends when the permeabilities return to their resting state *(right side of graphs)*. Phases 0 to 4 are discussed in the text.

eventually to return to its stable, negative resting membrane potential (*Phase 4*).

The specialized Ca^{2+} channels in cardiac muscle cell membranes are called *slow Ca^{2+} channels* (or *L-type Ca^{2+} channels*) because they take much longer to open than the Na⁺ channels, and they stay open much longer. As shown in Figure 19-5, Na⁺ permeability increases and then decreases (Na⁺ channels open and then inactivate) within a few milliseconds. Ca^{2+} permeability, in comparison, is slow to increase (Ca^{2+} channels are slow to

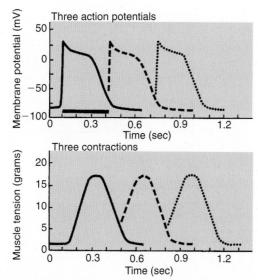

FIGURE 19-6 The first of three cardiac action potentials *(solid line, top)* causes a cardiac contraction *(solid line, bottom)*. Note that the action potential and contraction have similar durations. The *heavy horizontal bar* under the first action potential shows the duration of the absolute refractory period. The *dashed line* and *dotted line* in the top graph show the earliest possible occurrence of a second and a third action potential, each occurring right after the absolute refractory period for the preceding action potential. The *dashed line* and *dotted line* in the bottom graph depict the corresponding cardiac contractions. Because of the long refractory period, each contraction is almost over before the earliest possible next contraction can begin. This guarantees a period of cardiac relaxation between contractions.

open) and Ca^{2+} permeability remains elevated for about 200 msec (the time Ca^{2+} channels stay open). In recognition of their much quicker responses, the Na^+ channels in cardiac muscle are sometimes called *fast Na^+ channels.*

The Ca^{2+} that enters a cardiac cell during an action potential triggers the release of additional Ca^{2+} from the sarcoplasmic reticulum. This process is called *calcium-triggered calcium release* (or *calcium-induced calcium release*). In less than 0.1 second, the contraction of free Ca^{2+} in the cytosol increases about 100-fold. As in skeletal muscle, this increase in cytosolic Ca^{2+} initiates concentration. When the Ca^{2+} channels close, at the conclusion of the action potential, most of the free, cytosolic Ca^{2+} is pumped back into the sarcoplasmic reticulum or pumped back across the cell membrane into the extracellular fluid. Both these processes involve active transport, because the Ca^{2+} is being pumped against its electrochemical gradient. Once the cytosolic Ca^{2+} concentration is returned to its low, resting level, the cardiac muscle relaxes. Figure 19-6 shows the relationship between action potentials and the resulting contractions in a cardiac muscle cell.

The Long Duration of the Cardiac Action Potential Guarantees a Period of Relaxation (and Refilling) Between Heartbeats

Na^+ channels become inactivated at the peak of the cardiac action potential. Na^+ cannot pass through an inactivated channel; therefore, as long as the Na^+ channels remain inactivated, another action potential cannot occur. The inactivated state ends, and Na^+ channels become susceptible to reopening only when the cell membrane potential returns to (or nearly to) its resting level. Thus, Na^+ inactivation guarantees that the upstroke of a second

action potential cannot occur until the first action potential is completed (or very nearly).

While the Na^+ channels are inactivated, the cell is *refractory* (resistant) with regard to the formation of an action potential. The time after the beginning of one action potential during which another action potential cannot be initiated is called the *absolute refractory period*. Because Na^+ inactivation lasts until the membrane potential returns to (or nearly to) its resting level, the refractory period lasts about as long as an action potential. Thus the refractory period in a cardiac muscle cell lasts 100 to 250 msec, whereas the refractory period in a nerve or skeletal muscle cell lasts only about 1 or 2 msec (see Figure 19-4).

The long refractory period in cardiac muscle guarantees a period of relaxation (and cardiac refilling) between cardiac contractions. Figure 19-6 *(top)* depicts the quickest possible succession of three action potentials in a cardiac muscle cell: the second action potential begins immediately after the conclusion of the refractory period for the first action potential. Likewise, the third action potential begins immediately after the conclusion of the refractory period for the second. The *bottom graph* in Figure 19-6 shows the pattern of muscle contraction that results from the three action potentials. Note that contractile strength reaches a peak late in the plateau phase of each action potential, and that the contractile strength decreases (the muscle begins to relax) during the repolarization phase of each action potential. As a result, the cardiac muscle cell becomes partially relaxed before the earliest possible subsequent contraction can begin; that is, each cardiac action potential produces a contraction that is distinctly separated from the preceding contraction. Because of its long refractory period, cardiac muscle cannot sustain a continuous contraction. Thus the heart has a guaranteed period of relaxation (and refilling) between heartbeats.

The pattern of changes in muscle tension depicted in the bottom of Figure 19-6 corresponds closely to the changes in the cytosolic Ca^{2+} concentration. This makes sense, considering that the increase in cytosolic Ca^{2+} concentration initiates muscle contraction, and the subsequent removal of Ca^{2+} from the cytosol permits the muscle to relax. Cytosolic Ca^{2+} concentration increases during the plateau of the action potential (because of Ca^{2+}-triggered Ca^{2+} release) and decreases back to its resting level during the repolarization phase of the action potential (as active transport pumps move Ca^{2+} back into the sarcoplasmic reticulum or out into the extracellular fluid).

In skeletal muscle cells, an action potential lasts only 1 to 2 msec. The membrane is repolarized (and the refractory period is over) even before the release of Ca^{2+} from the sarcoplasmic reticulum is finished, and many milliseconds before the released Ca^{2+} is pumped back into the sarcoplasmic reticulum. As a result, the cytosolic Ca^{2+} concentration reaches its peak level after the action potential is over, and the contractile tension resulting from the action potential also reaches its peak after the action potential is over. Because a contractile twitch lasts much longer than the refractory period in skeletal muscle, several action potentials can occur during the time of a single contractile twitch. Multiple action potentials in quick succession cause cytosolic Ca^{2+} concentration to build to a high level and stay there. The resulting contractile tension is stronger than the tension that results from a single action potential, and it is sustained for a longer time. In effect, the muscle twitches caused by successive action potentials "fuse" together. This phenomenon is called *temporal summation*. Fusion and temporal summation are the mechanisms that permit graded and prolonged tension development in skeletal muscle. In contrast, the long refractory period in cardiac muscle cells prevents the fusion and summation of cardiac contractions. Each contraction of the heart (each heartbeat) is followed immediately by a relaxation.

Atrial Cells Have Shorter Action Potentials Than Ventricular Cells

The previous description of cardiac ion channels, action potentials, and contractions is based on properties of normal ventricular cells. Atrial cells are basically similar, except that their action potentials are shorter than action potentials in ventricular cells. Like ventricular cells, atrial cells have fast Na^+ channels that open briefly at the beginning of an action potential and then become inactivated. Likewise, atrial slow Ca^{2+} channels open during the action potential, and K^+ channels close. The differences between atrial and ventricular cells are that atrial slow Ca^{2+} channels typically stay open a shorter time than those in ventricular cells, and atrial K^+ channels stay closed for a shorter time. As a result, the plateau of an atrial cell's action potential is shorter and not as "flat" as the plateau of a ventricular cell's action potential (see Figure 19-3, *bottom*). As a consequence of having a shorter action potential, atrial cells have a shorter refractory period than ventricular cells. Therefore the atrial cells are capable of forming more action potentials per minute than ventricular cells; that is, the atria can "beat" faster than the ventricles. The implications of this difference are discussed later in this chapter.

Specialized Ion Channels Cause Cardiac Pacemaker Cells to Depolarize to Threshold and Form Action Potentials

As mentioned, the cardiac pacemaker cells of the SA node spontaneously depolarize to threshold and then form action potentials. The spontaneous depolarization is called a *pacemaker potential,* and it is the key distinguishing feature of a pacemaker cell (Figure 19-7, *top*). The action potentials of cardiac pacemaker cells typically have a rounded appearance; they lack the very rapid (phase 0) depolarization seen in ventricular and atrial cells.

The spontaneous depolarizations and rounded action potentials of pacemaker cells are consequences of the particular ion channels found in these cells. Pacemaker cells lack the usual voltage-gated fast Na^+ channels. Instead, these cells have *pacemaker Na^+ channels* (also called *funny Na^+ channels*), which close during an action potential and then begin to open again, spontaneously, once an action potential has finished. The spontaneous opening of the pacemaker Na^+ channels causes a progressive increase in the cell's Na^+ permeability (see Figure 19-7, *second from bottom*). The increase in Na^+ permeability allows Na^+ to enter the cell from the extracellular fluid, which depolarizes the cell toward threshold. Pacemaker cells also have an unusual set of K^+ channels, which participate in their spontaneous depolarization. At the end of one action potential, K^+ permeability in pacemaker cells is quite high, because most K^+ channels are open. Then some K^+ channels begin to close (see Figure 19-7, *second from top*). As K^+ permeability decreases, less K^+ leaves the cells, which makes the cells progressively less negatively charged inside. Ca^{2+} channels also make a small contribution to the pacemaker potential. Late in the pacemaker potential, just before a pacemaker cell reaches threshold, slow Ca^{2+} channels begin to open, and Ca^{2+} permeability begins to increase (see Figure 19-7, *bottom*). The resulting entry of Ca^{2+} into the cell speeds its final approach to threshold. Thus the pacemaker potential is caused by the opening of pacemaker Na^+ channels, the closing of K^+ channels, and (late in the process) the opening of Ca^{2+} channels. These

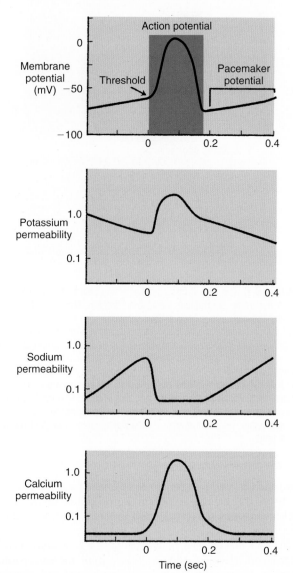

FIGURE 19-7 A cardiac pacemaker cell depolarizes spontaneously to threshold and initiates its own action potential *(top)*. The spontaneous depolarization (called the *pacemaker potential*) is the result of a spontaneous, progressive decrease in K^+ permeability *(second from top)* and an increase in Na^+ permeability *(second from bottom)*. An increase in Ca^{2+} permeability makes a late contribution to the depolarization toward threshold *(bottom)*. When threshold level is reached, an action potential is produced. The action potential is driven primarily by a large, prolonged increase in Ca^{2+} permeability. The absence of fast Na^+ channels in pacemaker cells causes the upstroke of the pacemaker action potential to be much slower than that seen in non-pacemaker cells. (Compare with Figure 19-5.)

spontaneous changes in Na^+, K^+, and Ca^{2+} channels in pacemaker cells are in contrast to the stable status of the ion channels in normal, resting atrial or ventricular cells.

When threshold is reached in a pacemaker cell, an action potential occurs. The upstroke of the action potential is quite slow compared with the rapid (phase 0) depolarization in a normal atrial or ventricular cell, because there are no fast Na^+ channels in pacemaker cells and therefore no sudden influx of Na^+. The ion primarily responsible for the action potential in a pacemaker cell is Ca^{2+}. When threshold is reached, many of the cell's slow Ca^{2+}

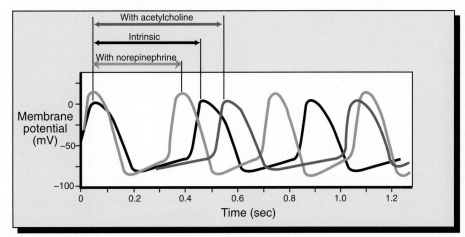

FIGURE 19-8 In the absence of neurohumoral influences, a pacemaker cell of the SA node spontaneously depolarizes to threshold and initiates a series of action potentials, three of which are shown by the *black line*. The interval between action potentials under these conditions determines the intrinsic, or spontaneous, heart rate (in this case, 0.43 sec between action potentials corresponds to a heart rate of 140 beats/min). Acetylcholine decreases the rate of depolarization and therefore lengthens the interval between action potentials (i.e., decreases heart rate). Norepinephrine increases the rate of depolarization and therefore shortens the interval between action potentials (i.e., increases heart rate).

channels open. The permeability to Ca^{2+} increases, and extracellular Ca^{2+} flows into the cell. The action potentials in pacemaker cells are often called slow action potentials, because they lack a rapid, phase 0 depolarization and because they are caused primarily by the opening of slow Ca^{2+} channels. In contrast, normal atrial or ventricular action potentials are called fast action potentials. Note, however, that all cardiac action potentials (whether "slow" or "fast") have a very long duration compared with action potentials in nerve or skeletal muscle cells.

Sympathetic and Parasympathetic Nerves Act on Cardiac Pacemaker Cells to Increase or Decrease the Heart Rate

Figure 19-8 shows how the neurotransmitters *norepinephrine* and *acetylcholine* affect the pacemaker cells of the heart. Norepinephrine exerts its effect by activating *β-adrenergic receptors* on the cell membranes of pacemaker cells. Activation of such receptors speeds up the ion channel changes that are responsible for the spontaneous depolarization of pacemaker cells. Because the pacemaker cells reach threshold more quickly in the presence of norepinephrine, there is a shorter interval between heartbeats. Therefore, heart rate is elevated above its intrinsic or spontaneous level.

Acetylcholine has the opposite effect. Acetylcholine activates *muscarinic cholinergic receptors* on the cell membranes of pacemaker cells, which slows the ion channel changes that are responsible for the pacemaker cell's spontaneous depolarization. Because the pacemaker cells take longer to reach threshold in the presence of acetylcholine, there is a longer interval between heartbeats. Therefore, heart rate is decreased below its intrinsic or spontaneous level.

Sympathetic neurons release norepinephrine at the SA node cells, and thus sympathetic nerve activity increases the heart rate. Epinephrine or norepinephrine, released from the adrenal glands and circulating in the bloodstream, has the same effect. Parasympathetic neurons release acetylcholine at the SA node cells, and thus parasympathetic activity decreases the heart rate. Figure 19-9 illustrates how sympathetic and parasympathetic neurons interact in the control of the heart rate. In the absence of

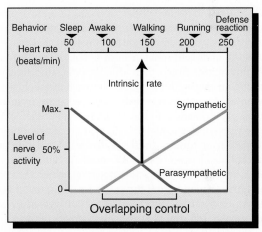

FIGURE 19-9 The upper scale shows that the heart rate of a normal, large dog ranges from 50 to 250 beats/min, depending on behavioral state. The graph illustrates that this wide range of heart rates is brought about by the interactions between sympathetic nerve activity, which speeds the heart above its intrinsic rate, and parasympathetic nerve activity, which slows the heart below its intrinsic rate. Sympathetic and parasympathetic nerves are simultaneously active over a considerable portion of the heart rate range (*overlapping control*). Note that the heart beats at its intrinsic rate (about 140 beats/min) either in the absence of any neural influence or when sympathetic and parasympathetic effects are equal and opposite.

norepinephrine and acetylcholine, the heart beats at its intrinsic rate. For a large dog, this rate is typically about 140 beats per minute (beats/min). Heart rates below the intrinsic rate are achieved by activation of parasympathetic neurons and release of acetylcholine. Accordingly, the graph in Figure 19-9 indicates that parasympathetic activity is high during awake rest (heart rate of 90 beats/min) and very high during sleep (heart rate of 55 beats/min). Heart rates above the intrinsic rate occur during exercise or emotional arousal and are achieved by activation of the sympathetic nerves to the heart and release of norepinephrine (or by circulating epinephrine or norepinephrine). The highest possible level of sympathetic activity, and therefore the highest possible heart rate, occurs during maximal exercise or a *defense alarm reaction ("fear, fight, or flight" response).*

Through variation in the levels of sympathetic and parasympathetic *tone*, the dog's heart rate is adjusted, over a wide range, as appropriate for each behavioral situation. When both systems are partially active, the resulting heart rate represents the outcome of a "tug-of-war" between sympathetic action to increase the heart rate and parasympathetic action to decrease the heart rate. Typically, the sympathetic and parasympathetic systems are both partially active during awake states, ranging from quiet rest (heart rate about 90 beats/min) to moderate exercise (heart rate about 175 beats/min). Parasympathetic activity predominates in the lower part of this range, and sympathetic activity predominates in the higher part. When sympathetic activity and parasympathetic activity are equal, their effects cancel, and the heart rate is at its intrinsic (spontaneous) level. Simultaneous activation of sympathetic and parasympathetic neurons appears to give the nervous system tight control over the heart rate under a wide variety of behavioral conditions.

Cells of the Atrioventricular Node Act as Auxiliary Pacemakers and Protect the Ventricles from Beating Too Fast

As with SA node cells, the cells of the AV node normally exhibit pacemaker activity and slow action potentials. As shown in Figure 19-10, the AV node cells spontaneously depolarize toward threshold, but much more slowly than SA node cells. Therefore, under normal circumstances, the SA node cells reach threshold first and initiate an action potential, which then propagates from cell to cell across the atria and into the AV node. Within the AV node, this action potential encounters cells that are slowly, spontaneously depolarizing toward threshold. The arriving action potential quickly depolarizes these AV node pacemaker cells to threshold, and they form an action potential, which then propagates into the AV bundle and the ventricles. Thus, under normal conditions, each cardiac action potential is triggered by an SA node pacemaker cell, and the pacemaker activity of the AV node cells is irrelevant.

Under certain abnormal conditions, AV node pacemaker function becomes critical for survival. For example, if the SA node is damaged and does not depolarize to threshold, the AV node pacemaker cells will initiate action potentials that propagate into the ventricles, causing them to contract. If not for this *auxiliary pacemaker function of AV node cells,* the heart with a damaged SA node would not beat at all. Because the AV node pacemaker cells depolarize more slowly than normal SA node cells, the heart rate resulting from AV node pacemakers is very low, about 30 to 40 beats/min in a resting dog, compared with 80 to 90 beats/min when the SA node cells are the pacemakers. Also, action potentials initiated by the AV node pacemakers usually do not propagate "backwards" into the atria; therefore atrial contractions are absent. Nevertheless, if the SA node fails as a pacemaker, ventricular contractions are initiated by the AV node frequently enough to sustain life temporarily. Thus, AV node cells are sometimes called the heart's *emergency pacemakers.*

Another important feature of the AV node cells is that they have longer refractory periods than normal atrial cells. The long refractory period of AV node cells helps protect the ventricles from being stimulated to contract at rates that are too rapid for efficient pumping. This *protective function of the AV node* is critical to an animal's survival when atrial action potentials

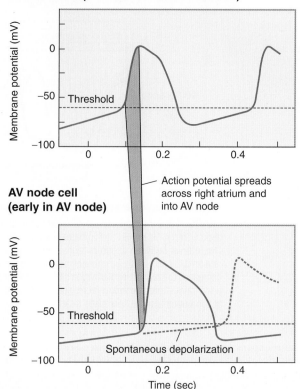

SA node cell (first one to reach threshold)

Action potential spreads across right atrium and into AV node

AV node cell (early in AV node)

Spontaneous depolarization

FIGURE 19-10 Both sinoatrial *(SA)* node cells and atrioventricular *(AV)* node cells exhibit pacemaker activity (spontaneous depolarization toward threshold). Normally the SA node cells depolarize more quickly and reach the threshold first *(top).* The resulting atrial action potential propagates into the AV node (as represented by *blue band*) and depolarizes the AV node cells quickly to their threshold, causing them to form an action potential *(solid line, bottom graph).* However, if the SA node pacemaker cells become nonfunctional or if atrial action potentials are not conducted into the AV node, the AV node cells eventually depolarize to threshold and initiate action potentials on their own *(dashed line, bottom graph).* In this way the AV node cells serve as an auxiliary (emergency) ventricular pacemaker.

are extremely frequent (see later discussion of atrial flutter/fibrillation). The long refractory period of the AV node cells plays an important role, even in a normal heart. When a normal action potential reaches the ventricles, it is prevented from "circling back" (and reactivating the atria) by the prolonged refractory state of the AV node cells.

Table 19-2 summarizes the four important electrical characteristics of the AV node previously discussed. Note that three of these characteristics are influenced by the nervous system. As indicated in the table, sympathetic activity increases the conduction velocity of the AV node cells, shortens their refractory period, and speeds their auxiliary pacemaker activity. Parasympathetic activation has the opposite effects. These sympathetic and parasympathetic effects are appropriate for different heart rates. For example, during exercise, when sympathetic activity is high and the SA node pacemakers are initiating heartbeats frequently, the speed of the whole process of cardiac contraction and relaxation must be increased. Thus it is appropriate that sympathetic action also increases the velocity of action potential conduction through the AV node, which shortens AV delay. In addition, sympathetic activation shortens the AV node refractory period, which allows each of the frequent atrial action potentials

TABLE 19-2 Electrical Characteristics of the Atrioventricular (AV) Node

Characteristic (Significance)	Sympathetic Effect*	Parasympathetic Effect[†]
Is the only conducting pathway between atria and ventricles (directs atrial action potentials into the rapidly conducting AV bundle and bundle branches)	—	—
Has a slow conduction velocity (creates AV delay)	Increases velocity (shortens AV delay)	Decreases velocity (lengthens AV delay)
Has a very long refractory period (protective effects: limits maximal rate to which atria can drive ventricles and prevents ventricular action potentials from re-exciting atria)	Shortens refractory period (appropriate for high heart rates)	Lengthens refractory period (appropriate for low heart rates)
Spontaneously depolarizes to threshold (acts as auxiliary pacemaker)	Faster depolarization (speeds auxiliary pacemaker)	Slower depolarization (slows auxiliary pacemaker)

*Through activation of β-adrenergic receptors on AV node cells.
[†]Through activation of muscarinic cholinergic receptors on AV node cells.

to be conducted to the ventricles. Finally, sympathetic activation enhances AV node auxiliary pacemaker activity, which provides the animal with a high enough ventricular rate to cope with some stress, even if the SA node pacemaker has failed. Conversely, when parasympathetic activation causes the SA node pacemakers to decrease the heart rate, all aspects of cardiac contraction and relaxation can proceed at a more leisurely pace. Under these conditions it is appropriate for AV node conduction velocity to be slowed and the AV node refractory period to be lengthened.

Sympathetic Nerves Act on All Cardiac Muscle Cells to Cause Quicker, More Forceful Contractions

Sympathetic neurons release norepinephrine in all regions of the heart, not only at the SA and AV nodes, and all cardiac muscle cells have β-adrenergic receptors that are activated by norepinephrine. Circulating epinephrine or norepinephrine (whether released from the adrenal medulla or administered as a drug) can also activate these same receptors. The effects of β-receptor activation on the SA and AV node cells have already been described (see Figure 19-8 and Table 19-2). In all other atrial and ventricular cells, β-receptor activation leads to taller, shorter action potentials and to stronger, quicker contractions. One reason for these effects is that activation of β receptors increases the number of L-type Ca^{2+} channels that open during the plateau (phase 2) of an action potential, which increases the amount of extracellular Ca^{2+} that enters the cell. Because Ca^{2+} entry is the primary depolarizing influence during the plateau, increased Ca^{2+} entry raises the plateau (makes the membrane potential more positive). A secondary consequence is to shorten the action potential. The action potential becomes shorter because of a complicated effect of the elevated plateau on the K^+ channels. Recall that K^+ channels close at the beginning of a cardiac action potential and then, after a time, reopen (see Figure 19-5). Reopening of the K^+ channels helps repolarize the cell to a resting state at the end of the action potential. The length of time before K^+ channels reopen depends on the membrane voltage during the plateau of the action potential. Specifically, when the membrane potential is more positive than normal during the plateau, the K^+ channels reopen sooner. This shortens the action potential and speeds repolarization. Overall, β-receptor activation makes each action potential taller and shorter. An action potential of higher amplitude propagates more quickly along each cell and from cell to cell, leading to faster conduction velocity. The shorter action potential

means a shorter refractory period, which permits more heartbeats per minute.

Because β-receptor activation opens more Ca^{2+} channels and increases the entry of extracellular Ca^{2+} into cardiac muscle cells during an action potential, it also increases the strength of the resulting contraction. The entry of more extracellular "trigger" Ca^{2+} creates a greater stimulus for the release of Ca^{2+} stores from the sarcoplasmic reticulum. Therefore the cytosolic Ca^{2+} concentration increases very rapidly and reaches an exceptionally high level during the action potential, which leads to a quicker, stronger contraction. In addition, the duration of the contraction is shortened, because β-receptor activation speeds up the pumps that move cytosolic Ca^{2+} back into the sarcoplasmic reticulum and out of the cell into the extracellular fluid. Thus, even though more Ca^{2+} than normal enters the cytosol during an action potential, its removal at the end of the action potential is faster than normal. Overall, β-receptor activation makes each cardiac contraction stronger, quicker, and shorter.

In summary, sympathetic nerves act (1) on the SA node pacemaker cells to increase the heart rate, (2) on the AV node cells to increase the conduction velocity and shorten the AV delay, and (3) on all cardiac cells to shorten the refractory period and make each cardiac contraction quicker, stronger, and shorter. All these changes cause the heart to pump more blood at a higher pressure, which is an animal's normal response during exercise or emotional arousal.

Because sympathetic effects on the heart are all brought about through activation of the β-adrenergic receptors on the cardiac muscle cells, the administration of a drug that activates β receptors (β-adrenergic agonist) has the same effects as sympathetic activation. Epinephrine, norepinephrine, and isoproterenol are common β-adrenergic agonists. Conversely, the administration of a drug that binds to and blocks β receptors reduces all the effects of sympathetic activation. Propranolol and atenolol are common β-adrenergic antagonists. Examples of their use are provided later.

Parasympathetic Effects Are Opposite to Those of Sympathetic Activation But Are Generally Restricted to the Sinoatrial Node, Atrioventricular Node, and Atria

Parasympathetic nerves affect the heart by the release of acetylcholine, which activates muscarinic cholinergic receptors on cardiac muscle cells. Qualitatively, all the effects of parasympathetic activation are opposite to those of sympathetic activation, because the effects of activating muscarinic cholinergic receptors are opposite to the effects of activating β-adrenergic receptors. Parasympathetic nerves have very powerful effects on the SA node pacemaker cells (see Figure 19-8) and on the AV node cells (see Table 19-2). In addition, parasympathetic nerves exert strong, antisympathetic influences on all the atrial cells. However, parasympathetic nerves have relatively weak effects on the ventricular muscle cells, because very few ventricular cells receive direct parasympathetic innervation. By contrast, all ventricular muscle cells receive direct sympathetic innervation. In summary, the predominant parasympathetic influences on the heart are exerted at the SA node (to decrease the rate), at the AV node (to slow conduction and lengthen the refractory period), and on all supraventricular cells (to lengthen the refractory period and make their contractions weaker and slower).

Parasympathetic neurons do exert a curious, indirect effect on ventricular muscle cells. In the ventricles, parasympathetic neurons release their acetylcholine onto sympathetic neuron terminals. This acetylcholine activates muscarinic cholinergic receptors that are located on the sympathetic neuron terminals. The effect of this activation is to inhibit the release of norepinephrine from the terminals, which weakens the effects of sympathetic activation on ventricular cells.

Parasympathetic effects on the heart can be mimicked by the administration of a *muscarinic cholinergic agonist* (e.g., acetylcholine or muscarine) and blocked by the administration of a *muscarinic cholinergic antagonist* (e.g., atropine). Some therapeutic applications are mentioned later.

Dysfunction in the Specialized Conducting System Leads to Abnormalities in Cardiac Rhythm (Arrhythmias)

Cardiac arrhythmias result either from problems with the formation of action potentials or from problems with the propagation (conduction) of action potentials. One example of a problem with action potential formation has already been mentioned: *sinus arrest,* in which the SA node completely fails to form action potentials. In a patient with sinus arrest, the auxiliary pacemaker function of the AV node keeps the ventricles beating, although at an abnormally low rate. Complete cessation of the SA node is the extreme case of the condition called *sick sinus syndrome.* In its more common and less extreme form, sick sinus syndrome is characterized by sluggish depolarization of the SA node pacemaker cells, which leads to an abnormally low intrinsic heart rate. Patients typically exhibit an abnormally low heart rate at rest (*bradycardia)* and an insufficient increase in heart rate during exercise. Specifically, in sick sinus syndrome, the intrinsic sinus rate is abnormally low.

Even though the problem in sick sinus syndrome is intrinsic to the sinus itself, one treatment strategy is to administer a cholinergic muscarinic antagonist drug (such as atropine) in order to block parasympathetic action on the heart. Table 19-3 illustrates the logic behind this treatment. In a normal, healthy large dog, the intrinsic rate of the heart is about 140 beats/min. However, resting heart rate is lower (about 90 beats/min) because parasympathetic tone slows the SA node pacemaker to a rate below its intrinsic rate. A drug that blocks parasympathetic effects on the heart would return the heart rate of a resting dog to 140 beats/min. A dog with a sick sinus has a low intrinsic heart rate, perhaps 80 beats/min. Parasympathetic tone makes the resting heart rate even lower, approximately 30 beats/min. A drug that blocks parasympathetic effects restores the heart rate to its intrinsic level, 80 beats/min. Therefore a dog with sick sinus syndrome treated with

TABLE 19-3 **Treatment of Sick Sinus Syndrome by Blocking Parasympathetic Effects on Heart Rate with a Cholinergic Muscarinic Antagonist**

Heart Rate (beats/min)	Normal Dog	Dog with Sick Sinus Syndrome
Intrinsic rate	140	80
Resting rate (with parasympathetic tone)	90	30
Resting rate after atropine	140	80

atropine has a heart rate that closely matches the rate of a normal resting dog.

Another possible therapeutic approach is to increase the heart rate by administering a β-adrenergic agonist drug (e.g., isoproterenol). Enough isoproterenol would be given to increase the resting rate from 30 to 80 beats/min.

If drug treatment of sick sinus syndrome is ineffective, an alternative way to increase the heart rate is through the use of an *artificial cardiac pacemaker.* Such a device periodically applies an electric shock to the heart, which depolarizes cardiac muscle to threshold. Shocks applied to the atria initiate atrial action potentials. If the AV node is functioning normally, these atrial action potentials are conducted to the ventricles, and the ventricles contract. For temporary or emergency treatment, the pacemaker electrodes can be inserted intravenously (e.g., via the jugular vein) and advanced into the right atrial chamber. For long-term treatment, a battery-powered electrical stimulator can be surgically implanted under the patient's skin and attached to electrodes that are either inserted into one of the heart's chambers or attached to the outside surface of the heart.

Atrioventricular Node Block Is a Common Cause of Cardiac Arrhythmias

Whereas sick sinus syndrome exemplifies a dysfunction of action potential *formation,* AV node block is a common dysfunction of action potential *conduction.* If damage to the AV node prevents *(blocks)* conduction of atrial action potentials into the ventricles, the atria continue to beat at a rate determined by the SA node pacemaker cells. The ventricles also continue to beat, but at a much lower rate. In such a case the ventricular action potentials and contractions are being initiated by auxiliary pacemaker cells low in the AV node (i.e., below the level of the block). Because the AV node pacemaker cells depolarize more slowly than the SA node pacemaker cells, the ventricles in a resting dog with AV node block typically beat at only 30 to 40 beats/min. Furthermore, these ventricular beats are not synchronized with the atrial contractions.

Three degrees of severity of AV node block are recognized. Complete block of the AV node, in which no atrial action potentials are conducted to the ventricles, is called *third-degree AV node block.* If action potentials are conducted sporadically from the atria to the ventricles, so that the AV node transmits some atrial action potentials but not all of them, the condition is called *second-degree AV node block.* In a patient with second-degree block, some atrial contractions are followed by ventricular contractions, and others are not. Strong parasympathetic activity can create or exaggerate second-degree AV node block because parasympathetic activity increases the refractory period of the AV node cells. For example, in quietly resting horses, parasympathetic tone is often so strong, and the AV node refractory period so long, that some atrial beats are not conducted to the ventricles. Therefore, if the pulse of a relaxed, resting horse is palpated, some "missing" ventricular contractions are likely to be noticed. During exercise the same horse does not show AV node block because parasympathetic activity has been decreased and sympathetic activity increased. Both these changes shorten the refractory period of the AV node and make it much more certain that every atrial action potential will be conducted to the ventricles.

Second-degree or third-degree AV node block often involves the electrical phenomenon known as *decremental conduction*. As mentioned, AV node cells have "slow" action potentials, characterized by a less rapid upstroke, a lower voltage amplitude, and a slower velocity of conduction than the action potentials in regular atrial or ventricular cells. All these differences make conduction of the action potential from cell to cell less reliable in the AV node than in regular atrial or ventricular tissue. When the AV node cells are in an electrically depressed state, an atrial action potential may simply die out within the AV node and not be conducted to the ventricles. This fading and eventual stoppage of a cardiac action potential in a slowly conducting region is called decremental conduction.

The mildest degree of AV node block is *first-degree block,* in which every atrial action potential is transmitted to the ventricles, but the action potential propagates even more slowly than normal through the AV node. Therefore, in first-degree block, the delay between atrial contraction and ventricular contraction is abnormally long. Because the AV node conduction velocity can be slowed by parasympathetic activity and sped by sympathetic activity, the behavioral state of the patient characteristically influences the severity of first-degree block.

AV node block can be caused by cardiac trauma, toxins, viral or bacterial infections, ischemia, congenital heart defects, or cardiac fibrosis. AV node block is sometimes caused by inadvertent damage of AV node tissue during a surgical repair of a ventricular septal defect.

AV node block must be treated if the resulting ventricular rate is too low to maintain adequate blood flow to the body. In such a patient, administration of a muscarinic cholinergic antagonist (e.g., atropine) may reduce the AV node refractory period and decremental conduction sufficiently to overcome the blocked state. The same effect might be achieved with a drug that mimics the effect of sympathetic nerves by activating β-adrenergic receptors (e.g., isoproterenol) (see Table 19-2). If drug treatment fails to correct AV node block, an artificial pacemaker is needed. In the case of AV node block, the pacemaker needs to be applied to the ventricles; pacing the atria would not be beneficial because atrial action potentials are not being reliably conducted to the ventricles.

Cardiac Tachyarrhythmias Result Either from Abnormal Action Potential Formation (by the Sinoatrial Node or Ectopic Pacemakers) or from Abnormal Action Potential Conduction ("Reentry")

Tachyarrhythmias are arrhythmias in which the atrial rate or the ventricular rate (or both) is abnormally high. An occasional extra atrial or ventricular beat is called a *premature contraction* (or *precontraction*). Occasional precontractions are common both in animals and in humans and usually have no clinical significance.

If the precontractions become frequent or continuous, the condition is called *tachycardia,* which means "rapid heart." Tachycardia is a heart rate that is more rapid than is appropriate for the behavioral circumstances (e.g., 160 beats/min in a resting dog). Tachycardia is a clinically significant sign.

Tachyarrhythmias result from abnormal pacemaker activity. The pacemaker initiating the rapid or "extra" beats can be the SA node itself. Alternatively, a region of abnormal cardiac muscle outside the SA node can act as a pacemaker by spontaneously depolarizing to threshold before the regular SA node pacemaker does. Any such region is called an *ectopic pacemaker.* Common causes of ectopic pacemaker activity include cardiac infection or trauma, reaction to a drug or toxin, electrolyte imbalances, myocardial ischemia, and myocardial infarction.

The tachyarrythmias are named for the site of the pacemaker at which they originate. Hence, if tachycardia appears to be caused by abnormally rapid depolarizations of SA node pacemaker cells, the condition is called *sinus tachycardia.* If tachycardia originates from an ectopic pacemaker within the atria, it is called *atrial tachycardia.* Atrial tachycardia is common in some canine breeds, including boxers and wolfhounds. *Junctional tachycardia* originates from ectopic pacemakers within the AV node or first part of the AV bundle. *Supraventricular tachycardia* is a collective term that encompasses sinus tachycardia, atrial tachycardia, and junctional tachycardia. If the ectopic pacemaker causing tachycardia is within the ventricles, the condition is called *ventricular tachycardia.* In this situation the ventricles beat at a rapid rate, as dictated by the ectopic ventricular pacemaker. In occasional patients, some of the action potentials initiated by an ectopic ventricular pacemaker may be conducted backward through the AV node and may cause atrial precontractions. Usually, however, the AV node does not conduct action potentials backward; the atria continue to beat at the rate dictated by the normal SA node pacemaker. In either case, ventricular contractions are not preceded in the normal way by atrial contractions. The major dysfunction associated with ventricular tachycardia is that the ventricles do not relax long enough between contractions for adequate filling, and this problem is exacerbated by the absence of appropriately timed atrial contractions.

An extremely rapid atrial tachycardia is called *atrial flutter.* Atrial flutter does not lead to ventricular flutter because of the long refractory period of the AV node cells; the AV node conducts some, but not all, of the frequent atrial depolarizations to the ventricles. This is an example of the AV node protecting the ventricles from beating at too rapid a rate. If atrial contractions become so rapid that they lose synchrony, the condition is called *atrial fibrillation.* Atrial fibrillation is characterized by the continuous, random passage of action potentials through the atria. Fibrillating atria appear to quiver; there is no effective, coordinated contraction, and no blood is pumped. Atrial fibrillation is common in horses and in certain breeds of dogs, including Doberman pinschers. Atrial fibrillation usually does not lead to ventricular fibrillation because of the protective effect of the AV node. The ventricles continue to contract with a synchronized, effective pumping stroke, in response to some, but not all atrial action potentials, at a rate that is limited by the refractory period of the AV node.

Synchronous ventricular contractions are essential for life. If the synchrony of ventricular contractions is disrupted and the ventricles begin to fibrillate, ventricular pumping stops. In *ventricular fibrillation ("V-fib"),* each tiny region of the ventricular wall contracts and relaxes at random, in response to action

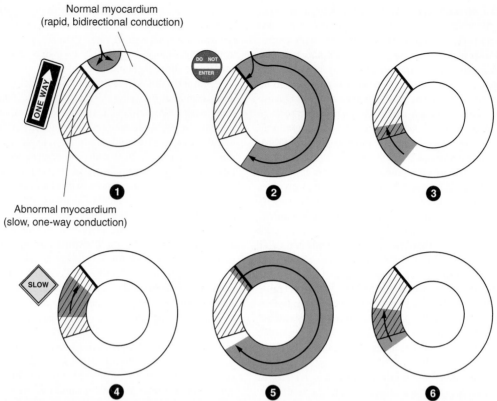

FIGURE 19-11 Cross section of a cardiac chamber (atrium or ventricle) is pictured at six different instants to illustrate how reentrant arrhythmias occur. A region of abnormal myocardium (cross-hatched area) conducts action potentials slowly and only in one direction (clockwise in this example). *Colored shading* indicates areas of heart where an action potential is underway. *1,* Normal action potential has just entered this ring of tissue, and only the *shaded area* is depolarized. *2,* Action potential propagates rapidly in both directions through the normal cardiac tissue but cannot propagate into the abnormal myocardium in a counterclockwise direction. *3,* The clockwise-going action potential can enter the abnormal region. *4,* While the action potential propagates slowly, in a clockwise direction through the abnormal region, the normal cardiac tissue repolarizes to a resting state (indicated by *lack of shading*). *5,* Action potential emerges from the abnormal region into normal cardiac tissue and propagates through the normal tissue for a second time. Meanwhile, the abnormal tissue repolarizes to a resting state. *6,* Action potential begins to move slowly through the abnormal region for a second time. States 4, 5, and 6 repeat themselves. Thus, the abnormal region functions as an ectopic pacemaker.

potentials that propagate randomly and continuously throughout the ventricles. The condition of ventricular fibrillation is synonymous with *sudden cardiac death*.

In most cases, ventricular fibrillation can be reversed only by electrical *defibrillation*. In this process a strong electrical current is passed briefly through the heart muscle. This current depolarizes all the cardiac cells simultaneously and holds them in a depolarized state for several milliseconds. It is hoped that when the current is turned off, all the cardiac muscle cells will simultaneously repolarize to a resting membrane potential, so that the normal pacemaker of the heart will again have a chance to initiate beats in an organized and synchronized manner. Sometimes it works; however, if the cardiac problems that caused ventricular fibrillation to develop in the first place are still present, fibrillation is likely to recur. Usually, defibrillation is performed by placing stimulating electrodes *(paddles)* on either side of the thorax. Therefore the stimulating current passes through, and depolarizes, the skeletal muscles of the thorax as well as the cardiac muscle of the heart. The resulting, involuntary contraction of the skeletal muscles causes the patient to "jump" at the moment of defibrillation.

Ectopic pacemaker activity typically arises when a region of ischemic or damaged cardiac muscle develops the abnormal, twin properties of slow conduction of action potentials and an ability to conduct action potentials in only one direction. Figure 19-11 illustrates how a region of slow, one-way conduction in the wall of one cardiac chamber can function as an ectopic pacemaker. The process begins with a normally originating action potential arriving at the region of slow, one-way conduction. The action potential can only enter the abnormal region from one side. If the one-way conduction through the abnormal muscle is so slow that all the normal, surrounding muscle is past its refractory period by the time the action potential emerges from the abnormal region, the emerging action potential can trigger another action potential in the normal muscle. If this second action potential then propagates around the cardiac chamber and back into the abnormal region, a self-perpetuating cycle can develop. The action potential again propagates slowly through the abnormal region, and again it emerges from the abnormal region after the normal muscle is past its refractory period. The result is a sequence of *reentrant* action potentials, each one initiating a contraction (an "extra" beat) as it propagates through the normal cardiac muscle. The reentrant pathway does not necessarily have to be all the way around the circumference of a cardiac chamber. A damaged, ischemic, or infarcted area of cardiac muscle can form the nonconducting center around which reentrant action potentials can travel. The passage of an action potential around and around a nonconducting center is called a *circus movement*. For the circus movement of the action potential to be self-regenerating, however, a portion of the circular, conducting pathway must have the twin properties of slow and one-way conduction. In effect, an area of slow, one-way conduction within a circular conducting pathway (and around a nonconducting center) functions as an ectopic pacemaker. Reentry of cardiac action potentials can lead to occasional precontractions, continuous tachycardia, or even fibrillation. In any of these cases, the resulting tachyarrhythmia is called a *reentrant arrhythmia*.

Common Antiarrhythmic Drugs Affect the Ion Channels Responsible for the Cardiac Action Potential

Whereas ventricular fibrillation is generally lethal without electrical defibrillation, other tachycardias can often be treated successfully with *antiarrhythmic drugs*. Because tachyarrhythmias result from extra cardiac action potentials, effective antiarrhythmic drugs must work by counteracting either the formation or the propagation of the extra action potentials.

Local anesthetics (e.g., quinidine, lidocaine, procaine) constitute one category of antiarrhythmic drugs. They act by binding to some of the voltage-gated Na^+ channels (fast Na^+ channels) in cardiac muscle cells and preventing them from opening. This counteracts membrane depolarization and action potential formation. In essence, blocking some of the Na^+ channels raises the threshold for action potential formation. This tends to "quiet" ectopic pacemakers and to stifle reentrant arrhythmias. Na^+ channel blockers such as lidocaine or procaine (Novocain) are called *local anesthetics* because, when applied to sensory neurons, they prevent the propagation of neural action potentials that would signal pain to the brain. The cardiac, antiarrhythmic effect of local anesthetics is not the result of their blockage of pain pathways.

A second category of antiarrhythmic drugs is the *calcium channel blockers*. Examples include verapamil, diltiazem, and nifedipine. These drugs bind to L-type (slow) Ca^{2+} channels and prevent them from opening, which decreases the entry of Ca^{2+} into cardiac muscle cells during an action potential. Because Ca^{2+} entry is the primary depolarizing influence during the plateau (phase 2) of the cardiac action potential, one major effect of a Ca^{2+} channel blocker is to lower the plateau (make the membrane potential less positive). A secondary consequence is to lengthen the action potential. The action potential is longer because of a complicated effect of the height of the plateau on K^+ channels, as discussed earlier in connection with sympathetic effects on cardiac action potentials. Drugs that lengthen the cardiac action potential also lengthen the refractory period, which makes it less likely that early extra action potentials will be formed in ectopic pacemakers or that they will propagate even if they are formed.

The calcium channel blockers have especially strong effects on the cells of the SA and AV nodes. As mentioned, Ca^{2+} entry through slow Ca^{2+} channels is the main event in the slow action potentials of these cells. Not surprisingly, therefore, the amplitude of slow action potentials is greatly reduced by Ca^{2+} channel blockers; these action potentials are also lengthened. The consequent increase in refractory period decreases the likelihood that early extra action potentials will form or propagate in SA or AV node

cells. The increased refractory period in the AV node is especially effective in protecting the ventricles from rapid rates in cases of persistent atrial flutter or fibrillation. Many of the extra atrial action potentials simply *die out* (through decremental conduction) in the AV node.

By reducing the entry of extracellular Ca^{2+} into cardiac muscle cells during an action potential, Ca^{2+} channel blockers not only suppress tachyarrhythmias, but also decrease the strength of cardiac contractions. Less entry of extracellular "trigger" Ca^{2+} means a less powerful stimulus for the release of stored Ca^{2+} from the sarcoplasmic reticulum. Therefore the cytosolic Ca^{2+} concentration does not increase as much as normal during the action potential, so there is a less forceful contraction. Some clinical situations in which it is desirable to decrease cardiac contractility are discussed in Chapter 21.

The *cardiac glycosides* (e.g., digitalis) constitute a third category of antiarrhythmic drugs. Cardiac glycosides act by inhibiting the Na^+,K^+ pump in cell membranes. As mentioned in Chapters 1 and 4, the Na^+,K^+ pump is an antiport carrier that uses energy from ATP to transport Na^+ out of cells and K^+ into cells. The pump also indirectly supplies energy to a Na^+,Ca^{2+} antiporter that helps to transport Ca^{2+} back out of cardiac cells after it enters during an action potential. Inhibition of the Na^+,K^+ pump with a cardiac glycoside has several important effects on cardiac function. The effects are listed here without much explanation because the mechanisms are quite complex. First, cardiac muscle cells do not repolarize fully at the end of an action potential; the resting membrane potential is not as negative as normal. As a consequence, some Na^+ channels remain inactivated, which makes the cells somewhat refractory with regard to the formation of subsequent action potentials. This tends to quiet ectopic pacemakers. Second, effects on the central nervous system lead to an increase in parasympathetic tone. This slows the heart rate, quiets atrial ectopic pacemakers, slows conduction through the AV node, and increases the refractory period of AV node cells. The overall effect is to suppress ectopic atrial action potentials or cause extra atrial action potentials to die out in the AV node and not to be conducted to the ventricles. A third effect of cardiac glycosides is to allow more Ca^{2+} than normal to accumulate inside cardiac cells, resulting in stronger cardiac contractions. In summary, the cardiac glycosides are antiarrhythmic and increase cardiac contractility.

Beta-adrenergic antagonists (e.g., propranolol) constitute a fourth class of antiarrhythmic drug. Beta (β) blockers, as they are called, bind to some of the β-adrenergic receptors on cardiac cells and prevent their activation by norepinephrine from sympathetic nerves or by epinephrine and norepinephrine from the adrenal medulla. Sympathetic activation tends to promote tachyarrhythmias by increasing heart rate, shortening refractory period, and speeding conduction of action potentials, especially through the AV node. Beta blockers reduce these effects and therefore reduce the likelihood that extra action potentials will form or propagate. An additional effect of β blockers is to reverse sympathetic-induced increases in cardiac contractility.

In summary, of the four categories of drugs used to treat tachyarrhythmias, three also have pronounced effects on cardiac contractility. The calcium channel blockers and β blockers decrease cardiac contractility, whereas cardiac glycosides increase contractility. Local anesthetics have little effect on contractility. This variety of effects allows a clinician to select the type of antiarrhythmic drug that is best matched to each patient's cardiac contractile state.

Electrical dysfunction of the heart has been discussed in considerable detail to illustrate how specific abnormalities in the specialized cardiac conduction system can result in specific and serious arrhythmias. Electrical dysfunction of the heart is encountered often in clinical practice, and its consequences are often serious or even lethal. Because electrical dysfunction is so important, Chapter 20 is devoted to an explanation of the electrocardiogram, which is the most commonly used tool for evaluating electrical dysfunction of the heart.

CLINICAL CORRELATIONS

THIRD-DEGREE ATRIOVENTRICULAR BLOCK

History. A 5-year-old male English bulldog has fainted several times during the past 3 weeks. On each occasion he collapses, is apparently unconscious for a few seconds, and then slowly recovers. These episodes occur most often during exertion. In general, he tends to be less active than normal, but he has no other obvious signs of illness.

Clinical Examination. The dog is moderately obese. There are no obvious neurological deficits. His mucous membranes appear normal; they are pink, and the capillary refill time is normal (1.5 seconds). Auscultation of the chest reveals a slow, regular heart rate of 45 beats/min. The femoral pulse rate is also 45 beats/min and strong. Thoracic radiography reveals a mildly enlarged heart, but the radiographs are otherwise within normal limits.

The electrocardiogram (ECG) reveals a disparity between the atrial rate (atrial depolarizations occurring regularly, 140 times/min) and the ventricular rate (ventricular depolarizations occurring regularly, 45 times/min). There is no consistent time interval between the atrial and ventricular depolarizations.

Comment. As will be discussed in Chapter 20, atrial and ventricular depolarizations produce characteristic voltage fluctuations at the body surface, which are detected by the ECG. The ECG of this dog shows a complete dissociation between atrial and ventricular depolarizations, which provides definitive diagnostic evidence of complete (third-degree) AV node block. The dog's atria are depolarizing 140 times/min in response to action potentials being initiated in the normal manner by pacemaker cells of the SA node. However, the atrial action potentials are not being conducted through the AV node. Ventricular action potentials are being initiated, at the slow rate of 45 times/min, by auxiliary pacemaker cells located below the blocked region of the AV node.

The low ventricular rate in this dog allows a longer-than-normal time for ventricular filling between beats. Therefore the volume of blood ejected with each beat (the stroke volume) is greater than normal. The increased stroke volume causes the femoral pulse to be very strong.

In a normal dog, sympathetic and parasympathetic nerves acting on the SA node pacemaker cells adjust the heart rate so that cardiac output is matched to the metabolic requirements of the body. In a dog with complete AV block, the ventricles do not respond to these autonomically mediated changes in SA node pacemaker rate. Typically, the rate of ventricular contractions is low at rest and does not increase much during exercise. Therefore, cardiac output does not increase enough during exertion to meet the increased metabolic needs of exercising skeletal muscle. As a consequence, arterial blood pressure decreases. The decreased arterial pressure during attempted exercise causes brain blood flow to fall below the level needed to sustain consciousness. The dog faints.

Treatment. Drug therapy for AV node block involves either blocking the effects of parasympathetic nerves on the AV node (with a muscarinic cholinergic antagonist drug such as atropine) or mimicking the effects of sympathetic activation (with cautious use of a β-adrenergic agonist such as isoproterenol or dopamine). The rationale for these treatments is based on the following physiology: AV node block occurs because atrial action potentials die out in the AV node (decremental conduction). Parasympathetic activation increases the tendency for decremental conduction because parasympathetic nerves act on AV node cells to increase their refractory period and to decrease the velocity with which action potentials spread from cell to cell. Therefore, blocking parasympathetic effects is occasionally effective in reversing AV node block. In contrast, sympathetic activation decreases the tendency for decremental conduction by decreasing the refractory period of AV node cells and increasing their conduction velocity. A sympathomimetic drug (one that mimics sympathetic effects by activating β-adrenergic receptors) has the same effect, and therefore may unblock the AV node. Even if administration of a sympathomimetic drug does not reverse the AV node block, it usually increases the rate of the auxiliary (emergency) pacemaker cells in the AV node or bundle, which are initiating the ventricular contractions. The increased ventricular rate improves cardiac output.

Many cases of third-degree AV block cannot be managed effectively with drugs, so an artificial ventricular pacemaker must be installed. The procedure is straightforward; pacemaker electrodes can be inserted into the right ventricle through a systemic vein (e.g., external jugular) with only sedation and local anesthesia. The electrode wires are attached to a battery-powered pacemaker unit that is then implanted under the skin.

PRACTICE QUESTIONS

1. An increase in heart rate could result from:
   a. An increase in sympathetic nerve activity to the heart.
   b. An abnormally rapid decrease in permeability of SA node cells to K^+ during diastole.
   c. An abnormally rapid increase in permeability of SA node cells to Na^+ during diastole.
   d. A decrease in parasympathetic nerve activity to the heart.
   e. All the above.

2. In which of the following arrhythmias will there be more atrial beats per minute than ventricular beats?
   a. Complete (third-degree) AV block
   b. Frequent premature ventricular contractions
   c. Sick sinus syndrome (sinus bradycardia)
   d. First-degree AV block
   e. Ventricular tachycardia

3. The normal pathway followed by a cardiac action potential is to begin in the SA node and then propagate:
   a. Across the atria in the bundle of His.
   b. Through the connective tissue layers that separate the atria and ventricles.
   c. Across the atria and to the AV node.
   d. From the left atrium to the right atrium.
   e. From the left atrium to the left ventricle and from the right atrium to the right ventricle.

4. Which statement is *true*?
   a. The refractory period of cardiac muscle cells is much shorter than their mechanical contraction.
   b. The cardiac action potential propagates from one cardiac cell to another through nexi, or gap junctions.
   c. Purkinje fibers are special nerves that spread the cardiac action potential rapidly through the ventricles.
   d. Ventricular muscle cells characteristically depolarize spontaneously to threshold.
   e. The permeability of ventricular muscle cells to Ca^{2+} is lower during the plateau of an action potential than it is at rest.

5. Which of the following types of drugs would be the best choice to treat a patient with both supraventricular tachycardia and inadequate cardiac contractility?
   a. Local anesthetic (fast Na^+ channel blocker)
   b. Muscarinic cholinergic antagonist
   c. Beta-adrenergic agonist
   d. Cardiac glycoside (inhibits Na^+,K^+ pump)
   e. Calcium channel blocker

6. During which phase of a normal ventricular action potential is it most likely that fast Na^+ channels are in an inactivated state, slow Ca^{2+} channels are open, and most K^+ channels are closed?
   a. Phase 0 (rapid depolarization)
   b. Phase 1 (partial repolarization)
   c. Phase 2 (plateau)
   d. Phase 3 (repolarization)
   e. Phase 4 (rest)

7. Which of the following is *true* for *both* cardiac muscle and skeletal muscle?
   a. The muscle forms a functional syncytium.
   b. An action potential in the muscle cell membrane is required to initiate contraction.
   c. Pacemaker cells spontaneously depolarize to threshold and initiate action potentials.
   d. Frequent action potentials in motor neurons can cause a sustained *(tetanic)* muscle contraction.
   e. Extracellular Ca^{2+} that enters the muscle cell during an action potential triggers the release of additional Ca^{2+} from the sarcoplasmic reticulum.

BIBLIOGRAPHY

Boron WF, Boulpaep EL: *Medical physiology*, ed 2, Philadelphia, 2009, Saunders.

Ettinger SJ, Feldman EC: *Textbook of veterinary internal medicine: diseases of the dog and cat*, ed 7, St Louis, 2010, Elsevier/Saunders.

Hall JE: *Guyton and Hall textbook of medical physiology*, ed 12, Philadelphia, 2011, Saunders.

Katz AM: *Physiology of the heart*, ed 5, Baltimore, 2010, Lippincott, Williams & Wilkins.

Koeppen BM, Stanton BA: *Berne & Levy physiology*, ed 6, Philadelphia, 2010, Mosby.

Levy MN, Pappano AJ: *Cardiovascular physiology*, ed 9, St Louis, 2007, Mosby.

Lilly LS, editor: *Pathophysiology of heart disease: a collaborative project of medical students and faculty*, ed 5, Baltimore, 2010, Lippincott, Williams & Wilkins.

Reece WO: *Dukes' physiology of domestic animals*, ed 12, Ithaca, NY, 2004, Comstock Publishing.

CHAPTER 20
The Electrocardiogram

KEY POINTS

1. An electrocardiogram is simply a graph, made by a voltmeter that is equipped to plot voltage as a function of time.
2. Atrial depolarization, ventricular depolarization, and ventricular repolarization cause characteristic voltage deflections in the electrocardiogram.
3. The electrocardiogram reveals the timing of electrical events in the heart.
4. Six standardized electrocardiographic leads are used in veterinary medicine.

5. Abnormal voltages in the electrocardiogram are indicative of cardiac structural or electrical abnormalities.
6. Electrical dysfunctions in the heart cause abnormal patterns of electrocardiogram waves.
7. In large animals there is considerable variability in the polarity and size of the electrocardiogram waves.

An Electrocardiogram Is Simply a Graph, Made By a Voltmeter That Is Equipped to Plot Voltage as a Function of Time

The *electrocardiogram* (ECG) is the most frequently used clinical tool for diagnosing electrical dysfunctions of the heart. In its most common application, two or more metal electrodes are applied to the skin surface, and the voltages recorded by the electrodes are displayed on a video screen or drawn on a paper strip. The physics of how the heart produces voltages that are detectable at the body surface is extraordinarily complex. However, it is not difficult to develop an intuitive model of how electrocardiography works; this intuitive model is adequate for most clinical applications.

An intuitive understanding of the ECG begins with the concept of an *electrical dipole* in a *conductive medium* (Figure 20-1). A dipole is a pair of electrical charges (a positive charge and a negative charge) separated by a distance. A common flashlight battery is a good example of a dipole. A battery has an excess of positive charges at one end (the "+" end) and an excess of negative charges at its other end (the "−" end), and the two ends are separated by a distance. If this dipole is placed in a conductive medium (e.g., a bowl containing a solution of sodium chloride in water), ionic currents will flow through the solution. Positive ions (Na^+) in the solution flow toward the negative end of the dipole, and negative ions (Cl^-) flow toward the positive end. The flow of ions creates voltage differences within the salt solution. These voltage differences can be detected by placing the electrodes of a simple voltmeter at the perimeter of the salt solution. In Figure 20-1 an electrode placed at point A is closer (more exposed) to the positive end of the dipole, and an electrode at point B is closer (more exposed) to the negative end of the dipole. Therefore the voltage at point A will be positive in comparison with the voltage at point B. The voltmeter would detect a positive voltage difference between point A and point B. Using *V* as an abbreviation for *voltage*, we would summarize this condition by saying, "V_{A-B} is positive." Points C and D are equally near (equally exposed to) the positive and negative ends of the dipole, so no voltage

difference would exist between electrodes placed at points C and D. We would say, "V_{C-D} is zero."

In Figure 20-2 the battery in the NaCl solution has been replaced with an elongated strip of cardiac muscle. Again, a voltmeter is set up to detect any voltage differences that are created at point A compared with point B, and at point C compared with point D. The voltage differences (A–B and C–D) are plotted for five different conditions. In *condition 1,* all the cells in the strip of cardiac muscle are at a resting membrane potential; each cell is charged negatively on its inside and positively on its outside. Because cardiac cells are electrically interconnected by gap junctions, the strip of cardiac muscle behaves electrically as if it were one large cell (a functional syncytium). From the outside, the strip of cells looks like one large cell that is symmetrically charged positively around its perimeter. Therefore, no dipole exists. There would be no voltage difference between point A and point B (i.e., V_{A-B} would be zero). There would also be no voltage difference between point C and point D (i.e., V_{C-D} would also be zero).

In *condition 2,* a pacemaker cell at the left end of the muscle strip has depolarized to threshold level and formed an action potential. The action potential is propagating from cell to cell, through the muscle strip, from left to right. In other words, the cells at the left end of the strip are depolarized and are at the plateau of their action potential, whereas the cells at the right end of the strip are still at a resting membrane potential. Under this condition, the outside of each depolarized cell is charged negatively, whereas the outside of each resting cell is still charged positively. The strip of muscle has created an electrical dipole, positive at its right end and negative at its left end. Therefore a positive voltage would exist at point A compared with point B. Note, however, that the voltage at point C compared with point D would still be zero, because neither of these points is closer to the positive end of the dipole. The graphs in Figure 20-2 summarize condition 2 by showing that V_{A-B} is positive at this time, and V_{C-D} is zero.

In *condition 3,* the entire muscle strip is depolarized; that is, all the cells are at the plateau of their action potential, with a

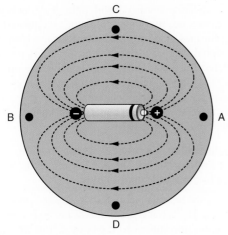

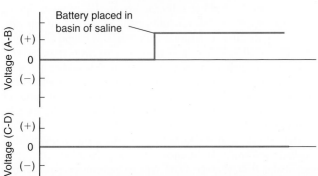

FIGURE 20-1 If an electric dipole (battery) is placed into a conductive medium (e.g., solution of NaCl in water), the charge difference between the two ends of the dipole (battery) will cause positive ions (Na^+) to flow within the solution, as indicated by the *dashed lines* and *arrows*. Negative ions (Cl^-) will flow in the opposite direction. These ionic currents will create voltage differences within the solution. A simple voltmeter can be used to detect these voltage differences, as shown in the lower graphs. In this example the ionic currents would create a positive voltage at point A compared with point B, because point A is "exposed to more positive" than is point B (i.e., voltage A–B is positive). No voltage difference would exist between point C and point D, because these two points are "equally exposed to positive" (i.e., voltage C–D is zero).

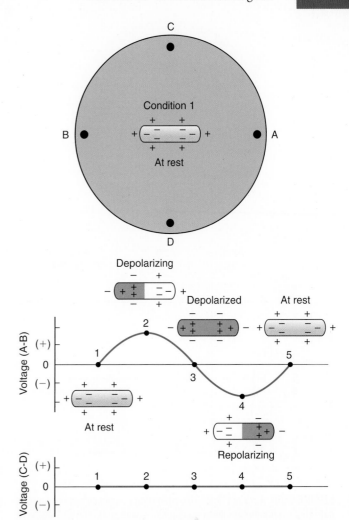

FIGURE 20-2 Strip of cardiac muscle cells in sodium chloride solution produces voltage differences between point A and point B during a phase of spreading depolarization or spreading repolarization, but not when all the cells are in a uniform state of polarization (i.e., not when all the cells are at rest or when all the cells are depolarized). No voltage difference is created between point C and point D. See text for a complete description.

uniform negative charge outside of each cell. Therefore, no voltage differences exist around the perimeter of the muscle strip. No dipole exists, so the recorded voltages (A–B and C–D) are both zero.

In *condition 4,* the muscle strip is repolarizing; cells at the left end have returned to a resting state, whereas cells at the right end are still at the plateau of their action potential. Under this condition, the outside of the muscle strip is charged negatively at its right end and positively at its left end. A dipole exists, with the voltage at point A being negative compared with point B. That is, V_{A-B} is negative. The dipole does not create a voltage difference between C and D, so V_{C-D} is still zero.

In *condition 5,* all the cells in the muscle strip have returned to a resting state (same as condition 1). Again, V_{A-B} is zero and V_{C-D} is zero.

Note that if the depolarization (in condition 2) had been spreading from right to left in the muscle strip (instead of from left to right), the voltage at point A compared with point B (V_{A-B}) would have been negative during depolarization. Likewise, if the repolarization (in condition 4) had been spreading from right to

TABLE 20-1 Sign (Polarity) of Voltages Created at Point A Compared with Point B (V_{A-B})*

	Depolarization	Repolarization
Approaching A	+	−
Going away from A	−	+

*When a strip of muscle within a conductive medium is depolarizing or repolarizing. The arrangement of muscle and electrodes is depicted in Figure 20-2.

left in the muscle strip, V_{A-B} would have been positive during repolarization. Table 20-1 summarizes these relationships.

Figure 20-3 takes the intuitive model of the ECG one step further by picturing the entire heart (rather than a strip of cardiac muscle) in the bowl of saline. The graphs below the drawing show the voltage differences that would be detected by electrodes at the perimeter of the basin during atrial depolarization.

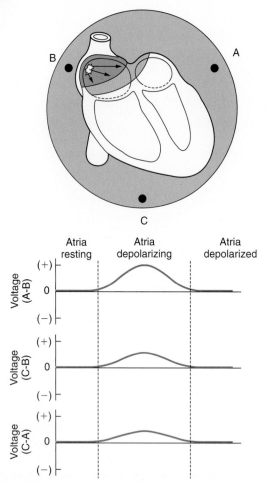

FIGURE 20-3 A resting heart, placed in sodium chloride solution, would not create voltage differences among electrodes A, B, and C. However, during depolarization of the atria, a positive voltage would be created at point A compared with point B. Atrial depolarization would also create positive voltages at point C compared with point B and at point C compared with point A. See text for a complete description.

The plots start at a time between cardiac contractions, when all the cells in the heart are at a resting membrane potential. Every cardiac cell is charged negatively on the inside of its membrane and positively on the outside. Therefore, all around the entire heart, viewed as one large cell, the charge would be positive, and no voltage differences would exist between any of the electrodes.

When the cells in the sinoatrial (SA) node depolarize to threshold level, they initiate an action potential that propagates from cell to cell outward from the SA node. As indicated by the arrows in the top diagram of Figure 20-3, the action potential propagates (spreads) simultaneously downward in the right atrium and leftward (across the right atrium and into the left atrium). At the moment depicted in Figure 20-3 *(top)*, the right atrial cells near the SA node are at the plateau of their action potential (i.e., negatively charged on their outside), whereas the cells in the left atrium and the cells in the inferior part of the right atrium are still at rest (i.e., positively charged on their outside). Therefore the depolarizing atria create an electrical dipole with its positive end angled downward and toward the left atrium. This dipole of atrial depolarization creates a voltage that is positive at point A compared with point B. Similarly, a voltage is created at

point C that is positive compared with point B. Atrial depolarization also creates a positive voltage at point C compared to point A, although the reason for this is admittedly not evident from the two-dimensional view of the atria depicted in Figure 20-3. The voltage differences created during atrial depolarization are summarized by the graphs in Figure 20-3. The graphs also show that, once the atria are completely depolarized (with every atrial cell at the plateau of its action potential), the voltage differences between all points return to zero.

Atrial Depolarization, Ventricular Depolarization, and Ventricular Repolarization Cause Characteristic Voltage Deflections in the Electrocardiogram

In Figure 20-4 the heart is pictured in its normal position in the thorax of a dog. The extracellular fluids of the body contain NaCl (and other salts) in solution, so the body can be imagined as a substitute for the bowl of saline shown in the previous figures. The positions of the left forelimb, right forelimb, and left hind limb in Figure 20-4 correspond with points A, B, and C in Figure 20-3. Figure 20-4, *A,* shows that, while atrial depolarization is in progress at the beginning of a heartbeat, there would be a positive voltage in the left forelimb compared with the right forelimb. This is simply a repetition of the idea illustrated in Figure 20-3, the left forelimb being equivalent to point A and the right forelimb equivalent to point B.

The deflection in the ECG trace during atrial depolarization is called the *P wave.* At the end of atrial depolarization (i.e., at the end of the P wave), the ECG voltage returns to zero. At this moment during a normal cardiac cycle, the action potential is propagating slowly, from cell to cell, through the atrioventricular (AV) node and the first part of the AV bundle. However, these tissues are so small that their depolarization generally does not create a voltage difference that is detectable at the body surface.

The next voltage differences that are detectable at the body surface are those associated with the depolarization of the ventricles. The first part of ventricular depolarization usually involves a depolarization that spreads from left to right (i.e., dog's left to dog's right) across the interventricular septum, as shown in Figure 20-4, *B.* This first phase of ventricular depolarization usually causes a small voltage difference *(Q wave)* between the left forelimb and the right forelimb, with the left forelimb being slightly negative compared with the right.

The next event in ventricular depolarization usually causes a large, positive voltage *(R wave)* at the left forelimb compared with the right, as depicted in Figure 20-4, *C.* To understand why this R wave is large and positive, recall that during ventricular depolarization, the left and right bundle branches conduct the spreading action potential to the ventricular apex. From there, Purkinje fibers carry the action potential rapidly up the inside walls of both ventricles. From there, the depolarization spreads from cell to cell, outward through the walls of both ventricles, as pictured by the small arrows in Figure 20-4, *C.* This outward-spreading action potential creates dipoles in each region of the ventricular wall. Therefore, each small arrow in Figure 20-4, *C,* can be considered a dipole, with its positive end pointing toward the outside wall of the ventricle (because the inside surfaces of each ventricle depolarize before the outside surface). The net electrical effect of depolarizations spreading outward through the walls of both ventricles is a large electrical dipole pointed diagonally downward (caudad) and toward the dog's left. This *net dipole* is depicted by the bold arrow in Figure 20-4, *C.* The net dipole points toward the left for two reasons. First, the cardiac axis is tilted toward the left (i.e.,

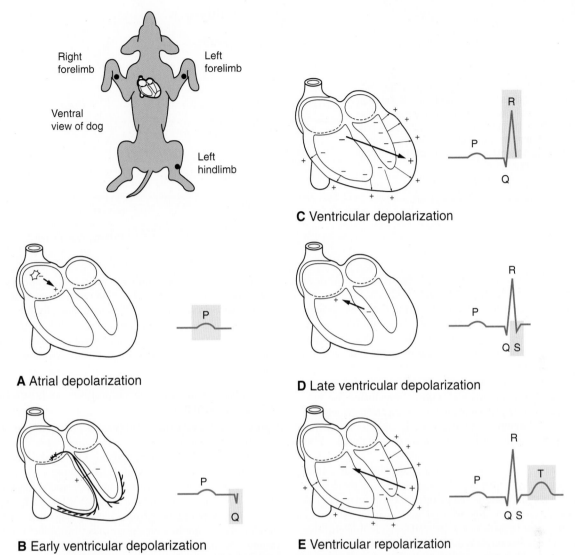

FIGURE 20-4 As a normal cardiac action potential is conducted through the atria and ventricles, a characteristic sequence of voltage differences is created between the left forelimb (analogous to point A in Figure 20-3) and the right forelimb (analogous to point B in Figure 20-3). See text for a complete description.

the normal orientation of the heart is with the ventricular apex angled toward the left wall of the thorax). Second, the left ventricle is much more massive than the right ventricle, so the dipoles created by depolarizations spreading outward in the massive wall of the left ventricle dominate electrically over the dipoles created by depolarizations spreading outward in the thinner wall of the right ventricle. The net result is a large, positive voltage (R wave) at the left forelimb compared with the right. The R wave is the predominant feature of a normal ECG. Abnormalities in the magnitude or polarity of the R wave have great diagnostic significance, as explained later.

As the depolarizations finish spreading outward through the walls of both ventricles, the voltage in the left forelimb compared with the right forelimb returns to zero and then often becomes slightly negative for a few milliseconds (as pictured in Figure 20-4, *D*). The physical basis of this small, negative S wave is obscure. After the S wave, the voltage in the left forelimb compared with the right forelimb returns to zero and stays there for a time, because all the cells throughout both ventricles are uniformly at the plateau of their action potential; no dipole exists.

Altogether, the process of *ventricular depolarization* produces a pattern of voltages in the ECG called the *QRS wave* (or *QRS complex*). The important feature to understand about the QRS complex is why its predominant component, the R wave, is normally large and positive.

Figure 20-4, *E*, shows that repolarization of the ventricular muscle causes a voltage deflection in the ECG called the *T wave*. Whereas the wave of *depolarization* spreads outward through the walls of both ventricles, the pattern of *repolarization* is not as predictable. Figure 20-4, *E*, illustrates one common pattern, in which the repolarization spreads inward through the walls of both ventricles; that is, the outside surface of the ventricles was the last ventricular tissue to depolarize but the first to repolarize. The inward-going repolarization creates dipoles, as depicted by the small arrows in Figure 20-4, *E*, with their negative end pointed toward the inside surface of both ventricles. The net dipole during this repolarization has its negative end pointed upward (craniad) and toward the dog's right, as depicted by the bold arrow in Figure 20-4, *E*. This net dipole creates a positive voltage in the left forelimb compared with the right forelimb

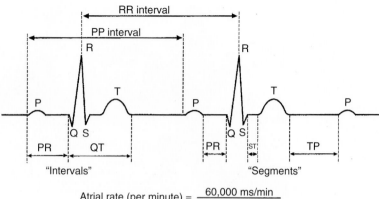

FIGURE 20-5 The time between various waves of the electrocardiogram corresponds to the timing of specific electrical events in the heart. See text for a complete description. The equations show how the atrial rate and the ventricular rate can be calculated from the P-P and R-R intervals, respectively. Of course, in a normally functioning heart, atrial rate = ventricular rate = heart rate.

$$\text{Atrial rate (per minute)} = \frac{60{,}000 \text{ ms/min}}{\text{P-P Interval (in ms)}}$$

$$\text{Ventricular rate (per minute)} = \frac{60{,}000 \text{ ms/min}}{\text{R-R Interval (in ms)}}$$

(T wave). The net dipole in Figure 20-4, *E,* points toward the dog's right, simply because the left ventricular wall is so much more massive than the right ventricular wall. That is, the repolarization proceeding from outside to inside in the massive walls of the left ventricle creates larger voltages (stronger dipoles) than the repolarization proceeding from outside to inside in the thinner walls of the right ventricle.

In many normal dogs ventricular repolarization proceeds in the same direction as the depolarization (from inside the ventricles to outside). This pattern of repolarization creates a negative voltage in the left forelimb compared with the right forelimb; that is, the T wave is negative. Whether positive or negative, T waves are caused by repolarization of the ventricles.

To summarize, the P wave is caused by atrial depolarization, the QRS complex by ventricular depolarization, and the T wave by ventricular repolarization. The pattern of ventricular repolarization varies from dog to dog, so the T wave may be positive or negative. Atrial repolarization does not cause an identifiable wave in the normal ECG, because atrial repolarization does not proceed in an orderly enough pattern or direction to create a significant net electrical dipole.

The Electrocardiogram Reveals the Timing of Electrical Events in the Heart

Because the predominant waves in an ECG correspond to specific electrical events in the heart, the time between these waves can be measured to determine the timing of events in the heart. Figure 20-5 indicates the conventions used to define the important *intervals* and *segments* in the ECG. The *PR interval* corresponds to the time between the start of atrial depolarization (start of P wave) and the start of ventricular depolarization (start of QRS complex). The PR interval is typically about 0.13 second in a large, resting dog. During this time the cardiac action potential is conducted slowly through the AV node. The duration of the QRS complex corresponds to the time it takes for the ventricles to depolarize, once the cardiac action potential emerges from the AV node and AV bundle. Typically this is less than 0.1 second. The *QT interval* (beginning of Q wave to end of T wave) corresponds to the time from the beginning of ventricular depolarization to the end of ventricular repolarization. This approximates the duration of an action potential in ventricular tissue. Typically the QT interval is about 0.2 second. The time between successive P waves *(PP interval)* corresponds to the time between atrial depolarizations (and thus atrial contractions). The PP interval can

be used to calculate the number of atrial contractions per minute (the atrial rate), as illustrated in Figure 20-5. Likewise, the time between successive R waves *(RR interval)* corresponds to the time between ventricular depolarizations (and thus ventricular contractions), so the RR interval can be used to calculate the ventricular rate. Of course, in a normal heart, the atrial rate equals the ventricular rate.

Six Standardized Electrocardiographic Leads Are Used in Veterinary Medicine

Figure 20-6 shows actual ECG records obtained from a normal dog. To obtain these recordings, electrodes were placed on the left forelimb, right forelimb, and left hind limb. Electrodes on these limbs are usually envisioned as forming a triangle around the heart (just as electrodes at points A, B, and C form a triangle around the heart in Figure 20-3). The various ECG tracings in Figure 20-6 were obtained by interconnecting these electrodes in standardized combinations prescribed by Willem Einthoven, inventor of the ECG. As shown in Figure 20-6, *B,* the voltage in the left forelimb compared with the right forelimb is called *lead I.* Note that lead I corresponds to the voltage measurements discussed with Figure 20-4. The same pattern of distinct P, R, and T waves is evident in the lead I tracing in Figure 20-6, as seen in Figure 20-4 (although the T wave happens to be negative in Figure 20-6).

In accordance with Einthoven's convention, the connections for the three standard limb leads are depicted in Figure 20-6 in the form of a triangle *(Einthoven's triangle).* The triangle indicates that to make a lead I ECG, the voltage is recorded in the left forelimb (labeled the + *electrode*) compared with the right forelimb (called the − *electrode*). Similarly, the diagram indicates that *lead II* is the voltage measured in the left hind limb compared with the right forelimb, and *lead III* is defined as the voltage in the left hind limb compared with the left forelimb. It is important to remember that the + and − signs on Einthoven's triangle are simply notations about how to hook up the electrodes. They indicate, for example, that lead I is obtained by measuring the voltage in the left forelimb compared with the right forelimb (not vice versa). The + and − signs on the triangle do not necessarily correspond to the orientation of the dipoles created in the heart.

As illustrated in Figure 20-6, *A,* the major ECG events (P, R, and T waves) are normally evident whether one is looking at tracings from leads I, II, or III. These *standard limb leads* simply provide different angles for viewing the electrical dipoles created

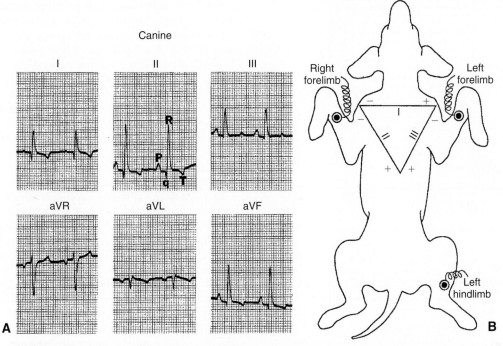

Canine

FIGURE 20-6 **A,** Six-lead electrocardiogram (ECG) from a normal dog. P, Q, R, and T waves (visible in all six leads) are labeled in lead II. There are no distinct S waves in these ECG recordings, and the T waves happen to be negative in leads I, II, aVL, and aVF. These are not abnormal signs. **B,** Einthoven's triangle (superimposed on ventral view of dog) depicts the standard conventions for interconnecting the three limb electrodes to obtain lead I, lead II, and lead III ECGs. See text for additional explanation. (*A,* From Tilley LP: *Essentials of canine and feline electrocardiography: interpretation and treatment,* ed 2, Philadelphia, 1985, Lea & Febiger.)

by the heart muscle as it depolarizes and repolarizes. Three additional electrical views are provided by the *augmented unipolar limb leads* (aV$_R$, aV$_L$, and aV$_F$). Lead aV$_R$ measures the voltage from the right forelimb electrode compared with the average voltage from the other two limb electrodes. Similarly, aV$_L$ and aV$_F$ measure the voltages from the left forelimb and left hind limb electrodes compared with the average voltage from the other two electrodes.

Leads I, II, and III are used routinely in veterinary electrocardiography. Recordings from the augmented unipolar limb leads (aV$_L$, aV$_R$, and aV$_F$) are often included as well. Special additional leads are sometimes recorded by placing ECG electrodes at standardized sites on the thorax. These *precordial (chest) leads* are used more often in human medicine than in veterinary medicine. They are helpful in evaluation of very specific cardiac electrical dysfunctions.

The standardized vertical calibration on an ECG is that two major divisions equal 1 millivolt (mV). Two standard chart speeds are used: 25 millimeters per second (mm/sec), whereby five major divisions on the horizontal axis (time) equal 1 second; or 50 mm/sec, whereby 10 major divisions on the horizontal axis equal 1 second. Using the faster chart speed (50 mm/sec) helps to spread out the ECG events in an animal with a rapid heart rate (e.g., a cat). Chart speed is a convention derived from older, analog, paper-readout (strip chart) ECG machines. Although ECG is now more commonly captured and stored digitally, the chart speed convention is still used to set the resolution of the digital display. Furthermore, many of these digital units can produce a permanent paper printout of their data that looks just like the older strip chart.

Abnormal Voltages in the Electrocardiogram Are Indicative of Cardiac Structural or Electrical Abnormalities

The ECG in Figure 20-7 was obtained from a dog with right ventricular hypertrophy. Note that the sequence of waves in the ECG appears to be normal; that is, each heartbeat begins with an upward-going P wave, which is followed by a QRS complex and a T wave (which happens to be positive in this dog). The atrial and ventricular rates are equal, at about 100 beats per minute (beats/min). An abnormality is evident, however, because the predominant polarity of the QRS complex recorded from lead I is negative. As mentioned, the QRS complex is caused by ventricular depolarization, and its dominant feature is normally a large, positive R wave. The R wave is normally positive as recorded from lead I, because the cardiac axis is normally angled to the left side of the thorax and because the left ventricular wall is much more massive than the right ventricular wall. Both these features have the effect of making the predominant direction of ventricular depolarization right-to-left (as shown in Figure 20-4, *C*). Therefore, reversal of this polarity suggests that the cardiac axis has shifted to the right, that the mass of the right ventricle has dramatically increased, or both. The abnormally high voltages of the QRS complex recorded from leads II and III are indicative of ventricular hypertrophy. The pronounced negative components in the QRS complexes recorded from leads II and III suggest that during part of ventricular depolarization, the predominant direction of depolarization is away from the left hind limb. This is consistent with a cardiac axis shifted to the right and a massive right ventricle. Substantial right ventricular hypertrophy is a common consequence of cardiac defects that increase the pressure that must be generated within the right ventricle during its

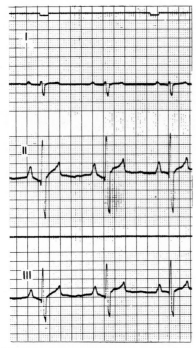

FIGURE 20-7 ECG from a dog with right ventricular hypertrophy. The chart speed is 50 mm/second; therefore, 10 major grid divisions on the horizontal axis equal 1 second. One-second timing marks are visible as small, downward deflections at the very top. Both the PP and the RR intervals are 0.6 second, so both atrial and ventricular rates are 100 per minute. The salient abnormalities are (1) predominantly negative QRS complexes recorded from lead I and (2) large-amplitude, bidirectional QRS complexes recorded from leads II and III. (From Ettinger SJ: *Textbook of veterinary internal medicine,* ed 3, Philadelphia, 1989, Saunders.)

contractions. Examples include pulmonic stenosis, patent ductus arteriosus, and ventricular septal defect (see Chapter 21).

Sometimes, ECG voltages are abnormally low. One common cause of low-voltage ECG waves is an accumulation of fluid in the pericardium. This condition is called *cardiac tamponade*. In a sense the pericardial fluid creates a short circuit for the ionic currents that would ordinarily flow outward toward the body surface. Therefore, voltages smaller than normal are created at the body surface.

An upward or downward shift of the ST segment, compared with the rest of the ECG, is often indicative of an area of ischemic or infarcted ventricular muscle. Typically, ischemic or infarcted ventricular muscle cells cannot maintain a normal, negative resting membrane potential; these cells are always more or less depolarized. Therefore, in between ventricular contractions, when normal ventricular cells are at a normal resting membrane potential, a voltage difference exists between the normal and ischemic (or infarcted) ventricular cells. This voltage difference creates an electrical dipole between normal, resting ventricular muscle and ischemic (or infarcted) ventricular muscle. Figure 20-8 *(bottom left)* shows the orientation of this dipole for the case of an ischemic area in the inferior (caudal) part of the ventricles. The dipole creates a negative voltage in lead II during ventricular rest (i.e., during the TP segment). When an action potential enters this ventricle, the normal ventricular tissue becomes depolarized, and a QRS complex is observed. The ischemic area cannot form action potentials; it simply remains depolarized. As a result, during the ST segment, the entire ventricle, normal and ischemic, is depolarized (Figure 20-8, *bottom right*). During the ST segment, there is no voltage difference (no dipole) between the injured area and the normal area. With no dipole present, the ECG voltage during the ST segment is close to a true zero level. However, the

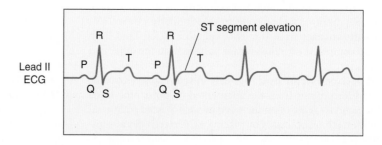

FIGURE 20-8 Voltage recorded during the ST segment is elevated compared with the baseline (TP segment) in this lead II ECG from a dog with an inferior (caudal) ventricular infarction. The drawings show why an ischemic or infarcted area of ventricle creates a net electrical dipole in the resting ventricle (during TP segment) but not in the depolarized ventricle (during ST segment).

During TP segment

During ST segment

Normal tissue
at resting
membrane potential

Ischemic area
depolarized

Whole ventricle
depolarized

ST segment is elevated in relation to the more negative voltage during the TP segment (ventricular rest). Thus, *ST segment elevation* (which is actually "TP segment depression") is indicative of an ischemic or infarcted area in the inferior (caudal) part of the ventricle. Ischemia or infarction in the anterior (cranial) ventricular area would cause *ST segment depression.*

Making a diagnosis solely on the basis of abnormal ECG voltage is risky. Theoretically, if the structural and electrical properties of a particular heart are known in detail, the appearance of the ECG can be predicted with certainty. However, the reverse situation is not strictly true. Several different cardiac defects may result in similar voltage abnormalities. Thus a voltage abnormality in an ECG cannot be ascribed with certainty to a particular cardiac defect. However, in conjunction with other clinical data (e.g., thoracic radiographs), ECG abnormalities are often strongly indicative of specific structural or electrical abnormalities in the heart.

Electrical Dysfunctions in the Heart Cause Abnormal Patterns of Electrocardiogram Waves

Figure 20-9 is an ECG from a dog with *premature ventricular contractions* (PVCs). This lead I strip begins with five normal beats (each QRS complex is preceded by a P wave and followed by a T wave). The P waves are evenly spaced, with a PP interval of 0.5 second (so heart rate is 120 beats/min). After five normal beats, a large-voltage complex of abnormal shape occurs without a preceding P wave. This is indicative of a premature ventricular depolarization (atrial depolarization could not produce such large voltage deflections). The predominant voltage in the abnormal complex is positive in lead I, indicating that the premature ventricular depolarization propagated predominantly in a right-to-left direction. The abnormal shape and long duration of the complex indicate that the premature depolarization did not spread across the ventricles by way of the rapidly conducting bundle branches and Purkinje fibers. In other words, the ectopic site that originated the premature depolarization was not within the AV bundle or bundle branches. Instead, the ventricular depolarization must have spread through more slowly conducting pathways. The abnormally large T wave associated with the premature beat further emphasizes this premature action potential spread across the ventricles with abnormal direction and speed.

If a premature ventricular depolarization originates from an ectopic pacemaker within the AV bundle or bundle branches, the pattern of ventricular depolarization and the pattern of ventricular repolarization would be normal; that is, the QRS complex and the T wave of the premature beat would look like the normal QRS and T waves. The QRS-T sequence would simply occur earlier than expected and would not be preceded by a P wave. Sometimes, premature contractions are initiated by ectopic pacemakers in the atria (*premature atrial contractions,* PACs). If an early atrial depolarization is conducted to the ventricles (i.e., if the AV node is not still refractory from the preceding atrial depolarization), the resulting ventricular depolarization and repolarization would follow normal ventricular pathways. Therefore, the ECG would show an earlier-than-expected P wave, followed by QRS-T sequence of normal size and shape.

Figure 20-10 shows additional examples of cardiac electrical dysfunctions, recorded from resting dogs. In the ECG in Figure 20-10, *A,* the R waves are evenly spaced and indicate a ventricular rate of 235 beats/min. This is fast for a resting dog. However, the pattern of ECG waves appears to be normal; each QRS complex is preceded by a clear, positive P wave and is followed by a positive T wave (which overlaps the next P wave). The most likely diagnosis is *sinus tachycardia* (rapid heart rate initiated by SA node pacemakers). Figure 20-10, *B,* shows the opposite extreme. The pattern of ECG waves is normal, but the heart rate is only 55 beats/min. The diagnosis is *sinus bradycardia* (the SA node is the pacemaker, but its rate is abnormally slow).

The ECG provides an easy way to diagnose AV node block. The ECG in Figure 20-11, *A,* looks normal, except that there is an abnormally long PR interval, which is indicative of abnormally slow conduction of the action potential through the AV node and AV bundle, and thus *first-degree AV node block.* In Figure 20-11, *B,* the P wave spacing indicates an atrial rate of 123 beats/min. Four of the P waves are followed by tall (but faintly visible) QRS complexes and large, negative T waves, but the other seven P waves are not followed by QRS-T sequences. Apparently some, but not all, atrial depolarizations are conducted through the AV node, which indicates a condition of *second-degree AV block.* The condition is not life threatening unless there are so many missed ventricular beats that cardiac output falls to dangerously low levels.

Figure 20-11, *C,* shows *third-degree (complete) AV node block* (and, incidentally, ST segment depression). Two large QRS complexes are visible, each followed by a negative T wave. The RR interval is about 2.9 seconds, indicating that the ventricular rate is only 21 beats/min. The QRS complexes are not immediately preceded by P waves. Small, evenly spaced, positive P waves are present, indicating a constant atrial rate of 142 beats/min, but

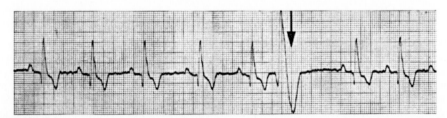

FIGURE 20-9 Lead I ECG of a dog showing five normal beats (normal P-QRS-T pattern) followed by one premature ventricular beat. A sixth P wave would be expected at the time marked by the *arrow.* This P wave is obscured by the large voltages associated with the premature ventricular beat. Also, the refractory period associated with the premature beat prevented the sixth normal ventricular beat from occurring; this creates a long pause (called the *compensatory pause*) between the premature beat and the next regular beat. In this and the remaining ECG examples, chart speed is 50 mm/sec (10 major grid divisions equal 1 second). (From Ettinger SJ: *Textbook of veterinary internal medicine,* ed 3, Philadelphia, 1989, Saunders.)

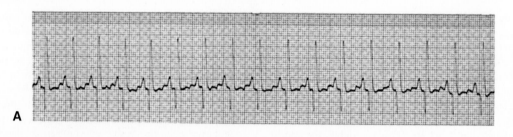

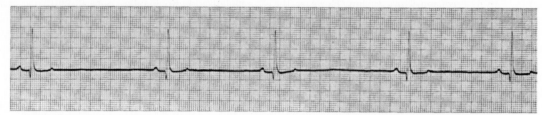

FIGURE 20-10 Sinus tachycardia **(A)** and sinus bradycardia **(B)** are evident in these otherwise-normal ECGs from two resting dogs. Chart speed is 50 mm/sec. (From Ettinger SJ: *Textbook of veterinary internal medicine,* ed 3, Philadelphia, 1989, Saunders.)

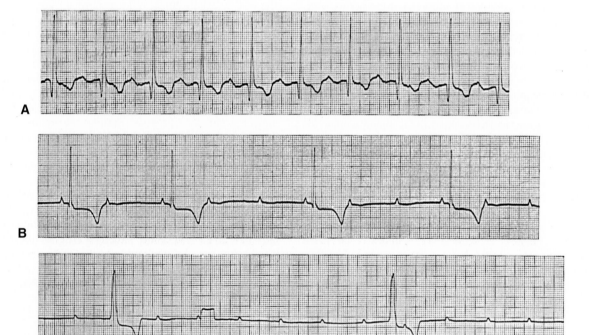

FIGURE 20-11 **A,** Example of first-degree AV node block (abnormally slow AV conduction). Each QRS complex is preceded by a positive P wave and followed by a negative T wave, which is normal. However, the PR interval is 0.2 second (normal for a dog is less than 0.14 second). **B,** Example of second-degree AV node block (sporadic AV conduction). The small, positive deflections are P waves. The broad, negative deflections are T waves, which follow the tall (but faintly visible) QRS complexes. Where P waves are followed by QRS-T complexes, the PR interval is normal. However, only every second or third P wave is followed by a QRS-T complex; that is, there are two or three atrial beats for every ventricular beat. **C,** Example of third-degree (complete) AV node block. Regularly spaced P waves are evident (although two of them are obscured by the two large QRS-T complexes). The QRS-T complexes are not immediately preceded by P waves. ST segment depression is also evident, but this is irrelevant to the diagnosis of AV block. The rectangular deflection one third of the way through the record is a voltage calibration signal (1 mV). Chart speed is 50 mm/sec. (From Ettinger SJ: *Textbook of veterinary internal medicine,* ed 3, Philadelphia, 1989, Saunders.)

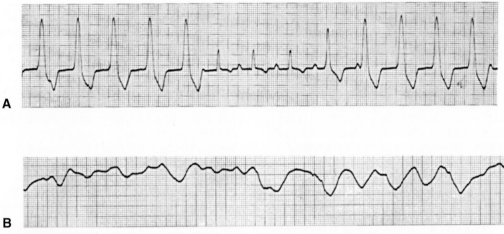

FIGURE 20-12 A, Example of ventricular tachycardia, which reverts briefly to a sinus rhythm. The ventricular rate is about 165 beats/min. This pattern would be typical for a dog with an ectopic ventricular pacemaker functioning at almost the same rate as the SA node pacemaker; some ventricular beats would be initiated by the ectopic pacemaker, and others would be initiated in the normal way through the AV node. **B,** Example of ventricular fibrillation. The random voltage fluctuations generated by the fibrillating ventricles would obscure any P waves that might be present, so it is not possible to determine whether the atria are beating normally or are also fibrillating. Chart speed is 50 mm/sec. (From Ettinger SJ: *Textbook of veterinary internal medicine,* ed 3, Philadelphia, 1989, Saunders.)

there is no synchronization between the P waves and the QRS complexes. Atrial action potentials are apparently being blocked at the AV node. The ventricles are beating slowly in response to an auxiliary pacemaker in the AV node or in the bundle of His.

Figure 20-12, *A,* shows an ECG record of a dog that is drifting in and out of ventricular tachycardia. The first five waves are abnormally shaped ventricular complexes, indicative of an ectopic ventricular pacemaker located outside the normal ventricular conduction system. No P waves are evident. Then there are three normal-appearing P-QRS-T sequences, which suggests that a normal rhythm is being established. However, the ectopic ventricular pacemaker usurps control again, and ventricular tachycardia returns.

Ventricular tachycardia degenerates frequently into ventricular fibrillation. The ECG in Figure 20-12, *B,* indicates ventricular fibrillation. The record shows fairly large, irregular voltage fluctuations with no discernible pattern. The atria may or may not be fibrillating; regularly occurring P waves may be present but obscured by the random electrical activity in the ventricles. However, ventricular fibrillation stops the heart from pumping blood, regardless of whether the atria continue to contract in a synchronized manner.

Atrial fibrillation, as with ventricular fibrillation, typically produces random voltage dipoles. However, because the atrial muscle mass is relatively small, the ECG voltages generated by atrial fibrillation are always much smaller than those seen in Figure 20-12, *B.* An ECG from an animal with atrial fibrillation would typically show normally shaped QRS-T sequences against a background of low-amplitude voltage fluctuations created by the fibrillating atria. In such a case the AV node is bombarded with very frequent action potentials from the fibrillating atria. Some of these action potentials are conducted to the ventricles, and others are blocked (because of the long refractory period of the AV node). Thus, in the case of atrial fibrillation, the QRS-T sequences would typically have normal shape but irregular spacing in time.

In Large Animals There Is Considerable Variability in the Polarity and Size of the Electrocardiogram Waves

The appearance of the normal ECG waves varies more, from animal to animal, among horses and cattle than among dogs and cats. For example, healthy cattle are likely to have QRS complexes (in any particular ECG lead) that are rather different in magnitude, duration, and shape, between individuals. This variability arises from the less consistent pathways followed by cardiac depolarizations in the atria and ventricles of large animals as compared to small animals. As a consequence, the ECG is less useful for diagnosing cardiac structural abnormalities (e.g., ventricular hypertrophy) in large animals than in small animals. Nevertheless, there is consistency in the basic sequence of electrical events in the hearts of normal animals, whether large or small. Each normal heartbeat begins with a depolarization of the SA node, and the consequent sequence of events (depolarization of the atria, depolarization of the ventricles, and repolarization of the ventricles) produces waves of voltage that are evident on an ECG. Therefore, the ECG is very useful in large animals for detecting and characterizing cardiac arrhythmias. Standardizing the placement of electrodes for particular ECG leads is usually not necessary for this purpose. Any ECG lead or electrode placement that yields clearly discernable P waves, QRS complexes, and T waves will suffice.

Sophisticated techniques are widely used in the analysis of ECGs both in human medicine and in many veterinary clinics. The purpose in this chapter is to introduce only enough complexity to establish a conceptual model for thinking about the ECG and to illustrate the usefulness of that model in the clinical diagnosis of cardiac electrical dysfunctions.

CLINICAL CORRELATIONS

DILATIVE CARDIOMYOPATHY WITH PAROXYSMAL ATRIAL TACHYCARDIA

History. An owner brings his 5-year-old male Saint Bernard to you because of a distended abdomen, weakness, coughing, and difficulty breathing. The owner believes these signs developed gradually over several weeks; however, before the last few weeks, there were occasional episodes when the dog suddenly seemed weak and very listless. The episodes lasted from a few minutes to about an hour.

Clinical Examination. Palpation reveals that the dog has muscle wasting and marked ascites (fluid in the abdominal cavity). The jugular veins are distended. The arterial pulse is rapid and irregular; there are frequent pulse deficits ("missing" beats). Thoracic radiography reveals an enlarged heart and an accumulation of fluid near the lung hilus.

You record the dog's ECG for several minutes. You note that P waves usually occur at a rate of 160 to 170 per minute and that each P wave is followed by a QRS-T complex. However, the ECG also shows frequent episodes when there are 210 to 230 P waves per minute. During these episodes, most P waves are followed by QRS-T complexes, but others are not. As a result, the QRS-T complexes occur irregularly, with about 180 per minute.

Echocardiography reveals severe dilation of all four cardiac chambers, particularly the atria. Even though the ventricles are enlarged, the ventricular walls are thinner than normal, a condition called *eccentric hypertrophy*. Ventricular contractions are weak.

Comment. The ECG indicates that this dog has atrial tachycardia. The information presented does not establish whether the atrial pacemaker is located in the SA node or somewhere else in the atria. It is likely that one atrial pacemaker area is initiating depolarizations at a rate of 160 to 170 per minute and that another atrial area intermittently preempts the first pacemaker by initiating depolarizations at the more rapid rate of 210 to 230 per minute. When the atrial rate is 160 to 170 per minute, the AV node conducts every atrial action potential to the ventricles, so that the ventricles also contract 160 to 170 times/min. However, when the atrial rate is 210 to 230 per minute, some of the atrial action potentials arrive at the AV node when the nodal cells are still refractory from the preceding action potential. These atrial action potentials are not conducted into the ventricles, which is why there are only about 180 ventricular contractions per minute. This is a case in which a second-degree AV node block, created by the relatively long refractory period of AV node cells, is beneficial, because it prevents the ventricles from beating too rapidly. The problem, when an arrhythmia triggers very frequent ventricular contractions, is that the time available between contractions becomes too short for adequate ventricular refilling. As ventricular rate increases, the volume of blood pumped with each beat (stroke volume) decreases, and so does cardiac output. At ventricular rates above 180 per minute, cardiac output could fall to such a low level that the dog would collapse.

This dog's primary problem is probably a chronic, progressive weakening of his heart muscle *(cardiomyopathy)*. All the clinical signs, including atrial tachycardia, can be attributed to a primary cardiomyopathy. Dilative cardiomyopathy is common in giant-breed dogs, especially males, and often (as in this case) there is no discernible cause.

Even though the cause of the cardiomyopathy could not be determined from the evidence available in this case, the sequence of dysfunctions that resulted from the cardiomyopathy can be inferred with near-certainty. Ventricular weakness caused heart failure; the cardiac output fell below normal, especially during exercise. The dog's body attempted to compensate for the heart failure by increasing blood volume, which increased both venous and atrial pressures far above normal. The elevated atrial pressure had the beneficial effect of "supercharging" the ventricles with an extra volume of blood before each contraction, which partially returned the volume of blood pumped by a ventricle with each heart beat *(stroke volume)* toward normal. However, the excessive volume and pressure of blood in the veins caused pulmonary edema (which led to coughing and difficulty breathing) and systemic edema (which led to fluid in the abdomen). Also, distention of the atria made the atrial cells more excitable electrically, which resulted in the formation of ectopic pacemakers and the onset of atrial tachycardia. The tachycardia limited the ventricular refilling time, causing further compromise in cardiac output. A vicious cycle began in which decreased cardiac output caused further venous congestion and atrial distention, which aggravated the arrhythmia, and so forth. The atrial tachycardia will likely progress to atrial fibrillation. The prognosis is poor without treatment.

This case of heart failure provides a good preview for the next several chapters, which deal in detail with the physiological mechanisms of cardiac and vascular control in both normal and heart failure states.

Treatment. A diuretic drug (e.g., furosemide) is administered to promote an increase in urine formation. The goal is to reduce the blood volume and venous and atrial pressures, thereby reducing the signs resulting from congestion and edema. Sometimes the paroxysmal atrial tachycardia resolves after diuretic-induced reductions in atrial size. If it does not, antiarrhythmic drugs (e.g., quinidine or lidocaine, and/or a cardiac glycoside such as digitalis) can be used to try to reduce the electrical excitability of atrial tissue.

PRACTICE QUESTIONS

1. In which of the following arrhythmias will the ECG characteristically show the same number of P waves and QRS complexes?
   a. Complete (third-degree) AV block
   b. First-degree AV block
   c. Ventricular tachycardia
   d. Atrial flutter
   e. All the above

2. The time required for the conduction of the cardiac action potential through the AV node would be approximately equal to the:
   a. RR interval.
   b. PR interval.
   c. ST interval.
   d. PP interval.
   e. QT interval.

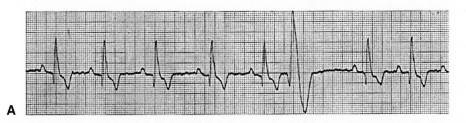

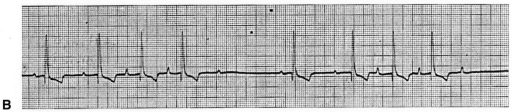

FIGURE 20-13 Lead I ECG recordings from two dogs. **A** is the basis for Practice Question 4. **B** is the basis for Practice Question 5. Chart speed is 50 mm/sec. (From Ettinger SJ: *Textbook of veterinary internal medicine*, ed 3, Philadelphia, 1989, Saunders.)

3. The T wave in a normal ECG is:
   a. Always negative.
   b. Always positive if the R wave is positive.
   c. Also known as the *pacemaker potential.*
   d. Caused by the delay between atrial and ventricular depolarization.
   e. Caused by ventricular repolarization.

4. The ECG in Figure 20-13, *A,* indicates:
   a. Sinus arrhythmia.
   b. Right ventricular hypertrophy.
   c. ST segment elevation.
   d. Premature ventricular contraction.
   e. Atrial fibrillation.

5. The ECG in Figure 20-13, *B,* indicates
   a. Second-degree AV block.
   b. Third-degree AV block.
   c. Sinus bradycardia.
   d. Ventricular tachycardia.
   e. ST segment elevation.

BIBLIOGRAPHY

Boron WF, Boulpaep EL: *Medical physiology*, ed 2, Philadelphia, 2009, Saunders.

Ettinger SJ, Feldman EC: *Textbook of veterinary internal medicine: diseases of the dog and cat*, ed 7, St Louis, 2010, Elsevier/Saunders.

Katz AM: *Physiology of the heart*, ed 5, Baltimore, 2010, Lippincott, Williams & Wilkins.

Levy MN, Pappano AJ: *Cardiovascular physiology*, ed 9, St Louis, 2007, Mosby.

Marr C, Bowen M, editors: *Cardiology of the horse*, ed 2, Philadelphia, 2011, Saunders.

Patteson MW: *Equine cardiology*, Oxford, UK, 1996, Blackwell Science.

Reece WO: *Dukes' physiology of domestic animals*, ed 12, Ithaca, NY, 2004, Comstock Publishing.

Tilley LP, Smith FWK, Oyama MA, Sleeper MM: *Manual of canine and feline cardiology*, ed 4, Philadelphia, 2008, Saunders.

CHAPTER 21
The Heart as a Pump

KEY POINTS

1. Each heartbeat consists of ventricular systole and ventricular diastole.
2. Cardiac output equals heart rate multiplied by stroke volume.
3. Increases in end-diastolic ventricular volume cause increases in stroke volume.
4. End-diastolic ventricular volume is determined by ventricular preload, ventricular compliance, and diastolic filling time.
5. Increases in ventricular contractility cause decreases in ventricular end-systolic volume.

6. Increasing the heart rate does not increase cardiac output substantially unless stroke volume is maintained.
7. Murmurs are abnormal heart sounds caused by turbulent flow through cardiac defects.
8. Some cardiac defects increase the heart's workload, which causes cardiac hypertrophy.
9. The pathophysiological consequences of cardiac defects are direct results of the abnormal pressures, volumes, and workloads created in the cardiac chambers.

Each Heartbeat Consists of Ventricular Systole and Ventricular Diastole

The heart is actually two pumps (two ventricles) that work together, side by side. Each ventricular pump works in a cycle, first relaxing and filling with blood and then contracting and ejecting some blood. In each *cardiac cycle* (heartbeat) the left ventricle takes in a volume of blood from the pulmonary veins and left atrium, then ejects it into the aorta. The right ventricle takes in a similar volume of blood from the systemic veins and right atrium, then ejects it into the pulmonary artery.

Figure 21-1 shows the events of a single cardiac cycle. A normal electrocardiogram (ECG) tracing is presented at the top of the figure. Atrial contraction is initiated by atrial depolarization, which is indicated by the P wave. Ventricular contraction is initiated by ventricular depolarization, which is indicated by the QRS complex. The period of ventricular contraction is called *ventricular systole.* Blood is ejected from the ventricles during ventricular systole. Each systole is followed by *ventricular diastole,* during which the ventricles relax and refill with blood before the next ventricular systole. Note that ventricular diastole corresponds to the period between a T wave and the subsequent QRS complex, when ventricular cells are at resting membrane potential.

The ventricles do not empty completely during systole. As shown in the graph of ventricular volume (see Figure 21-1, *second from top*), each ventricle of a large dog contains about 60 mL of blood at the end of diastole. This is called *end-diastolic volume.* During systole, about 30 mL of this blood is ejected from each ventricle, but 30 mL remains. This is called *end-systolic volume.* The volume of blood ejected from one ventricle in one beat is called *stroke volume,* expressed as follows:

Stroke volume = end-diastolic volume − end-systolic volume

The fraction of end-diastolic volume that is ejected during ventricular systole is called the *ejection fraction*, as follows:

$$\text{Ejection fraction} = \frac{\text{Stroke volume}}{\text{End-diastolic volume}}$$

In the example depicted in Figure 21-1, ejection fraction is 50%. Values between 50% and 65% are typical for resting dogs.

As shown in Figure 21-1, left ventricular pressure is low at the beginning of ventricular systole, but the powerful contraction of the ventricular muscle causes the ventricular pressure to increase rapidly. The increase in left ventricular pressure causes a momentary backflow of blood from the left ventricle to the left atrium, which closes the *left atrioventricular (AV) valve* (the *mitral valve*). Blood is not immediately ejected from the left ventricle into the aorta at the beginning of systole, because the *aortic valve* remains closed until the left ventricular pressure exceeds the aortic pressure. Therefore, ventricular volume remains unchanged during this first phase of systole, which is aptly named *isovolumetric contraction.*

When left ventricular pressure does rise above aortic pressure, the aortic valve is pushed open, and there is a *rapid ejection* of blood into the aorta. Rapid ejection is followed by a phase of *reduced ejection* of blood as both ventricular pressure and aortic pressure pass their peak *(systolic)* values and begin to decrease. (During the period of reduced ejection, the ventricular pressure actually falls below the aortic pressure, but ejection continues for a few moments, because the blood flowing out of the ventricle is carried along by the momentum imparted to it during rapid ejection.) As the ventricular pressure continues to decrease, ejection comes to an end. A momentary backflow of blood from the aorta into the left ventricle closes the aortic valve. The closure of the aortic valve demarcates the end of ventricular systole and the beginning of ventricular diastole.

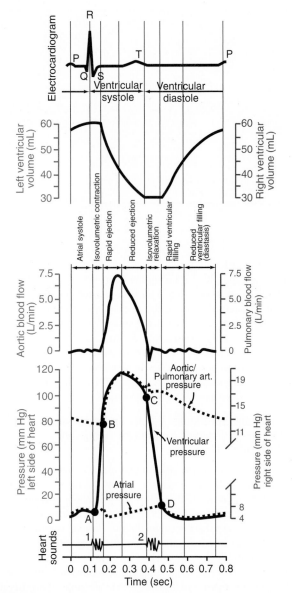

FIGURE 21-1 Events and terminology associated with one cardiac cycle (heartbeat) in a normal dog. Vertical scales on the left side of the graphs *(red)* are for the left side of the heart. Vertical scales on the right side of the graphs *(blue)* are for the right side of the heart. In the graph of *ventricular pressure,* point *A* indicates closure of the mitral and tricuspid valves (the atrioventricular valves); point *B* indicates opening of the aortic and pulmonic valves; point *C* indicates closure of the aortic and pulmonic valves; and point *D* indicates opening of the mitral and tricuspid valves. See text for details.

During the first phase of ventricular diastole, the ventricular muscle relaxes, and left ventricular pressure declines from a value near aortic pressure to a value near left atrial pressure. However, no filling of the ventricle can occur because the mitral valve remains closed until left ventricular pressure drops below left atrial pressure. This first phase of ventricular diastole is called *isovolumetric relaxation* because there is neither filling nor emptying of the ventricle.

When left ventricular pressure does fall below left atrial pressure, the mitral valve is pushed open, as blood begins to flow from the atrium into the ventricle. First, there is a period of *rapid ventricular filling,* which is followed by a phase of *reduced*

ventricular filling (diastasis). Diastasis persists until the sinoatrial node cells initiate an atrial action potential and atrial contraction *(atrial systole).* In a resting dog, as depicted in Figure 21-1, ventricular volume is nearly at its end-diastolic level even before atrial systole. Typically, 80% to 90% of ventricular filling occurs before atrial systole. Atrial systole simply "tops up" the almost-full ventricles. An important clinical consequence of this fact is that the ventricles in a resting animal can pump a nearly normal stroke volume even in the absence of properly timed atrial contractions (e.g., during atrial fibrillation). During exercise, however, atrial contractions make a relatively greater contribution to ventricular filling because the rapid heart rate in exercise leaves a shorter time for diastolic filling. Therefore, animals with atrial fibrillation typically exhibit exercise intolerance. Ventricular filling also becomes more dependent on atrial systole in patients with certain valve defects, such as narrowing of the mitral valve *(mitral stenosis).*

At the end of atrial systole, the atria begin to relax. The left atrial pressure drops slightly. Then, as the ventricles begin to contract, there is a momentary backflow of blood from the left ventricle to the left atrium. The backflow closes the mitral valve, which marks the end of ventricular diastole and the beginning of another left ventricular systole.

By definition, the cardiac cycle is divided into ventricular systole and ventricular diastole. Closure of the mitral valve marks the beginning of ventricular systole. Closure of the aortic valve marks the beginning of ventricular diastole. Note that atrial systole takes place during ventricular diastole.

The preceding six paragraphs discussed pressure changes in the left atrium, left ventricle, and aorta. However, all the events of the cardiac cycle also take place on the right side of the heart. Therefore, all the statements made about the left side of the heart also hold true for the right side of the heart; simply substitute "pulmonary artery" for "aorta," "pulmonic valve" for "aortic valve," and "tricuspid valve" for "mitral valve." As indicated in Figure 21-1, the ventricular volumes are similar for the left and right sides, and so are the blood flow rates. The pressures, however, differ greatly on the two sides. Systolic (peak) pressure in the right ventricle and pulmonary artery is only about 20 mm Hg, whereas systolic pressure on the left side of the heart reaches 120 mm Hg. This explains why there are different scales on the pressure axes in Figure 21-1 for the left and right sides of the heart.

The timing of the two major heart sounds is also shown in Figure 21-1 *(bottom).* The *first heart sound* (S1) is associated with the closure of the AV valves (the mitral and tricuspid valves). The actual closure of the valves does not make this sound; the valve leaflets are so light and thin that their closing would be almost silent. However, there is a momentary backflow of blood from the ventricles to the atria at the beginning of ventricular systole. When this backflow of blood is brought to a sudden stop against the closing valves, brief vibrations are created in the blood and in the cardiac walls. These vibrations create the heart sound.

The *second heart sound* (S2) is associated with closure of the aortic valve on the left side of the heart and the pulmonic valve on the right side of the heart. It is usually briefer, sharper, and higher pitched than the first heart sound. Again, what makes the sound is not the valve leaflets closing, but rather the reverberation produced when the momentary backflow of blood into the ventricles is brought to a sudden stop by closure of the valves. The closures of the aortic and pulmonic valves are normally simultaneous. Under certain circumstances, however, the two valves close at slightly different times, and the second heart sound is

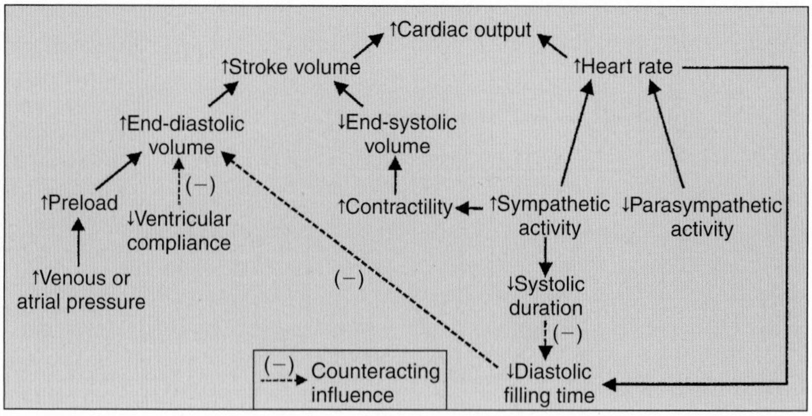

FIGURE 21-2 Summary of the control of cardiac output. The relationships shown here are described in detail in the text.

heard as two distinct sounds in quick succession; this condition is called a *split second heart sound*.

The AV valves close at the beginning of ventricular systole, and the aortic and pulmonic valves close at the end of ventricular systole. Therefore, ventricular systole is sometimes defined as the part of the cardiac cycle between the first heart sound and the second heart sound.

Two additional heart sounds can commonly be heard in large animals (and occasionally in dogs). The rush of blood into the ventricles during the rapid filling phase of early diastole can create sufficient turbulence and enough vibration of the ventricular walls to be heard as a *third heart sound* (S3). A *fourth heart sound* (S4), if audible, occurs right at the end of diastole, during atrial systole.

Cardiac Output Equals Heart Rate Multiplied by Stroke Volume

All the events diagrammed in Figure 21-1 occur during each heartbeat, and each heartbeat results in the ejection of one stroke volume of blood into the pulmonary artery and aorta. The number of heartbeats per minute is called the *heart rate*. Therefore, *cardiac output* (the total volume of blood pumped by each ventricle in 1 minute) is expressed as follows:

$$\text{Cardiac output} = \text{Stroke volume} \times \text{Heart rate}$$

This relationship emphasizes that cardiac output can be increased only if stroke volume increases, heart rate increases, or both increase. Therefore, to understand how the body controls cardiac output, you must understand how the body controls stroke volume and heart rate. Figure 21-2 summarizes the factors that affect stroke volume and heart rate. These factors are described in detail in the following three sections.

Increases in End-Diastolic Ventricular Volume Cause Increases in Stroke Volume

Stroke volume equals end-diastolic volume minus end-systolic volume. Therefore, as shown in Figure 21-2, stroke volume can be increased only by increasing end-diastolic volume (i.e., filling the ventricles fuller during diastole) or by decreasing end-systolic volume (i.e., emptying the ventricles more completely during systole), or both.

The effect of increasing end-diastolic ventricular volume (EDV) on stroke volume is plotted in Figure 21-3, *A*. The detailed physiological mechanisms underlying this relationship are complex. Basically, however, greater ventricular filling during diastole

places the ventricular muscle fibers in a more favorable geometry for the ejection of blood during the next systole. Also, stretching the ventricular muscle fibers during diastole causes a greater amount of calcium (Ca^{2+}) to be released from the sarcoplasmic reticulum during the subsequent systolic contraction, and this enhances the force of contraction. Resting conditions in a normal animal are somewhere around the middle of this *ventricular function curve*. Therefore, increases or decreases from normal ventricular end-diastolic volume result in approximately proportional increases or decreases in stroke volume.

End-Diastolic Ventricular Volume Is Determined By Ventricular Preload, Ventricular Compliance, and Diastolic Filling Time

Ventricular preload is the pressure within a ventricle during diastolic filling. Because ventricular pressure changes throughout filling (see Figure 21-1), the value of ventricular pressure at the end of diastole is usually accepted as a singular measure of preload. Normal values of preload (*end-diastolic ventricular pressure*) are about 5 mm Hg for the left ventricle and 3 mm Hg for the right ventricle. In a normal heart, ventricular pressure at the end of diastole is essentially equal to atrial pressure because the AV valves are open widely during late diastole. Also, because there are no valves between the veins and the atria, the atrial pressure is almost identical to the pressure within the nearby veins. Thus, pulmonary venous pressure, left atrial pressure, and left ventricular end-diastolic pressure are all essentially equivalent measures of left ventricular preload. Similarly, right ventricular end-diastolic pressure, right atrial pressure, and vena caval pressure are all essentially equivalent measures of right ventricular preload. In the clinic, right ventricular preload is measured by introducing a catheter into a peripheral vein (e.g., the jugular vein) and advancing it into the cranial vena cava (precava) or right atrium. Such a catheter is called a *central venous catheter*, and the pressure measured at its tip is called *central venous pressure*. Left ventricular preload is more difficult to measure clinically because there is no easy way to place a catheter tip into the left atrium or pulmonary veins.

Figure 21-3, *B,* shows that increases in preload are associated with increases in end-diastolic ventricular volume. The graph depicts a left ventricle that has a natural volume of 30 mL in a relaxed, nonpressurized state (i.e., when the preload equals 0 mm Hg). Increases in preload distend and fill the ventricle. A preload of 5 mm Hg brings about the normal left ventricular end-diastolic volume of 60 mL. However, ventricular tissue reaches its elastic

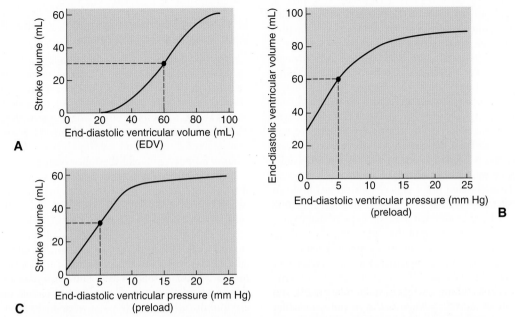

FIGURE 21-3 A, Increase in end-diastolic ventricular volume causes increased stroke volume. **B,** Increase in end-diastolic ventricular pressure (preload) causes increased end-diastolic ventricular volume. **C,** Combines the relationships of *A* and *B* to show that an increase in ventricular preload causes increased stroke volume. An upper limit is reached in each relationship (*A* to *C*) primarily because, at high levels of end-diastolic ventricular volume, the ventricular walls become stretched to their elastic limit. The numerical data are for the left ventricle of a large dog. The *points* and *dashed lines* indicate normal values for the resting state.

limit when the ventricular volume approaches 90 mL. Further increases in the preload do not cause much additional ventricular filling.

Increases in ventricular preload cause increases in end-diastolic volume (see Figure 21-3, *B*), and increases in end-diastolic volume cause increases in stroke volume (see Figure 21-3, *A*). Therefore, it follows that increases in preload cause increases in stroke volume (see Figure 21-3, *C*). Each of these relationships reaches an upper limit. Several factors are involved, but the main one (already mentioned) is that the ventricular walls become stretched to their elastic limit at high levels of end-diastolic ventricular volume. In a resting dog the normal values of ventricular preload, end-diastolic volume, and stroke volume are about midway between their minimum and maximum values (see Figure 21-3). Therefore a decrease below normal in preload will cause a decrease in both end-diastolic ventricular volume and stroke volume. This happens, for example, in response to hemorrhage (see Chapter 26).

The relationships among ventricular preload, end-diastolic volume, and stroke volume were first studied in detail by Ernest Henry Starling. The observation that changes in preload cause corresponding changes in end-diastolic ventricular volume and stroke volume is called *Starling's law of the heart*. The Starling mechanism is critical for moment-to-moment adjustments of stroke volume. For example, if the right ventricle begins, for any reason, to pump an increased stroke volume, the resulting additional pulmonary blood flow causes an increase in the pulmonary venous pressure, which increases left atrial pressure, which in turn increases left ventricular preload, which increases the filling of the left ventricle during diastole. The resulting increase in left ventricular end-diastolic volume leads to a greater stroke volume from the left ventricle. Thus an increase in right ventricular stroke

volume quickly results in a corresponding increase in left ventricular stroke volume. The reverse is also true.

The sequence just described has a potential for developing into a vicious circle, with runaway increases in stroke volume. Other control mechanisms prevent this from happening, as discussed in Chapter 25. The point here is that the Starling mechanism keeps the stroke volumes of the left and right ventricles balanced. If this equality were not maintained (and one ventricle pumped more blood than the other for several minutes), a large part of the body's blood volume would accumulate either in the lungs or in the systemic circulation.

An alternate name for Starling's law of the heart is *heterometric autoregulation*. This name implies self-control *(autoregulation)* of stroke volume as a result of different *(hetero)* initial volumes *(metric)*; that is, *heterometric* refers to different end-diastolic volumes.

End-diastolic ventricular volume is determined not only by preload but also by *ventricular compliance*. Compliance is a measure of the ease with which the ventricular walls stretch to accommodate incoming blood during diastole. A compliant ventricle is one that yields easily to preload pressure and readily fills with blood during diastole. Compliance is more rigorously defined as follows:

Compliance = Change in volume ÷ Change in pressure

Ventricular compliance therefore corresponds to the slope of a ventricular volume versus pressure curve, such as the one shown in Figure 21-3, *B*. This figure illustrates that a normal ventricle is quite compliant over the range of ventricular volumes up to and including the normal end-diastolic ventricular volume. Within this range, small changes in preload result in substantial changes in end-diastolic ventricular volume. At preloads higher than about 10 mm Hg, however, the ventricle becomes less compliant (stiffer). Inelastic connective tissue in the ventricular walls prevents increases in ventricular volume above about 90 mL.

Myocardial ischemia, certain cardiac diseases, or mere advancing age can cause the ventricular walls to become stiff and noncompliant even at normal preloads. Figure 21-4 shows a comparison of volume versus pressure curves for a normal ventricle and for a noncompliant ventricle. In the noncompliant ventricle, there is a smaller increase in ventricular volume for any given increase in ventricular preload. As a consequence, a larger-than-normal preload is needed to obtain a normal end-diastolic ventricular volume and a normal stroke volume. An elevated preload necessitates elevated atrial and venous pressure, which leads to edema (detailed in Chapters 23 and 26). Thus, stiffening of the left ventricle leads to elevated pressure in pulmonary veins and pulmonary edema; stiffening of the right ventricle leads to elevated pressure in the systemic veins and systemic edema.

In addition to preload and compliance, the third factor that affects ventricular end-diastolic volume is the length of time available for ventricular filling during diastole. Heart rate is the main determinant of *diastolic filling time*. At a normal resting heart rate, there is ample time for ventricular filling during diastole; in fact, ventricular filling is almost complete even before atrial systole occurs. As heart rate increases, however, diastolic duration decreases. At heart rates greater than about 160 beats/min, the shortness of diastolic filling time precludes achievement of normal end-diastolic ventricular volume. This limitation on ventricular filling would dramatically reduce stroke volume when heart rate is high if not for an additional, compensating influence brought about by the sympathetic nervous system, as discussed later.

Figure 21-2 *(left side)* provides a useful summary of the preceding discussion. End-diastolic ventricular volume is determined by ventricular preload, ventricular compliance, and diastolic filling time. An elevated preload increases ventricular filling. Decreased ventricular compliance or decreased diastolic filling time can limit ventricular filling.

Increases in Ventricular Contractility Cause Decreases in Ventricular End-Systolic Volume

Contractility refers to the pumping ability of a ventricle. With increased contractility, there is a more complete emptying of the ventricle during systole and therefore a decreased end-systolic volume (see Figure 21-2, *middle*). An increase in contractility brings about an increase in stroke volume without requiring an increase in end-diastolic volume. Figure 21-5 shows graphically that increased contractility brings about an increased stroke volume for any given end-diastolic volume.

Sympathetic nerve activity increases ventricular contractility through the action of the neurotransmitter norepinephrine, which activates β-adrenergic receptors on ventricular muscle cells. As discussed in Chapter 19, activation of β-adrenergic receptors leads to an increased influx of extracellular Ca^{2+} into cardiac cells during an action potential (and to several other effects); the overall result is that cardiac contractions are stronger, quicker to develop, and shorter. Epinephrine and norepinephrine released from the adrenal medulla and circulating in the blood can likewise activate β-adrenergic receptors and increase contractility, as can β-adrenergic agonist drugs (e.g., epinephrine, isoproterenol). The cardiac glycosides (e.g., digitalis) are another class of drugs that increases cardiac contractility, again by increasing the cytosolic Ca^{2+} concentration during an action potential.

If cardiac contractility becomes depressed, there is less-than-normal ventricular emptying during systole. End-systolic volume increases, and stroke volume decreases, as shown in Figure 21-5. A decrease in sympathetic activity causes a decrease in cardiac contractility, as do β-adrenergic antagonist drugs, which block the β-adrenergic receptors on cardiac muscle cells. Propranolol and atenolol are the β-adrenergic antagonists used most often to decrease cardiac contractility. As with β-adrenergic antagonists, calcium channel–blocking drugs also decrease cardiac contractility by making less Ca^{2+} available for the activation of

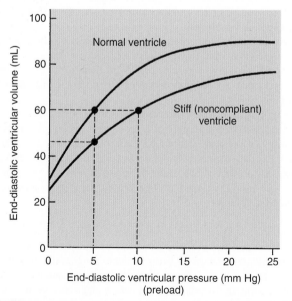

FIGURE 21-4 Stiff, noncompliant ventricle requires a higher filling pressure (higher preload) to reach a normal degree of filling (normal end-diastolic ventricular volume).

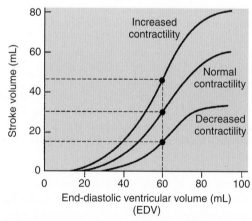

FIGURE 21-5 Increase in cardiac contractility is identifiable graphically as a leftward and upward shift of the ventricular function curve. Increase in contractility means that there will be a larger stroke volume for any given end-diastolic volume. Conversely, decrease in contractility (rightward and downward shift) means that there will be a smaller stroke volume for any given end-diastolic volume. With normal contractility and a normal end-diastolic volume of 60 mL, the end-systolic volume is 30 mL, and so the stroke volume is 30 mL *(middle dot)*. Increased contractility (with no change in end-diastolic volume) results in decreased end-systolic volume. For example, if end-systolic volume is reduced to 15 mL, the stroke volume increases to 45 mL *(upper dot)*.

the contractile proteins. Barbiturates, opioids, and some general anesthetics depress cardiac contractility as well; this must be kept in mind, particularly when administering such drugs to a patient who may already have compromised cardiac function. A decrease in cardiac contractility causes a decrease in stroke volume and therefore cardiac output. Consequently, the patient's blood pressure may fall to dangerously low levels.

A decreased cardiac contractility is the hallmark of the general clinical condition called *heart failure (myocardial failure)*. Although there are many forms of heart failure, they share one characteristic: a decrease in pumping ability of one or both ventricles. Heart failure can result from coronary artery disease, myocardial ischemia, myocardial infarction, myocarditis, toxins, or electrolyte imbalances.

Although ventricular contractility is usually the predominant factor affecting ventricular end-systolic volume, the effect of arterial blood pressure must also be considered. A substantial increase in arterial blood pressure impairs ventricular ejection because the left ventricular pressure during systole must exceed aortic pressure before ejection of blood from the ventricle can occur. Arterial pressure is called the *cardiac afterload*; this is the pressure against which the ventricle must pump in order to eject blood. The higher the afterload, the more difficult it is for the ventricle to eject blood. If arterial pressure is excessively high, ventricular ejection is impaired, end-systolic volume increases, and stroke volume decreases. This effect is minor for a normal heart and within the normal range of arterial pressure. However, high afterload can significantly limit stroke volume for a heart that is in failure.

Increasing the Heart Rate Does Not Increase Cardiac Output Substantially Unless Stroke Volume Is Maintained

Because cardiac output is equal to stroke volume multiplied by heart rate, cardiac output might be expected to be proportional to heart rate; that is, doubling the heart rate would be expected to double cardiac output (Figure 21-6, *dashed line*). However, if the heart rate is experimentally increased above its normal level with an electrical pacemaker, cardiac output increases somewhat, but not in proportion to the increase in heart rate. The reason, as

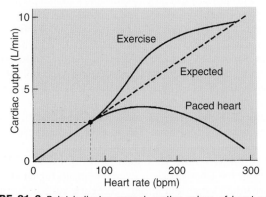

FIGURE 21-6 Point indicates normal, resting values of heart rate (80 beats/min) and cardiac output (2.4 L/min) for a dog. *Dashed line* shows the expected increase in cardiac output in proportion to increases in heart rate (assuming stroke volume remains constant). However, if the heart is paced to higher and higher rates, the observed increase in cardiac output is less than expected because stroke volume decreases *(lower solid line)*. In contrast, when a dog increases its own heart rate through sympathetic activation (e.g., during exercise), cardiac output increases even more than expected because stroke volume increases *(upper solid line)*.

mentioned earlier, is that increasing heart rate reduces diastolic filling time. The resulting reduction in end-diastolic volume reduces stroke volume, so cardiac output does not increase in proportion to heart rate (see Figure 21-6, *lower solid line*). In fact, at heart rates greater than about 160 beats/min, stroke volume decreases so much that cardiac output actually declines with further increases in heart rate. This problem was encountered when early versions of artificial cardiac pacemakers malfunctioned in ways that caused high ventricular rates. Decreases in stroke volume at high heart rates are also encountered in certain cardiac arrhythmias. In *paroxysmal atrial tachycardia,* for example, a rapid heart rate is originated by an ectopic atrial pacemaker. The tachycardia occurs typically in bursts or paroxysms. The high heart rate limits diastolic filling so much that cardiac output falls below normal. This causes the blood pressure to fall so low that the patient becomes lethargic and may even faint.

Although cardiac pacing does not cause a large increase in cardiac output, increases in heart rate in the course of normal daily activities are accompanied by substantial increases in cardiac output. An example is the increase in cardiac output that normally accompanies exercise. As shown in Figure 21-6 (*upper solid line),* the actual increase in cardiac output during progressively more intense exercise is even greater than would be expected on the basis of the associated increase in heart rate. The reason that cardiac output increases so much during exercise is that stroke volume also increases. During exercise, increases in heart rate are brought about by increases in sympathetic activity. This sympathetic activation also increases cardiac contractility, so the ventricles empty more completely with each beat. In addition, sympathetic activation shortens the duration of systole, which helps to preserve diastolic filling time. In summary, under sympathetic action, the heart not only contracts more frequently (increased rate) and more forcefully (increased contractility), but also contracts and relaxes more quickly (helping to preserve diastolic filling time).

Figure 21-7 illustrates how the shortening of systole helps to preserve diastolic filling time. When heart rate is 60 beats/min, each beat takes 1 second. This 1 second must include one systole and one diastole. Typically, systole lasts about ⅓ second, which leaves ⅔ second (plenty of time) for diastolic filling. If heart rate is increased to 120 beats/min, each beat lasts only ½ second. If systole remains at ⅓ second, there is only ⅙ second left for diastolic filling (not enough time). However, if the increase in heart rate occurs because of an increase in sympathetic activity, systole becomes shorter, which restores part of the lost diastolic filling time. Diastole is shorter under these conditions than at rest, but it is longer than it would have been if systole were not shortened. Thus, sympathetic activation is said to help preserve the diastolic filling time. Overall, sympathetic activation (especially when coupled with a decrease in parasympathetic activity) can dramatically increase cardiac output (Table 21-1).

It is useful at this point to review the control of cardiac output, as summarized in Figure 21-2. Cardiac output is determined by stroke volume and heart rate. Stroke volume is determined by end-diastolic volume and end-systolic volume. End-diastolic volume depends on preload, ventricular compliance, and diastolic filling time. End-systolic volume depends on contractility and, to a lesser extent, on arterial pressure or afterload (not shown in Figure 21-2). Sympathetic activation increases contractility. Heart failure decreases contractility, as do several drugs often used in veterinary practice. Increased heart rate acts directly to increase cardiac output, but it also decreases diastolic filling time,

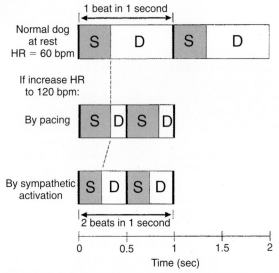

FIGURE 21-7 How shortening of systole (by sympathetic activation) helps to preserve diastolic filling time. *Top,* In this example, a large dog is resting very quietly with a heart rate *(HR)* of 60 beats per minute *(bpm)*. Systole *(S)* takes about one-third second, leaving two thirds of each beat for diastole *(D)* and filling. *Middle,* If HR is increased to 120 bpm by an artificial pacemaker, the duration of systole is unchanged, so diastolic duration (filling time) is greatly reduced. *Bottom,* If the same increase in heart rate is brought about by sympathetic activation, systole becomes shorter, which restores part of the lost diastolic filling time.

TABLE 21-1 Typical Cardiac Changes During Vigorous Exercise in a Large Dog

Measurement	Rest	Exercise
Ventricular end-diastolic volume (mL)	60	55
Ventricular end-systolic volume (mL)	30	15
Stroke volume (mL)	30	40
Ejection fraction (%)	50	73
Heart rate (beats/min)	80	240
Cardiac output (L/min)	2.4	9.6

which compromises the increased cardiac output. Heart rate is increased by sympathetic activation and parasympathetic withdrawal. Sympathetic activation also shortens systolic duration, which helps to preserve diastolic filling time. The aggregate effects of sympathetic activation on the heart are made evident by comparing cardiac function in a normal dog during rest and vigorous exercise (see Table 21-1).

Murmurs Are Abnormal Heart Sounds Caused By Turbulent Flow Through Cardiac Defects

Cardiac murmurs are abnormal heart sounds, and they often indicate the presence of cardiac abnormalities. Some murmurs are exaggerations of normal heart sounds; others are additional ("extra") heart sounds. Murmurs are caused by turbulent flow through cardiac defects. The underlying physical principle is that *laminar* or *smooth flow* of blood through the heart or blood vessels is quiet, whereas *turbulent flow* is noisy. An analogy is that a river does not make any sound as it flows smoothly through a

TABLE 21-2 Cardiac Valve Defects and Resulting Murmurs

Site of Defect	Nature of Defect	
	Incompetence or Insufficiency (Allows Regurgitation)	Stenosis (Narrow Valve Opening, Creates Restriction)
Atrioventricular valves	Systolic murmur	Diastolic murmur
Aortic or pulmonic valves	Diastolic murmur	Systolic murmur

broad, relatively flat channel. If the same river enters a channel that is restricted or drops steeply, a rapid or cataract forms. The flow becomes turbulent, and the turbulent flow makes noise.

The flow of blood through the heart and blood vessels is normally smooth, and therefore quiet, during the majority of the cardiac cycle. A moment of turbulent flow normally occurs at the beginning of ventricular contraction, on closure of the AV valves. A second moment of turbulent flow occurs at the end of ventricular systole, when the aortic and pulmonic valves close. The momentary turbulence and vibration associated with valve closure create the first and second heart sounds (S1 and S2) as discussed previously and as illustrated in Figure 21-1. On occasion (particularly in large animals), normal third and fourth heart sounds are faintly audible with the stethoscope, during rapid ventricular filling (S3) or during atrial systole (S4). In comparison, clinically important murmurs are louder and usually persist through a greater portion of the cardiac cycle. Sometimes, murmurs are even louder than the normal first and second heart sounds.

Table 21-2 lists cardiac valve defects that cause additional instances of turbulent flow and therefore murmurs. The table also indicates the timing of the murmurs in relation to the cardiac cycle. *Systolic murmurs* occur during ventricular systole; *diastolic murmurs* occur during ventricular diastole. *Continuous murmurs* occur throughout both systole and diastole. The timing of each murmur is easy to understand if two basic principles are kept in mind: murmurs are caused by turbulent blood flow, and blood flows in response to pressure differences. In other words, turbulent (noisy) flow through a cardiac defect occurs only if there is a substantial pressure difference from one side of the defect to the other.

Figure 21-8 indicates how these principles can be used to account for systolic murmurs. The numbers in the figure indicate the maximum pressures that normally exist in each cardiac chamber during ventricular systole. Note, for example, that the pressure in the left ventricle is normally much higher than the pressure in the left atrium during ventricular systole. The mitral valve is normally closed during ventricular systole, so no blood flows backward from the ventricle to the left atrium. If the mitral valve fails to close completely during ventricular systole, the large pressure difference between the left ventricle and the left atrium causes a rapid, backward flow of blood through the partially closed valve. This turbulent backflow creates a systolic murmur. A mitral valve that fails to close completely is said to be *insufficient* or *incompetent*. The backflow across the valve is called

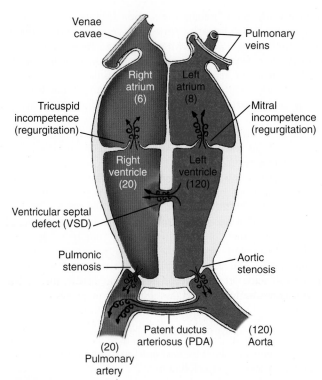

FIGURE 21-8 Schematic view of the heart showing cardiac defects that cause systolic murmurs. The *numbers in parentheses* indicate normal maximum pressures (mm Hg) during ventricular systole. The *swirled arrows* indicate the sites of turbulent (noisy) flow. See text for details.

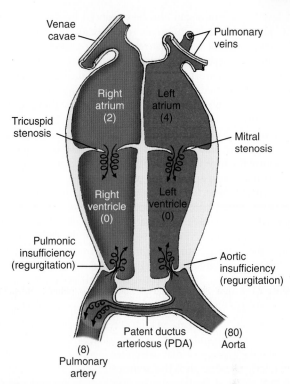

FIGURE 21-9 Cardiac defects that cause diastolic murmurs. The *numbers in parentheses* indicate normal minimum pressures (mm Hg) during ventricular diastole. The *swirled arrows* indicate the sites of turbulent (noisy) flow. See text for details.

regurgitation. Mitral regurgitation is present in about 8% of dogs over 5 years of age.

A *ventricular septal defect* (VSD) is a hole or cleft in the interventricular septum. Blood flows through a VSD from the left ventricle to the right ventricle during ventricular systole because systolic pressure is much higher in the left ventricle than in the right ventricle. Typically, the flow of blood through a VSD is turbulent, and a systolic murmur is created.

Systolic turbulence is also created if the aortic valve does not open widely enough. Blood ejected from the ventricle accelerates to a high velocity as it squeezes through the restricted aortic opening, and turbulence occurs. A valve that fails to open widely enough is called *stenotic;* the defect of *aortic stenosis* produces a systolic murmur. Likewise, *pulmonic stenosis* causes a systolic murmur. Aortic and pulmonic stenosis are common congenital defects in dogs.

A *patent ductus arteriosus* (PDA) is persistence after birth of the opening between the aorta and the pulmonary artery (see Chapter 51). A PDA produces a murmur during systole because the pressure in the aorta is much higher than the pressure in the pulmonary artery. Blood flows from the aorta into the pulmonary artery, and turbulence occurs. The murmur of a PDA is not restricted to systole, however, because the aortic pressure remains higher than the pulmonary artery pressure throughout diastole as well. Therefore the murmur of PDA is heard in both systole and diastole and is thus a *continuous murmur.* It is also called a *machinery murmur* because it characteristically sounds like the rumble of machinery. PDA is common in young dogs, especially females.

The site on the thorax from which a particular murmur can be heard *(auscultated)* best is often indicative of the particular

location and type of defect that causes the murmur. For example, the murmur of PDA is characteristically heard best over the left heart base. Occasionally, the turbulence caused by a cardiac defect will be so extreme as to cause a palpable thoracic vibration *(thrill).*

Animals sometimes have open pathways for blood flow between peripheral arteries and peripheral veins. These openings are called *arteriovenous fistulae.* Arteriovenous fistulae carry flow (and create turbulence) during both systole and diastole and therefore create continuous murmurs. The murmur of an arteriovenous fistula is most audible at the body surface close to the point of the fistula.

The numerical values in Figure 21-9 correspond to the minimum pressures that normally exist in the various cardiac chambers during ventricular diastole. These pressures form the basis for understanding why certain cardiac defects chacteristically produce diastolic murmurs. For example, a normal mitral valve opens widely during ventricular diastole, which creates a low-resistance pathway for blood to flow from the left atrium into the left ventricle. However, if the mitral valve fails to open widely *(mitral stenosis),* ventricular filling must occur through a stenotic (narrow) valve. This creates turbulent flow and a diastolic murmur. Mitral stenosis is a common murmur among humans who have developed calcification of the mitral valve as a result of rheumatic heart disease.

During diastole the normal aortic valve is closed, and no blood flows backward from the aorta into the left ventricle. If the aortic valve does not close tightly, blood flows backward (regurgitates) from the aorta to the left ventricle during diastole. Therefore, *aortic regurgitation* produces a diastolic murmur. The defect is called *aortic incompetence* or *aortic insufficiency.* Aortic regurgitation is common in horses but not in dogs.

Diastolic murmurs can also be produced by defects on the right side of the heart. Pulmonic regurgitation produces a diastolic murmur, but it is relatively rare. Tricuspid stenosis is uncommon, at least as a congenital defect. However, a heavy infestation of heartworms in the right side of the heart can create a stenosis at the tricuspid valve and a diastolic murmur.

Cardiac murmurs themselves are not harmful. They are clinically important, however, because the defects that cause the murmurs also have pathophysiological consequences. Cardiac defects typically lead to one or more of these consequences: (1) abnormally high or low blood flow to a region of the body, (2) abnormally high or low blood pressure in a region of the body, and (3) *cardiac hypertrophy* (enlargement of cardiac muscle).

It is not difficult to understand why cardiac defects lead to abnormal blood flows or abnormal blood pressures. For example, in the presence of a ventricular septal defect, the right ventricle receives blood from both the right atrium and the left ventricle, which leads to an abnormally high blood flow through the pulmonary circulation. In the presence of aortic stenosis, the left ventricle must generate an abnormally high systolic pressure to eject blood through the narrow valve opening. In the presence of mitral stenosis, blood dams up (and excessive pressure builds up) in the left atrium and pulmonary veins. It is more difficult to understand why some cardiac defects lead to cardiac hypertrophy. The underlying principle is that some cardiac defects increase the workload of one or both ventricles, and an increase in the workload of cardiac muscle leads to hypertrophy. Developing this concept more fully requires an understanding of cardiac energetics, as described next.

Some Cardiac Defects Increase the Heart's Workload, Which Causes Cardiac Hypertrophy

Cardiac defects often compromise the heart's ability to supply the systemic organs with the blood flow they need to support their metabolism. Compensating for such a *pump failure* frequently requires one or both ventricles to pump more blood than normal or to pump blood at a higher pressure than normal. These adaptations increase the workload of the heart. A persistent increase in cardiac workload leads, over several weeks, to cardiac hypertrophy. A ventricle that must pump more blood volume than normal will develop some hypertrophy, whereas a ventricle that must pump blood at a higher pressure than normal develops a huge hypertrophy. This observation is the basis for the clinical aphorism, "Pressure work is harder for the heart [i.e., causes more hypertrophy] than volume work." To understand the physiological reason of this difference, we must delve into cardiac muscle energetics. To get started, it is useful to consider the analogous case of skeletal muscle hypertrophy in response to increased workload (physical conditioning).

A skeletal muscle does work by exerting a force while shortening. The useful mechanical work *(external work)* done by a skeletal muscle is equal to the force developed by the contracting muscle, multiplied by the distance moved during one contraction, multiplied by the number of contractions (that is, work equals force multiplied by distance). Therefore, the external work done by a skeletal muscle can be increased by increasing the forcefulness of contraction, the distance moved, or the number of contractions. In weight lifting conditioning the emphasis is on performing a few very forceful contractions of skeletal muscle. In contrast, conditioning that involves repetitive, low-force contractions of skeletal muscle (e.g., running, swimming) emphasizes primarily the distance and duration components of skeletal

muscle work. Both "weight work" and "distance work" lead to skeletal muscle hypertrophy. However, a common observation is that weight work causes substantially more hypertrophy than does distance work. The basis for this difference is that weight work involves the generation of huge amounts of *internal work (wasted work)*, which appears as heat. This large expenditure of energy on internal work greatly increases the *total work* (external work plus internal work) being done during weight lifting as compared to distance running. It is the increase in total work of muscle, not just the external work, that is the primary stimulus for hypertrophy.

The heart does work by pumping blood. The useful mechanical work (external work) done by any pump is equal to the pressure generated by the pump, multiplied by the volume of fluid that is pumped in one pump stroke, multiplied by the number of pump strokes. Therefore the external work done by the left ventricle in 1 minute is equal to the pressure generated, multiplied by the stroke volume, multiplied by the heart rate. The pressure generated by the left ventricle can be approximated by the average (mean) pressure in the aorta, as follows:

Minute work of left ventricle =
Mean aortic pressure × Stroke volume × Heart rate

The external work done by the ventricle in one cardiac cycle is called the *stroke work*, as follows:

Stroke work of left ventricle =
Mean aortic pressure × Stroke volume

(The work of the right ventricle can be calculated in a similar way, but using mean pulmonary artery pressure.)

In accordance with the analogy to skeletal muscle conditioning, the average aortic pressure is analogous to the force developed by the contracting skeletal muscle; the stroke volume is analogous to the distance moved during one contraction; and the heart rate is analogous to the number of contractions. Obviously, the external work done by the left ventricle could be increased by increasing the pressure that the left ventricle generates, by increasing the stroke volume, or by increasing the heart rate. For example, a 50% increase in ventricular work can result from a 50% increase in the left ventricular pressure, a 50% increase in the left ventricular stroke volume, or a 50% increase in the heart rate. Any of these changes results, over a period of weeks, in left ventricular hypertrophy. However, an increase in the ventricular pressure causes a much more pronounced hypertrophy than does an increase in the stroke volume or heart rate. The basis for this difference is that increasing the pressure involves the generation of much more *internal work (wasted work)*, which appears as heat. This large expenditure of energy on internal work greatly increases the *total work* (external work plus internal work) being done by cardiac muscle. It is the total work of the cardiac muscle, not just the external work, that is the primary stimulus for hypertrophy.

Under normal resting conditions, about 85% of the metabolic energy consumed by the heart appears as heat, and only 15% appears as external work. A physicist would say that the heart has a "thermodynamic efficiency" of about 15%. However, the "cardiac efficiency" depends on the type of work being done by the ventricles. The heart becomes less efficient when the external work is increased by increasing the pressure. Conversely, the heart becomes more efficient when the external work is increased by an increase in the volume of blood pumped.

The dominant role of pressure in determining total ventricular energy consumption is evident from a comparison of the work done by the left and right ventricles. The stroke volume and heart rate are equivalent for the left and right ventricles, but the pressure generated is about five times higher in the left ventricle than in the right (mean aortic pressure is about five times higher than mean pulmonary artery pressure). Therefore the external work done by the left ventricle is approximately five times greater than the external work done by the right ventricle. However, the total metabolic energy consumption of the left ventricle is much more than five times greater than the energy consumption of the right ventricle, because the extra external work performed by the left ventricle is in the form of greater pressure. Consequently, the internal (wasted) work of the left ventricle is hugely greater than the internal (wasted) work of the right ventricle. Therefore, almost all the energy consumed by the heart is consumed by the left ventricle; almost all the coronary blood flow is delivered to the left ventricular muscle, and almost all the oxygen consumed by the heart is consumed by the left ventricle. Because of the high amount of pressure work done by the left ventricle compared with the right ventricle, the left ventricle develops much heavier and thicker muscle walls than the right ventricle.

A clinical observation from human medicine provides a further illustration of how an increase in the ventricular pressure work leads to ventricular hypertrophy. About 20% of adult humans have hypertension. In most of these patients, cardiac output is normal. Their arterial blood pressure is elevated because of an increased resistance to blood flow in the systemic arterioles. An elevated left ventricular pressure is required to force the cardiac output through these constricted systemic arterioles. The increased pressure work done by the left ventricle in hypertensive patients results in a striking left ventricular hypertrophy.

Up to a point, ventricular hypertrophy is an appropriate and beneficial adaptation to an increased workload imposed on the ventricular muscle. However, excessive hypertrophy is deleterious for three reasons. First, enlargement of the ventricular muscle restricts the opening of the aortic valve (or pulmonic valve, in the case of right ventricular hypertrophy). A vicious cycle develops. Ventricular hypertrophy leads to aortic or pulmonic stenosis, which necessitates that the ventricle generate an even greater systolic pressure to eject blood, which leads to more ventricular hypertrophy, and so on. A second complication of excessive hypertrophy is that the coronary circulation may be unable to provide enough blood flow to meet the increased metabolic demand of the massive ventricular muscle, particularly during exercise. Inadequate coronary blood flow is especially likely if the coronary vessels have become constricted because of coronary artery disease (atherosclerosis). As a result, patients with ventricular hypertrophy and coronary artery disease are at high risk for cardiac ischemia, myocardial infarction, ventricular arrhythmias, and sudden death during periods of exercise. This explains why the all-too-common combination of hypertension and coronary artery disease is such a serious problem in human medicine. Fortunately, coronary artery disease is rare in most animals. The third complication of cardiac hypertrophy is that the cellular growth factors that mediate the hypertrophy also predispose the cardiac muscle to apoptosis.

The Pathophysiological Consequences of Cardiac Defects Are Direct Results of the Abnormal Pressures, Volumes, and Workloads Created in the Cardiac Chambers

Figure 21-10 summarizes the consequences associated with some common cardiac defects. First, consider *mitral regurgitation*. With each contraction of the left ventricle, a normal volume of

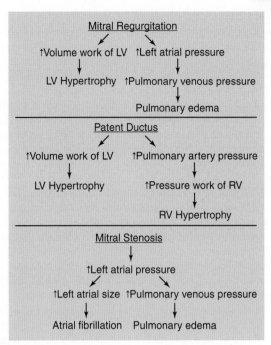

FIGURE 21-10 Pathophysiological consequences of several common cardiac defects. *LV,* Left ventricle; *RV,* right ventricle.

blood is ejected into the aorta, and an additional volume of blood is ejected backward (through the regurgitant valve) into the left atrium. As a result, there is an increase in the volume work performed by the left ventricle. Therefore, mild to moderate left ventricular hypertrophy develops. Also, in a heart with mitral regurgitation, the left atrium becomes distended, and left atrial pressure increases, as does pulmonary venous pressure. Elevated pressure in the pulmonary blood vessels forces water and electrolytes out of the bloodstream and into the pulmonary interstitial spaces, causing *pulmonary edema.* When left atrial pressures exceed about 20 mm Hg, pulmonary edema becomes so severe that the lungs' ability to transfer oxygen into the bloodstream is substantially reduced. The result is respiratory distress.

The consequences of mitral regurgitation are usually more noticeable during exercise than during rest. One reason is that despite the regurgitation, the left ventricle can usually adapt enough through hypertrophy and an increase in heart rate to maintain a normal cardiac output into the aorta (and therefore into the systemic circulation) at rest. Also, despite some pulmonary edema, the oxygenation of the blood is sufficient to meet the animal's needs during rest. During exercise, however, the output of the left ventricle into the systemic circulation must increase several-fold to supply adequate blood to exercising skeletal muscle. Also, the delivery of oxygen into the blood must increase several-fold. Despite the hypertrophy, the left ventricle may not be able to deliver adequate blood flow to the systemic circulation during exercise if mitral regurgitation is serious. Also, pulmonary edema may prevent delivery of enough oxygen into the blood to support the metabolism of the exercising animal.

Consider next the abnormalities associated with *aortic stenosis* (not shown in Figure 21-10). To eject a normal volume of blood with each beat through a stenotic aortic valve, the left ventricle must develop an abnormally high systolic pressure. This increases the pressure work of the left ventricle, which leads to a marked left ventricular hypertrophy. The hypertrophy has the desirable effect of increasing the contractility of the left ventricular muscle so that it can generate the increased pressure required to maintain normal cardiac output. As hypertrophy progresses, however, the ventricular muscle begins to impinge on the aortic outflow pathway, which further hampers the ability of the ventricle to eject blood. In a sense, the hypertrophic ventricular muscle "gets in its own way" or becomes muscle bound. The resulting limitation in aortic outflow is much more likely to be a problem during exercise than at rest. A patient with aortic stenosis may be able to function normally at rest but characteristically exhibits exercise intolerance.

Patent ductus arteriosus (PDA) is a defect that typically results in both left and right ventricular hypertrophy (Figure 21-10). In a typical patient with a PDA, the left ventricle pumps a near-normal volume of blood per minute to the systemic circulation and pumps two to three times that volume of blood per minute through the PDA. As a result, the volume work done by the left ventricle greatly exceeds normal amounts, which leads to left ventricular hypertrophy. The blood flowing through the PDA enters the pulmonary artery, and thus pulmonary arterial pressure exceeds normal levels. This in turn increases the pressure work that must be done by the right ventricle. The right ventricle receives a near-normal volume of blood back from the systemic circulation each minute, and the right ventricle must generate an elevated systolic pressure to eject this blood into the high-pressure pulmonary artery. The increased pressure work for the right ventricle is a powerful stimulus for hypertrophy, and pronounced right ventricular hypertrophy develops.

As a patient with PDA grows, exercise intolerance becomes evident. Despite hypertrophy, the left ventricle cannot supply both the increased blood flow needed by growing, exercising skeletal muscles, and also the blood that flows through the PDA. In patients with PDA the pulmonary artery and the pulmonary blood vessels must carry not only the blood that is pumped by the right ventricle (as in a normal animal), but also the blood that is pumped through the PDA. In a severe case, pulmonary blood flow can be more than four times greater than normal. The resulting increases in pulmonary vascular pressure can lead to pulmonary edema. Surgical repair of a PDA in a young animal leads to a rapid reversal of all these cardiovascular and pulmonary abnormalities.

An understanding of the preceding examples should make it easy to predict the pathological consequences of a *ventricular septal defect*. These consequences include increased volume work of the left ventricle, moderate left ventricular hypertrophy, increased volume and pressure work of the right ventricle, pronounced right ventricular hypertrophy, increased blood flow through the lungs, possible pulmonary edema, and probable exercise intolerance. It should also be clear why pulmonic stenosis leads to increased pressure work for the right ventricle and pronounced right ventricular hypertrophy (see Clinical Correlations).

Figure 21-10 also summarizes the pathological consequences associated with the diastolic murmur of *mitral stenosis*. The left atrial pressure must exceed normal levels to force a normal volume of blood through the stenotic mitral valve and into the left ventricle during each ventricular diastole. The elevated left atrial pressure distends the left atrium. There may be some hypertrophy of the atrial muscle. The atrium continues to function, however, mainly as a reservoir to collect and hold blood during ventricular systole, rather than as a pumping chamber to force blood into the ventricle during its diastole. One problem is that atrial action potentials tend to become discoordinated in a distended atrium, and atrial fibrillation is a common consequence.

Also, the increase in the left atrial pressure causes blood to back up and accumulate in the pulmonary blood vessels, so pulmonary edema is likely. It might seem that the backup of blood in the pulmonary vessels would eventually also increase the pressure in the pulmonary artery and thereby increase the pressure work of the right ventricle. In other words, mitral stenosis might be predicted to lead to right ventricular hypertrophy. This prediction is logical, but in practice, animals with greatly elevated left atrial pressures usually die from the effects of pulmonary edema before right ventricular pressures have had a chance to become high enough to induce right ventricular hypertrophy. Therefore, mitral stenosis does not generally lead to hypertrophy of either ventricle.

The defect of *aortic regurgitation* leads to left ventricular hypertrophy. With each systole, the left ventricle must eject an abnormally large volume of blood into the aorta. Of this, a normal volume of blood goes on into the systemic circuit; the rest is simply regurgitated back from the aorta into the left ventricle during diastole. Thus the volume work of the left ventricle is increased to above-normal levels, and left ventricular pressures may rise as well. Both these factors stimulate left ventricular hypertrophy. In severe cases of aortic regurgitation, diastolic ventricular pressure becomes elevated (because during diastole the left ventricle receives blood from both the left atrium and the aorta). This leads to increases in left atrial pressure, and pulmonary edema may develop.

Consideration of the abnormalities associated with cardiac defects is important for two reasons. First, these defects and their consequences are often encountered in veterinary medicine. Second, this discussion illustrates how the clinical signs and consequences of disease states can be understood and predicted in a rational way, on the basis of an understanding of basic principles of cardiac physiology.

CLINICAL CORRELATIONS

PULMONIC STENOSIS

History. A 6-month-old female schnauzer is referred to your clinic because of a heart murmur that was detected during a routine health care visit. The puppy is fairly active but is slightly smaller than her female littermates. She also tires more quickly than her littermates when they play together.

Clinical Examination. All physical parameters are normal except for a systolic heart murmur that can be heard best over the left third to fourth intercostal space. Femoral pulses are normal, and the jugular veins are not distended. Electrocardiography reveals that the dog is in normal sinus rhythm with a heart rate of 118 beats/min. The PR interval is normal. However, the major QRS deflection is negative in leads I and aV$_F$. Also, deep S waves are noted in leads II and III, and the QRS complexes are slightly prolonged as a result of the wide S waves. Thoracic radiographs show right ventricular enlargement; the right border of the cardiac silhouette is more rounded, and closer to the right thoracic wall, than normal.

A catheter is inserted into the jugular vein, and the following pressures are measured as the catheter is advanced through the right side of the heart and into the pulmonary artery: central venous pressure (mean right atrial pressure), 8 mm Hg (normal, 3 mm Hg); right ventricular systolic pressure, 122 mm Hg (normal, 20 mm Hg); and pulmonary artery systolic pressure, 16 mm Hg (normal, 20 mm Hg).

The jugular catheter is withdrawn until the catheter tip is in the right ventricle. Additional radiographs are then taken while a radiopaque dye is injected through the catheter. These radiographs reveal that the right ventricular outflow tract is narrowed just below the pulmonic valve and that the pulmonic valve does not open widely during ventricular systole.

Comment. The young age of this dog and the absence of other signs of illness suggest that the murmur results from a congenital cardiac abnormality. Murmurs are graded on a scale of I through VI, with VI being the most severe. This dog's murmur is graded IV. A systolic murmur can result from aortic or pulmonic stenosis, mitral or tricuspid regurgitation, or a ventricular septal defect (see Figure 21-8). On the basis of the location from which this murmur can be heard best, aortic or pulmonic stenosis is the most likely cause. All the additional clinical evidence supports a diagnosis of pulmonic stenosis.

The electrocardiogram indicates that the sinoatrial node is acting as the pacemaker and that the AV node is conducting each atrial action potential into the ventricles. However, the abnormalities observed in the polarities and shapes of the QRS complex are indicative of right ventricular hypertrophy, and the radiographs corroborate this finding. Pulmonic stenosis leads to right ventricular hypertrophy, because the right ventricle must generate much higher pressures than normal during systole in order to eject blood through the narrow outflow tract.

Normally, the pulmonic valve opens widely during systole, and the ventricular systolic pressure closely matches the pulmonary artery systolic pressure. In this dog, there is a difference of 106 mm Hg between right ventricular systolic pressure and the systolic pressure in the pulmonary artery just beyond the pulmonic valve. This difference indicates a severe pulmonic obstruction. The degree of obstruction can be visualized on the radiographs taken during dye injection.

Right ventricular hypertrophy is one of two adaptive responses that help this dog maintain a near-normal right ventricular stroke volume, despite the pulmonic stenosis. The other adaptive response is that the mean right atrial pressure is higher than normal (8 vs. 3 mm Hg). The right atrial pressure is elevated because blood backs up or accumulates in areas upstream from the stenosis (i.e., in the right ventricle, right atrium, and systemic veins). The elevated atrial pressure is adaptive because it increases the right ventricular preload, which increases the end-diastolic volume, which (according to Starling's law of the heart) helps keep the right ventricular stroke volume at a normal level, despite the stenosis. The right atrial pressure is not quite high enough in this dog to cause systemic edema or abdominal ascites (see Chapter 23). However, both these signs are sometimes seen in dogs with severe pulmonic stenosis because excessively elevated right atrial pressure leads to marked increases in blood pressure (hydrostatic pressure) within the systemic capillaries.

The combined effects of right ventricular hypertrophy and elevated right ventricular preload allow this dog's heart to pump a near-normal stroke volume during rest. However, the pulmonic obstruction limits the increase in the stroke volume that can occur during exercise. The resulting limitation in cardiac output accounts for this dog's lack of stamina during exercise. Over a prolonged period, such a limitation in cardiac output will likely stunt growth.

Treatment. Theoretically, the best treatment for pulmonic stenosis is to remove the obstruction surgically. A valve dilator can be used, or an artificial conduit can be installed across the stenotic valve. Although seriously affected dogs require such interventional treatment, dogs with mild to moderate pulmonic stenosis can lead sedentary lives without any treatment.

Some evidence indicates that the adverse effects of pulmonic stenosis can be minimized by the administration of β-adrenergic antagonists (e.g., propranolol) or calcium channel blockers (e.g., verapamil). Although the mechanism and efficacy of these drugs remain unclear, there is speculation that these drugs are beneficial because they limit ventricular contractility, which limits the work of the heart. Because an increase in cardiac work is the stimulus for hypertrophy, a drug that limits the increase in work also limits the hypertrophy. Although moderate hypertrophy can be adaptive (as explained earlier), excessive hypertrophy is detrimental for two reasons. First, the enlarged ventricular muscle can crowd the pulmonic outflow tract, worsening the stenosis. Second, the coronary circulation may be unable to deliver the increased amounts of blood flow required by the massive ventricular muscle.

OLDER HORSE WITH EXERCISE INTOLERANCE

History. A 22-year-old Thoroughbred mare is presented for exercise intolerance. The owner uses her for trail riding and some low-level eventing. The mare has had some mild arthritis during her career, but in the last 2 to 3 months she seems reluctant to work, takes longer to recover after rides, and seems lethargic. Vaccinations and deworming are current.

Clinical Examination. The mare appears to be slightly underweight. She is responsive but quiet (more quiet than normal, according to the owner). Her temperature is normal; pulse and respiration are slightly increased. Her mucous membranes are darker pink than normal (suggesting reduced blood flow), but capillary refill time is not abnormally long. She has a grade IV systolic murmur on the left side, most consistent with mitral regurgitation. Her lungs are normal on auscultation. No other abnormal findings are noted on physical examination. The mare is lunged for several minutes and reauscultated. No additional abnormalities are detected, except the mare's heart rate and respiratory rate seem to take longer than normal to return to their resting levels. A blood sample is taken for analysis.

Comment. Results of the complete blood count (CBC) and serum chemistry are within normal limits. Echocardiography reveals mitral regurgitation associated with fibrotic thickening of the mitral valve. The *chordae tendineae* are intact. There is some dilation (eccentric hypertrophy) of the left ventricle, but not of the left atrium.

Mitral valve thickening and insufficiency often develop with age, and mitral regurgitation is likely limiting this mare's left ventricular performance. The resulting tendency for inefficient pumping of blood into the systemic circulation can account for the decreased perfusion of the mucous membranes at rest and for the exercise intolerance and listlessness noticed by the owner. With each systolic contraction, the left ventricle is pumping blood both forward, into the aorta, and backward, through the leaky mitral valve and into the left atrium. The mild left ventricular hypertrophy and dilation are likely adaptive responses to this increased volume work. Animals with more severe mitral regurgitation also have left atrial dilation, associated with a much poorer prognosis than if there is no dilation or only left ventricular dilation.

Treatment. No medical treatment is indicated at this time. However, the owner needs to decrease the work by the mare. The mare should have only light, non-stressful activity. A follow-up examination is recommended in 3 to 6 months to assess the rate of progression of the mitral valve disease. If marked progression is noted at that time, the mare should be retired.

PRACTICE QUESTIONS

1. In the normal cardiac cycle:
   a. Ventricular systole and ventricular ejection begin at the same time.
   b. The second heart sound coincides with the beginning of isovolumetric relaxation.
   c. The highest left ventricular pressure is reached just as the aortic valve closes.
   d. Aortic pressure is highest at the beginning of ventricular systole.
   e. Atrial systole occurs during rapid ventricular ejection.

2. Figure 21-11 shows a plot of the changes in pressure and volume that occur in the left ventricle during one cardiac cycle. Which of the following is *true*?
   a. Point D marks the beginning of isovolumetric relaxation.
   b. Point B marks the closure of the aortic valve.
   c. Point C marks the opening of the mitral valve.
   d. Point A marks the beginning of isovolumetric contraction.
   e. Point D marks the beginning of ventricular systole.

3. Which statement is *true* for a normal heart?
   a. Sympathetic activation causes end-systolic ventricular volume to increase.
   b. An increase in ventricular preload causes end-diastolic ventricular volume to decrease.
   c. An increase in ventricular contractility causes systolic duration to increase.
   d. An increase in ventricular contractility causes the external work of the heart to decrease.
   e. Pacing the heart at a high rate causes stroke volume to decrease.

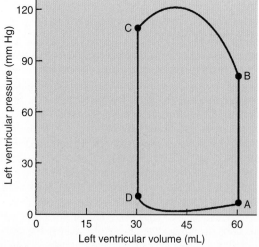

FIGURE 21-11 Closed loop depicts the changes in left ventricular pressure and volume that occur during one cardiac cycle. Practice Question 2 is based on this graph. The first step in understanding the figure is to determine whether the normal sequence of events proceeds clockwise or counterclockwise around the loop. To make this distinction, recall that the ventricles fill when ventricular pressure is low and they empty when ventricular pressure is high. Next, identify the phases of the cardiac cycle that correspond with each limb of the loop. Finally, determine what happens to the mitral and aortic valves at each corner of the loop. *Hint: A, B, C,* and *D* in this figure match the similarly labeled points in Figure 21-1 (on the graph of *ventricular pressure*).

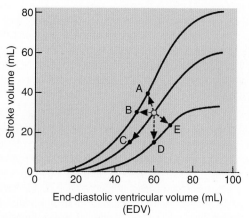

FIGURE 21-12 Practice Question 4 is based on this graph of three ventricular function curves.

4. Starting at the open circle in Figure 21-12, which point would be reached after the contractility decreased and the preload increased?
   a. Point A
   b. Point B
   c. Point C
   d. Point D
   e. Point E

5. You examine a 7-year-old poodle and find evidence of a systolic murmur (no diastolic murmur), pulmonary edema (indicated by rapid, noisy respiration and cough), left ventricular hypertrophy (no right ventricular hypertrophy), and exercise intolerance. The most likely explanation for the symptoms is:
   a. Mitral regurgitation.
   b. Mitral stenosis.
   c. Aortic regurgitation.
   d. Pulmonic stenosis.
   e. Ventricular septal defect.

BIBLIOGRAPHY

Boron WF, Boulpaep EL: *Medical physiology*, ed 2, Philadelphia, 2009, Saunders.

Ettinger SJ, Feldman EC: *Textbook of veterinary internal medicine: diseases of the dog and cat*, ed 7, St Louis, 2010, Elsevier/Saunders.

Hall JE: *Guyton and Hall textbook of medical physiology*, ed 12, Philadelphia, 2011, Saunders.

Katz AM: *Physiology of the heart*, ed 5, Baltimore, 2010, Lippincott, Williams & Wilkins.

Koeppen BM, Stanton BA: *Berne & Levy physiology*, ed 6, Philadelphia, 2010, Mosby.

Levy MN, Pappano AJ: *Cardiovascular physiology*, ed 9, St Louis, 2007, Mosby.

Marr C, Bowen M, editors: Cardiology of the horse, ed 2, Philadelphia, 2011, Saunders.

Smith FWK Jr, Keene BW, Tilley LP: *Rapid interpretation of heart and lung sounds: a guide to cardiac and respiratory auscultation in dogs and cats*, ed 2, St Louis, 2006, Saunders.

Tilley LP, Smith FWK, Oyama M, et al: *Manual of canine and feline cardiology*, ed 4, Philadelphia, 2008, Saunders.

CHAPTER 22

The Systemic and Pulmonary Circulations

KEY POINTS

1. Blood pressure represents a potential energy that propels blood through the circulation.
2. Vascular resistance is defined as perfusion pressure divided by flow.
3. The net resistance of the systemic circulation is called the *total peripheral resistance*.
4. Arterial pressure is determined by the cardiac output and the total peripheral resistance.
5. Blood flow to each organ is determined by perfusion pressure and by the organ's vascular resistance.

6. The pulmonary circulation offers much less resistance to blood flow than does the systemic circulation.
7. Arterial pressures are measured in terms of systolic, diastolic, and mean levels.
8. Pulse pressure increases when the stroke volume increases, heart rate decreases, aortic compliance decreases, or total peripheral resistance increases.

Blood Pressure Represents a Potential Energy That Propels Blood Through the Circulation

The *systemic circulation* has the aorta as its inlet point and the *venae cavae* as its outlet. The remainder of the circulation (i.e., right heart, pulmonary circuit, and left heart) is, by definition, the *central circulation*. Blood enters the central circulation from the *venae cavae* and leaves the central circulation through the aorta.

Figure 22-1 shows the normal pressure profile in the systemic circulation. This figure portrays the pressures that would be measured if a miniature pressure gauge were inserted into the various vessels that blood passes through in its journey through the systemic circulation. The blood pressure is highest in the aorta (typically, mean aortic pressure is 98 mm Hg) and lowest in the *venae cavae* (typically, 3 mm Hg). The difference between these pressures (i.e., 95 mm Hg) constitutes the driving force for the movement of blood, by bulk flow, through the systemic circulation. As discussed in Chapter 18, such a pressure difference between the inlet and outlet of a tube (or system of tubes) is called *perfusion pressure difference* (or more commonly, just *perfusion pressure*).

Aortic blood pressure can be thought of as the potential energy available to move blood; the decrease in pressure in the sequential segments of the systemic circuit represents the amount of this potential energy that is "used up" in moving blood through each segment. Pressure energy is used up through *friction,* which is generated as the molecules and cells of blood rub against each other and against the walls of the blood vessels. The energy used up through friction is converted to heat, although the actual increase in the temperature of the blood and blood vessels as a result of friction is very small.

The amount of the blood pressure energy used up in each of the sequential segments of the systemic circulation depends on the amount of friction or resistance that the blood encounters. The aorta and large arteries offer very little resistance to blood flow (very little friction), so the blood pressure decreases only a little in these vessels (from 98 to about 95 mm Hg). The greatest

pressure decrease (greatest loss of pressure energy through friction) occurs as blood flows through arterioles; that is, the resistance to blood flow is greater in the arterioles than in any other segment of the systemic circulation. The capillaries and the venules offer a substantial resistance to blood flow, but the resistance (and therefore the pressure decrease) is not as great in these vessels as it is in the arterioles. The large veins and the *venae cavae* are low-resistance vessels, so little pressure energy is expended in driving the blood flow through these vessels.

The pumping of blood by the heart maintains the pressure difference between the aorta and the *venae cavae*. If the heart stops, blood continues to flow for a few moments from the aorta toward the *venae cavae*. As this blood leaves the aorta, the aortic walls become less distended, and the blood pressure inside the aorta decreases. As extra blood accumulates in the *venae cavae,* they become more distended than before, and the blood pressure inside the *venae cavae* increases. Soon, there is no pressure difference between the aorta and the *venae cavae*. Blood flow in the systemic circuit ceases, and the pressure everywhere in the systemic circulation is the same. It has been demonstrated experimentally that this eventual pressure is about 7 mm Hg. This pressure, in a static circulation, is called the *mean circulatory filling pressure*. The mean circulatory filling pressure is greater than zero (i.e., above atmospheric pressure), because there is a "fullness" to the circulation; that is, even if the heart stops, blood still distends the vessels that contain it. The vessel walls, being elastic, recoil ("push back") against this distention, which accounts for the persistence of pressure in the circulation even if the heart stops. If a transfusion of blood is administered to an animal with the heart stopped, the vessels become more distended, and the mean circulating filling pressure rises above 7 mm Hg. Conversely, if blood is removed from an animal with the heart stopped, the pressure everywhere falls to a level below 7 mm Hg.

Consider what happens if the heart is restarted in an animal after the pressure has equalized everywhere at 7 mm Hg. With

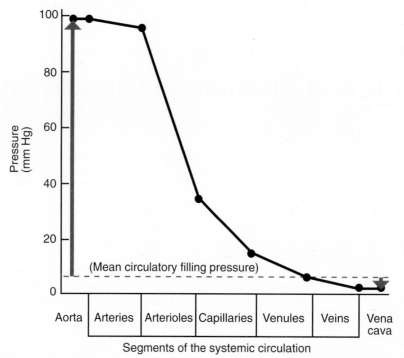

FIGURE 22-1 Graph of the blood pressures (hydrostatic pressures) that typically exist in the systemic circulation of a dog at rest *(solid black line)*. The blood pressure in the aorta and arteries is actually pulsatile, increasing with each cardiac ejection and falling between ejections. The values plotted here are the average (mean) values of those pulsatile pressures. Mean circulatory filling pressure *(dashed red line)* is the pressure that would persist throughout the systemic circulation if the heart were stopped. *Red arrows* show the contrasting directions and magnitudes of the pressure changes that would occur in the aorta and *venae cavae* if a stopped heart were restarted and cardiac output returned to normal (see text for details). All pressures are measured at heart level, with reference to atmospheric pressure (taken as zero).

each heartbeat, the heart takes some blood out of the *venae cavae* and this volume of blood is transferred (via the pulmonary circulation) into the aorta. The volume of blood in the *venae cavae* decreases, so the *venae cavae* become less distended and vena caval pressure drops below 7 mm Hg. The volume of blood in the aorta increases, so the aorta becomes more distended and aortic pressure rises above 7 mm Hg. As illustrated in Figure 22-1, the vena caval pressure drops about 4 mm Hg (from 7 to 3 mm Hg), and the aortic pressure rises about 91 mm Hg (from 7 to 98 mm Hg). It is important to understand why the pressure decreases only a little in the *venae cavae* but increases so much in the aorta, even though the volume of blood removed from the *venae cavae* with each heartbeat is the same as the volume of blood added to the aorta. The reason is that the veins are much more compliant (distensible) than the arteries; one can add or remove blood from veins without changing the venous pressure very much, whereas the addition or removal of blood from arteries changes the arterial pressure a great deal.

A compliant vessel readily distends when pressure or volume is added. It yields to pressure. By definition, *compliance* is the change in the volume within a vessel or a chamber divided by the associated change in distending (transmural) pressure, as follows:

$$\text{Compliance} = \frac{\Delta \text{Volume}}{\Delta \text{Transmural pressure}}$$

Compliance corresponds to the slope of a volume-versus-pressure graph. As illustrated in Figure 22-2, veins are about 20 times more compliant than arteries (over the range of pressures

typically encountered in the circulation). Therefore, veins can accept or give up a large volume of blood without incurring much of a change in pressure. Veins readily expand or contract to accommodate the changes in blood volume that occur with fluid intake (e.g., drinking) or fluid loss (e.g., sweating). Veins thus function as the major blood *volume reservoirs* of the body. In contrast, arteries function as *pressure reservoirs,* providing the temporary storage site for the surge of pressure energy that is created with each cardiac ejection. Arteries are tough vessels, with low compliance. Therefore, arteries can accommodate a large increase in pressure during a cardiac ejection and then sustain the pressure high enough between cardiac ejections to provide a continuous flow of blood through the systemic circulation.

Vascular Resistance Is Defined as Perfusion Pressure Divided by Flow

Everyday experience tells us that it is easier to force fluid through a large tube than through a small tube. For example, it is easier to drink a milk shake through a large-diameter straw than through a small-diameter straw. For a given driving force (perfusion pressure difference), the flow is higher in the large tube because it offers less resistance to flow (less friction) than the small tube. The precise definition of resistance is:

$$\text{Resistance} = \frac{\Delta \text{Pressure}}{\text{Flow}}$$

Where *Δ Pressure* is *perfusion pressure difference,* or simply *perfusion pressure* (i.e., the pressure at the tube inlet minus the pressure at its outlet). Figure 22-3 presents these concepts in pictorial and

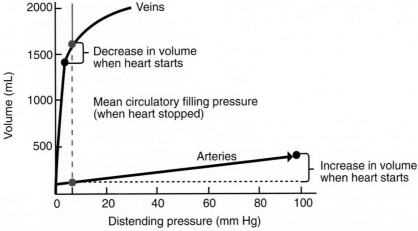

FIGURE 22-2 Typical relationships between volume (of blood) and distending pressure for veins and arteries. Veins are more compliant (easier to distend) than arteries, so they hold a greater volume of blood for a given distending pressure. This concept is illustrated for a distending pressure of 7 mm Hg *(vertical dashed red line),* which is a normal value for the mean circulatory filling pressure (the pressure that would exist in the circulation if the heart were stopped, as shown in Figure 22-1). For a distending pressure of 7 mm Hg, the veins contain about 1600 mL of blood and the arteries only 125 mL *(red circles).* When the heart is restarted, the venous volume decreases, and the arterial volume increases *(black circles).* Because the veins are much more compliant than the arteries, the venous pressure changes very little (decreases from 7 to 3 mm Hg), whereas the arterial pressure changes greatly (increases from 7 to 98 mm Hg).

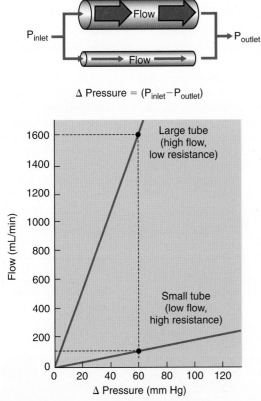

FIGURE 22-3 Relationship between fluid flow and perfusion pressure *(Δ Pressure)* for two tubes. The perfusion pressure is the pressure at the inlet *(P_{inlet})* of the tube minus the pressure at the outlet *(P_{outlet})*. In this example, the larger tube has twice the radius of the smaller tube. For a given perfusion pressure, the flow through the larger tube is 16 times greater than the flow through the smaller tube. That is, the resistance of the larger tube is one-sixteenth the resistance of the smaller tube.

graphic form. The dashed lines in this figure indicate that a perfusion pressure of 60 mm Hg causes a flow of 1600 milliliters per minute (mL/min) through the large tube. Thus the resistance of the large tube is 37.5 mm Hg/liter per minute (L/min). The same perfusion pressure (60 mm Hg) causes a flow of only 100 mL/min through the small tube. The resistance of the small tube is therefore 600 mm Hg/L/min. The resistance of the small tube is 16 times greater than the resistance of the large tube.

In the late 1800s the French physician J.L.M. Poiseuille demonstrated the dominant effect of radius on the resistance of a tube. He showed the following:

$$\text{Resistance of a tube} \cong \frac{8\eta l}{\pi r^4}$$

Where l is the length of the tube, r is the radius, η is the viscosity of the fluid flowing through the tube, and π has its usual meaning.

This equation *(Poiseuille's law)* emphasizes that radius (r) is the dominant factor influencing the resistance of a tube; resistance varies inversely with the fourth power of radius. Doubling the radius of a tube decreases its resistance by a factor of 16 (2^4). This explains why using a larger diameter straw makes it so much easier to drink a milk shake. Resistance is also influenced by the length (l) of the tube; it is harder to force fluid through a long tube than through a short tube of the same radius. The final determinant of resistance is the viscosity (η) of the fluid. The higher the viscosity of the fluid, the higher is the resistance to its flow through a tube. For example, honey is more viscous than water, so a tube offers a higher resistance to the flow of honey than to the flow of water.

As already described, the arterioles are the segment of the systemic circulation with the highest resistance to blood flow (see Figure 22-1). It may seem paradoxical that the arterioles are the site of highest resistance when the capillaries are smaller vessels. After all, Poiseuille's law and Figure 22-3 emphasize that a smaller tube has a much higher resistance than a larger tube. The resolution of this paradox is presented in Figure 22-4. It is true that each capillary has a smaller radius and therefore a greater resistance than each arteriole. However, each arteriole in the body distributes blood to many capillaries, and the *net resistance* of all those capillaries is less than the resistance of the single arteriole that delivers blood to them. It is only because each arteriole delivers blood to so many capillaries that the net resistance of the capillaries is less than the resistance of the arteriole.

Arterioles are the site not only of the highest resistance in the circulation, but also of adjustable resistance. Variation in arteriolar resistance is the main factor that determines how much blood flows through each organ in the body; an increase in arteriolar resistance in an organ decreases the blood flow through that organ, and vice versa. Arterioles change their resistance, moment to moment, by changing their radius. (The length of an arteriole does not change, at least not over the short term.) The walls of arterioles are relatively thick and muscular. Contraction of the arteriolar smooth muscle decreases the radius of arterioles, and this *vasoconstriction* substantially increases resistance to blood flow. Relaxation of the smooth muscle allows the radius of the vessels to increase, and this *vasodilation* substantially reduces the resistance to blood flow.

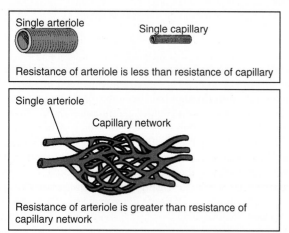

FIGURE 22-4 The resistance of a single arteriole is less than the resistance of a single capillary, because arterioles are larger in diameter. However, each arteriole supplies blood to a whole network of capillaries, and the resistance of an arteriole is greater than the resistance of the capillary network that it supplies with blood.

Figure 22-5 illustrates that a small change in the radius of arterioles in an organ brings about a large change in resistance and therefore in blood flow. In this example the arterial pressure is 93 mm Hg and the venous pressure is 3 mm Hg, so the perfusion pressure is 90 mm Hg. The brain blood flow is initially observed to be 90 mL/min. Based on the mathematical definition of resistance, the resistance of the brain blood vessels is 1000 mm Hg/L/min. Most of this resistance is provided by the brain arterioles. Next, consider the consequence of a slight vasodilation, such that the radius of the arterioles increases by 19% (e.g., from a radius of 1.00 to a radius of 1.19). Recall from Poiseuille's law that the resistance varies inversely as the fourth power of the radius. Because 1.19^4 equals 2.00, a 19% increase in radius cuts the resistance in half. Decreasing the brain's resistance by half (to 500 mm Hg/L/min) would double the brain blood flow (to 180 mL/min).

The Net Resistance of the Systemic Circulation Is Called the Total Peripheral Resistance

As with any other resistance, *systemic vascular resistance* (SVR), also called *total peripheral resistance* (TPR), is defined as a pressure difference (perfusion pressure) divided by a flow. In a calculation of the resistance of the systemic circulation, the perfusion pressure is the pressure in the aorta minus the pressure in the *venae cavae*. The flow is the total amount of blood that flows through the systemic circuit, which is equal to the cardiac output:

$$TPR = \frac{(\text{Mean aortic pressure} - \text{Mean vena caval pressure})}{\text{Cardiac output}}$$

For a typical dog at rest, the mean aortic pressure is 98 mm Hg, the mean vena caval pressure is 3 mm Hg, and the cardiac output is 2.5 L/min. Under these conditions, TPR is 38 mm Hg/L/min, which means that it takes a driving pressure of 38 mm Hg to force 1 L/min of blood through the systemic circuit.

Because the pressure in the *venae cavae* is usually close to zero, it is sometimes ignored in the calculation of TPR. The resultant simplified equation states that TPR is approximately equal to mean aortic pressure divided by the cardiac output. Usually, this equation is rearranged to form the statement that the mean aortic blood pressure (Pa) is approximately equal to the cardiac output (CO) multiplied by TPR:

$$Pa \cong CO \times TPR$$

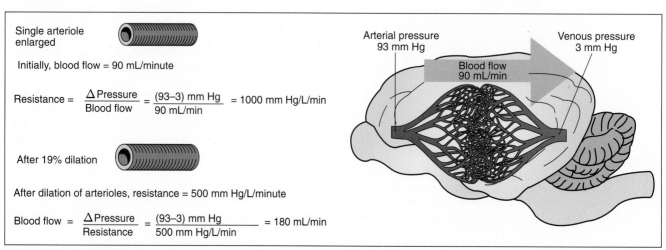

FIGURE 22-5 Example illustrating that a small arteriolar dilation (vasodilation) would substantially increase blood flow to an organ (brain, in this case).

This equation expresses one of the central concepts in cardiovascular physiology, namely that mean aortic blood pressure is determined by two, and only two, factors. Thus, if the aortic pressure is increased, it must be because the cardiac output increased, the TPR increased, or both. There are no other possibilities.

Arterial Pressure Is Determined by the Cardiac Output and the Total Peripheral Resistance

Three examples illustrate the application of the concept that the mean aortic blood pressure is determined by cardiac output and TPR. First, in the most common form of human essential hypertension, the cardiac output is normal. The blood pressure is elevated because of excessively constricted systemic arterioles, which increases TPR above normal. What remains unclear about human essential hypertension is why the arterioles are constricted. High blood pressure is a serious health problem in human medicine, because patients with uncontrolled hypertension often develop cardiac hypertrophy, and they are at high risk for cardiac arrhythmias, myocardial infarction, renal failure, and stroke. Naturally occurring hypertension is rare in veterinary species, although several techniques have been developed to induce hypertension in laboratory animals for research purposes.

Severe hemorrhage or dehydration is another condition in which the arterial pressure becomes abnormal, and it provides several distinct contrasts to chronic hypertension. For example, hemorrhage and dehydration are often encountered in veterinary medicine. Also, the arterial pressure is reduced in these conditions, not elevated. The cause of the decreased pressure is a decreased cardiac output. Hemorrhage or dehydration characteristically reduces the cardiac preload, which reduces the stroke volume and cardiac output. TPR is actually increased above normal because the body constricts the arterioles in the kidneys, splanchnic circulation, and resting skeletal muscle. Vasoconstriction in these organs minimizes the fall in arterial pressure and diverts the available cardiac output to the organs that are most critical for moment-to-moment survival, which include the brain, exercising skeletal muscle, and the heart (i.e., coronary circulation).

The response to vigorous exercise provides a third application of the concept that the mean aortic blood pressure is determined by the cardiac output and TPR. As in hemorrhage, exercise causes the cardiac output and TPR to change in opposite directions. In exercise, however, the cardiac output is elevated, and TPR is decreased. TPR decreases because the arterioles in the exercising skeletal muscle dilate, which increases skeletal muscle blood flow. During vigorous exercise, TPR decreases to about one-fourth of its resting value. The cardiac output increases about fourfold. The result is that the aortic pressure is negligibly changed. Figure 22-6 depicts the cardiovascular adjustments to vigorous exercise.

Blood Flow to Each Organ Is Determined by Perfusion Pressure and by the Organ's Vascular Resistance

If the equation that defines resistance is solved for flow, the result is:

$$\text{Flow} = \frac{\Delta\text{Pressure}}{\text{Resistance}}$$

As applied to the blood flow through any organ, this equation points out that the blood flow is determined by perfusion pressure (mean arterial pressure minus mean venous pressure) and by the resistance of the organ's blood vessels. There are no other factors. All the organs of the systemic circulation receive arterial blood flow via branches of the aorta, so all are exposed to essentially the same arterial pressure. Similarly, the venous blood from all the organs of the systemic circulation is collected into the *venae cavae*, so under normal circumstances, mean venous pressure is the same for all organs. Since all the systemic organs are exposed to nearly the same perfusion pressure, the differences in blood flow to the various organs result solely from their different vascular resistances. As explained earlier, the vascular resistance of an organ is determined primarily by the diameter of its arterioles. Thus, arteriolar vasodilation and vasoconstriction are the primary mechanisms that increase or decrease the blood flow in one organ relative to another organ.

Figure 22-6 illustrates how changes in the vascular resistance of various organs alter the distribution of cardiac output among the organs. In a typical dog at rest, the arteriolar resistances are similar in the splanchnic, renal, and skeletal vascular beds. Therefore, each of these beds receives about the same blood flow (indicated in Figure 22-6 by arrows of equal width). During exercise, skeletal muscle arterioles dilate greatly, almost doubling in diameter, which decreases their resistance to blood flow by a factor of almost 16. Therefore the skeletal muscle blood flow increases almost sixteenfold (from 0.5 to 7.8 L/min). Also during exercise, coronary arterioles dilate, so the coronary blood flow increases. Brain arterioles remain the same, so the brain blood flow is unchanged. By contrast, the arterioles in the splanchnic and renal circulations constrict slightly during exercise, which causes splanchnic and renal resistance to increase by about 20%. Therefore the splanchnic and renal blood flows decrease by about 20% (from 0.5 to 0.4 L/min).

This discussion of blood flow during exercise describes the responses of a normal dog with a healthy heart. Such a dog can readily increase its cardiac output enough to meet the increased blood flow needs of the skeletal and cardiac muscle. As a consequence, the arterial pressure (and hence the perfusion pressure) is very similar during rest and exercise. By contrast, a dog with heart failure cannot increase its cardiac output much above its resting level. Therefore the arterial pressure (and perfusion pressure) declines during exercise, and none of the organs receives the blood flow that it requires. This is why animals with heart failure exhibit weakness, fatigue, and exercise intolerance. (Additional complications of heart failure are discussed in Chapter 26.) The point for now is that the equation that relates blood flow, perfusion pressure, and vascular resistance is fundamental and inescapable; this relationship is profoundly important to an understanding of cardiovascular function and dysfunction.

The Pulmonary Circulation Offers Much Less Resistance to Blood Flow Than Does the Systemic Circulation

As with any other resistance, pulmonary resistance is calculated as a pressure difference (perfusion pressure) divided by a flow. The perfusion pressure that forces blood through the pulmonary circuit is the pressure in the pulmonary artery minus the pressure in the pulmonary veins. The flow that traverses the pulmonary circuit is equal to the cardiac output. Therefore:

$$\text{Pulmonary vascular resistance} = \frac{\begin{array}{c}(\text{Mean pulmonary artery pressure}\\ - \text{Mean pulmonary venous pressure})\end{array}}{\text{Cardiac output}}$$

For a typical dog at rest, the mean pulmonary arterial pressure is 13 mm Hg, the mean pulmonary venous pressure is 5 mm Hg,

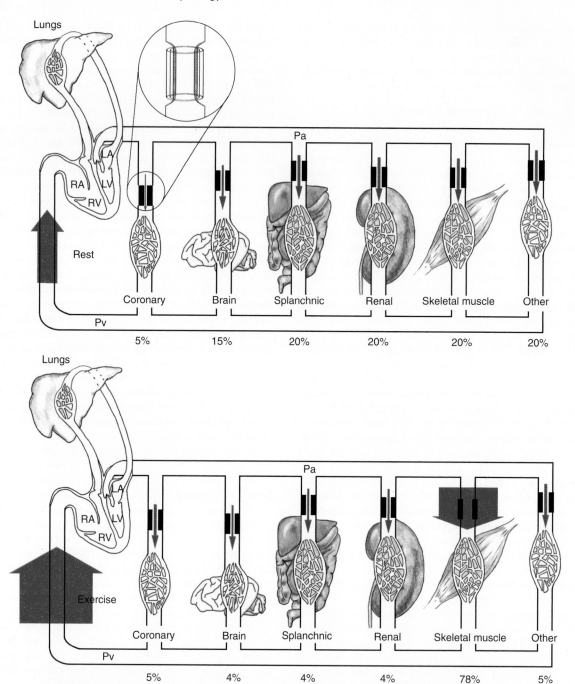

FIGURE 22-6 Cardiac output and its distribution compared during rest *(top)* and vigorous exercise *(bottom)* in a typical large dog. The width of the *red arrows* denotes the amount of blood flow. The flow of blood into the right side of the heart (which is equal to the cardiac output) is represented by the *very wide arrows* on the left. The cardiac output is 2.5 L/min at rest and increases to 10.0 L/min during exercise (fourfold increase). The entire cardiac output passes through the lungs and then is pumped by the left ventricle *(LV)* into the systemic arterial system *(horizontal tube across top)*. The systemic arteries deliver blood to each of the systemic vascular beds, which are grouped here into *Coronary, Brain, Splanchnic, Renal, Skeletal muscle,* and *Other*. In each systemic organ, blood must pass through high-resistance arterioles *(heavy bars)* before reaching the capillaries. The arterioles act as adjustable cuffs or constrictors (see magnified view, *top*). The proportion of the total cardiac output that passes through each organ is indicated by a percentage at the bottom. Because each organ is exposed to the same arterial pressure *(Pa)* and venous pressure *(Pv)*, the proportion of cardiac output that each organ receives is determined by its resistance. Resistance is determined primarily by the arteriolar diameter, which is indicated by the size of the opening between the heavy bars. During vigorous exercise, skeletal muscle arterioles dilate maximally, and the blood flow to the exercising muscles increases sixteenfold (from 0.5 L/min at rest to 7.8 L/min). Coronary arterioles also dilate, and the coronary blood flow increases about fourfold, which meets the increased demand by the heart muscle for oxygen. Vasoconstriction causes a small decrease in blood flow to the splanchnic and renal circulations. Blood flow to the brain is basically unchanged, although the percentage of total cardiac output received by the brain decreases. *RV,* Right ventricle; *LA,* left atrium; *RA,* right atrium.

and the cardiac output is 2.5 L/min. Thus, pulmonary resistance is 3.2 mm Hg/L/min. Note that this is only about $\frac{1}{12}$ the resistance of the systemic circulation.

The entire cardiac output passes through the lungs, so a fourfold increase in cardiac output during exercise also necessitates a fourfold increase in pulmonary blood flow. Pulmonary blood vessels are quite compliant, and they readily distend to accept the increase in blood flow. Because even a small increase in vessel radius greatly decreases resistance (in accordance with Poiseuille's law, as mentioned earlier), the resistance of the pulmonary blood vessels drops greatly during exercise. The decreased pulmonary resistance during exercise is advantageous because it allows the pulmonary flow to increase greatly without necessitating a large increase in the pulmonary arterial pressure.

Chapters 46 and 47 present additional details about the characteristics of pulmonary blood flow, including an explanation of the mechanisms that adjust the vascular resistance in various regions of the lungs so that the amount of blood that flows through each region of the lungs is appropriately matched to the amount of fresh air that is being delivered to the alveoli in that region (*ventilation-perfusion matching*).

Arterial Pressures Are Measured in Terms of Systolic, Diastolic, and Mean Levels

The pressures in the pulmonary artery and aorta are not constant but rather are *pulsatile,* as shown in Figure 21-1 and repeated in Figure 22-7. With each cardiac ejection, the pulmonary artery and aorta become distended with blood, which causes the pressures within these vessels to increase to peak values, called *systolic pressures*. Between cardiac ejections (i.e., during ventricular diastole), blood continues to flow out of the pulmonary artery and aorta into the pulmonary and systemic circulations, respectively. As the volume of blood in these large arteries decreases, the arteries become less distended, so arterial pressure decreases. Pressure continues to decrease until the next cardiac ejection begins. The minimal pressure reached before each new ejection is called the *diastolic pressure*. Figure 22-7 illustrates typical values for systolic and diastolic pressures.

The amplitude of the pressure pulsations in an artery is called the *pulse pressure,* specifically:

Aortic pulse pressure =
(Aortic systolic pressure − Aortic diastolic pressure)

and

Pulmonary artery pulse pressure =
(Pulmonary artery systolic pressure − Pulmonary artery diastolic pressure)

Typical values for pulse pressure are given in Figure 22-7. Note how much lower the systolic, diastolic, and pulse pressures are in the pulmonary artery than in the aorta. These differences illustrate why the pulmonary circulation is called the *low-pressure circulation,* whereas the systemic circulation is called the *high-pressure circulation.*

It is important to distinguish among systolic pressure, diastolic pressure, and pulse pressure; and to distinguish all of them from *mean pressure.* Mean aortic pressure is the average pressure in the aorta over the course of one or more complete cardiac cycles. Likewise, mean pulmonary artery pressure is the average pressure in that vessel. Obviously, the mean pressure in an artery is somewhere between the systolic (maximal) and diastolic (minimal) pressure levels. However, because the pressure waveforms in

arteries are not symmetric, the mean pressure is generally not exactly midway between the systolic and diastolic pressures.

A popular approximation is that mean pressure is about one third of the way up from diastolic toward systolic pressure; that is:

Mean arterial pressure $\cong$ Diastolic pressure $+ \frac{1}{3}$ Pulse pressure

Figure 22-7 reveals that this is *not* a valid approximation for the determination of mean pressure in the aorta. However, the approximation is a good one for pressures measured in the femoral artery or in most other major arteries distal to the aorta. The reason that the rule applies in the distal arteries but not in the aorta is that the waveform of the arterial pressure pulsations changes as the pulses move away from the heart. The pressure pulses become narrower and more sharply peaked. This pronounced asymmetry of the pressure pulses causes the mean level in distal arteries to be closer to the diastolic pressure than to the systolic pressure (see Figure 22-7).

For complex reasons, the pulse pressure typically *increases* as blood flows from the aorta into the distal arteries. However, the mean pressure necessarily *decreases* in accordance with the principle of the conservation of energy. As stated earlier, mean arterial pressure is a measure of the potential energy in the bloodstream, and this potential energy is used up (converted into heat by friction) as blood flows from the aorta through the systemic circulation. The aorta and large arteries offer only a small resistance to blood flow; mean arterial pressure decreases only 1 to 3 mm Hg between the aorta and the femoral artery (see Figure 22-7). Most of the resistance to blood flow is found in the arterioles and capillaries. Therefore the largest decrements in *mean pressure* occur in these segments of the systemic circulation (see Figure 22-1).

An important point to remember is that mean aortic pressure (not systolic, diastolic, or pulse pressure) must be used when calculating total peripheral resistance as:

$$\text{Total peripheral resistance} = \frac{\begin{array}{c}(\text{Mean aortic pressure}\\ - \text{Mean vena caval pressure})\end{array}}{\text{Cardiac output}}$$

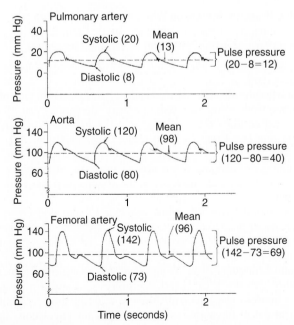

FIGURE 22-7 Blood pressure in the large arteries is pulsatile. The pressure patterns typical of the pulmonary artery, aorta, and femoral artery of the dog are shown.

Likewise, mean pulmonary artery pressure (not systolic, diastolic, or pulse pressure) must be used when calculating pulmonary vascular resistance as:

$$\text{Pulmonary vascular resistance} = \frac{\left(\begin{array}{c}\text{Mean pulmonary arterial pressure} \\ - \text{Mean pulmonary vein pressure}\end{array}\right)}{\text{Cardiac output}}$$

Unfortunately, the only way to measure a mean vascular pressure is by inserting a needle or catheter into the vessel of interest. The first direct measurement of mean arterial blood pressure was carried out by Stephen Hales, an English clergyman. In about 1730, Hales inserted a tube (catheter) into the femoral artery of a conscious horse and found that blood rose in the tube to a height of more than 8 feet. An 8-foot column of blood represents a pressure of more than 180 mm Hg, almost twice the mean arterial pressure expected in a normal resting animal. The high pressure undoubtedly reflected the physical and emotional distress of the horse, which was restrained upside down during the episode. In the present day, arterial catheterization (with anesthetic agents to reduce pain) is routine in human medicine (e.g., in cardiac catheterization laboratories) and is becoming more common in veterinary medicine. However, the lesson that physical or emotional distress can dramatically increase blood pressure is as relevant today as it was in Hales' time.

In human medicine, systolic and diastolic arterial pressures can be measured quite accurately with a blood pressure cuff and stethoscope. Mean arterial pressure can then be approximated using the equation given earlier. Blood pressure cuffs are less frequently used on veterinary species, but the pulse is often palpated by placing the fingertips over a major artery, such as the femoral artery. Palpation of an artery allows the clinician to sense the pulse pressure on the basis of the magnitude of the pulsations felt in the artery. A low pulse pressure is referred to as a *thready*, or weak, pulse. A high pulse pressure may be called a *bounding*, or strong, pulse.

Pulse Pressure Increases When the Stroke Volume Increases, Heart Rate Decreases, Aortic Compliance Decreases, or Total Peripheral Resistance Increases

Because the arterial pulse is so frequently palpated in patients, it is important for the veterinary clinician to understand the factors that typically influence pulse pressure. First, an increase in stroke volume tends to increase pulse pressure. Because cardiac ejections create the arterial pulsations in the first place, it is not surprising that larger ejections create larger pulsations. Figure 22-8, *A*, depicts this effect and shows that an increase in stroke volume also increases mean arterial pressure. Mean pressure increases because an increased stroke volume increases cardiac output.

A second factor that tends to increase pulse pressure is a decrease in heart rate. Between cardiac ejections, aortic pressure decreases as blood continues to run out of the aorta and through the systemic circulation. Aortic pressure falls to a minimal (diastolic) level before being boosted again by the next cardiac ejection. When heart rate decreases, there is a longer time between ejections and therefore a longer time for blood to run out of the aorta and into the systemic circulation. The blood pressure in the aorta falls to a lower level before the next cardiac ejection, and pulse pressure is increased (Figure 22-8, *B*).

A decrease in heart rate results in a decrease in cardiac output, so a decrease in heart rate decreases the mean arterial pressure (Figure 22-8, *B*).

Figure 22-8, *C*, shows the effect of a simultaneous increase in stroke volume and decrease in heart rate. In this example, cardiac output, which is stroke volume multiplied by heart rate, remains unchanged. Therefore, mean arterial pressure remains unchanged. However, pulse pressure is greatly increased as a result of the combined effects of an increase in stroke volume and a decrease in heart rate. Aerobic conditioning in humans, and in some animals, leads to increased stroke volume and decreased heart rate at rest. Therefore, in a well-trained athlete at rest, mean arterial pressure is typically normal, but pulse pressure is greater than normal. Palpation of the arteries of an athlete at rest reveals a strong, slow pulse.

A decrease in arterial compliance (stiffening of the arteries) is a third factor that tends to increase pulse pressure (see Figure 22-8, *D*). With each ventricular systole, the heart ejects blood into the aorta and large arteries, which distends these vessels. If these vessels become stiff, a greater increase in pressure is required to distend them. Arterial stiffening also decreases diastolic arterial pressure. This effect is more difficult to grasp intuitively but should not be surprising. Just as aortic pressure rises to higher-than-normal systolic levels when the heart ejects blood into a stiff aorta, so does aortic pressure fall to lower-than-normal diastolic levels when blood runs out of the stiff aorta between cardiac ejections. The higher systolic pressure and lower diastolic pressure are simply two direct consequences of the same phenomenon: decreased arterial compliance. The major arteries tend to become stiffer as a result of the normal aging process, which accounts for the increase in pulse pressure that is typical in older humans and some animals.

In general, cardiac output is not affected by arterial stiffening. A healthy ventricle is able to generate the higher systolic pressures needed to eject blood into a stiff arterial system, although ventricular hypertrophy is sometimes triggered. Moreover, arterial stiffening generally has very little effect on TPR because the arterioles remain normal. The arteries, although stiff, retain their large diameters, and therefore arterial resistance remains low. *Mean* arterial pressure, the product of cardiac output and TPR, is therefore generally unchanged by arterial stiffening.

Arteriolar vasoconstriction is a fourth factor that typically increases pulse pressure (Figure 22-8, *E*). In actuality, vasoconstriction does not affect pulse pressure directly but acts through a stiffening of the arteries. Vasoconstriction increases TPR, which causes blood to back up or accumulate in the large arteries. As the arteries become more distended, arterial pressure increases. Distention forces the arteries toward their elastic limit, so they also become stiffer than arteries under normal pressurization (Figure 22-9). This stiffening of the arteries causes pulse pressure to increase, for the reasons already explained. Moreover, because TPR is elevated, mean arterial pressure also increases.

Many human patients develop both stiffening of arteries (as a consequence of aging) and essential hypertension (caused by increased TPR). This combination produces dramatic increases in pulse pressure. As illustrated in Figure 22-8, *F*, an older person with severe hypertension might have a pulse pressure of 110 mm Hg (200 mm Hg systolic minus 90 mm Hg diastolic). Arterial hypertension and arterial stiffening both are less common in veterinary species.

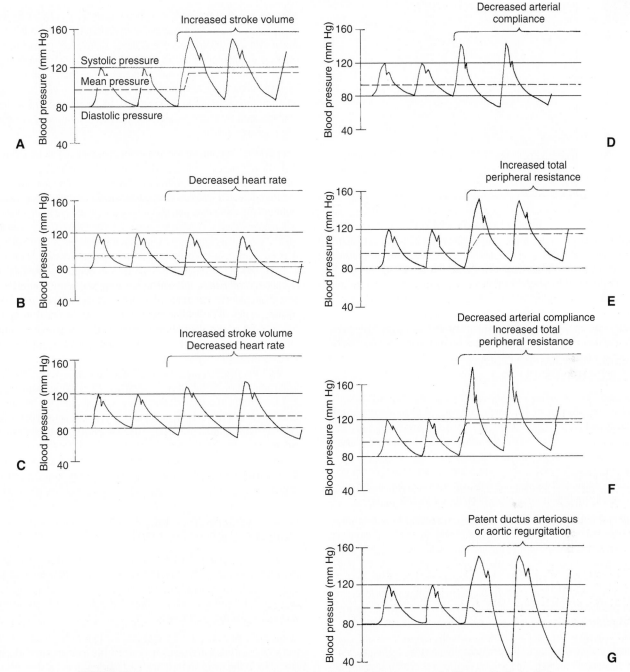

FIGURE 22-8 Various conditions that increase arterial pulse pressure are compared with regard to their effects on systolic pressure, diastolic pressure, and mean pressure (see text).

In summary, pulse pressure tends to be increased by increased stroke volume, decreased heart rate, decreased arterial compliance, or vasoconstriction.

Some of the cardiac defects that produce murmurs also cause characteristic changes in pulse pressure. For example, a patient with patent ductus arteriosus has a large left ventricular stroke volume, which elevates aortic systolic pressure. Aortic diastolic pressure is much lower than normal because, between cardiac ejections, blood runs out of the aorta by two pathways: into the

systemic circuit and through the open ductus. Pulse pressure is dramatically increased (Figure 22-8, *G*). Aortic regurgitation causes a similar, characteristic increase in pulse pressure. During diastole, blood leaves the aorta through two pathways: forward into the systemic circuit and backward (through the incompetent valve) into the left ventricle. Stroke volume is elevated because, with each systole, the left ventricle ejects both the blood that has returned to it through the normal pathway and also the regurgitant blood.

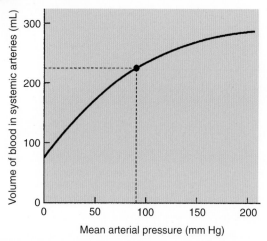

FIGURE 22-9 This volume-pressure graph shows that normal systemic arteries become stiffer (less compliant) when mean arterial pressure increases above its normal value *(dot)*. (Recall that compliance is equal to the slope of a volume-pressure curve.)

CLINICAL CORRELATIONS

CANINE HEARTWORM DISEASE WITH PULMONARY EMBOLISM

History. You examine a 6-year-old male beagle that has been a hunting companion of his owner for several years. The owner reports that the dog tires more easily than usual and has developed a cough that is worse during exercise. You treated this dog for a laceration when he was 3 years old, and your records indicate that the dog was otherwise in excellent health at that time. The owner acknowledges that the dog has not been given any immunizations or heartworm prophylactic medication for the past 2 years.

Clinical Examination. On physical examination of the dog, you notice the cough reported by the owner and an apparent, modest accumulation of fluid in the abdominal cavity *(ascites)*. You also auscultate a systolic murmur that is loudest over the left third and fourth intercostal spaces. The chest radiograph and electrocardiogram show evidence of right ventricular enlargement. In addition, the pulmonary vessels are more prominent than normal on the radiograph and are tortuous (twisted). You suspect canine heartworm disease. You obtain a blood sample, some of which you submit for an enzyme-linked immunosorbent assay (ELISA) to test for heartworm antigen. Additionally, you use a pipette to apply a sample of the buffy coat (from the centrifuge tube) onto a glass slide for microscopic examination. You see microfilaria of the type shed by adult canine heartworms *(Dirofilaria immitis)*, and the ELISA is positive for the presence of *D. immitis* antigen. You diagnose canine heartworm parasitism.

Comment. Mosquitoes transfer the microfilaria from the bloodstream of an infected dog to the bloodstream of a noninfected dog. The microfilaria develop into adult worms, which grow to a length of 10 to 20 cm while clinging to the walls of the pulmonary artery and its major branches. Heartworm infestation typically causes pulmonary arterial vessels to become enlarged and tortuous. In heavily infested dogs, adult worms also reside in the right ventricle and right ventricular outflow tract, where they cause pulmonic stenosis. The resulting turbulence during right ventricular ejection accounts for the murmur heard in this dog. The pulmonic

stenosis and the increased pulmonary resistance created by the worms also lead to right ventricular hypertrophy, exercise intolerance, and ascites (review the Clinical Correlation on pulmonic stenosis in Chapter 21 for an explanation of why these complications develop). An additional problem is that the adult worms release vasoactive substances into the circulation, which disrupt some of the normal mechanisms that adjust arteriolar diameter, control blood flow, and regulate arterial pressure. Heavily infested dogs become very ill.

Treatment. You advise the owner that the dog should be treated with an arsenic-containing medication that kills adult worms over several days. You also warn the owner that the treatment of severely infested dogs is risky. Dead adult worms break away from the right ventricle and pulmonary artery and lodge in smaller pulmonary vessels. These vascular occlusions *(pulmonary emboli)* restrict pulmonary blood flow and reduce cardiac output. Therefore, it is necessary to keep the dog in a quiet, unstressed state for 8 to 10 days after beginning treatment. In addition to restricting pulmonary blood flow, the emboli are likely to cause inflammation and blood clots in the lungs. Pulmonary edema is expected. Pulmonary blood vessels may break down, allowing blood to enter the airways of the lungs. Respiratory failure is possible. Anti-inflammatory drugs are sometimes administered to reduce these complications.

With the owner's consent, you keep the dog at your clinic for 2 days (to allow him to become accustomed to the surroundings) and then begin treatment. During the next week, the dog becomes even more lethargic than before and begins to cough up blood. The dog has a low-grade fever (102°-103° F), and his ascites becomes worse. However, his systolic murmur begins to fade. After 1 week, all the clinical signs have greatly improved. The dog is sent home for a prolonged period of recuperation. The long-term prognosis is good.

DUMMY FOAL: HYPOXEMIC ISCHEMIC ENCEPHALOPATHY

History. A 14-year-old Thoroughbred mare is presented for *dystocia* (difficult birth). The foal (a filly) was pulled with some difficulty. The filly was slow to stand and did not nurse voluntarily for several hours. The mare was *stripped* (milked) of colostrum, which was fed to the foal by nasogastric tube.

Clinical Examination. The foal has a slightly low temperature and increased pulse and respiratory rates. The mucous membranes are tacky to the touch (dehydrated) and dark pink in color (indicating poor perfusion and/or poor oxygenation). Capillary refill time is prolonged (consistent with poor perfusion). The foal has a marked murmur similar to that heard with a patent *ductus arteriosus*. Peripheral pulses are decreased (weak), and distal extremities are cool. Gastrointestinal motility is decreased. The foal appears mature physically, but she is acting dysmature when she attempts to stand, nurse, or lie down. Blood studies reveal that the foal is not septic, but she is hypoxemic, has evidence of poor kidney function, and is acidotic.

Comment. Hypoxemic ischemic encephalopathy (HIE) occurs when a foal receives decreased oxygen for some time. This can occur before, during, or after foaling. With a dystocia, after the water breaks and while the foal is being pulled, the oxygen supply to the foal is decreased. The foal must rely on anaerobic metabolism during the period of low oxygen, which results in acidosis.

Decreased oxygen also causes pulmonary blood vessels to constrict (*hypoxic pulmonary vasoconstriction,* discussed further in Chapter 46). The resulting increase in pulmonary vascular resistance causes blood to back up or accumulate in the pulmonary artery, right ventricle, and right atrium, and this increases the pressure in these chambers. If pressures in the right side of the heart exceed those in the left side, blood flow persists (from right to left) through the foramen ovale. (When a normal foal begins to breathe, pressures in the right side fall below those in the left side of the heart, so the foramen ovale closes.) The blood that flows through the foramen ovale in this foal reaches the aorta without passing through the lungs, and therefore without being oxygenated at all (*right-to-left shunt*).

Treatment. The foal needs oxygen to reverse the hypoxic pulmonary vasoconstriction and the consequent high pressure in the right heart, persistent flow through the foamen ovale, and hypoxemia. Supplemental oxygen can be provided by *nasal insufflation* (tube placed in nasal cavity for delivery of oxygen). Additionally, the foal will be given drugs, such as dopamine, to increase cardiac contractility, cardiac output, and blood pressure. This treatment, in addition to intravenous fluids, will likely improve blood flow to the vital organs, including the brain and kidneys. Improved respiratory and renal function will reverse the acidosis. Foals with HIE often develop other complications, which need to be addressed as they arise.

PRACTICE QUESTIONS

1. Which of the following is a correct comparison between segments of the systemic circulation?
   a. The aorta and large arteries have a higher compliance than the veins.
   b. The aorta and large arteries have a higher resistance to blood flow than the capillaries.
   c. The veins have a higher resistance to blood flow than the capillaries.
   d. The arterioles have a higher resistance to blood flow than the capillaries.
   e. If the heart is stopped, the pressure in the veins will become higher than the pressure in the aorta and large arteries.

2. If aortic compliance decreases while heart rate, cardiac output, and total peripheral resistance (TPR) remain unchanged:
   a. Pulse pressure will be unchanged.
   b. Pulse pressure will increase.
   c. Pulse pressure will decrease.
   d. One cannot know the effect on pulse pressure because stroke volume may have changed.
   e. One cannot know the effect on pulse pressure because mean aortic pressure may have changed.

3. Which of the following would cause mean aortic pressure to *increase*?
   a. Stroke volume increases from 30 to 40 mL, and heart rate decreases from 100 to 60 beats/min.
   b. Arterial compliance decreases.
   c. Cardiac output decreases.
   d. Arterioles throughout the body dilate.
   e. TPR increases.

4. The following measurements are made on a dog: heart rate, 80 beats/min; stroke volume, 30 mL; mean aortic pressure, 96 mm Hg; mean pulmonary artery pressure, 30 mm Hg; left atrial pressure, 5 mm Hg; and right atrial pressure, 12 mm Hg. The TPR of this dog (taking into account both arterial and atrial pressures) is exactly:
   a. 10.42 mm Hg/L/min
   b. 12.50 mm Hg/L/min
   c. 35.00 mm Hg/L/min
   d. 37.92 mm Hg/L/min
   e. 40.00 mm Hg/L/min

5. Which of the following would cause the largest *decrease* in coronary blood flow?
   a. Coronary arterioles constrict to half their normal diameter.
   b. Coronary arteries develop atherosclerosis, and lipid plaques plug up half their normal cross-sectional area.
   c. Mean aortic pressure decreases to half its normal level.
   d. The resistance to coronary blood flow doubles.
   e. The resistance to coronary blood flow decreases to $\frac{1}{4}$ its normal value.

6. A change from breathing normal air (21% O_2) to breathing a gas mixture with only 10% O_2 would cause pulmonary blood vessels to _____ and pulmonary vascular resistance to _____.
   a. Constrict; increase
   b. Constrict; decrease
   c. Dilate; increase
   d. Dilate; decrease
   e. Remain unchanged; remain unchanged

BIBLIOGRAPHY

Birchard SJ, Sherding RG: *Saunders manual of small animal practice,* ed 3, Philadelphia, 2006, Saunders.

Boron WF, Boulpaep EL: *Medical physiology,* ed 2, Philadelphia, 2009, Saunders.

Hall JE: *Guyton and Hall textbook of medical physiology,* ed 12, Philadelphia, 2011, Saunders.

Knottenbelt DC, Holdstock N, Madigan JE: *Equine neonatology: medicine and surgery,* New York, 2004, Saunders.

Koeppen BM, Stanton BA: *Berne & Levy physiology,* ed 6, Philadelphia, 2010, Mosby.

Levy MN, Pappano AJ: *Cardiovascular physiology,* ed 9, St Louis, 2007, Mosby.

Milnor WR: *Cardiovascular physiology,* New York, 1990, Oxford University Press.

Mohrman DE, Heller LJ: *Cardiovascular physiology,* ed 7, New York, 2010, Lange Medical Books/McGraw-Hill.

Tilley LP, Smith FWK, Oyama MA, Sleeper MM: *Manual of canine and feline cardiology,* ed 4, Philadelphia, 2008, Saunders.

CHAPTER 23
Capillaries and Fluid Exchange

KEY POINTS

1. Capillaries, the smallest blood vessels, are the sites for the exchange of water and solutes between the bloodstream and the interstitial fluid.
2. Lipid-soluble substances diffuse readily through capillary walls, whereas lipid-insoluble substances must pass through capillary pores.
3. Fick's law of diffusion is a simple mathematical accounting of the physical factors that affect the rate of diffusion.
4. Water moves across capillary walls both by diffusion (osmosis) and by bulk flow.
5. The Starling equation quantifies the interaction of oncotic and hydrostatic forces acting on water.
6. Several common physiological changes alter the normal balance of Starling forces and increase the filtration of water out of capillaries.
7. Edema is a clinically noticeable excess of interstitial fluid.

Capillaries, the Smallest Blood Vessels, Are the Sites for the Exchange of Water and Solutes Between the Bloodstream and the Interstitial Fluid

Because of their small size, the capillaries are sometimes called the *microcirculation*. They are also called the *exchange vessels*, because the exchange of water and solutes between the bloodstream and the interstitial fluid takes place across the walls of the capillaries. Each type of blood vessel in the body is structurally suited for its primary function, and the walls of the capillaries are especially well adapted for their exchange function.

Figure 23-1 shows the contrasting features of the walls of the various types of blood vessels in the systemic circulation. The distinguishing feature of the walls of the aorta and large arteries is the presence of a large amount of elastic material along with smooth muscle. These vessels are called the *elastic vessels;* elasticity is necessary because the aorta and large arteries must distend with each pulsatile ejection of blood from the heart. The arterial walls are also strong and quite stiff (low compliance). There is no contradiction in saying that the arteries are elastic and have low compliance. *Elasticity* denotes distensibility and an ability to return to the original shape after the distending force or pressure is removed. *Compliance* is a measure of how much force or pressure is required to achieve distention. The arteries are elastic, but a high pressure (systolic pressure) is required to distend them.

Small arteries, and particularly arterioles, have relatively thick walls with less elastic tissue and a predominance of smooth muscle, so they are called the *muscular vessels*. Contraction and relaxation of the smooth muscle enables these vessels to constrict or dilate, which varies their resistance to blood flow. The muscular vessels vary the total peripheral resistance and direct blood flow toward or away from particular organs or particular regions within an organ.

Capillaries are the smallest vessels, being about 8 μm in diameter and about 0.5 mm long. Capillaries are so small that red blood cells (7.5 μm in diameter) must squeeze through in single

file. Capillary walls consist of a single layer of endothelial cells. The small diameter of the capillaries and the thinness of their walls facilitate the exchange of water and solutes between the blood within capillaries and the interstitial fluid immediately outside the capillaries.

Venules and veins are larger than capillaries, and they have thicker walls. Venules and veins have both elastic tissue and smooth muscle in their walls. However, the walls of veins are not as thick or as muscular as the walls of arteries or arterioles. The primary role of veins is to serve as *reservoir vessels*. Veins are very compliant, and many veins in the body are normally in a state of partial collapse. Therefore, veins can accommodate substantial changes in blood volume without much change in venous pressure.

Capillaries form a network (see Figure 18-4). In most tissues the capillary network is so dense that each cell of the tissue is within 100 μm of a capillary. However, not all the capillaries of a tissue carry blood at all times. In most tissues the arterioles alternate between constriction and dilation, so blood flow is periodically reduced or even stopped in most capillaries. Also, in some tissues (e.g., intestinal circulation), tiny cuffs of smooth muscle encircle capillaries at the points where they branch off from arterioles. Contraction of these *precapillary sphincters* can reduce or stop the flow of blood in individual capillaries. When the metabolic rate of a tissue increases (and therefore its need for blood flow increases), the arterioles and precapillary sphincters still constrict periodically, but they spend more time in the dilated (relaxed) state. This increases the fraction of capillaries in which blood is flowing at any one time. At maximal metabolic rate (e.g., maximal exercise in a skeletal muscle), blood flows through all the capillaries all the time. Sending blood flow to all the capillaries not only increases the total blood flow through a tissue but also minimizes the distance between each cell of the tissue and the nearest capillary carrying blood by bulk flow. Both these effects speed up diffusional exchange between the capillary blood and the tissue cells.

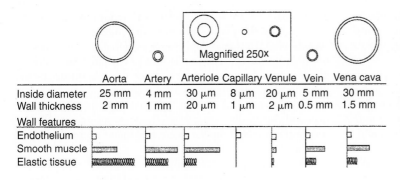

	Aorta	Artery	Arteriole	Capillary	Venule	Vein	Vena cava
Inside diameter	25 mm	4 mm	30 μm	8 μm	20 μm	5 mm	30 mm
Wall thickness	2 mm	1 mm	20 μm	1 μm	2 μm	0.5 mm	1.5 mm
Wall features							
Endothelium							
Smooth muscle							
Elastic tissue							

FIGURE 23-1 Each type of blood vessel in the systemic circulation is specifically suited to its particular function by its size, wall thickness, and wall composition. In this drawing, each type of vessel is shown in cross section. The drawings are to scale (note that the arteriole, capillary, and venule are magnified 250 times to make them visible). Also shown are the relative proportions of the three most important types of tissue found in blood vessel walls.

Typical continuous capillary

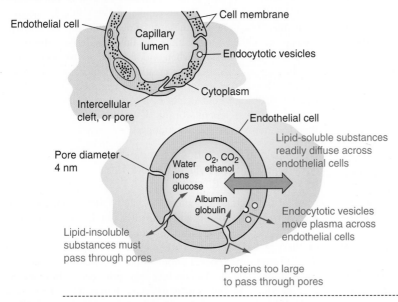

Discontinuous capillary (sinusoid)

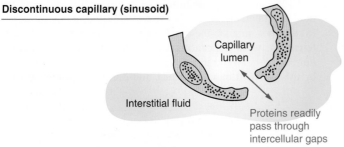

FIGURE 23-2 Capillaries in cross section. Typical continuous capillaries have small clefts, or pores, between endothelial cells *(top)*. Water and small, lipid-insoluble solutes move between the capillary plasma *(yellow)* and the interstitial fluid *(blue)* through these pores *(center)*. Plasma protein molecules are too large to pass through the pores. However, plasma proteins, along with other plasma constituents, are taken into endocytotic vesicles, which can deliver their contents into the interstitial fluid via exocytosis, although this is a relatively slow process. In contrast, lipid-soluble substances can diffuse directly, and very quickly, through the capillary endothelial cells. The size of the clefts between endothelial cells varies greatly from tissue to tissue, with the smallest being in brain capillaries and the largest being in the discontinuous capillaries, or sinusoids, such as those in the liver *(bottom)*.

Lipid-Soluble Substances Diffuse Readily Through Capillary Walls, Whereas Lipid-Insoluble Substances Must Pass Through Capillary Pores

The rate of diffusional exchange between capillary blood and the surrounding interstitial fluid depends both on the properties of the substances being exchanged and on the features of the capillary wall. Small, lipid-soluble substances (e.g., dissolved oxygen and carbon dioxide, fatty acids, ethanol, and some hormones) readily dissolve in the cell membranes of the endothelial cells that form the capillary walls. Such lipid-soluble substances can diffuse very rapidly through the endothelial cells from blood to interstitial fluid, or vice-versa. In contrast, lipid-insoluble substances (e.g., ions, glucose, and amino acids) do not dissolve in cell membranes and so cannot diffuse through the endothelial cells. Instead, such substances must pass through the *pores*, or *clefts*, that exist between the endothelial cells (Figure 23-2). These pores create tiny, water-filled channels between the capillary blood and the interstitial fluid. The diffusional movement of lipid-insoluble substances across capillary walls is much slower than the movement of lipid-soluble substances, because the lipid-insoluble substances are restricted to passage through the capillary pores, which constitute only about 1% of the total wall surface area of a typical capillary.

The capillaries in most tissues are called *continuous capillaries* because the endothelial cells form a continuous tube, except for the tiny, water-filled pores between the endothelial cells. In typical continuous capillaries, the diameter of the pores is about 4 nm, which is large enough to permit the passage of water and of all the small solutes in plasma and interstitial fluid. The plasma protein molecules, however, are a little too large to pass through pores of this size. Blood cells, of course, are far too large to pass through such small openings (see Figure 18-7).

The main route for the delivery of plasma proteins into the interstitial fluid is through the three-step process of *transcytosis*. The first step is *pinocytosis* (a form of *endocytosis*), which involves the invagination of the capillary endothelial cell membrane to form an intracellular vesicle that contains plasma, including plasma proteins (see Figure 23-2). Second, some of these vesicles cross the capillary endothelial cell from the side facing the bloodstream to the side facing the interstitial fluid. In the third step, these vesicles fuse with the membrane of the endothelial cell on the interstitial fluid side; the vesicles discharge their contents into the interstitial space. This third step is called *exocytosis*. The delivery of plasma constituents into the interstitial fluid by transcytosis is extremely slow, compared with the diffusion of lipid-soluble substances through endothelial cells, or the passage of small, lipid-insoluble substances through capillary pores.

The size of the capillary pores, or clefts, varies from tissue to tissue. Two extremes are found in the brain and the liver. In brain capillaries, the junctions between adjacent endothelial cells are so tight that only water and small ions (e.g., Na^+ and Cl^-) can pass through them; not even glucose or amino acid molecules can pass through these tiny pores. Yet brain neurons require glucose to carry out their normal metabolism. Glucose is moved across the brain capillary endothelial cells by means of specialized protein carrier molecules that are embedded in the cell membranes of the endothelial cells. The energy to drive this *facilitated diffusion* comes from the glucose concentration difference between the blood and the brain interstitial fluid. The tight junctions between endothelial cells in brain capillaries create a barrier between the bloodstream and the brain tissue that is called the *blood-brain barrier* (also discussed in Chapter 15). One function of the blood-brain barrier is to protect brain neurons from exposure to toxic substances that may be in the blood.

In the liver, the clefts between capillary endothelial cells are so large that these vessels are called *discontinuous capillaries* (or *sinusoids*). Even plasma proteins such as albumin and globulin can readily pass through these large clefts, which typically exceed 100 nm in width (see Figure 23-2, *bottom*). Large gaps between endothelial cells are an appropriate feature for capillaries in the liver because the plasma proteins are produced by liver cells (*hepatocytes*). The large gaps between endothelial cells permit the newly synthesized protein molecules to enter the bloodstream. The large gaps are also appropriate for the role of the liver in detoxification. Some toxins become bound to plasma proteins in the bloodstream, and then are removed from the blood by the liver and chemically changed into less toxic substances. Discontinuous (sinusoidal) capillaries are also found in the spleen and bone marrow.

Fenestrated capillaries ("capillaries with windows") present an additional variation on capillary pores. Fenestrae are holes or perforations through (not between) endothelial cells. Fenestrae are typically 50 to 80 nm in diameter, which is larger than the intercellular clefts of typical continuous capillaries but smaller than the clefts of discontinuous capillaries. Very fine diaphragms span most fenestrae, but these diaphragms do not prevent the passage of either lipid-soluble or lipid-insoluble substances. Fenestrae may be formed when endocytotic and exocytotic vesicles line up and merge, thus creating a temporary water-filled channel through an endothelial cell. Fenestrated capillaries are characteristically found in places where large amounts of fluid and solutes must pass into or out of capillaries (e.g., gastrointestinal tract, endocrine glands, kidneys).

Fick's Law of Diffusion Is a Simple Mathematical Accounting of the Physical Factors That Affect the Rate of Diffusion

Most of the factors that affect the rate of diffusional exchange between capillary blood and interstitial fluid have been mentioned. These factors include the distance involved, the size of the capillary pores (or fenestrae, when present), and the properties of the diffusing substance (i.e., lipid-soluble vs. lipid insoluble). The German physiologist Adolph Fick incorporated all these factors into an equation: *Fick's law of diffusion*. Figure 23-3 shows how Fick's law applies to the diffusional exchange between capillary fluid and interstitial fluid. The rate of diffusion of any substance (S) depends, first, on the *concentration difference*, that is, the difference between the concentration of the substance in capillary fluid and its concentration in interstitial fluid. Diffusion is driven by this concentration difference, and diffusion always proceeds

FIGURE 23-3 According to Fick's law, the four factors that affect the rate of diffusion of a particular substance S from the capillary plasma to the interstitial fluid next to a tissue cell are $[S]_c - [S]_i$, the concentration difference between the capillary plasma and interstitial fluid; A, area available for diffusion; Δx, distance involved; and D, diffusion coefficient for the substance.

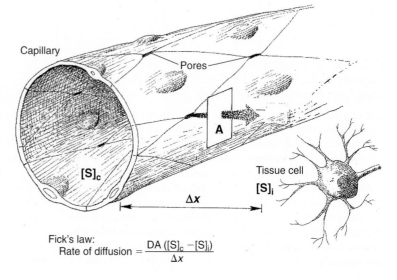

Fick's law:
$$\text{Rate of diffusion} = \frac{DA\,([S]_c - [S]_i)}{\Delta x}$$

from the area of higher concentration toward the area of lower concentration. Next, the rate of diffusion is determined by the *area available for diffusion*, the term *A* in the equation. For lipid-soluble substances, this area is equivalent to the total surface area of the capillaries. For lipid-insoluble substances, this area is much smaller, being equal to the area of the pores (or clefts) between capillary endothelial cells (plus the area of fenestrae, when present).

The term Δx in the equation represents the *distance* over which diffusion must occur. Functionally, Δx equals the distance from a tissue cell to the nearest capillary that is carrying blood by bulk flow (see Figure 23-3). The greater the distance from the tissue cells to the capillaries, the slower is the rate of diffusional exchange of substances between that cell and the capillary blood; therefore, Δx appears in the denominator in the equation.

The term *D* in the equation is a *diffusion coefficient*. The value of *D* increases with temperature because diffusion depends on the random (Brownian) motion of particles in solution, and the velocity of Brownian motion increases with temperature. *D* also depends on the molecular weight of the diffusing substance and on its solubility. For example, *D* for carbon dioxide is about 20 times greater than *D* for oxygen. As a result, carbon dioxide diffuses much more rapidly than does oxygen for a given concentration difference, area, and diffusion distance. This difference is inconsequential under normal physiological conditions. In certain disease states, however, the area available for diffusion decreases, and the diffusion distance increases. Under these conditions, the delivery of oxygen to the metabolizing cells of a tissue generally becomes critically impaired before the removal of carbon dioxide from the cells becomes inadequate.

Several of the factors that affect the rate of diffusion are physiologically adjustable. For example, in skeletal muscle at rest, the arterioles cycle between open and closed, and even when open, their diameter is small. Consequently, at any one moment, blood flows through only about one-fourth of the skeletal muscle capillaries. Blood sits still in the remainder of them. Nevertheless, this low and "part-time" blood flow through capillaries is adequate to deliver oxygen and nutrients to the resting skeletal muscle cells and to remove the small amounts of carbon dioxide and other waste products being produced by those cells. In contrast, during exercise, the metabolic rate of the skeletal muscle cells increases several-fold, as does their need for blood flow. During exercise, skeletal muscle arterioles dilate. Increasingly more of them remain open on a "full-time" basis as the level of exercise increases. Consequently, blood flow through the capillaries increases and becomes more continuous.

These changes act in three ways to speed the delivery of oxygen and metabolic substrates to the exercising muscle cells and to facilitate the removal of carbon dioxide and other metabolic waste products. First, when more capillaries carry blood, the area available for diffusion (*A* in Fick's diffusion equation) is increased. Second, because more capillaries carry blood, the distance between each exercising skeletal muscle cell and the nearest open capillary (Δx in the diffusion equation) is decreased. Third, the driving force for diffusion of oxygen (the oxygen concentration difference between the capillary blood and the interstitial fluid) is increased. The concentration difference is increased because (1) the greater blood flow brings more freshly oxygenated blood into the capillaries, and (2) the rapid utilization of oxygen by the exercising skeletal muscle cells decreases the concentration of oxygen within these cells and therefore within the surrounding interstitial fluid.

The same factors that increase the rate of oxygen diffusion during exercise also increase the rate of delivery of glucose and other nutrients. Furthermore, the same factors act to increase the rate at which carbon dioxide and other metabolic products are removed from the tissue cells and into the bloodstream. In the case of carbon dioxide and other metabolic products, the concentration is highest in the cells and lowest in the capillary plasma, so diffusional movement is from the cells toward the bloodstream.

Water Moves Across Capillary Walls Both by Diffusion (Osmosis) and by Bulk Flow

The exchange of water between the capillary plasma and the interstitial fluid merits special consideration for two reasons. First, the forces that govern water movement are more complicated than the simple diffusive forces that affect solute movement. Second, a particular imbalance in these forces causes an excessive amount of water to accumulate in the interstitial space, which leads to the important clinical sign, *edema*.

As the preceding discussion emphasized, solutes such as oxygen, carbon dioxide, glucose, electrolytes, and fatty acids move between the capillary plasma and the interstitial fluid by diffusion. Water also moves by diffusion; the diffusional movement of water is called *osmosis*. The physical prerequisites for osmosis are (1) the presence of a *semipermeable membrane* (a membrane that is permeable to water but not to specific solutes), and (2) a difference in the total concentration of the *impermeable solutes* on the two sides of the membrane.

The capillary wall constitutes a semipermeable membrane. Water can readily pass through capillary pores; however, the pores in continuous capillaries are too small to permit the passage of plasma proteins. As a consequence, the concentration of plasma proteins is normally much higher in the capillary plasma than in the interstitial fluid. Protein concentration is typically 7 grams per deciliter (g/dL) within the capillary plasma but only 0.2 g/dL in the interstitial fluid. These dissimilar protein concentrations create an osmotic imbalance. As a consequence, water molecules tend to move by osmosis from the interstitial fluid into the capillary blood plasma. (Remember that water moves by osmosis toward the side of the semi-permeable membrane with the higher concentration of impermeable solute.)

The tendency for water to move by diffusion is quantified as *osmotic pressure* (see Chapter 1). The normal osmotic pressure created by the proteins in the plasma is 25 mm Hg; that is, the osmotic effect of the plasma proteins is equivalent to a pressure of 25 mm Hg driving water into the capillaries. The osmotic pressure created by the plasma proteins is also called *plasma oncotic pressure* or *colloid osmotic pressure*. (The term *colloid* is used because the plasma proteins are not in a true solution but rather in a colloidal suspension.)

The plasma proteins in the interstitial fluid also exert an osmotic effect. However, because the concentration of plasma proteins in interstitial fluid is normally quite low, the oncotic pressure created in the interstitial fluid by these proteins is normally only about 1 mm Hg. The imbalance of oncotic pressures (higher in the capillary fluid than in the interstitial fluid) creates a net driving force for the diffusion (osmotic movement) of water from the interstitial fluid into the capillaries.

The movement of water into a capillary is called *reabsorption*. The movement of water in the opposite direction, from the capillary plasma into the interstitial fluid, is called *filtration*. The *oncotic pressure difference* normally favors reabsorption. Oncotic pressure difference is calculated by subtracting the oncotic pressure of interstitial fluid from the oncotic pressure of capillary blood (e.g., 25 mm Hg − 1 mm Hg = 24 mm Hg).

In addition to being affected by diffusional (osmotic) forces, water responds to hydrostatic pressure differences across the capillary wall. Hydrostatic pressure differences cause water to move by bulk flow; in this case the bulk flow occurs through the capillary pores. The hydrostatic pressure within the capillaries (capillary blood pressure) is higher at the arteriolar end of capillaries than at the venous end (see Figure 22-1). However, a representative average capillary hydrostatic pressure would be about 18 mm Hg. In contrast, interstitial fluid hydrostatic pressure is normally about −7 mm Hg. The negative sign simply means that interstitial fluid pressure is *less,* (although only slightly less) than atmospheric pressure. The negative interstitial fluid pressure (−7 mm Hg) together with the positive capillary hydrostatic pressure (18 mm Hg) creates a hydrostatic pressure difference of 25 mm Hg across the wall of a typical capillary. This hydrostatic pressure difference tends to force water out of the capillaries and into the interstitial spaces; that is, the *hydrostatic pressure difference* favors filtration.

In most capillaries of the systemic circulation, the hydrostatic pressure difference (which favors filtration) almost balances the oncotic pressure difference (which favors reabsorption). However, the balance is rarely perfect. Usually, the hydrostatic pressure difference slightly exceeds the oncotic pressure difference, so there is a small, net filtration of water out of the capillaries. This water would simply accumulate in the interstitial spaces and cause swelling there if not for the lymph vessels, which collect excess interstitial fluid and return it to the bloodstream through the subclavian veins (Figure 23-4).

Capillary hydrostatic pressure and interstitial fluid hydrostatic pressure are, by convention, always measured relative to atmospheric pressure. Thus, to say that interstitial pressure is normally "negative" does not imply that a vacuum exists in the interstitium but only that the interstitial pressure is slightly below atmospheric pressure. If all the interstitial spaces of the body had a hydrostatic pressure higher than atmospheric pressure, all parts of the body would bulge outward. The subatmospheric interstitial fluid pressure probably accounts for the fact that the skin normally stays snug against the underlying tissue and that some body surfaces normally have a concave shape (e.g., axillary space, orbits of the eyes).

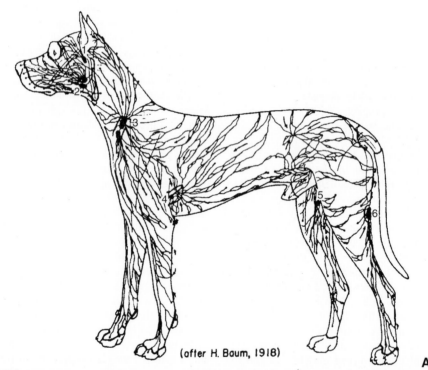

(after H. Baum, 1918)

A

FIGURE 23-4 Anatomical **(A)** and schematic **(B)** overviews of the lymphatic system. The lymphatic vessels collect excess interstitial fluid from tissues throughout the body (including the lungs) and carry it to the subclavian veins, where the lymph reenters the bloodstream. Lymph moves through lymph vessels via bulk flow. The driving force for this flow is interstitial fluid hydrostatic pressure minus subclavian vein pressure. Lymph flow is also promoted by the massaging action exerted on lymph vessels by contraction and relaxation of skeletal muscles and (in the lungs) by the pressure variations accompanying inspiration and expiration. The lymph vessels contain one-way valves, which prevent the backflow of lymph. Thus, massaging actions propel lymph in one direction only: toward the subclavian vein. In addition, some lymph vessels have smooth muscle in their walls, and the alternating contraction and relaxation of this smooth muscle also propels lymph flow toward the subclavian veins. The *numbers* in **A** identify the major lymph nodes. The *magnified inset* in **B** depicts the typical, net filtration of fluid out of a blood capillary and into the interstitial space. This excess interstitial fluid is collected and carried away by the lymph capillaries. Three red blood cells are depicted in the blood capillary. Plasma is indicated in *yellow,* interstitial fluid and lymph in *blue.* (**A** from Getty R: *Sisson and Grossman's the anatomy of the domestic animal,* vol 2, Philadelphia, 1975, Saunders.)

Continued

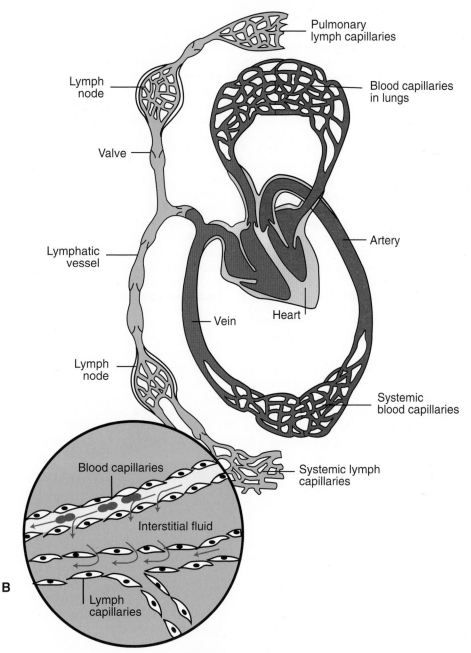

FIGURE 23-4, cont'd.

The Starling Equation Quantifies the Interaction of Oncotic and Hydrostatic Forces Acting on Water

The following equation expresses mathematically the interaction between osmotic pressures and hydrostatic pressures in determination of the net force (net pressure) acting on water:

$$\text{Net pressure} = (P_c - P_i) - (\pi_c - \pi_i)$$

Where P_c is capillary hydrostatic pressure, P_i is interstitial fluid hydrostatic pressure, π_c is capillary plasma oncotic pressure, and π_i is interstitial fluid oncotic pressure. Nominal values for these pressures in systemic tissues are as follows:

$P_c = 18$ mm Hg
$P_i = -7$ mm Hg
$\pi_c = 25$ mm Hg
$\pi_i = 1$ mm Hg

The solution of this equation, with nominal values inserted for each term, is:

$$\begin{aligned}\text{Net pressure} &= (18\text{ mm Hg} - -7\text{ mm Hg}) \\ &\quad - (25\text{ mm Hg} - 1\text{ mm Hg}) \\ &= +1\text{ mm Hg}\end{aligned}$$

A positive net pressure favors filtration (a negative net pressure would indicate that reabsorption is favored). The small magnitude of the net pressure (1 mm Hg) indicates that the hydrostatic and osmotic forces that affect water are almost in balance (i.e., there is only a slight tendency for filtration). The quantitative analysis of how oncotic and hydrostatic pressures affect water movement across capillary walls was first derived by Ernest Henry Starling (the same scientist for whom Starling's law of the heart is named). Therefore the oncotic and hydrostatic pressures that act on water are often called *Starling forces.* Furthermore, the tendency for the net oncotic effect to be closely balanced by the net hydrostatic effect is often referred to as the *balance of Starling forces.* Starling realized that the actual rate of water movement across capillary walls is affected both by the magnitude of the imbalance between hydrostatic and oncotic forces and by the permeability of the capillary wall to water. These ideas are expressed in the following equation, which indicates that the movement of water is equal to the permeability of the capillary wall (given as the filtration coefficient K_f) multiplied by the net difference between the hydrostatic and oncotic pressures:

$$\text{Transcapillary water flux} = K_f[(P_c - P_i) - (\pi_c - \pi_i)]$$

Examination of this equation reveals that the tendency for the filtration of water out of capillaries can be enhanced by (1) increasing the hydrostatic pressure difference between capillary blood and interstitial fluid, (2) decreasing the osmotic tendency for water to be reabsorbed, or (3) increasing the permeability of the capillary to water (i.e., increasing the filtration coefficient).

Several Common Physiological Changes Alter the Normal Balance of Starling Forces and Increase the Filtration of Water Out of Capillaries

An increase in capillary hydrostatic pressure (P_c) favors a greater filtration of water. Capillary hydrostatic pressure can be increased by an increase in arterial blood pressure or by a decrease in arteriolar resistance. An increase in arterial pressure causes more pressure to be transmitted down through the arterioles and into the capillaries. Likewise, a decrease in arteriolar resistance (e.g., a dilation of the arterioles) allows a greater portion of the arterial pressure to be transmitted into the capillaries. Capillary hydrostatic pressure can also be increased by a "backing up" (or "damming up") of venous blood. For example, an increase in central venous pressure causes blood to accumulate in the systemic capillaries and raises capillary pressure. An obstruction to venous outflow (e.g., too tight a dressing on a limb) also causes blood to back up in the capillaries of the limb, which increases capillary hydrostatic pressure.

The primary determinant of interstitial fluid hydrostatic pressure is the volume of fluid present in the interstitial space. An accumulation of interstitial fluid increases interstitial hydrostatic pressure. Removal of interstitial fluid decreases the pressure. As stated earlier, interstitial fluid hydrostatic pressure is usually slightly subatmospheric (e.g., −7 mm Hg). When interstitial fluid hydrostatic pressure rises above atmospheric pressure, the accumulation of interstitial fluid becomes clinically noticeable as a swelling, or *edema.*

The net oncotic pressure depends on the concentrations of proteins in the capillary plasma and in the interstitial fluid. The normal protein concentration in plasma is 7 g/dL, which results in a plasma oncotic pressure of 25 mm Hg. Any alteration in the concentration of proteins in the capillary plasma alters the plasma oncotic pressure.

Similarly, changes in the interstitial protein concentration alter interstitial fluid oncotic pressure. In most organs of the systemic circulation protein molecules do not readily pass through the capillary pores or clefts. As already described, the main route for the delivery of plasma proteins into the interstitial fluid is through the three-step process of *transcytosis.* An increase in the rate of vesicle formation and discharge increases the delivery of plasma proteins into the interstitial space and therefore increases

interstitial fluid oncotic pressure. In addition, abnormal circumstances (e.g., tissue inflammation) can cause the capillary pores to open wide enough that plasma proteins can pass through.

Plasma proteins are removed from the interstitial space through lymph flow. The smallest lymphatic vessels (*lymphatic capillaries*) are structured much like blood capillaries. One difference is that the clefts between the endothelial cells of lymphatic capillaries are large enough to readily accommodate the passage of plasma protein molecules. Therefore, when excess interstitial fluid flows into lymph capillaries, any plasma proteins that are present in the interstitial fluid are also carried into the lymph capillaries. The lymphatic fluid, containing these plasma proteins, flows to the thorax, where the fluid reenters the bloodstream at the subclavian veins (see Figure 23-4).

The role of lymphatic flow in counteracting the accumulation of excessive interstitial fluid is especially important in the lungs. Lung capillaries are more permeable to plasma proteins than are most capillaries in the systemic circulation. As a result, the oncotic pressure of interstitial fluid in the lungs is normally rather high (nominally 18 mm Hg). Capillary hydrostatic pressure in the lungs is generally about 12 mm Hg. (This value is lower than the capillary hydrostatic pressure in systemic capillaries because pulmonary arterial pressure is so much lower than systemic arterial pressure.) Interstitial hydrostatic pressure in the lungs is generally about −4 mm Hg (the same as intrapleural pressure). Summation of these Starling forces for lung capillaries yields the following:

$$\begin{aligned}\text{Net pressure} &= (P_c - P_i) - (\pi_c - \pi_i) \\ &= (12 \text{ mm Hg} - -4 \text{ mm Hg}) \\ &\quad - (25 \text{ mm Hg} - 18 \text{ mm Hg}) \\ &= +9 \text{ mm Hg}\end{aligned}$$

A net pressure of +9 mm Hg indicates that there is a substantial driving force for filtration of fluid out of the capillaries and into the lung interstitial spaces. The lung interstitial spaces would fill rapidly with water, and pulmonary edema would develop, were it not for the well-developed system of lymph vessels in the lungs. These vessels continuously remove interstitial fluid and prevent its excessive accumulation.

Edema Is a Clinically Noticeable Excess of Interstitial Fluid

Edema is a common clinical problem. Edema results either from excessive filtration of fluid out of capillaries or from depressed lymphatic function. One common cause is increased venous pressure. Increased venous pressure can result from the application of a too-tight dressing on the extremity of an animal. The resulting constriction of the veins impedes the outflow of venous blood from the limb. Blood backs up in the limb veins, which increases venous pressure. Blood then backs up in the capillaries and increases capillary hydrostatic pressure. As shown in Figure 23-5, the increase in capillary hydrostatic pressure leads to excessive filtration of capillary fluid into the interstitial space. When this accumulation of fluids becomes clinically noticeable, the patient is said to exhibit edema.

Other causes of increased venous pressure are severe pulmonic stenosis (see Clinical Correlation for Chapter 21) and severe heartworm disease (see Clinical Correlation for Chapter 22). In these conditions, an excessive volume of blood accumulates in the right atrium and systemic veins. The resulting increase in venous pressure causes blood to back up in the systemic

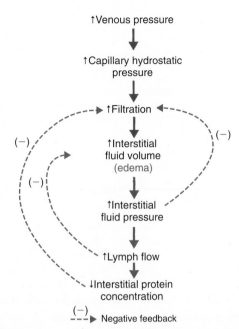

FIGURE 23-5 Increase in venous pressure leads to increase in interstitial fluid volume (edema). The *dashed lines (negative feedback)* indicate the counteracting effects of the three safety factors against edema. First, an increase in interstitial fluid hydrostatic pressure reduces the rate of filtration back toward normal. Second, an increase in lymph flow reduces interstitial fluid volume back toward normal. Third, a decrease in interstitial fluid protein concentration reduces the rate of filtration back toward normal.

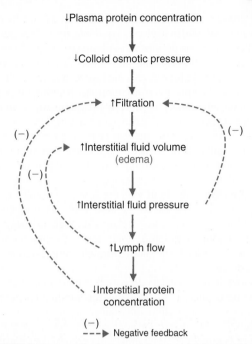

FIGURE 23-6 Decrease in plasma protein concentration leads to edema, but the degree of edema is limited by the same three safety factors as shown in Figure 23-5.

capillaries and this increases capillary hydrostatic pressure and leads to edema, as shown in Figure 23-5.

Whatever the cause of an increase in venous pressure, three factors *(safety factors)* limit the degree of the resulting edema. All three safety factors depend on an increased interstitial fluid volume leading to an increase in interstitial fluid hydrostatic pressure. The first safety factor is that the increased interstitial fluid pressure acts directly to oppose or limit filtration. Interstitial fluid pressure does not need to rise above capillary hydrostatic pressure to limit edema. Any increase in interstitial fluid pressure (e.g., from a normal value of −7 to +2 mm Hg) helps to change the net balance of the Starling forces in the direction of reducing excessive filtration.

The second safety factor against edema is that increased interstitial fluid pressure promotes lymph flow. Lymph flow removes edema fluid from the tissue and therefore helps to limit the degree of edema.

The third safety factor is an indirect consequence of increased lymph flow. Recall that interstitial fluid normally contains a small amount of plasma protein, usually the result of transcytosis. This protein exerts a small but significant oncotic pressure that favors filtration. Under the circumstance of increased capillary hydrostatic pressure, the increased capillary filtration delivers fluid into the interstitial space that is relatively free of proteins. Meanwhile, the elevated lymph flow carries away not only interstitial fluid but also the proteins that were originally present in the interstitial fluid. Therefore, the combination of increased filtration and increased lymph flow leads to a reduction in the interstitial protein concentration. The resulting decrease in interstitial fluid oncotic pressure helps reduce the excess filtration back toward normal.

To summarize, an increase in venous pressure leads to an increase in capillary hydrostatic pressure, which increases filtration. Edema develops. Three safety factors then come into play to reduce filtration back toward normal and to limit the degree of edema. A steady-state degree of edema is eventually reached, in which interstitial fluid is removed by lymph vessels as fast as it is filtered.

The *systemic edema* that results from an increase in systemic venous pressure is often most noticeable in the dependent regions of the body, such as the lower extremities in human patients or the abdominal organs in humans or animals. When edema develops in the abdominal organs, excess interstitial fluid tends to ooze out of the edematous tissues and accumulate in the peritoneal space. Excessive fluid in the peritoneum is called *ascites*.

Marked systemic edema and ascites is common in patients with right ventricular heart failure. By contrast, failure of the left ventricle leads to *pulmonary edema*. Ineffective pumping by the left ventricle results in increased blood volume and increased pressure in the left atrium and pulmonary veins. This elevated pressure extends back into the pulmonary capillaries, which increases capillary filtration in the lung tissue. In severe cases of pulmonary edema, some of the excess interstitial fluid oozes into the alveoli and bronchial airways. Such a patient typically coughs up a frothy fluid. Excess edema fluid may also ooze into the intrapleural space, which is called *pleural effusion*. The consequences of heart failure are discussed more fully in Chapter 26.

A decreased plasma protein concentration *(hypoproteinemia)* is another common cause of edema (Figure 23-6). One cause of hypoproteinemia is a decrease in the rate of plasma protein production by the liver. This occurs in malnutrition and leads to the clinical syndrome of *kwashiorkor*. Victims of kwashiorkor typically look emaciated, except that the abdomen is grossly distended by edema and ascites. Another cause of abnormally low plasma protein concentration is an increase in the rate of loss of plasma proteins from the body. Protein loss occurs in kidney disease. For example, in *nephrotic syndrome,* the kidney glomerular capillaries become permeable to plasma proteins. Plasma proteins leave the bloodstream and enter the urinary tubules (nephrons) of the kidney. A chronic loss of proteins in the urine reduces the plasma protein concentration. Therefore the presence of substantial amounts of plasma protein in the urine is an alarming clinical sign.

Severe burns also cause the loss of plasma proteins from the body. The capillaries of burned skin become very permeable to both fluid and proteins. Substantial amounts of plasma can leave the body through these damaged capillaries. The presence of plasma proteins in the fluid weeping from a burn site accounts for the typical yellow color of that fluid. If the water and electrolytes lost through burns are replaced through drinking or an intravenous administration of fluids, and if the plasma proteins are not also replaced, the plasma protein concentration in the blood decreases.

Whether it results from decreased production or increased loss, hypoproteinemia leads to a decrease in plasma colloid osmotic pressure. This alters the balance of the Starling forces in a direction that favors excessive filtration of fluid from the capillaries (see Figure 23-6). Interstitial fluid accumulates and edema is noticed. However, the same three safety factors that limit edema in the case of increased venous pressure (see Figure 23-5) also operate in the case of decreased plasma protein concentration. The degree of edema is limited by (1) an increased interstitial fluid pressure, (2) an increased lymph flow, and (3) a decreased interstitial protein concentration.

Another cause of edema is lymphatic obstruction. Clinically, this situation is called *lymphedema.* The passage of lymph through lymph nodes can be impaired by inflammation of the nodal tissue or cancerous tumors growing within the nodes. Also, in certain parasitic diseases, microfilariae lodge in the lymph nodes and obstruct lymph flow. Filarial parasites cause the pronounced edema seen in cases of *elephantiasis.* Lymphedema also occurs as a secondary consequence of surgical procedures that damage lymph nodes. A common example of this in human medicine is the edema of the arm that follows radical mastectomy. The removal of axillary lymph nodes during radical mastectomy creates scar tissue that impairs lymphatic drainage from the arm.

Figure 23-7 traces the causes of edema after lymphatic obstruction and shows why lymphedema is clinically so troublesome. Lymphatic obstruction decreases lymph flow. Interstitial fluid accumulates in the tissues, instead of being removed by the lymph, and edema results. The accumulation of edema fluid raises interstitial fluid pressure, which acts as a safety factor by reducing capillary filtration. However, the second and third safety factors discussed earlier are absent in the case of lymphedema because these factors depend on an increase in lymph flow. In lymphedema a decreased lymph flow is the causative problem, so there cannot be an increased lymph flow (second safety factor) to compensate for the edema. Moreover, when lymph flow is impaired, plasma proteins accumulate in the interstitial fluid instead of being carried away by the lymph. Therefore the third safety factor that protects against edema (decreased interstitial fluid oncotic pressure) is also compromised in lymphedema.

Another cause of edema is physical injury or an allergic reaction to antigen challenges. Physical trauma, such as a scratch or a cut on the skin, results in a localized bump or swelling. A similar swelling is observed when the skin reacts to an irritating agent or antigen challenge (e.g., response to an insect bite). An allergic swelling can also occur in bronchial tissue during an asthmatic

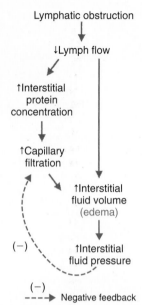

FIGURE 23-7 Lymphatic obstruction leads to edema. Lymphedema is clinically troublesome because only one of the normal three safety factors is operative to limit the degree of edema.

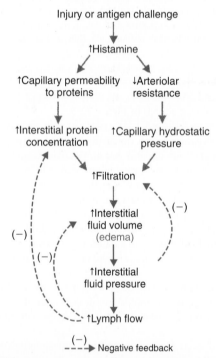

FIGURE 23-8 Histamine mediates the changes that lead to edema in response to a physical injury or an antigen challenge. The normal three safety factors against edema are intact and help to limit the degree of edema. Treatment with an antihistamine (a drug that blocks histamine receptors on arterioles and capillaries) also helps to reduce edema in these cases.

reaction. The edema of asthma can be life threatening because it limits airflow to the lungs. As shown in Figure 23-8, an injury or antigen challenge leads to the release of the chemical *histamine* from mast cells in the affected tissue. Histamine has two effects that cause edema. First, histamine increases the permeability of capillaries to proteins. As proteins leave the bloodstream and accumulate in the interstitial space of the damaged tissue, they increase the interstitial fluid oncotic pressure, which promotes filtration of fluid. Second, histamine relaxes arteriolar smooth muscle. The arterioles dilate, and the resulting decrease in arteriolar resistance allows more of the arterial blood pressure to impinge on the capillaries. This leads to an increase in the capillary hydrostatic pressure, which promotes filtration. Although histamine promotes excess filtration and edema through two mechanisms, all three safety factors that protect against edema are intact and act to limit the degree of edema.

Other situations also cause edema, but the examples discussed here cover some of the most common causes of clinical edema. These examples also reinforce an understanding of the interplay of the osmotic (oncotic) and hydrostatic forces that act on water to govern its filtration out of capillaries or its reabsorption into capillaries.

CLINICAL CORRELATIONS

ACUTE PROTEIN-LOSING ENTEROPATHY IN A HORSE

History. You are called to a home a few miles from your clinic by parents who are concerned about their daughter's 4-year-old Quarter Horse mare. They report that the horse is listless and has had diarrhea for 2 days.

Clinical Examination. You arrive at the client's home to find that the horse is stabled in a small barn with poor ventilation and no access to pasture. Low-quality grass hay is stacked in the barn. On physical examination, you find the horse to be somewhat emaciated, with dry mucous membranes, a foul-smelling diarrhea, and an elevated heart rate (tachycardia). When you pinch a section of the horse's skin, it falls back to the normal position slowly, which indicates dehydration. The horse's temperature is within a normal range.

You take a blood sample and then begin an intravenous administration of polyionic fluid (lactated Ringer's solution). You tell the clients that you will return later. Analysis of the blood sample indicates a hematocrit of 55% (normal range for the horse, 35% to 45%) and a plasma protein concentration of 4.5 g/dL (normal range, 5.9 to 7.8 g/dL). You become concerned that the administration of fluids, without replacement of plasma proteins, will exacerbate the horse's hypoproteinemia, so you arrange to obtain plasma from a donor horse. You return with the plasma and find that the sick horse is still listless. Edema is now evident along the horse's ventral abdomen and in the limbs.

Comment. *Acute enteropathy* (intestinal disorder) often causes diarrhea. The loss of water and solutes leads to dehydration; blood volume and interstitial fluid volume are both reduced. The hematocrit (fraction of cells in blood) is typically elevated because fluid is being removed from the bloodstream but blood cells are not. In some forms of enteropathy (called *protein-losing enteropathy*) the capillaries in the intestine become leaky to plasma proteins. Albumin, in particular, moves from the bloodstream into the intestinal lumen and is eliminated in the feces.

This horse has a severe shortage of plasma proteins. The shortage of plasma proteins probably resulted from a combination of poor nutrition (which depresses the production of plasma proteins by the liver) and protein-losing enteropathy. The deficit of plasma proteins in this horse is even more severe than might be suspected on the basis of the plasma protein concentration of 4.5 g/dL, because this value is the net result of two opposing

processes. The loss of protein in the diarrhea lowered the plasma protein concentration, but the loss of water (dehydration) decreased plasma volume and therefore increased the concentration of the remaining proteins in the plasma.

The development of edema in this horse was predictable. The administration of intravenous fluids added water and electrolytes to the circulating blood volume, but this reduced the concentration of the plasma proteins remaining in the bloodstream. As a result, plasma oncotic pressure decreased even further, and this led to excess filtration of water out of capillaries and into the interstitial space. The result was edema, especially in the dependent regions of the body (ventral abdomen and legs). Restoration of a normal plasma protein concentration would reverse the edema.

Treatment. Bacterial or parasitic infections are a common cause of protein-losing enteropathy. If this horse had a fever, an infectious cause would be more likely. Acute enteropathy without fever (as in this case) is often self-limiting. Therefore the aim of treatment should be to remedy the dehydration, the electrolyte loss, and the plasma protein deficit. Intravenous administration of plasma, in addition to polyionic fluids, is usually effective. In some cases, antibiotics are also indicated, because enteropathy involves inflammation of the intestinal wall, which can allow transmural migration of bacteria (and toxic bacterial products) from the gastrointestinal tract into the peritoneum. Important steps for long-term health in this horse would include better nutrition, regular deworming, and improved stable management.

PRACTICE QUESTIONS

1. Which of the following will *not* cause pulmonary edema?
   a. An increase in pulmonary capillary permeability to protein
   b. A blockage of pulmonary lymph vessels
   c. An increase in left atrial pressure
   d. A constriction of pulmonary arterioles
   e. Left-sided heart failure

2. A patient with a form of protein-losing kidney disease has a plasma colloid osmotic pressure of 10 mm Hg. The patient has edema but is not getting any worse. Blood pressure and heart rate are normal. Which of the following is probably preventing further edema?
   a. Increased interstitial fluid hydrostatic pressure
   b. Increased capillary hydrostatic pressure
   c. Decreased lymph flow
   d. Increased plasma sodium ion concentration
   e. Increased interstitial fluid oncotic pressure

3. The following parameters were measured in the microcirculation of a skeletal muscle during a period of vigorous exercise:
   P_c (capillary hydrostatic pressure) = 34 mm Hg
   P_i (interstitial fluid hydrostatic pressure) = 10 mm Hg
   π_c (capillary plasma oncotic pressure) = 24 mm Hg
   π_i (interstitial fluid oncotic pressure) = 3 mm Hg
   Which of the following is *true*?
   a. These conditions would favor filtration.
   b. These conditions would favor reabsorption.
   c. These conditions would favor neither filtration nor reabsorption.
   d. It is not clear what these conditions favor because the concentration of plasma protein is not specified.

4. The rate of diffusion of glucose molecules from capillary blood to interstitial fluid is most directly affected by the:
   a. Voltage difference between capillary blood and interstitial fluid.
   b. Interstitial fluid hydrostatic pressure.
   c. Size and number of capillary pores.
   d. Amount of oxygen in the blood.
   e. Hematocrit.

5. During a 30-minute hemorrhage, a horse loses a substantial volume of blood. The horse's mean arterial pressure decreases from 90 to 75 mm Hg, and the heart rate increases from 40 to 90 beats/min. The skin becomes cold and the mucous membranes become pale, suggesting marked vasoconstriction. Because hemorrhage involves the loss of whole blood (both plasma and cells), you might expect that, soon after such a hemorrhage, the horse's remaining blood would still have a normal composition. However, you take a blood sample and discover that the hematocrit is abnormally low (only 28%). Which of the following would *most likely* account for the decrease in hematocrit observed after the hemorrhage?
   a. Arteriolar constriction has caused capillary hydrostatic pressure to increase above normal.
   b. Low capillary hydrostatic pressure has caused interstitial fluid to be reabsorbed into the bloodstream.
   c. Many blood cells have been filtered out of capillaries and into the interstitial fluid.
   d. Excess capillary filtration has caused interstitial fluid pressure to increase above normal.
   e. Excess capillary filtration has caused capillary colloid osmotic pressure to increase above normal.

BIBLIOGRAPHY

Boron WF, Boulpaep EL: *Medical physiology*, ed 2, Philadelphia, 2009, Saunders.

Ettinger SJ, Feldman EC: *Textbook of veterinary internal medicine: diseases of the dog and cat*, ed 7, St Louis, 2010, Elsevier/Saunders.

Hall JE: *Guyton and Hall textbook of medical physiology*, ed 12, Philadelphia, 2011, Saunders.

Koeppen BM, Stanton BA: *Berne & Levy physiology*, ed 6, Philadelphia, 2010, Mosby.

Levy MN, Pappano AJ: *Cardiovascular physiology*, ed 9, St Louis, 2007, Mosby.

Mohrman DE, Heller LJ: *Cardiovascular physiology*, ed 7, New York, 2010, Lange Medical Books/McGraw-Hill.

Mortillaro NA, Taylor AE, editors: *The pathophysiology of the microcirculation*, Boca Raton, Fla, 1994, CRC Press.

Renkin EM: Microcirculation and exchange. In Patton HD, Fuchs AF, Hille B, et al, editors: *Textbook of physiology*, ed 21, Philadelphia, 1989, Saunders.

Robinson NE, Sprayberry KA: *Current therapy in equine medicine*, ed 6, Philadelphia, 2009, Saunders.

Scallan J, Huxley VH, Korthuis RJ: *Capillary fluid exchange: regulation, function, and pathology*, San Rafael, Calif, 2010, Morgan & Claypool Life Sciences.

Wilson DA: *Clinical veterinary advisor: the horse*, Philadelphia, 2011, Saunders.

CHAPTER 24

Local Control of Blood Flow

KEY POINTS

1. Vascular resistance is affected by intrinsic and extrinsic control mechanisms.
2. Metabolic control of blood flow is a local mechanism that matches the blood flow of a tissue to its metabolic rate.
3. Autoregulation is a relative constancy of blood flow in an organ despite changes in perfusion pressure.
4. Many chemical signals act locally (as paracrines) to exert important control on vascular resistance.
5. Regardless of the status of arterioles, mechanical compression can reduce blood flow to a tissue.

Vascular Resistance Is Affected by Intrinsic and Extrinsic Control Mechanisms

As described in Chapter 22, the blood flow through any organ or tissue is determined by the perfusion pressure (arterial pressure minus venous pressure) and by the resistance of the blood vessels of the organ (and by no other factors), as follows:

$$\text{Blood flow} = \text{Perfusion pressure} \div \text{Vascular resistance}$$

Normally, all the organs of the systemic circulation are exposed to the same perfusion pressure. Therefore, differences in blood flow to the various organs result from their different vascular resistances. The vascular resistance of an organ is determined mainly by the diameter of its arterioles. Thus, arteriolar vasodilation and vasoconstriction are the mechanisms that increase or decrease the blood flow in one organ relative to another organ.

In general, the factors that affect arteriolar resistance can be divided into intrinsic and extrinsic factors. *Extrinsic control* involves mechanisms that act from outside an organ or tissue, through nerves or hormones, to alter arteriolar resistance. *Intrinsic control* is exerted by local mechanisms within an organ or tissue. For example, as described in Chapter 23, histamine is released from mast cells of a tissue in response to injury or during an allergic reaction. Histamine acts locally on the arteriolar smooth muscle to relax it. Dilation of the arterioles decreases arteriolar resistance and therefore increases blood flow to the tissue. Histamine is an example of a *paracrine:* a substance released from one type of cell that acts on another cell type in the vicinity. Paracrine signaling molecules move by diffusion, which is why paracrine signaling is only effective over very short distances. A second example of intrinsic control is the arteriolar dilation and increased blood flow during exercise in skeletal muscle. This example illustrates the general phenomenon of *metabolic control* of blood flow: tissues tend to increase their blood flow whenever their metabolic rate increases.

Although the arterioles in all tissues are affected by both intrinsic and extrinsic mechanisms, intrinsic mechanisms predominate over extrinsic mechanisms in the control of arterioles in the brain, heart (i.e., coronary circulation), and working skeletal muscle. By contrast, extrinsic mechanisms predominate over intrinsic mechanisms in the control of blood flow to the kidneys, splanchnic organs, and resting skeletal muscle. Skin is an example of an organ in which both intrinsic and extrinsic control mechanisms have strong influences. In general, local (intrinsic) control dominates extrinsic control in the *critical organs:* those that must have sufficient blood flow to meet their metabolic needs on a second-by-second basis for an animal to survive. Extrinsic control dominates intrinsic control in organs that can withstand temporary reductions in blood flow (and metabolism) to make extra blood available for the critical organs.

Metabolic Control of Blood Flow Is a Local Mechanism That Matches the Blood Flow of a Tissue to Its Metabolic Rate

Metabolic control of blood flow is the most important local control mechanism. For example, metabolic control accounts for the huge increase in blood flow through a skeletal muscle as it goes from rest to maximal exercise. The functional significance of metabolic control of blood flow is that it matches the blood flow in a tissue to the metabolic rate of the tissue. An increase in tissue blood flow in response to increased metabolic rate is called *active hyperemia* (*hyper* means "elevated," *emia* refers to blood, and *active* implies an increased metabolic rate).

Metabolic control of blood flow works by means of chemical changes within the tissue. When the metabolic rate of a tissue increases, its consumption of oxygen increases, and there is an increased rate of production of metabolic products, including carbon dioxide, adenosine, and lactic acid. Also, some potassium ions (K^+) escape from rapidly metabolizing cells, and these ions accumulate in the interstitial fluid. Therefore, as the metabolism of a tissue increases, the interstitial concentration of oxygen decreases, and the interstitial concentrations of metabolic products and K^+ increase. All these changes have the same effect on arteriolar smooth muscle: they relax it (Table 24-1). The arterioles dilate, vascular resistance decreases, and more blood flows through the tissue.

TABLE 24-1 Chemical Signals Important in Local Control of Systemic Arterioles*

Chemical Signal	Source	Effect
Signals Related to Metabolism		
Oxygen	Delivered by arterial blood; consumed in aerobic metabolism	Vasoconstriction. (Rapid metabolism depletes O_2, which causes vasodilation.)
Carbon dioxide	Produced by aerobic metabolism	Vasodilation
Potassium ions (K^+)	Released from rapidly metabolizing cells	Vasodilation
Adenosine	Released from rapidly metabolizing cells	Vasodilation
Metabolic acids (e.g., lactic acid)	Produced by anaerobic metabolism	Vasodilation
Other Local Chemical Signals (Paracrines)		
Endothelin-1 (ET1)	Endothelial cells	Vasoconstriction
Nitric oxide (NO)	Endothelial cells and some parasympathetic nerve endings	Vasodilation
Thromboxane A_2 (TXA_2)	Platelets	Vasoconstriction (also increases platelet aggregation)
Prostacyclin (PGI_2)	Endothelial cells	Vasodilation (also decreases platelet aggregation)
Histamine	Mast cells	Vasodilation (also increases capillary permeability)
Bradykinin	Globulins in blood or tissue fluid	Vasodilation (also increases capillary permeability)

*Some of these chemical signals have different effects on pulmonary blood vessels than on systemic vessels. A high level of oxygen, for example, causes dilation of pulmonary vessels, whereas the effect in systemic vessels is vasoconstriction. See Chapter 46 for more details.

Low levels of oxygen and high concentrations of metabolic products and K^+ also cause relaxation of the precapillary sphincters (in the tissues that have them), and this opens more of the capillaries in the tissue to blood flow. As explained in Chapter 23, the opening of more capillaries decreases the diffusion distance between fresh, oxygenated blood and the metabolizing cells of the tissue. Opening more capillaries also increases the total capillary surface area for diffusional exchange. The net result of the increased blood flow, the decreased diffusion distance, and the increased total capillary surface area is a more rapid delivery of oxygen and other metabolic substrates to the tissue cells and a more rapid removal of metabolic waste products from the tissue.

Metabolic control of blood flow involves negative feedback. The accumulation of metabolic products and the lack of oxygen initiate vasodilation, which increases blood flow. The increased blood flow removes the accumulating metabolic products and delivers additional oxygen. A new balance is reached when the increased blood flow closely matches the increased metabolic needs of the tissue. Figure 24-1 summarizes the major features of metabolic control of blood flow.

Reactive hyperemia is a temporary increase above normal in the flow of blood to a tissue after a period when blood flow was restricted. In this case the increased flow (hyperemia) is a response (reaction) to a period of inadequate blood flow. Mechanical compression of blood vessels is one cause of inadequate blood flow, and release of that mechanical compression elicits reactive hyperemia. This can be easily demonstrated in any accessible nonpigmented epithelial tissue. For example, press a finger against nonpigmented skin hard enough to occlude the blood flow. Maintain the pressure for about 1 minute, and then release. After release of the pressure, the previously compressed skin will appear

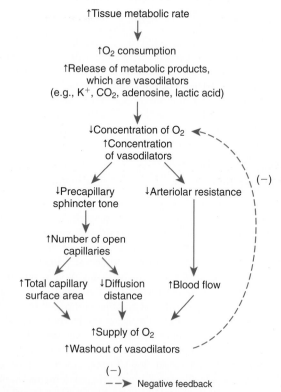

FIGURE 24-1 Metabolic control of blood flow is a local (intrinsic) mechanism that acts within a tissue to match the blood flow to the tissue with the metabolic activity of the tissue. As a tissue becomes more active metabolically, the metabolic control mechanism increases blood flow and thereby regulates the concentration of oxygen and metabolic products in the tissue.

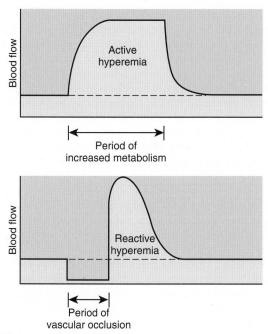

FIGURE 24-2 Both active hyperemia and reactive hyperemia involve increases above normal in blood flow. Both phenomena are brought about by the mechanisms for the local, metabolic control of blood flow.

darker (redder) for a short time, because blood flow will become greater than normal after the compression is released.

The same metabolic control mechanisms that account for active hyperemia also explain reactive hyperemia. During the period when mechanical compression restricts blood flow, metabolism continues in the compressed tissue; metabolic products accumulate, and the local concentration of oxygen decreases. These metabolic effects cause dilation of the arterioles and a decrease in arteriolar resistance. When the mechanical obstruction to flow is removed, blood flow increases above normal until the "oxygen debt" is repaid and the excess metabolic products have been removed from the compressed tissue. Figure 24-2 compares active and reactive hyperemia.

Autoregulation Is a Relative Constancy of Blood Flow in an Organ Despite Changes in Perfusion Pressure

Metabolic control mechanisms also participate in the phenomenon known as *blood flow autoregulation*. Autoregulation is evident in denervated organs and organs in which local control of blood flow is predominant over neural and humoral control (e.g., in coronary circulation, brain, and working skeletal muscle).

Figure 24-3 summarizes an experiment that demonstrates autoregulation in the brain. Initially, the perfusion pressure (arterial pressure minus venous pressure) in this animal is 100 mm Hg, and the blood flow to the brain is 100 milliliters per minute (mL/min) (point A). When perfusion pressure is increased suddenly to 140 mm Hg, brain blood flow rises initially to 140 mL/min but returns toward its initial level over the next 20 to 30 seconds. Eventually, blood flow reaches a stable level of about 110 mL/min (point B). Conversely, if the perfusion pressure is decreased suddenly from 100 to 60 mm Hg, blood flow in the brain decreases initially to 60 mL/min but returns toward its initial level over the next 20 to 30 seconds (see *dashed lines* in the top and middle graphs of Figure 24-3). Eventually, blood flow reaches a stable level of about 90 mL/min (point C). These stable responses are

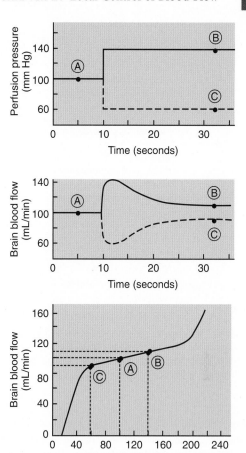

FIGURE 24-3 The experiment summarized here demonstrates autoregulation of blood flow in the brain. Perfusion pressure was artificially set to various levels *(top)*, and the resulting changes in brain blood flow were measured *(middle)*. The steady-state values of blood flow were then plotted against perfusion pressure *(bottom)*. Points A, B, and C are discussed in the text.

plotted in the bottom graph. The remainder of the bottom graph is obtained in a similar way; that is, perfusion pressure is set artificially to various levels, ranging from 40 to 220 mm Hg, and the resulting steady-state levels of blood flow are plotted.

Over a considerable range of perfusion pressure (about 60 to 190 mm Hg), relatively little change occurs in steady-state blood flow to the brain; that is, brain blood flow is autoregulated. The range of perfusion pressures over which flow remains relatively constant is called the *autoregulatory range*. Autoregulation fails at very high and very low perfusion pressures. Extremely high pressures result in marked increases in blood flow, and extremely low pressures result in marked decreases in blood flow. Nevertheless, over a considerable range of perfusion pressure, autoregulation keeps blood flow in the brain relatively constant.

Figure 24-4 shows how the metabolic control mechanisms previously described can account for the phenomenon of autoregulation. If the metabolic rate of an organ does not change but perfusion pressure is increased above normal, the increased pressure forces additional blood flow through the organ. The additional blood flow accelerates the removal of metabolic products from the interstitial fluid and increases the rate of oxygen delivery to the interstitial fluid. Therefore the concentration of vasodilating metabolic products in the interstitial fluid decreases,

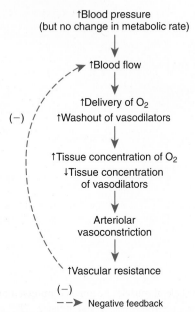

FIGURE 24-4 The same metabolic mechanism that is responsible for active hyperemia and reactive hyperemia can also account for autoregulation, in which blood flow to an organ stays relatively constant despite changes in perfusion pressure.

and the concentration of oxygen in the interstitial fluid increases. These changes cause the arterioles of the tissue to constrict, which increases the resistance to blood flow above normal. The consequence is that blood flow decreases back toward its initial level, despite the continuation of the elevated perfusion pressure.

To summarize, metabolic control mechanisms bring about active hyperemia (the increase in blood flow in an organ in response to an increased metabolic rate, in the absence of any blood pressure change). The same metabolic mechanisms can also account for reactive hyperemia (the increase in blood flow above normal in an organ after a period of flow restriction). In addition, the same metabolic mechanisms can account for autoregulation (the relative constancy of blood flow in an organ when there has been no change in metabolic rate but blood pressure has either increased or decreased). Other mechanisms also contribute to autoregulation, and the reader may encounter discussions of these under the terms *myogenic hypothesis* and *tissue pressure hypothesis*. However, metabolic control plays a major role in autoregulation of blood flow in the critical tissues of a body (brain, coronary vessels, and exercising skeletal muscle).

Many Chemical Signals Act Locally (as Paracrines) to Exert Important Control on Vascular Resistance

As already described, metabolic control of blood flow is mediated by chemical changes that occur when tissue metabolism increases. In addition to the signaling molecules that mediate metabolic control of blood flow, there are many other chemicals that act locally, within a tissue, to affect vascular resistance and therefore blood flow. Some of these locally acting (*paracrine*) chemical signals are listed in Table 24-1.

Endothelin-1 (ET1) is released from endothelial cells in response to a variety of mechanical or chemical stimuli, especially those that traumatize the endothelium. Endothelin-1 causes vascular smooth muscle to contract, which results in vasoconstriction and a decrease in blood flow. *Nitric oxide* (NO), another

signaling molecule released from endothelial cells, has the opposite effect. NO relaxes vascular smooth muscle, which results in vasodilation. One stimulus for NO release is an increase in blood flow velocity past the endothelium. The NO acts locally to dilate vessels, especially small arteries, which allows them to accommodate an increased blood flow without such high flow velocities. In some tissues, most notably the erectile tissues of the external genital organs (penis and clitoris), parasympathetic nerve endings release NO and the neurotransmitter acetylcholine. The acetylcholine stimulates endothelial cells to release additional NO. The NO from the nerve endings, augmented by the NO from the endothelial cells, dilates local blood vessels, which causes engorgement of the tissues with blood, and therefore erection.

Thromboxane A_2 (TXA$_2$) and *prostacyclin* (PGI$_2$) act antagonistically in the control of vascular smooth muscle and also in the control of platelet aggregation. Thus the relative balance between TXA$_2$ and PGI$_2$ is more important than the absolute level of either chemical alone. Under normal conditions the balance ensures adequate blood flow to tissues and prevents platelet aggregation. If blood vessels become traumatized or rupture, the balance shifts in favor of TXA$_2$. The resulting vasoconstriction and platelet aggregation are critical in minimizing blood loss. In some pathological states, imbalances develop between TXA$_2$ and PGI$_2$. Depending on the direction of the imbalance, the result is either excessive vasoconstriction and blood coagulation or excessive vasodilation and bleeding.

Histamine, which is released from mast cells, is another locally acting vasodilator. The role of histamine in the vascular responses to tissue injury or antigen challenge is described in Chapter 23 (see Figure 23-8). *Bradykinin* is another signaling chemical that causes vasodilation. Bradykinin is a small polypeptide that is split away by the proteolytic enzyme *kallikrein* from globulin proteins that are present in plasma or tissue fluid. Bradykinin may also be formed in sweat glands when they are activated by acetylcholine that is released from sympathetic nerve endings. The resulting vasodilation of skin blood vessels, together with the evaporation of sweat, promotes heat loss from the skin. Both histamine and bradykinin exert their vasodilating effects, at least in part, by stimulating the formation of NO.

Regardless of the Status of Arterioles, Mechanical Compression Can Reduce Blood Flow to a Tissue

Mechanical compression can reduce blood flow in a tissue by literally squeezing down on all its blood vessels. The example of compressing skin blood vessels for a minute and then releasing the compression has been mentioned as a way to trigger a readily visible reactive hyperemia. Long-term mechanical pressure on the skin must be avoided, however, because a prolonged period of subnormal blood flow (ischemia) leads to irreversible tissue damage (infarction) and cell death (necrosis). Pressure sores are an unfortunate and common example of this sequence. Three other specific instances of mechanical compression are also described because of their clinical importance.

Figure 24-5 illustrates the effect of mechanical compression on blood flow through the coronary vessels. The top tracing shows the changes in arterial (aortic) blood pressure during one complete cardiac cycle and the beginning of a second one. The periods of ventricular systole and ventricular diastole are labeled at the bottom of the figure. One would expect that blood flow through the coronary circulation would be highest during ventricular systole (when the aortic pressure is highest) and that flow would be lowest during diastole (when the aortic pressure is lowest). However, the tracings of left coronary blood flow indicate that

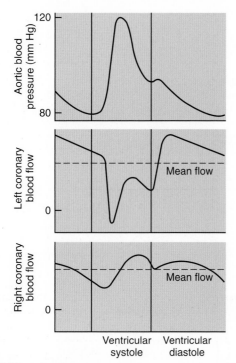

FIGURE 24-5 Coronary blood flow to the left ventricular muscle is greatly reduced during ventricular systole because the left ventricular muscle contracts so forcefully that it compresses the left ventricular blood vessels. Coronary blood flow to the right ventricular muscle is less affected by mechanical compression because the contractions of the right ventricle are less forceful that those of the left ventricle.

blood flow through the left ventricular wall is actually depressed during systole and much higher during diastole. Flow even reverses (blood flows backward, *toward* the aorta) momentarily near the beginning of systole. The fact that left coronary blood flow is much lower during systole, even though the perfusion pressure is higher, implies that the resistance of the coronary vessels must be substantially higher during systole than during diastole.

Left coronary resistance is high during systole because the contracting left ventricular muscle squeezes down on the coronary blood vessels. The coronary vessels are not constricted in this way during diastole because the ventricular muscle is relaxed. Therefore, coronary vascular resistance decreases dramatically (and blood flow increases) during diastole. The bottom tracing in Figure 24-5 indicates that mechanical compression has relatively little influence on blood flow through the right ventricular wall. That is, the magnitude of right coronary blood flow closely follows the changes in arterial pressure (being highest during systole and lowest during diastole). Right coronary flow is not restricted by mechanical compression during systole because the right ventricle contracts with much less force than the left ventricle. The right ventricle simply does not develop sufficient compressive force to constrict its own blood vessels.

Most of the blood that is needed to support left ventricular metabolism must be delivered during ventricular diastole, when the vessels are not compressed. This fact has great clinical significance. In a resting animal with a low heart rate, there is adequate time during diastole for the coronary vessels to supply the amount of blood needed by the ventricular tissue. During exercise, heart rate and cardiac contractility both increase, which greatly increases the metabolic rate of the ventricular muscle cells.

To support the increased metabolic rate, the ventricular tissue needs much more blood flow than at rest. However, the duration of diastole is reduced during exercise, so there is less time available for delivery of this increased flow. Nevertheless, normal, healthy coronary vessels have a sufficiently low resistance (during diastole) to supply the needed blood flow, even during maximal exercise. The situation is different, however, in animals with coronary artery disease. In animals whose coronary vessels are narrowed because of atherosclerosis, blood flow cannot increase enough to supply the needs of the vigorously working ventricular muscles. This is why ventricular ischemia develops during exercise in patients with coronary artery disease. Ischemic areas of the ventricle fail to contract normally. Ischemia can also cause arrhythmias or even ventricular fibrillation (sudden death). Coronary artery disease is more common in humans than in veterinary species, so this scenario is more likely to occur in the veterinarian than in the veterinarian's patients.

Mechanical compression caused by muscle contraction can also restrict blood flow through skeletal muscles. The blood vessels within skeletal muscles become compressed during strenuous, sustained contractions of the muscle. The compression reduces blood flow through the muscle, which can create ischemia. Ischemic muscles cannot contract with normal vigor. Ischemia also activates sensory nerve endings in the muscle, which causes pain. Activation of these muscle ischemia receptors also triggers a reflex increase in arterial pressure. The high arterial pressure is advantageous because it helps to force blood flow through the skeletal muscle blood vessels, despite the compressive effects of the muscle contraction. The high arterial pressure of ischemic exercise is risky for patients with coronary artery disease, however, because high arterial pressure imposes a tremendous increase in workload on the heart. This is why patients with coronary artery disease are cautioned against types of exercise that involve strenuous, sustained muscle contractions, such as weightlifting.

Mechanical compression has important effects on the pulmonary circulation. Pulmonary vessels are more compliant than their counterparts in the systemic circulation. Greater compliance makes the pulmonary vessels more distensible, but also makes them more susceptible to narrowing under the influence of mechanical compression. Moreover, because pulmonary arterial pressure is much lower than systemic arterial pressure, there is less intravascular pressure in a pulmonary vessel to oppose any external force acting to compress the vessel. Most pulmonary vessels travel within the tissues that comprise the walls of the airways, including the very thin walls of alveoli. Figure 24-6 shows how an abnormal elevation in airway pressure can compress pulmonary blood vessels. This could happen during surgery if a patient has a tracheal tube inserted into its airway and if the tracheal tube is attached to a source of elevated pressure. The elevated pressure could be generated by a mechanical respirator that is not adjusted properly or by an anesthetist when he or she squeezes the bag that is attached to the tracheal tube. In either case, the pressures generated in the tracheal tube are transmitted through the airways and into the alveoli. An increase in airway pressure exerts a compressing force on the pulmonary blood vessels.

Alveolar pressures exceeding 10 to 15 mm Hg compress pulmonary blood vessels sufficiently to raise the resistance to blood flow through the lungs. As a result, blood ejected by the right ventricle dams up in the pulmonary arteries. This causes pulmonary arterial pressure to increase. An elevated pulmonary arterial pressure helps force blood through the compressed vessels.

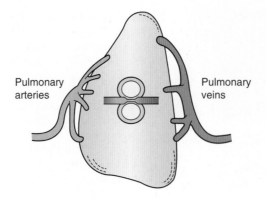

Magnified views of pulmonary capillaries passing between alveoli

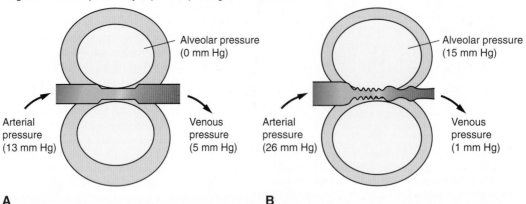

Alveolar pressure
(0 mm Hg)

Arterial
pressure
(13 mm Hg)

Venous
pressure
(5 mm Hg)

Alveolar pressure
(15 mm Hg)

Arterial
pressure
(26 mm Hg)

Venous
pressure
(1 mm Hg)

A   **B**

FIGURE 24-6 Pulmonary blood vessels are susceptible to mechanical compression, which can be created by abnormally high pressure within the airways. **A**, Under normal conditions pulmonary arterial pressure is about 13 mm Hg and the venous pressure is about 5 mm Hg. The pressure within the pulmonary capillary depicted here would be intermediate between these two values. The pressure just outside the capillary (in the alveolar air space) is even lower; alveolar pressures typically vary between −1 mm Hg (during inspiration) and +1 mm Hg (during expiration). Because the pressure inside pulmonary vessels is greater than the pressure outside, the vessels are not compressed. **B**, If alveolar pressure increases to 15 mm Hg or higher, the pulmonary vessels become compressed. The resulting increase in pulmonary vascular resistance causes pulmonary blood flow to decrease, pulmonary arterial pressure to increase, and pulmonary venous pressure to decrease.

However, the increased pulmonary artery pressure also imposes an increased workload on the right ventricle. If the pressure in the airways is not excessively high, the right ventricle can generate a big enough increase in pulmonary arterial pressure to restore pulmonary blood flow almost to normal. However, with extremely high airway pressures, the right ventricle may be unable to raise pulmonary arterial pressure high enough to sustain flow. Under these conditions, pulmonary blood flow falls substantially below normal. Because the left heart can only pump as much blood as it receives via the pulmonary circulation, left ventricular output also decreases. The consequences can be fatal. The veterinary clinician must be mindful of the risks of high airway pressures whenever a patient is intubated and attached to a mechanical respiratory device.

CLINICAL CORRELATIONS

PATENT DUCTUS ARTERIOSUS

History. A 3-month-old female Welsh corgi is brought to your clinic by its owner, who has noticed a "rumbling noise" in the dog's chest. The dog is smaller than her littermates and less playful. The dog coughs occasionally, but the cough does not produce fluid.

Clinical Examination. The dog appears to be in good health except for the occasional cough. The mucous membranes are pink, and the capillary refill time is normal (1.5 seconds). However, when you place your hand on the anterior left chest, you feel an abnormal vibration *(thrill)* with each heartbeat. With a stethoscope, you can auscultate a cardiac murmur that is loudest during systole but continues throughout both systole and diastole *(continuous murmur)*. The murmur is heard most loudly at the ventral third intercostal space on the left side. Expiratory sounds are slightly louder than normal. The heart rate is 152 beats/min, which you consider to be above normal for a dog of this size and age. While you are listening to the heart with the stethoscope, you palpate the femoral pulses, which are synchronized with the heart rate and very strong.

The electrocardiogram indicates that the dog has sinus tachycardia; the atrial and ventricular rates are both 152 beats/min. The R waves are abnormally large in leads II and III (2.5 and 3.5 mV, respectively). The QRS complex in lead I shows a large negative deflection followed immediately by a slightly larger positive deflection.

Thoracic radiographs show a generalized enlargement of the heart. The initial portion of the pulmonary artery is also substantially larger than normal, and the pulmonary blood vessels appear generally to be more prominent than normal.

An echocardiogram confirms the presence of a *patent ductus arteriosus.*

Comment. A murmur in a young, otherwise-healthy dog is most likely the result of a congenital cardiac abnormality. A continuous murmur can occur only if a defect causes turbulent flow throughout both systole and diastole. Because flow can occur only when there is a pressure gradient, the defect in this dog must be in a location where there is a substantial pressure gradient throughout the cardiac cycle. No single intracardiac defect meets this criterion; that is, a stenotic or regurgitant valve produces either a systolic murmur or a diastolic murmur, but not both. A valve that is both stenotic and regurgitant produces two murmurs: one in systole and one in diastole. In such a case, however, there are brief moments during the cardiac cycle when no pressure gradient exists across the valve, so there are moments of silence between the systolic murmur and the diastolic murmur. (Admittedly, if the heart rate is high, these moments of silence are very brief, and the two murmurs can be mistaken for a continuous murmur, particularly in the case of combined aortic stenosis and regurgitation.)

The most common cardiac defect that causes turbulent flow throughout both systole and diastole is a *patent ductus arteriosus* (PDA). This vessel is normal in the fetus but should close shortly after birth. The flow through a PDA is continuous because aortic pressure is higher than pulmonary artery pressure throughout the cardiac cycle. The resulting murmur is usually heard best in the left third intercostal space. All the other clinical signs in this dog are consistent with the diagnosis of PDA. The prominence of the pulmonary vessels on the radiographs indicates that pressure and flow are abnormally high in the pulmonary artery and its branches. In a dog with a PDA the pulmonary artery receives blood flow from both the right ventricle and the aorta, which increases both pulmonary arterial pressure and pulmonary flow.

The radiographs and electrocardiograms indicate that this dog has both right and left ventricular hypertrophy. The large R waves in leads II and III indicate left ventricular hypertrophy, and the large negative deflection during the QRS complex in lead I suggests that the right ventricle is hypertrophic as well. The left ventricle becomes hypertrophic in a dog with PDA because it is called on to pump three to five times the normal cardiac output. (It pumps a near-normal volume of blood to the organs of the systemic circulation and two to four times that much through the PDA.) The flow through the PDA is large because the PDA offers little resistance to flow. The demand on the left ventricle to pump so much blood (increased volume work) leads to left ventricular hypertrophy. The volume of blood pumped by the right ventricle is almost normal; it only needs to pump the blood that returns through the venae cavae from the systemic organs. However, the right ventricle must develop higher systolic pressures than normal to eject this blood into the pulmonary artery because pulmonary artery pressure is higher than normal, as explained earlier. This increase in pressure work leads to right ventricular hypertrophy.

Because the PDA carries so much blood away from the aorta, dogs with PDA tend to have an abnormally low aortic pressure. Diastolic pressure is particularly reduced because of the rapid outflow of blood from the aorta during ventricular diastole. Therefore, PDA is typically associated with low mean aortic pressure but elevated pulse pressure (review Figure 22-8, *G*).

Two mechanisms work together to keep blood flow to the systemic organs almost normal despite the fact that a large fraction of cardiac output is "lost" through the PDA. First, reflex mechanisms (discussed in Chapter 25) increase sympathetic activity to the heart, which increases heart rate and contractility above normal. These sympathetic effects keep left ventricular output (and aortic pressure) sufficiently high to supply blood to the systemic organs, despite the PDA. Second, metabolic control mechanisms cause the systemic organs to vasodilate, which keeps their blood flow almost normal despite the subnormal aortic pressure.

The compensatory mechanisms just described allow most dogs with a PDA to maintain a nearly normal blood flow to the systemic organs at rest. Several months may pass before the dog's owner notices limitations in the dog's activity or growth. Eventually, however, the heart cannot increase its output sufficiently to supply the systemic blood flow needed by the muscles during exercise, so as time passes, a puppy with a PDA becomes less playful and energetic than its normal littermates. Also, if the heart is unable to supply the blood flow needed by metabolically active tissues, the owner may notice some stunting of growth. In any case, a dog with a widely open ductus has a poor long-term prognosis, unless treated.

Treatment. You show the dog's owner a diagram of the fetal circulation and explain that the *ductus arteriosus* normally closes and seals itself within 1 to 6 weeks after birth, but that the *ductus* fails to close spontaneously in about 1 of every 700 newborns (the condition is four times more common in female pups than in male pups). Treatment involves closure of the *ductus,* either by ligation during open-chest surgery or by insertion of a specially designed plug during a cardiac catheterization procedure. Most dogs treated before age 6 months go on to lead completely normal lives. However, you inform the owner that PDA is hereditary and that this puppy should probably not be used for breeding.

The owner elects to have the dog treated surgically, and the surgery is successful. The murmur and cough disappear immediately. Within 1 week the dog is noticeably more energetic. At age 6 months, the dog has "grown into" her enlarged heart, and all physical findings are within normal limits.

ENDOTOXEMIA IN A FOAL

History. A 3-day-old Tennessee Walking Horse filly presents with progressive signs of lethargy, diarrhea, decreased eating, and weakness. The owners report that the filly appeared to be normal at birth, and shortly thereafter, she nursed briefly. Her condition did not cause them great concern until about a day ago.

Clinical Examination. The filly is markedly dehydrated. Although the environment is not cold, the filly has subnormal rectal temperature, suggesting that she can no longer thermoregulate. She has increased heart rate and respiratory rate. Her mucous membranes are dark red and exhibit prolonged capillary refill time, and her distal extremities feel cool. These signs indicate poor perfusion, low blood pressure, and hypoxia. She has hypermotile gut sounds and diarrhea. She only supports herself voluntarily for short periods of time. You suspect that the foal has an infection and is likely septic (bacteria and endotoxins in the blood). You submit a venous blood sample for immunoglobulin status (IgG), complete blood count (CBC) and biochemical profile, and culture. You also collect an arterial blood sample for measurement of blood gases.

Comment. This foal likely has acquired an infection from either ingestion or inhalation of contaminated liquid. Foals are frequently infected with gram-negative bacteria, and if they have not received adequate protection from antibodies in colostrum, the bacteria proliferate and release endotoxins. Circulating in the bloodstream, the bacteria and endotoxins stimulate the production of a large number of chemical mediators that cause inflammation, increased capillary permeability, intravascular coagulation, cardiac depression, poor perfusion, and hypoxia. These chemical mediators include host proinflammatory intercellular signaling molecules (i.e., cytokines and chemokines), procoagulants, adhesion molecules, enzymes, and acute phase proteins (plasma concentrations change in association with inflammatory states). An additional complication is hypoproteinemia, resulting both from impaired intestinal absorption of nutrients and from loss of protein in the diarrhea.

Treatment. The bacterial infection must be treated aggressively with appropriate antibiotics. Additional treatments would include nutritional support, oxygen, and intravenous fluid therapy. The fluid therapy would include a combination of plasma (to counteract hypoproteinemia) and electrolytes (to correct dehydration). Glucose (dextrose in water) can also be given intravenously to prevent hypoglycemia. The foal must be monitored closely so that she does not become overhydrated, as she will then develop edema due to hypoproteinemia. Pulmonary edema would further jeopardize the oxygenation of blood and the delivery of adequate oxygen to the tissues. Additional drug treatments may be needed to enhance cardiac function and support blood pressure. In cases such as this one, foals are encouraged to nurse, or else are provided with milk, provided they do not develop ileus (a type of intestinal obstruction). Alternatively, parenteral (non-oral, often intravenous) nutrition can be provided. Anti-inflammatory medications can be helpful; however, they must be used with caution, as they can cause renal (kidney) failure or gastric and colonic ulcers. Prognosis is guarded in these cases because of the severity of disease and the lasting damage that it can cause in multiple organ systems (also including lungs and joints).

PRACTICE QUESTIONS

1. The increase in coronary blood flow during exercise is:
   a. Called Starling's law of the heart.
   b. Caused by activation of parasympathetic nerves to the heart.
   c. Caused by compression of the coronary blood vessels during systole.
   d. Closely matched to the metabolic requirements of the heart.
   e. Called reactive hyperemia.

2. A dog with an arterial blood pressure of 120/80 mm Hg has a cerebral blood flow of 100 mL/min. When blood pressure is increased to 130/100 mm Hg, the cerebral blood flow increases to 105 mL/min. This is an example of:
   a. Active hyperemia.
   b. Autoregulation.
   c. Reactive hyperemia.
   d. The blood-brain barrier.
   e. Hypoxic vasoconstriction.

3. Local, metabolic control of blood flow through skeletal muscle:
   a. Characteristically dominates over neurohumoral control.
   b. Characteristically is subservient to neurohumoral control.
   c. Can either dominate or be subservient to neurohumoral control, depending on whether the muscle is exercising or resting.
   d. Depends primarily on changes in the resistance of the veins within the muscle.
   e. Depends on the release of histamine from mast cells within the skeletal muscle.

4. In response to an increase in perfusion pressure, the arterioles of an autoregulating organ _____, and the vascular resistance of the organ _____.
   a. constrict; increases
   b. constrict; decreases
   c. dilate; increases
   d. dilate; decreases

5. When a young dog with a PDA attempts vigorous exercise:
   a. Arterioles in the exercising skeletal muscle constrict.
   b. Oxygen concentration in the skeletal muscle interstitial fluid decreases.
   c. Left ventricular output decreases.
   d. Right ventricular output decreases.
   e. Mean arterial pressure increases to very high levels.

6. Which of the following characteristically acts as a paracrine to cause vasoconstriction in systemic arterioles?
   a. Carbon dioxide
   b. Nitric oxide
   c. Prostacyclin (PGI_2)
   d. Endothelin-1 (ET1)
   e. Bradykinin

BIBLIOGRAPHY

Boron WF, Boulpaep EL: *Medical physiology,* ed 2, Philadelphia, 2009, Saunders.

Ettinger SJ, Feldman EC: *Textbook of veterinary internal medicine: diseases of the dog and cat,* ed 7, St Louis, 2010, Elsevier/Saunders.

Hall JE: *Guyton and Hall textbook of medical physiology,* ed 12, Philadelphia, 2011, Saunders.

Kittleson MD, Kienle RD: *Small animal cardiovascular medicine,* St Louis, 1998, Mosby-Year Book.

Koeppen BM, Stanton BA: *Berne & Levy physiology,* ed 6, Philadelphia, 2010, Mosby.

Levy MN, Pappano AJ: *Cardiovascular physiology,* ed 9, St Louis, 2007, Mosby.

Mohrman DE, Heller LJ: *Cardiovascular physiology,* ed 7, New York, 2010, Lange Medical Books/McGraw-Hill.

Mortillaro NA, Taylor AE, editors: *The pathophysiology of the microcirculation,* Boca Raton, Fla, 1994, CRC Press.

Robinson NE, Sprayberry KA: *Current therapy in equine medicine,* ed 6, Philadelphia, 2009, Saunders.

Smith BP: *Large animal internal medicine,* ed 4, St Louis, 2009, Mosby Elsevier.

Tilley LP, Smith FWK, Oyama MA, Sleeper MM: *Manual of canine and feline cardiology,* ed 4, Philadelphia, 2008, Saunders.

Wilson DA: *Clinical veterinary advisor: the horse,* Philadelphia, 2011, Saunders.

CHAPTER 25

Neural and Hormonal Control of Blood Pressure and Blood Volume

KEY POINTS

1. Neurohumoral mechanisms regulate blood pressure and blood volume to ensure adequate blood flow for all body organs.
2. The autonomic nervous system affects the cardiovascular system through the release of epinephrine, norepinephrine, and acetylcholine.
3. The arterial baroreceptor reflex regulates arterial blood pressure.

4. The atrial volume receptor reflex regulates blood volume and helps to stabilize blood pressure.
5. The cardiovascular state of conscious subjects is determined by an ongoing and ever-changing mixture of reflex effects and psychogenic responses.

Neurohumoral Mechanisms Regulate Blood Pressure and Blood Volume to Ensure Adequate Blood Flow for All Body Organs

The influences of the nervous system and hormones on the cardiovascular system are referred to collectively as the *neurohumoral mechanisms* of cardiovascular control. The neurohumoral mechanisms are also called *extrinsic control mechanisms* because they act on organs from the outside. As described in Chapter 24, the mechanisms of cardiovascular control that act locally, within individual tissues, are referred to as *intrinsic control mechanisms*. The local, or intrinsic, mechanisms predominate over extrinsic mechanisms in the control of blood flow to the "critical" organs, which include the heart (i.e., coronary circulation), brain, and working (exercising) skeletal muscle. In contrast, neurohumoral, or extrinsic, control mechanisms predominate over the intrinsic mechanisms in the control of blood flow to the "noncritical" organs, which include the kidneys, the splanchnic organs, and resting skeletal muscle. The noncritical organs are those that can withstand temporary reductions in blood flow (and metabolism) to make extra blood flow available for the critical organs, whose optimal function on a moment-to-moment basis may be necessary for survival (e.g., in a life-threatening situation involving "fight or flight").

Neurohumoral mechanisms also control the heart rate and cardiac contractility. This allows cardiac output to be adjusted to provide adequate blood flow for all the systemic organs, or at least for the critical organs. An important distinction is that cardiac muscle is under neurohumoral control, whereas the coronary blood vessels are primarily under local control. When neurohumoral mechanisms increase the heart rate and cardiac contractility, the cardiac metabolic rate also increases. The increased metabolic rate acts via local metabolic control mechanisms to dilate coronary arterioles, which increases coronary blood flow.

To appreciate the importance of neurohumoral control mechanisms, consider what would happen in their absence. For example, what would occur during exercise if all the body organs relied on local control mechanisms to adjust their blood flow? At the onset of exercise, metabolic control mechanisms would cause vasodilation in the exercising skeletal muscles. Vascular resistance would decrease in the exercising muscles, and the blood flow through the muscles would increase. However, decreasing the vascular resistance in skeletal muscles would lower the total peripheral resistance (TPR). As a consequence, arterial blood pressure would decrease. This would decrease the perfusion pressure for all the systemic organs, and blood flow would therefore decrease below normal levels in the brain, kidneys, splanchnic organs, and so forth. The decreased blood flow in these organs would trigger autoregulatory responses, and these organs would vasodilate. However, the vasodilation would lower the TPR even further, which would reduce arterial pressure even more. This in turn would limit the increase in skeletal muscle blood flow. The end result would be some increase in blood flow in the exercising muscle and decreased blood flow elsewhere, but none of the organs (including skeletal muscle) would be receiving sufficient blood flow to meet their metabolic needs. Arterial pressure would be dangerously low, and the animal would exhibit profound exercise intolerance.

Neurohumoral control mechanisms allow an animal to avoid these complications. First, cardiac output is increased sufficiently to meet the increased need for blood flow in the exercising muscle (and in the coronary circulation) while keeping all the other organs supplied with a normal blood flow. If cardiac output cannot be increased sufficiently to meet all these needs, the control mechanisms take the additional step of temporarily reducing blood flow in the noncritical organs and making this extra flow available to the critical organs.

How do the neurohumoral control systems "know" when cardiac output is sufficiently high to meet the needs of all the organs and when to initiate vasoconstriction in the noncritical organs? An indirect strategy is used: cardiac output is increased enough to keep arterial pressure at a normal level. As long as arterial pressure is maintained at the normal level, local metabolic control mechanisms can successfully match blood flow to metabolic need in each individual organ. If cardiac output cannot be sufficiently increased to keep arterial pressure from falling, neurohumoral mechanisms initiate vasoconstriction in the noncritical organs. Thus, neurohumoral control mechanisms will deprive noncritical organs of an ideal level of blood flow if the critical organs are in need of more blood flow than can be supplied by the heart.

There are many important neurohumoral control mechanisms, but four are emphasized in the following presentation. The first two of these are *cardiovascular reflexes*. The *arterial baroreceptor reflex* works to regulate arterial pressure through the continual adjustment of cardiac output and vascular resistance (in the noncritical organs). The *atrial volume receptor reflex* works in conjunction with the arterial baroreceptor reflex to regulate arterial pressure and to adjust cardiac preload. The other two neurohumoral mechanisms described in this chapter are the *defense-alarm reaction* (the "fight or flight response") and *vasovagal syncope* (the "playing dead" reaction). These responses exemplify *psychogenic influences* on the cardiovascular system.

The Autonomic Nervous System Affects the Cardiovascular System Through the Release of Epinephrine, Norepinephrine, and Acetylcholine

The autonomic nervous system is the "neuro" arm of neurohumoral control. Sympathetic and parasympathetic neurons influence the cardiovascular system through the release of the neurotransmitters norepinephrine and acetylcholine. In addition, sympathetic nerves affect the cardiovascular system by stimulating the release of epinephrine and norepinephrine from the adrenal medulla. The adrenal secretions enter the bloodstream as hormones and circulate throughout the body. Chapter 13 contains additional, basic information about the autonomic nervous system.

Whether acting as neurotransmitters or as hormones, epinephrine, norepinephrine, and acetylcholine exert their cardiovascular effects by activating receptor proteins located in the membranes of cardiac muscle cells or of the smooth muscle cells (or in some cases the endothelial cells) in the walls of blood vessels. The receptors activated by epinephrine and norepinephrine are called *adrenergic receptors* (named after the *adrenal gland*). There are two major types: *α-adrenergic receptors* and *β-adrenergic receptors*. The α-adrenergic receptors are subdivided into α_1 and α_2. There are three subtypes of β-receptors: β_1, β_2, and β_3, with the first two of these being important in cardiovascular control.

Acetylcholine activates *cholinergic receptors*. There are two major types: *muscarinic cholinergic receptors* and *nicotinic cholinergic receptors*. The main cardiovascular effects of acetylcholine are mediated through muscarinic cholinergic receptors located on cardiac, smooth muscle, or endothelial cells. Of five subtypes of muscarinic receptors, the M_2 and M_3 receptor subtypes have the greatest cardiovascular importance.

Table 25-1 summarizes the main cardiovascular consequences of the activation of adrenergic and cholinergic receptors. α-Adrenergic receptors (both α_1 and α_2) are located in the cell membranes of the smooth muscle cells of the arterioles in all organs and in the smooth muscle cells of the abdominal veins. These adrenergic receptors are innervated by postganglionic sympathetic neurons, which release the neurotransmitter norepinephrine. Circulating epinephrine or norepinephrine can also activate the adrenergic receptors. Activation of these α-adrenergic receptors leads to constriction of the arterioles or the veins.

Arteriolar vasoconstriction increases the resistance and decreases the blood flow through an organ. If one or more major body organs are vasoconstricted, the *total peripheral resistance* (TPR) increases. TPR (along with cardiac output) determines arterial blood pressure, so widespread α-adrenergic vasoconstriction in the body leads to an increase in arterial blood pressure. The increase in arterial pressure increases the driving force for blood flow in all organs of the systemic circulation. In effect, the sympathetic nervous system can vasoconstrict some organs and thereby direct more blood flow to other, non-vasoconstricted organs.

The major role of veins is to act as reservoirs for blood. *Venoconstriction* displaces venous blood toward the central circulation, which increases central venous pressure, right ventricular preload, and (by the Starling mechanism) stroke volume. Venoconstriction in the abdominal organs is particularly effective in increasing central venous pressure. Venoconstriction causes a relatively small increase in the resistance to blood flow through an organ because the veins, whether dilated or constricted, offer much less resistance to blood flow than do the arterioles.

Sympathetic control of the heart is exerted through the β_1-adrenergic receptors, which are found on every cardiac muscle cell. These beta receptors are activated by norepinephrine or epinephrine. Chapters 19 and 21 discuss the effects of activation of the cardiac β-adrenergic receptors. In brief, pacemaker rate increases, cell-to-cell conduction velocity increases, and refractory period decreases. In addition, contractility is increased, so the cardiac contractions are quicker and stronger. The overall effect is increased heart rate and increased stroke volume.

β_2-Adrenergic receptors are found on the arterioles, particularly in the coronary circulation and in skeletal muscles. The activation of arteriolar β_2-adrenergic receptors causes relaxation of the vascular smooth muscle and dilation of the arterioles. However, these β_2-adrenergic receptors are not innervated by the sympathetic nervous system, so they are not activated directly by sympathetic nerves. Instead, they respond to circulating epinephrine and norepinephrine (released from the adrenal medulla). The adrenal medulla releases epinephrine and norepinephrine in situations that involve trauma, fear, or anxiety. Dilation of arterioles in the coronary circulation and in skeletal muscles is appropriate in such "fear, fight, or flight" response situations because the dilation results in an anticipatory increase in blood flow to the heart and skeletal muscle. Appropriately for its role in emergency situations, β_2-adrenergic vasodilation can overpower α-adrenergic vasoconstriction in the coronary circulation and in skeletal muscles.

Parasympathetic effects on the heart are mediated via the neurotransmitter acetylcholine, which activates cholinergic muscarinic receptors of the M_2 type. Cardiac muscle cells of the sinoatrial and atrioventricular nodes are densely innervated by postganglionic parasympathetic neurons. Atrial cells also receive strong parasympathetic innervation. In these parts of the heart, activation of cardiac M_2 receptors has effects basically opposite to those of the activation of β_1-adrenergic receptors. Parasympathetic activation powerfully slows the cardiac pacemakers, decreases cell-to-cell conduction velocity, and increases refractory period. Curiously, ventricular muscle cells receive very little direct parasympathetic innervation. Therefore, parasympathetic activation has only a minor, direct effect on ventricular contractility. However, parasympathetic neurons do exert an interesting, indirect effect on ventricular muscle cells. Most parasympathetic neurons in the ventricles release their acetylcholine onto sympathetic

TABLE 25-1 Receptors Involved in Autonomic Control of the Cardiovascular System

Receptor Type	Location	Usual Activator	Effect of Activation	Function
α Adrenergic				
α_1 and α_2	Arterioles (all organs)	Norepinephrine from sympathetic neurons, or circulating epinephrine and norepinephrine	Vasoconstriction	Decreases blood flow to organs; increases total peripheral resistance **(major effect)**
	Veins (abdominal organs)	Norepinephrine from sympathetic neurons, or circulating epinephrine and norepinephrine	Venoconstriction	Displaces venous blood toward heart
β Adrenergic				
β_1	Heart (all cardiac muscle cells)	Norepinephrine from sympathetic neurons, or circulating epinephrine and norepinephrine	Increased pacemaker rate; faster speed of conduction; decreased refractory period; quicker, stronger contractions	Increases heart rate, stroke volume, and cardiac output **(major effects)**
β_2	Arterioles (coronary and skeletal muscle)	Circulating epinephrine and norepinephrine [β_2 receptors not innervated]	Vasodilation	Increases coronary blood flow; increases skeletal muscle blood flow
Muscarinic Cholinergic				
M_2	Heart (all cardiac muscle cells, but sparse direct innervation of ventricular muscle cells)	Acetylcholine from parasympathetic neurons	Opposite of β_1	Decreases heart rate and cardiac output **(major effect)**
	Sympathetic nerve endings at ventricular muscle cells	Acetylcholine from parasympathetic neurons	Inhibition of norepinephrine release from sympathetic neurons	Decreases magnitude of sympathetic effects on ventricular muscle cells
M_3	Arterioles (coronary)	Acetylcholine from parasympathetic neurons	Vasodilation (mediated via nitric oxide)	Increases coronary blood flow (minor effect)
	Arterioles (genitals)	Acetylcholine from parasympathetic neurons	Vasodilation (mediated via nitric oxide)	Causes engorgement and erection
	Arterioles (skeletal muscle)	Acetylcholine from specialized sympathetic neurons	Vasodilation (mediated via nitric oxide)	Increases muscle blood flow (in anticipation of exercise)
	Arterioles (most other organs)	[Receptors not innervated; normal activator unknown]	Vasodilation (mediated via nitric oxide)	Function unknown

neuron terminals, rather than directly onto ventricular muscle cells. This acetylcholine activates muscarinic cholinergic receptors on the sympathetic neuron terminals, which inhibits the release of norepinephrine from the terminals and thus weakens the effects of sympathetic activity on ventricular cells. By decreasing heart rate and by opposing sympathetic effects on ventricular contractility, parasympathetic activation can profoundly decrease cardiac output.

Cholinergic muscarinic receptors of the M_3 type are found on the endothelial cells and also on the smooth muscle cells of most arteries and arterioles. Activation of M_3 receptors on smooth muscle cells causes them to contract. However, this *vasoconstrictor* effect is usually overridden by a *vasodilatory* effect of activating the M_3 receptors on the vascular endothelial cells. In this strange arrangement, activation of M_3 receptors on endothelial cells causes the synthesis of *nitric oxide,* which then diffuses out of the endothelial cells and into the nearby smooth muscle cells, where it causes vasodilation. The vasodilatory effect of stimulating the M_3 receptors on endothelial cells is stronger than the vasoconstrictor effect of stimulating the M_3 receptors on smooth muscle cells.

The M_3 receptors on vascular endothelial cells are innervated in three organs. Parasympathetic neurons innervate vascular M_3 receptors in the coronary circulation, where the effect of parasympathetic activation is vasodilation. This vasodilatory effect is minor, however, and the function of this innervation is unclear. In the blood vessels of the external genital organs, parasympathetic neurons release both acetylcholine and nitric oxide. The acetylcholine activates M_3 receptors on the endothelial cells to stimulate the release of additional nitric oxide from endothelial cells. The nitric oxide relaxes vascular smooth muscle, which causes vasodilation, engorgement of the organs with blood, and therefore erection. The third tissue in which vascular M_3 receptors are innervated is skeletal muscle. In some species (e.g., cats and dogs) but not in others (e.g., primates), the M_3 receptors of skeletal muscle blood vessels are innervated by special postganglionic sympathetic neurons that release acetylcholine as a neurotransmitter (rather than the usual, norepinephrine). These *sympathetic cholinergic neurons* appear to be activated specifically in anticipation of muscular exercise and during the "fear, fight, or flight" (defense-alarm) reaction. The resulting vasodilation increases blood flow through the skeletal muscle just before and during the initiation of exercise. Although primates do not have sympathetic cholinergic vasodilatory nerves, they can bring about an anticipatory vasodilation of skeletal muscle arterioles through activation of β_1-adrenergic receptors by circulating epinephrine and norepinephrine, as mentioned earlier.

To summarize, arteries and arterioles throughout the body have M_3 adrenergic receptors, and these blood vessels dilate when exposed to acetylcholine (with nitric oxide serving as the mediator). But acetylcholine-releasing autonomic neurons only innervate the blood vessels in the heart, the external genitalia, and (in some species) skeletal muscle. The functional significance of the M_3 receptors on arteries and arterioles in other organs is unclear because no neurons (either sympathetic or parasympathetic) appear to innervate them, and neither acetylcholine nor any other muscarinic receptor agonist normally circulates in the bloodstream.

Of all the autonomic influences on the cardiovascular system just mentioned, three stand out as most important. The first is α_1- and α_2-adrenergic vasoconstriction in the arterioles of all body organs, which is brought about by the sympathetic nervous system. The second is β_1-adrenergic excitation of cardiac muscle, which is brought about by the sympathetic nervous system and results in an increased heart rate and stroke volume. The third is the decrease in heart rate brought about by parasympathetic activation of cardiac M_2 receptors.

The Arterial Baroreceptor Reflex Regulates Arterial Blood Pressure

Arterial blood pressure is monitored by pressure-sensitive nerve endings known as *baroreceptors*. The baroreceptors send afferent impulses to the central nervous system (CNS), which reflexively alters cardiac output and vascular resistance (in noncritical organs) to keep blood pressure at a set point. The reflex is called the *arterial baroreceptor reflex.*

The arterial baroreceptors are specialized nerve endings that are embedded in the walls of the carotid arteries and aortic arch (Figure 25-1). The baroreceptors are concentrated at the origin of each internal carotid artery in enlarged parts of the arteries called the *carotid sinuses.* Similar nerve endings are found in the wall of the aortic arch, especially at the origin of its major branches. These nerve endings are sensitive to stretch *(distention)* of the arterial wall. In effect, they sense arterial pressure because blood pressure is the natural force that distends these arteries. Therefore, these nerve endings are called *baroreceptors* (literally, "pressure sensors") even though the actual physical factor being sensed is not pressure but rather stretch.

With every systolic ejection from the heart, blood distends the aorta and arteries, including the carotid sinuses, which causes the baroreceptors to initiate neural impulses (action potentials). Figure 25-2 illustrates that the frequency of these action potentials is proportional to the arterial blood pressure. The tracing on

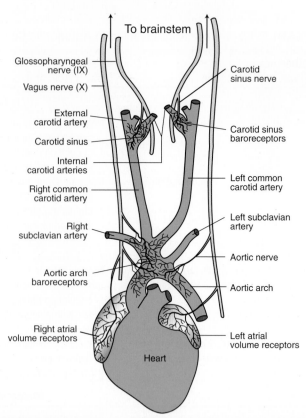

FIGURE 25-1 Arterial baroreceptors are located in the walls of the carotid sinuses and in the walls of the aortic arch and its major branches. The atrial volume receptors are located in the walls of the right and left atria. See text for a description of the neural pathways followed by the baroreceptor and volume receptor afferents.

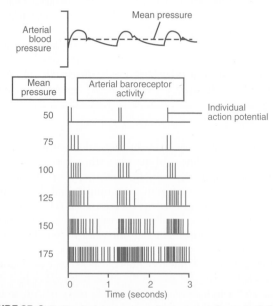

FIGURE 25-2 Each arterial pressure pulse causes action potentials to be generated in baroreceptor afferent neurons. The number of action potentials generated per heartbeat increases dramatically with increases in mean arterial pressure.

the top shows the pulsatile arterial pressure on three successive heartbeats. The mean level of arterial pressure is indicated by the dashed line. The tracings below depict the typical patterns of action potentials that would be seen in a baroreceptor afferent neuron for various levels of *mean arterial pressure* (MAP). When MAP is lower than normal (e.g., 50 mm Hg), there are only one or two action potentials with each heartbeat. These action potentials occur during the rapid upstroke of the pressure wave, because the baroreceptors are sensitive to the rate of change of pressure as well as to mean pressure. When MAP is at a higher level (e.g., 75 mm Hg), more action potentials are formed during each heartbeat, but the action potentials still tend to occur during the rapid pressure increase at the beginning of the cardiac ejection. The higher the MAP, the more action potentials are formed in each heartbeat. Thus the arterial baroreceptors signal increases in pressure by increasing their action potential frequency. Because the baroreceptors are active when arterial pressure is normal (MAP near 100 mm Hg), they can also signal a decrease in arterial pressure by decreasing their action potential frequency.

The afferent neurons from the aortic arch baroreceptors join the vagus nerves (see Figure 25-1). In some species the aortic baroreceptor afferents form a distinct bundle within the vagal nerve sheath, called the *aortic depressor nerve*. The stretch receptors in the carotid sinuses have their afferents in the carotid sinus nerves (Hering's nerves), which join the glossopharyngeal (ninth cranial) nerve. By way of these afferent neurons, the brain receives beat-by-beat information about the level of arterial blood pressure.

Figure 25-3 summarizes the reflex consequences of a decrease in blood pressure, which decreases afferent baroreceptor activity. The brain responds to a decrease in the afferent activity from the baroreceptors by increasing sympathetic activity. In the heart, sympathetic activation results in increased stroke volume and heart rate, which increases cardiac output. The increase in cardiac output helps to restore blood pressure toward normal. The sympathetically driven increase in heart rate is augmented by a simultaneous reduction in parasympathetic activity to the sinoatrial node. Thus the baroreceptor reflex uses reciprocal changes in sympathetic and parasympathetic activity to control heart rate. Sympathetic activity is also increased to the arterioles of all organs, but the consequent vasoconstriction is most pronounced in the noncritical organs (kidney, splanchnic organs, and resting skeletal muscle) because these are the organs in which neurohumoral control of arterioles predominates over local (metabolic)

control. Vasoconstriction in the noncritical organs increases the resistance to blood flow through these organs and therefore increases total peripheral resistance (TPR). The increase in TPR helps to restore arterial blood pressure back toward its normal level. The fact that resistance increased in the noncritical organs has the effect of preserving adequate blood flow in the critical organs.

To understand fully the function of the baroreceptor reflex, it is important to recognize that the reflex does not *reverse* disturbances that alter blood pressure but only *minimizes* them. Also, it is important to distinguish between cause and effect when thinking about the baroreflex. What *causes* blood pressure to decrease *below normal* is a decrease *below normal* in cardiac output, TPR, or both. *There is no other way to lower blood pressure.* If TPR falls below normal and causes blood pressure to decrease below normal, the *compensatory response* of the baroreceptor reflex is (1) to increase cardiac output above normal through increased sympathetic (and decreased parasympathetic) activation of the heart and (2) to minimize the decrease in TPR by initiating a sympathetic vasoconstriction in the noncritical organs. After compensation by the baroreceptor reflex, cardiac output is above normal. TPR is still *below* normal, but not as far below normal as in the uncompensated state. Blood pressure is still below normal, but not as far below normal as in the uncompensated state. Similarly, if the initiating disturbance is that cardiac output falls below normal, the compensatory response of the baroreceptor reflex is to increase TPR *above* normal and to restore cardiac output *toward* normal. Blood pressure is still below normal, but not as far below normal as in the uncompensated state.

All the reflex responses just described for a decrease in arterial blood pressure occur in reverse in response to an increase in arterial blood pressure above its normal level. Thus the *baroreflex* acts to counteract and minimize both decreases and increases in blood pressure.

The baroreflex responds quickly, initiating compensations for disturbances in blood pressure within 1 second. The reflex is also very powerful. For example, a hemorrhage that would decrease blood pressure by 40 to 50 mm Hg if there were no baroreflex decreases blood pressure by only 10 to 15 mm Hg in an animal with intact baroreflexes. The baroreflex also acts to maintain blood pressure close to normal during changes in posture or activity. In a dog without baroreflexes, changes in posture are accompanied by large, uncontrolled variations in blood pressure,

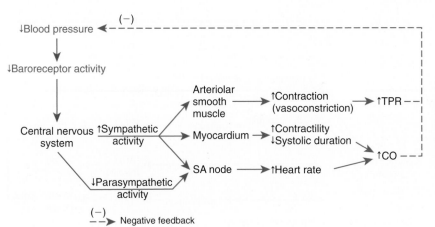

FIGURE 25-3 The arterial baroreceptor reflex responds to decreases in blood pressure *(top left)* by increasing cardiac output *(CO)*, total peripheral resistance *(TPR)*, or both *(far right)*. These reflex effects offset the initial fall in blood pressure *(dashed line)*. *SA,* Sinoatrial.

as shown in Figure 25-4. By minimizing fluctuations in blood pressure, the baroreflex helps ensure an adequate driving force for blood flow to the critical organs.

Although the baroreceptor reflex is essential for the moment-to-moment stability of blood pressure, it does not appear to be the major mechanism responsible for setting the long-term level of arterial blood pressure, because baroreceptors slowly adapt or *reset* to the prevailing level of arterial pressure. In other words, the baroreceptors come to accept whatever the prevailing blood pressure is as if it were the normal pressure. For example, in an animal or a human who has been hypertensive for a few days or weeks, the baroreflex functions to regulate blood pressure at the elevated level rather than to restore blood pressure toward its normal level. Also, the baroreflex can become reset in a downward direction during a period of sustained hypotension. For example, in chronic heart failure, in which arterial pressure may be below normal for days or weeks, the baroreflex appears to regulate blood pressure at a depressed level rather than to push it back toward its normal level.

In summary, the baroreflex responds quickly and powerfully to counteract sudden changes in blood pressure, but it has little influence on the long-term level of blood pressure over days or weeks.

The Atrial Volume Receptor Reflex Regulates Blood Volume and Helps to Stabilize Blood Pressure

The *atrial volume receptor reflex* is initiated by specialized sensory nerve endings that are located primarily in the walls of the

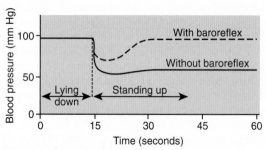

FIGURE 25-4 The baroreflex is essential for normal, moment-to-moment stability of blood pressure. Dogs in which baroreflexes are eliminated exhibit much larger swings in blood pressure in response to postural changes than do dogs with intact baroreflexes.

left and right atria (see Figure 25-1). These nerve endings are activated by stretch, but they are called *volume receptors* because the volume of blood in each atrium determines how much the atrial wall is stretched. For example, a decrease in the total blood volume of an animal (e.g., hemorrhage) results in a decrease in the amount of blood in the major veins and in the atria. When atrial volume decreases, atrial pressure decreases, as does the stretch on the atrial walls. This decreases the frequency of action potentials generated in atrial stretch receptors. Conversely, increases in blood volume result in increased atrial stretch and an increased frequency of action potentials generated by the atrial stretch receptors. Therefore, these atrial stretch receptors are sensitive detectors of atrial blood volume and, indirectly, of total blood volume. Additional stretch-sensitive nerve endings, which act in concert with the atrial volume receptors, are located in the walls of the pulmonary veins.

Figure 25-5 summarizes the reflex consequences of a decrease in blood volume, which decreases atrial volume receptor activity. The CNS responds reflexively to the decrease in afferent activity from the atrial volume receptors by increasing sympathetic efferent activity to the heart and systemic arterioles and decreasing parasympathetic efferent activity to the heart. In this respect, the atrial volume receptor reflex and the baroreceptor reflex exert synergistic effects; that is, a decrease in blood volume leads (via the atrial volume receptor reflex) to the same responses that are triggered by the baroreflex in response to a decrease in arterial blood pressure. In both cases the reflex responses include an increase in cardiac contractility, a decrease in systolic duration, and an increase in heart rate as well as arteriolar vasoconstriction in the noncritical organs. By initiating these responses, the atrial volume receptor reflex helps to combat the decrease in arterial blood pressure that would otherwise result from a decreased blood volume. In this regard, the atrial volume receptor reflex augments the effectiveness of the baroreceptor reflex as a regulator of blood pressure.

The atrial volume receptor reflex acts in three additional ways to help restore lost blood volume (see Figure 25-5). First, the reflex acts through the hypothalamus to increase the sensation of thirst. If water is available, the animal drinks. This provides the fluid necessary to increase blood volume back toward normal. Second, the atrial volume receptor reflex acts through the hypothalamus and pituitary gland to increase the release of *antidiuretic hormone* (ADH, also known as *arginine vasopressin*). ADH is synthesized in hypothalamic neurons, which transport it to the

FIGURE 25-5 The atrial volume receptor reflex responds to a decrease in blood volume by decreasing sodium and water loss in the urine and by increasing oral water intake. The reflex also helps support blood pressure by increasing cardiac output and total peripheral resistance (similar to baroreflex). *ADH,* Antidiuretic hormone.

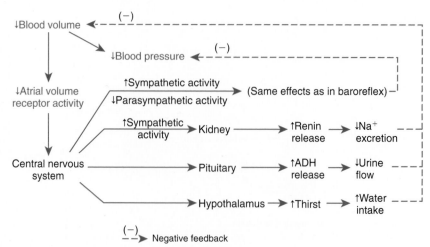

posterior pituitary gland. From there, ADH is released into the bloodstream (see Chapter 33). ADH acts on the kidneys to decrease urine production. The third way in which the atrial volume receptor reflex helps to restore lost blood volume is to stimulate the release of the hormone *renin* from the kidneys. Renin acts to increase the production of the hormone *angiotensin II,* which acts to increase production of the hormone *aldosterone,* which acts to decrease the amount of sodium excreted by the kidneys; that is, activation of the *renin-angiotensin-aldosterone system* causes the body to conserve available sodium.

The combination of decreased sodium excretion (by the actions of renin) and decreased urine flow (by the actions of ADH) results in the conservation of body fluid. The conservation of body fluid, combined with an increased water intake, eventually restores blood volume back toward normal.

Although not diagrammed in Figure 25-3, the arterial baroreceptor reflex also responds to decreases in arterial pressure by increasing thirst, ADH release, and renin release. An increase in arterial pressure above normal initiates the opposite effects. Thus the arterial baroreceptor reflex and the atrial volume receptor reflex are synergistic partners in the interrelated tasks of regulating arterial pressure and blood volume.

The Cardiovascular State of Conscious Subjects Is Determined by an Ongoing and Ever-Changing Mixture of Reflex Effects and Psychogenic Responses

The baroreceptor reflex and the atrial volume receptor reflex are only two of several important cardiovascular reflexes. They are primarily responsible for the regulation of blood pressure and blood volume, and they illustrate several properties common to all cardiovascular reflexes. First, these reflexes originate from changes detected by peripheral sensory receptors. Second, the reflexes occur at a subconscious level, through neural pathways that primarily involve cardiovascular centers in the brainstem and midbrain. Consequently, cardiovascular reflexes persist in unconscious and anesthetized subjects, although the strength and character of the reflexes are altered by anesthesia. Finally, the reflexes use sympathetic and parasympathetic neurons as well as hormonal and behavioral responses to bring about cardiovascular changes.

In conscious subjects, neurohumoral control of the cardiovascular system involves both cardiovascular reflexes and psychogenic effects. Psychogenic responses originate from conscious perceptions or emotional reactions. They are eliminated by unconsciousness or general anesthesia. They involve neural pathways of the midbrain and forebrain, including the limbic system and cerebral cortex. Psychogenic responses are often triggered by sensory stimuli. For example, the sights, sounds, and smells of a veterinary clinic may trigger perceptions and emotions that cause increases in heart rate and blood pressure in both animal patients and their human companions. Psychogenic responses can also occur without any obvious sensory triggers. For example, anxiety about a future event can increase heart rate and blood pressure, at least in humans. Cardiovascular reflexes and psychogenic reactions use the same sympathetic and parasympathetic neurons and some of the same hormonal responses to bring about cardiovascular changes.

Two important psychogenic responses are the defense-alarm reaction and vasovagal syncope (the "playing dead" reaction). The *defense-alarm reaction* ("fear, fight, or flight" response) is an emotional and behavioral response to a threatening situation, physical injury, or trauma. The cardiovascular component of this reaction involves increased sympathetic activity and decreased parasympathetic activity. Typically, the sympathetic activation is sufficiently strong to cause the release of epinephrine and norepinephrine from the adrenal medulla. The cardiovascular responses during a defense-alarm reaction therefore include an increased heart rate, increased stroke volume, vasoconstriction in noncritical organs (kidneys, splanchnic organs, resting skeletal muscle), vasoconstriction in skin, vasodilation in coronary vessels and in working skeletal muscle, and increased blood pressure. The cardiovascular responses during the defense reaction are enhanced by other circulating hormones, including ADH and angiotensin II. The resulting elevated blood pressure helps to ensure adequate blood flow for the critical organs (exercising skeletal muscles, heart, and brain).

During a defense-alarm reaction, the baroreceptor reflex is reset by the CNS so that it regulates blood pressure at an elevated level rather than acting to oppose the increased pressure. This is analogous to resetting the cruise control on a car so that it regulates speed at an elevated level rather than acting to oppose an increased speed. Thus it is more accurate to say that the baroreceptor reflex regulates blood pressure at a variable set point (set by the CNS) than to say that the baroreflex regulates arterial pressure at any single "normal" pressure.

It is important to recognize that the defense-alarm reaction is simply the extreme form of a continuum of states of emotional arousal. Sleep is at the opposite end of this cardiovascular and emotional continuum. In quiet rest or sleep, sympathetic activity is minimal and parasympathetic activity is maximal. During a full-blown defense-alarm reaction, sympathetic activity is maximal and parasympathetic activity is minimal. Between these extremes lie all the levels of emotional arousal experienced by animals and humans, from moment to moment, during ordinary and extraordinary daily activities. Cardiovascular variables, such as heart rate and blood pressure, are sensitive to these changes in emotional state (Figure 25-6). For example, a large dog may normally have a heart rate of 70 beats/min while resting at home; but it would be entirely normal for the same dog to have a heart rate of 120 beats/min while "resting" in a clinic, if the dog is apprehensive in that setting. Another important point for the clinician to remember is that emotional responses are subjective. Situations that severely agitate one animal may cause only a mild alerting response in another animal. The clinician must evaluate heart rate, blood pressure, and other cardiovascular signs with respect to the particular patient's emotional state.

Vasovagal syncope is another psychogenic response that may be encountered in veterinary practice. This response is also called "playing dead" or "playing possum" (i.e., behaving like an opossum). In response to certain threatening or emotional situations, some humans and animals experience a psychogenic decrease in blood pressure and may faint. In many ways, this

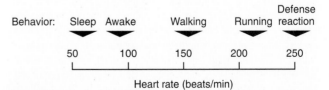

FIGURE 25-6 The defense-alarm reaction is simply the extreme on a continuum of emotional and physical arousal. Cardiovascular variables (e.g., heart rate, plotted here for a typical large dog) respond sensitively to every change along this arousal scale.

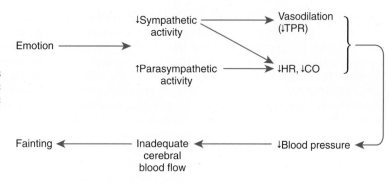

FIGURE 25-7 Vasovagal syncope ("playing dead" reaction) is an emotional response that involves decreases in sympathetic activity and increases in parasympathetic activity. *CO,* Cardiac output; *HR,* heart rate; *TPR,* total peripheral resistance.

response is the opposite of the defense-alarm reaction. As shown in Figure 25-7, vasovagal syncope involves a decrease in sympathetic activity and an increase in parasympathetic activity. These neural changes bring about a vasodilation in the noncritical organs, with a consequent decrease in TPR. Heart rate and cardiac output also decrease, so there is a large drop in arterial blood pressure. The expected compensatory reflex responses do not take place because emotional state appears to override the baroreceptor reflex in this case. If blood pressure falls so low that there is inadequate cerebral blood flow, the patient faints. The term *vasovagal syncope* denotes *vaso*dilation, *vagal* (parasympathetic) activation, and *syncope* (fainting). It is not clear why some animals respond to a threatening situation with a defense-alarm reaction, whereas others exhibit vasovagal syncope.

CLINICAL CORRELATIONS

INTRAOPERATIVE HEMORRHAGE

History. Four hours after abdominal surgery for a splenic sarcoma, a 30-kg, 9-year-old male Labrador retriever is observed to be severely lethargic and recumbent. An abnormally large amount of blood had been lost during the surgical removal of the spleen because the dog had a hereditary blood-clotting defect (von Willebrand's disease).

Clinical Examination. The dog's gums are pale, and his capillary refilling time is abnormally prolonged (3 sec). His extremities are cool to the touch. The femoral pulse is rapid and weak. An electrocardiogram indicates sinus tachycardia at a rate of 185 beats/min. The hematocrit (packed cell volume) is 38%, and the plasma protein concentration is 5.6 g/dL; both values are below normal. A jugular catheter is inserted, and central venous pressure is measured and found to be –1 mm Hg (normal, 0 to +3 mm Hg). Despite the intravenous administration of 600 mL of lactated Ringer's solution during surgery, the dog has not produced any urine. About 100 mL of blood-tinged fluid is removed from the abdomen by *abdominocentesis.*

Comment. This case illustrates the clinical signs that are typical of hemorrhage. Most of the blood in a dog is in the systemic veins, so most of the blood missing after hemorrhage is missing from the veins. The result is an abnormally low central venous pressure, as observed in this dog. The decreased central venous pressure causes a decreased ventricular preload and a decreased ventricular end-diastolic volume. This leads to decreases in stroke volume (Starling's law of the heart), cardiac output, and arterial blood pressure. Inadequate cardiac output and blood pressure lead to behavioral depression.

Neurohumoral compensation for the hemorrhage is initiated by the atrial volume receptor reflex and the arterial baroreceptor reflex. Heart rate is increased by the combination of increased sympathetic activation and decreased parasympathetic activation. The combination of high heart rate and low stroke volume accounts for the rapid but weak (low pulse pressure) femoral pulse. Sympathetic activity also causes vasoconstriction in the mucous membranes, resting skeletal muscle, splanchnic organs, and kidneys (noncritical organs and tissues). The reduced blood flow in these tissues accounts for the pale gums, the slow refilling of capillaries, the cool limbs, and the lack of urine production by the kidneys. Urine formation by the kidneys is also being depressed by the combined hormonal effects of ADH and the renin-angiotensin-aldosterone system.

Hemorrhage does not directly reduce either the hematocrit or the plasma protein concentration, because whole blood is being lost. However, two factors caused the hematocrit and plasma protein concentration to decrease in this dog. First, the fluid administered intravenously during surgery (lactated Ringer's solution) contained neither red blood cells nor plasma proteins, so the cells and proteins remaining in the bloodstream were diluted by the addition of the fluid. Second, the hemorrhage reduced not only venous and arterial pressures but also capillary hydrostatic pressure, which changed the balance of hydrostatic and oncotic forces (Starling forces) across the capillary walls in favor of reabsorption. The interstitial fluid that was reabsorbed into the bloodstream contained no red blood cells and almost no plasma proteins. This caused a further dilution of the cells and proteins in the blood.

Treatment. Therapy for this dog involves measures to stop ongoing blood loss and to restore the lost blood volume. In this dog the hemorrhage is predominantly seepage from small intraabdominal vessels as a result of the coagulation defect. Transfusions of fresh blood or plasma, or concentrated preparations of clotting proteins, would promote clotting and limit subsequent hemorrhage. After measures are taken to promote clotting, additional crystalloid solutions (e.g., lactated Ringer's solution) can be infused into this dog because the hematocrit and plasma protein concentration are not dangerously low. If crystalloid solutions are administered, the hematocrit and plasma protein concentration should be monitored closely to avoid the hypoxia that results from too much dilution of the red blood cells, or the edema that results from too much dilution of the plasma proteins. Renal function should be monitored closely because the combination of hypoxia and reflex vasoconstriction can lead to ischemic damage of kidney tissue, resulting in renal failure.

PRACTICE QUESTIONS

1. Vasovagal syncope:
   a. Involves decreased blood pressure and heart rate.
   b. Involves increased sympathetic activity.
   c. Involves decreased cardiac parasympathetic activity.
   d. Prepares an animal for "fight or flight."
   e. Involves constriction of splanchnic arterioles.

2. The dilation of arterioles that occurs during steady-state exercise in active skeletal muscles could be eliminated by:
   a. Pharmacological blockade of action potentials in all autonomic nerves innervating the muscles.
   b. Complete surgical removal of sympathetic innervation of the skeletal muscles.
   c. Administration of a muscarinic cholinergic blocking agent.
   d. Administration of a β-adrenergic blocking agent.
   e. None of the above.

3. A drug is injected intravenously into a dog and causes a transient increase in mean arterial pressure and a transient decrease in heart rate. The baroreceptor nerves are cut; the drug is reinjected and now causes a greater increase in blood pressure but no change in heart rate. These results are most consistent with the primary action of the drug being to:
   a. Activate the muscarinic cholinergic (M_3) receptors of arterioles.
   b. Activate the α-adrenergic receptors of arterioles.
   c. Activate $β_1$-adrenergic receptors of the pacemaker cells of the SA node.
   d. Increase the synthesis of nitric oxide in arterioles.
   e. Decrease the activity of arterial baroreceptors.

4. A dog has had a hemorrhage. The heart rate is increased above normal, and the skin is cold. The mucous membranes are pale. In this situation (compared with normal):
   a. The baroreceptor nerves are firing at a higher rate.
   b. The sympathetic nerves to the heart are firing at a decreased rate.
   c. The sympathetic nerves to the blood vessels of the skin and mucous membranes are firing at an increased rate.
   d. The parasympathetic fibers to the blood vessels are firing at an increased rate.
   e. The release of renin by the kidney is decreased.

5. Blood (250 mL) is taken from a vein of a dog. Mean arterial pressure does not decrease measurably. Nevertheless, it is likely that:
   a. Stimulation of atrial stretch receptors has decreased.
   b. Stroke volume has increased.
   c. Stimulation of aortic arch baroreceptors has increased.
   d. Total peripheral resistance has decreased.
   e. Secretion of ADH by the pituitary has decreased.

BIBLIOGRAPHY

Boron WF, Boulpaep EL: *Medical physiology*, ed 2, Philadelphia, 2009, Saunders.

Chapleau MW, Abboud FM: *Neuro-cardiovascular regulation: from molecules to man*, New York, 2001, New York Academy of Sciences.

Ettinger SJ, Feldman EC: *Textbook of veterinary internal medicine: diseases of the dog and cat*, ed 7, St Louis, 2010, Elsevier/Saunders.

Katz AM: *Physiology of the heart*, ed 5, Baltimore, 2010, Lippincott, Williams & Wilkins.

Kittleson MD, Kienle RD: *Small animal cardiovascular medicine*, St Louis, 1998, Mosby-Year Book.

Levick RJ: *An introduction to cardiovascular physiology*, ed 5, New York, 2010, Hodder Arnold Publishers.

Levy MN, Pappano AJ: *Cardiovascular physiology*, ed 9, St Louis, 2007, Mosby.

Shepherd JT, Vatner SF, editors: *Nervous control of the heart*, Amsterdam, 1996, Harwood Academic.

Silverstein D, Hopper K: *Small animal critical care medicine*, St Louis, 2009, Saunders Elsevier.

Tilley LP, Smith FWK, Oyama MA, Sleeper MM: *Manual of canine and feline cardiology*, ed 4, Philadelphia, 2008, Saunders.

Zucker IH, Gilmore JP: *Reflex control of the circulation*, Boca Raton, Fla, 1991, CRC Press.

CHAPTER 26
Integrated Cardiovascular Responses

KEY POINTS

1. Both Starling's mechanism and the arterial baroreflex help compensate for heart failure.
2. Serious complications secondary to heart failure include exercise intolerance, edema, salt and water retention, kidney failure, uremia, septic shock, and decompensation.
3. The immediate cardiovascular effects of hemorrhage are minimized by compensations initiated by the atrial volume receptor reflex and the arterial baroreceptor reflex.
4. The blood volume lost in hemorrhage is restored through a combination of capillary fluid shifts and hormonal and behavioral responses.
5. In large animals, the transition from a recumbent to a standing posture elicits the same cardiovascular responses as hemorrhage.
6. The initiation of exercise involves an interplay of local and neural changes that increases cardiac output and delivers increased flow to exercising muscle.

Chapters 18 to 25 describe the various elements of cardiovascular function and control. An understanding of these individual elements is not sufficient, however, to provide a basis for the diagnosis and treatment of cardiovascular dysfunction. The veterinary clinician must understand the *interaction* of these elements in both normal and abnormal situations. Therefore this chapter discusses three fundamentally important, *integrated* cardiovascular responses: (1) the response to heart failure, (2) the response to hemorrhage, and (3) the response to exercise. In addition to elucidating important, integrated responses, this discussion provides a review and summary of key concepts of cardiovascular physiology.

Both Starling's Mechanism and the Arterial Baroreflex Help Compensate for Heart Failure

There are many types and causes of *heart failure.* Some clinicians use the term very broadly to refer to any condition in which a problem in the heart limits its ability to deliver a normal cardiac output to the body tissues. Such conditions would include various valve defects, arrhythmias, and even heartworm infestation. A more restrictive definition, and one favored by physiologists, is that *heart failure* is any condition in which a depressed *cardiac contractility* limits the ability of the heart to deliver a normal cardiac output. The broader definition of heart failure encompasses virtually any problem with the heart as a pump; a common synonym is *pump failure.* The more restrictive definition, as used in this chapter, equates heart failure with *myocardial failure,* a depressed contractility of the heart muscle itself.

A depressed cardiac contractility can result from coronary artery disease, cardiac hypoxia, myocarditis, toxins, drug effects, or electrolyte imbalances. If the decrease in contractility affects both sides of the heart, the condition is called *bilateral heart failure.* In other circumstances, failure may be restricted primarily to either the left ventricle or the right ventricle and thus is called *left-sided heart failure* or *right-sided heart failure.*

Ventricular function curves provide a helpful way to envision the consequences of heart failure and the compensations for heart failure. In Figure 26-1 the curve labeled *Normal* indicates the relationship between stroke volume and preload for a normal ventricle (for a review, see Figure 21-3, *C*). The curve labeled *Initially severe failure* shows that a ventricle in failure has a depressed contractility (i.e., a smaller stroke volume for any given preload). If a normal heart suddenly goes into severe failure, stroke volume changes from its normal value (shown by point 1) to the low value (shown by point 2). For purposes of illustration, imagine that these curves define the function of the left ventricle and that the left ventricle is the one that fails. A decrease in left ventricular stroke volume causes a decrease in left ventricular output, which results in a decrease in mean arterial blood pressure. If there is inadequate compensation for this fall in blood pressure, severe exercise intolerance is certain, inadequate perfusion of the critical organs is likely, and death is a strong possibility. However, several mechanisms react rapidly, within seconds to minutes, to compensate for heart failure and to minimize its adverse effects.

One compensation for heart failure is *Starling's mechanism.* If the left ventricle suddenly decreases its stroke volume, the right ventricle (at least for a few heartbeats) maintains a higher stroke volume than the failing left ventricle. The excess blood pumped by the right ventricle has to "go somewhere," and most of the excess accumulates in the pulmonary veins and left atrium. In effect, blood backs up or dams up behind (i.e., upstream of) the left ventricle. The resulting increase in left atrial pressure creates an increase in left ventricular preload, which leads to an increase in left ventricular end-diastolic volume and, by Starling's mechanism, an increase in stroke volume. This improvement in stroke volume is depicted in Figure 26-1 as a transition from point *2* to point *3.* The sequence of events, whereby an increase in preload helps offset the initial fall in stroke volume, is also diagrammed in Figure 26-2 *(top left loop).* Note that the compensation by Starling's mechanism does not return stroke volume to its normal value because contractility remains severely depressed; however, without this compensation severe heart failure would be fatal.

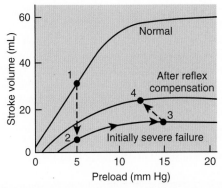

FIGURE 26-1 Ventricular function curves depicting the consequences and compensations for heart failure in terms of changes in preload (end-diastolic ventricular pressure) and stroke volume. See text for details.

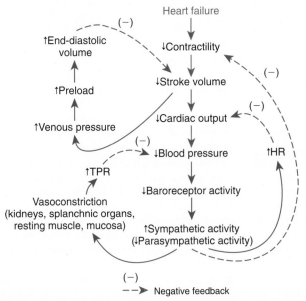

FIGURE 26-2 Consequences *(red arrows)* and compensations *(green arrows)* for heart failure. The changes described here include those presented graphically in Figure 26-1. See text for details. *HR,* Heart rate; *TPR,* total peripheral resistance.

The arterial baroreflex is another mechanism that reacts rapidly to compensate for heart failure. Even after compensation by Starling's mechanism, left ventricular output remains below normal, as does arterial blood pressure. Therefore, baroreceptor activity is below normal. The central nervous system (CNS) responds reflexively by increasing sympathetic efferent activity to the heart and blood vessels and by decreasing parasympathetic activity to the heart.

The sympathetic effect on the heart increases ventricular contractility. Contractility is not restored to normal but is brought to a higher level than existed in the absence of reflex compensation. Graphically, the effect of the baroreflex is to move the failing ventricle to a function curve that is intermediate between the *Normal* curve and the curve of *Initially severe failure* (see point 4 in Figure 26-1). Note that the increase in contractility also brings stroke volume back toward (but not reaching) its normal level.

The reflexive increase in sympathetic activity raises heart rate above normal and decreases systolic duration; these changes also

help to restore cardiac output and arterial pressure toward normal despite the persistently depressed stroke volume. Finally, sympathetic activation causes vasoconstriction, particularly in the noncritical organs, which increases total peripheral resistance (TPR) above normal. This also helps to return arterial pressure toward its normal level.

The net effect of the compensations by way of Starling's mechanism and the baroreflex is that arterial blood pressure can be maintained near its normal level, at least when the animal is at rest, despite a severe ventricular failure. Figure 26-2 summarizes these reflex effects. Note that after compensation by Starling's mechanism and the baroreflex, contractility, stroke volume, cardiac output, and blood pressure remain at least somewhat below normal. By contrast, preload, sympathetic activity, heart rate, and TPR are above normal.

Serious Complications Secondary to Heart Failure Include Exercise Intolerance, Edema, Salt and Water Retention, Kidney Failure, Uremia, Septic Shock, and Decompensation

Even though Starling's mechanism and the baroreflex can compensate to a remarkable degree for severe heart failure, important secondary complications often develop. These complications make heart failure a serious clinical problem, even in cases where compensatory mechanisms can maintain cardiac output and arterial pressure at near-normal levels when the animal is at rest.

Heart failure causes *exercise intolerance*. In a normal animal the ability of the heart to increase cardiac output during exercise depends on sympathetically mediated increases in stroke volume and heart rate. In a patient with heart failure, however, sympathetic activation is being harnessed to restore cardiac output toward normal in the resting state. Therefore the patient has a limited ability to invoke an effective, further increase in sympathetic activity. The failing heart cannot provide the increased cardiac output required to meet the blood flow requirements of exercising skeletal muscle. In the absence of an adequate increase in cardiac output, metabolic vasodilation in the exercising muscle results in a large decrease in arterial pressure and inadequate blood flow to all organs, including the exercising muscle. The patient exhibits lethargy and weakness; even mild exercise leads quickly to exhaustion.

Edema is another serious complication secondary to heart failure. As noted, blood dams up in the atrium and veins behind a failing ventricle. In the case of left ventricular failure, left atrial pressure increases, as does pressure in the pulmonary veins and pulmonary capillaries. The increase in pulmonary capillary hydrostatic pressure leads to an increase in the filtration of capillary fluid into the interstitial spaces of the lungs. *Pulmonary edema* develops. The excess of interstitial fluid slows the transfer of oxygen from the lung alveoli into the lung capillaries and can result in inadequate oxygenation of the blood *(hypoxemia)*. In extreme cases, interstitial fluid leaks into the intrapleural space *(pleural effusion)* or into the alveolar air spaces, which causes a further reduction in lung function. The resulting hypoxia in critical organs can be fatal. In a patient with right ventricular failure the increase in venous pressure occurs in the systemic circulation. Therefore the resulting edema occurs in the systemic organs, particularly in dependent extremities and in the abdomen. The cause-and-effect sequence by which heart failure leads to edema is summarized in Figure 26-3 *(top left)*.

Whether the edema is in the lungs or in the systemic circulation, its degree is limited by the three safety factors previously

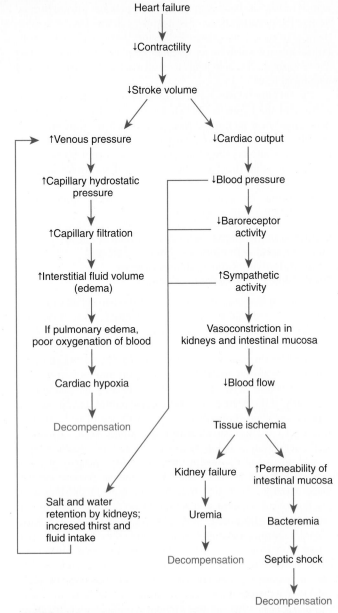

Heart failure

↓Contractility

↓Stroke volume

↑Venous pressure

↑Capillary hydrostatic pressure

↑Capillary filtration

↑Interstitial fluid volume (edema)

If pulmonary edema, poor oxygenation of blood

Cardiac hypoxia

Decompensation

↓Cardiac output

↓Blood pressure

↓Baroreceptor activity

↑Sympathetic activity

Vasoconstriction in kidneys and intestinal mucosa

↓Blood flow

Tissue ischemia

Kidney failure

Uremia

Decompensation

↑Permeability of intestinal mucosa

Bacteremia

Septic shock

Decompensation

Salt and water retention by kidneys; incresed thirst and fluid intake

FIGURE 26-3 Heart failure leads to exercise intolerance. Additional, life-threatening complications secondary to heart failure are diagrammed here, including edema, salt and water retention and increased fluid intake, kidney failure, uremia, and septic shock. Vicious cycles develop in which the effects of heart failure make the heart failure worse (decompensation). See text for details.

discussed (see Figure 23-5). These safety factors would probably keep the edema of heart failure well controlled were it not for an additional factor that exaggerates the elevation of venous pressure in heart failure. As long as arterial pressure remains subnormal in a patient with heart failure, the baroreceptor reflex and some mechanisms involving the kidneys work to raise blood volume above normal. These volume-increasing mechanisms include increased thirst (which raises fluid intake), increased release of antidiuretic hormone (ADH) from the pituitary (which decreases the amount of fluid lost in the urine), and activation of the renin-angiotensin-aldosterone system (which decreases sodium loss in the urine). These effects of the baroreflex were mentioned briefly

in Chapter 25; the mechanisms involving the kidneys are described in more detail in Chapters 41 and 43.

The point for now is that the patient with severe heart failure experiences a substantial and persistent increase in blood volume. The excess blood accumulates particularly in the veins upstream from the failing ventricle, which exaggerates the increases in venous pressure and capillary filtration. The normal safety factors against may be overwhelmed. This is why one of the main goals in the clinical treatment of heart failure is to counteract the buildup of excessive blood volume and interstitial fluid volume. *Diuretic drugs* are the main therapies used for this purpose (see Chapter 43).

Severe, persistent heart failure leads to several additional adverse effects. The baroreceptor reflex responds to an abnormally low arterial pressure in heart failure by initiating arteriolar vasoconstriction, primarily in the kidneys, splanchnic organs, and resting skeletal muscle (the noncritical organs). In severe heart failure the skin and mucous membranes are also vasoconstricted. Vasoconstriction in these organs helps compensate for heart failure by permitting the available cardiac output to be routed to the critical organs (brain, heart, and working skeletal muscle). However, persistent vasoconstriction leads to the additional complications of kidney failure, uremia, and septic shock.

Vasoconstricted kidneys cannot form urine in a normal manner and therefore do not rid the body of the excess volume of blood and interstitial fluid that accumulates in heart failure. Persistent vasoconstriction damages kidney tissue and leads to a buildup of nitrogenous and acidic waste products in the body. The condition is called *uremia*, which literally means "urine in the blood." To make matters worse, after a prolonged period of intense vasoconstriction, damage to the kidney tissue becomes irreversible. At this stage, uremia, acidosis, and salt and water retention may persist even if clinical treatment is temporarily successful in returning cardiac output and blood pressure close to normal. For this reason, *renal failure* often is the terminal event in chronic heart failure.

Intense and prolonged vasoconstriction in the splanchnic circulation can also have lethal consequences. The mucosa of the gastrointestinal tract is particularly susceptible to ischemic damage. Normally, the intestinal mucosa creates a barrier between the contents of the intestinal lumen and the bloodstream. Ischemic damage to the intestinal mucosa allows bacteria and bacterial toxins to pass into the bloodstream or the peritoneum. The resulting bacteremia or peritonitis can cause septic shock and death. The causes and consequences of renal and splanchnic ischemia are summarized in Figure 26-3 *(bottom right)*.

Cardiac decompensation is an additional (and frequently terminal) complication secondary to heart failure. The basic concept of decompensation is that when heart failure reaches a certain degree of severity, the body's attempted compensations for heart failure end up making the heart failure worse. Vicious decompensatory cycles develop and can lead to death within a few hours unless there is vigorous medical intervention.

The specific mechanisms of the *decompensatory cycles* are very complex, but three examples illustrate the concept. As previously explained, in the case of left ventricular failure, the damming up of blood in the left atrium is compensatory because it increases left ventricular preload, which helps boost stroke volume back toward normal. However, the increased left ventricular preload leads to the secondary complication of pulmonary edema. If severe, pulmonary edema interferes with the oxygenation of blood. One tissue that depends critically on an adequate supply of oxygen is cardiac muscle; hypoxia depresses the contractility of cardiac muscle. Thus a vicious cycle can develop: severely depressed ventricular contractility → severe pulmonary edema → inadequate oxygenation of blood → hypoxia of the left ventricular muscle → further depression of ventricular contractility.

For a second example of a vicious decompensatory cycle, consider again the effects of the baroreflex on the kidneys. Renal vasoconstriction is compensatory for heart failure in that it helps increase TPR, which helps raise arterial pressure back toward normal, which helps keep perfusion pressure high enough to deliver adequate blood flow to the critical organs. However, as already mentioned, intense and prolonged renal vasoconstriction leads to kidney failure and an accumulation of acidic and nitrogenous waste products in the blood (uremia). Uremia depresses cardiac contractility. Thus, another vicious cycle can develop: severe ventricular failure → intense and prolonged renal vasoconstriction → damage to kidney tissues → uremia → metabolic waste products accumulate in cardiac muscle → further depression of ventricular contractility.

A third vicious decompensatory cycle results from the fact that septic shock depresses cardiac contractility. The cycle is: severe ventricular failure → intense and prolonged splanchnic vasoconstriction → ischemic damage to intestinal mucosa → bacteria and endotoxins pass through the damaged mucosa, from intestines into bloodstream → bacteremia causes further depression of ventricular contractility.

Other decompensatory cycles develop in cases of severe, prolonged heart failure, but these three examples (which are illustrated in Figure 26-3) show why decompensation is such a serious development.

Careful clinical diagnosis and prompt treatment of heart failure are imperative, even if compensatory mechanisms have maintained blood pressure near its normal level when the patient is at rest. In evaluating the severity of heart failure and the extent of compensation, it is clinically useful to group the signs of heart failure into two categories. The first category is referred to as *backward heart failure*. The signs of backward heart failure include the changes in the circulation *upstream* from the failing ventricle: increased atrial pressure, increased venous pressure, excessive capillary filtration, edema, and the functional changes secondary to edema (e.g., respiratory failure). The category *forward heart failure* refers to the consequences of heart failure *downstream* from the failing ventricle: decreased cardiac output, decreased arterial blood pressure, and the consequences of excessive vasoconstriction in the systemic organs, especially the kidneys and intestines.

The Immediate Cardiovascular Effects of Hemorrhage Are Minimized by Compensations Initiated by the Atrial Volume Receptor Reflex and the Arterial Baroreceptor Reflex

Figures 26-4 and 26-5 summarize the cardiovascular responses to hemorrhage. The curve labeled *Normal* in Figure 26-4 shows that the maintenance of a normal stroke volume depends on the maintenance of a normal level of ventricular preload. When hemorrhage occurs, blood is lost from the whole cardiovascular system, but particularly from the veins, which are the blood reservoirs of the body. Hemorrhage therefore decreases venous volume, venous pressure, atrial pressure, ventricular preload, and ventricular end-diastolic ventricular volume. In the absence of any compensation,

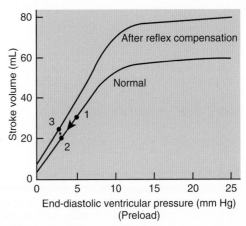

FIGURE 26-4 Direct effect of hemorrhage is to decrease ventricular preload, which decreases stroke volume (transition from *point 1,* which is normal, to *point 2*). A reflex increase in sympathetic activity increases ventricular contractility above normal *(upper curve),* which restores stroke volume *toward normal* (transition from *point 2* to *point 3*).

ventricular stroke volume decreases from point 1 in Figure 26-4 to point 2.

Note that no specification was made in the preceding paragraph about whether the itemized sequence of events was affecting the right heart or the left heart. The distinction is irrelevant because the right and left hearts are part of a series circuit. Therefore, the volumes of blood pumped by the right and left ventricles must always come into balance within a few beats. Specifically, if hemorrhage lowers right ventricular preload (and therefore right ventricular output), the consequence will be decreased venous return to the left heart, which will decrease left ventricular preload (and therefore left ventricular output).

Figure 26-4 shows that the normal ventricular function curve is rather steep to the left of point 1 (the normal operating point). Therefore a 40% hemorrhage results in approximately 40% reductions in venous pressure, atrial pressure, ventricular preload, and stroke volume. In the absence of compensations, cardiac output and mean arterial pressure (MAP) would also decrease by 40%. MAP would then be inadequate to sustain normal function in the critical organs, and the animal would die. With intact compensatory mechanisms, however, a normal animal can withstand a 40% hemorrhage without death and have only about a 10% decrease in MAP.

The immediate compensations for hemorrhage are initiated by the arterial baroreflex and atrial volume receptor reflex. Hemorrhage decreases MAP, which decreases the activity of arterial baroreceptors. The baroreflex response is to increase sympathetic activity and to decrease parasympathetic activity. The increased sympathetic activity acts on the heart to increase cardiac contractility. This helps restore stroke volume back toward normal, despite a persistent, subnormal preload and end-diastolic volume. The effect of this sympathetic compensation is diagrammed in Figure 26-4 as point 3. Although stroke volume is returned toward normal, it remains low; after compensation for a 40% hemorrhage, the stroke volume may remain 25% below normal.

Additional compensations help restore MAP closer to normal despite the persistence of low stroke volume. First, heart rate increases above normal, which brings cardiac output back to within about 20% of its normal level. In addition, sympathetic vasoconstriction in the noncritical organs raises TPR above

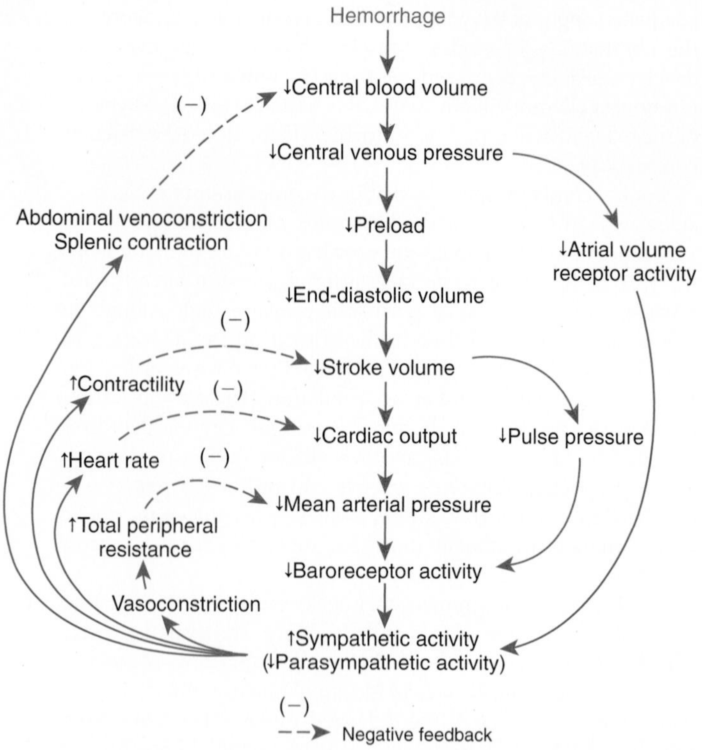

FIGURE 26-5 Summary of the consequences of hemorrhage *(red arrows)* and the rapid compensations initiated by the arterial barore-flex and atrial volume receptor reflex *(green arrows)*. The changes described here include those portrayed graphically in Figure 26-4.

normal, resulting in a MAP that remains within approximately 10% of its normal level, despite a persistent 20% drop in cardiac output. Review the compensations described thus far by locating them on Figure 26-5.

You may wonder why baroreflex compensatory actions continue if MAP is returned most of the way toward normal. Compensatory baroreflex responses are sustained because baroreceptors are responsive to changes in pulse pressure as well as to changes in MAP, and pulse pressure remains low. There are two reasons for the subnormal pulse pressure: (1) the persistent decrease in stroke volume and (2) the increase in heart rate above normal. Thus, even if MAP is returned substantially toward normal after compensation for a hemorrhage, baroreceptor activity (action potential frequency) remains below normal.

The atrial volume receptor reflex also contributes to the sustained increase in sympathetic activity after hemorrhage. Hemorrhage leads to a persistent decrease in central venous pressure and atrial pressure. Therefore the activity of the atrial volume receptors is decreased below normal. The CNS responds to this decreased afferent activity from atrial volume receptors by elevating sympathetic efferent activity and by decreasing cardiac parasympathetic efferent activity. Thus, as illustrated in Figure 26-5, the atrial volume receptor reflex and the arterial baroreflex work synergistically to compensate for hemorrhage.

In severe hemorrhage the reflex increases in sympathetic activity affect not only the heart and resistance vessels but also the veins. The abdominal veins in particular are constricted when sympathetic activation is intense. Sympathetic venoconstriction displaces blood from the abdominal veins and moves it toward the central circulation, which helps to restore the low central venous pressure, atrial pressure, and preload back toward normal (see Figure 26-5, *left side*). Sympathetic activation also constricts the blood vessels within the spleen and the muscular capsule

around the spleen. Some of the blood that is sequestered in the spleen is expelled into the abdominal veins, and then it moves toward the heart. In species that have large spleens (e.g., dog and horse), splenic contraction can mobilize a volume of blood equal to 10% of the total blood volume. An additional, adaptive feature of the blood sequestered in the spleen is that it has a higher-than-normal hematocrit. The mobilization of these sequestered red blood cells helps to offset the fall in hematocrit that is a normal consequence of interstitial fluid reabsorption after hemorrhage (as described next).

The arterial baroreceptor reflex and the atrial volume receptor reflex act within a few seconds to restore blood pressure toward its normal level after a hemorrhage. Other compensations come into play in the minutes and hours after hemorrhage to restore the lost fluid volume.

The Blood Volume Lost in Hemorrhage Is Restored Through a Combination of Capillary Fluid Shifts and Hormonal and Behavioral Responses

Hemorrhage causes both venous and arterial pressures to fall below normal, so capillary hydrostatic pressure also falls below normal throughout the body. This alters the balance of hydrostatic and oncotic pressures acting on water in a direction that favors reabsorption of interstitial fluid back into the capillaries (Figure 26-6). The volume of interstitial fluid that can be reabsorbed by this process in 1 hour is approximately 10% of the volume lost in the hemorrhage. However, the rate of reabsorption of interstitial fluid becomes limited after 3 to 4 hours. As interstitial fluid is reabsorbed, there is a decrease in interstitial fluid hydrostatic pressure (it becomes even more negative than normal), and this opposes further reabsorption. Also, as interstitial fluid is reabsorbed, the interstitial fluid protein concentration increases because proteins in the interstitial fluid are not reabsorbed. The

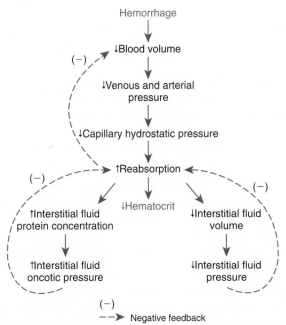

FIGURE 26-6 During the first 3 to 4 hours after a hemorrhage, interstitial fluid is reabsorbed into the bloodstream, which helps compensate for the lost blood volume. A complication is that the hematocrit decreases. Reabsorption is limited by decreases in interstitial fluid hydrostatic pressure and by increases in interstitial fluid oncotic pressure.

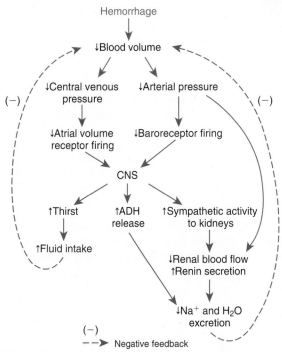

FIGURE 26-7 Behavioral and hormonal responses after hemorrhage include increased fluid intake and decreased salt and water loss in the urine, which lead to the eventual restoration of the blood volume lost in the hemorrhage. *ADH,* Antidiuretic hormone; *CNS,* central nervous system.

resulting increase in interstitial fluid oncotic pressure also opposes further reabsorption. Despite these limits, the reabsorption of interstitial fluid is an important compensation for hemorrhage in the first few hours.

The interstitial fluid that is reabsorbed into the bloodstream after a hemorrhage contains neither plasma proteins nor blood cells. Therefore the proteins and cells remaining in the bloodstream after the hemorrhage become diluted as interstitial fluid is reabsorbed. As a consequence the concentration of plasma proteins in blood decreases, and so does the hematocrit. This is why a decreasing hematocrit over a few hours in an otherwise normal patient is presumptive evidence that a hemorrhage has occurred recently or is continuing to occur. In the absence of an obvious hemorrhage, such a patient should be examined for evidence of internal bleeding.

Figure 26-7 illustrates how the atrial volume receptor reflex and the arterial baroreceptor reflex participate in the eventual, complete restoration of blood volume after a hemorrhage. As mentioned, hemorrhage leads to a decrease in the activity of both atrial volume receptors and arterial baroreceptors. One reflexive response to the decreased receptor activity is activation of sympathetic nerves, and some of the effects of the sympathetic activation have already been described (see Figure 26-5). Sympathetic activity (coupled with a decrease in arterial pressure) also acts on the kidneys to increase their release of the hormone renin. As mentioned in Chapter 25, renin works through the renin-angiotensin-aldosterone system to decrease sodium excretion by the kidneys. Decreased activity of the baroreceptors and atrial volume receptors also triggers increased ADH secretion from the pituitary gland. ADH circulates to the kidneys, where it reduces urine formation. Through the combined actions of renal

vasoconstriction, the renin-angiotensin-aldosterone system, and ADH, sodium excretion and water excretion are both decreased. Note that these actions *conserve* the available body fluid volume after hemorrhage, but they do not *restore* it to normal. The actual restoration of body fluid volume after hemorrhage requires increased fluid intake. The baroreceptor reflex and the atrial volume receptor reflex act through the hypothalamus to increase the sensation of thirst. If water is available, fluid intake increases until the lost body fluid volume is restored to normal. This may take 1 to 2 days.

The final compensations for hemorrhage involve the restoration of the lost plasma proteins and blood cells. The plasma proteins are synthesized by the liver, and the blood cells are produced by the bone marrow. The time required may be several days for the plasma proteins and a few weeks for the blood cells.

The preceding discussion focused on the effects of severe hemorrhage. All the same compensations occur to a lesser degree after mild hemorrhage. For example, when a human donates blood, about 10% of the blood volume (0.5 L) is removed. All the compensations just described are evident after this 10% hemorrhage.

In Large Animals, the Transition from a Recumbent to a Standing Posture Elicits the Same Cardiovascular Responses as Hemorrhage

You can understand the reason for this if you consider the effect of gravity on blood contained within blood vessels of the body. In a standing subject, gravity increases the distending pressure in the dependent vessels (those below heart level), particularly in the leg vessels. The gravitational effect does not cause much accumulation of blood in the arteries and arterioles because these vessels are not easily distensible (i.e., they have low compliance). However, the gravitational effect causes a significant distention of the dependent veins because of their much greater compliance. The extra blood that pools in the dependent veins is blood that would otherwise have returned to the central circulation. Therefore, in an upright subject, there is a decrease in central blood volume and central venous pressure, just as there would be after hemorrhage. In a normal human the assumption of an upright posture is equivalent to a 10% hemorrhage, and it triggers all the compensatory responses already described for hemorrhage. In small animals the gravitational effect of standing is negligible. In some large animals, such as horses and cattle, the volume of blood that pools in the leg veins is minimized by the relatively small size of veins in the extremities.

The Initiation of Exercise Involves an Interplay of Local and Neural Changes That Increases Cardiac Output and Delivers Increased Flow to Exercising Muscle

As discussed in Chapter 24, local metabolic control mechanisms dilate skeletal muscle arterioles during exercise. As reviewed in Figure 26-8 (top), metabolic products accumulate in exercising muscle, and the local oxygen concentration decreases. The

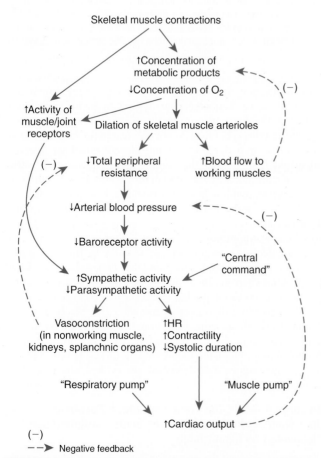

FIGURE 26-8 Cardiovascular responses to exercise involve a complex interplay of local metabolic control mechanisms with central command, reflexes, and the blood-pumping effects of muscle contraction and respiration. The overall result is increased blood flow in exercising muscle, decreased blood flow in the noncritical organs, decreased total peripheral resistance, increased cardiac output, and (normally) maintenance of arterial blood pressure near its normal level. *HR,* Heart rate.

metabolic products and hypoxia both cause dilation of the arterioles within the exercising muscle. This vasodilation is a local response, not dependent on nerves or hormones. The result is an increased blood flow to the exercising muscle (*active hyperemia*). The increased blood flow delivers more oxygen and removes some of the accumulated metabolic vasodilating products. In this way, muscle blood flow is matched to metabolic rate.

Metabolic control of blood flow in exercising muscle can succeed only if arterial blood pressure is maintained at a level sufficient to provide the needed additional blood flow. This necessitates a substantial increase in cardiac output and, in extreme exercise, vasoconstriction in the noncritical organs (which makes more blood flow available for the exercising muscle and other critical organs). These adjustments are brought about by three neural mechanisms: central command, the exercise reflex, and the arterial baroreflex.

Central command is a psychogenic effect. In preparation for exercise (and continuing during exercise) the CNS increases sympathetic activity to the heart and blood vessels and decreases parasympathetic activity to the heart. The sympathetic and parasympathetic changes are graded, depending on the intensity of the exercise. In effect, central command represents a "guess" by the brain as to the levels of sympathetic and parasympathetic activity that will be needed during the exercise to match cardiac output to the needs of the systemic organs.

The *exercise reflex* is the second mechanism that helps set the level of sympathetic and parasympathetic activity during exercise. The exercise reflex is initiated by specialized nerve endings within muscles and joints. An increase in muscular work and in the movement of the body joints activates these muscle and joint receptors. The resulting increased afferent neural activity initiates a reflex increase in sympathetic (and decrease in parasympathetic) efferent drive. Although the mechanism for excitation of the muscle and joint receptors is not completely understood, it is clear that the activation of these receptors is necessary to keep blood pressure from falling during exercise.

The *arterial baroreceptor reflex* is the third major controller of sympathetic and parasympathetic activity during exercise. The baroreflex serves to fine-tune autonomic drive to the heart and arterioles to keep arterial pressure at its set point. If central command and the exercise reflex do not raise sympathetic activity to a sufficiently high level during a particular bout of exercise, arterial pressure falls below normal. The arterial baroreceptors detect this low pressure, and the baroreflex responds by increasing sympathetic activity. Conversely, if central command and the exercise reflex raise sympathetic activity too high for the level of exercise, arterial pressure rises above normal. The response of the baroreflex is to decrease sympathetic activity.

In effect, central command and the exercise reflex initiate the autonomic adjustments for exercise, and the arterial baroreflex performs the fine-tuning to keep arterial pressure near its set point (see Figure 26-8).

Two additional, nonneural mechanisms also help to increase the cardiac output during exercise. The first of these is the *muscle pump* (Figure 26-9). When skeletal muscles contract, they tend to squeeze the blood vessels contained within them. One consequence of this is the tendency for a muscle to restrict its blood flow during a sustained contraction (see Chapter 24). If the contractions are rhythmical, however, each contraction causes blood to be expelled out of the muscle veins and thus toward the central circulation. Minimal backflow of blood occurs from the central circulation into the veins during muscular relaxation because the

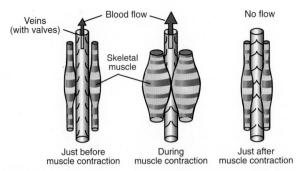

Veins (with valves) — Blood flow — No flow

Skeletal muscle

Just before muscle contraction | During muscle contraction | Just after muscle contraction

FIGURE 26-9 During dynamic exercise, the rhythmical contractions of the skeletal muscles squeeze venous blood back toward the central circulation. This so-called muscle pump helps increase central venous pressure in an exercising animal.

veins have one-way valves within them. Thus, by massaging the veins, exercising muscles exert a pumping action that displaces venous blood toward the central circulation and increases central venous pressure. The consequence is an increase in ventricular preload above the level that would otherwise exist.

The second nonneural mechanism that helps to increase cardiac output during exercise is the *respiratory pump.* Vigorous exercise involves an increase in the rate and the depth of respiration. During each inspiration, a subatmospheric pressure is generated within the intrapleural space. This negative pressure distends the airways of the lungs and expands them. It also increases the distending pressure on the central veins and the heart. Distention of the central veins and heart helps promote the flow of blood from the abdominal veins into the central veins and heart. In addition, the diaphragm muscle moves caudally during inspiration and compresses the abdominal organs. The resulting increase in intraabdominal pressure "squeezes" blood out of the abdominal veins and toward the central veins. Overall, the respiratory pumping action helps to increase venous return, central venous volume, and ventricular preload during exercise.

Cardiac output in well-conditioned humans and many animal species can increase to six times its resting level during vigorous exercise, as a result of the combined effects of sympathetic and parasympathetic responses, the muscle pump, and the respiratory pump. Note, however, that the success of the mechanisms that increase cardiac output during exercise depends on the heart's ability to respond normally both to increased sympathetic drive and to increases in preload. As mentioned earlier, during heart failure the autonomic mechanisms available to increase cardiac contractility and heart rate are invoked simply to maintain a normal cardiac output at rest. Therefore the autonomic nervous system in a patient with heart failure has a limited ability to bring about further increases in cardiac output during the initiation of exercise. For this reason, patients with heart failure typically exhibit exercise intolerance.

Maximal exercise ability in normal humans and animals appears to be limited by cardiac output. That is, the respiratory system can oxygenate as much blood as the heart can deliver to the lungs, and skeletal muscle can take up and metabolize as much oxygen as the heart can deliver to it. When cardiac output has reached a maximal level, however, oxygen transport from the lungs to the skeletal muscle also is maximized. This sets the upper limit to the level of exercise that can be sustained.

CLINICAL CORRELATIONS

EXERCISE INTOLERANCE SECONDARY TO CONGESTIVE HEART FAILURE

History. An 8-year-old female Great Dane has been diagnosed previously with idiopathic dilative cardiomyopathy. Severe, generalized cardiac enlargement was evident on thoracic radiographs. The dog has been losing weight and is unable to complete daily walks with her owners.

Clinical Examination. Femoral pulses are weak but regular at 140 beats/min. The mucous membranes are pale, and the capillary refill time is prolonged. Heart sounds are muffled, and a murmur is heard on the left side over the atrioventricular valve. Respiratory rate is greater than normal (45 breaths/min). Auscultation reveals increased bronchovesicular (respiratory) sounds. The abdomen is distended, and the abdominal organs are difficult to palpate. The electrocardiogram shows sinus tachycardia with broad, high-voltage QRS complexes. Thoracic radiography reveals a greatly enlarged heart and moderate pulmonary edema. Echocardiography reveals dilation of all four cardiac chambers. Ejection fraction is below normal, and there is mitral regurgitation.

Additional diagnostic tests are conducted to help assess the degree of complications secondary to the heart failure. The percentage saturation of hemoglobin in arterial blood is 78% (normal, 95% to 100%), the difference in oxygen content between arterial and venous blood is 8.5 mL of O_2 per deciliter of blood (normal, 4 to 6 mL), the serum creatinine concentration is 3 mg/dL (normal, <1 mg/dL), urine specific gravity is 1.036 (high normal), and central venous pressure is 14 mm Hg (normal, 0 to 3 mm Hg).

When persuaded to exercise, the dog appears to become tired after walking less than 1 minute. Her legs begin to tremble, and then she collapses. Her pulse rate is 180 beats/min, and her mucous membranes are dark and cyanotic (blue).

Comment. Chronic heart failure secondary to cardiomyopathy is common in large dogs older than 4 years of age. Often the cardiomyopathy is idiopathic (of unknown cause). The case presented here is fairly typical of advanced heart failure. All the clinical findings are either direct consequences of the heart failure or consequences of attempts by the body to compensate for the heart failure (see Figures 26-1, 26-2, and 26-3). In brief, ventricular failure (decreased contractility) leads to decreased stroke volume, cardiac output, and blood pressure.

Compensations for the heart failure involve reflex decreases in parasympathetic activity, increases in sympathetic activity, and increases in the release of ADH and renin. Heart rate is increased, which helps raise cardiac output back toward normal. Pulse pressure, judged by palpation of the femoral pulse, is reduced (because heart rate is high and stroke volume is low). There is decreased blood supply to the mucosa, splanchnic organs, kidneys, and resting skeletal muscle because of vasoconstriction. This helps support arterial pressure and reserves the available cardiac output for the heart and brain. The vasoconstriction is evident in the pale color and slow refilling of the mucous membranes. Renal vasoconstriction reduces the rate of urine formation. Urinary loss of salt and water is further reduced by the actions of ADH and the renin-angiotensin-aldosterone system. The urine that does form has a high solute concentration (high specific gravity). Metabolic products (e.g., creatinine) that are normally eliminated by the kidneys accumulate in the blood. The resulting uremia, if severe, can further depress cardiac function and initiate the vicious cycle of decompensation.

Salt and water retention increases blood volume above normal. Most of the excess blood volume is in the veins, so venous and atrial pressures are above normal. The elevated atrial pressure (preload) increases ventricular end-diastolic volume above normal, which helps the failing heart to pump a larger stroke volume than it otherwise would. However, the excessive volume and pressure of blood in the veins also cause systemic edema (distended abdomen caused by ascites) and pulmonary edema (visible on the radiograph). Pulmonary edema impairs the ability of the lungs to oxygenate blood. Therefore the hemoglobin saturation and the oxygen content of arterial blood are both below normal in this dog. The tissues of the body respond to the low rate of oxygen delivery by unloading as much oxygen as they can from the blood as it flows through the tissue. This makes the arteriovenous difference in oxygen content greater than normal. The general inadequacy of cardiovascular transport leads to poor gastrointestinal function and metabolic stresses on the tissues of the dog, and weight loss occurs.

Despite many compensatory mechanisms, this dog is unable to deliver a normal amount of well-oxygenated blood to the body tissues, even at rest. When the dog tries to exercise, cardiac output increases very little. Therefore, when exercise-induced vasodilation occurs in the exercising muscles and total peripheral resistance decreases, blood pressure falls dramatically. There is a further decrease in blood flow in the tissues of the systemic circulation that were already vasoconstricted (e.g., mucous membranes), and these tissues become hypoxic and cyanotic. Inadequate blood flow in the exercising skeletal muscles leads to hypoxia and acidosis, and the dog collapses.

Treatment. The ideal treatment strategy for this dog is to improve the contractile performance of the myocardium. Theoretically, β-adrenergic agonists or cardiac glycosides could be administered to increase cardiac contractility. However, currently available drugs are either ineffective or only mildly effective in dogs with severe, chronic heart failure. One reason is that dogs in heart failure have already engaged adrenergic drive to the heart through activation of their sympathetic nervous systems. Therefore, treatment emphasizes symptomatic therapy, with the goals of controlling pulmonary congestion and improving cardiac output. Diuretics or venodilators reduce venous pressures and are usually effective in controlling signs of congestion (venous distention and edema). Such drugs must be used cautiously, however, because they create the risk of lowering preload and therefore exacerbating the low cardiac output. Arteriolar vasodilators can augment the output of a failing heart by reducing the afterload (arterial pressure) against which the heart must eject blood. An appropriate initial treatment for this dog includes a diuretic (furosemide) and a cardiac glycoside (digitalis). If digitalis fails to improve cardiac contractility in this advanced case of cardiomyopathy, an arteriolar vasodilator (hydralazine) or a mixed vasodilator-venodilator (enalapril) can be added to the furosemide regimen.

Despite therapy, the prognosis for a dog with such severe, chronic heart failure is poor.

COW WITH "HARDWARE DISEASE"

History. A 4-year-old, pregnant Holstein cow is presented for lethargy, poor appetite, and edema. She is due to calve in 2 months. The producer noticed that over the last few weeks the cow has seemed progressively more lethargic and reluctant to move. He observed swelling below her jaw and in her brisket. She has lost 75 to 125 pounds.

Clinical Examination. The cow appears depressed. She is dehydrated. Her mucous membranes are dark (indicating poor perfusion), and capillary refill time is prolonged. She has marked brisket and submandibular edema. Her jugular veins are prominent. She grunts when she moves. Her temperature, pulse, and respiratory rates are all increased. Her heart sounds are muffled (as if heard through fluid), and she has a murmur ("washing machine" murmur). She has increased bronchovesicular (respiratory) sounds dorsally, but the sounds are muffled ventrally. Peripheral pulses are weak. Rumen contractions are decreased (one every 1 to 3 minutes). Feces are scant. Blood is submitted for a complete blood count and chemistry profile. Results indicate that the white blood cell count is low and serum creatinine concentration is increased. Fibrinogen, globulins, and total protein are all increased. Calcium and potassium levels are low.

An electrocardiogram reveals decreased amplitude of QRS complexes and ST segment elevation. Echocardiography reveals excessive fluid and gas in the pericardial space. Fibrin tags are also present. The right atrium and right ventricle appear to collapse during diastole, which is consistent with *cardiac tamponade* (excessive pericardial fluid pushing in on the heart). The left ventricle also contracts less forcefully and less completely than normal during systole (*decreased left ventricular free wall motion*).

With guidance from the echocardiogram, a sample of pericardial fluid is obtained. The fluid is reddish in color (rather than clear) and has a distinct, bad odor. Laboratory analysis reveals elevated protein concentration and an elevated count of white blood cells (primarily neutrophils) in the pericardial fluid. Culture reveals that both aerobic and anaerobic bacteria are present.

Comment. This cow has traumatic reticuloperitonitis with pericarditis. *Traumatic reticuloperitonitis* (TRP), or "hardware disease," is common in cattle. Cattle are indiscriminate eaters, and they accidentally swallow sharp metal objects that get mixed into their feed. Metal objects settle in the reticulum of the rumen. Contractions of the reticulum may push sharp objects through the wall of the reticulum and into the peritoneum. Bacteria follow and cause peritonitis. Subsequently, the sharp object may penetrate the diaphragm, which is located just cranial to the reticulum, and may then move on to penetrate the pericardium. The consequence is pericarditis (inflammation of the pericardium). Sequelae include formation of scar tissue (seen as fibrin tags), pericardial bacterial infection, and accumulation of inflammatory fluid in the pericardium. The pericardial fluid presses on the cardiac chambers, restricting their filling during diastole, and this causes pump failure.

Evidence of congestive pump failure in this cow includes poor perfusion (weak pulses, dark mucous membranes, and prolonged capillary refill time), cardiac abnormalities (subnormal right atrial and ventricular filling, decreased left ventricular motion), elevated heart rate, distended jugular veins, edema, and lethargy.

Treatment. Prognosis is poor in this case because of the combination of pericardial infection and congestive pump failure. The producer could try to treat the infection, in hopes of delivering a live calf. Because the cow is already in pump failure with very limited cardiac output, however, it is likely that the calf is not receiving sufficient blood flow and oxygen. The calf could die in utero and could be aborted by the cow.

PRACTICE QUESTIONS

1. During experimental trials on a new artificial aortic valve, a dog is anesthetized and placed on cardiac bypass for 1 hour (i.e., a heart-lung machine is substituted for the dog's own heart and lungs). After successful installation of the artificial valve, the dog is taken off bypass, and the normal circulation is restored. Ten minutes later, the dog's central venous pressure is 20 mm Hg, mean arterial pressure is 90 mm Hg, and heart rate is 130 beats/min. The cardiac output is not measured, but the surgeon suspects that it is too low and therefore the patient's tissues are not being adequately supplied with blood. Which of the following measures would be most likely to improve the delivery of blood to the patient's tissues?
   a. Transfusion with 500 mL of whole blood
   b. Administration of isoproterenol (selective β-adrenergic agonist)
   c. Increasing the heart rate by electrical pacing
   d. Administration of norepinephrine (nonselective α/β-adrenergic agonist)
   e. Administration of a β-adrenergic antagonist, such as propranolol

2. One of the nerves leading to a dog's heart is stimulated for 1 minute while left atrial pressure, heart rate, and left ventricular output are measured (Figure 26-10). During this stimulation:
   a. Venous return to the left atrium transiently exceeds left ventricular output.
   b. The increase in left ventricular output at the beginning of stimulation can be explained by Starling's law of the heart.
   c. Stroke volume is lower after 15 seconds of stimulation than before stimulation.
   d. The effects of the nerve stimulation are similar to those caused by sympathetic activation of the heart.
   e. The progressive decline in left ventricular output during the stimulation is probably caused by a progressive increase in ventricular end-diastolic volume.

3. One hour after a severe hemorrhage, a dog's arterial pulse pressure, mean pressure, and hematocrit are all below normal. Which of the following statements is *true*?
   a. The diminished pulse pressure reflects decreased aortic compliance.
   b. The diminished mean pressure probably results from decreased total peripheral resistance (TPR).
   c. The diminished hematocrit probably results from reabsorption of interstitial fluid into the bloodstream.
   d. Under these conditions, the action potential frequency of the arterial baroreceptors is greater than normal.
   e. Under these conditions, sympathetic activity is probably less than normal.

4. When a sheep is held in a vertical, head-up position, arterial pressure decreases because:
   a. The baroreceptor reflex causes an increase in TPR.
   b. Valves in the leg veins promote the return of blood to the heart.
   c. The respiratory pump promotes movement of abdominal venous blood into the thorax.
   d. Central blood volume is increased.
   e. Right atrial pressure is decreased.

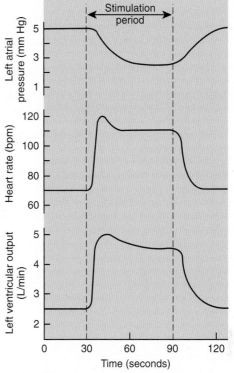

FIGURE 26-10 Cardiovascular data for Practice Question 2.

5. During exercise in a normal animal:
   a. TPR is decreased.
   b. Cardiac output is increased.
   c. Stroke volume is increased.
   d. Blood pressure is nearly normal.
   e. All the above are true.

BIBLIOGRAPHY

Boron WF, Boulpaep EL: *Medical physiology*, ed 2, Philadelphia, 2009, Saunders.

Dunlop RH, Malbert CH: *Veterinary pathophysiology*, Oxford, 2004, Wiley-Blackwell.

Ettinger SJ, Feldman EC: *Textbook of veterinary internal medicine: diseases of the dog and cat*, ed 7, St Louis, 2010, Elsevier/Saunders.

Hinchcliff KW, Geor RJ, Kaneps AJ, editors: *Equine exercise physiology: the science of exercise in the athletic horse*, Philadelphia, 2008, Saunders Elsevier.

Katz AM, Konstam MA: *Heart failure: pathophysiology, molecular biology, and clinical management*, ed 2, Baltimore, 2008, Lippincott, Williams & Wilkins.

Klabunde RE: *Cardiovascular physiology concepts*, ed 2, Baltimore, 2011, Lippincott, Williams & Wilkins.

Levick RJ: *An introduction to cardiovascular physiology*, ed 5, New York, 2010, Hodder Arnold Publishers.

Levy MN, Pappano AJ: *Cardiovascular physiology*, ed 9, St Louis, 2007, Mosby.

Mohrman DE, Heller LJ: *Cardiovascular physiology*, ed 7, New York, 2010, Lange Medical Books/McGraw-Hill.

Noble A, Johnson R, Thomas A: *The cardiovascular system: basic science and clinical conditions*, ed 2, New York, 2010, Churchill Livingstone Elsevier.

Radostits OM, Gay CC, Hinchcliff KW, et al: *Veterinary medicine—a textbook of the diseases of cattle, horses, sheep, pigs and goats,* ed 10, Philadelphia, 2007, Saunders Elsevier.

Silverstein D, Hopper K: *Small animal critical care medicine,* St Louis, 2009, Saunders Elsevier.

Smith BP: *Large animal internal medicine,* ed 4, St Louis, 2009, Mosby Elsevier.

Tilley LP, Smith FWK, Oyama MA, Sleeper MM: *Manual of canine and feline cardiology,* ed 4, Philadelphia, 2008, Saunders.

Ware WA: *Cardiovascular diseases in small animal medicine,* updated ed, London, 2011, Manson Publishing.

Xiang L, Hester RL: *Cardiovascular responses to exercise,* San Rafael, Calif, 2012, Morgan & Claypool Life Sciences.

Zachary JF, McGavin MD: *Pathologic basis of veterinary disease,* ed 5, St Louis, 2011, Mosby Elsevier.

CHAPTER 27

Regulation of the Gastrointestinal Functions

KEY POINTS

1. The gastrointestinal tract, or gut, supplies the body with nutrients, electrolytes, and water by performing five functions: motility, secretion, digestion, absorption, and storage.
2. Intrinsic and extrinsic control systems regulate various functions of the gut.
3. The intrinsic neuronal control system of the gastrointestinal tract is the enteric nervous system.
4. The intrinsic hormonal control system of the gut consists of five hormones including secretin, gastrin, cholecystokinin, gastric inhibitory polypeptide, and motilin.

5. The immune system of the gut is extensive and interacts with the regulatory systems of the gastrointestinal tract to control the various functions of the gut.
6. The extrinsic neuronal control system of the gut is comprised of two nerves: the vagus and the splanchnic.
7. The extrinsic hormonal control system of the gut is limited to one hormone: aldosterone.

The Gastrointestinal Tract, or Gut, Supplies the Body with Nutrients, Electrolytes, and Water by Performing Five Functions: Motility, Secretion, Digestion, Absorption, and Storage

The *digestive system* consists of two parts, the gastrointestinal (GI) tract and the major digestive accessory glands, which include the liver and pancreas (Figure 27-1). This chapter focuses on the control systems that regulate the various functions of the GI tract. The control systems that regulate the functions of the liver and pancreas will be discussed in Chapter 29.

The GI tract, also known as the gut, is a tube-like structure that extends from the mouth to the anus. Histologically, this tube consists of four main layers: (1) the mucosa, which comprises epithelial cells (enterocytes, endocrine cells, and others), the lamina propria, and the muscularis mucosae; (2) the submucosa; (3) two muscle layers, an inner thick circular layer and an outer thin longitudinal layer; and (4) a serosal layer (Figure 27-2).

Functionally, the GI tract supplies the body, including the gut itself, with *nutrients, electrolytes,* and *water*. To supply the body with these substances, the gut performs five functions: *motility, secretion, digestion, absorption,* and *storage*. On the basis of the needs of the various organ systems in the body, the GI tract orchestrates and controls these five functions through two control systems, intrinsic and extrinsic. The intrinsic control system elements are located between the different layers of the gut, whereas the extrinsic control system resides outside the wall of the GI tract. Each of these systems consists of two components, namely, *nerves* and *endocrine secretions* (Figure 27-3).

Intrinsic and Extrinsic Control Systems Regulate Various Functions of the Gut

The intrinsic control system has two components: the *enteric nervous system* (ENS) and gut hormones, which include *gastrin, gastric inhibitory peptide* (GIP), *cholecystokinin* (CCK), *secretin,*

and *motilin*. The extrinsic control system elements that regulate gut functions consist of the *vagus* and *splanchnic nerves* and the hormone *aldosterone*.

The secretions of the intrinsic and extrinsic control systems of the gut are *regulatory* and *not digestive* in nature (Box 27-1). That is, they regulate the activity of cells and tissues of the GI tract, but are not secreted into the gut lumen. They reach their target tissues by four different routes (Figure 27-4). *Endocrine* secretions are deposited close to blood vessels, and then blood cells carry the secretions to their target tissues. *Paracrine* denotes peptides secreted from cells with subsequent diffusion through the interstitial space to contact and affect other cells. *Autocrine* secretions of a given cell modify or regulate functions of the same cell. *Neurocrine* refers to secretion by enteric neurons of neuromodulators or *regulatory peptides* that affect nearby muscle cells, glands, or blood vessels. The endocrine and paracrine cells of the gut are columnar in shape with a wide base and a narrow apex (Figure 27-5). The narrow apex of the cell is exposed to the lumen of the gut, which allows it to "sample" or "taste" the luminal contents and respond to such stimuli by releasing hormones and/or other regulatory substances/peptides. The endocrine and paracrine cells have wide bases that contain secretory granules (storage forms of hormones and paracrine substances). This design allows cells to spread their secretions in a much wider area.

In addition to the previously mentioned control systems, the GI tract contains the highest number of immune cells and immune mediators in the body. Those cells and mediators interact with the intrinsic control system of the gut, both nerves and endocrine cells, to regulate some functions of the GI tract, including motility and secretion. However, because of their unique nature, the immune cells will not be discussed as part of the intrinsic control system, although they are located in the GI tract. Instead, they will be discussed at the end of this section.

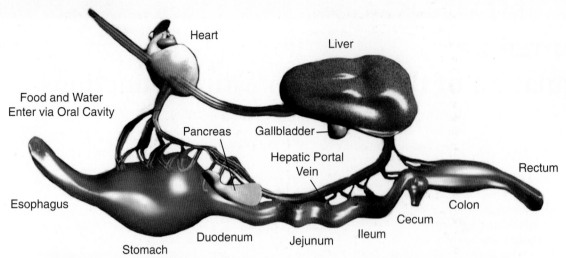

FIGURE 27-1 The digestive system consists of two parts: the GI tract, which consists of esophagus; stomach; small (duodenum, jejunum, and ileum) and large intestine (cecum, colon, and rectum); and the accessory digestive glands, which include the liver and pancreas.

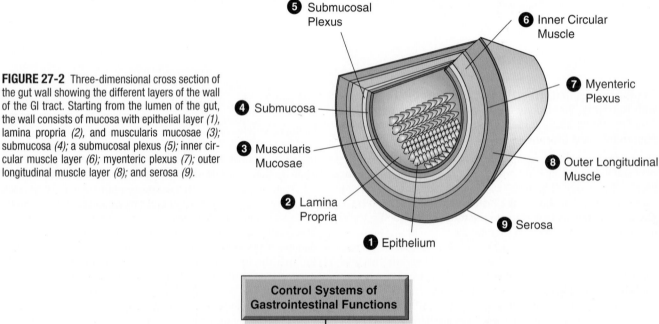

FIGURE 27-2 Three-dimensional cross section of the gut wall showing the different layers of the wall of the GI tract. Starting from the lumen of the gut, the wall consists of mucosa with epithelial layer *(1),* lamina propria *(2),* and muscularis mucosae *(3);* submucosa *(4);* a submucosal plexus *(5);* inner circular muscle layer *(6);* myenteric plexus *(7);* outer longitudinal muscle layer *(8);* and serosa *(9).*

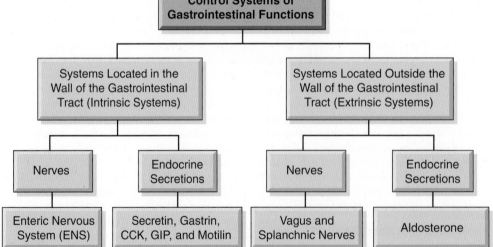

FIGURE 27-3 A diagram summarizing the various systems that control the different functions of the GI tract: intrinsic and extrinsic control systems. Each system contains nerves and endocrine secretions. *CCK,* Cholecystokinin; *GIP,* gastric inhibitory peptide (or glucose-dependent insulotropic peptide).

BOX 27-1 The Regulatory Molecules of the Various Gastrointestinal Functions

Hormones
Aldosterone
Cholecystokinin
Secretin
Gastric inhibitory polypeptide or glucose-dependent insulinotropic peptide
Gastrin
Motilin

Hormone Candidates
Enteroglucagon
Pancreatic Polypeptide
Peptide YY

Neurocrines
Adenosine triphosphate (ATP)
Calcitonin gene-related peptide (CGRP)

Enkephalins
Galanin
Gastrin releasing peptide (GRP)
Neuropeptide Y (NPY)
Neurotensin (NT)
Nitric oxide
Peptide histidine isoleucine (PHI)
Pituitary adenylate cyclase–activating peptide (PACAP)
Secretin or 5-Hydroxytryptamine (5-HT)
Substance K
Substance P (Sub P)
Vasoactive intestinal peptide (VIP)

Paracrines
Histamine
Somatostatin

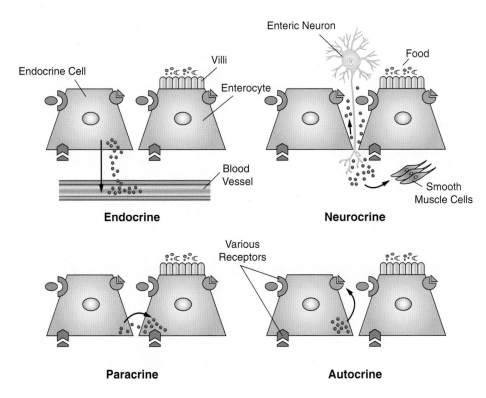

FIGURE 27-4 The four different routes by which endocrine or paracrine secretions of the gut reach their target tissue. Endocrine secretions reach the target tissue by the blood. Paracrine secretions reach the target tissue by diffusion through the interstitial space, whereas autocrine secretions of the paracrine cell modify the function of the same cell. The enteric neurons secrete contents via vesicles located on axon branches of these neurons, namely, from varicosities.

The Intrinsic Neuronal Control System of the Gastrointestinal Tract Is the Enteric Nervous System

The enteric nervous system (ENS) is a component of the autonomic nervous system (ANS). The other two ANS components are the sympathetic and parasympathetic systems. The ENS controls the majority of the GI functions *independent* from the central nervous system (CNS).

Anatomically, the ENS consists of two main ganglionated plexuses, termed the *submucosal (Meissner)* and *myenteric (Auerbach)* plexuses. The submucosal plexus is located under the submucosal layer of the gut, and the myenteric plexus resides between the inner circular muscle layer and the outer longitudinal muscle layer (Figure 27-6). The enteric plexuses communicate with each other through *interneurons* and with the CNS through vagal, pelvic, and splanchnic nerves.

In general, the enteric neurons consist of sensory *(afferent)* neurons, interneurons, and motor *(efferent)* neurons. Sensory input comes from mechanoreceptors within the muscular layers and chemoreceptors within the mucosa. Mechanoreceptors monitor distention of the gut wall, whereas chemoreceptors in

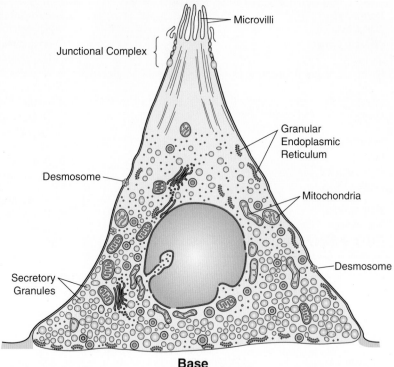

FIGURE 27-5 The endocrine cell of the gut is columnar in shape with a narrow apex (to allow sensing of the luminal contents of the gut), and a wide base (to allow a large area for spreading the secretions).

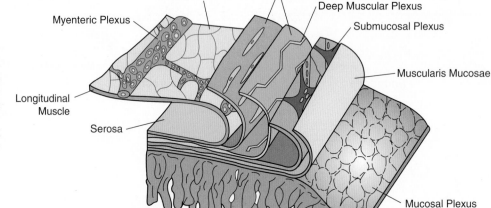

FIGURE 27-6 The ENS, the major controller of gut functions, consists of two main ganglionated plexuses: the submucosal, which is located under the submucosal layer, and the myenteric, which resides between the inner thick circular muscle layer and the outer thin longitudinal muscle layer of the gut wall.

the mucosa monitor chemical conditions in the gut lumen. Enteric motor nerves supply vascular muscle, gut muscle, and glands within the gut wall. Efferent neurons of the ENS may be stimulatory or inhibitory. The nature of their action is largely determined by the type of neurocrine substance they secrete and the nature of the receptors activated (Table 27-1).

Unlike classical neurons, the enteric neurons release their neurotransmitter/neuromodulator molecules from vesicles located in swellings along often extensive branches of the axon, not just at the level of the distal synaptic terminals. These swellings are referred to as *varicosities* (Figure 27-7). The varicosities contain regulatory peptides, substances collectively known as

neurocrines. These substances are secreted in response to action potentials, and they affect the activities of nearby smooth muscles or glandular cells. The presence of varicosities in the enteric neurons allows these neurons to activate a wider area in the vicinity of the axon compared with most other types of neurons, which release their neurotransmitters in a more focused and localized area at the distal synaptic terminal.

Depending on the species, the number of enteric neurons may reach 100 million. This number, in some cases, is more than the number of neurons in the spinal cord. To simplify the study of these neurons and to understand their physiological importance, four main classification methods have been used. These methods

TABLE 27-1 Gastrointestinal Hormones

Hormone	Production Site	Action	Release Stimulus
Secretin	Duodenum and upper jejunum	Stimulates bicarbonate secretion and inhibits acid secretion (nature's anti-acid)	Acid, fat, and protein
Gastrin	Stomach and duodenum	Stimulates acid secretion and growth of stomach epithelium (marker for cancer)	Protein, increased high gastric acidity
Cholecystokinin	Duodenum, jejunum, and ileum	Stimulates pancreatic enzyme secretion and gallbladder contractions; inhibits food intake and gastric emptying	Fats and proteins
Gastric inhibitory polypeptide	Duodenum and jejunum	Inhibits gastric secretions and stimulates insulin secretion	Fat and glucose
Motilin	Duodenum and jejunum	Induction of phase III of the MMC during fasting (digestive state)	Acetylcholine

MMC, Migrating motor complex.

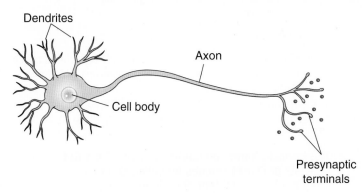

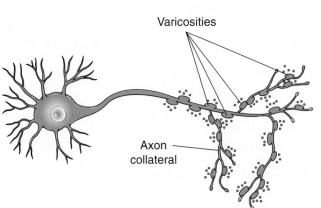

FIGURE 27-7 Unlike a typical neuron *(beige)* that releases neurotransmitters or neuromodulators from the synaptic terminal, enteric neurons *(green)* secrete their neurotransmitters/neuromodulators from varicosities or bulge-like structures located on often lengthy axonal collaterals or branches of these neurons. Although the effect of the classical neuron is focused to a certain area, the effect of the enteric neuron is spread to affect a wide area.

depend on the *morphology* (different shapes) of enteric neurons, the types of neurotransmitters or peptides they may contain (also known as their *chemical coding*), the electrical properties of the enteric neurons or *electrophysiology,* and the *function* (e.g., sensory, motor, inhibitory, and excitatory) of the enteric neurons.

On the basis of their morphology, three main types of enteric neurons exist: *Dogiel type I, II,* and *III* (Figure 27-8). These classifications are named for Alexander Dogiel, the histologist who initially described them. Dogiel type I neurons have small, irregular cell bodies with multiple short dendrites. Dogiel type II neurons have large, oval-shaped cell bodies with one or two long dendrites. Dogiel type III neurons have large cell bodies with different shapes and multiple dendrites.

Electrophysiologically, there are two types of enteric neurons. In the first, a fast (e.g., millisecond) action potential is evoked; these are referred to as *S-type* (S for synaptic) neurons. The second type of enteric neuron has a longer lasting action potential (e.g., seconds) compared with the S-type. Such neurons are referred to as *AH neurons* (AH for the long after hyperpolarization phase).

The enteric neurons contain many peptides and neurotransmitters, which can be detected by various immunohistochemical methods. The enteric neurons can be classified on the basis of these chemical contents. For example, some enteric neurons contain the neurotransmitter acetylcholine. Such neurons are called *cholinergic neurons* and are generally stimulatory to gut activities. Other enteric neurons contain adrenaline (also known as *epinephrine*). These neurons are called *adrenergic neurons* and are generally inhibitory to gut activities.

Finally, the enteric neurons can be classified on the basis of their function: excitatory, inhibitory, sensory, or motor. *Excitatory* neurons cause an increase in secretion if they innervate a

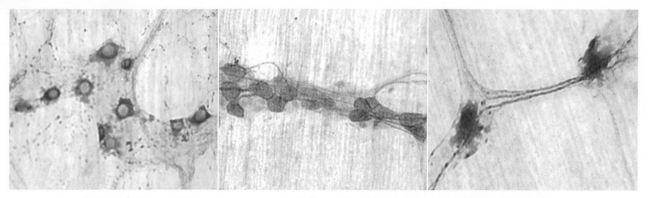

Dogiel type I   Dogiel type II   Dogiel type III

FIGURE 27-8 On the basis of their shape (morphology), the enteric neurons are classified into three types: Dogiel type I, Dogiel type II, Dogiel type III. Dogiel type I neurons have a small cell body with short dendrites and have a motor function. Dogiel type II neurons have large cell bodies with one or two long dendrites, and have a sensory function. Dogiel type III neurons have multiple shapes and functions.

BOX 27-2 Relationship of Enteric Neuron Function to Electrophysiology, Morphology, and Chemical Coding

Function
Motor
S-type
Dogiel type I

Sensory
AH-type
Dogiel type II

Excitatory
Acetylcholine (Ach)
Substance P (Sub P)

Inhibitory
Nitric oxide (NO)
Vasoactive intestinal peptide (VIP)

---

gland or cause muscle contraction if they innervate a muscle. *Inhibitory* neurons cause a decrease in secretion or muscle relaxation. *Sensory* neurons detect luminal pH and pressure or temperature in the gut wall. *Motor* neurons innervate muscles and sphincters and cause contraction or relaxation.

In general, Dogiel type I neurons and S-type enteric neurons are considered motor neurons, whereas Dogiel type II and AH neurons are considered sensory neurons (Box 27-2). The *excitatory enteric neurons* of the gut contain acetylcholine (Ach) and/or substance P (sub P), whereas the *inhibitory enteric neurons* of the gut contain vasoactive intestinal peptide (VIP) and/or nitric oxide (NO). The inhibitory enteric neurons of the gut are also referred to as *guards* (organizers or regulators). These neurons are required to control spurious excitation or contraction if either of these processes occurs.

In addition to the three neuronal components of the ENS, myenteric, and submucosal plexuses and interneurons, there is a special type of cell in the gut that is referred to as the *interstitial cell of Cajal* (ICC; see Figure 28-1). The multiple arms or projections of these specialized smooth muscle cells contact both adjacent smooth muscle cells and enteric neurons. This interaction, in addition to the pacemaker-like activity of the ICCs, plays a critical role in gut muscle contraction and motility. The role of the ICCs in GI motility is discussed in more detail in the next chapter.

The Intrinsic Hormonal Control System of the Gut Consists of Five Hormones Including Secretin, Gastrin, Cholecystokinin, Gastric Inhibitory Polypeptide, and Motilin

The GI endocrine system consists of specialized cells that are dispersed among the other epithelial cells lining the gut. The GI tract contains millions of epithelial cells, which are referred to as *enterocytes, enterochromaffin cells,* and *endocrine cells.* The enterocytes have an absorptive function, whereas the enterochromaffin cells are secretory in nature. They were named originally for their staining characteristics in histological preparations. We now know these enterochromaffin cells secrete *peptides* or *hormones* that help regulate gut motility, food digestion, and nutrient absorption. For example, one type of enterochromaffin cell secretes *serotonin,* a regulatory molecule that affects gut motility; another secretes *cholecystokinin* (CCK), which causes gallbladder contraction among other things. These endocrine cells of the gut are all similar morphologically, but each secretes only one type of hormone or regulatory molecule. They are typically distinguished by a capital letter name, such as *I cells* for CCK production and *G cells* for gastrin production.

As we have seen from the discussion of endocrine, neurocrine, paracrine, and autocrine actions in the gut, there is a large variety of molecules that influence the activities of various gut functions; most of these molecules are peptides. For a gut peptide to be called a hormone it must fulfill certain criteria. These criteria consist of five characteristics. First, the gut hormone must be secreted by one cell in the gut and must affect another cell. Second, the vehicle that transports gut hormones from the secreting cell to the target cell must be the blood (endocrine route). Third, the release of gut hormones must be stimulated by food. Fourth, it is not necessary for gut hormones to be secreted under neuronal control. Fifth, a synthetic form of the hormone (e.g., as synthesized by a drug company), must be capable of mimicking the actions of the natural hormone.

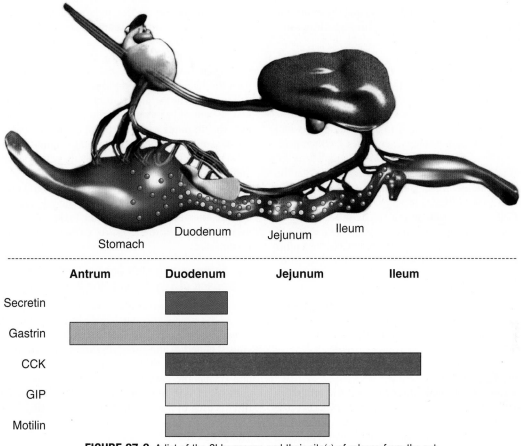

Stomach   **Duodenum**   **Jejunum**   **Ileum**

	Antrum	Duodenum	Jejunum	Ileum
Secretin				
Gastrin				
CCK				
GIP				
Motilin				

FIGURE 27-9 A list of the GI hormones and their site(s) of release from the gut.

If a gut peptide fulfills these criteria, it is termed a *gut hormone;* otherwise, it retains reference as a gut peptide. Therefore, all gut hormones are also considered gut peptides, whereas not all gut peptides are gut hormones. The gut peptides that fulfill the previous criteria are *secretin, gastrin, CCK, gastric inhibitory polypeptide* (also known as *glucose-dependent insulinotropic peptide* [GIP]), and *motilin.* The following section discusses each of the hormones individually in more detail. A list of these hormones, their secretion sites, and their most important functions are summarized in Table 27-1 and Figure 27-9. In addition, there are candidate hormones that do not completely fulfill the previous criteria. These candidate hormones are pancreatic polypeptide, peptide YY, and enteroglucagon (one family member being glucagon-like peptide-1 [GLP-1]).

Secretin

In 1902, Bayliss and Starling discovered secretin, the first gut peptide hormone to be identified. Secretin is secreted by the S-cells of the duodenum and upper jejunum in response to fat, protein, gastric acid, bile acids, and herbal extracts. Functionally, secretin stimulates exocrine pancreatic and biliary secretions of water, bicarbonate, gastric mucus, and pepsinogen; endocrine pancreatic secretions of insulin, glucagon, and somatostatin; and pancreatic growth. In addition, secretin inhibits gastric acid secretion (functioning as a sort of *nature's anti-acid*), as well as motility of the intestine and gastric mucosal growth. The regulation of secretin functions is controlled by the action of hormones such as CCK or by hormonal-neuronal interaction, such as CCK

and the vagus nerve. Pathologically, hypersecretinemia can be found in cases of duodenal ulcer, renal failure, chronic pancreatitis, and esophageal small cell carcinoma.

Gastrin

Gastrin (G) was discovered in 1905 by John Sidney Adkins as a hormone that is secreted by the G cells of the gastric pylorus, antrum, and duodenum. Gastrin is secreted in response to the presence of protein and gastric distention. Its major action is to increase gastric acid secretion. Depending on the number of amino acids in the peptide chain, gastrin has two different forms, G-17 (also known as *little gastrin*) and G-34 (also known as *big gastrin*). These forms are equipotent. The gastric antrum produces G-17 in response to food (90% of gastrin production in the gut is G-17), whereas the duodenum produces G-34 between meals. If the sixth tyrosine residue from the C-terminus is sulfated, then gastrin is called *Gastrin II.* However, if this residue is not sulfated, then the peptide is called *Gastrin I.*

Gastrin I and II bind to the cholecystokinin-2 (CCK_2) receptor (also called the *CCK-B receptor*), a G-protein–coupled receptor (see Chapter 1), with an affinity similar to CCK. This binding results in stimulation of gastric acid secretion and hyperplasia of the enterochromaffin-like (ECL) cells, a type of endocrine cell of the gastric mucosa. Increased plasma levels of gastrin, independent of food or increased gastric acidity, can be used as a diagnostic tool for cases of pernicious anemia or gastrinoma (a tumor that secretes gastrin). In addition, gastrin increases acid secretion indirectly by stimulation of histamine release from the ECL, which can activate histamine-2 (H_2) receptors on acid-secreting gastric parietal cells. Therefore, one of the ways that the inhibition of gastric acid secretion can be affected is through drugs that block the H_2 receptor, such as cimetidine.

Cholecystokinin

In 1928, Ivy and Oldberg discovered cholecystokinin (CCK), which is a hormone that is secreted by the endocrine I cells and the enteric neurons of the duodenum and jejunum in response to fat and protein. Its major action is to stimulate gallbladder emptying and the secretion of pancreatic enzymes. CCK controls many GI functions by activating two G-protein–coupled receptors: CCK_1, formerly known as *CCK-A* (alimentary) receptor, which is distributed mainly in the alimentary tract, and CCK_2, formerly known as *CCK-B* (brain) receptor, which is distributed mainly in the CNS. Sulfation (adding a sulfate group) of CCK affects the binding of the peptide to its receptors. Sulfated CCK has a 100 to 1000 times greater binding affinity to CCK_1 receptors than the non-sulfated form of CCK or gastrin. Sulfated CCK, non-sulfated CCK, and gastrin bind to CCK_2 receptors with equal affinity.

Physiologically, CCK controls many GI-related functions. For example, CCK causes gallbladder and smooth muscle contraction while increasing pancreatic secretion, and it inhibits gastric emptying and food intake.

Gastric Inhibitory Polypeptide

In 1969, Brown and his colleagues discovered gastric inhibitory polypeptide (GIP). GIP is referred to as an *enterogastrone* because of its ability to reduce the rate of stomach emptying. Enterogastrone is a collective term that refers to any hormone or regulatory substance that slows the movement of ingesta, particularly from the stomach to intestine. The name *glucose-dependent insulinotropic peptide* is also given to GIP because its secretion is stimulated by the presence of glucose in the duodenum and one of its actions is to stimulate the secretion of insulin from the endocrine pancreas. This hormone is secreted by the K cells of the proximal small intestine in response to fat and glucose. Functionally, GIP inhibits gastric acid secretion and stimulates insulin secretion.

Motilin

In 1973, Brown and colleagues discovered motilin. This peptide is secreted by the M (or Mo) cells of the duodenum and, to a lesser extent, by the jejunum. Motilin works on both muscles and nerves to regulate the *migrating motor complex* (MMC), the basic pattern of intestinal motility present during the period between meals that is interrupted by feeding. The MMC is discussed further in Chapter 28. In addition, motilin stimulates gastric emptying during the between-meal period and secretion of pepsinogen, a protein-digesting enzyme of the stomach. Clinically, drugs that mimic the actions of motilin are used to treat gut motility disorders (hypokinetic disorders), including delayed gastric emptying.

The Immune System of the Gut Is Extensive and Interacts with the Gastrointestinal Regulatory Systems to Control the Various Functions of the Gut

The mucosa of the gut is exposed to numerous microorganisms and antigens (e.g., contaminated food or toxins). Such harmful agents require a local defense system (immune system) to control their numbers and to limit their access to the body. The majority of the immune cells in the body reside in the gut mucosa. These immune cells defend the GI milieu in two ways. First, the immune cells of the gut respond to antigenic stimulation similar to any other immune cells in the body including the creation of antigenic memory, neutralization, and the synthesis of antibodies and recruitment of killer cells. Second, the immune cells of the gut respond by secreting inflammatory mediators such as prostaglandins, histamine, and cytokines, which interact directly with the ENS and GI endocrine and paracrine cells. This interaction results in the modulation of gut functions such as motility and secretion. For example, when bad food or toxins enter the gut, the immune cells become sensitized and start secreting prostaglandins, cytokines, and other immune mediators. These substances will then interact directly with the ENS, endocrine, and paracrine systems of the gut to evoke responses such as increased fluid secretion, dilution of toxin, and increased motility in order to move the harmful material quickly through the system. Therefore, the microbe or toxin will be washed and will eventually pass in the feces. As a result of these actions, the gut is protected.

The Extrinsic Neuronal Control System of the Gut Is Comprised of Two Nerves: the Vagus and the Splanchnic

In addition to the intrinsic control system of the GI tract, two extrinsic systems also participate in the regulation of gut functions. Similar to the intrinsic systems, the extrinsic systems also consist of nerves and endocrine secretions. The extrinsic innervations that control the functions of the GI tract consist of vagus and splanchnic nerves, whereas the extrinsic hormonal system consists of one hormone, aldosterone. The following sections discuss each of these systems in more detail.

The Vagus Nerve

Anatomically, the vagus nerve has two components: parasympathetic efferents (nerve fibers that send orders from the brain to the gut) and vagal afferents (nerve fibers that send information from the gut to the brain). Functionally, the vagus nerve consists of two general types of nerve fibers, *afferents* (sensory), which carry the signal from the organs to the CNS, and *efferents* (motor), which carry orders from the CNS to the organs. Specific vagal fiber types most relevant to the GI tract are: (1) *general visceral afferents* (GVA), which innervate the abdominal viscera, including the GI tract, as well as the pharyngeal mucosa; (2) *special visceral afferents* (SVA), which carry signals from taste buds of the oral cavity; and (3) *general* and *special visceral efferents* (GVE and SVE) projecting from the CNS to parasympathetic ganglia near organs and to the pharynx, respectively.

The cell bodies of the GVA and SVA are located in the inferior vagal ganglion (nodose ganglion), and the cell bodies of the GVE and SVE are located in the dorsal motor nucleus of the vagus (DMV) and nucleus ambiguus, respectively. The DMV is located in the dorsal vagal complex of the hindbrain, along with the nucleus of the solitary tract (Figure 27-10). The nucleus of the solitary tract receives vagal GVA input from the GI tract and vagal SVA input from oral cavity taste buds.

The vagus nerve innervates the GI tract via two main branches: the left and right vagi (Figure 27-11). The left vagus branches into celiac and left gastric nerves, whereas the right vagus branches into hepatic, right gastric, and accessory celiac nerves. Vagotomy of some of these branches can be used as an optional treatment for gastric/peptic ulcers.

Furthermore, the vagus nerve communicates with the ENS of the gut, which also communicates with the dorsal vagal complex of the CNS, through *vagal afferents*. These GVAs are *intravillus*

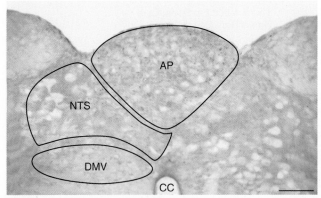

FIGURE 27-10 A photomicrograph depicting the various areas of the dorsal vagal complex (DVC) of the hindbrain, which controls various GI functions. These areas include the *nucleus tractus solitarius* (NTS, synaptic target of gut general and special visceral afferents, or sensory portion of the vagus nerve), dorsal motor nucleus of the vagus (DMV, the location of cell bodies for the gut general visceral efferent, or motor portion of the vagus nerve), and area postrema (AP, emitting center). The dorsal portion of a transverse section of the caudal medulla is depicted with the central canal (CC) representing the midline.

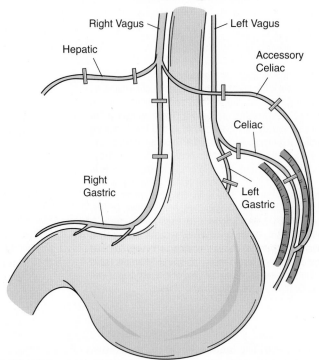

Selective Vagotomies

FIGURE 27-11 A schematic showing the location of both vagi along the esophagus and their branches. The right vagus provides hepatic, right gastric, and accessory celiac branches; and the left vagus provides a celiac and left gastric branch. The *thin rectangles* along the branches represent potential locations for vagotomy in the treatment of gastric/peptic ulcers.

arbors (IVA), *interganglionic laminar endings* (IGLE), and *intramuscular arrays* (IMA) (Figure 27-12). The IVAs reach the villi of the gut mucosa and function as chemoreceptors, providing information to the CNS about the chemical condition of the gut lumen. The IMAs and IGLEs act as mechanoreceptors, and stretch or tension receptors, which provide the CNS with information

about the physical situation in the gut. The vagal GVEs that communicate with the gut ENS are parasympathetic preganglionic neurons that synapse on neurons of the submucosal or myenteric plexuses. In general, this parasympathetic efferent control is stimulatory (i.e., they increase gut blood flow, motility, and glandular secretions).

The Splanchnic Nerve

The splanchnic nerve supplies the GI tract with both *sympathetic efferent* and *spinal afferent* innervations. The sympathetic preganglionic neuronal cell bodies are located in the thoraco-lumbar region of the spinal cord, and the cell bodies of afferents to the spinal cord lie in the dorsal root ganglia (see Figure 27-12). Postganglionic sympathetic cell bodies reside in the celiaco-mesenteric ganglia (CMG), and synapse at the target organ. The CMG, solar in shape, consist of two major ganglia, celiac and cranial (superior) mesenteric, as well as smaller ganglia with no specific names. These ganglia reside between the celiac and cranial mesenteric arteries, representing branches of the aorta. In general, the sympathetic neurocrine secretions are inhibitory in nature.

Splanchnic nerves, carrying visceral and spinal afferents, are distributed in the mucosa, muscularis, serosa, and mesentery of the gut. They carry signals to the CNS regarding the presence of pathological conditions in the gut. Such signals include the distention of the gut wall, inflammation, or the presence of noxious chemicals or substances in the lumen of the gut with associated colic or abdominal pain. These painful stimuli evoke sympathetic responses in the GI tract, including the inhibition of gut motility and increased glandular secretions.

The Extrinsic Hormonal Control System of the Gut Is Limited to One Hormone: Aldosterone

Only one known hormone is secreted outside the GI tract but still participates in controlling some of the functions of the GI tract: *aldosterone.*

Aldosterone

In 1953, Simon and Tait isolated aldosterone. This hormone is a steroid hormone (mineralocorticoid) that is secreted by the outer zona glomerulosa section of the adrenal cortex following stimulation by a low-salt (low sodium) diet, angiotensin, adrenocorticotropic hormone, or high potassium levels. The main function of aldosterone is to act on the distal convoluted tubules and collecting ducts of the kidney causing secretion of potassium and reabsorption of sodium and water, with attending increase in blood pressure.

In the GI tract, aldosterone stimulates sodium and water reabsorption from the gut and salivary glands in exchange with potassium ions. In addition, although it is species-dependent, aldosterone promotes increased absorption of water and sodium in the proximal colon and decreased absorption in the distal colon.

This chapter has focused on the neural and secretory sources of control that regulate the functions of the GI tract. In subsequent chapters, these control mechanisms will be discussed with respect to their integrated actions in the control of the digestive system.

Acknowledgment

The authors thank Dr. Deidra Quinn Gorham and Dr. Carol S. Williams from the College of Veterinary Medicine, Tuskegee University for assistance with drawing the pictures in Figures 27-1,

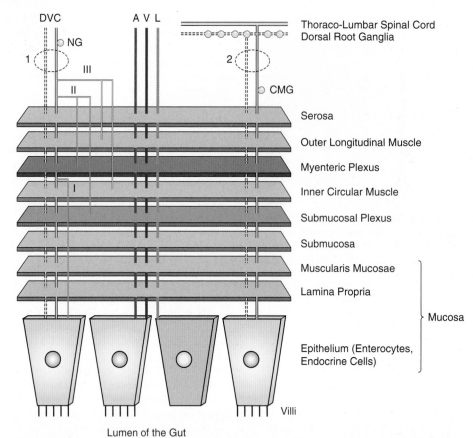

FIGURE 27-12 A schematic showing the layers of the gut and the locations of the innervations that regulate the various functions of the gut. Starting from the lumen of the GI tract, the layers of the gut are mucosa (consists of enterocytes, lamina propria, and muscularis mucosae); submucosa (SM); muscularis, which consists of two muscle layers, inner circular muscle (CM) and outer longitudinal muscle (LM); and serosa. The functions of the gut are regulated by two neuronal control systems. The intrinsic system, also referred to as the ENS, consists of two plexuses: submucosal plexus (SP) resides under the SM, and myenteric plexus (MP) resides between the CM and LM. The extrinsic system consists of the vagus nerve *(1)* and the splanchnic nerve *(2)*. Each of these nerves consists of two components (*dashed circles* around them): afferent and efferent. The vagal afferents (*solid yellow line* in *1,* with cell bodies in the nodose ganglia [NG]) consists of three types: intravillus arbors (IVA = I), interganglionic laminar endings (IGLE = II), and intramuscular arrays (IMA = III). They communicate the signals generated by the intestinal contents or regulatory peptides (e.g., stretch, movement, temperature, acidity, or chemical content) with the dorsal vagal complex *(DVC)* in the CNS. Spinal afferents (*dashed yellow line* in *2,* with cell bodies in the dorsal root ganglia along the thoraco-lumbar area of the spinal cord) synapse in the spinal cord gray matter. The orders of the brain to the gut are carried by the vagal parasympathetic efferents (*dashed yellow line* in *1,* with cell bodies in the dorsal motor nucleus of the vagus) and the sympathetic efferents (*solid yellow line* in *2,* with presynaptic cell bodies in the thoraco-lumbar area of the spinal cord and postsynaptic cell bodies in the celiaco-mesenteric ganglia *(CMG)*. A, Artery; L, lacteal or lymphatic vessel; V, vein.

and 27-9, and editorial corrections, respectively. Some of the information presented in this chapter was collected with support from the National Institutes of Health (NIH 1SC1GM092285-01A1) and The Birmingham Racing Commission.

PRACTICE QUESTIONS

1. The functions of the GI tract are *mainly* controlled by:
   a. The central nervous system.
   b. The enteric nervous system.
   c. The endocrine system.
   d. The enterochromaffin system.
   e. The hormonal and central nervous systems.

2. The extrinsic innervation of the gut consists of:
   a. The enteric nervous system.
   b. The myenteric and submucosal plexuses.
   c. Sympathetic (splanchnic) and parasympathetic (vagus) nerves.
   d. Sympathetic (vagus) and parasympathetic (splanchnic) nerves.
   e. The pelvic nerve.

3. The AH neurons of the enteric nervous system are:
   a. Dogiel type I with a sensory function.
   b. Dogiel type I with a motor function.
   c. Dogiel type II with a sensory function.
   d. Dogiel type II with a motor function.
   e. Dogiel type III with multiple functions.

4. Which one of the following is one of the criteria for a gut peptide to be called a gut hormone:
   a. It must be released by the gut and affect the gut.
   b. It must be secreted under a neuronal control.
   c. It must be secreted by the Q cells.
   d. It must travel through nerves.
   e. It must cause a pathological effect.

5. One of the following answers contains a non-hormone:
   a. CCK, GIP, and secretin
   b. CCK, motilin, and secretin
   c. CCK, gastrin, and secretin
   d. CCK, gastrin, and GRP
   e. CCK, gastrin, and motilin

6. Only one of the following statements is correct:
   a. Acetylcholine stimulates secretin.
   b. Fat stimulates gastrin.
   c. Carbohydrates stimulate CCK.
   d. Protein and glucose stimulate GIP.
   e. Protein stimulates motilin.

7. Only one of these statements is correct:
   a. The stomach and colon secrete most gut hormones.
   b. The duodenum secretes most gut hormones.
   c. The jejunum secretes most gut hormones.
   d. The ileum secretes most gut hormones.
   e. The colon secretes most gut hormones.

8. Cholecystokinin and gastrin:
   a. Share all of the same receptors.
   b. Share CCK_1 receptors.
   c. Share CCK_2 receptors.
   d. Share gastrin I receptors.
   e. Share gastrin II receptors.

9. The neurotransmitters in the gut are:
   a. NO and Ach as excitatory, and substance P and VIP as inhibitory.
   b. NO and Ach as inhibitory, and VIP and substance P as inhibitory.
   c. NO and VIP as excitatory, and Ach and substance P as inhibitory.
   d. NO and VIP as inhibitory, and Ach and substance P as excitatory.
   e. NO and substance P as inhibitory, and Ach and VIP as excitatory.

BIBLIOGRAPHY

Furness JB: The enteric nervous system: normal functions and enteric neuropathies, *Neurogastroenterol Motil* 20(Suppl 1):32–38, 2008.

Johnson LR: Regulation: peptides of the gastrointestinal tract. In Johnson LR, editor: *Gastrointestinal physiology*, ed 6, St Louis, 2001, Mosby.

Sayegh AI, Reeve JR Jr, Lampley ST, et al: Role for the enteric nervous system in the regulation of satiety via cholecystokinin-8, *J Am Vet Med Assoc* 226(11):1809–1816, 2005.

Sayegh AI, Ritter RC: Morphology and distribution of nitric oxide synthase-, neurokinin-1 receptor-, calretinin-, calbindin-, and neurofilament-M-immunoreactive neurons in the myenteric and submucosal plexuses of the rat small intestine, *Anat Rec A Discov Mol Cell Evol Biol* 271(1):209–216, 2003.

Wood JD: Enteric nervous system: reflexes, pattern generators and motility, *Curr Opin Gastroenterol* 24(2):149–158, 2008.

CHAPTER 28
Motility Patterns of the Gastrointestinal Tract

KEY POINTS

1. Slow waves of electrical depolarization are a unique feature of gut smooth muscle.
2. When slow waves reach sensitized smooth muscle cells, action potentials and contraction result.
3. Coordinated motility enables the lips, tongue, mouth, and pharynx to grasp food and propel it down the gastrointestinal tract.
4. Motility of the esophagus propels food from the pharynx to the stomach.
5. The function of the stomach is to process food into a fluid consistency and release it into the intestine at a controlled rate.
6. The proximal stomach stores food awaiting further gastric processing in the distal stomach.
7. The distal stomach grinds and sifts food entering the small intestine.
8. Control of gastric motility differs in the proximal and distal stomach.
9. The rate of gastric emptying must match the small intestine's rate of digestion and absorption.
10. Between meals, the stomach is cleared of indigestible material.
11. Vomiting is a complex reflex coordinated from the brainstem.
12. Motility of the small intestine has digestive and interdigestive phases.
13. The ileocecal sphincter prevents movement of colon contents back into the ileum.
14. Motility of the colon causes mixing, retropulsion, and propulsion of ingesta.
15. The colon is an important site of storage and absorption in all animals.
16. Despite large anatomical differences in the colons of herbivores compared to omnivores and carnivores, there are similarities in motility.
17. The anal sphincter has two layers with separate innervation.
18. The rectosphincteric reflex is important in defecation.
19. Major differences between avian and mammalian digestive systems include, in birds, both the lack of teeth and the separation of gastric functions into distinct anatomical regions.

The walls of the gastrointestinal (GI) tract, at all levels, are muscular and capable of movement. Movements of the GI muscles have direct actions on ingesta in the gut lumen. GI movements have several functions: (1) to propel ingesta from one location to the next; (2) to retain ingesta at a given site for digestion, absorption, or storage; (3) to break up food material physically and mix it with digestive secretions; and (4) to circulate ingesta so that all portions come into contact with absorptive surfaces.

The dynamics of fluid movement in the gut are not as well understood as in other organ systems, particularly the cardiovascular system. The heart and great vessels behave in a manner similar to that of most mechanical pumping systems: a central pump pushes fluid through a conduit of relatively fixed diameter. Because of this configuration, the cardiovascular system more or less conforms to physical laws that are well established and studied reasonably easily; sophisticated quantitative analyses of cardiovascular function can be made clinically. In contrast to the situation in the heart, the fluid pump and the conduit are the same organ in the gut. This makes study of the fluid dynamics of the gut extremely complex. At this time, the mathematically defined physical laws of fluid dynamics, as applied to the gut, are of little clinical usefulness. Therefore the physiology of GI motility is usually applied clinically on a qualitative, rather than a quantitative, basis.

Movement of the gut wall is referred to as *motility*, and motility may be of a propulsive, retentive, or mixing nature. The time it takes material to travel from one portion of the gut to another is referred to as the *transit time*. An increase in propulsive motility decreases the transit time, whereas an increase in retentive motility increases the transit time. Selectively increasing retentive motility and reducing propulsive motility are important aspects of diarrhea therapy.

Slow Waves of Electrical Depolarization Are a Unique Feature of Gut Smooth Muscle

The first level of control of GI motility lies in the intrinsic electrical properties of the smooth muscle mass. These electrical properties consist of spontaneously undulating waves of partial depolarization that sweep over the gut smooth muscle. The origin of this electrical activity is from specialized smooth muscle cells referred to as the *interstitial cells of Cajal* (ICC). The ICC form an interconnecting lattice of cells that surrounds the circular and longitudinal layers of muscle over the entire length of the gut. These cells are very similar in structure and function to the Purkinje cells of the heart. The ICC exhibit rhythmical and spontaneous oscillation in their transmembrane electrical potentials, as illustrated in Figure 28-1. They are connected to one another and to cells of the general smooth muscle mass by *tight junctions* or *nexuses*. These connections allow for the flow of ions from cell to cell. The resulting ionic movements lead to the propagation of waves of partial cell membrane depolarization across large numbers of cells. Within the ICC, fluctuations in intracellular calcium concentrations appear responsible for the spontaneous

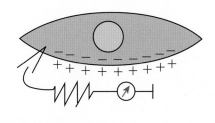

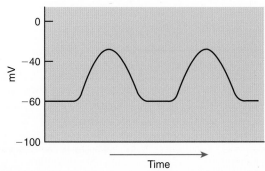

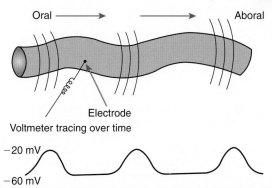

FIGURE 28-2 Partial membrane depolarizations of GI smooth muscle cells occur in a coordinated manner, creating waves of depolarization that sweep over large segments of muscle. Electrodes placed on or near the surface of the muscle record changes in potential as waves of depolarization pass toward or away from them. Coordinated changes in membrane potential among cells are necessary for these waves to be measured because random changes among cells would cancel each other out, and no changes would be recorded by electrodes placed extracellularly.

FIGURE 28-1 Spontaneous changes in membrane polarity of the interstitial cells of Cajal, specialized gastrointestinal (GI) smooth muscle cells that are responsible for spontaneous electrical rhythmicity in gut muscle. The upper illustration represents a single cell with a voltmeter measuring the transmembrane electrical potential. The graph illustrates spontaneous changes in electrical potential (in millivolts, mV) that would be measured across the cell membrane.

changes in membrane polarization. Figure 28-1 illustrates the concept of a fluctuating membrane potential in a single ICC. The property of spontaneous electrical rhythmicity, in combination with their electrical connection to the smooth muscle mass, imparts to the ICC their role as electrical "pacemakers" of the gut.

In GI smooth muscle cells, the baseline membrane potential is usually –70 to –60 millivolts (mV). Under the influence of the ICC, the membrane potential fluctuates from this baseline level by as much as 20 to 30 mV. Thus, under resting conditions, the depolarization is only partial, and the membrane potential never reaches 0 mV. The smooth muscle cells are connected to the ICC and to each other by nexuses, allowing the changes in membrane potential to be spread, or *propagated,* over large areas of muscle. The ICC initiate these changes and thus determine their origin and direction of propagation. Under normal conditions in the small intestine, changes in membrane potential begin high in the duodenum and are propagated aborally (away from the mouth) along the length of the small intestine (Figure 28-2). These aborally moving waves of partial depolarization are called *slow waves* or the *basic electrical rhythm* of the gut. In the dog, slow waves occur about 20 times per minute in the small intestine. In the stomach and colon, slow waves occur less frequently, about five times per minute. However, the slow waves are present throughout the smooth muscle portions of the GI tract. The frequency of slow waves varies among domestic species, but their presence does not vary.

The slow waves are an intrinsic property of the GI smooth muscle and associated ICC. The presence of the slow waves depends only on the ICC, whereas the amplitude and, to a lesser extent, the frequency of the slow waves can be modulated by the ENS. The link between slow waves and muscle contractions, however, is under control of nervous, endocrine, and paracrine factors, as discussed next.

When Slow Waves Reach Sensitized Smooth Muscle Cells, Action Potentials and Contraction Result

Slow waves have an important relationship with muscle contractions, but they are not the direct stimuli for contractions. Slow waves are constantly passing over GI smooth muscle, whether it is actively contracting or not. GI smooth muscle cells, as with other muscle cells, contract in association with action, or spike, potentials. These potentials are characterized by complete depolarization of the membrane for a short time, in contrast to the slow waves, which are characterized by incomplete depolarization (see Chapter 4). Action potentials in the GI smooth muscle occur only in association with slow waves. Thus the presence of slow waves is necessary but not sufficient to cause muscle contractions. When slow waves pass over an area of smooth muscle without eliciting action potentials, no contractions occur. When slow waves pass over an area of smooth muscle and action potentials are superimposed on the slow waves, gut muscle contracts. Control and coordination of smooth muscle activity is achieved by influencing the likelihood that action potentials will be superimposed on slow waves. Such control is a function of peptides and regulatory substances produced by the ENS and enteric endocrine and paracrine cells.

Smooth muscle control and coordination are achieved by modulation of the baseline electrical potential in the smooth muscle cells. Peptides and other regulatory molecules from ENS neurons or endocrine/paracrine cells are released in the vicinity of the smooth muscle cells, affecting membrane ion channels and influencing the baseline membrane potential (see Chapter 27 for a discussion of gut peptides and other regulatory molecules). Excitatory molecules elevate the baseline (bring it closer to zero), and inhibitory molecules lower the baseline (make it more negative). The position of the baseline influences how close the overall potential will come to 0 mV at the crest of a slow wave. When the membrane potential of a smooth muscle comes close to zero, action potentials occur and muscle contracts (Figure 28-3). Regulatory molecules (neurocrines, paracrines, and hormones) that are excitatory elicit smooth muscle contraction by elevating the baseline, whereas inhibitory substances inhibit muscle contraction by lowering the baseline.

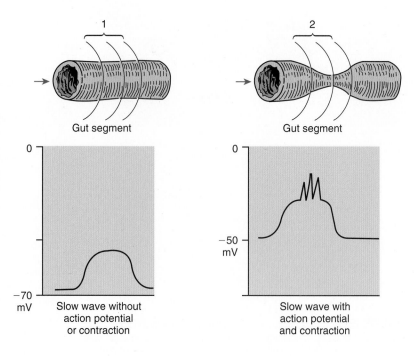

FIGURE 28-3 *1,* No muscle contraction occurs in the absence of action potentials. *2,* Muscle contracts when the crest of the slow waves reaches a critical point of depolarization, allowing action potentials to occur. The probability of action potentials occurring during the passage of a slow wave over a segment of gut muscle is influenced by the degree of baseline depolarization. Norepinephrine lowers the baseline (increases its absolute value), whereas acetylcholine raises the baseline (decreases its absolute value). *mV,* Millivolts.

The integrated actions of the slow waves, ENS, and endocrine/paracrine system appear to function to synchronize the contractions of the GI muscle mass. For the muscle to perform efficiently, all or many of the muscle cells in one layer of a segment of gut must be synchronized to contract simultaneously. This can best be visualized by considering the circular muscle layer. The contents of the circle cannot be "squeezed" effectively unless all the muscles of the circumference contract simultaneously; it would have little effect on luminal pressure if one portion of the circle contracted while another portion relaxed. In any discrete area of gut, slow waves pass simultaneously over the entire circumference of the smooth muscle. If that area has been sensitized by an excitatory regulatory molecule, the entire circumference of circular muscle will contract in synchrony.

Muscle contractions can occur at a frequency no higher than the frequency of the slow waves. As an example of frequency modulation, consider the activity of muscle in the stomach of the dog. Slow waves in the canine stomach occur about five times per minute. The crest of each slow wave may or may not be accompanied by action potentials. Therefore, during a given minute, the muscle in a localized area may not contract at all or may contract up to five times. If the passing slow waves generate no action potentials, the muscle does not contract at all. In a given minute, if action potentials are associated with one slow wave, the muscle contracts once. Action potentials on two slow waves result in two contractions, and so on, up to a maximum of five contractions per minute, but no more than five, because there are no more slow waves.

The motility patterns of the gut vary in their complexity, as described in the following sections. In the stomach and colon, motility patterns are relatively complex compared with the small intestine. In all cases, motility patterns are programmed into the ENS and coordinated in conjunction with the slow waves.

Coordinated Motility Enables the Lips, Tongue, Mouth, and Pharynx to Grasp Food and Propel It Down the Gastrointestinal Tract

Before digestion can begin, food must be directed into the GI tract. To ingest food, quadruped animals must first grasp it with the lips, teeth, or tongue. This involves highly coordinated activity of small, voluntary skeletal muscles. The muscles of the face, lips, and tongue appear to be among the most delicately controlled voluntary muscles of most domestic animals. The exact method of food *prehension* varies greatly among different species. For example, horses use their lips extensively, whereas cattle often use their tongues for grasping food. In all domestic animals, however, prehension is a highly coordinated process involving direct control by the central nervous system (CNS). Problems of prehension may develop because of abnormalities in the teeth, jaws, muscles of the tongue and face, cranial nerves, or CNS. The facial nerve, the glossopharyngeal nerve, and the motor branch of the trigeminal nerve control the muscles of prehension.

Mastication, or chewing, involves the actions of the jaws, tongue, and cheeks and is the first act of digestion. It serves not only to break food particles down to a size that will pass into the esophagus but also to moisten and lubricate food by thoroughly mixing it with saliva. Abnormalities of the teeth are a common cause of digestive disturbances in animals.

Deglutition, or swallowing, involves voluntary and involuntary stages and occurs after food has been well masticated. In the voluntary phase of swallowing, food is molded into a bolus by the tongue and then pushed back into the pharynx. When food enters the pharynx, sensory nerve endings detect its presence and initiate the involuntary portion of the swallow reflex.

The involuntary actions of the swallow reflex occur primarily within the pharynx and esophagus. The *pharynx* is the common opening of both the respiratory and the digestive tract. The major physiological function of the pharynx is to ensure that air, and only air, enters the respiratory tract and that food and water, and only food and water, enter the digestive tract. The involuntary portion of the swallow reflex is the action that directs food into the digestive system and away from the upper airway. This reflex involves the following series of highly coordinated actions (Figure 28-4). Breathing stops momentarily. The soft palate is elevated, closing the pharyngeal opening of the nasopharynx and preventing food from entering the internal openings of the nostrils. The tongue is pressed against the hard palate, closing off the oral opening of the pharynx. The hyoid bone and larynx are pulled

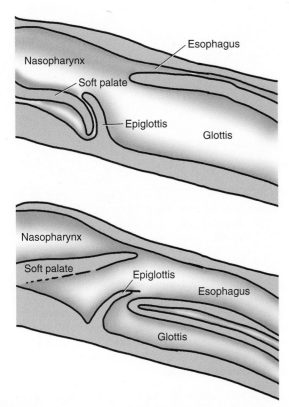

FIGURE 28-4 Midline cross-sectional schematics showing the position of the structures of the larynx and pharynx during breathing *(top)* and swallowing *(bottom)*.

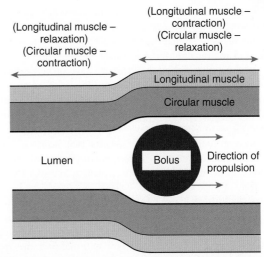

FIGURE 28-5 Peristalsis consists of a moving ring of luminal constriction preceded by an area of luminal distention. The area of constriction is created by contractions of the circular muscle, whereas the dilation is created by contractions of the longitudinal muscle. The net action is to propel a bolus of ingesta.

forward; this action pulls the glottis under the epiglottis, blocking the laryngeal opening. Concurrently, the arytenoid cartilages constrict, further closing the opening of the larynx and preventing the movement of food into the respiratory system. When all openings to the pharynx are closed, a wave of muscular constriction passes over the walls of the pharynx, pushing the bolus of food toward the opening of the esophagus. As the food reaches the esophagus, the upper esophageal sphincter relaxes to accept the material.

The complex reactions of deglutition are controlled by lower motor neurons located in various centers of the brainstem. Efferent nerve fibers from these centers travel in the facial, vagus, hypoglossal, and glossopharyngeal nerves, as well as the motor branch of the trigeminal nerve. Clinically, problems with prehension, mastication, and deglutition frequently are related to neurological lesions, either peripherally in the cranial nerves or centrally in the brainstem.

Motility of the Esophagus Propels Food from the Pharynx to the Stomach

The *esophagus,* as with other tubular portions of the gut, contains an outer longitudinal and inner circular layer of muscle. The esophagus is unique compared with other areas of the gut in that much of its muscular wall is composed of striated skeletal muscle fibers. In most domestic animals the entire length of esophageal musculature is striated. In horses, primates, and cats, however, a portion of the distal esophagus is smooth muscle. The striated muscle portions of esophagus are under control of somatic (not parasympathetic) motor neurons in the vagus nerve, whereas the smooth muscle portions are under direct control of the ENS and

indirect control of the autonomic nervous system. A myenteric plexus exists throughout the entire length of the esophagus. In the area of striated muscle, the myenteric plexus probably serves a sensory function and acts to coordinate the movements of the striated muscle portion with the esophageal smooth muscle segments and stomach.

In terms of motor activity, the esophagus may be viewed as consisting of an upper sphincter, body, and lower sphincter. The upper esophageal sphincter is called the *cricopharyngeal muscle.* This muscle and the upper end of the esophagus are attached to the cricoid cartilage of the larynx. When deglutition is not taking place, the muscle compresses the end of the esophagus against the cartilage of the larynx, tightly closing the upper esophageal opening. During deglutition the cricopharyngeal muscle relaxes and the larynx is pulled forward. The ventral portion of the upper end of the esophagus is attached to the larynx and the dorsal portion to the cervical spine. Because of these attachments, the forward motion of the larynx in conjunction with the relatively fixed nature of the cervical spine tends to pull open the upper esophageal orifice passively (see Figure 28-4).

The body of the esophagus serves as a relatively simple conduit, rapidly transferring food from the pharynx to the stomach. Food is propelled through the esophagus by propulsive movements known as *peristalsis.* Peristalsis consists of a moving ring of constriction in the wall of a tubular organ. In the esophagus, these rings start at the cranial end and progress toward the stomach. The rings reduce or obliterate the esophageal lumen, thus pushing the bolus of food ahead of them in much the same manner as a person would push material out of a soft rubber tube by stripping it with the fingers. In addition to the constriction of the circular muscles, there may be some contraction of longitudinal muscles just ahead of, or aboral to, the ring of circular muscle contraction. This longitudinal muscle activity increases the size of the esophageal lumen to accommodate the advancing food bolus (Figure 28-5). Peristalsis is a universal type of GI propulsive motility that exists at all levels of the gut.

During deglutition the upper esophageal sphincter relaxes as the pharynx constricts; food is pushed into the upper portion of the esophageal body, and a wave of peristalsis propels the material toward the stomach. As the food bolus reaches the distal end of the esophagus, the lower sphincter relaxes, and the ingested matter enters the stomach. If the esophagus is not cleared of food material by the primary wave of peristalsis, secondary peristaltic waves are generated. One or more secondary waves are almost always adequate for pushing material into the stomach and clearing the esophagus. If food or foreign bodies become lodged in the esophagus, secondary waves of peristalsis may lead eventually to muscle spasms that constrict tightly around the lodged material. These spasms frequently interfere with therapeutic attempts to remove obstructing objects in the esophagus.

When deglutition is not taking place, the body of the esophagus is relaxed, but the upper and lower sphincters remain constantly constricted. The constriction of these sphincters is important because of the differences in external pressure applied to the esophagus at different points along its length. During the inspiratory phase of breathing, the portion of the esophagus within the thorax is subjected to less-than-atmospheric pressure. If the two esophageal sphincters were not tightly closed, inspiration would cause aspiration of air from the pharynx and reflux of ingesta from the stomach into the body of the esophagus, in the same manner as inspiration draws air into the lung. Stomach contents would be drawn into the esophagus because inspiratory pressures in the thorax are lower than intraabdominal pressure. It is particularly important that the lower esophageal sphincter remain closed during inspiration because the mucosa of the esophagus is not equipped to resist the caustic actions of gastric contents; thus movement of stomach contents into the esophagus would cause damage to the esophageal mucosa.

In many species the action of the lower esophageal sphincter is aided by the anatomical nature of the attachment of the esophagus and stomach. The esophagus enters the stomach obliquely, allowing distention of the stomach to block the esophageal opening in a valve-like manner. During deglutition the longitudinal muscle of the esophagus contracts, shortening the esophagus and opening the valve at the junction with the stomach. This anatomical arrangement, along with the lower esophageal sphincter, is particularly well developed in the horse, making reflux of stomach material into the esophagus extremely rare in this species. In many cases, when the intragastric pressure of the horse is pathologically raised, the stomach ruptures before vomiting or esophageal reflux takes place.

The Function of the Stomach Is to Process Food into a Fluid Consistency and Release It into the Intestine at a Controlled Rate

Among animals there is tremendous diversity in the anatomy and motility patterns of the stomach. The following discussion applies best to the animals with the simplest stomachs, such as the dog and cat, but is probably also a reasonable description of the activity of the somewhat more complex stomachs of the pig, horse, and rat. The complex motility patterns of the ruminant stomach are discussed in Chapter 31.

The function of the stomach is to serve food to the small intestine. There are two important aspects of this function: rate of delivery and consistency of material. The stomach serves both as a storage vat to control the rate of delivery of food to the small intestine and as a grinder and sieve that reduces the size of food particles and releases them only when they are broken down to a consistency compatible with small-intestinal digestion.

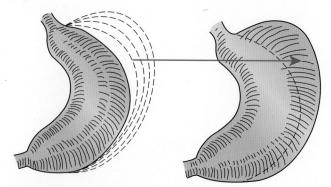

FIGURE 28-6 Adaptive relaxation refers to the stretching of the stomach wall that occurs as the organ fills during eating. This stretching results from muscle relaxation and is accompanied by little or no change in intraluminal pressure.

The stomach is divided into two physiological regions, each of which has a different impact on gastric function. The *proximal region,* at the esophageal end of the stomach, serves a storage function, retaining food as it awaits eventual entry into the small intestine. The *distal region* serves a grinding and sieving function, breaking solid pieces of food down into particles small enough for small-intestinal digestion.

The Proximal Stomach Stores Food Awaiting Further Gastric Processing in the Distal Stomach

The major muscular activity in the proximal region of the stomach is of a weak, continuous-contraction nature. These *tonic* contractions tend to shape the gastric wall to its contents and provide gentle propulsion of material into the distal stomach. The major muscular reflex of the proximal stomach is *adaptive relaxation* (Figure 28-6). This reflex is characterized by relaxation of the muscles as food enters the stomach. Because of this relaxation, the stomach can dilate to accept large quantities of food without an increase in intraluminal pressure. Thus the proximal stomach serves as a food storage area. Because of the rather passive muscular activity of the proximal stomach, little mixing occurs there. In fact, food boluses tend to become layered in the stomach in the order in which they were swallowed. As the stomach empties, tension on the wall of the proximal stomach increases slightly, pushing food distally in the stomach, where it can be processed for transport into the duodenum.

The Distal Stomach Grinds and Sifts Food Entering the Small Intestine

The muscular activity of the distal stomach and *pylorus* (sphincterlike junction between stomach and duodenum) is completely different from that of the proximal stomach. In the distal stomach, known as the *antrum,* there is intense slow-wave activity, and muscular contractions are frequently present. Strong waves of peristalsis begin at about the middle of the stomach and migrate, with the slow waves, toward the pylorus. As the waves of peristalsis near the pylorus, the pylorus constricts, blocking the gastric exit of all but the smallest particles (Figure 28-7). Particles leaving the stomach during the digestive phase of activity are less than 2 mm in diameter. Particles too large to pass the pylorus are crushed and ejected back into the antrum by the passing wave of peristalsis. Thus the peristaltic actions of the distal stomach walls serve not only to propel food but also, and perhaps more importantly, to grind and mix it.

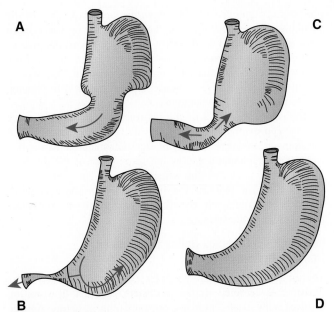

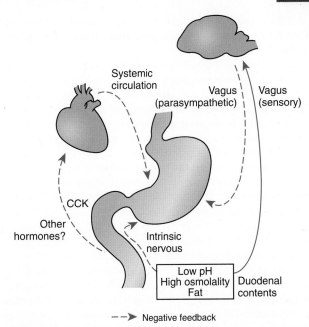

- - ▸ Negative feedback

FIGURE 28-7 Grinding and churning activity of the distal stomach. **A,** Wave of peristalsis begins at the junction of the proximal and distal areas of the stomach and moves toward the pylorus. **B,** As the peristaltic wave approaches the pylorus, the pylorus constricts, causing some of the ingesta to be crushed within the peristaltic ring and propelled back toward the proximal stomach. **C,** As the peristaltic wave reaches the pylorus, some finely ground and liquefied material passes through into the duodenum, but the majority of material has been propelled back into the stomach. **D,** Between contractions, no gross movement of gastric contents occurs. (From Johnson LR, editor: *Gastrointestinal physiology,* St Louis, 1985, Mosby).

FIGURE 28-8 Inhibitory arcs of the enterogastric reflex. Low pH, high osmolality, and the presence of fat in the duodenum stimulate vagal, enteric neuronal, and hormonal reflexes that inhibit stomach emptying. After the duodenal pH and osmolality have moderated and some of the fat has been absorbed, the inhibitory influences on the stomach are removed. *CCK,* Cholecystokinin.

Control of Gastric Motility Differs in the Proximal and Distal Stomach

The motility of the stomach, as in other smooth muscle portions of the gut, is under the control of regulatory molecules from the ENS and endocrine/paracrine systems. Fibers of the vagus nerve synapse on nerve cell bodies of the extensive gastric myenteric plexus and thereby exert a high degree of control over the ENS and thus over gastric motility. The effects of vagal stimulation on the proximal and distal regions of the stomach are opposite; in the proximal stomach, vagal activity suppresses muscular contractions and leads to adaptive relaxation, whereas in the distal stomach, vagal stimulation causes intense peristaltic activity. Vagal stimulation of distal antral motility is mediated by acetylcholine, but vagal inhibition of proximal stomach motility is not. The identity of the inhibitory mediator is not well established, but it may be vasoactive intestinal peptide.

Vagal action on the stomach is stimulated by events occurring within the CNS, as well as within the stomach and intestine. The anticipation of food consumption causes vagal stimulation of the stomach and thus primes the stomach to receive a meal. Reactions of the GI tract that originate in the CNS in response to anticipated food intake are often referred to as the *cephalic phase* of digestion. Reactions to the cephalic phase are then augmented as food enters the stomach. In response to food in the stomach, vagal activity increases as sensory receptors in the stomach create a positive feedback loop.

The exact role of hormones in regulation of gastric motility is not completely established. *Gastrin,* which is secreted from cells

in the gastric antrum, appears to enhance gastric motility. *Cholecystokinin* (CCK), *secretin,* and *gastric inhibitory peptide* (GIP) appear to suppress gastric motility, at least in the dog. The roles of the various GI hormones are difficult to determine from available information, because many of the experimental results reported have been in response to administration of GI hormones at amounts far greater than those normally occurring.

The Rate of Gastric Emptying Must Match the Small Intestine's Rate of Digestion and Absorption

The rate at which food leaves the stomach must match the rate at which it can be digested and absorbed by the small intestine. Because some types of foods can be digested and absorbed more rapidly than others, the rate at which the stomach empties must be regulated by the contents of the small intestine. Thus there are reflexes that regulate gastric emptying and allow the stomach to serve as a storage site. The afferent receptors of these reflexes are in the duodenum and are activated by low pH, high osmolality, and the presence of fat. Separate sensory receptors apparently exist for each of these stimuli, but these receptors have not been identified anatomically.

Many reflexes occur within the GI system. Their names usually reflect the site of origin of the afferent stimulus and the site of the efferent response. Thus, reflex control of gastric emptying by the duodenum is referred to as the *enterogastric reflex* ("entero" referring to the intestine).

The arc of the enterogastric reflex probably involves both the CNS and the ENS, as well as the endocrine/paracrine system (Figure 28-8). The extrinsic reflex pathway appears to involve afferent fibers of the vagus nerve, which receive stimuli in the duodenum. These stimuli are integrated in the brainstem, and the response is mediated by vagal efferent fibers to the stomach.

The enteric reflex arc involves receptors in the duodenum and nerve fiber connections in the ENS that directly affect gastric emptying.

A contribution of the GI endocrine system to the enterogastric reflex has long been suspected, but the exact hormones responsible for the reflex are not known. CCK and secretin may be important. Both hormones are secreted by cells in the duodenum; CCK is secreted in response to fat and secretin in response to low pH; both appear to have suppression of gastric emptying as secondary effects. Gastric inhibitory peptide is a hormone produced in the duodenum in response to the presence of carbohydrate. In the dog, gastric inhibitory peptide may function as an inhibitor of gastric emptying, although stimulation of insulin secretion is probably its major action.

Enterogastric reflexes control gastric emptying by regulating stomach motility. The manner in which motility affects gastric emptying of solids is different from that for liquids. The rate at which solids are expelled from the stomach is regulated by the rate at which they are broken down into particles small enough to pass through the pylorus. This in turn is controlled by the motility of the antrum, or distal stomach; the greater the motility of the antrum, the faster material is broken down. Thus, antrum motility regulates the rate of release of solid material from the stomach. Liquid material leaves the stomach more quickly than solid matter, and the release of liquid may be less dependent on antral motility than on the motility of the proximal stomach.

Minimal mixing activity occurs in the proximal stomach. Therefore, liquids and solids tend to separate, the liquids moving to the outside and the solids to the center of the mass of food in the proximal stomach. Increased tension in the wall of the stomach body forces liquid into the antrum. Liquid may leave the antrum quickly, dependent on the activity of the pylorus. On the other hand, increased tension in the stomach body has little effect on the transport of solid material, because such material cannot leave the gastric body until sufficient space has been made available in the antrum. Thus, motility of the stomach body appears primarily responsible for the liquid-emptying rate, whereas motility of the antrum is most responsible for the solid-emptying rate. The effect of the pylorus itself on gastric emptying is not as great as might be expected; removal of the pylorus results in a slight increase in the liquid-emptying rate and little increase in the rate of emptying of solid material. It appears that the distal portion of the antrum can account for much of the sieving action usually attributed to the pylorus. The rate of emptying of an isotonic liquid from the stomach is exponential and dependent on the initial volume of the liquid meal. Under usual circumstances, a liquid meal in the canine stomach has a half-life of about 18 minutes and is essentially gone by 1 hour after ingestion. Solid material is emptied more slowly, and its rate depends on its fat content. Low-fat meat meals are usually gone from the stomach in 3 to 4 hours after ingestion.

Between Meals, the Stomach Is Cleared of Indigestible Material

Some types of ingested materials, such as bone and indigestible foreign objects, cannot be reduced to particles less than 2 mm in diameter. During the digestive phase of gastric motility, such material does not leave the stomach. To clear the stomach of indigestible debris, a particular type of motility occurs between meals. This motility pattern is called the *interdigestive motility complex*. This motility pattern in the stomach is similar to, and probably continuous with, the *migrating motility complex* of the small intestine. The latter will be discussed in the next section. In association with the interdigestive motility complex, the pylorus relaxes as strong waves of peristalsis sweep over the antrum, forcing less digestible material into the duodenum. This type of motility appears to have a "housekeeping" function in clearing the stomach of indigestible material.

The peristaltic waves of the interdigestive motility complex occur at approximately 1-hour intervals during the periods when the stomach is relatively empty of digestible material. Eating disrupts the complex and causes the resumption of the digestive motility pattern. Herbivores, which eat almost constantly, have a slightly different pattern; the interdigestive motility complex occurs at approximately hourly intervals, even with digestible food present in the stomach.

Vomiting Is a Complex Reflex Coordinated from the Brainstem

Vomiting is a complex reflex activity, and its integration, or coordination, is centered in the brainstem. The act of vomiting involves many striated muscle groups and other structures outside the GI tract. Vomiting is associated with the following actions:

1. Relaxation of the muscles of the stomach and lower esophageal sphincter and closing of the pylorus.
2. Contraction of the abdominal musculature, creating an increase in intraabdominal pressure.
3. Expansion of the chest cavity while the glottis remains closed; this action lowers intrathoracic pressure and thus the pressure in the body of the esophagus.
4. Opening of the upper esophageal sphincter.
5. Antiperistaltic motility (peristaltic motility propelling ingesta toward the mouth) in the duodenum, which may precede the previous actions; thus vomiting may include ingesta of intestinal origin.

The efferent limb of this reflex arc involves motor fibers in many different peripheral nerves.

Afferent stimulation of the vomiting reflex comes from a large number of receptors. Of particular importance are mechanoreceptors in the pharynx and tension receptors and chemoreceptors in the gastric and duodenal mucosa. Stimulation of these receptors sends signals to the *vomit center* in the brainstem. Thus, noxious tactile or chemical stimulation of the GI mucosa can result in vomiting, clearing, or attempting to clear the offending stimulus from the GI tract. Direct irritation of GI structures, however, is not the only stimulus for vomiting. The vomit center receives afferent input from a variety of organs; thus vomiting is not always an indication of a primary GI problem.

An important structure outside the GI tract that supplies afferent input in the vomit center is the *chemoreceptor trigger zone*. This is an area of the brainstem that lies in contact with the third ventricle. The chemoreceptor trigger zone is sensitive to the presence of some drugs and toxins in the blood. When stimulated, this zone sends signals to the vomit center and induces vomiting. Some of the products of inflammation stimulate the chemoreceptor trigger zone. Thus, inflammatory disease, even outside the GI tract, can sometimes lead to vomiting.

The semicircular canals of the inner ear are other important structures that supply afferent input to the vomit center. Constant stimulation of the semicircular canals may induce vomiting, as occurs in motion sickness. Other sites in the body also may stimulate the vomit center; thus vomiting is a rather nonspecific sign of disease.

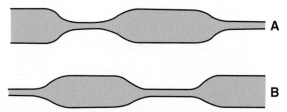

FIGURE 28-9 Segmentation in the small intestine. **A,** Areas of circular muscle constriction close the lumen and divide the gut into dilated segments containing ingesta. **B,** At periodic intervals the areas of constriction and dilation alternate, exerting a mixing and circulating action on the ingesta.

Motility of the Small Intestine Has Digestive and Interdigestive Phases

Motility of the small intestine occurs in two distinct phases: (1) during the digestive period after food intake and (2) during the interdigestive period when little food is present in the gut. In the digestive phase there are two primary motility patterns: propulsive and nonpropulsive. The *nonpropulsive* pattern is referred to as *segmentation*. Segmentation results from localized contractions of circular muscle. Portions of small intestine, usually 3 to 4 cm long, contract tightly, dividing the gut into segments of constricted and dilated lumen. Within a few seconds, the constricted portions relax and new areas constrict (Figure 28-9). This action tends to "milk" gut contents back and forth within the small intestine, mixing them with digestive juices and circulating them over the absorptive mucosal surfaces. This type of motility does not contribute much to the net aboral propulsion of ingesta. In fact, segmentation tends to slow down the aboral movement of material because of closure of the intestinal lumen in the constricted segments.

Propulsive activity during the digestive phase consists of peristaltic contractions that migrate down the gut in phase with the slow waves. Digestive-phase peristaltic contractions pass over short segments of intestine and then die out. Thus, ingesta are pushed down the gut for a short distance and then subjected to additional segmentation contractions and mixing activity. The interaction of segmentation and peristaltic motility has caused some authors to describe the movement of ingesta during digestive-phase motility as "two steps forward, one step back."

The interdigestive phase of small-intestinal motility is characterized by waves of powerful peristaltic contractions that sweep over a large length of small intestine, sometimes traversing the entire organ. These waves are referred to as the *migrating motility complex* (MMC) or, alternatively, the *migrating myoelectric complex*. The MMC begins in the duodenum as groups of slow waves that stimulate intense action potential and muscular contraction activity. The complex migrates down the intestine at the rate of the slow waves. Some of the MMCs die out before reaching the ileum, but some travel the entire length of the small intestine.

The MMC is the basic motor activity in the gut during a fasting or the period between meals, which may be referred to as interdigestive states. Meal consumption interrupts the MMC. The MMC typically lasts 80 to 120 min and consists of three successive phases: phase I (60-70 min), which has no contractions; phase II (20-30 min), which has intermittent and irregular contractions; and phase III, which has strong peristaltic contractions that last 3 to 10 minutes and that start from the stomach and lower esophagus and migrate distally to reach the colon.

The MMC probably has a "housekeeping" function and serves to push undigested material out of the small intestine. The MMC is also important in controlling the bacterial population in the upper gut. Normally the duodenum harbors a relatively small population of bacteria, and the population increases distally into the ileum, which has a moderately large number of bacterial organisms. The colon is heavily colonized by numerous species of bacteria. It is important for digestive function that this relative distribution of bacteria be maintained within the gut. The MMC may help to impede the migration of bacteria from the ileum to the duodenum.

The Ileocecal Sphincter Prevents Movement of Colon Contents Back into the Ileum

The *ileocecal sphincter* is at the junction of the small and large bowel and prevents the retrograde movement of colon contents into the ileum. It consists of a well-developed ring of circular muscle that remains constricted at most times. In addition to the muscular sphincter, in many species there is a flap of mucosa that acts as a one-way valve, further blocking movement of colon contents into the ileum. During periods of peristaltic activity in the ileum, the sphincter relaxes, allowing movement of material into the colon. When colonic pressure increases, the ileocecal sphincter constricts more tightly.

Motility of the Colon Causes Mixing, Retropulsion, and Propulsion of Ingesta

The colon has multiple functions, including (1) absorption of water and electrolytes, (2) storage of feces, and (3) fermentation of organic matter that escapes digestion and absorption in the small intestine. The relative importance of these functions varies with the species, and tremendous differences in colon size and shape exist among animals. The major determinant of colon size is the importance of colonic fermentation to the energy needs of the animal. Some species, such as the horse and rabbit, make extensive use of fermentation products for nutritional needs and have large and complex colons. (The ruminant's fermentation chamber is in the stomach.) Other species, such as the dog and cat, do not rely on fermentation products and have relatively simple colons. Figure 28-10 illustrates differences in colonic anatomy among four species with different needs for fermentative digestion.

Considerable similarity appears to exist in colon motility patterns among animals, despite the anatomical diversity. *Mixing* activity is prominent in the colons of all species because mixing and circulating are important to both absorptive and fermentative functions. Mixing is achieved by segmentation contractions along with other types of motility. In many species, such as the horse and pig, colonic segmentation is pronounced and in some areas results in the formation of sacculations, known as *haustra,* which are visible even after death.

A particular characteristic of colonic motility is *retropulsion,* or *antiperistalsis*. This type of peristaltic contraction migrates orally, the opposite of normal peristaltic movement. Such motility results from colonic slow-wave activity that is somewhat more complex than that of the small intestine. In the colon, as in the small intestine, the slow waves originate in the ICC. The colonic ENS, however, can influence the ICC in such a manner as to shift the site of origin of slow waves and the direction of their propagation. Under resting conditions in the colon, slow waves originate from *pacemakers* in one or more central sites. The pacemakers are not anatomical structures; rather, they are areas

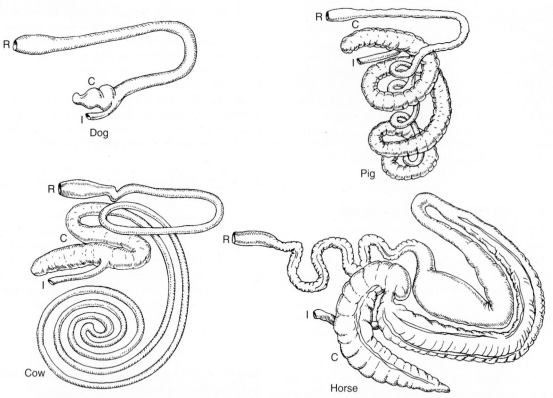

FIGURE 28-10 Variations of colon anatomy of four mammals. Animals with simple colons, such as the dog, are not dependent on colonic fermentation to supply energy needs. Horses, which have tremendous colonic development, rely on colonic fermentation for a large portion of their energy needs. In animals such as pigs and cattle, the importance of colonic fermentation to digestive needs is intermediate between that of the horse and dog, and this intermediate position is noted in their colon development. *C*, Cecum; *I*, ileum; *R*, rectum.

defined by activities of the ENS. Thus the pacemakers are not always the same areas; they can disappear and form in different locations in response to the need for different motility patterns. Antiperistaltic contractions occur in the segments in which slow waves migrate in an oral direction. Antiperistaltic contractions are retropulsive and impede the movement of ingesta, causing intense mixing activity and forcing material to accumulate in the proximal portions of the colon. Retropulsion appears to be particularly strong near the pacemakers, and the pacemakers therefore represent sites of high resistance to the flow of colonic ingesta.

Because of continued inflow of material from the ileum into the colon, some ingesta escape the retropulsive, antiperistaltic motility, move into areas of propulsive, peristaltic activity, and proceed along the colon. In addition, there are periods of intense propulsive activity that involve the entire colon. These are called *mass movements* and frequently involve the distal translocation of the entire colonic content.

The Colon Is an Important Site of Storage and Absorption in All Animals

The colon of the dog and cat is a relatively simple organ consisting of a short cecum, an ascending part, a transverse part, and a descending part. During the resting phase, there is a colonic pacemaker at about the junction of the transverse and descending colons (Figure 28-11). This gives rise to antiperistaltic activity in the proximal colon, with resultant accumulation of ingesta in the

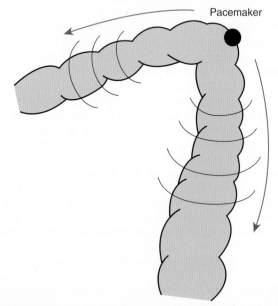

FIGURE 28-11 A pacemaker is present at the junction of the transverse and descending parts of the colon of the cat and probably in other mammals with similar colonic anatomy. Slow waves and peristaltic activity emanate in both directions from the pacemaker. Retrograde, or reverse, peristalsis in the proximal portions of the colon causes ingesta to be retained there, promoting the storage and absorptive functions of the colon.

cecum and ascending colon areas. Moderate peristaltic activity usually occurs in the descending colon, whereas the distal colon and rectum are usually constricted and empty.

Material entering the carnivore colon is of a fluid consistency. It is thoroughly mixed in the ascending and transverse colons, and much of the water and many of the electrolytes are absorbed. By the time it reaches the descending colon, it is semisolid and becoming feces.

Despite Large Anatomical Differences in the Colons of Herbivores Compared to Omnivores and Carnivores, There Are Similarities in Motility

There are important similarities in motility among various species, even those with extensive anatomical differences. The purpose of this discussion is to describe the similarities in motility between species with simple colons and those with complex colons. Chapter 31 provides a more extensive discussion of the highly developed colons of herbivores.

The equine hindgut, as an example of an herbivore hindgut, is complex and highly developed (see Figure 28-10). The cecum is large and separated into haustra. The equine cecum is unique among ceca of most species, even other herbivores, because a distinct, sphincterlike orifice joins it to the colon. The colon is divided into a large and a small portion, and the large colon is folded on itself so that three distinct flexures exist. The longitudinal muscles of the cecum and most areas of the colon are not evenly dispersed around the circumference of the gut. Instead, they form discrete bands, or teniae, that course along the longitudinal axis of the gut. The teniae divide the haustra longitudinally, giving the equine cecum and large colon a sacculated appearance.

Motility in the equine cecum consists of active segmentation and mixing, along with occasional mass movements that appear to transfer large amounts of ingesta to the colon. Motility in the colon consists of segmentation, antiperistalsis, and peristalsis. A colonic pacemaker appears to exist at the pelvic flexure and creates an area of high resistance to flow that results in prolonged retention of material in the ventral portions of the large colon. The pelvic flexure pacemaker in the equine colon is similar in function to the colonic pacemaker in the transverse colon of the dog and cat. Little is known about regulation of motility in the equine small colon. The characteristic ball-shaped form of equine feces probably represents intense segmentation-type motility in the small colon, where the feces are formed (see Chapter 31).

In ruminants and swine, the hindgut consists of a cecum of intermediate complexity, a spiral colon, and a straight colon. Compared with other species, less is known about the hindgut motility of animals with spiral colons. There seems to be an area of high flow resistance at the flexure, or central point, of the spiral colon. This site of flow resistance may represent a pacemaker that generates antiperistaltic motility in the centripetal portion of the colon.

The Anal Sphincter Has Two Layers with Separate Innervation

The anal opening is constricted by two sphincters: an *internal sphincter* of smooth muscle, which is a direct extension of the circular muscle layer of the rectum; and an *external sphincter* of striated muscle. The internal anal sphincter usually remains tonically contracted and is responsible for anal continence. The internal sphincter receives parasympathetic innervation from the

sacral spinal segments through the pelvic nerve and sympathetic innervation from the lumbar spinal segments through the hypogastric nerve. In most species, sympathetic stimulation results in constriction of the sphincter, and parasympathetic stimulation results in relaxation.

The external sphincter maintains some degree of tonic contraction, but the consistent tone of the anus is primarily regulated by the internal sphincter. The external sphincter is innervated by general somatic efferent fibers that have cell bodies in the cranial sacral spinal segments and course in the pudendal nerve.

The Rectosphincteric Reflex Is Important in Defecation

The entry of feces into the rectum is accompanied by the reflex relaxation of the internal anal sphincter, followed by peristaltic contractions of the rectum. This is known as the *rectosphincteric reflex* and is an important part of the act of defecation (Figure 28-12). The reflex normally results in defecation, but in trained animals its effects can be blocked by voluntary constriction of the external anal sphincter. When defecation is voluntarily suppressed, the rectum soon relaxes to accommodate the fecal bolus, and the internal anal sphincter regains its tone. In humans, and presumably in dogs and cats, relaxation of the rectum and constriction of the internal sphincter is associated with fading of the urge to defecate, until another bolus of feces enters the rectum.

Uninhibited animals respond to the presence of feces in the rectum with a number of voluntary actions associated with defecation. In carnivores the diaphragm and abdominal muscles contract to increase intraabdominal pressure, and striated muscles of the anal canal relax as the animal assumes the defecation posture. These acts are important for complete evacuation of the rectum.

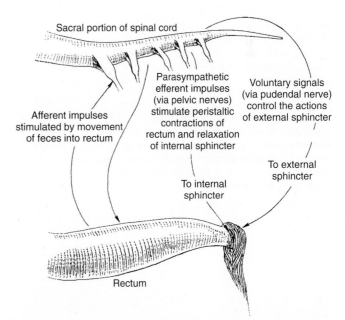

FIGURE 28-12 Arcs of the rectosphincteric reflex. The reflex is initiated by the movement of feces into the rectum and results in peristaltic movements of the rectal wall and relaxation of the internal anal sphincter. Fecal passage is the normal effect of the reflex, but voluntary constriction of the external anal sphincter can prevent the passage of feces and eventually override the reflex, apparently enabling trained animals to suppress the urge to defecate.

Major Differences Between Avian and Mammalian Digestive Systems Include, in Birds, Both the Lack of Teeth and the Separation of Gastric Functions into Distinct Anatomical Regions

Important anatomical differences exist between the digestive systems of birds and mammals. These differences affect motility functions more than other aspects of digestion, such as secretion, digestion, and absorption. Therefore the digestive tract of birds is covered in this chapter as a separate topic. In other chapters of this section, aspects of avian digestion are integrated into the general discussion.

Figure 28-13 illustrates the general anatomy of the avian digestive system. The pharynx of birds is simpler than that in mammals, with birds having no soft palate. There are no teeth, although in carnivorous species, the beak is modified for tearing food into pieces small enough to swallow. The esophagus has a large diameter so as to accommodate unmasticated food. An outpouching of the esophagus is known as the *crop*. The extent of development of the crop varies widely among avian species. The glandular portion of the stomach is the *proventriculus,* which is separated from the muscular stomach, known as the *ventriculus* or *gizzard,* by a short isthmus. The small intestine varies greatly in length among avian species but is generally rather short compared with that of mammals of similar size. The ceca are usually paired and vary tremendously in development among avian species. In some carnivorous species, such as the hawk, the ceca are rudimentary, whereas in some of the nonflying herbivores, such as the ostrich, cecal development is extensive (see Figure 28-13). The colon and rectum are very simple; the rectum ends in the cloaca, which is a

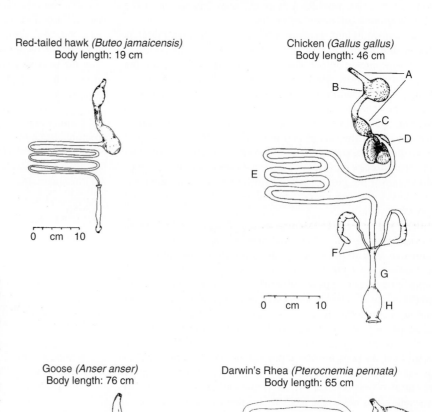

Red-tailed hawk *(Buteo jamaicensis)*
Body length: 19 cm

Chicken *(Gallus gallus)*
Body length: 46 cm

Goose *(Anser anser)*
Body length: 76 cm

Darwin's Rhea *(Pterocnemia pennata)*
Body length: 65 cm

FIGURE 28-13 Comparative anatomy of the digestive tracts of four avian species. Note the variation in crop and cecal development. The carnivorous red-tailed hawk has a small crop and rudimentary ceca. The chicken has a well-developed crop, and the rhea has tremendous cecal development. *A,* Esophagus; *B,* crop; *C,* proventriculus; *D,* gizzard or ventriculus; *E,* small intestine; *F,* ceca; *G,* rectum; *H,* cloaca. (From Stevens CD: *Comparative physiology of the vertebrate digestive system,* Cambridge, UK, 1988, Cambridge University Press.)

common passageway for digestive, urinary, and reproductive discharges.

The crop performs a storage function. In some species the crop is little more than a pouch in the esophagus, whereas in others, such as the chicken, there is a distinct sphincter-like opening between the esophagus and crop. In general, ingesta do not begin to accumulate in the crop until the gizzard is full. The crop is richly populated with mucus-secreting cells, but no digestive glands are present. However, digestive glandular secretions originating from the salivary glands and proventriculus are present in the crop. In many species it appears that ingesta and secretions pass in a retrograde manner up the esophagus from the gizzard and proventriculus to the crop. The motility of the crop is under regulation of vagal impulses. Crop motility and rate of emptying are coordinated so as to release ingesta at a rate matching the emptying rate of the proventriculus and gizzard. In some avian species the crop also functions as a storage place for food being transported to the young. In this case, food is swallowed into the crop and later regurgitated as feed for offspring.

The proventriculus is a low-volume organ with a glandular epithelium resembling that of the stomach of mammals (see Chapter 29). Motility functions of the proventriculus are to propel ingesta and digestive secretions into the gizzard for mixing and grinding. The gizzard is a muscular organ that grinds and liquefies ingesta. In addition, particle-size discrimination occurs in the gizzard; small particles are passed into the duodenum, whereas large particles are retained for further comminution or ejected back into the proventriculus for further addition of digestive secretions. In carnivorous birds, concretions of bone, hair, feathers, and other indigestible material accumulate in the gizzard and are occasionally ejected orally in an action known as *egestion.* In grain-eating birds, small stones or gravel are swallowed and retained in the gizzard to aid in the comminution of ingesta. This inorganic material is referred to as *grit,* and its presence increases digestive efficiency, although it is not essential. The mucosa of the gizzard is covered by a tough coating known as *koilin.* This coating is composed of glandular secretions and desquamated cells. It protects the mucosa from the physical grinding actions of the gizzard.

The motility and function of the various stomach areas of birds are easily comparable with gastric motility and function in mammals. The crop and proventriculus function in much the same manner as the fundus and body of the mammalian stomach, with storage and secretory functions. The gizzard functions in much the same way as the antrum of the mammalian stomach, with grinding and particle-size discrimination functions. The major functional differences between birds and mammals include the physical separation of the stomach compartments in birds and the advanced grinding function of the gizzard.

The motility patterns of the avian small intestine appear to be generally similar to those in mammals. The motility of the hindgut also shares some characteristics of other animals. Reverse peristalsis is a dominant characteristic of the avian colon and rectum, moving ingesta into the ceca. Urinary excretions arriving at the cloaca become incorporated with ingesta and move in a retrograde manner into the ceca, thus facilitating reabsorption of the remaining water and electrolytes from urine. Cecal motility is characterized primarily by mixing and reverse peristalsis, with occasional mass movements resulting in the evacuation of the ceca. These mass movements in avian species are followed by defecation.

CLINICAL CORRELATIONS

EQUINE RABIES

History. Owners report that their horse has not "been itself" for the past few days. Today the animal is extremely lethargic and stands with forelegs wide apart and head held low. The nostrils are soiled, and the owners report that water and feed come out of the nostrils when the animal attempts to eat or drink.

Clinical Examination. From the history and presenting signs, you recognize that the horse may have paralysis of muscles of the pharynx and larynx. Because these lesions are typically associated with rabies in horses, you don a pair of plastic gloves and sleeves and proceed with your examination. To assess the function of the swallow reflex, you attempt to pass a stomach tube. You observe that the swallow reflex appears to be diminished, but that with some persistence the tube can be passed. This indicates that there is no physical obstruction in the pharynx or esophagus and that the problem is functional. These findings support, but do not confirm, a diagnosis of rabies.

Comment. Rabies in herbivorous animals may take a number of forms. One of the most common signs in cattle and horses is paralysis of the pharynx and larynx as a result of viral lesions in the brainstem nuclei supplying the appropriate cranial nerves. If rabies is suspected, no one should come into direct contact with the excretions of the animal, especially saliva.

Treatment. In this horse, treatment should consist of oral fluid and electrolyte therapy administered through an indwelling stomach tube. If there is no response to this conservative therapy, and if the animal's condition appears to deteriorate, euthanasia is necessary, and the animal's head should be submitted for evaluation for a positive diagnosis of rabies.

PRACTICE QUESTIONS

1. A unique feature of gastrointestinal (GI) smooth muscle cells is that:
   a. Their resting transcellular electrical potential has the positive pole on the outside surface of the cell membrane.
   b. Action potentials, or spikes of membrane depolarization, are not associated with muscle contractions.
   c. Muscle contractions are stimulated by partial depolarization of the membrane.
   d. There are spontaneous, rhythmical undulations in the electrical potential across the cell membrane.
   e. Contraction of the muscles is never influenced by nervous activity.

2. The interstitial cells of Cajal are:
   a. Modified neurons capable of generating contraction.
   b. Modified neurons capable of generating only action potentials.
   c. Modified neurons capable of generating only slow waves.
   d. Modified smooth muscle cells capable of generating only slow waves.
   e. Modified smooth muscle cells capable of generating only action potentials.

3. The term *slow waves* as applied to the gut refers to:
   a. Slowly moving fronts of electrical activity that are propagated down the enteric nervous system.
   b. Slowly moving fronts of electrical activity that result from coordinated changes in cell membrane potential occurring throughout the smooth muscle of the intestinal wall.
   c. Slowly moving fronts of ingesta that proceed down the intestine in response to peristaltic movement.
   d. Slowly moving fronts of action potentials that are constantly passing over the gut smooth muscle.
   e. Slowly moving fronts of peristaltic contractions that pass uniformly over the entire small intestine during the digestive period.

4. An animal is presented to you with aspiration pneumonia (the result of food material entering the lower respiratory tract). Which of the following lesions would be a likely cause?
   a. Loss of myenteric plexus function in the pharynx and upper esophagus
   b. Loss of slow-wave activity in the pharynx and upper esophagus
   c. A lesion in the brainstem
   d. A lesion in the trachea
   e. None of the above

5. The term *cephalic phase* is used in reference to a number of activities occurring in the GI tract. In general, the term means:
   a. The early phases of digestion, when food is nearest the head.
   b. Any actions stimulated directly by the presence of food in the stomach.
   c. Any actions stimulated directly by the presence of food in the mouth.
   d. Digestive events stimulated by the presence of food in the GI tract, but requiring reflexes integrated in the central nervous system.
   e. Digestive events that occur before the ingestion of food and in response to central nervous system stimulation that is brought on by the anticipation of eating.

6. Conditions in the duodenum, such as low pH or high fat concentration, can reflexively inhibit gastric emptying. Which reflex arc is involved in this inhibition?
   a. Parasympathetic nervous system
   b. GI enteric nervous system
   c. GI endocrine system
   d. All the above

7. Which of the following best describes the motility of the proximal region of the monogastric stomach?
   a. Rhythmic segmentation
   b. Peristalsis
   c. Retropulsion
   d. Adaptive relaxation

8. Which of the following is characteristic of the interdigestive phase of small intestinal motility?
   a. Migrating motility complexes consisting of waves of peristaltic contractions that pass over the entire length of the small intestine
   b. Rhythmic segmentation
   c. Short waves of peristalsis that die out after a few centimeters
   d. Complete relaxation of small intestinal smooth muscle

9. Which of the following aspects of colon physiology is common to many species, irrespective of interspecies anatomical differences in colon structure?
   a. Rapid flow of ingesta
   b. Adaptive relaxation
   c. Retropulsion, or antiperistalsis
   d. Haustra formation

10. Colonic "pacemakers":
    a. Are anatomically distinct structures composed of specialized smooth muscle cells.
    b. Shift in their sites under the influence of the ENS.
    c. Are involved in segmentation, but not peristalsis.
    d. Control defecation.

11. The rectosphincteric reflex is integrated in the:
    a. Brainstem.
    b. ENS.
    c. Lumbar spinal cord.
    d. Sacral spinal cord.

BIBLIOGRAPHY

Bharucha AE, Fletcher JG: Recent advances in assessing anorectal structure and functions, *Gastroenterology* 133(4):1069–1074, 2007.

Clouse RE, Diamant NE: Motor function of the esophagus. In Johnson LR, editor: *Physiology of the gastrointestinal tract*, vol 1, ed 4, Amsterdam, 2006, Elsevier Science & Technology Books.

Denbow DM: Gastrointestinal anatomy and physiology. In Whittow GC, editor: *Sturkie's avian physiology*, ed 5, San Diego, 2000, Academic Press.

Duke GE: Alimentary canal: anatomy, regulation of feeding and motility. In Sturkie PD, editor: *Avian physiology*, ed 4, New York, 1986, Springer-Verlag.

Hanani M, Farrugia G, Komuro T: Intercellular coupling of interstitial cells of Cajal in the digestive tract, *Int Rev Cytol* 242:249–282, 2005.

Hanani M, Freund HR: Interstitial cells of Cajal: their role in pacing and signal transmission in the digestive system, *Acta Physiol Scand* 170(3):177–190, 2000.

Hasler WL: Motility of the small intestine and colon. In Yamada T, editor: *Textbook of gastroenterology*, vol 1, ed 5, Hoboken, 2008, Wiley-Blackwell.

Hasler WL: The physiology of gastric motility and gastric emptying. In Yamada T, editor: *Textbook of gastroenterology*, vol. 1, ed 5, Hoboken, 2008, Wiley-Blackwell.

Hasler WL: Small intestinal motility. In Johnson LR, editor: *Physiology of the gastrointestinal tract*, vol 1, ed 4, Amsterdam, 2006, Elsevier Science & Technology Books.

Horowitz B, Ward SM, Sanders KM: Cellular and molecular basis for electrical rhythmicity in gastrointestinal muscles, *Annu Rev Physiol* 61:19–43, 1999.

Kahrilas PJ, Pandolfino JE: Esophageal motor function. In Yamada T, editor: *Textbook of gastroenterology*, vol 1, ed 5, Hoboken, 2008, Wiley-Blackwell.

Kerlin P, Zinsmeister A, Phillips S: Relationship of motility to flow of contents in the human small intestine, *Gastroenterology* 82:701, 1982.

Makhlouf GM, Murthy KS: Smooth muscle of the gut. In Yamada T, editor: *Textbook of gastroenterology*, vol 1, ed 5, Hoboken, 2008, Wiley-Blackwell.

Makhlouf GM, Murthy KS: Cellular physiology of gastrointestinal smooth muscle. In Johnson LR, editor: *Physiology of the gastrointestinal tract*, vol 1, ed 4, Amsterdam, 2006, Elsevier Science & Technology Books.

Merritt AM: Normal equine gastroduodenal secretion and motility, *Equine Vet J Suppl* 29:7–13, 1999.

Rasmussen OO, Christiansen J: Physiology and pathophysiology of anal function, *Scand J Gastroenterol Suppl* 216:169–174, 1996.

Sanders KM, Koh SD, Ward SM: Organization and electrophysiology of interstitial cells of Cajal and smooth muscle cells in the gastrointestinal tract. In Johnson LR, editor: *Physiology of the gastrointestinal tract*, vol 1, ed 4, Amsterdam, 2006, Elsevier Science & Technology Books.

Sarna S: Function and regulation of colonic contractions in health and disease. In Johnson LR, editor: *Physiology of the gastrointestinal tract*, vol 1, ed 4, Amsterdam, 2006, Elsevier Science & Technology Books.

Shaker R: Pharyngeal motor function. In Johnson LR, editor: *Physiology of the gastrointestinal tract*, vol 1, ed 4, Amsterdam, 2006, Elsevier Science & Technology Books.

Stevens CE, Hume ID: *Comparative physiology of the vertebrate digestive system*, ed 2, Cambridge, UK, 1996, Cambridge University Press.

Weisbrodt NW: Gastric emptying. In Johnson LR, editor: *Gastrointestinal physiology*, ed 7, St Louis, 2007, Mosby.

Weisbrodt NW: Motility of the large intestine. In Johnson LR, editor: *Gastrointestinal physiology*, ed 7, St Louis, 2007, Mosby.

Weisbrodt NW: Motility of the small intestine. In Johnson LR, editor: *Gastrointestinal physiology*, ed 7, St Louis, 2007, Mosby.

Weisbrodt NW: Regulation: nerves and smooth muscle. In Johnson LR, editor: *Gastrointestinal physiology*, ed 7, St Louis, 2007, Mosby.

Weisbrodt NW: Swallowing. In Johnson LR, editor: *Gastrointestinal physiology*, ed 7, St Louis, 2007, Mosby.

CHAPTER 29
Secretions of the Gastrointestinal Tract

KEY POINTS

The salivary glands
1. Saliva moistens, lubricates, and partially digests food.
2. Salivary secretions originate in the gland acini and are modified in the collecting ducts.
3. Salivary glands are regulated by the parasympathetic nervous system.
4. Ruminant saliva is a bicarbonate-phosphate buffer secreted in large quantities.

Gastric secretion
1. Depending on the species, there may be two general types of gastric mucosa: glandular and nonglandular.
2. The gastric mucosa contains many different cell types.
3. The gastric glands secrete hydrochloric acid.
4. Pepsin is secreted by gastric chief cells in an inactive form and is subsequently activated in the stomach lumen.
5. The parietal cells are stimulated to secrete by the action of acetylcholine, gastrin, and histamine.

The pancreas
1. Pancreatic exocrine secretions are indispensable for the digestion of the complex nutrients: proteins, starches, and triglycerides.
2. Acinar cells secrete enzymes, whereas centroacinar cells and duct cells secrete an electrolyte solution rich in sodium bicarbonate.
3. Pancreatic cells have cell surface receptors stimulated by acetylcholine, cholecystokinin, and secretin.

Bile secretion
1. The liver is an acinar gland with small acinar lumina known as *canaliculi*.
2. Bile contains phospholipids and cholesterol maintained in aqueous solution by the detergent action of bile acids.
3. The gallbladder stores and concentrates bile during the periods between feeding.
4. Bile secretion is initiated by the presence of food in the duodenum and stimulated by the return of bile acids to the liver.

Digestion and absorption can take place only in the aqueous milieu of digestive secretions. Synthesis and secretion of these fluids represent a well-controlled process regulated by endocrine, paracrine, and neural events. The total volume of digestive secretions is large, with the daily amount substantially larger than the volume of fluid ingested over a similar period. In addition, most of the digestive secretions have a relatively large concentration of electrolytes. This large outpouring of fluid and electrolyte into the gut makes reabsorption of these secretions imperative if fluid and electrolyte homeostasis of the body is to be maintained. Indeed, one of the major life-threatening ramifications of digestive diseases is the loss of water and electrolytes from the body caused by inadequate reabsorption of digestive secretions.

THE SALIVARY GLANDS

Saliva Moistens, Lubricates, and Partially Digests Food

As food is chewed, it is mixed with salivary secretions that allow it to be molded into well-lubricated boluses that facilitate swallowing. In addition, saliva may have antibacterial, digestive, and evaporative cooling functions, depending on the species.

The antibacterial activity of saliva results from antibodies and antimicrobial enzymes known as *lysozymes*. Initially, you may think that the antibacterial properties of saliva are inefficient because the mouth normally contains a large, thriving population of bacteria. However, saliva aids in keeping this population in check, and animals with impaired salivary function are prone to infectious diseases of the oral cavity.

In omnivorous animals, such as rats and pigs, saliva contains a starch-digesting enzyme known as *salivary amylase*. This enzyme is usually absent from the saliva of carnivorous animals, such as cats. The saliva of some species also contains a fat-digesting enzyme known as *lingual lipase*. This enzyme is frequently present in young animals, such as calves, while they are on a milk diet; the enzyme disappears as they mature.

Salivary enzymes probably have their major digestive effect in the proximal stomach, because food is not retained in the mouth long enough to permit extensive digestion. The lack of mixing activity in the proximal stomach may be essential for the starch-digesting function of saliva. This is because the amylase enzyme is functional at neutral to slightly basic pH, which characterizes saliva. The low pH of the distal stomach probably inactivates the enzyme; therefore it may be important that food entering the stomach initially not be mixed with gastric secretions, so as to allow the salivary enzymes some time to work before being inactivated by gastric acid. Some birds have salivary amylase that is active in the environment of the crop.

The evaporative cooling function of saliva is covered in Chapter 53.

Salivary Secretions Originate in the Gland Acini and Are Modified in the Collecting Ducts

The salivary gland is a typical *acinar* gland composed of an arborizing system of collecting ducts that end in cellular evaginations known as *acini* (Figure 29-1). The cellular epithelium of the acini is functionally distinct from that of the collecting ducts. Saliva is initially secreted into the lumen of the acini. The glandular cells

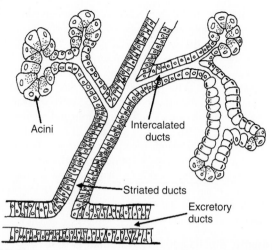

FIGURE 29-1 Schematic illustration of the salivary gland. Saliva is initially secreted by the acinar cells and is then modified as it passes through the intercalated, or collecting, ducts. Modification of acinar secretions by duct epithelia is a physiological phenomenon common among several types of glands, including the pancreas.

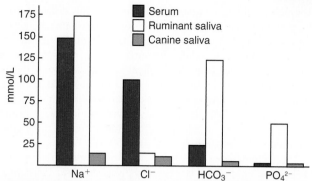

FIGURE 29-2 Electrolyte composition of blood serum and of canine and ruminant saliva. Note that the electrolyte concentration of canine saliva is much lower than that of serum, in contrast to the concentration in ruminant saliva. Also note the high concentrations of bicarbonate (HCO_3^-) and phosphate (PO_4^{2-}) in ruminant saliva; these ions give ruminant saliva its alkalizing quality.

lining the acini secrete water, electrolytes, enzymes, and mucus. As the newly formed saliva progresses through the collecting ducts, its composition is modified. The duct epithelium reabsorbs electrolytes, especially sodium and chloride, in a manner similar to that in the proximal tubules of the kidneys. The final product, saliva, is hypotonic and has a sodium concentration substantially less than that of extracellular fluid. The extent to which the acinar secretion is modified in the collecting ducts depends on the rate of saliva production. At high rates of salivary flow, there is little modification, which results in higher tonicity and electrolyte concentration, in comparison to low rates of flow.

Most mammals have at least three pairs of salivary glands: the *parotid* glands, which lie just under the ear and behind the vertical ramus of the mandible; the *mandibular* glands, which are in the intramandibular space; and the *lingual* glands, which lie in the base of the tongue. Each of these glands drains into a main duct that has a single opening into the mouth. In addition to these major glands, there are minor glands in the tongue and buccal mucosa. These small, indistinct glands often have numerous secretory ducts emptying into the mouth. The concentration of mucus is different in the secretions of the various salivary glands. The parotid gland secretes watery, or *serous*, saliva, whereas many of the minor glands secrete highly mucous saliva. Other glands secrete a mixed type of saliva containing both mucous and serous material. Avian salivary glands secrete a copious amount of mucus to lubricate unmasticated food for swallowing.

Salivary Glands Are Regulated by the Parasympathetic Nervous System

Autonomic, parasympathetic nerve fibers of the facial and glossopharyngeal nerves end on the secretory cells of the salivary gland acini and stimulate the cells through cholinergic receptors. All phases of salivary activity are stimulated by this mechanism, including electrolyte, water, and enzyme secretion. The anticipation of eating can initiate a parasympathetic response that results in salivary secretion. In Pavlov's famous experiment, parasympathetic stimulation of the salivary gland was evoked in dogs by the sound of a ringing bell. The dogs had been trained to anticipate

eating after hearing the bell. This well-known experiment was one of the first demonstrations that the central nervous system (CNS) could regulate digestive functions. Chewing and stimulation of taste buds, in addition to the anticipation of eating, are afferent stimuli for salivation.

Salivary secretory cells also contain β-adrenergic receptors that are activated by sympathetic nerve stimulation or circulating catecholamines. This form of stimulation probably has little association with normal digestive activity but is related to the salivation and drooling seen in carnivores preparing to attack. Among digestive glands, the salivary glands are unique because there is no endocrine regulatory component.

Ruminant Saliva Is a Bicarbonate-Phosphate Buffer Secreted in Large Quantities

The normal composition of ruminant parotid saliva is quite different from the saliva of monogastric animals. Bovine and canine saliva are compared in Figure 29-2. Ruminant saliva is isotonic and, compared with blood serum, has high concentrations of bicarbonate and phosphate and a high pH. This well-buffered solution is necessary for neutralizing acids formed by fermentation in the rumen, and ruminants secrete it in enormous quantities. An adult cow may secrete 100 to 200 L of saliva per day. This volume is approximately equivalent to the extracellular fluid volume of most adult cattle. It is obvious that much of the water and electrolytes secreted in saliva must be reabsorbed rapidly and recirculated through the total body water, or the cow would die of dehydration. In abnormal circumstances, such as blockage of the esophagus, in which the flow of saliva is diverted from the gastrointestinal (GI) tract, cattle quickly become dehydrated and acidotic.

In general, the salivary glands of domestic animals are seldom involved in disease processes and infrequently require veterinary attention.

GASTRIC SECRETION

Depending on the Species, There May Be Two General Types of Gastric Mucosa: Glandular and Nonglandular

Most domestic, monogastric animals have only glandular mucosa in the stomach, but horses and rats have an area in the proximal portion of their stomachs that is covered by nonglandular, stratified squamous epithelium. This area is visibly different from the glandular area, to which it adjoins with a sharp line of demarcation. The function of the nonglandular area of gastric mucosa is unclear. The nonglandular area may serve as a place where a small amount of fermentative (rumenlike) digestion could occur. Because there is little mixing activity in the proximal stomach, food in the nonglandular area would be protected from the secretions of the gastric glands. These acid secretions kill bacteria, and thus their presence would prevent fermentation. Fermentative digestion is discussed in detail in Chapter 31.

The glandular area of the stomach is divided into three regions: *cardiac mucosa, parietal mucosa,* and *pyloric mucosa.* These areas contain glands of similar structure but with different types of secretions, as described later. In most species the cardiac mucosa forms a narrow band around the gastric opening of the esophagus. In the pig, however, the cardiac mucosa covers a substantial portion of the proximal stomach.

The Gastric Mucosa Contains Many Different Cell Types

The glandular mucosa of the stomach has frequent invaginations, or pores, known as *gastric pits.* The size of the pits is such that the pores leading into them can be seen with a hand-held magnifying glass. At the base of each pit is a narrowing, or isthmus, that continues into the opening of one or more gastric glands (Figure 29-3).

The major surface areas of the stomach, as well as the lining of the pits, are covered with *surface mucous cells.* These cells produce thick, tenacious mucus that is a special characteristic of the stomach lining. The mucous cells and their associated secretion are important for protecting the stomach epithelium from the acid conditions and grinding activity present in the lumen. When the mucous cells are injured, stomach ulcers result.

Each region of the mucosa contains glands with characteristic cell types. Within the parietal area, the glands contain *parietal cells.* These cells are clustered in the neck, or proximal area, of the gland. Their function is to secrete hydrochloric acid (HCl). Distributed among the parietal cells in the neck of the gland is another type of cell, the *mucous neck cells.* These mucous cells secrete thin mucus, less viscous than that of the surface mucous cells. The mucous neck cells, in addition to their secretory function, appear to be the progenitor cells for the gastric mucosa. They

are the only cells of the stomach lining capable of division. As they divide, they migrate either down into the glands or up into the pits and onto the surface epithelium. As they migrate, the mucous neck cells differentiate into any of the several types of mature cells of the gastric surface and glands. In the base of the gastric glands is yet a third type of cell, the *chief cells.* These cells secrete *pepsinogen,* the precursor to the digestive enzyme *pepsin.*

The glands of the cardiac and pyloric mucosal regions resemble those of the parietal area in structure but contain different cell types. The cardiac glands secrete only mucus. Their mucus is alkaline and probably serves to protect the adjacent esophageal mucosa from the acid secretions of the stomach. The pyloric glands have no parietal cells but contain the gastrin-producing G cells. According to most reports, pyloric glands do secrete pepsinogen.

The Gastric Glands Secrete Hydrochloric Acid

When the gastric glands are stimulated maximally, the HCl solution secreted into the lumen is isotonic and has a pH of less than 1. Both the hydrogen (H^+) and the chloride (Cl^-) ions are secreted by the parietal cells but apparently by different cellular mechanisms. H^+ is secreted through an H^+,K^+-ATPase (adenosine triphosphatase) enzyme located on the luminal surface of the cell. This enzyme, sometimes referred to as a *proton pump,* exchanges H^+ for potassium ions (K^+), pumping one K^+ into the cell for each H^+ secreted into the lumen. In the exchange process, one molecule of adenosine triphosphate (ATP) is hydrolyzed to adenosine diphosphate (ADP), representing an expenditure of energy. The K^+ cations that accumulate within the cells are released back into the lumen in combination with Cl^- anions. This allows the recycling of K^+ ions as they are pumped back into the cells in exchange for H^+, resulting in the net secretion of H^+ and Cl^-, with little net movement of K^+.

Hydrogen ions for secretion come from the dissociation of intracellular carbonic acid (H_2CO_3), leaving a bicarbonate ion (HCO_3^-) in the cell for each H^+ secreted into the lumen (Figure 29-4). Carbonic acid originates from water and carbon dioxide through the action of *carbonic anhydrase,* an enzyme found in high concentration in the gastric mucosa.

As hydrogen cations are secreted, bicarbonate anions accumulate in the cell. To counterbalance this accumulation, bicarbonate

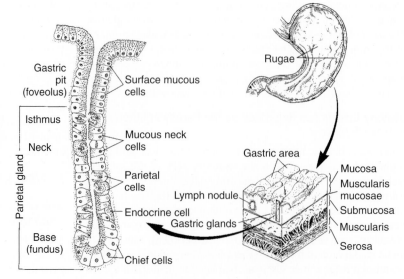

FIGURE 29-3 Anatomical illustration of glands of the stomach body. Other portions of the glandular stomach mucosa have similar structures but may differ somewhat in the cell types present in the glands. The gland openings are large enough to be seen with a hand-held magnifying glass.

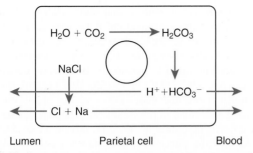

FIGURE 29-4 Electrolyte movements during gastric acid secretion. The production of hydrogen and bicarbonate ions from water and carbon dioxide is stimulated by the action of the enzyme carbonic anhydrase, the activity of which is high in the gastric mucosa.

anions are exchanged for chloride anions at the cell's nonluminal surface. In this manner, additional chloride is made available to the cell for secretion into the glandular lumen, and bicarbonate is secreted into the blood. During periods of intense secretion by the gastric glands, large amounts of bicarbonate are released into the blood. This transient and mild alkalization of the blood during digestion is known as the *alkaline tide*. Normally, the alkaline tide is reversed when bicarbonate in the blood is consumed indirectly during the neutralization of gastric secretions as they enter the intestine (see the section on pancreatic secretions later in this chapter). Thus, on a total-body basis, gastric acid production results in only small and transient changes in blood pH. In disease states, however, in which the secretions of the stomach are prevented from entering the intestine or are lost from the body because of vomiting, the pH of the blood can rise to dangerously high values.

Pepsin Is Secreted by Gastric Chief Cells in an Inactive Form and Is Subsequently Activated in the Stomach Lumen

Pepsin is usually described as a single compound, but it is actually a family of protein-digesting enzymes that are secreted from the gastric glands. They are formed in the chief cells as inactive proenzymes called *pepsinogens*. Pepsinogens are stored in the chief cells as granules until secreted into the lumen of the gastric glands. After secretion, pepsinogens are exposed to the acid contents of the stomach, resulting in cleavage of a small portion of the protein molecule, which leads to activation of the enzymes.

Digestive enzymes that are synthesized and stored as inactive proenzymes and activated in the lumen of the gut are known by the general name of *zymogens*. The general pattern of zymogen formation and activation is necessary because the active enzymes could digest and destroy the cells that synthesize them.

The Parietal Cells Are Stimulated to Secrete by the Action of Acetylcholine, Gastrin, and Histamine

Gastric acid secretion is stimulated by the anticipation of eating and the presence of undigested food in the stomach. When an animal anticipates eating, parasympathetic vagal impulses stimulate cells of the enteric nervous system (ENS), which in turn release acetylcholine (ACh) into the vicinity of G cells and parietal cells. These secretory cells have ACh receptors on their surfaces and respond by secreting gastrin and HCl, respectively. Gastrin circulates in the bloodstream and eventually finds its way to the parietal cells, which have gastrin receptors, in addition to ACh receptors, on their surfaces. The combined actions of gastrin

and ACh on the parietal cells result in high rates of HCl flow. The response of the stomach to anticipatory stimuli originating in the brain is referred to as the *cephalic phase* of gastric secretion.

Food entering the stomach initiates the second phase, or *gastric phase,* of gastric secretion. Distention of the stomach by food stimulates stretch receptors, providing afferent stimulation of the ENS; the system responds by direct nervous (ACh) stimulation of the G and parietal cells. In addition, food acts as a buffer, raising the stomach pH. This removes the inhibiting effect of acid on G-cell secretion, further stimulating the production of gastrin, which leads to even greater enhancement of acid production by the parietal cells.

Histamine plays a role as an amplifying substance in gastric acid secretion. Parietal cells have surface receptors for gastrin, ACh, and histamine. They are stimulated maximally when all three receptors are occupied. Histamine is secreted by *mast cells* and *enterochromaffin-like cells* in the parietal mucosa. The histamine-secreting cells are stimulated to secrete by gastrin and ACh. Thus the effects of gastrin and ACh on gastric acid secretion are amplified through their stimulation of histamine secretion.

As gastric secretion and digestion proceed, the pH of the stomach decreases. When the stomach pH falls to about 2, gastrin secretion is suppressed, and at a pH of 1, gastrin secretion is completely abolished. Thus the gastrin stimulus to the parietal cells is removed, and acid secretion is reduced.

The intestinal environment also influences the secretion of gastric acid. As acid contents from the stomach flow into the duodenum and the duodenal pH is reduced, gastric acid production is suppressed. The exact mechanism by which duodenal acidification exerts negative feedback on the parietal cells is unclear. The hormone *secretin*, produced in the duodenum, may be involved, as well as neuronal reflexes acting through the ENS.

The secretion of pepsinogen appears to be under the same regulatory influences as the secretion of HCl. However, regulation of pepsin secretion has been researched much less than regulation of HCl secretion.

THE PANCREAS

Pancreatic Exocrine Secretions Are Indispensable for the Digestion of the Complex Nutrients: Proteins, Starches, and Triglycerides

The pancreas is composed of two functionally separate types of glandular tissue. A small but important portion of the pancreatic tissue is arranged into discrete islets within the parenchyma of the gland. These cells are collectively called the *endocrine pancreas* because they secrete hormones into the bloodstream; the endocrine pancreas is discussed in Chapter 34. The great majority of the pancreatic tissue is involved with the elaboration of digestive secretions. This portion is known as the *exocrine pancreas* because its secretions are delivered into the intestinal lumen; the exocrine pancreas is the subject of this section.

Acinar Cells Secrete Enzymes, Whereas Centroacinar Cells and Duct Cells Secrete an Electrolyte Solution Rich in Sodium Bicarbonate

The exocrine pancreas is a typical acinar gland in which the end-pieces, or acini, are connected by an arborizing system of ducts; thus the gland conceptually resembles a bunch of grapes. Its general structure resembles the salivary gland, as illustrated in Figure 29-1. The cells of the acini contain a generous portion of rough endoplasmic reticulum, on which large amounts of secretory proteins, the digestive enzymes, are synthesized. Each pancreatic acinar cell can produce all of the more than 10 different enzymes secreted by the pancreas. Chapter 30 discusses the functions of the major digestive enzymes of the pancreas (see Table 30-1). Protein-digesting enzymes, which are potentially harmful to the pancreatic cells, are synthesized as zymogens in the same manner as pepsinogen synthesis in the gastric glands. After synthesis, the enzymes and proenzymes are stored in vesicles, or *zymogen granules,* near the cellular apex. When the cells are stimulated, the zymogen granules fuse with the plasma membrane and release their contents into the lumen of the gland and eventually into the duodenal lumen, where they are converted to the activated form of the enzyme.

Specialized cells near the junction of the acini and ducts are called *centroacinar cells.* The function of these cells, and to a lesser degree the duct epithelial cells, is to modify the electrolyte composition of the fluid secreted by the acinar cells. The electrolyte makeup of the acinar secretion initially resembles extracellular fluid, having a relatively high concentration of sodium and chloride. The centroacinar cells have on their luminal surface a chloride-bicarbonate exchange protein that transports bicarbonate out of the cell in exchange for chloride, thus greatly enriching the bicarbonate concentration of pancreatic fluid. This exchange protein does not require an energy input, and its action is driven by a high intracellular concentration of bicarbonate. This system is facilitated by electrolyte transport proteins on the *basolateral surface* of the cell (see Chapter 30). These transport proteins consist of Na^+,K^+-ATPase, an Na^+-HCO_3^- co-transporter, an H^+-Na^+ exchanger, and an H^+-ATPase. The Na^+-HCO_3^- co-transporter, in combination with carbonic anhydrase, generates bicarbonate within the cell, thus driving the chloride-bicarbonate exchange at the luminal membrane. The H^+ remaining from the dissociation of carbonic acid is removed from the cell at the basolateral membrane by Na^+-H^+ exchange and by the H^+-ATPase pump. The net result is that pancreatic fluid is a bicarbonate-rich, alkaline fluid that neutralizes the acid ingesta arriving in the duodenum from the stomach. In addition, the H^+ ions transported into the basal interstitial fluid of the pancreas are absorbed into the blood, balancing the "alkaline tide" that was created by gastric acid secretion.

In broad generality, the ion transport activities of the pancreatic duct cells are similar, but directionally opposite, to those of the parietal cells, as illustrated in Figure 29-4. The overall effect of the two secretory cell types is to mix hydrochloric acid with ingesta in the stomach and to neutralize the acid with sodium bicarbonate in the duodenum.

The ducts of the pancreatic lobules coalesce in an arborizing pattern to form either one or two main pancreatic ducts, depending on the species. The pancreatic duct or ducts may empty directly into the duodenum or, as in sheep, into the common bile duct. In the latter case, the pancreatic secretions enter the intestinal lumen along with bile.

Pancreatic Cells Have Cell Surface Receptors Stimulated by Acetylcholine, Cholecystokinin, and Secretin

When binding sites on the surfaces of pancreatic acinar, centro-acinar, or duct cells are occupied, the cells are stimulated to secrete. Each type of cell appears to have receptors for ACh as well as for cholecystokinin (CCK) and secretin. ACh, released from nerve endings near the cells, stimulates secretion, as do CCK and secretin arriving in the blood. CCK is the primary hormonal stimulus for acinar cells, whereas secretin is the primary

hormonal stimulus for centroacinar and duct cells. It appears, however, that maximal stimulation of the cells occurs when all receptors are occupied. Thus, acinar cells secrete most actively in the presence of all three ligands: ACh, CCK, and secretin. In this manner, secretin is said to *potentiate,* or increase, the action of CCK on acinar cells, and CCK potentiates the action of secretin on centroacinar and duct cells.

Nerve fibers ending in the vicinity of pancreatic acinar glands originate from cell bodies in the ENS, traveling outside the gut wall and into the pancreas. These neurons are stimulated to release ACh by impulses arriving from other neurons of the ENS, or by parasympathetic fibers arriving through the vagus nerve. Vagal stimulation of pancreatic secretion may arise as the result of several stimuli. The sight and smell of food induce centrally integrated vagal responses, leading to pancreatic secretion. This is known as the *cephalic phase* of pancreatic secretion, which is analogous in concept to the cephalic phase of salivary and gastric secretion. Distention of the stomach causes a vagovagal reflex stimulating pancreatic secretion, called the *gastric phase* of pancreatic secretion. The effects of the cephalic and gastric phases of pancreatic secretion are to "ready" the intestine for the imminent arrival of food by prior stimulation of pancreatic secretions.

The third phase, or *intestinal phase,* of pancreatic secretion is the most intense and involves endocrine as well as neuronal stimuli. This phase commences as food material from the stomach enters the duodenum. This leads to distention of the duodenum, which appears to produce enteric nerve impulses, resulting in ACh stimulation of pancreatic secretory cells. This stimulation reinforces and enhances the vagally mediated neuronal stimulation of the cephalic and gastric phases. The endocrine portion of the intestinal phase of pancreatic secretion occurs in response to the chemical stimulation that results from the presence of gastric contents in the duodenum. Peptides in the duodenal lumen, arising from the digestion of food protein, stimulate CCK production from endocrine cells in the duodenum. Fats in gastric ingesta also stimulate CCK secretion, whereas the low pH of material entering the duodenum from the stomach stimulates the secretion of secretin.

This stimulatory pattern is logical and results in a coordinated pattern of digestion. Proteins (peptides) and fats stimulate, through CCK, the secretion of protein-digesting and fat-digesting enzymes. These enzymes function best in an alkaline environment, and so the acid secretions of the stomach must be neutralized in order for these enzymes to be effective. Acid conditions in the duodenum stimulate pancreatic bicarbonate secretion through secretin, leading to alkalization of the ingesta. As food is digested and absorbed and acid is neutralized, the stimuli for pancreatic secretion are removed, and the amount of secretion diminishes to low, basal rates.

BILE SECRETION

One function of the liver is being a secretory gland of the digestive system. Its secretion, bile, has an important role in fat digestion.

The Liver Is an Acinar Gland with Small Acinar Lumina Known as *Canaliculi*

The liver is composed of *plates,* or one-cell–thick layers of hepatocytes that are bathed on either side by blood from the hepatic sinusoids. Between each row of cells is a small space created by cavitations in the plasma membranes of two apposing cells. The portions of the plasma membranes lining the spaces are isolated

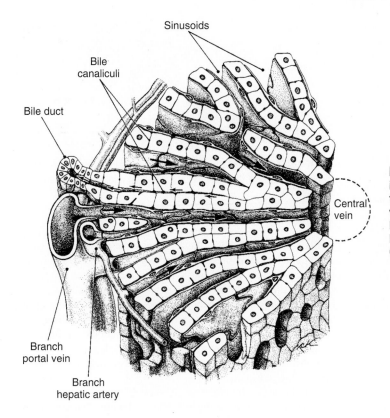

FIGURE 29-5 Hepatic microanatomy is complex and can be visualized in several ways. Note the relationship of the bile canaliculi to the bile ducts; the biliary system may be viewed as an acinar gland with the bile canaliculi forming a long, narrow acinus. (Modified from Ham AW: Textbook of *histology*, ed 5, Philadelphia, 1965, Lippincott. In Fawcett DW: *Bloom and Fawcett: a textbook of histology*, ed 12, Chapman & Hall, New York, 1994.)

from the remainder of the plasma membrane by tight junctions, which seal off the spaces from the surrounding extracellular environment. Within the plates of cells, these spaces join to form channels, or *canaliculi,* that connect to the *bile ductules.* Bile is secreted from the hepatocytes into the canaliculi, from which it flows into the bile duct system. From a functional standpoint, the canaliculi may be perceived as acini lined by hepatocytes and emptying into the biliary duct system, as illustrated in Figure 29-5. The bile duct epithelium is metabolically active and capable of altering the composition of canalicular bile by adding additional water and electrolytes, especially bicarbonate. In this function, the bile duct epithelial cells function in a manner similar or identical to the centroacinar and duct cells of the pancreas. In fact, they even respond to secretin by increasing their bicarbonate secretion.

Bile Contains Phospholipids and Cholesterol Maintained in Aqueous Solution by the Detergent Action of Bile Acids

Hepatocytes form bile acids from cholesterol. The chemical changes necessary to convert cholesterol to cholic acid, a representative bile acid, are shown in Figure 29-6. Cholesterol is almost totally insoluble in water, but the chemical changes involved in the conversion of cholesterol to bile acids result in a molecule with a water-soluble (*hydrophilic,* or "water-loving") side and a lipid-soluble (*hydrophobic,* or "water-hating") side. This combination hydrophobic-hydrophilic attribute is the characteristic property of a detergent. Because of this dual solubility, detergents can render lipids soluble in water. The function of the bile acids is to emulsify dietary lipids and to solubilize the products of fat digestion.

Bile acids are produced in the smooth endoplasmic reticulum of the hepatocytes. As they are secreted from the cells into the lumen of the canaliculi, bile acids "dissolve away" some of the cell

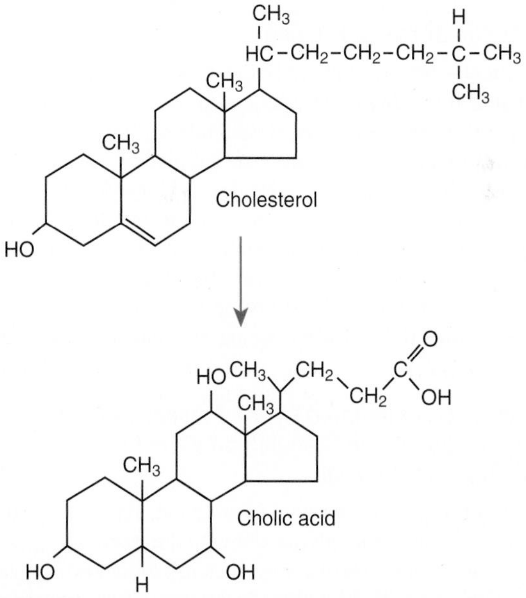

FIGURE 29-6 Conversion of cholesterol to cholic acid, a representative bile acid. Note the presence of two additional hydroxyl groups on the ring structure of cholic acid compared with cholesterol. These hydroxyl groups enhance the water solubility and detergent action of the bile acid molecule. Other bile acids differ from cholic acid in the number and position of hydroxyl groups.

membrane components: phospholipids and cholesterol. These constituents—phospholipids, cholesterol, and bile acids—are the major functional components of bile and are important for the digestion and absorption of fats. The mechanism by which bile aids in fat digestion is discussed in Chapter 30.

Bile acids are secreted into the canaliculi as their sodium salts. The presence of bile acid salts and sodium in the canaliculi draws water, by osmosis, from the cells into bile. The electrolyte composition of canalicular bile usually resembles that of plasma but may be somewhat lower in chloride. As bile flows through the bile ducts, water and electrolytes are added. Bicarbonate may be secreted by the duct cells, so the bicarbonate concentration of bile is often higher than that in blood serum.

In addition to bile acids, phospholipids, and cholesterol, bile contains other lipid-soluble organic substances. Of these, the *bile pigments* are present in the highest concentration. Bile pigments are breakdown products of heme porphyrin, a portion of the hemoglobin molecule. The principal bile pigment is *bilirubin,* which is produced during the normal process of red blood cell turnover. Bilirubin gives bile its characteristic green color. In the lumen of the gut, bilirubin is converted by bacterial action to other compounds. These secondary compounds are responsible for the characteristic brown color of the feces of nonherbivorous animals. Bile pigments serve no useful digestive function: the body simply uses bile, and ultimately feces, as a route for the excretion of these waste products.

The liver serves as an excretory organ for many lipid-soluble substances in addition to bilirubin. The detergent action of the bile acids makes the liver an ideal excretory organ, in comparison with the kidney, for these types of compounds. Substances metabolized and secreted by the liver include many important drugs and toxins. This is important clinically because the actions of these agents can be potentiated by impaired liver function.

The Gallbladder Stores and Concentrates Bile During the Periods Between Feeding

When there is little or no food in the intestinal lumen, the *sphincter of Oddi,* at the union of the common bile duct and duodenum, is closed. With this sphincter closed, bile cannot enter the intestine and is diverted instead into the gallbladder. The gallbladder epithelium absorbs sodium, chloride, and bicarbonate from bile; water is absorbed passively. Thus, in the gallbladder the organic constituents of bile are concentrated, and the volume of bile is reduced. In species that have no gallbladder, such as horses and rats, the sphincter of Oddi is apparently nonfunctional, and bile is secreted into the intestine during all phases of the digestive cycle.

Bile Secretion Is Initiated by the Presence of Food in the Duodenum and Stimulated by the Return of Bile Acids to the Liver

When food, especially fat-containing food, reaches the duodenum, the GI endocrine cells are stimulated to secrete CCK, which in turn causes relaxation of the sphincter of Oddi and contraction of the gallbladder. These actions force stored bile into the intestine. Bile acids aid in the digestion and absorption of fats in the jejunum (see Chapter 30) but are not absorbed themselves until they reach the ileum. After absorption in the ileum, the bile acids travel via the hepatic portal vein to the liver. In the liver, bile acids are almost completely absorbed from the portal blood. As a result, almost no bile acids reach the posterior *venae cavae,* and they are consequently found only in low concentrations in the systemic circulation. The flow of bile acids from liver to intestine to portal blood to liver and back to intestine is known as *enterohepatic circulation* (Figure 29-7).

Bile acids arriving at the liver, by way of the portal circulation, stimulate further bile synthesis. Thus a positive feedback system

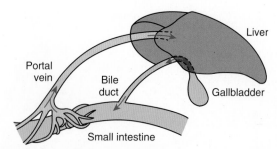

FIGURE 29-7 Bile acids and other molecules circulate in an enterohepatic cycle. Phases of the cycle include the portal vein, biliary system, and intestinal lumen.

is initiated when the gallbladder contracts: the absorption of gallbladder bile from the intestine stimulates additional bile synthesis by the hepatocytes. Rapid bile synthesis and secretion continue as long as the sphincter of Oddi is open and the gallbladder is contracted. When fats have been digested and absorbed, the stimulus for CCK secretion is removed, resulting in closure of the sphincter of Oddi and diversion of bile to the gallbladder. Because bile acids are no longer reaching the intestine, they are no longer being absorbed, and thus the stimulus for bile secretion is reduced, and bile flow slows down.

In addition to the effect of CCK on bile secretion, secretin influences secretion from the bile duct epithelium. Secretin stimulates water and bicarbonate secretion from the bile ducts in a manner similar to that of its effects on the duct cells of the pancreas. Thus, bile may participate in the neutralization of stomach acids.

CLINICAL CORRELATIONS

HORSE IN PAIN WITH WEIGHT LOSS

History. A 4-year-old Thoroughbred mare presents for weight loss, inappetence, grinding of teeth, and low-grade colic. She is off the track now but was winning until 1 month ago, and thus the trainer is concerned.

Clinical Examination. The mare seems to be quieter than expected. Her temperature, pulse, and respiration are normal. She appears thin for a horse from the track, and the trainer thinks the mare has lost 100 to 150 pounds in the last month. Her hair coat is poor. Your examination reveals no other abnormal findings.

With this history, gastric ulcers are a likely differential diagnosis. You discuss this with the trainer and decide to perform gastroscopy before doing any other diagnostic tests.

Comment. On endoscopy the mare has several ulcers along the junction of the squamous and glandular sections of the gastric epithelium. In addition, she has two large and a few small ulcers on the nonglandular squamous compartment of the stomach. The squamous epithelium of the equine stomach has no mucus-secreting glands, in contrast to the glandular mucosa. The thick alkaline mucus that coats the glandular surface is an important component of the stomach epithelium's natural defense against acid damage. The lack of surface mucus makes the squamous portion of the equine stomach particularly prone to ulcer development. Ulcers are likely the cause of this horse's weight loss, colic, and poor performance. She will be treated, and her management will be modified to encourage healing of the ulcers.

Horses continuously secrete hydrochloric acid (HCl) in the stomach, in contrast to many other species that can modulate acid secretion based on food intake. Horses are thus suited to be constant grazers with access to food 24 hr/day. This mare is kept in the stall 24 hr/day unless she is being worked, and she is given a high-grain low-hay diet. Thus, she eats two high-grain meals per day, and she only has a small amount of grass hay, which she typically eats quickly. When horses do not eat, the pH of the stomach decreases rapidly. Furthermore, being inside all the time adds to her stress, making this mare more prone to gastric ulcers. Histamine and gastrin also stimulate HCl secretion, whereas somatostatin inhibits it. Therefore, treatment is multifactorial, aimed at changing the management to increase the pH of the stomach as well as administering drugs to help decrease acid secretion.

The parietal cells secrete HCl through H^+,K^+-ATPase (proton pump). Omeprazole, a once-daily medication, inhibits the proton pump. Other anti-ulcer medications include histamine type 2 receptor antagonists, such as cimetidine and ranitidine, which block histamine attachment to stimulatory receptors on the surface of parietal cells, decreasing HCl release. Another way to protect the stomach from acid damage is to coat the gastric lining with medications such as sucralfate, which forms a protective barrier between the mucosa and luminal contents.

Treatment. A common treatment choice in this case currently is omeprazole, which specifically decreases HCl secretion. Treatment depends on the severity of the ulcers and the inciting cause. In many cases, treatment may be recommended for up to 28 days. Additional management changes to enhance healing would include increasing the time per day the mare spends eating. Pasture would be ideal, particularly alfalfa forage, which has inherent buffering capacity. Gradually decreasing the amount of grain fed daily and increasing the amount of forage would also be beneficial. Although these management changes are ideal, they can be difficult to maintain because of the typical management of these horses.

PANCREATITIS IN A DOG

History. A 10-year-old female spayed overweight beagle escaped from the backyard. She was found by the owners in the neighbor's trashcan, eating discarded food. This was 2 days after a festive holiday, during which she had been given additional treats, including more fat than normal. About 12 hours after the dog had gotten into the garbage, she was depressed, and not eating as well. Twenty-four hours after eating the trash, she was vomiting and had diarrhea, as well as a fever.

Clinical Examination. The clients take the dog to their veterinarian. The veterinarian determines that the dog has a fever of 103.9, and she has a painful abdomen on palpation, particularly on the right side. She is still vomiting and has continued to have diarrhea. She is dehydrated. Blood work demonstrates an increased white cell count, demonstrating inflammation. Additionally, her amylase, lipase, and serum pancreatic lipase immunoreactivity (cPLI) are markedly increased. Abdominal radiographs demonstrate decreased contrast and a ground glass appearance in the region of the pancreas. Ultrasound of the pancreas demonstrates enlargement and some localized peritoneal fluid.

Comment. This dog has pancreatitis, which was likely triggered by the increased ingestion of fatty food. With a normal functioning pancreas, many of the enzymes are made in the inactive form (zymogens) and stored in intracellular zymogen granules. They are activated by cleavage of the amino-terminal polypeptide chain. Zymogens are normally not activated until they reach the small intestine. Cells in the duodenum have enteropeptidase, which cleaves the peptide from trypsinogen to activate trypsin. The latter cleaves the activation peptide from other digestive zymogens, thus providing considerable control over enzyme activity. Lysosomes are intracellular organelles that represent the cell's digestive system, and contain enzymes capable of activating trypsinogen. Normally, the zymogens (in zymogen granules) and lysosomes are kept separately from each other. During pancreatitis the zymogen granules and lysosomes can fuse, and their contents can mix together in intracellular vacuoles, leading to premature, increased, intracellular activation of zygomens. Such abnormal activation leads to local damage of pancreatic cells. Other regulation of pancreatic function is associated with inhibitors, such as pancreatic secretory trypsin inhibitor (PSTI). PSTI protectively inhibits trypsin if premature trypsinogen activation occurs within the acinar cell or duct system. However, if the pH is low, which occurs in the abnormal fusion vacuoles, this mechanism of regulation does not work. Additionally, if there is premature intracellular activation of trypsinogen, trypsin, and zymogens, this causes additional activation of other zymogens, thus leading to additional pancreatic damage. With pancreatitis, whether it is mild or more severe, many inflammatory mediators are also released, including TNF-alpha, IL-1, IL-2, IL-6, IL-8, IL-10, IFN-alpha, IFN-gamma, and platelet activating factor. Inflammation can be controlled by plasma protease inhibitors, including alpha macroglobulins, as well as alpha proteinase inhibitors. If these inhibitors are severely depleted, free proteases activate the coagulation, fibrinolytic and complement cascades. This can lead to shock, disseminated intravascular coagulation (DIC), and death. The exact causes of pancreatitis are not known. It is more prevalent in obese dogs.

Treatment. Stabilization of patients with fluid/electrolyte therapy is recommended. Additionally, analgesics and antibiotics are often recommended. Both parenteral and enteral feeding, after vomiting ceases, have been recommended. Prognosis varies, depending on cause, severity, and chronicity of disease.

PRACTICE QUESTIONS

1. In monogastric animals, saliva produced during periods of rapid secretion has a higher electrolyte concentration than saliva produced during periods of slow salivary secretion. From your understanding of salivary gland physiology, which appears to be the most likely explanation?
   a. During periods of slow salivary secretion, the acinar cells are inactive, and low-electrolyte saliva is secreted by the duct cells.
   b. Parasympathetic stimulation of the acinar cells results in the elaboration of a more electrolyte-rich saliva.
   c. Gastrin stimulation increases the electrolyte concentration of saliva.
   d. During rapid secretion, fluid produced by the acinar cells is exposed to the actions of the duct cells for a shorter time than during slow rates of secretion.
   e. Different cell types within the acinus are responsible for salivary production, depending on the type of stimulus.

2. Some nutritionists are experimenting with a drug that increases salivary secretion in cattle. What effect do you think this would have on rumen pH?
   a. Increase rumen pH
   b. Decrease rumen pH
   c. Have no effect on rumen pH

3. Inhibition of the enzyme carbonic anhydrase is likely to have what effect on gastric pH?
   a. Decrease gastric pH
   b. Increase gastric pH
   c. Have no effect on gastric pH

4. Which of the following is *not* a potential stimulus for gastric acid secretion?
   a. Norepinephrine secretion resulting from stimulation of sympathetic nerves.
   b. Vagal nerve activity resulting from the sight of food.
   c. The presence of undigested protein in the pyloric antrum.
   d. Acetylcholine release stimulated by gastric stretch receptors acting on nerves of the ENS.
   e. Histamine release from cells in the gastric mucosa.

5. Which of the following is *not* a natural ligand for receptors in the pancreas?
   a. Cholecystokinin
   b. Acetylcholine
   c. Gastrin
   d. Secretin

BIBLIOGRAPHY

Barrett K: *Gastrointestinal physiology*, Columbus, Ohio, 2006, McGraw-Hill.

Chandra R, Liddle RA: Neural and hormonal regulation of pancreatic secretion, *Curr Opin Gastroenterol* 25(5):441–446, 2009.

Del Valle J, Todisco A: Gastric secretion. In Yamada T, editor: *Textbook of gastroenterology*, vol 1, ed 5, Philadelphia, 2009, Lippincott, Williams & Wilkins.

Esteller A: Physiology of bile secretion, *World J Gastroenterol* 14(37):5641–5649, 2008.

Johnson LR: *Gastrointestinal physiology*, ed 7, Philadelphia, 2007, Mosby Physiology Monograph Series (Elsevier).

Keating N, Keely SJ: Bile acids in regulation of intestinal physiology, *Curr Gastroenterol Rep* 11(5):375–382, 2009.

Kopic S, Geibel JP: Update on the mechanisms of gastric acid secretion, *Curr Gastroenterol Rep* 12(6):458–464, 2010.

Monte MJ, Marin JJ, Antelo A, et al: Bile acids: chemistry, physiology, and pathophysiology, *World J Gastroenterol* 15(7):804–816, 2009.

Owyang C, Williams JA: Pancreatic secretion. In Yamada T, editor: *Textbook of gastroenterology*, vol 1, ed 5, Philadelphia, 2009, Lippincott Williams & Wilkins.

Schubert ML: Gastric secretion, *Curr Opin Gastroenterol* 26(6):598–603, 2010.

Stevens CE, Hume ID: *Comparative physiology of the vertebrate digestive system*, ed 2, Cambridge, UK, 1995, Cambridge University Press.

Weinman SA, Jalil S: Bile excretion and cholestasis. In Yamada T, editor: *Textbook of gastroenterology*, vol 1, ed 5, Philadelphia, 2009, Lippincott, Williams & Wilkins.

Williams DA, Steiner JM: Canine exocrine pancreatic disease. In Ettinger SJ, Feldman EC, editors: *Textbook of veterinary internal medicine: diseases of the dog and cat*, ed 6, St Louis, 2005, Elsevier.

Williams JA: Regulation of acinar cell function in the pancreas, *Curr Opin Gastroenterol* 26(5):478–483, 2010.

CHAPTER 30

Digestion and Absorption: The Nonfermentative Processes

KEY POINTS

1. Digestion and absorption are separate, but related, processes.
2. The small-intestinal mucosa has a large surface area and epithelial cells with "leaky" junctions between them.
3. The intestinal surface microenvironment consists of glycocalyx, mucus, and an unstirred water layer.

Digestion

1. Breaking down food particle size by physical action is an important part of the digestive process.
2. Chemical digestion results in the reduction of complex nutrients into simpler molecules.
3. Luminal-phase carbohydrate digestion results in the production of short-chain polysaccharides.
4. Luminal-phase digestion of carbohydrates applies only to starches, because sugars are digested in the membranous phase.
5. Proteins are digested by a variety of luminal-phase enzymes.
6. Membranous-phase digestive enzymes are a structural part of the intestinal surface membrane.
7. Membranous-phase digestion occurs within the microenvironment of the unstirred water layer, intestinal mucus, and glycocalyx.
8. A specific membranous-phase enzyme exists for the digestion of each type of polysaccharide.
9. Complete digestion of peptides to free amino acids takes place both on the enterocyte surface and within the cells.

Intestinal absorption

1. Specialized nutrient transport systems exist in the apical and basolateral membranes.
2. Secondary and tertiary active transport mechanisms utilize the transcellular sodium ion electrochemical gradient as their source of energy.
3. Passive transport occurs either through specialized channels in cell membranes or directly through the tight junctions.
4. The products of membranous-phase digestion are absorbed by sodium co-transport.

Absorption of water and electrolytes

1. There are at least three distinct mechanisms of sodium absorption.
2. There are three major mechanisms of chloride absorption.
3. Bicarbonate ion is secreted by several digestive glands and must be recovered from the gut if body acid-base balance is to be maintained.
4. Potassium is absorbed primarily by passive diffusion through the paracellular route.

5. The major mechanisms of electrolyte absorption are selectively distributed along the gut.
6. All intestinal water absorption is passive, occurring because of the absorption of osmotically active solutes.

Intestinal secretion of water and electrolytes

1. Passive increases in luminal osmotic pressure occur during hydrolytic digestion and result in water secretion.
2. Active secretion of electrolytes from the crypt epithelium leads to intestinal water secretion.

Gastrointestinal blood flow

1. Water and solute movement between the lateral spaces and villous capillaries is subject to the same forces that govern water and solute movement between the extracellular and vascular fluids in other tissues.
2. Absorbed nutrients enter the capillaries by diffusion from the lateral spaces.
3. A countercurrent, osmotic-multiplier system may increase the osmolality of blood at the tips of the villi, further promoting absorption of water into the blood.
4. Disturbances in the venous drainage from the intestine can greatly affect the mechanisms of capillary absorption in the villi.

Digestion and absorption of fats

1. Detergent action as well as enzymatic action is necessary for the digestion and absorption of lipids.
2. Lipids are absorbed through the apical membrane by carrier proteins and simple diffusion.
3. Bile acids are reabsorbed from the ileum by a sodium co-transport system.
4. Absorbed lipids are packaged into chylomicrons before leaving the enterocytes.

Growth and development of the intestinal epithelium

1. The length of intestinal villi is determined by the relative rates of cell loss at the tips and cell replenishment at the base.

Digestion in the neonate

1. During the first few hours of life, proteins are not digested but are absorbed intact.
2. The major intestinal disaccharidase switches from lactase to maltase with maturity.

Pathophysiology of diarrhea

1. Diarrhea occurs when there is a mismatch between secretion and absorption.

Digestion and Absorption Are Separate, but Related, Processes

Digestion is the process of breaking down complex nutrients into simple molecules. In contrast, *absorption* is the process of transporting those simple molecules across the intestinal epithelium (Figure 30-1). The two processes are the result of different biochemical events occurring within the gut. Both processes are necessary for the assimilation of nutrients into the body; absorption cannot occur if food is not digested, and the process of digestion is fruitless if the digested nutrients cannot be absorbed.

Disturbances of nutrient assimilation are common in veterinary medicine and may be caused by a variety of diseases, with some affecting digestion and others affecting absorption. The overt signs of failure of nutrient assimilation are often similar, but the biochemical lesions and specific therapies associated with *maldigestive* disease can be quite different from those associated with *malabsorptive* disease. Therefore, diagnosing the cause of failure of nutrient assimilation is a frequent challenge faced by veterinary clinicians, a challenge that requires a thorough understanding of the physiology of nutrient digestion and absorption. This chapter first reviews the structural characteristics of the small-intestinal epithelium that are of particular importance to the digestive and absorptive processes.

The Small-Intestinal Mucosa Has a Large Surface Area and Epithelial Cells with "Leaky" Junctions Between Them

Contact between the small-intestinal mucosa and the luminal contents is facilitated by an extensive intestinal surface area. Three levels of surface convolutions serve to expand the surface area of the small intestine (see Figure 27-2). First, large folds of mucosa known as *plicae circulares* add to the intestinal surface area of some animals, but these are not present in all species. Second, the mucosal surface is covered with fingerlike epithelial projections

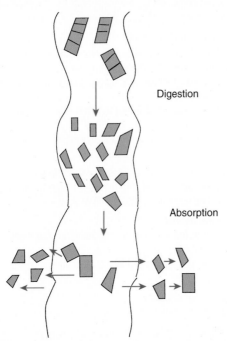

FIGURE 30-1 Digestion is the process of reducing macromolecules to their constituent monomers. Absorption is the transport of the resultant monomers across the intestinal epithelium into the bloodstream.

Digestion

Absorption

known as *villi*. These structures are present in all species and increase the intestinal surface area by tenfold to fourteenfold compared with a flat surface of equal size. Third, the villi themselves are covered with a brushlike surface membrane known as the *brush border*. The brush border is composed of submicroscopic *microvilli* that further enlarge the surface area (Figure 30-2). At the base of the villi are glandlike structures known as *crypts of Lieberkühn* (Figure 30-3). The villi and crypts are covered with a continuous layer of cellular epithelium.

The epithelial cells covering the villi and crypts are called *enterocytes*. Each enterocyte has two distinct types of cell membranes (Figure 30-4). The cell surface facing the lumen is called the *apex* and is covered by the *apical membrane*. The apical membrane contains the microvilli. Under the light microscope, the microvilli give the cell surface its brushlike appearance. This appearance has led to the term *brush border*, which is synonymous with *apical membrane*. Attached to the apical membrane are many *glycoproteins*. These specialized proteins are synthesized within the enterocytes and transferred to the apical membrane. They are the enzymes and transport molecules responsible for the digestive and absorptive functions of the intestinal epithelium. Under the intense magnification of the electron microscope these proteins, which extend into the intestinal lumen, give the microvilli a fuzzy appearance (see Figure 30-2). This rich area of glycoproteins on the surface of the apical membranes is given the name *glycocalyx*. The apical membrane is a complex cellular membrane with an unusually high protein content.

The remaining portion of the enterocyte plasma membrane, that part not facing the gut lumen, is called the *basolateral membrane*, referring to the base and sides of the cell. This membrane is not especially unusual and indeed has many similarities to cell membranes of other tissues. Although the basolateral membrane is not in direct contact with ingesta in the gut lumen, it serves an important role in intestinal absorption; nutrients that are absorbed into the enterocytes through the apical membrane must exit the cell through the basolateral membrane before gaining access to the bloodstream.

The attachments between adjacent enterocytes are called *tight junctions*. These connections serve a special function in the process of digestion and absorption. The tight junctions form a narrow band of attachment between adjacent enterocytes. The band is near the apical end of the cells and divides the apical membrane from the basolateral membrane. The junctions may be called "tight," but from a molecular standpoint, they are rather loose. This is especially true in the duodenum and jejunum, where the tight junctions are loose enough to allow the free passage of water and small electrolytes. Recent evidence indicates that the relative impermeability, or "tightness," of the tight junctions is not constant and can be altered by neurohumoral regulatory substances in the gut. These selective changes in permeability can affect the rates of water and ion movement across the gastrointestinal (GI) epithelium, depending on the physiological needs for secretion or absorption. However, the tight junctions are never permeable enough to permit the passage of organic molecules.

The narrow band of tight junctions leaves the majority of the basolateral membrane unattached to its neighboring membrane on the adjacent enterocyte. This arrangement creates a potential space between enterocytes. This area between the lateral surfaces of the enterocytes is called the *lateral space*. The lateral spaces are normally distended and filled with extracellular fluid (ECF). At the end of the lateral spaces nearest the apical membrane, the ECF

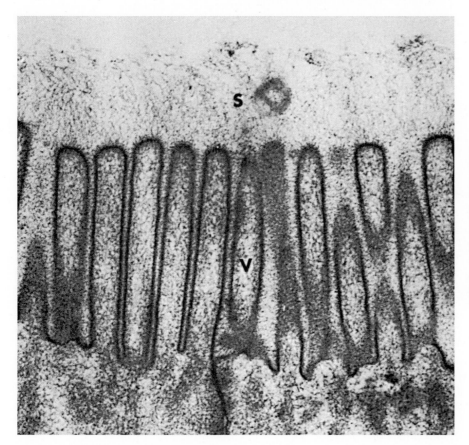

FIGURE 30-2 Electron micrograph of the microvilli of the intestinal brush border. The brush border is composed of the apical membranes of enterocytes. Note the indistinct array of molecular material *(S)* that radiates away from the microvilli *(V);* membranous-phase digestion occurs within this array of molecular material, which includes the membrane-bound digestive enzymes. (From Johnson LR, Christensen J, Jacobsen ED, et al, editors: *Physiology of the gastrointestinal tract,* ed 2, New York, 1987, Raven Press.)

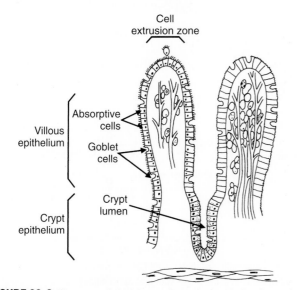

FIGURE 30-3 The one-cell-thick layer of intestinal epithelium is continuous over the villi and the crypts of Lieberkühn.

The Intestinal Surface Microenvironment Consists of Glycocalyx, Mucus, and an Unstirred Water Layer

Liberally interspersed among the enterocytes are *goblet cells,* which secrete a rich layer of mucus that covers the mucosa. At the brush border surface, the mucus blends into the glycocalyx, with the two layers forming a viscous coating that tends to trap molecules near the apical membrane. In addition to the mucus and glycocalyx layers, there is an area near the intestinal surface known as the *unstirred water layer.* With respect to the unstirred water layer, the intestine can be likened to a large stream or river; that is, the water in the center flows relatively rapidly, whereas the water near the edge or bank is quiet and flows slowly. Because of the same fluid-friction phenomenon that causes the water on the banks of rivers to be less turbulent and to flow at a slower rate than water in center stream, the water very near the intestinal surface is quiet and flows at a much slower rate than water in the central part of the lumen. The unstirred water layer, mucus, and glycocalyx form an important diffusion barrier through which nutrients must pass before entering the enterocytes.

DIGESTION

Breaking Down Food Particle Size by Physical Action Is an Important Part of the Digestive Process

The overall process of digestion is the physical and chemical breaking down of food particles and molecules into subunits suitable for absorption. Physical reduction of food particle size is important not only because it allows food to flow through the relatively narrow digestive tube, but also because it enlarges the surface area of the food particles, thus increasing the area exposed

is separated from the fluid of the intestinal lumen only by the tight junctions. At the opposite end of the lateral spaces, the ECF is separated from the blood only by the basement membrane of the intestinal capillaries. Both the tight junctions and the capillary endothelium are permeable barriers that allow the free passage of water and small molecules. Thus, there is relatively free flow of water and most electrolytes among the fluid in the lumen of the intestine, the ECF in the lateral spaces, and the blood.

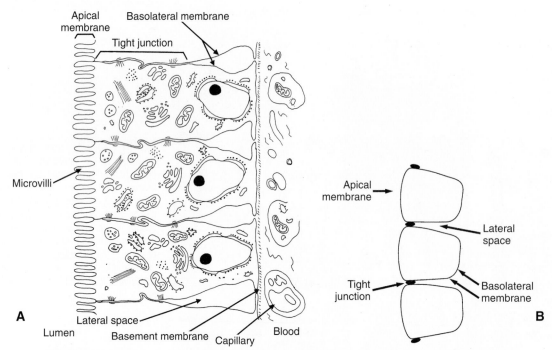

FIGURE 30-4 Understanding the anatomical relationships of the enterocytes, tight junctions, apical membrane, basolateral membrane, and lateral spaces is critical to an understanding of the physiology of intestinal absorption. **A**, Anatomic illustration of the intestinal epithelium. **B**, Stylized sketch of the epithelium, including a capillary containing formed elements of blood. It is important to understand the relationship between part *A* and part *B* of this diagram.

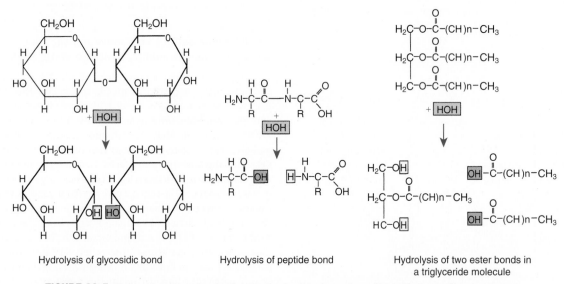

Hydrolysis of glycosidic bond   Hydrolysis of peptide bond   Hydrolysis of two ester bonds in a triglyceride molecule

FIGURE 30-5 Major polymeric molecules forming food nutrients can be split into their constituent monomers by the insertion of a water molecule. This process, referred to as *hydrolysis,* is the major action of the digestive enzymes.

to the actions of digestive enzymes. Physical reduction of food particle size begins with mastication (chewing) but is completed by the grinding action of the distal stomach. In the distal stomach the physical action of grinding is aided by the chemical actions of pepsin and hydrochloric acid. The chemical actions of these stomach secretions break down connective tissue and thus aid in breaking apart food particles, especially foods of animal origin. The reduction of food particle size by physical means is essentially complete when food leaves the stomach, as described in Chapter 28 in the discussion of motility of the distal stomach.

Chemical Digestion Results in the Reduction of Complex Nutrients into Simpler Molecules

Chemical digestion of each major nutrient is accomplished by the process of *hydrolysis,* the splitting of a chemical bond by the insertion of a water molecule. Glycosidic linkages in carbohydrates, peptide bonds in proteins, ester bonds in fats, and phosphodiester bonds in nucleic acids are all cleaved by hydrolysis during digestion. Figure 30-5 illustrates hydrolytic splitting of these various chemical bonds.

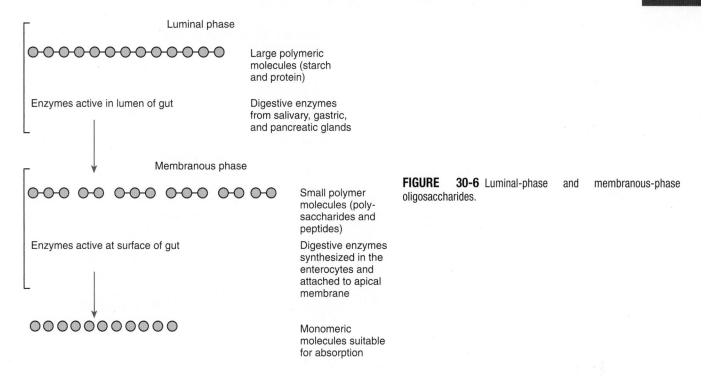

FIGURE 30-6 Luminal-phase and membranous-phase oligosaccharides.

Hydrolysis in the digestive tract is catalyzed by the action of enzymes. There are two general classes of digestive enzymes: those that act within the lumen of the gut, and those that act at the membrane surface of the epithelium. Enzymes acting within the lumen originate from the major GI glands, including the salivary gland, gastric glands, and especially the pancreas. The secretions of these glands become thoroughly mixed with ingesta and exert their actions throughout the lumen of their associated gut segments; thus the actions they catalyze are referred to as the *luminal phase* of digestion. In general, luminal-phase digestion results in the incomplete hydrolysis of nutrients, resulting in the formation of short-chain polymers from the original macromolecules (Figure 30-6).

The hydrolytic process is completed by enzymes that are chemically bound to the surface epithelium of the small intestine. These enzymes break the short-chain polymers resulting from luminal-phase digestion into monomers that can be absorbed across the epithelium. This final phase, which occurs at the epithelial membrane surface, is referred to as the *membranous phase* of digestion. Membranous-phase digestion is followed closely by absorption.

Luminal-Phase Carbohydrate Digestion Results in the Production of Short-Chain Polysaccharides

Carbohydrates are nutrients containing carbon, hydrogen, and oxygen atoms arranged as long chains of repeating simple-sugar molecules. Dietary carbohydrates originate primarily from plants. There are three general types of plant carbohydrates: fibers, sugars, and starches. *Fibers,* the structural parts of plants, form an important energy source for herbivorous animals; however, plant fibers are not subject to hydrolytic digestion by mammalian enzymes and therefore cannot be digested directly by animals (see Chapter 31).

Sugars are energy-transport molecules in plants. Sugars, or *saccharides,* may be *simple* (made up of a single molecular unit, monosaccharides) or *complex* (made up of two or more repeating saccharide subunits, polysaccharides). *Glucose, galactose,* and

fructose are the most important simple sugars in animal diets. These monosaccharides are present, preformed in small quantities, in normal diets; however, most monosaccharides absorbed from the gut arise from the enzymatic hydrolysis of more complex carbohydrates. Complex sugars are referred to as *disaccharides, trisaccharides,* and *oligosaccharides,* depending on the number of repeating simple-sugar subunits. Oligosaccharides contain several monomer units, usually between 3 and 10. Important complex sugars in animal diets are *lactose,* or milk sugar, and *sucrose,* or table sugar. Lactose is a disaccharide composed of glucose and galactose, whereas sucrose is a disaccharide composed of glucose and fructose. Other important complex sugars are *maltose, isomaltose,* and *maltotriose;* these three sugars are composed of two or three repeating glucose units (Figure 30-7). They are seldom present preformed in the diet but rather are formed in the gut as intermediate products of starch digestion.

Starch is an energy-storage carbohydrate of plants that forms the major energy-yielding nutrient in the diets of many omnivorous animals, such as pigs, rats, and primates. There are two chemical forms of starch, *amylose* and *amylopectin.* Both are long-chain glucose polymers, but amylose is a straight-chain molecule containing glucose monomers linked by $\alpha[1\text{-}4]$ glycosidic linkages. Amylopectin also contains glucose chains joined by $\alpha[1\text{-}4]$ glycosidic linkages, but the amylopectin chains are branched, having an $\alpha[1\text{-}6]$ linkage at each branch point (see Figure 30-7). Although the chemical structure of starch is limited to these two molecular types, the physical structure and encapsulation of starches vary among plant sources. This variation results in the unique characteristics of starches from different sources, such as wheat, corn, and barley.

Luminal-Phase Digestion of Carbohydrates Applies Only to Starches, Because Sugars Are Digested in the Membranous Phase

The enzyme involved in luminal starch digestion is α-amylase, which is actually a mixture of several similar molecules. This enzyme arises from the pancreas in all species, as well as from the salivary glands of some species (see Chapter 29). The α[1-4] linkages of either amylose or amylopectin are attacked by α-amylase. Characteristic of luminal-phase digestion, α-amylase does not break off, or *cleave,* single glucose units from the ends of the chain. Rather, the starch chains are broken in their midsections, resulting in the production of polysaccharides of intermediate chain length, known as *dextrins.* These chains continue to be attacked until disaccharide (maltose) and trisaccharide (maltotriose) units are formed.

This digestive process proceeds for amylopectin in the same way as it does for amylose, except that the α[1-6] linkages at the chain branch points of amylopectin are not hydrolyzed. Because these branch points are not hydrolyzed, branch-chain oligosaccharides, known as *limit dextrins,* as well as an α[1-6]-linked disaccharide, known as *isomaltose,* are formed (see Figure 30-7). The end result of luminal-phase carbohydrate digestion is the creation of many disaccharides, trisaccharides, and oligosaccharides from large starch molecules. These complex sugars are not hydrolyzed further in the luminal phase.

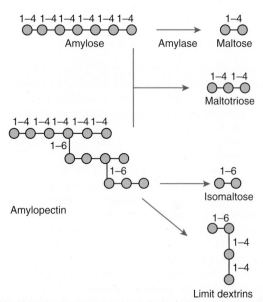

FIGURE 30-7 Two major forms of dietary starch are amylose and amylopectin. Amylose is composed of repeating glucose units joined by α[1-4] linkages. Amylopectin is a similar molecule, except that it has branch points formed by α[1-6] linkages. Because of the different linkage points, various polysaccharides result from luminal-phase digestion, as illustrated.

Proteins Are Digested by a Variety of Luminal-Phase Enzymes

Proteins are a source of amino acids, which are essential components of all animal diets. Dietary proteins come from both plant and animal sources. The general pattern of protein digestion is similar to that of carbohydrate digestion, in that large molecular proteins are broken down into small peptide chains by luminal digestion. Subsequent digestion of the peptide chains to individual amino acids occurs to a large extent by membranous-phase digestion, although unlike in carbohydrate digestion, a portion of free monomers, that is, amino acids, is released in the luminal phase.

A major difference between protein digestion and carbohydrate digestion is in the number of different enzyme types involved. The relatively larger number of enzymes involved in protein digestion is expected, considering that starch molecules are made up of only one type of monomer, glucose, and protein molecules are made up of a variety of amino acids. Therefore, only bonds between glucose molecules need to be broken in the case of starch. On the other hand, proteins are made up of infinite combinations of up to 20 individual types of amino acids; the various proteolytic enzymes are necessary for digestion because they differ in their efficiency in cleaving peptide bonds between specific types of amino acids.

The major luminal-phase proteolytic enzymes are listed in Table 30-1. Most proteolytic enzymes are *endopeptidases,* meaning that they break proteins at internal points along the amino acid chains, resulting in the production of short-chain peptides from complex proteins. Endopeptidases produce essentially no free amino acids. Two *exopeptidases,* which release individual amino acids from ends of peptide chains, are secreted also from the pancreas and are active in luminal-phase digestion.

The proteolytic enzymes are secreted from the stomach glands or pancreas in the form of inactive *zymogens* (see Chapter 29), which are activated in the stomach or intestinal lumen, respectively. These enzymes must be secreted in an inactive form; otherwise, the active enzymes would digest the cells in which they are synthesized. Activation of the zymogens occurs in the gut lumen. The proteolytic zymogens of the stomach, *pepsinogen* and *chymosinogen,* are activated by hydrochloric acid (HCl) in the stomach lumen. Pepsinogen is also activated by pepsin in an autocatalytic feedback loop. *Trypsinogen* from the pancreas is activated by *enterokinase,* an enzyme elaborated by duodenal mucosal cells. The active enzyme, *trypsin,* then serves as an autocatalytic agent to activate additional trypsinogen as well as the other pancreatic protein-digesting enzymes. Figure 30-8 illustrates the cascade of intraluminal zymogen activation.

TABLE 30-1 Luminal-Phase Enzymes of Protein Digestion

Enzyme	Action	Source	Precursor	Activator
Pepsin	Endopeptidase	Gastric glands	Pepsinogen	Hydrochloric acid, pepsin
Chymosin (rennin)	Endopeptidase	Gastric glands	Chymosinogen	?
Trypsin	Endopeptidase	Pancreas	Trypsinogen	Enterokinase, trypsin
Chymotrypsin	Endopeptidase	Pancreas	Chymotrypsinogen	Trypsin
Elastase	Endopeptidase	Pancreas	Proelastase	Trypsin
Carboxypeptidase A	Exopeptidase	Pancreas	Procarboxypeptidase A	Trypsin
Carboxypeptidase B	Exopeptidase	Pancreas	Procarboxypeptidase B	Trypsin

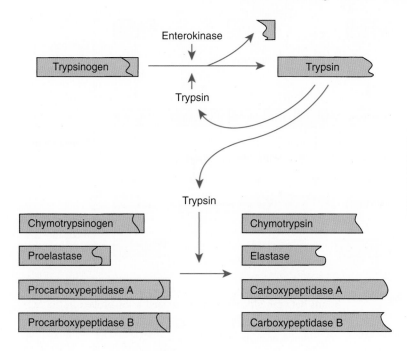

FIGURE 30-8 Activation of pancreatic zymogens. Note that trypsinogen is activated by trypsin as well as by the duodenal enzyme enterokinase. The autocatalytic action of trypsin on trypsinogen forms a positive feedback loop that ensures the rapid and complete activation of trypsinogen in the gut. Trypsin then activates the other zymogens.

Luminal-phase protein digestion begins in the stomach. Gastric digestion of protein is facilitated not only by the stomach enzymes but also by HCl, which has hydrolytic properties of its own. The acid environment of the stomach is suited to the action of pepsin, which has its optimal activity at pH 1 to 3. Gastric hydrolysis of protein is probably important to the physical as well as the chemical digestion of protein, because most connective tissue of animal origin is protein; digestion of connective tissue aids in breaking food down into particles small enough to pass the pylorus. Although stomach action is important in initiating protein digestion, it is not essential; animals without stomachs can digest proteins, provided they have a functional pancreas and are fed small, frequent meals of soft, moist food. Luminal-phase digestion of proteins is completed in the small intestine by the action of pancreatic enzymes.

Membranous-Phase Digestive Enzymes Are a Structural Part of the Intestinal Surface Membrane

Membranous-phase digestion, as with its luminal counterpart, occurs because of the hydrolytic action of enzymes. The difference between the two phases is that membranous-phase enzymes are chemically bound to the surface membrane of the intestine. They constitute a large and important portion of the glycocalyx. The substrates for these enzymes must diffuse into the glycocalyx before hydrolysis can occur. These membrane-bound digestive enzymes are synthesized within the enterocytes and subsequently transported to the luminal surface of the apical membrane. They remain attached to the surface by a short anchor segment, whereas the large, catalytic portion of the enzyme molecule projects away from the surface, toward the gut lumen.

Membranous-Phase Digestion Occurs Within the Microenvironment of the Unstirred Water Layer, Intestinal Mucus, and Glycocalyx

As previously described, the unstirred water layer, mucus, and glycocalyx form a diffuse zone separating the mucosal surface from the lumen of the intestine. The membranous-phase digestive enzymes project from the apical membrane into this surface layer.

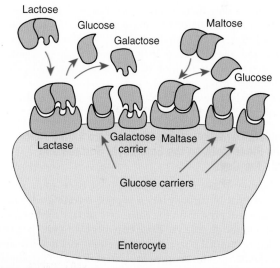

FIGURE 30-9 Relationship of membranous-phase digestion to absorption. The enzymes responsible for digestion and the carrier molecules responsible for absorption are both part of the apical membrane. The products of digestion are thus formed in the immediate vicinity of the carrier proteins, avoiding long diffusion distances. Specific enzymes and carrier molecules are present for the various substrates, as illustrated.

The quiet surface layer forms a microenvironment in which membranous-phase digestion occurs. Peptides and polysaccharides in the intestinal lumen must diffuse into the surface layer before membranous-phase digestion can take place. Furthermore, most of the products of membranous-phase digestion never diffuse away from the surface environment back into the lumen of the intestine; instead, they are absorbed, soon after formation, into the underlying epithelial cells. This arrangement is efficient because it ensures that the final products of carbohydrate and protein digestion are formed near their site of absorption, avoiding the need for long diffusion distances (Figure 30-9).

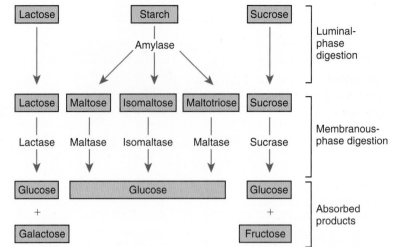

FIGURE 30-10 Luminal-phase and membranous-phase digestion of carbohydrate. Note that specific enzymes exist for each polysaccharide, and that a limited number of monomers are formed eventually from a relatively large number of starches and polysaccharides.

A Specific Membranous-Phase Enzyme Exists for the Digestion of Each Type of Polysaccharide

The membranous-phase enzymes of carbohydrate digestion have as their substrates dietary complex carbohydrates, such as sucrose and lactose, as well as the polysaccharide products of luminal-phase starch digestion, including maltose and isomaltose. The specific membranous-phase enzymes are named according to their substrates and include *maltase, isomaltase, sucrase,* and *lactase.* The sole product of maltose and isomaltose digestion is glucose, whereas in addition to glucose, fructose and galactose are produced from the digestion of sucrose and lactose, respectively. All polysaccharides are digested to monosaccharides before absorption (Figure 30-10).

Complete Digestion of Peptides to Free Amino Acids Takes Place Both on the Enterocyte Surface and Within the Cells

Membranous-phase digestion of peptides is, in some respects, similar to that of carbohydrates; peptide-digesting enzymes, or *peptidases,* are present on the enterocyte surface membrane and extend into the glycocalyx. These enzymes hydrolyze the peptide products of luminal-phase protein digestion, yielding free amino acids. Some of the longer-chain peptides are incompletely digested, yielding dipeptides and tripeptides. A large portion of dietary amino acids is absorbed directly in the form of dipeptides and tripeptides. This mode of absorption contrasts with that of carbohydrates, in which only monomeric, simple sugars may pass the apical membrane. Dipeptides and tripeptides that are absorbed intact are subsequently hydrolyzed by the action of intracellular peptidases, which results in the formation of free amino acids that are then available for passage into the blood. Thus the final digestion of peptides to free amino acids may occur at either of two sites: on the surface membrane of the enterocyte or within the cell. In either case, the final product of protein digestion is free amino acid (Figure 30-11).

INTESTINAL ABSORPTION

Absorption refers to the movement of the products of digestion across the intestinal mucosa and into the vascular system for distribution. To better understand the physiologically eloquent and clinically important processes of intestinal absorption, the reader might need to review the processes of diffusion across

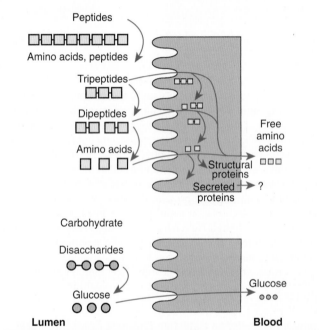

FIGURE 30-11 Membranous-phase digestion of peptides and carbohydrates. Note that tripeptides and dipeptides may be hydrolyzed to their constituent amino acids either on the apical membrane or within the enterocyte. In carbohydrate digestion, however, all disaccharide hydrolysis occurs at the apical membrane. Regardless of the site at which the final hydrolysis of peptides occurs, the product absorbed into the blood is free amino acid (see Figure 30-16).

membranes, the difference in composition of intracellular and extracellular fluid (see Chapter 1), the electrical polarity across cell membranes, the function of the sodium-potassium (Na^+,K^+) adenosine triphosphatase (ATPase) pump, and the function of selective ion channels (see Chapters 1 and 4).

In considering intestinal absorption, keep in mind that molecules move across membrane barriers in response to chemical and electrical gradients. When molecules can freely penetrate a membrane, their movement across it is completely determined by the laws of diffusion and differences in chemical and electrical gradients: molecules flow to areas of lower concentration and charged particles move to areas of opposite charge. However, charged ions (especially cations) and most organic nutrient molecules do not freely penetrate the GI epithelium. Therefore, they do not move in accordance with the laws of diffusion unless there is some mechanism to facilitate their transport across membranes.

Specialized Nutrient Transport Systems Exist in the Apical and Basolateral Membranes

Specialized *transport mechanisms* exist for the movement of molecules across membranes in the intestinal epithelium. These mechanisms are interactions of events involving specific proteins that lie embedded in the matrix of the cell membranes of the epithelial cells. These proteins provide the *transport pathway* for the passage of ions and organic molecules across the plasma membranes of cells. As discussed here, there are many transport pathways. In general, the different pathways are polarized within the enterocytes, meaning that specific transport pathways exist on either the apical or the basolateral membrane, but not both. The transport pathway proteins chemically interact with specific organic nutrients and inorganic ions to affect their transport across the membrane. The transport mechanisms can be classified as active transport, secondary active transport, tertiary active transport, and passive transport.

Active transport involves the direct consumption of metabolic energy. During active transport, energy stored as ATP is expended to move ions or molecules across membranes against an electrical or chemical gradient. In the large and small intestine, the active transport pathway of greatest importance is the Na^+,K^+-ATPase pump. This protein pathway lies on the basolateral membrane and uses energy from the hydrolysis of one molecule of ATP to drive three ions of sodium out of the cell, in exchange for the entry of two potassium ions into the cell. This important transport pathway exists in a wide variety of cells, in addition to enterocytes. The Na^+,K^+-ATPase pump is the mechanism by which (1) the interior of cells is kept electrically negative with respect to the extracellular fluid and (2) the concentration of sodium is kept very low in the intracellular fluid (see Chapter 1).

Secondary and Tertiary Active Transport Mechanisms Utilize the Transcellular Sodium Ion Electrochemical Gradient as Their Source of Energy

Just as a large stone resting atop a hill represents potential energy, so does the electrochemical gradient of sodium ions (Na^+) across the enterocyte membrane. Gravity imparts potential energy to the stone, whereas diffusion forces impart potential energy to Na^+ outside cells. Transport mechanisms that harness the potential energy of the sodium gradient are referred to as *secondary active transport*. Various transport pathway proteins exist for secondary active transport.

One type is referred to as a *co-transport* protein or *symport*. The characteristic of a co-transport protein is that it has binding sites for one or more Na^+ ions as well as an additional binding site for some other specific molecule. For example, the glucose co-transport protein has one binding site for glucose and two for Na^+. Co-transport proteins exist in the apical membrane of enterocytes. When the binding sites are unoccupied, they face the intestinal lumen. When all binding sites are occupied, a change in molecular configuration results in the translocation of binding sites, with their ligand molecules, to the interior of the cell. When this happens, the Na^+ ions along with the co-transported molecule are released into the intracellular fluid. Thus, there is transport of sodium and another molecule, such as glucose, across the apical membrane. When the ligand molecules are

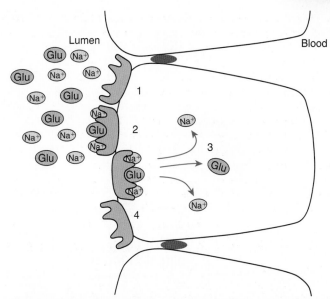

FIGURE 30-12 Co-transport is made possible by the allosteric transformation of transport proteins that lie in the apical membrane. The co-transport protein has two binding sites for sodium ions *(Na⁺)* and one for glucose *(Glu)*. When all three binding sites are occupied, the protein changes configuration in such a way as to transport the three ligands into the cell. The favorable gradient for sodium movement is maintained by the continuous action of the Na^+,K^+-ATPase pump (see Figure 30-13).

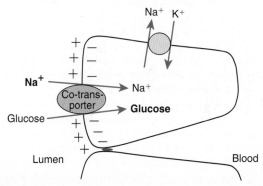

FIGURE 30-13 During co-transport, glucose is transported against an unfavorable concentration gradient. This diagram illustrates that the large sodium concentration difference across the apical membrane provides energy to transport glucose against its concentration gradient. The sodium concentration gradient, created by the action of the Na^+,K^+-ATPase pump, provides energy to drive this reaction.

released, the protein assumes its original configuration so that the binding sites are again on the extracellular surface of the apical membrane, ready to transport additional molecules (Figure 30-12).

This process proceeds only as long as there is an electrochemical gradient for the Na^+. When this gradient is large, as is normally the case, it can provide the energy to "pull" the co-transported molecule, such as glucose, from an area of lower concentration to one of higher concentration, as illustrated in Figures 30-13 and 30-14. Although the movement of a molecule against its concentration gradient represents expenditure of energy, there is no direct expenditure of metabolic energy by the sodium co-transport process. The energy expenditure is indirect and

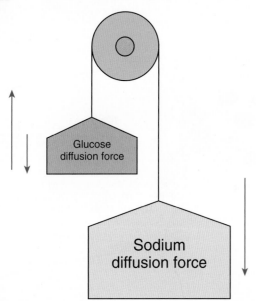

FIGURE 30-14 Secondary transport is an important concept. The tremendous sodium concentration difference between intracellular and extracellular fluid could be likened to the force of gravity; a pervasive force that affects many relationships in our environment. Movement of most ions, glucose, and many other organic molecules across the intestinal epithelium is driven by the strength of the sodium concentration difference.

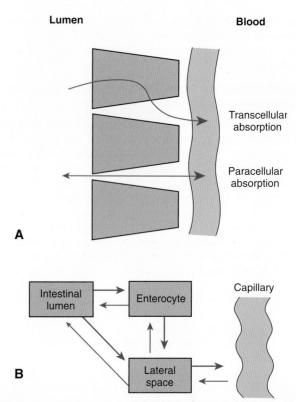

FIGURE 30-15 Transcellular and paracellular absorption. **A,** Substances move from the intestinal lumen to the capillary by either transcellular (through the enterocyte) or paracellular (through the tight junction) absorption. **B,** Intestinal lumen, enterocytes, and lateral spaces form three separate pools that may contain nutrients in different concentrations. Note that nutrients move into the capillaries from the lateral spaces and that reverse transport (from the capillary to the intestinal lumen) is possible for some substances.

results from the direct expenditure of energy by the Na$^+$,K$^+$-ATPase pump in creating and maintaining the sodium electrochemical gradient. This is the definition of secondary active transport, with glucose transport being secondary to the active transport of sodium. Many organic nutrients, including glucose, amino acids, several vitamins, and bile acids, are absorbed by sodium co-transport processes.

In addition to sodium co-transport, there are other types of secondary active transport pathways. These pathway proteins are known as *exchangers* or *antiports*. Exchangers are usually involved with ion transport and are similar to co-transport proteins in that they have binding sites for selected ions. The difference between exchangers and co-transport proteins is that for exchangers, the binding sites for the two different ligands are on opposite sides of the plasma membrane. For example, an important exchanger is the sodium/hydrogen (Na$^+$/H$^+$) exchanger in the apical membrane. The protein has a binding site for Na$^+$ and another for H$^+$. When the sites are unoccupied, the Na$^+$ site faces the intestinal lumen, and the H$^+$ site faces the interior of the enterocyte. When both sites are occupied, the protein flips, transporting H$^+$ out of and Na$^+$ into the cell, thus explaining the name *exchanger,* with H$^+$ exchanged for Na$^+$. As with co-transport, the force driving the exchange is the Na$^+$ electrochemical gradient across the cell membrane.

Another form of active transport, tertiary active transport, occurs via transport pathway proteins and is driven by electrochemical gradients that are established by secondary active transport. The best example of tertiary active transport is the chloride/bicarbonate (Cl$^-$/HCO$_3^-$) exchanger. This mechanism occurs in response to gradients established by the Na$^+$/H$^+$ exchanger, a secondary active transport mechanism. The Cl$^-$/HCO$_3^-$ exchanger is discussed in more detail later, in the section on absorption. In essence, the term tertiary is used because the Na$^+$,K$^+$-ATPase system (primary) establishes the gradient that drives the Na$^+$/H$^+$ exchanger (secondary), which then establishes the gradient that drives the Cl$^-$/HCO$_3^-$ exchanger (tertiary).

Passive Transport Occurs Either Through Specialized Channels in Cell Membranes or Directly Through the Tight Junctions

Ion channels, which are protein constituents of cell plasma membranes, are the transport pathways of passive diffusion into cells. Ions move through the channels in a completely passive manner, responding only to electrochemical gradients. No metabolic energy is directly required to effect ion movement. The only regulatory influence the cell can exert over this form of transport is in opening or closing of the channels (see Chapter 1).

A second form of passive molecular movement through the intestinal epithelium is through the tight junctions. As previously mentioned, the "tight" junctions are not so tight, especially in the duodenum and upper jejunum. In these areas the tight junctions are freely permeable to water and small, inorganic ions. Thus, water and ions move across the tight junctions in response to osmotic pressure and electrochemical gradients. Movement of materials through the tight junctions is called *paracellular* (around the cells) *absorption,* in contrast to absorption through the apical membrane, which is called *transcellular* (through the cells) *absorption.* Transcellular absorption and paracellular absorption work in a complementary manner to produce an efficient absorptive process (Figure 30-15).

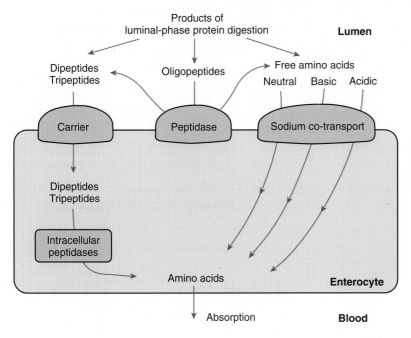

FIGURE 30-16 At least three different sodium co-transport proteins exist for the transport of amino acids: those for neutral, basic, and acidic amino acids. A sodium co-transport process might be involved in the absorption of dipeptides and tripeptides, but this possibility is not well established.

The Products of Membranous-Phase Digestion Are Absorbed by Sodium Co-Transport

Sodium co-transport proteins for glucose and galactose are located in the apical membrane, in proximity to the membranous-phase digestive enzymes. Because these saccharide monomers are produced by the action of membranous-phase enzymes on polysaccharides, they move very short distances to binding sites on co-transport proteins. When both the glucose-binding (or galactose-binding) sites and the sodium-binding sites on these proteins are occupied, absorption occurs as previously described in the description of transport proteins.

In the initial phases of digestion of a starch-containing meal, the glucose concentration at the apical membrane is very high because there is ample substrate. Sodium is also readily available as a result of its presence in the various GI secretions. At this time, movement of both sodium and glucose into the enterocytes is down a concentration gradient. As digestion and absorption proceed, the glucose concentration at the apical membrane diminishes. Thus, toward the end of the digestive and absorptive process, the concentration of glucose at the luminal surface of the enterocyte apical membrane becomes small. At this point the concentration of glucose within the enterocyte can be higher than in the intestinal lumen, thus creating an unfavorable concentration gradient for glucose absorption. However, the transcellular sodium concentration gradient is maintained, driving the continued absorption of glucose (see Figure 30-14). The process of glucose absorption by this mechanism is very efficient, and little free glucose escapes the absorptive process.

To complete the process of carbohydrate absorption, the glucose must move through the basolateral membrane, into the lateral spaces, and then into the capillaries. Movement of glucose through the basolateral membrane occurs by *facilitated diffusion,* in which there is a transport pathway protein, but the direction of transport is driven only by the concentration gradient for glucose. As the intracellular glucose concentration in the enterocytes increases because of the action of sodium-glucose co-transport from the gut lumen, glucose diffuses from the cells

into the lateral spaces. From the lateral spaces, it diffuses through the capillary basement membrane into the blood.

Absorption of the products of membranous-phase protein digestion occurs in a manner similar to that of carbohydrates. Sodium co-transport systems exist for free amino acids and might also exist for dipeptides and tripeptides. At least three co-transport proteins are necessary for absorption of free amino acids. The mechanism of transport for dipeptides and tripeptides might also involve sodium co-transport, but this issue is not established with certainty (Figure 30-16).

ABSORPTION OF WATER AND ELECTROLYTES

Conservation of the body's supply of water and electrolytes, primarily sodium, potassium, chloride, and bicarbonate, is a high priority for sustaining life. The gut plays a major role in this conservation, not only because it is the portal of entry for replenishment of the nutrients, but also because water and electrolytes in GI secretions must be efficiently reclaimed to maintain body composition. The most immediate clinical ramifications of GI disease usually involve the loss of water and electrolytes. This section discusses the absorption of the major ions and electrolytes sequentially.

There Are at Least Three Distinct Mechanisms of Sodium Absorption

The first pathway of sodium absorption is through sodium co-transport proteins, as previously discussed. This secondary active transport pathway is not only the mechanism for glucose and amino acid absorption (Figure 30-17, *A*), but also a major means of sodium absorption.

The second sodium absorption mechanism is through the Na^+/H^+ exchanger (see Figure 30-17, *B*), mentioned previously as an example of an ion exchanger, or antiport. Through this mechanism, intracellular H^+ is exchanged for luminal Na^+ across the apical membrane. The H^+ for this exchange is formed by the action of carbonic anhydrase, which generates HCO_3^- as well as

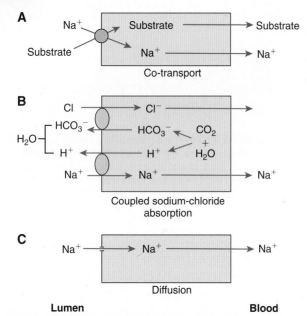

FIGURE 30-17 Three mechanisms of sodium (Na^+) absorption. **A**, Sodium co-transport with organic molecules is a major means of sodium uptake during active digestion and absorption. **B**, Chloride-coupled sodium absorption is also an important means of sodium absorption and requires the action of carbonic anhydrase and the existence on the apical membrane of bicarbonate-chloride (HCO_3^-/Cl^-) and sodium-hydrogen (Na^+/H^+) exchange mechanisms. **C**, Simple diffusion of sodium across the apical membrane may occur because of the large, favorable concentration gradient, but it is a relatively minor means of sodium absorption. CO_2, Carbon dioxide; H_2O, water.

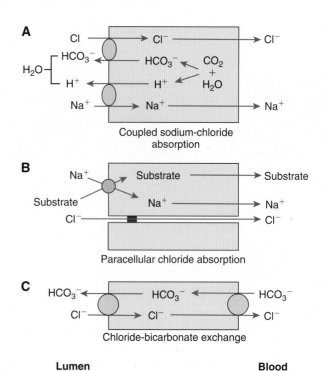

FIGURE 30-18 Three mechanisms of chloride (Cl^-) absorption. **A**, Chloride-coupled sodium absorption is directly related to sodium (Na^+) uptake. **B**, Paracellular chloride absorption is indirectly related to sodium absorption that occurs during co-transport. **C**, Chloride-bicarbonate (Cl^-/HCO_3^-) exchange occurs especially in areas where bicarbonate secretion into the intestinal lumen is important.

H^+. As H^+ is exchanged for Na^+, HCO_3^- concentrations build up in the cell. The resulting transcellular HCO_3^- gradient drives the action of the Cl^-/HCO_3^- exchanger, which results in the exchange of intracellular HCO_3^- for luminal Cl^-. Because of the close connection between Na^+ and Cl^- absorption by these pathways, this transport mechanism is often called *coupled sodium chloride transport,* as illustrated in Figure 30-17, *B.* One must appreciate, however, that it is only the intracellular balance of H^+ and HCO_3^- that couples the two exchange pathways. There are instances in which the intracellular pH is such that Na^+/H^+ exchange occurs without Cl^-/HCO_3^- exchange, and vice versa.

Coupled sodium chloride absorption is usually most active in the ileum and colon, where the sodium concentration in the gut is usually relatively low compared with that in the duodenum and jejunum. As usual, sodium entering the enterocytes is transported across the basolateral membrane to the lateral spaces by the action of the Na^+,K^+-ATPase pump. Chloride, however, remains in the enterocyte until its concentration is high enough to promote the diffusion of chloride through special channels, or gates, in the basolateral membranes. The rate of absorption of sodium and chloride by the coupled mechanism appears to depend on the permeability of the chloride channels; when the permeability is high, chloride passes rapidly out of the enterocyte, allowing continued chloride absorption. Conversely, when chloride channels are relatively closed, the intracellular chloride concentration rises, diminishing chloride absorption by the creation of an unfavorable concentration gradient across the apical membrane.

The third mechanism of sodium absorption is by simple diffusion through ion channels in the apical membrane (see Figure 30-17, *C*). The large electrochemical gradient that can exist for sodium across the enterocyte apical membrane allows direct, uncoupled movement of sodium across the membrane when the ion channels are open. Although some sodium absorption probably occurs by this mechanism, its overall importance in body sodium homeostasis is probably not great.

There Are Three Major Mechanisms of Chloride Absorption

One mechanism of chloride absorption is coupled sodium chloride absorption, as discussed previously in relation to sodium (Figure 30-18, *A*). Another mechanism is paracellular chloride absorption, which occurs in association with sodium co-transport of glucose and amino acids (see Figure 30-18, *B*). Paracellular chloride transport occurs because of an electrical gradient. Sodium co-transport leads to the net movement of positive electrical charges (Na^+) across the apical membrane, because neither glucose nor most amino acids are charged molecules. As the sodium cations are transferred to the lateral spaces, the spaces develop a positive polarity with respect to the gut lumen. Chloride from the gut lumen passes directly into the lateral spaces through the tight junctions because these junctions are readily permeable to small anions. This provides a major mechanism for the absorption of Cl^- while maintaining electrical neutrality, although a small electrical potential is maintained across the gut surface, the lumen being negative with respect to the lateral spaces.

The last mechanism of chloride absorption is by direct exchange for bicarbonate (see Figure 30-18, *C*) without coupled sodium absorption. With this mechanism, there is a net movement of bicarbonate into the gut lumen, resulting in an increase in luminal pH. This can be particularly important in the colon of large herbivores where large concentrations of fermentation acids are created and require buffering.

Bicarbonate Ion Is Secreted by Several Digestive Glands and Must Be Recovered from the Gut if Body Acid-Base Balance Is to Be Maintained

Much bicarbonate is in essence "absorbed" by the neutralization of HCl from the stomach. Sodium bicarbonate entering the intestine reacts with HCl to form water, carbon dioxide, and sodium chloride, effectively resulting in the absorption of bicarbonate (HCO_3^-) and hydrogen (H^+) ions. (See Chapter 28 for an explanation of the counterbalancing effects of gastric acid secretion and pancreatic bicarbonate secretion.) However, considerable bicarbonate remains in the intestine after the neutralization of stomach acid. This remaining bicarbonate is reabsorbed, primarily in the ileum and colon via an ion-exchange mechanism.

Bicarbonate anions in the gut are electrically balanced, primarily with sodium cations, and reabsorbed essentially as sodium bicarbonate. In the absorptive process, H^+ and HCO_3^- ions are first generated within the enterocytes from water and carbon dioxide. H^+ is then exchanged for Na^+ across the apical membrane. Within the cell, Na^+ is electrically balanced by the remaining HCO_3^-, whereas the HCO_3^- remaining in the gut lumen is neutralized by the secreted H^+ (Figure 30-19). The result is that sodium is transferred through the membrane. However, luminal bicarbonate is converted to water and carbon dioxide in the gut lumen, whereas bicarbonate anion is regenerated intracellularly. The net effect is the absorption of sodium bicarbonate.

Potassium Is Absorbed Primarily by Passive Diffusion Through the Paracellular Route

Potassium (K^+), although a highly important ion in the body, is present in abundance in most animal diets. This is in contrast to sodium (Na^+), which is present in nutritionally inadequate amounts in most natural animal feeds. Therefore, frequently the K^+ concentration in the material entering the intestinal lumen is relatively high compared with Na^+ concentration. In addition, dietary potassium is concentrated in the gut lumen because of the absorption of other nutrients, electrolytes, and water, unaccompanied by active potassium absorption. Thus, K^+ concentration within the gut lumen increases as digestion and absorption of other osmotically active molecules proceeds.

As K^+ reaches relatively high concentrations in the intestinal lumen, a concentration gradient favorable for the diffusion of potassium across the intestinal epithelium is created. Furthermore, the concentration gradient is enhanced by the normally

low K^+ concentration in the lateral spaces. The primary mechanism of potassium absorption is paracellular passive diffusion, which occurs in response to this concentration gradient (Figure 30-20). A clinical ramification of this absorptive mechanism is that potassium absorption is directly coupled to water absorption. That is, the movement of water out of the intestinal lumen results in an increase in the luminal K^+ concentration, which in turn drives K^+ absorption. In diarrhea conditions, in which net absorption of water is impaired, K^+ absorption is impaired as well, because potassium in the gut lumen is diluted so that a concentration gradient favorable for passive diffusion of K^+ never develops. In addition to passive diffusion, it appears that an H^+,K^+-ATPase pump exists in the distal colon. This transport pathway may be important for recovering the last remaining potassium from the colonic ingesta of animals with diets low in potassium.

The Major Mechanisms of Electrolyte Absorption Are Selectively Distributed Along the Gut

The activity of the assorted electrolyte absorption mechanisms discussed earlier varies along the length of the gut. The distribution of activity is listed in Table 30-2.

All Intestinal Water Absorption Is Passive, Occurring Because of the Absorption of Osmotically Active Solutes

Water moves through the intestinal mucosa by either the paracellular or the transcellular route, but always by osmosis. The general discussion of osmosis in Chapter 1 should be reviewed by those who do not have a clear understanding of the process. The intestinal mucosa is freely permeable to water, allowing it to move in

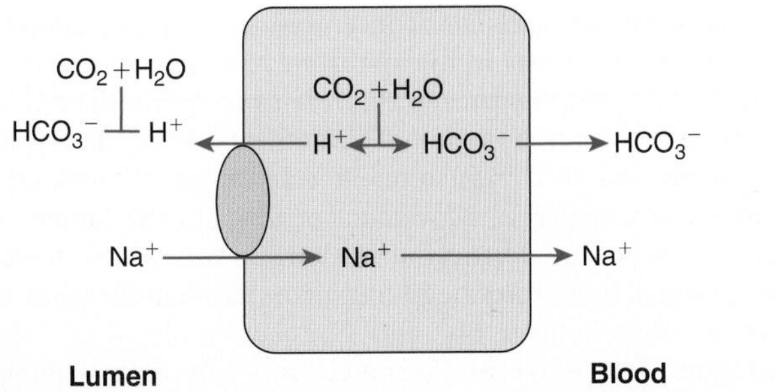

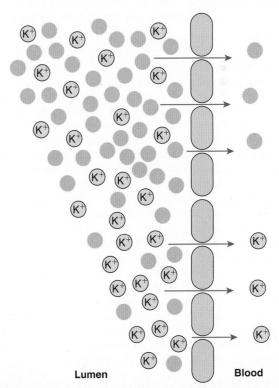

FIGURE 30-20 Potassium *(K⁺)* is absorbed by simple diffusion through the paracellular route. Water absorption in the upper intestine increases K⁺ concentration in the lower intestine, creating a favorable diffusion gradient for potassium. Note that the removal of water *(solid blue circles)* in the upper part results in a relative increase in the number of K⁺ ions in the lower part.

FIGURE 30-19 Absorption of bicarbonate *(HCO₃⁻)* is facilitated by sodium-hydrogen *(Na⁺/H⁺)* exchange at the apical membrane. The bicarbonate ion is regenerated by the action of carbonic anhydrase.

TABLE 30-2 Distributions of Electrolyte Absorptive Mechanisms Throughout the Gut

Mechanism	Duodenum	Jejunum Upper	Jejunum Middle	Jejunum Lower	Ileum	Colon
Sodium co-transport	+++++	++++	+	+	−	−
Chloride-coupled sodium absorption	+	+	+	+	++	+++
Chloride-bicarbonate exchange	−	−	−	−	++	+++
Bicarbonate absorption	−	−	−	−	++	+++
Potassium absorption	−	−	−	−	+	+++

whatever direction is dictated by changes in osmotic pressure. As electrolytes and other soluble nutrients are actively absorbed, water is drawn along passively from lumen to intestinal capillaries. Water may move also into the intestinal lumen at times when the intraluminal osmotic pressure is high, as discussed later.

INTESTINAL SECRETION OF WATER AND ELECTROLYTES

In addition to the water and electrolytes that are secreted into the intestine by the pancreas, liver, and other glandular organs, a considerable portion of GI water and electrolyte secretion occurs directly from the intestinal surface. All water secretion is osmotic, but the osmotic gradient driving water secretion may occur in response to either passive or active processes.

Passive Increases in Luminal Osmotic Pressure Occur During Hydrolytic Digestion and Result in Water Secretion

Food entering the intestine may be hyperosmotic because of its composition, such as salty foods and foods with high sugar content. Alternatively, food may become hyperosmotic after digestion. Digestion of foods creates many osmotically active molecules from one giant precursor molecule; thus the osmotic activity of ingesta is increased initially by digestion. When starchy meals, for example, first enter the duodenum, intraluminal digestion creates thousands of osmotically active disaccharide and trisaccharide molecules from single starch molecules. These osmotically active saccharide molecules draw water from the lateral spaces into the intestinal lumen. Water in the lateral spaces is quickly replaced by water from the intestinal capillaries, so water is essentially drawn into the intestine from the vascular system. As digestion proceeds, the saccharide molecules are absorbed, thus reducing the number of particles and lowering the osmotic pressure of the intestinal lumen. As solute molecules are absorbed, water follows them osmotically back through the epithelium and into the blood vascular system. *The cardinal rule of water movement in the intestine is that water moves in whatever direction necessary to keep ingesta iso-osmotic,* entering the gut when ingesta is hyperosmotic and leaving the gut when ingesta is hypo-osmotic. This fact has important clinical implications in the pathophysiology of diarrhea, as discussed later.

Active Secretion of Electrolytes From the Crypt Epithelium Leads to Intestinal Water Secretion

In contrast to the absorptive function of the villous cells, the crypt cells have a secretory function. This secretory function appears to use a chloride transport mechanism. The mechanism seems to be similar to coupled sodium chloride transport, as occurs in the

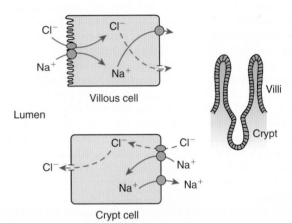

FIGURE 30-21 Water and electrolyte secretion in the crypts is affected by the secretion of chloride *(Cl⁻)* from the apical membrane of crypt enterocytes. Sodium *(Na⁺)* moves into the lumen by the paracellular route and electrically balances Cl⁻ secretion. Water follows osmotically, the net effect being secretion of a sodium chloride (NaCl) solution into the crypt lumen. In the crypts the coupled NaCl absorption mechanism appears to exist on the basolateral membrane, with Cl⁻ gates present on the apical membrane. The opening of Cl⁻ gates on the crypt cell apical membranes initiates crypt secretion. The membrane position of the coupled NaCl transport process reverses itself, moving from the basolateral membrane to the apical membrane as the cells mature and move up the villi.

villous enterocytes, except that the direction of transport is reversed. In the crypt cells the coupled sodium chloride transport mechanism is on the basolateral membrane, in contrast to its position on the apical membrane of the villous cells. The effect of this arrangement is to pump Na⁺ and Cl⁻ into the crypt enterocytes from the lateral spaces. As these ions are transported into the enterocytes, Na⁺ is quickly pumped out by the Na⁺,K⁺-ATPase pump. In contrast, Cl⁻ is trapped within the cells, reaching relatively high intracellular concentrations. Under appropriate stimuli, Cl⁻ channels in the apical membranes of the crypt cells are opened, and the pent-up chloride from within the cells flows down its concentration gradient into the lumen of the crypt. (Ion channels and their regulation in cellular membranes are discussed in Chapter 1.) Movement of Cl⁻ into the lumen of the crypts creates an electrical attraction for Na⁺, which move into the luminal fluid from the lateral spaces through the paracellular route. Water follows Na⁺ and Cl⁻ osmotically; thus chloride, sodium, and water are secreted from the crypt epithelium (Figure 30-21).

You may find the concept of ion transport processes jumping from one side of the cell to another intuitively "unappealing," especially when you consider that the cells of the intestinal crypts will eventually mature and migrate up the villi to assume absorptive, as opposed to secretive, roles. Consider, however, that ion transport mechanisms are simply proteins inserted into the cell membranes. As with other cellular proteins, they are synthesized within the cell under the direction of genetic code. The state of maturity and cellular differentiation dictates the membrane position into which the newly synthesized proteins are directed. The differential distribution of membrane proteins to one side of a cell or another is called *polarization*. Enterocytes are said to be "polarized" with respect to membrane function.

The triggering mechanism that activates water secretion from the crypts is the opening of the chloride gates in the crypt enterocyte apical membrane. Much study has been devoted to determining the factors controlling the opening of the chloride gates in crypt cells. One important factor in regulating chloride gates appears to be the activity of the adenylate cyclase enzyme and the intracellular concentration of cyclic adenosine $3',5'$-monophosphate (cyclic AMP, or cAMP). (The role of adenyl cyclase and cAMP in cellular regulation is discussed in Chapter 1.) As cAMP concentrations rise, chloride gates open, and secretion of water and electrolytes is stimulated. Vasoactive intestinal peptide originating from effector neurons of the mucosal plexus is probably an important normal regulator of cAMP and chloride gates in crypt apical membranes. Of perhaps greater medical significance than the normal regulation of this process is the existence of pathological, or abnormal, activators of crypt cell adenyl cyclase (see later section on the pathophysiology of diarrhea).

The physiological function of water and electrolyte secretion by the crypts is to maintain an appropriate hydration and ionic environment for digestion and absorption. Ingesta must be kept sufficiently moist to allow for the mixing of nutrients with digestive enzymes and for the circulation of digested nutrients in contact with absorptive surfaces. In addition, a constant supply of sodium must be available to promote the sodium co-transport necessary for the absorption of several nutrients. The regulated process of water and electrolyte secretion from the crypts ensures the continual availability of water and sodium in the gut lumen.

GASTROINTESTINAL BLOOD FLOW

Water and Solute Movement Between the Lateral Spaces and Villous Capillaries Is Subject to the Same Forces That Govern Water and Solute Movement Between the Extracellular and Vascular Fluids in Other Tissues

Water and all other nutrients, whether they are absorbed through the transcellular or paracellular routes, enter the extracellular fluid of the lateral spaces before entering the vascular system. Therefore the movement of extracellular fluid components into capillaries is of particular importance to intestinal absorption. The physical laws determining the distribution of water between the intravascular and extravascular fluid are the same in the villi as in other tissues. These Starling laws (which can be reviewed in Chapters 1 and 23) simply state that the movement of water is determined by the algebraic sum of osmotic and hydrostatic (created by water pressure) forces.

Absorbed Nutrients Enter the Capillaries by Diffusion from the Lateral Spaces

The collective action of the various intestinal absorptive mechanisms concentrates solutes (nutrients) in the lateral spaces. When

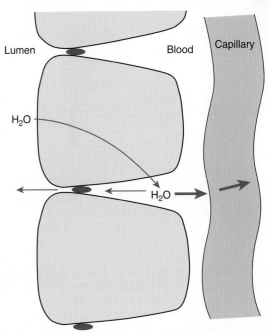

FIGURE 30-22 Water *(H₂O)* enters the lateral spaces because of osmotic effects created by absorbed solutes, thus creating a hydrostatic pressure head in the lateral spaces. Under pressure, the lateral-space solution can exit through the tight junctions or through the basement membrane of the capillaries. Under normal conditions the route of least resistance is into the capillaries, resulting in little movement of water from the lateral space into the intestinal lumen.

the concentrations of individual solutes in the lateral spaces exceed their concentrations in blood, a gradient favoring the diffusion of nutrients from lateral spaces into the capillaries is established. The movement of solutes by diffusion into the capillaries creates an osmotic force that draws water into the capillaries (water follows solute). In addition, the oncotic force (the osmotic force exerted by plasma proteins; see Chapters 1 and 23) also tends to draw water into the capillary lumen. Moreover, hydrostatic pressure in the lateral spaces may force water directly into the capillaries. Lateral-space hydrostatic pressure can be created by the osmotic effect of absorbed solutes. As these solutes attract water from the intestinal lumen, the lateral spaces become distended, developing a small amount of hydrostatic pressure. There are two exits for the relief of this pressure: the tight junctions and the capillary endothelium, with the endothelium presenting the route of least resistance to water flow. Thus, water under slight pressure within the lateral spaces tends to flow into the capillaries rather than into the intestinal lumen (Figure 30-22).

A Countercurrent, Osmotic-Multiplier System May Increase the Osmolality of Blood at the Tips of the Villi, Further Promoting Absorption of Water into the Blood

The villous vascular system consists of an arteriole rising up the central portion of the villi and dividing at the tip into many capillaries, which course down the outer portion of the villous stroma between the mucosa and artery. This arrangement provides for direct countercurrent flow of blood; that is, blood coming down the venules passes close to blood flowing in the opposite direction up the arteriole. Because blood in the venules contains absorbed nutrients, its osmolarity could be expected to be slightly higher than that of blood entering the villi in the arteriole. This slight difference in osmolarity can be multiplied and perpetuated by the

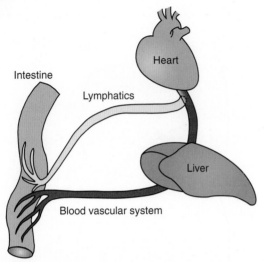

FIGURE 30-23 All blood exiting the gut flows through the liver before returning to the heart. Lymphatic drainage from the gut bypasses the liver, entering the bloodstream through the thoracic duct.

countercurrent flow characteristics of the arterial and venous blood supplies. These conditions create a potential for the creation of an osmotic gradient along the villi; some researchers calculate osmolalities near the tips of the villi to be as high as 600 mOsm, approximately twice that of blood entering the base of the villi. (The characteristics of a countercurrent osmotic multiplier are further explained in Chapter 43 in reference to the renal loop of Henle.) The existence of the villous countercurrent osmotic multiplier is still somewhat controversial, and its presence may depend on the species in question. The effect of this osmotic-multiplier system would be to accentuate all the osmotic forces that result in the movement of water from lumen to lateral spaces and from lateral spaces to capillaries.

Disturbances in the Venous Drainage from the Intestine Can Greatly Affect the Mechanisms of Capillary Absorption in the Villi

With the exception of blood from the terminal colon and rectum, all venous blood from the GI tract is collected into the hepatic portal vein and passes through the liver before entering the vena cava and returning to the heart (Figure 30-23). Because of this system, the nutrient-rich blood leaving the intestine may be modified by the liver. The liver can thus regulate the nutrient concentration of blood reaching general body tissues, keeping it relatively constant. This particular vascular arrangement of the GI system results in the passage of blood through two capillary beds, one in the gut wall and one in the liver, before its return to the heart. In most tissues, arterial hydrostatic pressure forces blood through the capillary beds. In the liver, however, this is not the case, because most of the arterial hydrostatic pressure has been dissipated during flow of blood through the intestinal capillaries. The following two circumstances tend to overcome this problem and allow hepatic blood flow to occur:

1. The capillaries (referred to as *sinusoids*) of the liver are comparatively large and thus offer little resistance to flow; therefore they can function in a low-pressure system.
2. The venous outflow of the liver goes directly into the thoracic vena cava.

The bellows-like action of the thorax transmits a negative pressure to the thoracic vena cava, which tends to aspirate blood

from the hepatic veins and abdominal vena cava. Under normal circumstances, these conditions allow blood to flow readily from the intestine through the liver. However, small changes in circulatory function can have a large impact on GI blood flow. If the pumping capacity of the heart becomes reduced, it cannot remove returning venous blood quickly. Accumulation of blood and an increase in pressure in the thoracic vena cava result. This increase in pressure interferes with the flow of blood out of the liver, which in turn reduces blood flow out of the intestine. This sequence of events makes the GI system particularly susceptible to right-sided heart failure, in which the heart's pumping action is compromised.

Diffuse liver disease, in addition to right-sided heart failure, can also interfere with GI blood flow. In this condition the resistance to blood flow through the liver is increased because of pressure on the sinusoids. Small rises in hepatic flow resistance can have large effects on intestinal blood flow because the pressure gradient across the hepatic portal vein is normally small. When the flow of blood out of the intestine is impaired, hydrostatic pressure in the capillaries of the villi is increased; the higher pressure tends to offset the osmotic and hydrostatic forces promoting water absorption, and thus water absorption is impaired.

DIGESTION AND ABSORPTION OF FATS

Detergent Action as Well as Enzymatic Action Is Necessary for the Digestion and Absorption of Lipids

Lipids, or fats, present a special digestive problem to the animal because they do not dissolve in water, the major medium in which most body processes, including digestion, occur. Detergent action is necessary to emulsify or dissolve lipids so that they may be subjected to the actions of water-soluble hydrolytic enzymes in the gut. The problem of solubility makes the mechanics of digestion and absorption of lipids somewhat different from that of proteins and carbohydrates. For that reason, lipid assimilation is discussed here in a separate section.

Lipids make up a large portion of the diets of carnivores and omnivores, whereas they usually form a minor portion of the natural diets of adult herbivores. Nonetheless, it appears that herbivorous species have the capacity to digest and absorb lipids in quantities considerably higher than found in their natural diets, and frequently, supplemental lipids are added to the diets of performance horses and high-producing dairy cows. The neonates of all mammalian species have a high capacity for lipid digestion and absorption because milk has a high fat content.

The primary dietary lipid is *triglyceride,* which may originate from either plant or animal sources. Other important dietary lipids are *cholesterol* and *cholesteryl ester* from animal sources, waxes from plant sources, and *phospholipids* from both plant and animal sources. Figure 30-24 illustrates the structures of these dietary lipids. In addition, the lipid-soluble vitamins A, D, E, and K are absorbed along with the other dietary lipids.

Lipid assimilation can be divided into four phases: (1) emulsification, (2) hydrolysis, (3) micelle formation, and (4) absorption. *Emulsification* is the process of reducing lipid droplets to a size that forms stable suspensions in water or water-based solutions. In the gut the emulsification phase begins in the stomach as the lipids are warmed to body temperature and subjected to the intense mixing, agitating, and sieving actions of the distal stomach. This distal-stomach activity tends to break lipid globules up into droplets that pass into the small intestine. In the small intestine, emulsification is completed by the detergent action of

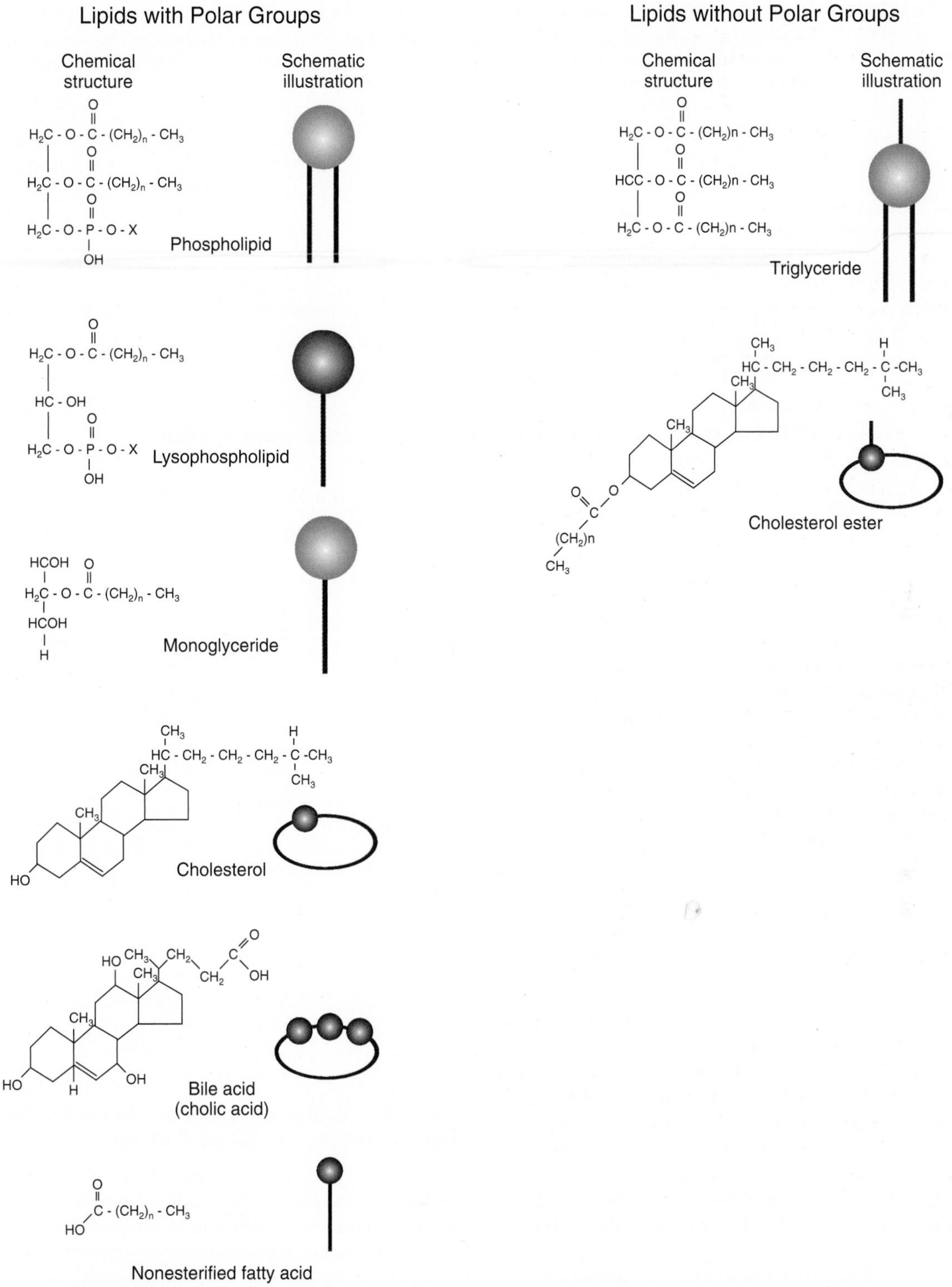

Lipids with Polar Groups

Chemical structure	Schematic illustration

$$H_2C - O - \overset{\overset{O}{\|}}{C} - (CH_2)_n - CH_3$$
$$H_2C - O - \overset{\overset{O}{\|}}{C} - (CH_2)_n - CH_3$$
$$H_2C - O - \overset{\overset{O}{\|}}{P} - O - X$$
$$\overset{|}{OH}$$

Phospholipid

$$H_2C - O - \overset{\overset{O}{\|}}{C} - (CH_2)_n - CH_3$$
$$HC - OH$$
$$H_2C - O - \overset{\overset{O}{\|}}{P} - O - X$$
$$\overset{|}{OH}$$

Lysophospholipid

$$HCOH \quad \overset{O}{\|}$$
$$H_2C - O - C - (CH_2)_n - CH_3$$
$$HCOH$$
$$\overset{|}{H}$$

Monoglyceride

Cholesterol

Bile acid (cholic acid)

$$\underset{HO}{\overset{O}{\|}}{C} - (CH_2)_n - CH_3$$

Nonesterified fatty acid

Lipids without Polar Groups

Chemical structure	Schematic illustration

$$H_2C - O - \overset{\overset{O}{\|}}{C} - (CH_2)n - CH_3$$
$$HCC - O - \overset{\overset{O}{\|}}{C} - (CH_2)n - CH_3$$
$$H_2C - O - \overset{\overset{O}{\|}}{C} - (CH_2)n - CH_3$$

Triglyceride

Cholesterol ester

FIGURE 30-24 Chemical structures and their schematic representations for lipid molecules involved in fat digestion and absorption. *n*, Number of carbon atoms in fatty-acid chains; *X*, phospholipid head group, most often choline.

bile acids and phospholipids. (See Chapter 29 for a discussion of bile formation and secretion.) These bile products reduce the surface tension of the lipids and allow the droplets to become even further divided and reduced in size (Figure 30-25).

While in the bile-coated, or emulsified-droplet, stage, the lipids are subject to the actions of hydrolytic enzymes.

Hydrolysis of triglyceride, the major dietary lipid component, occurs because of the combined action of the pancreatic enzymes *lipase* and *co-lipase*. Lipase is an enzyme secreted, in its active form, from the pancreas. However, lipase cannot directly attack the emulsified lipid droplets in the gut because it cannot penetrate the coat of bile products surrounding the droplets. The function

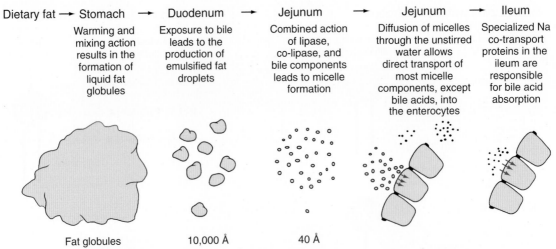

FIGURE 30-25 Sites and reactions involved in fat digestion and absorption. Å, Angstroms.

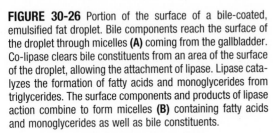

FIGURE 30-26 Portion of the surface of a bile-coated, emulsified fat droplet. Bile components reach the surface of the droplet through micelles **(A)** coming from the gallbladder. Co-lipase clears bile constituents from an area of the surface of the droplet, allowing the attachment of lipase. Lipase catalyzes the formation of fatty acids and monoglycerides from triglycerides. The surface components and products of lipase action combine to form micelles **(B)** containing fatty acids and monoglycerides as well as bile constituents.

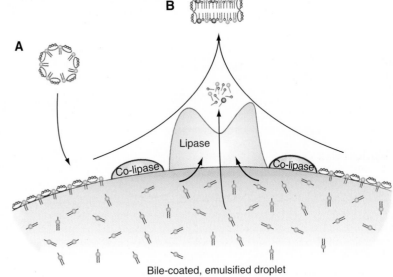

Bile-coated, emulsified droplet

of co-lipase, a relatively short peptide, is to "clear a path" through the bile products, giving lipase access to the underlying triglycerides. Lipase cleaves the fatty acids off each end of the triglyceride molecule but does not attack the central fatty acid, resulting in the formation of two *free* (or *nonesterified*) *fatty acids* and a *monoglyceride* from each molecule of triglyceride hydrolyzed (Figure 30-26).

Other lipid-digesting pancreatic enzymes are *cholesterol esterase* and *phospholipase*. The products of these enzymes are nonesterified fatty acids, cholesterol, and lysophospholipids.

The products of hydrolytic lipid digestion (fatty acids, monoglycerides, etc.) combine with bile acids and phospholipids to form *micelles,* small water-soluble aggregations of bile acids and lipids. Micelles are considerably smaller than the emulsified fat droplets from which they are derived (see Figure 30-25). The soluble micelles allow the lipids to diffuse through the gut lumen into the unstirred water layer and into close contact with the absorptive surface of the apical membrane (Figure 30-27; see Figure 30-26).

Lipids Are Absorbed Through the Apical Membrane by Carrier Proteins and Simple Diffusion

The process of lipid absorption into the enterocytes is incompletely understood. As the micelles come close to the surface of the enterocytes, the various lipid components diffuse the short distance through the glycocalyx to the apical membrane by means of special *fatty acid–binding proteins* (not shown in Figure 30-27). Fatty acids in the micelles appear to be taken up and transported across the apical membrane by special fatty acid–binding proteins in the apical membrane. Other micellar components appear to simply diffuse into the apical membrane; they include such lipids as monoglycerides, cholesterol, and vitamin A. The apical membrane, as with other cellular membranes, is composed primarily of phospholipids (see Chapter 1). The highly hydrophobic products of lipid digestion are soluble in the phospholipid matrix of the membrane and thus may diffuse freely through the apical membrane and into the cell. Figure 30-27 illustrates lipid absorption from micelles.

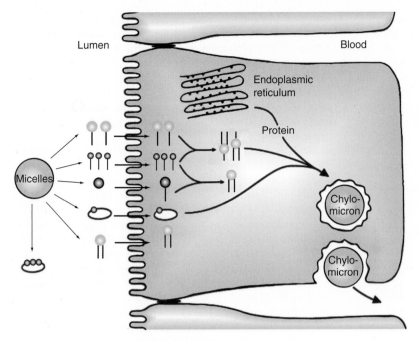

FIGURE 30-27 Lipid absorption from micelles with subsequent formation of chylomicrons. As micelles come close to the apical membrane, lipid constituents, except bile acids, are transported through the membrane into the cell. When in the enterocyte, triglycerides are re-formed from fatty acids and monoglycerides. Triglycerides are then packaged into the core of chylomicrons for transport out of the cell. The chylomicron surface is coated with phospholipids, cholesterol, and proteins.

Bile Acids Are Reabsorbed from the Ileum by a Sodium Co-Transport System

All components of the micelle diffuse into the enterocytes except the bile acids. Bile acids remain in the lumen of the gut, being separated from the other micellar elements as absorption proceeds. By the time bile acids reach the ileum, they are in a relatively free state, devoid of other lipids. Localized in the ileum is a specific bile acid transport system. This system operates by sodium co-transport and results in the nearly complete reabsorption of bile acids. After absorption, bile acids are transported directly back to the liver by the portal vasculature. The liver efficiently extracts bile acids from the portal blood, so normally the concentration of bile acids in the nonportal blood (systemic circulation) is small. The bile acids extracted by the liver are recycled into the bile. This recycling process occurs repeatedly, so the entire mass of bile acids within the body is circulated through the intestine several times per day.

Absorbed Lipids Are Packaged into Chylomicrons Before Leaving the Enterocytes

After passing the apical membrane, the absorbed lipids are quickly picked up by carrier molecules and transported within the cell to the endoplasmic reticulum. When they're on the smooth endoplasmic reticulum, the major lipids are re-esterified to form triglyceride and phospholipids. The re-esterified lipids are then packaged with cholesterol, minor dietary lipids, and proteins from the rough endoplasmic reticulum into structures known as *chylomicrons*. Chylomicrons are spherical structures with a core of triglyceride and cholesterol ester and a surface of phospholipid and cholesterol. The phospholipid and cholesterol are arranged with their *hydrophobic* (water-repelling) ends facing the core lipids and their *hydrophilic* (water-attracting) ends facing the surface of the chylomicron particle (Figure 30-28). This arrangement of surface lipid makes the chylomicron water soluble. A small number of special protein molecules are also present on the chylomicron surface. These proteins help to stabilize the surface and to direct the metabolism of the particle.

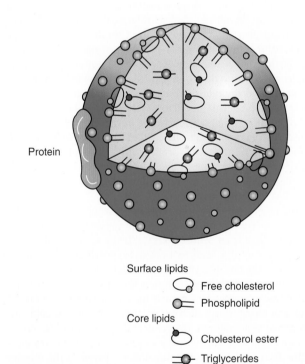

Surface lipids
⬯— Free cholesterol
●— Phospholipid

Core lipids
⬯— Cholesterol ester
⊙—⊙ Triglycerides

FIGURE 30-28 Chylomicron structure. Special proteins and lipids with polar groups form the surface coat, whereas nonpolar lipids form the core of the particle.

After their formation, chylomicrons are expelled from the basolateral membrane into the lateral spaces. Unlike most other nutrients entering the lateral spaces, chylomicrons are too large to pass through the basement membrane of the intestinal capillaries. Thus, chylomicrons cannot be absorbed through the intestinal blood system. Rather, they travel through the intestinal lymphatics, which eventually form a major abdominal lymph duct that passes through the diaphragm and into the *thoracic duct.* The major lymph-collecting vessel of the body, the thoracic duct, empties into the vena cava. Through this means, chylomicrons eventually reach the blood vascular system. During absorption of a fatty meal, the character of intestinal lymph changes from water-clear to milky white because of the presence of chylomicrons. After a fatty meal, this milky white color can even be seen in blood plasma. In normal animals this white color in blood plasma, known as *lipemia*, is transient, disappearing within 1 to 2 hours after digestion of the meal. The metabolic fate of the chylomicrons is discussed in Chapter 32.

GROWTH AND DEVELOPMENT OF THE INTESTINAL EPITHELIUM

The Length of Intestinal Villi Is Determined by the Relative Rates of Cell Loss at the Tips and Cell Replenishment at the Base

Division and replication of enterocytes occur in the crypts only. Crypt enterocytes are highly mitotic and regenerate rapidly. In fact, the intestinal crypt cells are among the most rapidly regenerating cells of the body, representing the single greatest need for protein synthesis in nongrowing animals. As crypt cells multiply, they migrate upward onto the villi, pushing other villous cells ahead of them, so there is a continuous progression of cells migrating up the villi. As the cells migrate they mature, changing from relatively undifferentiated cells in the crypts to highly specialized absorptive cells on the villi. As the cells reach the tips of the villi, they are lost because of age and exposure to gut contents. The length of villi is determined by the rate at which cells are lost at the tips and the rate at which they are replaced by cells from the crypts. An increase in cell loss at the villi tips, relative to crypt cell replication, results in shortening of the villi. Conversely, fast replication of crypt cells, relative to cell loss, leads to lengthening of the villi. The time taken for an enterocyte to migrate from its site of origin in the crypt to the tip of a villus varies with species and physiological state; on average, however, the turnover time of enterocytes is 4 to 7 days.

The rate of cell replication in the crypts appears to be stimulated by several GI hormones. When appetite and feed intake increase, there is an overall increase in the secretion of GI hormones. This in turn leads to a rise in crypt cell proliferation. An increase in the rate of crypt cell replication adds cells to the villus at a rate faster than they are lost at the tips, resulting in longer villi. Appetite and feed intake may increase because of conditions of greater energy need, such as lactation, exercise, and cold environmental temperatures. The greater villi length provides greater digestive and absorptive capacity to match the need created by higher feed intake. Thus the functional capacity of the intestine is adjusted to match the nutrient needs of the animal.

DIGESTION IN THE NEONATE

During the First Few Hours of Life, Proteins Are Not Digested but Are Absorbed Intact

In general, a major function of digestion is to break down proteins by hydrolysis. Under most circumstances, this process is a benefit to the animal not only from a nutritional and digestive standpoint, but also from a toxicologic and allergic standpoint; potentially toxic or allergenic proteins are broken down before they are absorbed into the body. In the special case of some neonates, however, there is a need to absorb proteins intact. In most livestock species, including horses, cattle, sheep, and swine,

essentially no antibodies are passed through the placenta from the dam to fetus. Thus, young livestock are born without the immunological protection of their mother's antibodies. In these species, antibodies from the mother must be acquired through ingestion of colostrum, the special mammary secretion present at birth. In these animals the digestive tract at birth is altered from the adult state, so the antibody proteins are absorbed intact rather than after digestion. There are three primary alterations, as follows:

- Acid secretion from the stomach is delayed for several days after birth.
- A similar delay appears in the development of pancreatic function, and thus acid and trypsin digestion of proteins is avoided.
- A specialized intestinal epithelium present at birth only is capable of engulfing soluble proteins in the intestinal lumen and discharging them into the lateral spaces.

The fetal intestinal epithelium has the same villous structure as the mature epithelium, but the villi are covered with special enterocytes capable of protein absorption. Immediately after birth, this special epithelium starts to disappear, and it is essentially gone after 24 hours. The loss of the protein-absorptive function in the neonate is referred to as *gut closure.*

The Major Intestinal Disaccharidase Switches from Lactase to Maltase with Maturity

Lactose from milk is the major carbohydrate in the diets of neonatal and young mammals; thus all mammals are born with high intestinal lactase activity. In contrast, maltase activity, necessary for digesting the products of luminal starch digestion, is weak or absent for several weeks after birth. As animals progress toward weaning, lactase activity wanes and maltase activity increases, allowing the animals to shift from lactose to starch as a carbohydrate source. In many species of adult animals, lactase activity is practically nonexistent.

PATHOPHYSIOLOGY OF DIARRHEA

Diarrhea refers to an increase in frequency of defecation or fecal volume. Volume often increases in diarrhea primarily because of increased water content. The amount of water passed in feces is the algebraic sum of GI water input and water absorption. As discussed earlier, water in the gut results from (1) ingested water, (2) water secreted by glands of the GI system, and (3) water secreted or lost directly through the mucosal epithelium. Under most circumstances the amount of water secreted into the gut greatly exceeds the amount ingested. Normally, the amount absorbed is just slightly less than the sum of the amounts secreted and ingested, leaving a small remainder for passage in the feces (Figure 30-29, *A*).

Diarrhea Occurs When There Is a Mismatch Between Secretion and Absorption

The amount of water in the feces is the result of the balance between secretion and absorption. *Malabsorptive diarrhea* occurs when absorption is inadequate to recover a sufficient portion of secreted water, as illustrated in Figure 30-29, *C*. Malabsorptive diarrhea usually occurs because of the loss of GI epithelium. In most instances, such losses occur because of viral, bacterial, or protozoal infections. Viral infections often cause particularly severe destruction of villous epithelium. These infections result in the loss of enterocytes from the villi. As noted previously, villous length is determined by the relative rates of cell loss and cell replacement (Figure 30-30).

Intestinal infections result in decreased villous length because the rate of cell loss is higher than the rate of cell replacement. Short villi cause impaired absorption for two reasons: (1) there is an absolute loss of absorptive intestinal surface area and (2) the cells that are lost are the mature cells from the upper regions of the villi. It is these mature cells that possess the enzymes of membranous-phase digestion and the transport proteins for sodium co-transport; loss of these cells results in impairment of digestion and absorption of nutrients. Because nutrient absorption is necessary for the osmotic absorption of water, water absorption is diminished when nutrient absorption is impaired.

Secretory diarrhea occurs when the rate of intestinal secretion increases and overwhelms the absorptive capacity. Most cases of hypersecretory diarrhea result from inappropriate secretion from the small intestinal crypts. This occurs when the normal secretory mechanism of the crypt epithelium (as discussed earlier) is abnormally stimulated. Toxins known as *enterotoxins* are produced by some types of pathogenic bacteria. These toxins bind to enterocytes and stimulate adenyl cyclase activity and the production of cAMP within the cells, resulting in opening of the chloride gates and the secretion of water and electrolytes from crypt epithelium. If the stimulation is mild, the gut may respond with an increase in absorption, and diarrhea does not result. However, when the secretion exceeds the capacity of the gut to increase absorption, as illustrated in Figure 30-29, *B*, diarrhea results. Hypersecretory diarrhea has devastating effects on the water, electrolyte, and acid-base status of animals, especially neonates. Hypersecretory diarrhea caused by enterotoxin-producing *Escherichia coli* is an extremely common disease of neonatal calves and pigs. This disease causes large economic losses in the cattle and swine industries as a result of treatment costs and death.

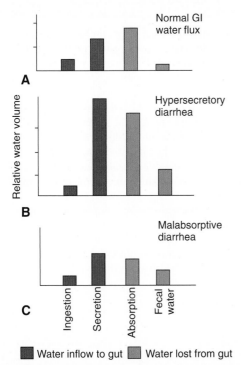

FIGURE 30-29 Pathophysiology of diarrhea. The bars represent the relative amounts of water entering or leaving the gut. Fecal volume is the sum of the water ingested and the water secreted minus the water absorbed. Therefore, fecal volume depends not on the amount of water entering the gut, but rather on the balance between water influx and efflux.

CLINICAL CORRELATIONS

DIARRHEA WITH DEHYDRATION AND ACIDOSIS IN A CALF

History. You are asked to examine a 2-day-old calf. The owner reports that the calf appeared normal the night before, but this morning she is recumbent and will not rise. In addition, she shows no interest in suckling a bottle.

Clinical Examination. The calf's body temperature is subnormal. The mouth is dry, and the eyes are sunken into the orbits. The ears, tail, and distal legs are cool to the touch. The tail and perineum of the calf are wet. As you remove your thermometer, the calf passes a stream of liquid feces. The feces are almost clear and slightly yellow, with the consistency of water. Simple laboratory tests indicate that the packed cell volume is 50% (normal, 30% to 35%) and the serum total-solids concentration 7.5% (normal, 5.5% to 6.5%).

Comment. The calf has diarrhea, and the physical examination and laboratory findings indicate a state of advanced dehydration. Loss of body fluid volume is so severe that the calf appears to be in or near a state of hypovolemic shock. Although you cannot be

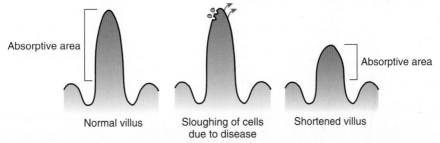

FIGURE 30-30 Shortening of villi caused by increased cell loss. Many infectious diseases result in an increased rate of cell sloughing from the villi. As cells are lost, the villus shrinks to fill in the gap in the epithelial coat. If villous height is to be maintained in the presence of rapid loss of enterocytes, the rate of recruitment of new cells, generated in the crypts, must be increased. Therefore, when the rate of cell loss exceeds the capacity for cell replacement, shortened villi with reduced absorptive surfaces and relatively immature enterocytes appear.

certain from your examination of the calf at the farm, the severity of dehydration, the rapidity of onset, and the age of the calf all suggest a hypersecretory diarrhea caused by enterotoxigenic *E. coli* bacteria. Animals with such clinical signs are usually severely acidotic, although blood pH is seldom measured in field cases. Diarrhea, acidosis, and dehydration occur because toxins produced by the bacteria stimulate opening of chloride gates in the apical membranes of crypt cells, stimulating copious secretion of water and electrolytes, including bicarbonate. The sodium co-transport system on the villi is unaffected by the bacterial toxin, but the simultaneous presence of glucose and sodium in the lumen is necessary to promote co-transport, which can offset some of the fluid and electrolyte losses caused by hypersecretion from the intestinal crypts.

Treatment. Vascular volume expansion and correction of acidosis are primary concerns in such cases. This calf should receive 2 L of alkalizing fluids by rapid intravenous (IV) administration, with an additional 2 L or more over the next 24 hours. Frequently, the response of calves to such treatment is remarkable, and calves that appear almost dead can often be saved by vigorous fluid therapy. After the initial replacement of lost fluids by IV therapy, further dehydration caused by ongoing fluid losses can be prevented by oral administration of fluids containing glucose and sodium.

JUVENILE PANCREATIC ATROPHY IN A DOG

History. You are presented with a thin, 3-year-old German shepherd. The owners report that the dog appeared normal until 6 months ago. At that time they noticed that he started losing weight and began to eat his own feces. Recently the weight loss has become more severe, even though he has had a good appetite and seems normal otherwise. Lately, the owners have noted that the dog seems to pass a large amount of feces, which is soft and gray with a claylike consistency.

Clinical Examination. Physical examination reveals an extremely thin dog with a dull, uneven hair coat. Other physical findings are unremarkable, and the dog seems bright and friendly. You hospitalize the animal for further testing and note that he readily eats two cans of commercial dog food per day. Laboratory analysis of feces collected over a 24-hour period reveals that the dog is passing 25 g of fat in the feces per day (normal, <5 g, assuming normal diet).

Comment. This degree of fat malabsorption is characteristic of *pancreatic exocrine insufficiency*. Because there is insufficient pancreatic lipase, fats cannot be hydrolyzed to fatty acids for absorption and thus pass unabsorbed through the gut. Other laboratory tests for assessing pancreatic exocrine function include (1) examination of blood for the presence of orally administered markers that require pancreatic enzymes for digestion and absorption and (2) direct examination of feces for the presence of pancreatic enzymes or undigested nutrients. Currently, the most definitive laboratory test for the diagnosis of pancreatic exocrine insufficiency is serum *trypsin-like immunoreactivity*. Under normal conditions, a very small proportion of the trypsinogen synthesized by the pancreatic acinar cells escapes into the peripheral bloodstream, and a similar small portion of trypsin is absorbed from the intestine. Although these concentrations are too small to have an effect on the body, they can be measured in blood. The assay is based on an antibody reaction and the quantitative result is referred to as trypsin-like immunoreactivity. A low value for *trypsin-like immunoreactivity* is indicative of pancreatic exocrine insufficiency.

Treatment. Feeding highly digestible diets mixed with commercially prepared pancreatic enzymes is usually successful in promoting adequate nutrient absorption in animals with *juvenile pancreatic atrophy*. Digestion may not be completely normal but is sufficient for the dog to attain a normal body weight. Treatment must be continued for life. You may question how orally administered pancreatic enzymes can survive intact through the proteolytic environment of the stomach. Undoubtedly, portions are destroyed, but sufficient enzyme appears to make it through the stomach to be effective.

PRACTICE QUESTIONS

1. Finding triglycerides and starch in the feces of a thin dog with a normal feed intake would suggest:
   a. Malabsorption.
   b. Maldigestion.

2. Which statement about the tight junctions is *false?*
   a. Tight junctions encircle the enterocyte near its apical end.
   b. Tight junctions form the dividing line between the apical membrane and the basolateral membrane.
   c. Tight junctions are impermeable to water.
   d. Tight junctions separate the lateral space from the intestinal lumen.
   e. Tight junctions are the only points that attach enterocytes together.

3. Which of the following molecules is consumed during the process of hydrolytic digestion?
   a. Glucose
   b. Alanine
   c. Dipeptides
   d. Fatty acids
   e. Water

4. A drug that blocks the activity of the Na^+,K^+-ATPase pump could be expected to have what effect on sodium-glucose co-transport?
   a. Increased sodium-glucose co-transport
   b. Decreased sodium-glucose co-transport
   c. No effect on sodium-glucose co-transport

5. During sodium absorption by glucose co-transport:
   a. Chloride is absorbed by the paracellular route.
   b. Chloride absorption is not affected.
   c. Chloride is absorbed in exchange for bicarbonate.
   d. Chloride absorption is coupled with potassium absorption.
   e. Chloride is absorbed in exchange for hydrogen ion.

6. Before entering the intestinal capillaries, all nutrients pass through the:
   a. Apical membrane.
   b. Tight junction.
   c. Lateral space.
   d. Basolateral membrane.
   e. Enterocyte cytoplasm.

BIBLIOGRAPHY

Barrett K: *Gastrointestinal physiology*, Columbus, Ohio, 2006, McGraw-Hill.

Ganapathy V, Ganapathy ME, Leibach FH: Protein digestion and assimilation. In Yamada T, editor: *Textbook of gastroenterology*, vol 1, ed 5, Philadelphia, 2009, Lippincott Williams & Wilkins.

Hall EJ: Clinical laboratory evaluation of small intestinal function, *Vet Clin North Am Small Anim Pract* 29(2):441–469, 1999.

Johnson LR: Digestion and absorption. In Johnson LR, editor: *Gastrointestinal physiology*, ed 7, St Louis, 2007, Mosby.

Johnson LR: Fluid and electrolyte absorption. In Johnson LR, editor: *Gastrointestinal physiology*, ed 7, St Louis, 2007, Mosby.

Keely SJ, Montrose MH, Barrett KE: Electrolyte secretion and absorption: small intestine and colon. In Yamada T, editor: *Textbook of gastroenterology*, vol 1, ed 5, Philadelphia, 2009, Lippincott Williams & Wilkins.

Lundgren O: Enteric nerves and diarrhea, *Pharmacol Toxicol* 90(3):109–120, 2002.

Nagy B, Fekete PZ: Enterotoxigenic *Escherichia coli* (ETEC) in farm animals, *Vet Res* 30(2–3):259–284, 1999.

Naylor JM: Oral electrolyte therapy, *Vet Clin North Am Food Anim Pract* 15(3):487–504, 1999.

Rao MC: Oral rehydration therapy: new explanations for an old remedy, *Annu Rev Physiol* 66:385–417, 2004.

Shi X, Summers RW, Schedl HP, et al: Effects of solution osmolality on absorption of select fluid replacement solutions in human duodenojejunum, *J Appl Physiol* 77(3):1178–1184, 1994.

Shirazi-Beechey SP, Moran AW, Bravo D, Al-Rammahi M: Nonruminant nutrition symposium: intestinal glucose sensing and regulation of glucose absorption: implications for swine nutrition, *J Anim Sci* 89(6):1854–1862, 2011.

Sibley E: Carbohydrate assimilation. In Yamada T, editor: *Textbook of gastroenterology*, vol 1, ed 5, Philadelphia, 2009, Lippincott Williams & Wilkins.

Stevens CE, Hume ID: *Comparative physiology of the vertebrate digestive system*, ed 2, Cambridge, UK, 1995, Cambridge University Press.

Sun W, Lo C, Tso P: Intestinal lipid absorption. In Yamada T, editor: *Textbook of gastroenterology*, vol 1, ed 5, Philadelphia, 2009, Lippincott Williams & Wilkins.

CHAPTER 31

Digestion: The Fermentative Processes

KEY POINTS

1. Fermentation is the metabolic action of bacteria.
2. The sites of fermentative digestion must be conducive to microbial growth.

Microbial ecosystem of fermentative digestion
1. The microbes responsible for fermentative digestion include bacteria, fungi, and protozoa.
2. Cooperation and interplay among the many species of microbes give rise to a complex ecosystem in the forestomach and hindgut.

Substrates and products of fermentative digestion
1. Plant cell walls are important substrates for fermentative digestion and significant nutrient sources for many species.
2. Nutrients other than cell walls are also subject to fermentative digestion.
3. Anaerobic conditions in the rumen result in metabolic activities leading to the production of volatile fatty acids.
4. Volatile fatty acids are important energy substrates for the host animal.
5. Fermentative digestion of protein results in the deamination of a large portion of amino acids.
6. When protein and energy availability in the forestomach are well matched, rapid microbial growth and efficient protein utilization result.
7. Microbial protein can be synthesized in the rumen from nonprotein nitrogen sources.

Reticulorumen motility and maintenance of the rumen environment
1. The physiological functions of the reticulorumen maintain an environment favorable to fermentation patterns that are beneficial to the host.
2. Rumen fermentation is maintained by selectively retaining actively fermenting material while allowing unfermentable residue to pass on to the lower digestive tract.
3. Digestibility and physical characteristics of feed have important influences on both the rate of particle passage from the rumen and the rate of feed intake.

4. Rumination, or cud chewing, has an important effect on the reduction of particle size and the movement of solid material through the rumen.
5. Water moves through the rumen at a much faster rate than particulate matter.
6. Rumen dilution rate has important influences on fermentation and microbial cell yield.

Control of reticulorumen motility
1. Reticulorumen motility is controlled by the central nervous system and affected by intraluminal conditions.

Omasal function
1. Passage of material from the reticulum to the omasum occurs during reticular contraction.

Volatile fatty acid absorption
1. Volatile fatty acids, representing 60% to 80% of the energy needs of the animal, are absorbed directly from the forestomach epithelium.

Rumen development and esophageal groove function
1. Significant changes in forestomach size and function occur with dietary changes in early life.
2. The esophageal groove diverts the flow of ingested milk past the forestomach and into the abomasum.

Function of the equine large hindgut
1. The equine hindgut has a great capacity for fermentation.
2. The types of substrate and fermentation patterns are essentially identical for forestomach and hindgut fermentation.
3. The motility functions of the cecum and colon retain material for fermentation and separate particles by size.
4. The rate of fermentation and volatile fatty acid production in the equine colon is similar to that in the rumen.
5. Hindgut anatomy and function vary greatly among the many species of veterinary interest.

Fermentation Is the Metabolic Action of Bacteria

In fermentative digestion, molecular substrates are broken down by the action of bacteria and other microorganisms. Enzymatic hydrolysis of large molecules is an essential part of fermentative digestion, just as it is for glandular digestion. The major difference between the two processes is that the enzymes of fermentative digestion are microbial in origin, rather than coming from the host animal. Other major differences between fermentative and glandular digestion involve the rate of reactions and the extent of alteration of the substrate molecules. In general, fermentative

digestion is much slower than glandular digestion, and the substrates are altered to a much greater degree.

The Sites of Fermentative Digestion Must Be Conducive to Microbial Growth

Fermentative digestion occurs in specialized compartments that are positioned either before or after the stomach and small intestine. Fermentative compartments positioned before the stomach are called *forestomachs* and are most highly developed in the ruminants and camelids. The size and development of the forestomach fermentation compartments vary greatly among species; many species have distinct forestomachs that are less developed than those of ruminants. Some species, including the horse and rat, have no anatomically distinct forestomach; however, some fermentative digestion may occur in a nonglandular portion of the proximal stomach.

Fermentation compartments positioned distal to the small intestine are the cecum and colon, often collectively called the *hindgut*. As with the forestomach, great anatomical differences exist in the hindgut of various species. This variation can be so extensive that the cecum and colon may appear to be functionally different organs in different species; however, when the variations are evaluated critically, important similarities can be seen in hindgut function among species.

The forestomach and hindgut can support fermentative digestion because their pH, moisture, ionic strength, and oxidation-reduction conditions are maintained in a range compatible for the growth of suitable microbes. In addition, the flow of ingesta through these areas is comparatively slow, allowing microbes time to maintain their population size. The importance of these factors can be illustrated through comparison of the forestomach and colon to the stomach and small intestine. In the stomach, bacterial numbers are kept low by the acid pH, whereas in the small intestine, bacterial numbers are kept in check by the constant flushing action of ingesta and secretions. In contrast, the pH in the forestomach and large colon is close to neutral, and the flow rate is comparatively slow.

In general, the fermentative patterns of the hindgut appear to be similar to those of the forestomach, although forestomach fermentation, especially that of the rumen, appears to be the better studied of the two. The following discussion focuses on rumen digestion but includes comments on hindgut digestion. Digestion in the equine cecum and colon is discussed at the end of the chapter.

MICROBIAL ECOSYSTEM OF FERMENTATIVE DIGESTION

The Microbes Responsible for Fermentative Digestion Include Bacteria, Fungi, and Protozoa

The bacterial population associated with fermentative digestion is vast, with at least 28 functionally important species occurring in the rumen. Box 31-1 lists some of the major species found in the rumen and their preferred substrates. Total bacterial numbers in the forestomach or hindgut normally range from 10^{10} to 10^{11} cells per gram of ingesta. Most of these bacteria are strict anaerobes that cannot survive in the presence of oxygen, although facultative organisms are also present. In the rumen, fungi are

---

BOX 31-1 Grouping of Rumen Bacterial Species According to Type of Substrates Fermented

Major Cellulolytic Species
Bacteroides succinogenes
Ruminococcus flavefaciens
Ruminococcus albus
Butyrivibrio fibrisolvens

Major Hemicellulolytic Species
Butyrivibrio fibrisolvens
Bacteroides ruminicola
Ruminococcus species

Major Pectinolytic Species
Butyrivibrio fibrisolvens
Bacteroides ruminicola
Lachnospira multiparus
Succinivibrio dextrinosolvens
Treponema bryantii
Streptococcus bovis

Major Amylolytic Species
Bacteroides amylophilus
Streptococcus bovis
Succinimonas amylolytica
Bacteroides ruminicola

Major Ureolytic Species
Succinivibrio dextrinosolvens
Selenomonas species
Bacteroides ruminicola
Ruminococcus bromii
Butyrivibrio species
Treponema species

Major Methane-Producing Species
Methanobrevibacter ruminantium
Methanobacterium formicicum
Methanomicrobium mobile

Major Sugar-Utilizing Species
Treponema bryantii
Lactobacillus vitulinus
Lactobacillus ruminis

Major Acid-Utilizing Species
Megasphaera elsdenii
Selenomonas ruminantium

Major Proteolytic Species
Bacteroides amylophilus
Bacteroides ruminicola
Butyrivibrio fibrisolvens
Streptococcus bovis

Major Ammonia-Producing Species
Bacteroides ruminicola
Megasphaera elsdenii
Selenomonas ruminantium

Major Lipid-Utilizing Species
Anaerovibrio lipolytica
Butyrivibrio fibrisolvens
Treponema bryantii
Eubacterium species
Fusocillus species
Micrococcus species

From Church DC, editor: *The ruminant animal: digestive physiology and nutrition*, Englewood Cliffs, NJ, 1988, Prentice-Hall.

present, and research suggests that fungi may play an important role in the digestion of plant cell walls.

There is also a large population of protozoa in the rumen as well as in the cecum and colon. Protozoal numbers average about 10^5 to 10^6 cells per gram of rumen contents. Although this number is considerably smaller than the number of bacteria, the relatively larger size of the individual protozoa compared with bacteria results in a total rumen protozoal cell mass approximately equal to the bacterial cell mass, under most dietary conditions. Most of the rumen protozoa are ciliated and belong to the genus *Isotricha* or *Entodinium*, although flagellate species are also present, especially in young ruminants. As with the other organisms of the rumen, the protozoa are anaerobic.

The digestive abilities, or capacities, of protozoa and bacteria are similar; thus either type of organism can perform most of the fermentative functions of the rumen. Protozoa ingest large numbers of bacteria and hold rumen bacterial numbers in check. However, none of the actions of protozoa appears essential to rumen function because ruminants can survive well without protozoa. Thus the role of protozoa in the total ecological picture of the rumen is uncertain. One potentially important function of protozoa involves their ability to slow down the digestion of rapidly fermentable substrates, such as starch and some proteins. Protozoa are capable of ingesting particles of starch and protein and storing them in their bodies, protected from bacterial action. The starch and protein remain engulfed until digested by the protozoa, or until the protozoa die or are swept from the rumen into the lower digestive tract. Thus, protozoa may have the effect of delaying or prolonging the digestion of these substrates. Especially in the case of starch, this protozoal effect may be beneficial to the host through modulation or delay of the digestion of rapidly fermentable substrate.

Cooperation and Interplay Among the Many Species of Microbes Give Rise to a Complex Ecosystem in the Forestomach and Hindgut

The digestive process in the rumen or colon involves the interplay among the many species of bacteria and other microbes. The ecosystem of fermentative digestion is extremely complex, with the waste products of one microbial species serving as substrate for another. For example, *Ruminococcus albus* and *Bacteroides ruminicola* appear to exist synergistically. *R. albus* digests cellulose (is *cellulolytic*) but cannot digest protein. *B. ruminicola*, on the other hand, can digest protein but cannot digest cellulose. When the microbes are grown together, cellulose digestion by *R. albus* provides hexoses for the energy needs of *B. ruminicola*, and protein digestion by *B. ruminicola* provides ammonia and branch-chain fatty acids for the growth needs of *R. albus*.

In addition to substrate needs, growth factor needs are also supplied synergistically within the rumen ecosystem. For example, B vitamins are necessary for the growth of several rumen microbes, but these nutrients are generally not necessary in ruminant diets. The synergistic effect of B vitamins results from cross-feeding between species of those microbes that produce various B vitamins and those microbes that require them.

Despite tremendous ecological complexity, however, the entire pattern of fermentation may be viewed as a holistic process, without consideration of the roles and interactions of individual microbial species. Fermentative digestion is examined here from this viewpoint, with the actions of the entire rumen biomass considered as an overall digestive process, irrespective of the specific needs and actions of individual microbial species.

SUBSTRATES AND PRODUCTS OF FERMENTATIVE DIGESTION

Plant Cell Walls Are Important Substrates for Fermentative Digestion and Significant Nutrient Sources for Many Species

Forages, or the foliage of plants, are both the major feedstuff of large herbivores and an important substrate for fermentative digestion. Some appreciation of the physical and chemical nature of plants is important to an understanding of the fermentative digestion of forages. This understanding may be aided by a brief comparison of plant and animal tissue structure.

At the cellular level, a major difference between plants and animals is the existence of a *cell wall* in plants. The cell wall is a complex of various carbohydrate molecules. The structural parts of plants, the leaves and stems, contain a large portion of cell-wall material. This material gives the plants their rigid framework and protects them from weather and other elements during growth. The cell-wall structure of plants can be roughly compared to the connective tissue structure of animals. Long, fiberlike molecules of *cellulose* have a strength-giving role similar to that of collagen, whereas *hemicellulose, pectin,* and *lignin* cement the cellulose together, much as hyaluronic acid and chondroitin sulfate do in animal connective tissue. With the exception of lignin, all these cell-wall molecules are carbohydrate.

Cellulose is composed of nonbranching chains of glucose monomers joined by $\beta[1\text{-}4]$ glycosidic linkages, in contrast to the $\alpha[1\text{-}4]$ linkages in starch. Pectin and hemicellulose are chemically more heterogeneous than cellulose, being composed of various proportions of several sugars and sugar acids. None of the cell-wall materials is subject to hydrolytic digestion by mammalian glandular digestive enzymes. However, cellulose, hemicellulose, and pectin are subject to the hydrolytic action of a complex of microbial enzymes known as *cellulase*. This enzyme system releases monosaccharides and oligosaccharides from the complex carbohydrates of cell walls, but the released saccharides are not directly available for absorption by the animal. Rather, they are further metabolized by the microbes, as discussed later.

Lignin, a heterogeneous group of phenolic chemicals, is resistant to the action of either mammalian or microbial enzymes, and only a small portion of lignin is digested by either process. Lignin is important not only because it is indigestible itself, but also because it tends to encase the cell-wall carbohydrates, reducing their digestibility by protecting them from the action of bacterial cellulase. The lignin concentration of plants increases with age and ambient temperature; thus young, cool-season plants are more digestible than mature plants grown in hot weather.

Nutrients Other Than Cell Walls Are Also Subject to Fermentative Digestion

The fermentative digestion of plant cell-wall material and its importance to herbivore digestion are well known. In addition, however, essentially all protein and carbohydrate nutrients that can provide substrate for energy and growth in mammals can also support the similar needs of microbes. Therefore, almost all dietary protein and carbohydrate are potentially subject to fermentative digestion. This fact is especially important in ruminants, in which food is exposed to fermentative digestion in the forestomach before its arrival at sites of glandular digestion. This temporal arrangement leads to the fermentative digestion of many nutrients that would otherwise have been available to the animal through glandular digestion. Thus, forestomach fermentative digestion, which provides for the efficient use of plant cell walls, can potentially lead to the inefficient use of other nutrients because of microbial alteration.

Anaerobic Conditions in the Rumen Result in Metabolic Activities Leading to the Production of Volatile Fatty Acids

When carbohydrate material enters the rumen or colon, it is attacked by hydrolytic microbial enzymes. In the case of insoluble carbohydrates, attack requires the physical attachment of bacteria to the surface of the plant particle, with the enzymes themselves part of the surface coating of the bacteria. Enzymatic action liberates glucose, other monosaccharides, and short-chain polysaccharides into the fluid phase, outside the microbial cell bodies. Although free in solution, these products of microbial enzyme action do not become immediately available to the host animal; rather, they are quickly subjected to further metabolism by the microbial mass. Glucose and other sugars are absorbed into the cell bodies of the microbes.

Within the microbial cells, glucose enters the glycolytic, or *Embden-Meyerhof,* pathway. This is the same glycolytic pathway that exists in mammalian cells, and as in mammalian tissues, catabolism of glucose through this pathway yields two molecules of pyruvate for each molecule of glucose metabolized. In the process, two molecules of oxidized nicotinamide adenine dinucleotide (NAD) are reduced to NAD hydrogen (NADH), and two molecules of adenosine triphosphate (ATP) are formed from adenosine diphosphate (ADP). The potential energy represented by the ATP formed in this reaction is not directly available to the host animal but is the major source of energy for maintenance and growth of microbes.

If fermentative digestion were to occur under aerobic conditions, which it does not, the pyruvate produced by the glycolytic process would enter the citric acid (Krebs) cycle and would be metabolized to carbon dioxide and water, as occurs under the aerobic conditions in mammalian cells. Furthermore, in an aerobic system, the NADH produced would be oxidized in the cytochrome oxidase system with additional production of ATP and the regeneration of NAD. However, fermentative digestion is not an aerobic system; on the contrary, it proceeds in a reductive, highly anaerobic environment. Therefore a different mechanism must be provided for the oxidation of NADH and other reduced cofactors. If such a mechanism were not available, all the oxidized cofactors present would soon be reduced, and metabolism would come to a halt. Because no atmospheric oxygen is available, some other compound must serve as an "electron sink" for the oxidation of enzyme cofactors.

In fermentative digestion, pyruvate can act as an electron sink, being further reduced to provide for regeneration of NAD and the general removal of excess electrons, with an additional yield of ATP. Also, carbon dioxide can be reduced to methane, accepting electrons for the regeneration of NAD. Figure 31-1 illustrates the metabolic pathways of these reactions. These pathways lead to the major end products of the fermentative digestion of carbohydrate, the *volatile fatty acids* (VFAs). The primary VFAs are *acetic acid, propionic acid,* and *butyric acid;* the VFAs are often referred to as their dissociated ions: acetate, propionate, and butyrate, respectively. Other quantitatively minor but metabolically important VFAs are valeric acid, isovaleric acid, isobutyric acid, and 2-methylbutyric acid. Figure 31-2 shows the chemical structures of the VFAs.

Production of propionic acid from pyruvate results in the efficient regeneration of NAD with no net production of NADH.

In fact, production of available oxygen by the *randomizing branch* of the propionic acid pathway leads to oxidation of excess NADH originating from the acetic or butyric acid pathways (see Figure 31-1). The production of acetic acid leads to the efficient generation of ATP but, in contrast to the production of propionic acid, does not result in the regeneration of NAD from NADH. In the acetic acid pathway, excess NADH is produced. In this case, NAD is regenerated by the formation of free hydrogen, which is subsequently used to reduce carbon dioxide to methane and water (see Figure 31-1, *lower portion*).

Thus a direct relationship exists between acetic acid production and methane production; as the amount of pyruvate entering the acetic acid pathway increases, there must be a concomitant rise in methane production. Likewise, a reciprocal relationship exists between methane production and propionic acid production; as pyruvate is diverted to propionic acid production, there is less need for methane synthesis. These relationships are shown in the stoichiometric equations of Box 31-2. These reactions do not, however, fully describe the flow of hydrogen, or reducing substances, in rumen or colonic metabolism. The chemical reactions of fermentation are extremely complex and interdependent, and NADH can donate its electrons to reactions other than those described in Box 31-2, such as the synthesis of microbial protein and the saturation of unsaturated fatty acids.

In the rumen, methane production is facilitated by methanogenic bacteria, such as *Methanobacterium ruminantium.* This fragile bacterium is sensitive to changing conditions in the rumen. When conditions are unfavorable for the survival of *M. ruminantium,* methane production is reduced, shifting the metabolic pathways toward propionic acid production. Some conditions that suppress methanogenic species are high levels of feed intake,

---

BOX 31-2 Theoretical Stoichiometric Carbon-Hydrogen Balance Equations Describing Conversion of Glucose in Rumen

Case 1

Glucose $\rightarrow$ 2 acetate + 2 CO_2 + 8 H

Glucose $\rightarrow$ Butyrate + 2 CO_2 + 4 H

Glucose + 4 H $\rightarrow$ 2 propionate + 2 H_2O

CO_2 + 8 H $\rightarrow$ CH_4 + H_2O

Net*

3 glucose $\rightarrow$ 2 acetate + butyrate + 2 propionate + 3 CO_2 + CH_4 + 2 H_2O

Case 2

3 glucose $\rightarrow$ 6 butyrate + 2 propionate + CO_2 + CH_4 + 24 H

Glucose $\rightarrow$ Butyrate + 2 CO_2 + 4 H

Glucose + 4 H $\rightarrow$ 2 propionate + 2 H_2O

3 CO_2 + 24 H $\rightarrow$ 3 CH_4 + 6 H_2O

Net*

5 glucose $\rightarrow$ 6 acetate + butyrate + 2 propionate + 5 CO_2 + 3 CH_4 + 6 H_2O

From Van Soest PJ: *Nutritional ecology of the ruminant,* Ithaca, NY, 1982, Cornell University Press.

*Note that, in Case 1, the acetate/propionate ratio is 1:1 and the methane/glucose ratio 1:3; in Case 2, however, the acetate/propionate ratio is 3:1 and the methane/glucose ratio 3:5.

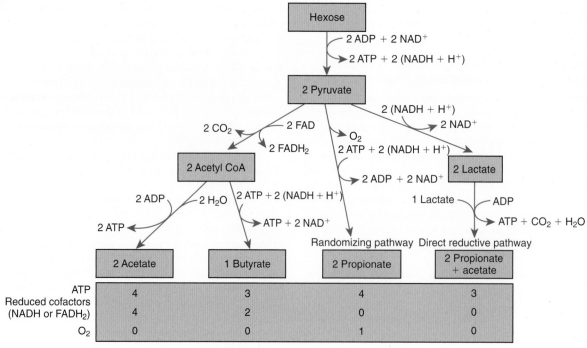

FIGURE 31-1 Pathways of volatile fatty acid (VFA) production by the rumen or colonic biomass. The production of methane is necessary for the production of oxidized cofactors in the pathways leading to acetate and butyrate production, but not in the pathways leading to propionate production. The production of oxygen by the randomizing pathway results in the net production of oxidized cofactors. *ADP,* Adenosine diphosphate; *ATP,* adenosine triphosphate; *NAD,* nicotinamide adenine dinucleotide; *FAD,* flavin adenine dinucleotide; *H,* hydrogen; *CoA,* coenzyme A; *CO₂,* carbon dioxide.

use of finely ground or pelleted feeds, and high-grain or high-starch diets. Under these circumstances the rate of methane production is reduced, resulting in a lower rate of acetic acid production with a concomitant increase in the propionic acid production rate.

The proportional rates at which acetic acid, propionic acid, and butyric acid are produced are reflected in their relative concentrations in the rumen fluid. The relative concentrations of the VFAs have important nutritional and metabolic consequences, and although seldom measured for medical purposes, VFA concentrations are frequently reported in research literature. Typically, the ruminal acetic/propionic/butyric acid concentration ratio in ruminants ranges from 70 : 20 : 10 for animals eating high-forage diets to 60 : 30 : 10 for animals eating high-grain diets. One must remember that these values represent relative proportions and not absolute amounts. The total amount of VFA produced with a high-starch diet is usually much higher than that produced with a high-fiber diet, such that total acetic acid production may be higher with a high-starch diet than with a high-fiber diet, even though the acetic acid production relative to the other VFAs may be reduced. Figure 31-3 illustrates this principle.

Volatile Fatty Acids Are Important Energy Substrates for the Host Animal

One can appreciate the elegance and beauty of the symbiotic relationship represented by fermentative digestion by considering the metabolism of VFAs. These molecules are the end products, indeed, the waste products, of anaerobic microbial metabolism, just as carbon dioxide is the waste product of aerobic metabolism. If the VFAs were allowed to accumulate, they would suppress or alter the fermentative process by lowering the pH of the gut or forestomach. However, the host animal maintains conditions for fermentation both by buffering pH changes and by removing VFAs from the gut by absorption. The benefit derived by the host is from the chemical energy that is contained in the VFAs. These bacterial "waste products" represent spent compounds within the framework of the anaerobic fermentation system, but they still contain considerable energy that can be derived from aerobic metabolism. In ruminants and other large herbivores, the VFAs are the major energy fuels, to a large extent serving the role played by glucose in omnivorous monogastric animals. The metabolic fates of the VFAs are discussed further in Chapter 32.

Fermentative Digestion of Protein Results in the Deamination of a Large Portion of Amino Acids

To this point, the discussion of fermentative digestion has centered primarily on carbohydrates, but as previously mentioned, other energy-yielding substrates are subject to microbial attack as well. Proteins are particularly vulnerable because they are composed of carbon compounds that can be further reduced to provide energy for anaerobic microbes. As proteins enter fermentative areas of the gut, they are attacked by extracellular microbial proteases. The majority of these enzymes are "trypsin-like" endopeptidases that form short-chain peptides as end products. These peptides are formed extracellularly and are absorbed into the microbial cell bodies, much as glucose is formed from carbohydrate and then absorbed. Within the microbial cells, the peptides

can be used to form microbial protein or can be further degraded for the production of energy through the VFA pathways (Figure 31-4).

To enter the VFA pathways, the individual amino acids are first deaminated to yield *ammonia* (NH_3) and a carbon skeleton. The carbon structures of many of the amino acids can fit directly into various steps of the pathways leading to the production of the three major VFAs. The three *branch-chain amino acids* (BCAAs) are exceptions, however, and lead to the production of branch-chain VFAs by the following reactions:

$$Valine + 2\,H_2O \rightarrow Isobutyrate + NH_3 + CO_2$$

$$Leucine + 2\,H_2O \rightarrow Isovalerate + NH_3 + CO_2$$

$$Isoleucine + 2\,H_2O \rightarrow 2\text{-}Methylbutyrate + NH_3 + CO_2$$

These branch-chain VFAs are important growth factors for several species of bacteria, as described later.

Although many species of rumen microbes appear capable of using preformed amino acids for the synthesis of protein, several species cannot do so. These species must synthesize amino acids from ammonia and the various carbon metabolites of the VFA pathways. For synthesis of the BCAAs, the branch-chain VFAs are required. Among the microbial species that require ammonia and branch-chain fatty acids are some of the important cellulose-digesting bacteria.

When Protein and Energy Availability in the Forestomach Are Well Matched, Rapid Microbial Growth and Efficient Protein Utilization Result

Because a large part of preformed dietary protein is fermented in the rumen, ruminant animals depend, to a large extent, on microbial protein to meet their own protein needs. Microbial protein reaches the abomasum and small intestine when microbes are washed out of the rumen and into the lower tract. Digestive efficiency is optimized in ruminants when the growth rate of the microbial mass is maximal, resulting in maximal delivery of microbial protein to the host animal. These conditions are best met by rapidly growing populations of microbes. The microbial growth rate depends on the supply of nutrients and the rate at which microbes are washed from the rumen. Here we consider the effect of nutrient supply on microbial growth rate; factors affecting the rate of microbial removal are discussed later.

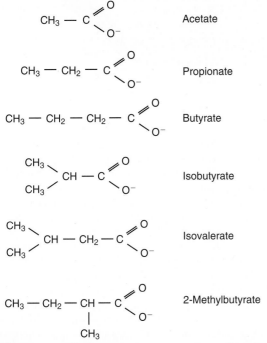

FIGURE 31-2 Chemical structures of the major volatile fatty acids (VFAs) produced by fermentative digestion.

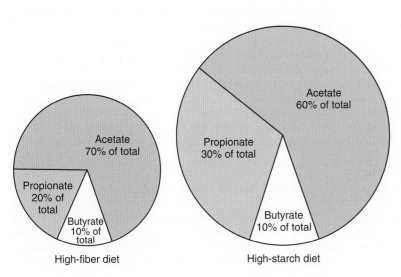

High-fiber diet High-starch diet

FIGURE 31-3 VFA production on high-fiber and high-starch diets. Although the percentage of acetate is lower on the high-starch diet, the total amount of acetate produced is greater on the high-starch diet. In contrast, propionate increases in both amount and proportion on the high-starch diet.

FIGURE 31-4 Protein metabolism by rumen microbes. Protease enzymes on the microbe surfaces generate peptides that are then taken up by many types of organisms. Absorbed peptides contribute to an intracellular pool of amino acids from which microbial proteins are synthesized **(A)**. Another source of amino acids is from intracellular synthesis **(B)**, using ammonia (NH_3) and volatile fatty acid (VFA). Many microbes appear capable of deriving their amino acids from either extracellular peptides or intracellular synthesis; however, several types of bacteria seem incapable of using peptides for an amino acid source and are thus dependent on an extracellular source of ammonia **(C)** for amino acid synthesis. Amino acids not used for protein synthesis can be metabolized to VFA and ammonia **(D)**.

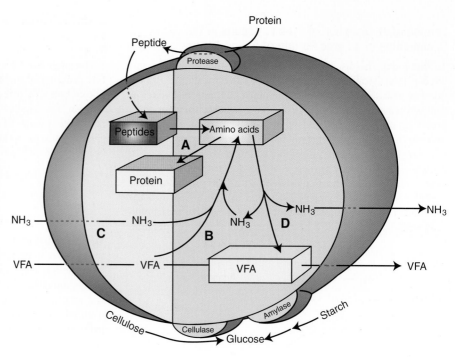

The overall reaction in the rumen may be greatly simplified, for the purposes of this discussion, to Equation 1:

$$glucose + peptide = microbes + VFA + NH_3 + CH_4 + CO_2 \quad (1)$$

Glucose and peptide represent ruminally available carbohydrate and protein, respectively. In this context, *available* means available to the microbes for fermentation. Carbohydrate or protein that is not susceptible, or accessible, to microbial attack is classified as *unavailable* and is not included in Equation 1. Glucose was chosen to represent carbohydrate, and peptide to represent protein, because all carbohydrates must be broken down to simple sugars, and proteins to peptides, before becoming available to bacteria. The term *peptide* in this equation could be replaced by other forms of nitrogen, but for now, the discussion is confined to peptide as a nitrogen source. Peptide is the only nitrogen-containing substrate on the left in the equation, but there are two nitrogen-containing products on the right: microbes (as protein) and NH_3 (ammonia). Both substrates, glucose and peptide, contain carbon, oxygen, and hydrogen and thus can contribute to the formation of microbial carbon, VFA, CH_4, and CO_2.

Equation 1 always balances, but the distribution of products varies according to the relative concentrations of substrates, as illustrated in Figure 31-5. For microbial cells to be produced, both energy and nitrogen are required. Energy can come from either glucose or peptide, but nitrogen must come from peptide. When glucose and peptide availability are appropriately matched (Figure 31-5, A), energy for cellular growth comes primarily from glucose, with peptides directed toward microbial protein synthesis. Under these conditions, the products of Equation 1 favor microbial cells with little ammonia production. Glucose fermentation with accompanying VFA production must be high to meet the large energy demands necessary to support the rapid growth of the microbial mass. Ammonia production is low because most peptide nitrogen is being incorporated into microbial protein.

When the availability of glucose is high relative to peptide (Figure 31-5, B), there is ample energy but insufficient nitrogen to support adequate protein synthesis, and thus microbial replication is not maximal. In this case, microbial energy utilization becomes inefficient as energy is used for the maintenance of nondividing cells, rather than for the energy-requiring synthetic processes of growing cells. The maintenance energy needs of the microbes still drive some fermentation of glucose with moderate VFA production, but production of both microbial cells and ammonia is limited because of lack of nitrogen.

When peptide availability exceeds glucose availability (Figure 31-5, C), there is ample nitrogen to support growth, but growth is limited because of insufficient energy supplies. These conditions force the microbes to use peptides to meet energy needs instead of for protein synthesis. Microbial growth rate is low, and VFA production is moderate, because fermentation is driven only by the maintenance energy needs of the microbes. Much of the VFA production comes from the carbon portions of the peptides, whereas the amine groups are shunted to ammonia production; thus the products of Equation 1 favor ammonia.

The relationship between available glucose (carbohydrate) and peptide (or nitrogen) has a tremendous effect on the production of microbial cells and thus a profound impact on the nutrition of the host. This relationship, as illustrated in Figure 31-5, is quantified by expressing microbial growth in terms of grams of microbial dry matter produced per mole of energy-producing substrate used. This value, referred to as *microbial yield*, is usually designated by a capital Y subscripted with the abbreviation of the energy substrate to which it is referenced. A convenient but somewhat theoretical substrate with which to reference microbial cell yield is ATP. Microbial yield is then written as $Y_{ATP} = x$, where x is the number of grams of microbial dry matter produced per mole of ATP used. The value of Y_{ATP} varies between about 10 and 20 g of microbes per mole of ATP. Nitrogen availability, from either peptide or nonprotein sources, has an important effect on the Y_{ATP} value. When microbial growth is limited by *low* nitrogen

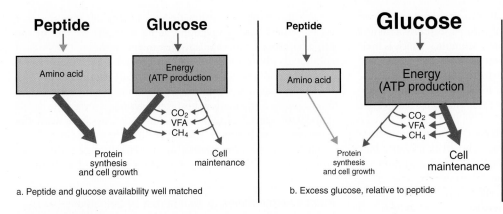

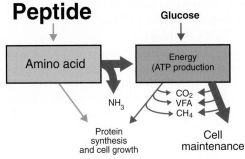

a. Peptide and glucose availability well matched

b. Excess glucose, relative to peptide

c. Excess peptide, relative to glucose

FIGURE 31-5 The efficiency with which dietary energy is used for protein synthesis in the rumen depends on the balance between energy and nitrogen sources. The proportion of energy used for protein synthesis and cell maintenance (as indicated by the size of the *arrows*) changes in relation to the balance of peptide (nitrogen) and glucose supplies. *ATP,* Adenosine triphosphate; *VFA,* volatile fatty acid.

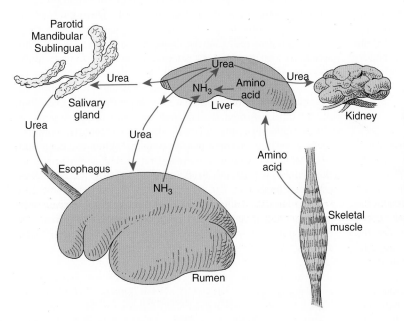

FIGURE 31-6 Interorgan nitrogen cycling in ruminants. The diagram shows the effects of rumen ammonia *(NH₃)* concentration on the formation and utilization of urea. When rumen ammonia concentrations are high, the net movement of nonprotein nitrogen is toward the liver, resulting in high urea production rates and poor nitrogen conservation. When rumen ammonia concentrations are low, the net movement of nonprotein nitrogen is from liver to rumen, resulting in protein production from endogenous urea.

availability, a large portion of available ATP is used for maintenance rather than cell growth; thus the number of cells produced per ATP is small, and the Y_{ATP} value is low.

Microbial Protein Can Be Synthesized in the Rumen from Nonprotein Nitrogen Sources

If sufficient carbohydrate is available, most rumen microbes, even those capable of utilizing preformed peptides, can synthesize protein from ammonia (see Figure 31-4). Thus, protein can be produced in the rumen from such nonprotein sources as ammonia, nitrates, and urea. From a nutritional and economic point of view, this capability has been exploited by the inclusion of inexpensive nonprotein nitrogen sources in place of expensive protein in ruminant diets, allowing the microbes to synthesize protein for the amino acid needs of the host. This process also can be exploited physiologically by the recycling of endogenous urea.

Urea, the nitrogenous waste product of protein catabolism, is formed in the liver. In ruminant animals, hepatic urea production is from two sources: (1) nitrogen arising from the deamination of endogenous amino acids and (2) nitrogen absorbed as ammonia from the rumen (Figure 31-6). Ammonia absorption from the rumen is proportional to the ruminal ammonia production rate, which is subject to the influences of ruminal carbohydrate and protein availability, as discussed earlier. Ammonia, which is toxic at moderate concentrations, is absorbed from the rumen and delivered to the liver through the hepatic-portal blood vascular system. The liver extracts ammonia from the portal blood efficiently; thus little of the potentially toxic ammonia reaches the systemic circulation.

In monogastric animals, urea is excreted from the body almost exclusively by the kidneys. In ruminants, however, urea also may be excreted into the rumen (see Figure 31-6). Such excretion can occur by direct absorption of urea into the rumen from the blood or by excretion of urea into saliva. In either case, the urea reaches the rumen, where it is quickly transformed to ammonia, and enters the general pool of rumen nitrogen from which microbial proteins are synthesized.

The direction of nonprotein nitrogen flow, either into the rumen as urea or out of the rumen as ammonia, depends on rumen ammonia concentrations. During times of high nitrogen availability in the rumen, relative to carbohydrate availability, this system results in high blood urea concentrations and the extensive loss of precious nitrogen through urinary excretion, making ruminants nutritionally inefficient under these dietary conditions. However, during times of high carbohydrate availability relative to nitrogen availability, the major flow of urea nitrogen is from the blood into the rumen. Under these circumstances, in which ruminal ammonia concentrations are low, most of the blood urea is from endogenous protein catabolism. A portion of this urea, which in monogastric animals would be unavailable for protein synthesis, is excreted into the rumen, where it can be resynthesized into protein that will contribute eventually to the amino acid needs of the host. Thus, under conditions of low dietary protein, ruminants are efficient conservers of nitrogen.

RETICULORUMEN MOTILITY AND MAINTENANCE OF THE RUMEN ENVIRONMENT

The Physiological Functions of the Reticulorumen Maintain an Environment Favorable to Fermentation Patterns That Are Beneficial to the Host

The host animal has no direct control over the metabolism of the microbes in its gut. However, important physiological factors influence the gastrointestinal (GI) fermentation process. For the host to ensure that the proper type of fermentation patterns occur, it must maintain within the rumen (or colon) conditions that promote the growth and favorable metabolic patterns of the most beneficial bacteria and other microbes. The following requirements must be met by the host for proper fermentation to occur:

1. Substrate for fermentation must be supplied.
2. Temperature must be maintained at or near 37° C.
3. Ionic strength (osmolality) of the rumen fluid must be kept within an optimal range (near 300 mOsm).
4. A negative oxidation-reduction potential must be maintained (−250 to −450 mV).
5. Indigestible waste (solid material) must be removed.
6. The rate of removal of microbes must be compatible with the regeneration times of the most favorable microbes.
7. Acid products of anaerobic fermentation (VFAs) must be buffered or removed.

The first of these requisites, delivery of substrate, requires only eating; others (e.g., temperature, ionic strength) are met by the same homeostatic mechanisms that maintain these physiological conditions within the host body in general. Maintenance of an appropriate oxidation-reduction potential requires only that oxygen be kept away from the fermentation site. The remaining requisites for fermentation, however, have necessitated the development of special physiological functions associated with the forestomach (or hindgut). These specialized functions include the motility patterns characteristic of the reticulorumen, the direct absorption of VFA, and the production of copious amounts of saliva.

Rumen Fermentation Is Maintained by Selectively Retaining Actively Fermenting Material While Allowing Unfermentable Residue to Pass on to the Lower Digestive Tract

The walls of the reticulorumen are muscular, possess an extensive intrinsic nervous system, and are capable of highly complex and coordinated motility patterns. These motility patterns are necessary for the critical function of the rumen, which is the selective retention of actively fermenting material accompanied by the simultaneous release of unfermentable residue. An understanding of reticulorumen anatomy is necessary to appreciate the effects of reticulorumen motility patterns. Figure 31-7 illustrates the division of the reticulorumen into compartments, or *sacs*. These divisions are created by muscular pillars that project into the lumen of the organ. The reticular fold and rumen pillars, in addition to the walls themselves, are motile. During reticulorumen contractions the pillars alternately elevate and relax, either accentuating or reducing the divisions within the lumen of the reticulorumen. Students accustomed to studying the reticulorumens of embalmed specimens may find it difficult to visualize the extent of rumen movement. At times during contractions, the excursions of the walls and pillars are so great that the total shape of the reticulorumen is distorted; sacs and compartments are almost obliterated, and pillars elevate to the extent that compartmental divisions become nearly complete. When the magnitude of these contractions is recognized, it is not difficult to appreciate the tremendous effect that reticulorumen motility has on the flow of rumen ingesta.

Two patterns of reticulorumen motility are generally described: primary (or mixing) contractions and secondary (or *eructation*) contractions. The complexity, sequential pattern, and highly

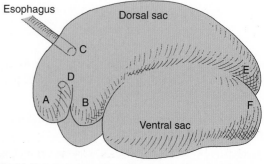

FIGURE 31-7 Rumen anatomy. *A*, Reticulum; *B*, cranial sac; *C*, cardia; *D*, reticulo-omasal orifice; *E*, caudal-dorsal blind sac; *F*, caudal-ventral blind sac.

coordinated nature of these motility patterns are illustrated and described in Figure 31-8. More important than knowing the exact sequence of contractions, however, is understanding the influence this pattern has on the flow of ingesta through the rumen. To illustrate the primary pattern of motility and describe its effect on ingesta flow, consider the path of a single bolus of feed material as it passes through the rumen. Assume this material is forage such as grass, hay, or ensilage. The animal chews the feed to create an initial reduction in particle size and to form it into a bolus by mixing it with saliva. The swallowed bolus enters the rumen at the cardia, which is at the dorsal portion of the reticulum near the junction of the reticulum and the cranial ventral sac (Figure 31-9, A). The viscous nature of saliva causes the feed material to initially remain in a bolus as it enters the rumen. Air bubbles trapped in the bolus give it a relatively low specific gravity, compared to surrounding ingesta, so it remains suspended in the area near the cardia (Figure 31-9, B). As a primary rumen contraction begins, there is a biphasic, or double contraction of the reticulum. The first of these contractions is relatively weak. The second follows very quickly after the first and is extremely forceful, nearly obliterating the lumen of the reticulum and creating a strong and rapid flow of fluid ingesta. Material in the dorsal portion of the reticulum, including the recently swallowed bolus of feed, is washed back into the rumen by this flow of liquid ingesta (Figure 31-9, C). A caudal-moving contraction of the dorsal sac follows the reticular contraction, continuing to move the recently swallowed bolus and other material further back into the dorsal sac. A subsequent cranial-moving contraction of the dorsal sac serves to mix the dorsal sac ingesta, creating a mass of tangled forage fibers representing a large collection of relatively recently swallowed material (Figure 31-9, D).

This mass of material tends to remain in the dorsal rumen due to buoyancy. Microbial action creates small bubbles of gas that adhere to the plant material accounting for its buoyancy and giving it a low *functional specific gravity*. As time passes, however, microbial action tends to cause the material to break apart. The small particles that remain become less buoyant because there is less fermentable substrate from which microbes can generate gas bubbles. The functional specific gravity of these particles increases due to the lack of gas bubbles and the material begins to sink in the rumen as small particles (Figure 31-9, E). The material in the dorsal sac, especially in animals on a diet with a large portion of forage, is typically a relatively solid mass of tangled forage fibers while the material in the ventral sac is a suspension of small particles that is much more fluid and water like. The interface between the two areas is not distinct and is composed of a "mushy," or slurry-like transition zone, a zone of intermediate-sized particles with intermediate functional specific gravity. Contractions of the ventral sac tend to push the more buoyant material back up into the dorsal sac, while allowing the smallest and least buoyant particles to spill over the cranial ruminal pillar into the cranial ventral sac (Figure 31-9, F).

Subsequent to the contractions of the ventral sac is a contraction of the cranial ventral sac, which further separates material based on functional specific gravity and results in small particles with the highest functional specific gravity flowing back into the reticulum (Figure 31-9, G). At this point material has made a complete circuit of the rumen, entering at the cardia and passing through the dorsal, ventral, and cranial ventral sacs and back to the reticulum. As the reticulum contracts at the beginning of a primary cycle, the reticulo-omasal orifice relaxes and dense (high

functional specific gravity) material near the bottom of the reticulum is forced through the opening and into the omasum (Figure 31-9, H).

The overall effect of the transit of feed through the rumen, particularly forage feed, is a reduction in particle size associated with the loss of fermentable portions of the plant structure. Long forage material is reduced by initial mastication to particles of 1 to 2 cm or shorter. Most of the material in the dorsal rumen is of similar particle size. Particle size diminishes in the more ventral portions of the rumen. Most particles that move through the reticulo-omasal orifice are 2 to 3 mm long. The selection of small particles for passage into the omasum occurs even though the reticulo-omasal orifice, when dilated for food passage, is probably about 2 cm in diameter, indicating that size discrimination is not based on the size of the reticulo-omasal orifice.

The discussion above applies to the effects of the primary (or mixing) pattern of motility. *Secondary* (or *eructation*) *contractions* occur as an added sequence of events at the end of a primary sequence of contractions. In general they occur in association with every second or third set of primary contractions. Secondary contractions consist of a cranial-moving wave that starts in the caudal-dorsal blind sac and continues over the dorsal sac (see Figure 31-8, segments 17 through 21). The function of the secondary contraction is to force gas toward the cranial portion of the rumen. The pattern begins with a contraction of the caudo-ventral blind sac, expressing trapped gas in that compartment into the dorsal sac. The secondary contraction continues with a forward-moving contraction of the dorsal sac that moves gas toward the cardia, while cranial sac relaxation and cranial pillar elevation allows liquid ingesta to move away from the cardia so that gas can enter the esophagus and be eructated. Secondary contractions are important because large amounts of gas, primarily CO_2 and CH_4, are formed during fermentation and must be removed rapidly to prevent distention of the rumen.

In general, one to three reticulorumen contractions occur per minute. Contractions occur most frequently during eating and disappear entirely during deep sleep. The rate and strength of contractions depend on the character of the diet: coarse, fibrous feeds stimulate the most frequent and strongest contractions. Secondary contractions usually occur in association with half the primary contractions, although this relationship is variable and depends on the rate of gas formation.

Digestibility and Physical Characteristics of Feed Have Important Influences on Both the Rate of Particle Passage from the Rumen and the Rate of Feed Intake

As indicated earlier, feed does not leave the rumen until it is broken down into small particles. Microbial action and remastication (as discussed later) are primarily responsible for particle size reduction in the rumen, and the rate of breakdown of fiber is chiefly a function of its digestibility. Poorly digestible fiber takes longer to be broken down sufficiently to sink into the ventral sac, compared with fiber of greater digestibility. This means that poorly digestible fiber remains in the rumen longer than fiber of greater digestibility. Because there are fixed limits to the volume of the rumen, the rate of feed intake cannot exceed the rate of ingesta outflow; therefore, intake of poorly digestible feeds is always less than intake of highly digestible feeds.

Feed preparation can influence this relationship. Chopping or grinding of poorly digestible forages increases their rate of passage from the rumen because less particle size reduction is necessary

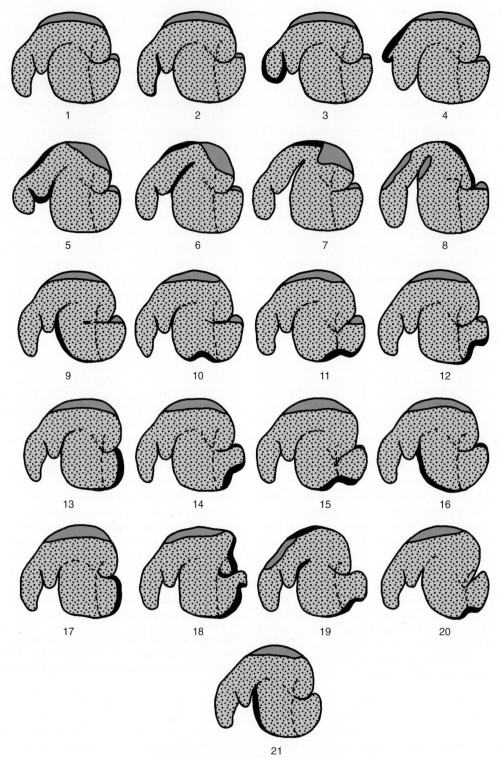

FIGURE 31-8 *See legend on opposite page.*

FIGURE 31-8 Contraction sequence in the reticulorumen. These drawings were derived by taking tracings directly from radiographs. The *open regions* represent the rumen gas cap (zone), whereas the stippled region represents ingesta. The *heavy lines* indicate portions of the wall that are actively contracting. Drawings *1* through *16* represent the sequence of events in a primary contraction in a normally fed sheep. Drawings *17* through *21* represent the sequence of events in a secondary or eructation contraction. *1,* Resting stage. *2,* Initiation of sequence with elevation of reticuloruminal fold. *3,* End of first phase of reticular contraction. *4,* End of second phase of reticular contraction; note dilation of cranial sac. *5* to *7,* Contraction of cranial sac followed by contraction of cranial pillar and dorsal sac. *8,* Contraction of caudal-dorsal blind sac and caudal pillar, causing cranial displacement of gas cap toward reticulum, under cranial pillar, and into caudal-ventral blind sac. *9,* Contraction of longitudinal pillar and cranial ventral rumen; in anorectic sheep, the sequence frequently ceases at this point, and the occurrence of the remaining steps in the sequence varies according to the degree of filling of the reticulorumen. *10* to *12,* Wave of contraction migrating caudally onto the caudal-ventral blind sac, associated with a ventral displacement of the caudal pillar. *13,* Contraction of the pole of the caudal-ventral blind sac displacing gas cap around the caudal pillar. *14* to *16,* Cranial migration of contraction if no secondary contraction sequence occurs. *17,* When a secondary contraction follows a primary, the terminal contraction of the caudal-ventral blind sac may be maintained over a prolonged period or may be repeated simultaneously with a second contraction of the caudal pillar. *18,* Contraction of caudal pillar and dorsal blind sac start to push gas cap cranially; contraction starts to move cranially across caudal-ventral blind sac. *19,* Contraction has moved rapidly across dorsal rumen, and cranial pillar has moved for the second time; eructation, if it occurs, occurs at this point. *20* and *21,* Contraction migrates cranially onto ventral rumen, causing contraction of ventral coronary pillars and second ventral displacement of the caudal pillar; cycle terminates with a contraction of the cranial ventral rumen. (From Ryckebusch Y, Thivend P: *Digestive physiology and metabolism in ruminants,* Westport, Conn, 1980, AVI Publishing.)

before pieces can pass into the omasum. Chopping or grinding also usually increases the amount of material that an animal can eat because the rumen throughput is increased. Often, however, digestibility is decreased by chopping or grinding of forages, because the duration of exposure to microbial action is reduced as a result of rapid passage of feed through the rumen. Thus, physical form (length) and digestibility each have an effect on rate of passage from the rumen and also on feed intake. In general, forage material of relatively high digestibility has a rumen half-life of approximately 30 hours, whereas poorly digestible material has a half-life of up to 50 hours.

Rumination, or Cud Chewing, Has an Important Effect on the Reduction of Particle Size and the Movement of Solid Material Through the Rumen

Rumination is the act of remasticating rumen ingesta. The initial act of rumination is regurgitation, which occurs just before the initiation of a primary rumen contraction. When regurgitation occurs, there is an extra contraction of the reticulum, which takes place just before the regular biphasic reticular contraction that initiates the primary cycle. Simultaneous with the extra reticular contraction, the cardia relaxes, and there is an inspiratory excursion of the ribs with the glottis closed. The latter action creates a negative pressure within the thorax, favoring the movement of food into the esophagus. When food enters the esophagus, a reverse peristaltic wave propels the material cranially into the mouth. As soon as the food bolus reaches the mouth, excess water is expressed by action of the tongue, the water is swallowed, and remastication of the material begins. The duration of remastication depends on the character of the diet, with coarse material requiring more time for remastication than finely ground or highly digestible feeds.

Regurgitated material comes from the dorsal portion of the reticulum, where particle size and functional specific gravity are intermediate. Thus the ingesta selected for remastication are not the coarsest material in the rumen, but rather the material that has already been through the digestive actions of the dorsal sac. This appears to be an efficient system in which some of the structural material of the plant is softened by soaking and removed or weakened by microbial action during the initial phases of digestion in the dorsal sac. The partially fermented material is then subjected to remastication, causing further comminution and exposing additional fermentable substrate that may not have been directly exposed to previous microbial action.

Rumination may also aid the particle separation process: as the regurgitated bolus reaches the mouth, it is squeezed by the tongue and cheeks before mastication begins. Water and small particles are expressed from the bolus by this squeezing action and are swallowed before mastication of the remaining bolus. This action tends to separate small particles from large particles. The small particles, when reswallowed, sink into the reticulum where they are subject to passage to the omasum whereas the larger particles, when swallowed after remastication, are ejected back into the more cranial portions of the rumen.

Rumination occurs when the animal is not actively eating, usually during times of rest, but not during deep sleep. The time spent ruminating depends on the type of diet; it ranges from almost none for high-grain diets to a maximum of about 10 hours per day for high-forage diets. The feed intake level also influences the amount of rumination time, with high intakes stimulating greater rumination.

Water Moves Through the Rumen at a Much Faster Rate Than Particulate Matter

The flow of water has important effects on rumen dynamics. For small particles and soluble material to exit the rumen, liquid must constantly be washing through all sections of the rumen and moving through the reticulo-omasal orifice. This means that

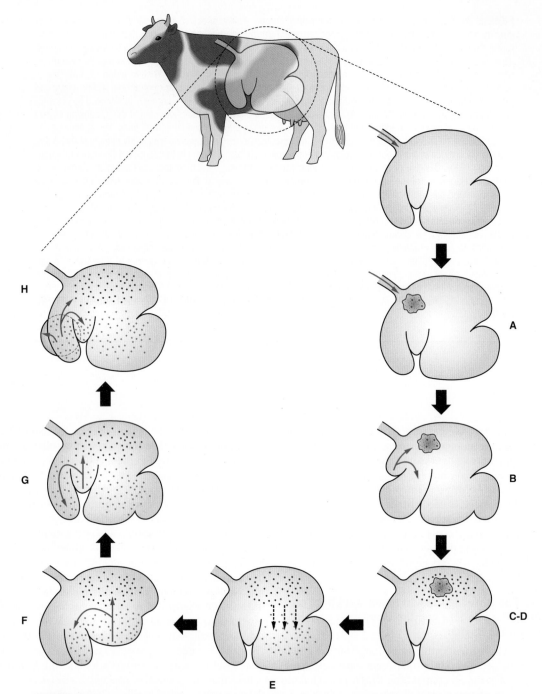

FIGURE 31-9 The sequential figures illustrate the pattern of flow of feed material through the reticulorumen from its arrival at the cardia *(A)* to its exit via the reticulo-omasal orifice *(H)*. Details of the sequential flow pattern are given in the text.

water must be constantly flowing through the mass of solid material. In effect, the reticulorumen functions as a giant strainer or sieve, holding the fermenting mass of particulate matter while water flows through it and washes small particles and soluble material away. Therefore the transit rate of water must be considerably greater than the transit rate of particulate matter through the rumen. The relative differences in the rates of movement of solid-phase and liquid-phase material through the rumen can be appreciated from their respective rumen half-lives: 30 to 50 hours for particulate matter and about 15 to 20 hours for liquid.

The rate of liquid flow through the rumen is often measured as the dilution rate, which is expressed as the percentage of total liquid that leaves the rumen in an hour. The term *dilution rate* comes from the way liquid turnover is measured; some soluble marker substance is mixed into the rumen, and its concentration is measured as soon as it is thoroughly dispersed into the liquid phase. Samples are then taken over time, and the rate at which the marker substance becomes diluted is measured. The rate of dilution depends on the rate at which water that contains marker leaves the rumen and is replaced with new, unmarked water; thus the dilution rate is an indirect measure of the rate of water flow through the rumen. Normal dilution rate values vary with diet and feed intake and are usually in the range of 5% to 30% per hour. One other point should be appreciated from the concept of dilution rate: water leaves the rumen only as it is replaced from some other source.

Almost all water that enters the rumen does so through the esophagus, from salivary flow, drinking, or succulent feeds. Thus the dilution rate depends on rates of salivation and drinking. The salivation rate is influenced by the chewing time and feed type; feeds such as long-stemmed dry roughages, which require relatively high rates of mastication, stimulate high rates of both salivary flow and dilution. Salivation occurs during rumination as well as during initial mastication; therefore those feeds that stimulate high rumination rates, such as forages, also stimulate high dilution rates. Conversely, feeds that do not stimulate extensive rumination (e.g., concentrates) result in relatively low dilution rates. The rate of drinking is influenced by (1) the rate of feed intake and (2) the salt, or electrolyte, content of the diet. Thus, high rates of intake or diets with high electrolyte contents stimulate high dilution rates.

Little water enters the rumen by way of the mucosa. The mucosa of the forestomachs is stratified squamous epithelium and is aglandular; thus there is no direct fluid secretion. Some water can enter the rumen through osmosis, but under normal conditions, the amount appears to be minimal. Normal rumen osmolality is about 280 mOsm/kg, slightly less than the 300-mOsm/kg osmolality of blood and extracellular fluid. Thus the usual osmotic flow of water is out of the rumen. After consumption of relatively digestible feeds, rumen osmolality increases briefly because of VFA production; however, it appears that osmolalities in excess of 340 mOsm/kg are necessary for water to flow osmotically into the rumen. Under normal conditions, osmolalities this high are not sustained for long, and thus there is usually little osmotic flow of water into the rumen.

Rumen Dilution Rate Has Important Influences on Fermentation and Microbial Cell Yield

Small particles, including microbes, leave the rumen with the liquid phase. Therefore, high dilution rates result in rapid removal of microbes and reductions in microbial cell concentrations. Because high microbe concentrations suppress microbial cell division, the growth of microbes is stimulated by high dilution rates. High growth rates are nutritionally desirable because a larger portion of the energy available to the microbes is used for growth instead of for maintenance, as occurs in older, relatively stable microbial populations. Thus, high dilution rates usually increase Y_{ATP} values, provided that adequate protein is available to support cell growth.

In addition to its effect on Y_{ATP}, the dilution rate may affect the microbial makeup of the rumen biomass and also may have some influence on the fermentation pattern. The rate of microbial washout increases with the dilution rate. At high dilution rates, microbial species with slow growth rates diminish in population size because their replication rate is not great enough to match the rate at which they are removed. Thus, selection pressure favors species with faster growth rates during times of high rumen dilution rates. Exceptions to this pattern occur because some microbes are able to attach themselves to the particulate matter in the solid and slurry zones. Such microbes then exit the rumen according to the kinetics of particle size reduction rather than dilution rate.

In general, the changes occurring in the rumen microbial population with high dilution rates appear to favor acetic acid production and to increase the acetic/propionic acid ratio.

CONTROL OF RETICULORUMEN MOTILITY

Reticulorumen Motility Is Controlled by the Central Nervous System and Affected by Intraluminal Conditions

In the dorsal vagal nucleus of the brainstem, there is a motility control center for the regulation of reticuloruminal motility. This center sends action potentials along fibers to the forestomach by way of the vagus nerve. There is an extensive enteric nervous system within the reticulorumen, but vagal innervation is necessary for coordination of normal motility patterns. When the vagal nerves are destroyed, motility of the rumen musculature ceases initially but returns within several days; however, the motility that develops after vagotomy is erratic, uncoordinated, and incapable of supporting the normal flow of ingesta through the reticulorumen. Vagotomized ruminants do not survive.

The dorsal vagal nucleus receives afferent stimuli that affect the control of forestomach motility. Important afferent signals come from the lumen of the reticulorumen and monitor distention, ingesta consistency, pH, VFA concentration, and ionic strength. Rumen volume, or distention, appears to be monitored by stretch receptors in the walls and especially in the pillars. Moderate distention increases rumen motility and rumination. Increased motility and rumination have the effect of raising the rate at which particles are broken down, leading to a higher passage rate. Thus, rumen throughput is enhanced when increased intake expands rumen volume. Severe distention, as occurs pathologically in bloat, causes cessation of rumen motility.

The consistency of ingesta also has an important influence on rumen motility. Consistency is determined largely by diet type. When the diet consists of succulent plants, grain, or finely chopped forage, there is little material in the solid zone, or rumen mat, and the slurry zone is fluid. This type of fluid ingesta offers little resistance to the movement of the rumen pillars; thus the rumen musculature has to apply relatively little force to mix and circulate the rumen contents. Tension receptors in the reticuloruminal muscle appear to monitor the force necessary to move the pillars through the ingesta. Highly fluid rumen ingesta are associated with low muscle tension and have a negative influence on reticulorumen motility. At the other dietary extreme, when animals are eating dry, long-stem hay, the rumen contents are solid and create a large and highly interwoven rumen mat. Resistance to movement of the pillars through the solid mass of ingesta is high and leads to stimulation of tension receptors, resulting in a positive feedback on motility. The motility rate is directly related to the rate of particle breakdown; this arrangement appears to be a self-regulatory mechanism that increases the rate of particle comminution when animals consume diets with large particle size.

Chemoreceptors in the walls of the rumen and reticulum monitor pH, VFA concentration, and ionic strength (or osmolality). The pH of the reticulorumen is normally slightly acid, reflecting the acidity of the VFAs, but extreme acid conditions are undesirable. Increasing VFA concentrations or decreasing pH results in a suppression of rumen motility. The normal rumen pH is in the range of 5.5 to 6.8, depending on the type of diet. When the rumen pH falls much below 5.0, motility is severely depressed. This response appears to be protective because fermentation tends to be enhanced by motility-induced mixing; thus suppression of motility slows down fermentation, allowing VFA absorption to catch up with VFA production.

Osmolality may influence rumen motility as well, although motility appears less sensitive to osmotic changes than it does to pH changes. Normal osmolality in the rumen is about 280 mOsm, but the osmolality increases during active fermentation. Osmotically active solutes in the rumen include organic acids as well as salivary and dietary electrolytes. As organic acid formation increases during fermentation, osmolality also increases, tending to reduce motility. The rumen epithelium creates a relatively impermeable barrier to water, so wide swings in rumen osmolality can occur without large shifts in water between the rumen and the vascular compartment. At abnormally high osmolalities, however, water can be drawn into the rumen.

OMASAL FUNCTION

Passage of Material from the Reticulum to the Omasum Occurs During Reticular Contraction

The *omasum* is composed of a body and a canal. The body is filled with multiple muscular folds, or leaves, that project from the greater curvature into the lumen. The canal, which is located on the lesser curvature, connects the reticulum to the abomasum. Ingesta move into the omasum during reticular contractions. The reticulo-omasal orifice usually remains open, but dilates especially during the second phase of the reticular contraction, during which ingesta flow rapidly into the omasal canal. After the reticular contraction, the reticulo-omasal orifice closes briefly as the canal contracts, forcing newly arrived ingesta up into the leaves. Intermittently, the body and leaves of the omasum contract, forcing the material from the body of the organ into the canal and on into the abomasum.

Proper functioning of the omasum and reticulum appears to be particularly important to the passage of ingesta out of the rumen. Occasionally, traumatic injury resulting from ingested foreign bodies causes severe adhesions of the reticulum and omasum to the body wall. In addition, damage to vagal fibers entering the organs may occur. In such cases, motility of the rumen proper may continue normally, but the ability to move food out of the forestomachs and into the abomasum is severely impaired. The rumen becomes greatly distended with finely comminuted feed, and the entire rumen becomes a slurry zone. Despite the distended rumen, little movement of ingesta occurs into the abomasum, and the animals eventually suffer severe inanition. This condition is variably known as *omasal transport failure* and vagal indigestion; usually, little can be done to correct it.

The structure of the omasum, with its many leaves and large mucosal surface area, suggests that it has an absorptive function, but the exact nature of this function is still incompletely understood. One important possibility is that it exists to remove residual VFAs and bicarbonate from ingesta before material is transported to the abomasum. VFAs appear to cause unfavorable reactions in the abomasum, so it is important that the major portion of them be removed before abomasal entry. Also, it appears desirable to absorb, before abomasal entry, any bicarbonate remaining in the ingesta. Bicarbonate remaining in ingesta and entering the abomasum would only neutralize abomasal hydrochloric acid, increasing the work load of the abomasal glands in order to maintain appropriate abomasal pH.

VOLATILE FATTY ACID ABSORPTION

Volatile Fatty Acids, Representing 60% to 80% of the Energy Needs of the Animal, Are Absorbed Directly from the Forestomach Epithelium

VFAs are bacterial waste products and, if allowed to accumulate, will suppress fermentation. Furthermore, the VFAs are extremely important energy substrates for the host, supplying 60% to 80% of the dietary energy to ruminants with most types of diets. Therefore the presence of an efficient and high-capacity mechanism for VFA absorption is important to both digestion and host metabolism. The forestomach epithelium supplies such a system, absorbing almost all the VFAs, with only small amounts escaping to the lower digestive tract. In addition, the absorptive process helps maintain rumen pH by removing acid from the forestomach ingesta and contributing bicarbonate in the process.

The epithelium responsible for this tremendous absorption is structurally much different from other absorptive epithelia of the GI system. However, the nature of the rumen epithelium may give it functional characteristics similar to those of the absorptive epithelium of the small intestine and colon. The forestomach surface is of the stratified squamous type and, as with the stratified squamous epithelium of the skin and other surfaces, consists of several layers of cells of varying maturity. The deepest layer is the *stratum basale,* from which cells divide and migrate into the stratum spinosum. Cells of the stratum spinosum begin the process of keratinization and continue into the *stratum granulosum,* which is covered by the outermost and most keratinized layer, the *stratum corneum.* Although the forestomach epithelium seems completely different from the columnar epithelium of the small intestine, an interesting similarity between forestomach and intestinal epithelia is noted when the cellular attachments and intercellular spaces of the forestomach are examined (Figure 31-10).

The cells of the stratum granulosum are tightly joined by junctions that may functionally resemble the tight junctions of the enterocytes (see Chapter 30). Deeper in the epithelium, the cells of the stratum spinosum and stratum basale are separated by intercellular spaces that increase in size as the basement membrane is approached. These intercellular spaces are reminiscent of the lateral spaces of columnar absorptive epithelia. If these observations are combined with the existence of the intercellular bridges that characterize the forestomach epithelium, an interesting analogy to columnar absorptive epithelia can be constructed. VFAs, electrolytes, and water apparently are initially absorbed through the stratum corneum and passed cell to cell by way of intercellular bridges to the cells of the stratum spinosum and stratum basale, from which the absorbed substances are passed into the intercellular spaces before entering the capillaries.

This arrangement of the forestomach epithelium is very similar to the three-compartment characteristics of the columnar absorptive epithelia, with solutes passing from ruminoreticular lumen to cell contents and ultimately to lateral spaces. Although the keratinized cells of the stratum corneum do not appear to retain adequate metabolic machinery (e.g., mitochondria) to maintain appropriate gradients for diffusion, the cells of the stratum spinosum and stratum basale are metabolically active. Because of the intercellular bridges, absorbed solute can be transferred directly from the outer keratinized cells to the deeper, more metabolically active cells. Thus the metabolic activity deep in the epithelium appears to maintain conditions for absorption at the epithelial surface.

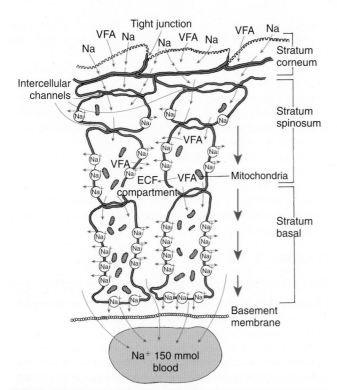

FIGURE 31-10 The stratified squamous epithelium of the rumen, although anatomically much different, shares functional similarities with the columnar epithelium of the intestine. Note the tight junctions of the cells of the stratum corneum and the lateral space–like compartment between adjacent cells of the stratum spinosum and stratum basale. Although the cells of the stratum spinosum are metabolically inactive, the intercellular channels allow the metabolic actions of the stratum basale to be reflected in the more superficial layers. *VFA,* Volatile fatty acid; *Na,* sodium; *ECF,* extracellular fluid. (Modified from Steven DH, Marshall AB: Organization of the rumen epithelium. In Phillipson AT, editor: *Physiology of digestion and metabolism in the ruminant,* Newcastle upon Tyne, UK, 1970, Oriel Press.)

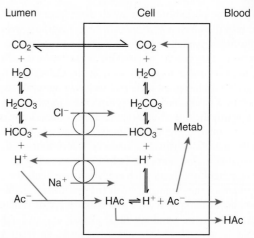

FIGURE 31-11 VFA absorption is promoted by the conversion of VFA anions *(Ac⁻)* to free acids *(HAc)* in the microenvironment near the epithelial surface. This diagram illustrates two proposed means, one intracellular and one extracellular, by which hydrogen ions could be locally generated to effect the formation of VFA free acids; both mechanisms could exist simultaneously. (From Stevens CE, Argenzio RA, Roberts MC: Comparative physiology of mammalian colon and suggestions for animal models of human disorders, *Clin Gastroenterol* 15(4):763-785, 1986.)

The molecular mechanism of VFA absorption is incompletely understood but seems to involve local alterations in pH near the absorptive surface. Differences in pH can have an important influence on VFA absorption because of shifts in the dissociation state of the VFA molecules. The pKa of the VFA is approximately 4.8, well below the normal pH of the rumen; thus most of the VFAs exist in the rumen in the dissociated, or ionic, form. However, sodium-hydrogen ion exchange by the epithelial cells may decrease the local pH at the absorptive surface. Such a drop in pH would lead to a shift in the VFA from the ionic to the free-acid state. Cell membranes are permeable to VFA free acids, and absorption proceeds because of the concentration gradient between the lumen and cells. The high CO_2 tension in the rumen, caused by the production of fermentation gases, may also enhance the conversion of VFA to the free-acid state. As shown in Figure 31-11, when one VFA molecule is absorbed, one molecule of bicarbonate (HCO_3^-) is generated in the lumen; thus VFA absorption helps buffer rumen pH both by generating base and by removing acid.

All the VFAs appear to be absorbed by the same mechanism, but they are handled differently within the epithelial cells. Some acetate seems to be completely oxidized within the cells, with the remainder absorbed unchanged. Most propionate is absorbed, but a small portion is converted to lactate by the epithelial cells. Butyrate is modified extensively, and essentially all molecules are changed to β-hydroxybutyrate before absorption. β-Hydroxybutyrate is an important metabolite known as a *ketone body.* Ketone bodies are metabolites that frequently have special medical significance (see Chapter 32). In ruminants the rumen itself is a significant source of ketone bodies. In monogastric animals, however, ketone bodies arise exclusively from the partial oxidation of long-chain fatty acids.

The rumen epithelium is arranged in *papillae,* fingerlike projections that increase the absorptive surface area. Although they serve the same area-expanding function as the villi of the small intestine, papillae are much larger and easily visible to the unaided eye. The size and shape of the papillae are quite dynamic and responsive to changes in diet. Papillary growth is stimulated by VFAs, especially butyrate and propionate. Diets with high digestibility result in high rumen VFA concentrations, which stimulate the growth of long papillae. In contrast, animals receiving little feed or diets of low digestibility have short rumen papillae. It is important to adapt ruminants gradually when changing them from diets of low digestibility to high digestibility; this may allow time for sufficient adjustment of papillary size so that VFA absorption will match VFA production.

RUMEN DEVELOPMENT AND ESOPHAGEAL GROOVE FUNCTION

Significant Changes in Forestomach Size and Function Occur with Dietary Changes in Early Life

At birth the forestomach is about equal in size to the abomasum in both lambs and calves, a stark contrast to the normal adult proportions, in which the forestomach accounts for more than 90% of the total stomach volume. Enlargement of the forestomach occurs rapidly after birth, but the rate depends on diet type. When young ruminants are given access to solid feeds soon after birth, the forestomach development rate is maximal.

In cattle the period of forestomach development is arbitrarily divided into the *nonruminant period,* from birth to 3 weeks, and the *transitional period,* from 3 to 8 weeks. Approximate adult distribution of stomach proportions is achieved usually by 8 weeks, if calves have access to solid feeds. Calves can be seen eating grain and forage as early as 2 weeks of age and frequently ruminate by 3 weeks, indicating considerable forestomach development by this time. Withholding solid feed dramatically reduces the rate of rumen development. In calves that are given diets of only milk or milk substitute ("replacer"), forestomach development remains rudimentary for 14 to 15 weeks or longer.

Development of forestomach epithelium parallels the general development of the organ. At birth the epithelium is thin, with small or nonexistent papillae. Exposure of the epithelium to VFAs appears to stimulate papillary development and general organ development as well. Highly digestible feeds, such as concentrates, result in the greatest VFA production and fastest epithelial development. Some dietary forage may aid in muscular development of the forestomachs, but calves and lambs in the transitional period should receive most of their solid feed as grain because their energy needs are high compared with their ability to ferment forages.

The forestomach is sterile at birth but is quickly colonized by environmental bacteria, mostly facultative organisms. As bacterial fermentation proceeds in the anaerobic confines of the forestomach, the electromotive force decreases; the typical reductive environment of the rumen is created by bacterial action. This environment creates conditions necessary for the growth and establishment of the strict anaerobes. The development of forestomach bacterial flora occurs independently of any special inoculation process, and indeed, it is impossible to prevent it from occurring except by raising calves under gnotobiotic conditions. Protozoal inoculation, in contrast to bacterial inoculation, seems to require some exposure to other cattle; calves raised in complete isolation do not develop protozoal fauna. It appears that aerosol spread of protozoa can occur because no direct physical contact among cattle is necessary to establish a protozoal fauna.

The Esophageal Groove Diverts the Flow of Ingested Milk Past the Forestomach and into the Abomasum

For proper rumen development in the suckling animal, it is important for milk to be diverted away from the developing rumen. This is accomplished by the actions of the *reticular groove* (also called the *esophageal groove*). This structure is a gutterlike invagination traversing the wall of the reticulum from the cardia to the reticulo-omasal orifice. When stimulated, muscles of the groove contract, causing it to shorten and twist. The twisting action causes the lips of the groove to close together, forming a nearly complete tube from the cardia to the omasal canal. When the groove is contracted, milk entering the cardia is directed into the omasum, with 10% or less entering the rumen. Milk quickly traverses the omasum and enters the abomasum.

Reticular groove closure is a reflex action, with brainstem efferent impulses arriving through the vagus nerve. Afferent stimuli arise centrally and from the pharynx. Anticipation of suckling invokes central stimulation of reticular groove closure, which may be considered a cephalic phase. Fluid, especially sodium-containing fluid in the pharynx, stimulates afferent fibers that reinforce the cephalic phase of groove closure. The posture of the calf or lamb when suckling does not appear to have much influence on reticular groove function, but rapid drinking from an open pail, in contrast to suckling from a nipple, frequently results in inefficient groove function and spillage of milk into the rumen. Milk in the rumen results in the formation of improper fermentation patterns.

The reticular groove has its primary function in suckling animals, and the activity of the groove reflex appears to diminish after weaning and with advancing age. However, the groove reflex is stimulated by antidiuretic hormone (ADH; see Chapter 43), indicating that it may have some physiological function in adult life. ADH is secreted by the posterior pituitary in response to dehydration or increases in plasma osmolality. ADH is associated with thirst, and because it stimulates the reticular groove, a large portion of the water consumed by drinking in water-deprived animals may bypass the rumen. This may be a functional mechanism to ensure that water arrives quickly at the site of most rapid absorption, the small intestine.

FUNCTION OF THE EQUINE LARGE HINDGUT

The Equine Hindgut Has a Great Capacity for Fermentation

A general function of the cecum and colon, as mentioned in Chapter 30, is to recover fluid and electrolytes from ingesta leaving the ileum. In many herbivorous species, this function has been expanded to include fermentative digestion. Absorptive and fermentation functions complement each other in the colons of nonruminant herbivores. This arrangement leads to an elegantly interactive system of fermentation and absorption; however, it also results in an interdependence between the two processes, meaning that disturbances in fermentation can result in important abnormalities in absorption, and vice versa.

The Types of Substrate and Fermentation Patterns Are Essentially Identical for Forestomach and Hindgut Fermentation

Structural and nonstructural carbohydrates as well as proteins form the major substrates for hindgut fermentation. However, the passage of material through the stomach and small intestine before its arrival at the cecum and colon may have some important effects on fermentative digestion. First, hindgut fermentation may be aided by prior gastric action. The effects of soaking and acid exposure on plant particles in the stomach may increase their susceptibility to microbial attack and thus raise their rate of digestion in the hindgut. Second, some of the readily available carbohydrate, particularly sugars and starches, may be digested and absorbed before the other material arrives in the cecum. Most evidence indicates, however, that glandular digestion of carbohydrate in the horse is not extremely efficient and that substantial amounts of starch and sugars reach the cecum. Further, cell-wall carbohydrate appears to interfere with the digestion or absorption of nonstructural carbohydrate, so that diets high in cell-wall content result in relatively little starch digestion and absorption in the equine small intestine. Even with a high-grain diet, up to 29% of dietary starch may reach the cecum and colon.

Protein as well as carbohydrate is absorbed in the small intestine, potentially leading to a deficiency of nitrogen for colonic microbes. However, there is extensive urea recycling into the colon and cecum, similar to that occurring in the rumen (see Figure 31-6). Thus, urea plus protein escaping small-intestinal digestion supplies the nitrogen needs of the microbes. In contrast to ruminants, horses do not have an efficient means of recovering the microbial protein synthesized in the hindgut, and most of it passes out in the feces. Some experiments have shown a small amount of amino acid absorption from the equine cecum or colon, but the amount does not compare with microbial protein availability in the ruminant.

The Motility Functions of the Cecum and Colon Retain Material for Fermentation and Separate Particles by Size

The functions of the equine hindgut in maintaining fermentation are similar to those of the rumen: favorable conditions must be maintained to support optimal fermentation. As in the rumen, these conditions are (1) substrate supply, (2) control of pH and osmolality, (3) anaerobiosis, (4) retention of fermenting material, and (5) continual removal of waste products and the residue of spent fermentation substrate. Separation of fermenting material from residue appears to be accomplished by selective retention of particles according to size, just as in the rumen; however, the means by which the cecum and colon accomplish size separation and discriminate passage are quite different from those of the forestomach. Anatomical characteristics and motility patterns in the cecum and colon are responsible for selective retention of long particles, allowing sufficient exposure for microbial digestion to occur. In general, the fermentative digestive process in the horse is not as efficient as that in the ruminant, and digestible energy values for forages are usually lower for horses than for cattle.

Before the motility of the equine cecum and colon is discussed, a brief review of the anatomy of the equine hindgut is important. Figure 31-12 shows the equine digestive system, separated from its mesenteric attachments and laid out in linear fashion. The hindgut commences with the cecum, which is separated from the large colon by a well-defined orifice. The large colon is folded on itself three times, forming four major anatomical divisions: the *right ventral* and *left ventral* and the *left dorsal*

and *right dorsal* colon segments. Ingesta enter the right ventral colon and course to the left ventral colon, from which the material enters the left dorsal portion through the *pelvic flexure.* From the left dorsal colon, material moves to the right dorsal colon before entering the small colon. (Anatomy textbooks describe the arrangement of the large colon in the abdomen.) For the purposes of physiological study, the reader should note in Figure 31-12 the tremendous size and volume of the cecum and colon compared with the small intestine. The differences in diameter that occur throughout the colon should also be noted, particularly the reductions in diameter that occur at the pelvic flexure and at the junction of the large and small colons. The saclike evaginations that occur in the wall of the cecum and most segments of the colon are called *haustra.* Functionally, the equine hindgut can be divided into four sections: cecum, ventral colon, dorsal colon, and small colon.

Ingesta reach the cecum after a relatively short time in the stomach and small intestine. A large portion of soluble ingesta usually reaches the cecum by 2 hours after ingestion, whereas solids take somewhat longer, depending on particle size and consistency. The material in the cecum and throughout the large colon has a high water content and a slurrylike consistency.

The majority of cecal motility is of a mixing nature, with frequent low-amplitude contractions that transport ingesta from haustrum to haustrum and back in a mixing pattern. The mixing action of the cecum maintains the cecal contents in a homogeneous state. About once every 3 to 4 minutes, there is a strong contraction of cecal muscles in a mass movement type of action (see Chapter 28 for a description of *mass movement*) in which the *body* and *apex* of the organ shorten and constrict, lifting ingesta into the *base.* Constriction of the base forces material through the *cecocolic orifice* and into the right ventral colon. The motility pattern functionally separates the cecum from the ventral colon. In contrast to some other species, in horses there is no retrograde flow of material from the colon back into the cecum, so the composition of ingesta in these two organs usually differs somewhat.

Three types of motility patterns exist in the right and left ventral colon: *haustral segmentation, propulsive peristalsis,* and *retropulsive peristalsis.* Segmentation serves a mixing function that aids in promoting fermentation and bringing VFAs in contact with the mucosa for absorption. Mixing occurs throughout the ventral colon, and the right and left segments may be regarded as one functional unit with homogeneous ingesta. Propulsive activity, or aboral peristalsis, in the ventral colon originates near the cecum and appears to occur as a continuation of the cecal mass movements. Peristaltic activity in the proximal ventral colon propels ingesta distally into the left ventral colon. In the left ventral colon, retropulsive or antiperistaltic movements resist the flow of ingesta and result in the retention and mixing of material in the ventral colon, allowing time for microbial digestion and preventing the washout of microbes. In addition, the retropulsive actions of the left ventral colon aid in creating differential flow rates of liquid and particulate matter through the colon. The antiperistaltic motility appears to originate from a pacemaker in the *pelvic flexure,* the area of restricted diameter where the left ventral and left dorsal colons meet.

The motility of the ventral colon can be roughly compared with that of the stomach, with the pelvic flexure and distal left ventral colon acting as the pylorus and antrum, respectively. The pumping action of cecal mass movements, combined with the propulsive action of the proximal ventral colon, continually

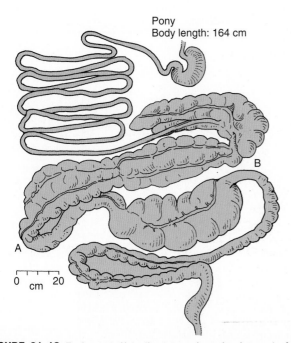

Pony
Body length: 164 cm

0 cm 20

FIGURE 31-12 Equine gut. Note the tremendous development of the colon compared with the small intestine. Note also the relative areas of constriction at the junctions of the ventral and dorsal colons *(A)* and the large and small colons *(B).* (From Stevens CE: Comparative physiology of the digestive system. In Swenson MJ, editor: *Dukes' physiology of domestic animals,* ed 9, Ithaca, NY, 1977, Cornell University Press.)

moves ingesta toward the pelvic flexure. In the distal ventral colon, however, antiperistaltic activity and the narrow diameter of the pelvic flexure impede the movement of material, causing it to be retained in the ventral colon. The squeezing action of the pelvic flexure mimics the action of the pylorus in selectively retaining relatively large particulate matter while allowing liquid and small particles to pass. As particle size is reduced by fermentative action and the mixing activity of the colon, particles eventually become small enough to flow with the fluid phase and leave the colon. The action of the pelvic flexure is not as efficient as that of the pylorus, and some large particles do escape the ventral colon. In addition, there are periods during which propulsive movements occur in the left ventral colon and pelvic flexure. These factors allow the movement of particulate matter into the left dorsal colon.

The actions of the dorsal colon appear to mimic those of the ventral colon. Impedance to ingesta flow is created by the size restriction at the junction of the right dorsal colon and small colon. In addition, retropulsive motility may originate in the area of the distal right dorsal colon, near the junction with the small colon. These actions tend to impede the movement of ingesta through the dorsal colon, subjecting the material to another round of fermentative digestion, as occurred in the ventral colon. The delay in the flow of ingesta created by the combined actions of the ventral and dorsal colons results in significant retention of material, with most particulate matter taking from 24 to 96 hours to pass the large colon. The efficiency of the large colon in retaining and separating ingesta of different particle sizes can be understood from Figure 31-13.

Understanding the motility of the equine colon is important because problems of colon impaction in horses are common. Impactions usually occur near or within the pelvic flexure, probably because the pelvic flexure is a site of flow restriction and differential flow of solid and liquid material. One can easily

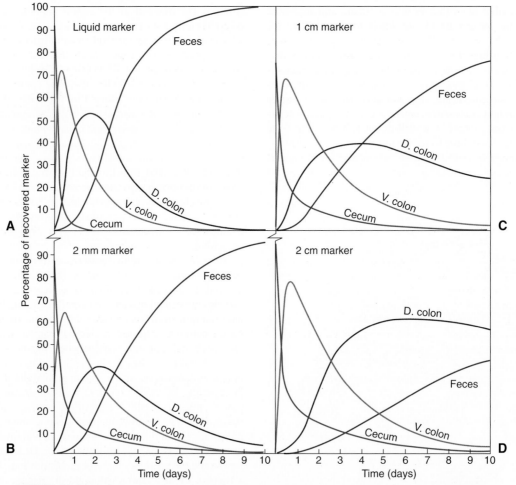

FIGURE 31-13 Retention of liquid and particles of various sizes in the compartments of the equine large intestine. Marker liquid **(A)** and marked particles of various sizes (**B**, 2 mm; **C**, 1 cm; **D**, 2 cm) were placed in the cecum of ponies, and the distribution of marked materials among colon segments was measured at 2-hour intervals. The lines of the graph were mathematically fitted to the data. Each line indicates the percentage of marker in a given segment at any time. Note in graph **A** that at 7 days after infusion, almost all the liquid marker had been recovered in the feces, with little or none remaining in the intestinal segments. Increasing particle size has a relatively small effect on the movement of particles out of the cecum. In contrast, as particle size increases, there is significant retention of material in the colon and slow passage to the feces. *D*, Dorsal; *V*, ventral. (From Argenzio RA, Lowe JE, Pickard DW, et al: Digesta passage and water exchange in the equine large intestine, *Am J Physiol* 226(5):1035-1042, 1974.)

appreciate how the normal motility pattern could allow solid material to accumulate in this area and cause obstructions.

Although general understanding of small colon motility is limited, it appears to consist primarily of segmentation and propulsion. The characteristic fecal balls of horses are formed by segmentation within the small colon.

The Rate of Fermentation and Volatile Fatty Acid Production in the Equine Colon Is Similar to That in the Rumen

In the equine colon, efficient means of buffering and VFA absorption must be present. Salivary buffering, as occurs in ruminants, cannot aid in buffering the colon. In the horse, large quantities of fluid, rich in bicarbonate and phosphate buffers, are secreted by the ileum and transferred to the cecum, thus mimicking the actions of the salivary glands in ruminants. Also, because of the glandular nature of the colonic mucosa, bicarbonate and other electrolytes are added more directly to the lumen fluid in the cecum and colon than in the rumen.

Large fluxes of water traverse the cecal and colonic mucosa during the course of digestion. When horses are meal-fed, feed starts to enter the cecum about 2 hours after eating, and VFA production rapidly commences. As ingesta are transported from the cecum, VFA production continues in the large colon. During the period of active VFA production, large quantities of water enter the hindgut from the blood through the mucosa. Although this water flux may be a response to increased osmolality created by the generation of osmotically active VFA molecules, it is more likely a response to direct fluid secretion from the crypts of the colonic epithelium (see Chapter 30). Secretion of fluid containing sodium, bicarbonate, and chloride from the colonic mucosa appears to occur in response to high concentrations of VFA in the lumen. This secretory response, in combination with the ileal secretions, is responsible for buffering of the lumen contents. Figure 31-14 illustrates the magnitude of water fluxes that occur during hindgut digestion in the pony. Note that considerable inward and outward movement of water occurs across the mucosa in each of the major fermentation compartments, ventral and dorsal colons, and cecum. Inward (into the lumen) water movement results from mucosal secretion, whereas outward water movement occurs in association with absorption of VFA.

The molecular mechanisms of VFA absorption in the equine colon appear to be identical to those in the rumen (see Figure 31-11). Note in Figure 31-11 that sodium absorption accompanies VFA absorption and that bicarbonate is generated in the lumen. The absorption of VFA and sodium leads to osmotic absorption of water, probably through the transcellular pathway. (See Chapter 30 for a review of the dynamics of water and electrolyte absorption in the gut.)

The function of the small colon is to recover water, electrolytes, and VFAs that were not absorbed in the large colon. VFA production appears minimal in the small colon, but considerable absorption of water, sodium, and phosphate occurs there.

The large water and electrolyte fluxes in the colon make horses vulnerable to colonic diseases, resulting in fluid and electrolyte losses that are more characteristic of small-intestinal disease in many other animals.

Hindgut Anatomy and Function Vary Greatly Among the Many Species of Veterinary Interest

All the variations in hindgut anatomy and function among the species are beyond the scope of this discussion, but you should

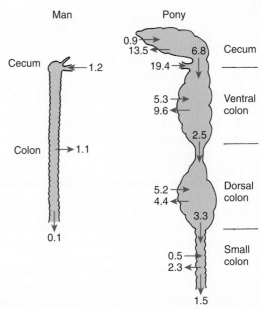

FIGURE 31-14 Net movement of water through the large intestine of a 70-kg man and a 160-kg pony. Values are in liters per day. Note the relatively large amount of fluid delivered to the pony's colon from the ileum (19.4 L/day) compared with the human colon. Also note the inward and outward movement of fluid in the various compartments of the pony's large intestine. (From Argenzio RA, Lowe JE, Pickard DW, Stevens CE: Digesta passage and water exchange in the equine large intestine, *Am J Physiol* 226(5):1035-1042, 1974.)

remember that rabbits, rats, guinea pigs, swine, and some large birds, in addition to Equidae, depend on hindgut fermentation for a significant portion of their energy needs. Also, ruminants have a reasonably extensive hindgut, and fermentative digestion occurs there, even after material has been through the rumen.

Scientific understanding of colonic function in general is not as advanced as that of small-intestinal function. This dichotomy probably exists because in humans, diseases of the small intestine are more frequent and severe than diseases of the colon. However, interest in colonic physiology and pathophysiology has increased among basic scientists and physicians. Veterinary physiologists have long been interested in colonic function and have become leaders in the exploration of this area.

CLINICAL CORRELATIONS

GRAIN ENGORGEMENT TOXEMIA

History. In mid-January a cattle feeder has asked you to examine a feedlot full of 400-kg steers. The steers have been on free-choice grain from a self-feeder for several weeks. Three days ago a blizzard prevented the caretaker from delivering feed to the feeders, and they were empty for 36 hours. Yesterday the feeders were filled, and all the steers ate ravenously. Today, two of the 40 steers are dead, and many appear lethargic and uncoordinated and have diarrhea.

Clinical Examination. Two steers are isolated for physical examination; they are lethargic and must be coaxed to move. Their heart rates are all above 100 beats/min (normal, <80 beats/min), and their body temperatures are less than 101.0° F (normal, 101.5°

to 103.0° F). Their rumens appear distended, and there is no evidence of rumen motility. The eyes are sunken in the orbits, and the oral mucosa is dry and sticky, indicating clinical dehydration. Necropsy examination of a dead steer reveals a greatly distended rumen filled with grain and fluid. A pH-paper test indicates that the rumen fluid pH of the dead animal is below 4.5 but above 3 (normal, 5.5-7.0).

Comment. Ruminants may be fed large amounts of grain if they are accustomed to it and receive it on a regular and frequent basis. In this case, even though the steers had been accustomed to a high-grain diet, the lack of grain for more than a day, followed by a large grain intake, set up conditions for *grain engorgement toxemia.*

In grain engorgement there is an abundant supply of starch, leading to the rapid growth and proliferation of rumen streptococci. These bacteria produce VFA rapidly, causing the rumen pH to diminish. As the rumen pH becomes lower, conditions become unfavorable for the growth and survival of cellulose-fermenting organisms and favorable for the growth of lactic acid–producing bacteria. This leads to the accumulation of lactic acid, a stronger acid than the VFAs. Thus, rumen pH becomes even lower, killing many of the normal microflora. Some of the lactic acid is absorbed, leading to a reduced blood pH and a life-threatening situation. Moreover, the large ruminal concentration of lactic acid and VFA results in a high osmotic pressure, drawing water out of the vascular fluid compartment and into the rumen. This leads to systemic hypovolemia, which may proceed to hypovolemic shock.

Treatment. This is a life-threatening situation, and the farmer will likely lose additional steers. Treatment is aimed at expanding the intravascular fluid volume, correcting the systemic acidosis, and reestablishing a normal rumen environment. Severely affected steers should be evaluated to determine whether their prognosis is good enough to warrant the expense of therapy; if not, euthanasia should be employed. Initial treatment should consist of rapid intravenous administration of large quantities of alkalizing fluid. After the correction of fluid and acid-base disturbances, ideally the rumen should be emptied, either by intubation with a large-bore stomach tube or by rumenotomy. In some cases, oral administration of an antifermentation agent, such as oil of turpentine, mineral oil, or an antibiotic, along with an alkalizing agent, is an acceptable alternative to emptying the rumen. After the rumen environment is brought back to normal, it may be helpful to re-inoculate the rumen with material taken from the rumen of a normal animal.

IMPACTION COLIC

History. You are presented with a 20-year-old gelding that has been showing signs of abdominal discomfort (colic) for 16 hours. When left alone in the stall, the horse lies down, frequently preferring to lie on his back. There is little fresh manure in the stall. When taken out of the stall, the gelding leads normally, but then lies down and rolls on release from the lead rope.

Clinical Examination. The heart rate is slightly elevated, at 60 beats/min; respiratory rate and temperature are normal. The hydration state, as well as the color and perfusion of the mucous membranes, is normal. Simple laboratory evaluation reveals the packed cell volume to be 41% (normal, 35% to 45%) and the plasma total solids to be 7.8 g/dL (normal, 6.5 to 8.0 g/dL). Borborygmi (intestinal sounds) are softer and less frequent than normal, especially on the left side. Examination by rectal palpation reveals the pelvic

flexure to be firm with a doughlike consistency; normally, the contents of the pelvic flexure have a fluid consistency. When you examine the teeth, you find that the molar surfaces are irregular, and one of the molars has a crack extending from the table surface to below the gum line.

Comment. The pelvic flexure is a site of flow restriction and particle size separation. As water moves through the pelvic flexure, large forage particles accumulate and are retained for further fermentation and mixing in the ventral colon. A horse with poor teeth may not chew its forage adequately; as a result, many large particles may be swallowed. These particles tend to accumulate in the pelvic flexure and may cause an impaction and obstruction, as occurred in this case.

Treatment. Treatment involves the oral administration of softening agents, such as mineral oil. Drugs such as dioctyl sodium sulfosuccinate, which stimulate water secretion from the intestinal mucosa, are also beneficial. Prevention in this case involves correction of the dental problems so that forage is more thoroughly chewed. Feeding pelleted feeds may also be beneficial.

PRACTICE QUESTIONS

1. In which of the following respects is fermentative digestion *different* from glandular digestion?
   a. Enzymes are not involved in fermentative digestion.
   b. Chemical bonds are not split by hydrolysis in fermentative digestion.
   c. Only carbohydrates are digested by fermentative digestion.
   d. Substrates are more extensively altered in fermentative digestion than in glandular digestion.
   e. Proteins are digested to amino acids by fermentative digestion and to dipeptides by glandular digestion.

2. In a comparison of hindgut fermentation and forestomach fermentation, which of the following statements is *true*?
   a. The microbial populations are considerably different, but the products of digestion are the same.
   b. The microbial populations are the same, but the products of digestion are considerably different.
   c. Both the microbial populations and the digestion products are similar.
   d. Structural carbohydrates of plants are not digested by hindgut fermentation.
   e. A nitrogen source is not required by the microbes of the hindgut.

3. The three VFAs—acetate, propionate, and butyrate—are:
   a. Net-reaction products of the fermentative action of the entire rumen biomass.
   b. The individual products of cellulose, starch, and hemicellulose digestion, respectively.
   c. The individual products of bacterial, protozoal, and fungal digestion, respectively.
   d. Volatile products that leave the rumen with the gas phase during eructation.
   e. Intermediate metabolites that are passed between microbial species.

4. Matching protein and energy availability in the rumen is an important nutritional goal in feeding ruminants. Which of the following completions of this statement concerning protein and energy availability in the rumen is *false*? Diets well matched in available protein and energy result in:
   a. The most efficient use of energy for microbial growth.
   b. Maximal delivery of protein to the host.
   c. Minimal breakdown of protein in the rumen.
   d. Loss of a minimal amount of dietary amino acids due to formation of excess ammonia.
   e. Optimal rumen ammonia concentrations.

5. Which of the following statements is *true* of both methane and propionate?
   a. They are waste products of anaerobic fermentation but contain potential energy that is recoverable by the host.
   b. They are highly oxidized molecules.
   c. They are eructed from the rumen.
   d. Their formation results in the generation of NAD from NADH.
   e. They are toxic to monogastric animals.

BIBLIOGRAPHY

Argenzio RA: Functions of the equine large intestine and their interrelationship in disease, *Cornell Vet* 65(3):303–330, 1975.

Aschenbach JR, Penner GB, Stumpff F, Gäbel G: Ruminant nutrition symposium: role of fermentation acid absorption in the regulation of ruminal pH, *J Anim Sci* 89(4):1092–1107, 2011.

Cheeke PR, Dierenfeld ES: *Comparative animal nutrition and metabolism*, Wallingford, UK, 2010, CAB International.

Church DC, editor: *The ruminant animal: digestive physiology and nutrition*, Prospect Heights, Ill, 1993, Waveland Press.

Forbes JM, France J, editors: *Quantitative aspects of ruminant digestion and metabolism*, Wallingford, UK, 1993, CAB International.

Gäbel G, Aschenbach JR, Müller F: Transfer of energy substrates across the ruminal epithelium: implications and limitations, *Anim Health Res Rev* 3(1):15–30, 2002.

Hungate RE: *The rumen and its microbes*, New York, 1966, Academic Press.

McDonald IW, Warner ACI, editors: *Digestion and metabolism in the ruminant*, Armidale, Australia, 1975, University of New England Publishing.

Penner GB, Steele MA, Aschenbach JR, McBride BW: Ruminant nutrition symposium: molecular adaptation of ruminal epithelia to highly fermentable diets, *J Anim Sci* 89(4):1108–1119, 2011.

Phillipson AT, editor: *Physiology of digestion and metabolism in the ruminant*, Newcastle upon Tyne, UK, 1970, Oriel Press.

Reynolds CK, Kristensen NB: Nitrogen recycling through the gut and the nitrogen economy of ruminants: an asynchronous symbiosis, *J Anim Sci* 86(14 Suppl):E293–305, 2008.

Russell JB: *Rumen microbiology and its role in ruminant nutrition*, Ithaca, NY, 2002, Cornell University Press.

Ryckebusch Y, Thivend P: *Digestive physiology and metabolism in ruminants*, Westport, Conn, 1980, AVI Publishing.

Sejrsen K, Hvelplund T, Nielsen MO, editors: *Ruminant physiology: digestion, metabolism and impact of nutrition on gene expression, immunology and stress*, Wageningen, The Netherlands, 2006, Wageningen Academic Publishers.

Stevens CE, Hume ID: *Comparative physiology of the vertebrate digestive system*, ed 2, Cambridge, UK, 1995, Cambridge University Press.

Van Soest PJ: *Nutritional ecology of the ruminant*, ed 2, Ithaca, NY, 1994, Cornell University Press.

Von Engelhardt W, Leonhard-Marek S, Breves G, Giesecke D, editors: *Ruminant physiology: digestion, metabolism, growth and reproduction*, Albany, NY, 1995, Delmar Publishers.

CHAPTER 32
Postabsorptive Nutrient Utilization

KEY POINTS

1. Homeostatic mechanisms balance the supply and demand of almost all nutrients.

The furnace

1. The tricarboxylic acid (or Krebs) cycle is the major energy-yielding pathway of fuel utilization in the body.

The fuels

1. The major metabolic fuels consist of glucose, amino acids, fatty acids, and ketone bodies.
2. Glucose is the central fuel in the energy metabolism of most animals.
3. Amino acids are important fuels in addition to being the building blocks of protein.
4. Fatty acids are the major form of energy storage in the animal body.
5. Ketone bodies are fat-derived, water-soluble metabolites that serve as glucose substitutes.

Nutrient utilization during the absorptive phase

1. During the absorptive phase, the liver takes up glucose and converts it into glycogen and triglyceride.
2. The conversion of glucose to fatty acids is an irreversible process.
3. Transport of fatty acids out of the liver is through chylomicron-like particles known as very-low-density lipoproteins.
4. Amino acids can be classified into groups on the basis of metabolic characteristics.
5. Amino acids are extensively modified during absorption.
6. Many amino acids are removed by the liver on "first pass," never reaching the systemic circulation.
7. Some amino acids taken up by the liver are used for protein synthesis.
8. Most amino acids taken up by the liver are converted to carbohydrates.
9. Not all amino acids are subject to hepatic destruction.
10. Metabolism at the tissue level is coordinated with hepatic metabolism and results in the deposition of fuel into storage tissues during the absorptive period.
11. Insulin promotes the synthesis of protein and the deposition of glycogen in muscle.
12. Insulin-stimulated uptake of amino acids by muscle results in a net increase in muscle protein synthesis.
13. During the absorptive phase, triglyceride accumulation in adipose tissue occurs by two mechanisms: uptake from very-low-density lipoproteins and direct lipid synthesis from glucose.

Nutrient utilization during the postabsorptive phase

1. Hepatic metabolism switches from glucose utilization to glucose production during the postabsorptive phase.
2. Fuel mobilization in peripheral tissues occurs when the blood insulin concentration declines.
3. Muscle reacts to a metabolic demand for glucose by mobilizing amino acids to support hepatic gluconeogenesis.
4. Muscle release of amino acids is related to reduced glucose and amino acid uptake.
5. The complex pattern of muscle amino acid catabolism and release is necessary to accommodate the liver's limited capacity for uptake of branch-chain amino acids and to facilitate the removal of amino nitrogen from the muscle.
6. The reaction of adipose tissue during the postabsorptive phase is to mobilize fatty acids.

Nutrient utilization during prolonged energy malnutrition or complete food deprivation

1. During prolonged periods of fasting or undernutrition, glucose and amino acids are conserved by extensive utilization of fats and ketone bodies for energy production.
2. A large portion of the fatty acids released from adipose tissue is taken up directly by the liver.
3. Hepatic ketone body formation is promoted by low glucose availability, a high glucagon/insulin ratio, and a ready supply of fatty acids.
4. Glucagon plays an important role in the excessive production of ketone bodies in diabetes mellitus.
5. Fatty acids cannot be used for glucose synthesis.
6. Ketone bodies are formed in the mitochondria from acetyl coenzyme A.
7. Hepatic very-low-density lipoproteins may be synthesized from adipose-derived fatty acid as well as from newly synthesized fatty acid.
8. Hormonal conditions direct the distribution of very-low-density lipoprotein fatty acids in the body.
9. Changes in growth hormone concentrations may aid in shifting peripheral fuel utilization from glucose and amino acids to ketone bodies and fatty acids.

Special fuel considerations of ruminants

1. Ruminants exist in a perpetual state of gluconeogenesis because of their unique digestive process.

The rate of absorption of nutrients from the gut is not constant, but rather fluctuates greatly with food intake. Meals are digested at a rate dependent on their chemical composition, regardless of the animal's nutrient needs. The nature of digestion dictates that nutrient absorption from the gut is rapid during digestion and then ceases during interdigestive periods. In other words, the gut is not a storehouse for nutrients, and digestion is not modulated by the animal's nutritional demands. Nutrient needs are not well matched to the wide fluctuations that occur in nutrient absorption from the gut. In fact, a vital need exists for a constant, steady supply of fuel-providing nutrients to maintain the basal metabolic functions of the body. In addition, the periods when the animal's metabolic needs are greatly elevated often do not coincide with times of rapid absorption of nutrients from the gut. Therefore, animals must have a sophisticated system for maintaining the supply of nutrients, particularly energy-supplying nutrients, and buffering both the short-term and the long-term "feast or famine" effects associated with the absorptive and postabsorptive periods of digestion.

Homeostatic Mechanisms Balance the Supply and Demand of Almost All Nutrients

This chapter focuses on supply regulation of the major energy-supplying nutrients; however, other nutrients, including vitamins and minerals, also are subject to homeostatic regulatory mechanisms. Although many of these mechanisms directly involve the digestive system, a complete discussion is beyond the scope of this book. The homeostatic mechanisms regulating the supply of minerals and vitamins are described in select references of the Bibliography.

Energy-supplying nutrients are referred to as *metabolic fuels,* and the physiological mechanisms for maintaining the supply of fuels and matching it to demand constitute *fuel homeostasis.* Fuel homeostasis is maintained by several mechanisms: the insulin-glucagon axis, the hypothalamic-pituitary axis, and the central nervous system (CNS). This chapter discusses some of the ways in which fuel is stored during the absorptive period of digestion and subsequently mobilized when needed to supply energy requirements. You may want to review Chapter 1 and the section on insulin and glucagon in Chapter 34 before reading this chapter.

THE FURNACE

The Tricarboxylic Acid (or Krebs) Cycle Is the Major Energy-Yielding Pathway of Fuel Utilization in the Body

The Krebs cycle is the pathway through which all body fuels are eventually "burned." In this cycle carbon compounds from the various body fuels are completely oxidized to carbon dioxide and water. Much of the energy released in this process is captured as ATP, the direct source of chemical energy for most physiological processes. The substrate for oxidation in the Krebs cycle is *acetate,* a two-carbon compound that enters the Krebs cycle in an activated form known as *acetyl-CoA.* Figure 32-1 illustrates that glucose and fatty acids are the sources of acetate for oxidation. Selecting between these two sources of acetate is a major function of fuel homeostasis.

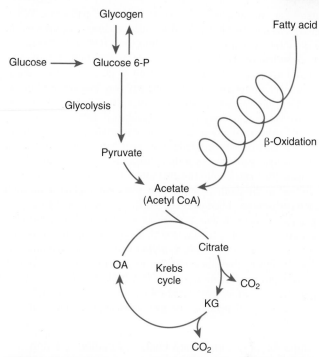

FIGURE 32-1 Relationship of the three major oxidative, catabolic pathways. *P,* Phosphate; *OA,* oxaloacetic acid; *KG,* α-ketoglutarate; *CO_2,* carbon dioxide.

THE FUELS

The Major Metabolic Fuels Consist of Glucose, Amino Acids, Fatty Acids, and Ketone Bodies

Glucose, amino acids, fatty acids, and ketone bodies are the compounds that can be directed into the Krebs cycle for energy production. Fuel homeostasis is the coordinated process by which these fuels are stored, mobilized, and interconverted to assure a continuous supply of energy for the body.

Glucose Is the Central Fuel in the Energy Metabolism of Most Animals

Glucose, the digestion product of carbohydrate, is the basic metabolic fuel during periods of adequate nutrition in omnivorous monogastric animals, such as dogs and rats. Although there are other important fuels in the body, glucose has special significance because under most conditions it is the only fuel that is consumed by the CNS. Therefore, maintaining a steady supply of glucose for brain metabolism is of paramount importance to the body. It is not surprising that an elegant system of homeostasis exists to regulate the availability of glucose to the brain and other tissues. This system of maintaining glucose availability is a major focus of this chapter.

Glucose can be stored in the body as glycogen, a highly branched starch found in liver and skeletal muscle. Glycogen is the only direct storage form of glucose in the body. Directing glucose to and from glycogen depots is a major function of fuel homeostasis. Glucose is released from glycogen through the process of *glycogenolysis.*

The first step through which glucose is used as a fuel is through *glycolysis,* the series of biochemical steps that initiate the oxidation of glucose. Through glycolysis, each molecule of glucose is converted to two molecules of *pyruvate,* a key molecule that stands at the junction of several metabolic pathways. When glucose is completely oxidized for fuel, pyruvate is converted to acetate (acetyl CoA) and passes into the *Krebs cycle,* the site of its complete oxidation. For the study of fuel homeostasis, you should appreciate that the conversion of glucose to pyruvate is reversible. Therefore any metabolic pathway that can lead to the production of pyruvate can also lead to the creation of glucose. Figure 32-1 illustrates a key relationship between pyruvate, acetate, and oxaloacetic acid. The conversion of pyruvate to acetate is irreversible while the conversion of pyruvate to oxaloacetate can flow in either direction. Thus any metabolic pathway that can lead to the creation of pyruvate or oxaloacetate can lead to the synthesis of glucose. Creation of glucose through such pathways is called *gluconeogenesis.* The process of gluconeogenesis occurs in the liver and to a small extent also in the kidneys. It occurs in no other tissues. Another pathway for glucose oxidation is the *pentose-phosphate pathway.* This is a quantitatively minor pathway that does not have great impact on fuel homeostasis. However, it is an important metabolic pathway in erythrocytes (RBCs), which have an absolute need for glucose, although these cells' overall need for energy is small compared with the rest of the body.

Amino Acids Are Important Fuels in Addition to Being the Building Blocks of Protein

Amino acids are important fuels. These monomers, the building blocks of proteins, are also carbon-containing compounds that can provide energy to the body. In addition, they are important substrates for gluconeogenesis, indicating that most amino acids can be converted to glucose when the available glucose supply is limited. Although it is sometimes said that there is no storage site of amino acids in the body, the protein of skeletal muscle could be considered to have an amino acid storage function in addition to its locomotor functions.

Fatty Acids Are the Major Form of Energy Storage in the Animal Body

Fatty acids are stored in adipose tissue in the form of *triglycerides* (also called *triacylglycerols*), which consist of three fatty acid molecules linked to a glycerol molecule by ester bonds (see Figure 30-24). Triglycerides are an ideal form of energy storage for animals. They are highly reduced molecules (there is little oxygen compared with the amount of carbon and hydrogen), which means they are a concentrated energy source, having more than twice the caloric value per gram than carbohydrates or amino acids. In addition, adipose tissue contains little water compared with protein or glycogen, the storage forms of the other two potential fuels. Thus, adipose tissue is undiluted by bulky water, allowing it to be a concentrated form of energy storage that permits animals to carry with them a maximal amount of energy at a minimal amount of weight. Fats, however, have a metabolic disadvantage; they are not water soluble. Therefore, special transport systems are needed to enable fats to be distributed among the tissues through the blood and lymph systems. In addition, fatty acids cannot be converted to glucose, so they cannot, under usual circumstances, contribute to the energy supply of the CNS. However, fatty acids can be converted to *ketone bodies.*

Ketone Bodies Are Fat-Derived, Water-Soluble Metabolites That Serve as Glucose Substitutes

Although glucose cannot be formed from fat, the fat-derived ketone bodies do have some glucoselike attributes. For example,

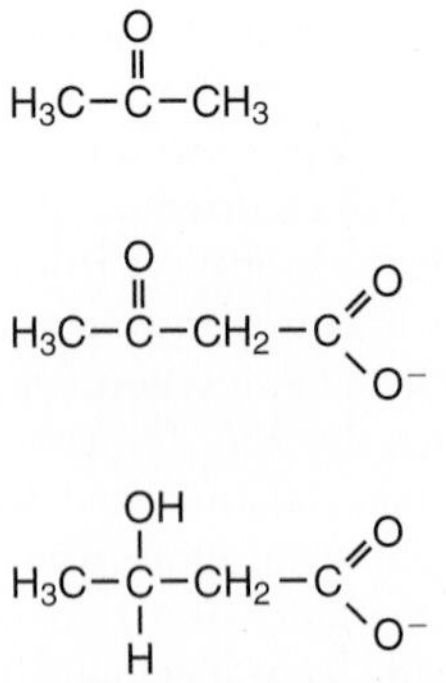

FIGURE 32-2 Physiological ketone bodies.

ketone bodies can pass the blood-brain barrier. During prolonged periods of dietary energy deprivation, they can provide a large portion of the energy supply to the CNS, at least in some species. It does appear, however, that ketone bodies cannot totally replace glucose in this function, and that a small amount of glucose is always needed by the CNS.

In monogastric species, ketone bodies are formed exclusively in the liver and are used by a wide variety of tissues. Some tissues, including cardiac muscle, use ketone bodies instead of glucose. In ruminants the ketone body β-hydroxybutyrate is formed from butyrate in the rumen epithelium. Thus, in ruminants, ketone bodies are not only products of fatty acid metabolism, but also products of normal digestion. Elevated serum concentrations of ketone bodies are characteristic of several diseases associated with abnormalities of fuel homeostasis. This fact might lead one to conclude that ketone bodies are abnormal, or even toxic, metabolites. In fact, when present in physiological concentrations, ketone bodies are important fuels that occupy an integral part of the scheme of fuel homeostasis. Figure 32-2 illustrates the chemical structure of the three major ketone bodies.

NUTRIENT UTILIZATION DURING THE ABSORPTIVE PHASE

The discussions in this chapter will divide fuel metabolism into three phases: (1) an absorptive phase associated with the active digestion and absorption of nutrients from the gut, (2) a postabsorptive phase that occurs during intermeal intervals when nutrients are not being absorbed from the gut, and (3) a prolonged energy deficiency or food deprivation phase.

During the absorptive phase as nutrient absorption takes place, metabolic events in the liver and peripheral organs are coordinated to direct nutrients into storage molecules and storage sites. Figure 32-3 illustrates the general scheme of metabolism during the absorptive phase.

During the Absorptive Phase, the Liver Takes up Glucose and Converts It into Glycogen and Triglyceride

When a meal is ingested, insulin secretion begins even before maximal absorption of glucose is achieved. This secretion is stimulated by the action of gastric inhibitory peptide (see Chapter 27) and perhaps other enteric hormones. Early insulin secretion ensures that the liver and other tissues will be "primed" and ready for the arrival of glucose from the gut. A large portion of the glucose absorbed postprandially is taken up by the liver as portal blood traverses the hepatic sinusoids. Under the influence of insulin, glucose in the liver is directed into glycogen synthesis.

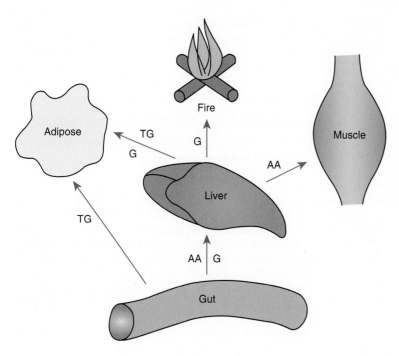

FIGURE 32-3 Metabolism during the absorptive period is characterized by the movement of potential fuels into depot sites and the utilization of glucose *(G)* as a fuel. *AA,* Amino acid; *TG,* triglyceride.

The net effect is that glucose from the digestion and absorption of carbohydrate is stored in the liver during absorptive periods. This process moderates the flow of glucose from the gut to the general circulation and keeps blood glucose concentrations from becoming excessively high during the digestion of a carbohydrate meal. Insulin exerts its stimulatory effect on hepatic glycogen synthesis by stimulating intracellular metabolic pathways that lead to the formation of glycogen. These effects are discussed further in reference to the counterbalancing effects of glucagon.

The amount of glycogen that can be stored in the liver is limited and, under normal conditions, probably never exceeds 10% of the total weight of the liver. In humans, this represents about 100 g of glycogen, and a proportionately similar limit likely exists for the storage of glycogen in the livers of other species. This amount of glycogen does not account for all the glucose taken up by the liver during the digestion and absorption of a large carbohydrate meal; therefore, some additional mechanism must exist for the disposal of excess glucose. If there were no such alternatives for glucose disposal, blood glucose concentrations could rise out of control after glycogen stores had reached their maximum. Fatty acid synthesis offers an alternative mechanism for glucose removal.

The Conversion of Glucose to Fatty Acids Is an Irreversible Process

The synthesis of fatty acids from glucose begins with glycolysis. This pathway leads to the production of two pyruvate molecules for each molecule of glucose consumed. Pyruvate can then enter the mitochondria to be activated to *acetyl coenzyme A* (acetyl CoA) for entry into the Krebs cycle, as discussed previously. However, the Krebs cycle is for energy generation, and during the absorptive period, there is more than enough acetyl CoA and Krebs cycle activity to provide for energy needs; therefore the excess acetyl CoA must be shunted away from the Krebs cycle. The excess acetyl CoA combines with *oxaloacetate* to form *citrate* in what is essentially the first reaction of the Krebs cycle. Instead of continuing through the Krebs cycle reactions, however, during

the absorptive period much of the citrate is transported out of the mitochondria into the cytosol. When in the cytosol, each citrate molecule contributes two carbons toward the synthesis of fatty acids. The remaining portion of the citrate molecule cycles back into the mitochondria for further use. Citrate serves as a carrier molecule to transport two-carbon units out of the mitochondria because acetyl CoA cannot pass the mitochondrial membrane directly (Figure 32-4).

Several important steps in this conversion of glucose to fatty acids are promoted by insulin and are discussed in detail later. It is important to recognize that the conversion of glucose to fatty acids is irreversible; thus carbohydrate can form fat, but fat cannot form carbohydrate. The discussion here concerns hepatic metabolism, and the liver is an important site of fatty acid synthesis in several species. Direct synthesis of fatty acids also occurs in adipose tissue. The relative importance of liver and adipose tissue as sites of fatty acid synthesis varies with species, as discussed later.

Transport of Fatty Acids out of the Liver Is Through Chylomicron-Like Particles Known as Very-Low-Density Lipoproteins

When formed in the liver, fatty acids must be transported either to adipose tissue for storage or to other tissues (e.g., muscle) for direct utilization for energy production. Because fatty acids are insoluble in blood, some special transport mechanism for their distribution is necessary. This mechanism is through the hepatic formation of triglyceride-rich serum lipoproteins, also known as *very-low-density lipoproteins* (VLDLs); these triglyceride-rich lipoproteins are much less dense than other lipoproteins in blood serum. In the synthesis of VLDLs, fatty acids are first esterified to form triglycerides, and the triglycerides are wrapped in a coat of phospholipid, cholesterol, and specific proteins (Figure 32-5). This is essentially the same mechanism by which fatty acids are transported out of the enterocytes after absorption from the gut. In the latter case the lipoproteins are called *chylomicrons.* The VLDLs of the liver are smaller than chylomicrons but have a similar structure and function. The mechanisms by which VLDLs and chylomicrons deliver fatty acids to peripheral tissues are further discussed in relation to peripheral tissues.

Amino Acids Can Be Classified into Groups on the Basis of Metabolic Characteristics

The discussion of amino acid absorption and metabolism becomes complicated because not all amino acids are subject to the same reactions. For this discussion the amino acids are divided into two groups, each containing two subgroups (Table 32-1). The major groups are the "nutritionally dispensable" amino acids and the "nutritionally indispensable" amino acids. Within the dispensable amino acid group, glutamate, aspartate, alanine,

glutamine, and asparagine are separated out as *transport amino acids;* within the indispensable amino acid group, leucine, isoleucine, and valine form a special subgroup known as the *branch-chain amino acids* (BCAAs). The transport amino acids are utilized in several reactions in which amino groups are transferred from molecule to molecule or organ to organ.

Amino Acids Are Extensively Modified During Absorption

The profile of amino acids in the portal vein is considerably different from that of the diet, indicating that amino acid destruction and transformation occur during the absorptive process. Essentially all the glutamate and much of the aspartate in the diet are removed by the intestinal epithelial cells during absorption, so the portal blood is almost devoid of glutamate and contains little aspartate. Much of the nitrogen from glutamate and aspartate is transferred to pyruvate to form the amino acid alanine, which is present in high concentrations in portal blood. The metabolism of the transport amino acids in the intestinal epithelium is a good example of both the way in which amino groups can be gained and lost and how the metabolism of amino acids interfaces with the metabolism of carbohydrate. Glutamate and aspartate are similar to two Krebs cycle intermediates,

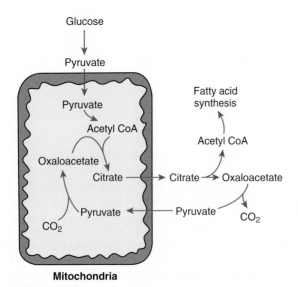

Mitochondria

FIGURE 32-4 Hepatic synthesis of fatty acid from carbohydrate requires the passage of carbohydrate carbons through the mitochondria. Citrate forms a shuttle to transport the carbons of acetyl coenzyme A *(acetyl CoA)* out of the mitochondria because acetyl CoA cannot pass directly through the mitochondrial membrane. The formation of citrate from oxaloacetate and acetyl CoA is the first reaction of the Krebs cycle; thus fatty acid formation is an alternative to Krebs cycle oxidation when there is more than enough acetyl CoA to provide cellular energy through Krebs cycle activity.

TABLE 32-1 Metabolic Classification of Amino Acids

Indispensable Amino Acids		Dispensable Amino Acids	
Branch-Chain Amino Acids	**Others**	**Transport Amino Acids**	**Others**
Leucine	Arginine*	Alanine	Cysteine
Isoleucine	Histidine	Glutamine	Glycine
Valine	Lysine	Glutamate	Proline
	Methionine	(Glutamic acid)	Tyrosine[†]
	Phenylalanine	Asparagine	Serine
	Threonine	Aspartate	
	Tryptophan	(Aspartic acid)	

*Indispensable for cats, but not required in the diets of many other species.
[†]Dietary adequacy depends on a supply of phenylalanine.

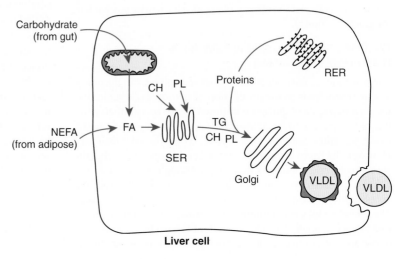

Liver cell

FIGURE 32-5 Formation of very-low-density lipoprotein *(VLDL).* Fatty acids *(FA)* for triglyceride *(TG)* formation may come from synthesis by carbohydrate or amino acids or from adipose tissue FA arriving at the liver in the form of nonesterified fatty acids *(NEFA).* Note the similarity to chylomicron formation (see Figure 30-27). *CH,* Cholesterol; *PL,* phospholipid; *SER,* smooth endoplasmic reticulum; *RER,* rough endoplasmic reticulum.

α-ketoglutarate and oxaloacetate, differing only by the presence of an amino group or a keto-oxygen. Carbohydrates and amino acids having this relationship are said to be *analogues;* thus, α-ketoglutarate is the keto-analogue of glutamate, and pyruvate is the keto-analogue of alanine (Figure 32-6). All amino acids can form keto-analogues, and all keto-analogues can be readily converted back to their parent amino acids.

Many Amino Acids Are Removed by the Liver on "First Pass," Never Reaching the Systemic Circulation

The hepatic-portal circulation is arranged in such a way that all nutrients leaving the gut via the blood pass through the liver before entering the systemic circulation (see Figure 30-23). This arrangement places the liver in a "sentinel" position, from which

it can modify the nutrient composition of portal blood before the blood is distributed to other tissues. The function of the liver in modifying portal blood composition is well illustrated in the case of amino acid absorption. Many of the amino acids absorbed into portal blood are removed as the blood passes the liver, so they never reach the general circulation. Figure 32-7 illustrates that in the dog, only about 23% of the amino acids reaching the liver during the absorptive period pass into the general circulation; the liver thus helps keep blood amino acid concentrations stable during periods of amino acid absorption. The blood amino acid concentration, as with the blood glucose concentration, is usually kept relatively constant.

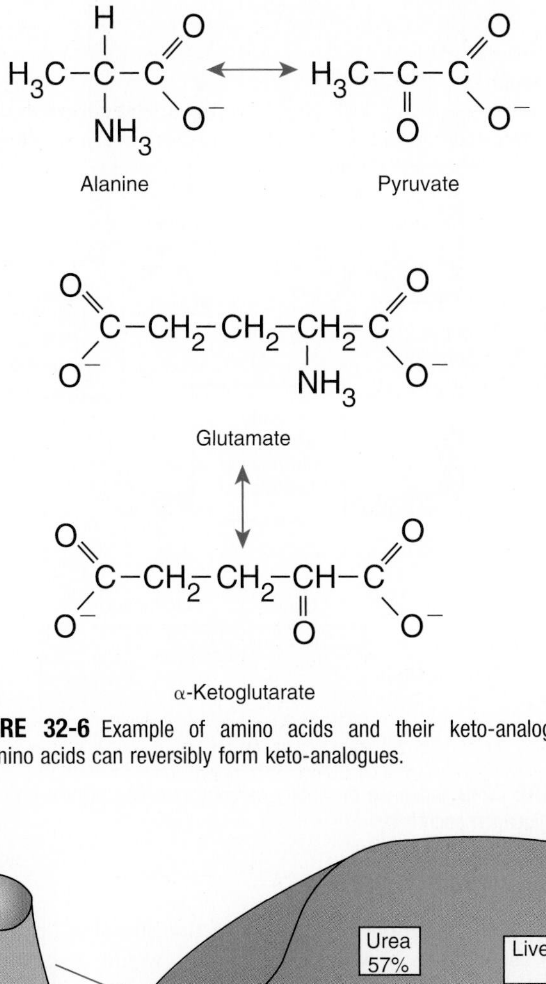

Some Amino Acids Taken up by the Liver Are Used for Protein Synthesis

The liver is an important site of protein synthesis, and thus its priority position for amino acid uptake seems reasonable. Figure 32-7 shows that approximately 20% of the portal blood amino acid supply is used for protein synthesis in the liver, although this proportion varies with dietary protein intake. Almost all the serum proteins are synthesized in the liver, including such critical proteins as albumin and the blood-clotting factors. Although the liver-derived serum proteins serve many important functions, one function they *do not* serve is that of amino acid transport. The direct amino acid supply for protein synthesis in non-hepatic tissue comes from free amino acids in the blood, not from preformed serum proteins.

Most Amino Acids Taken up by the Liver Are Converted to Carbohydrates

Most amino acids entering the liver undergo *deamination,* which means the amino groups are removed and the molecules converted to their keto-analogues. The keto-analogues enter the pathways of carbohydrate metabolism, from which they may be completely metabolized for energy, converted to glucose or glycogen, or shunted to fatty acid synthesis. All these reactions proceed in the same manner as previously described for carbohydrate metabolism. Figure 32-8 illustrates the sites at which the various amino acids enter the carbohydrate pathways.

Deamination of amino acids for the production of carbohydrate or energy may seem like a waste of expensive dietary protein; in some species, however, the deamination of amino

FIGURE 32-6 Example of amino acids and their keto-analogues. All amino acids can reversibly form keto-analogues.

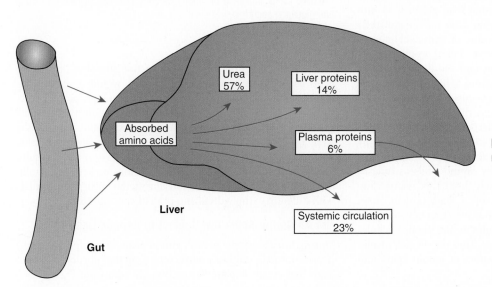

FIGURE 32-7 Fate of dietary amino acids reaching the canine liver.

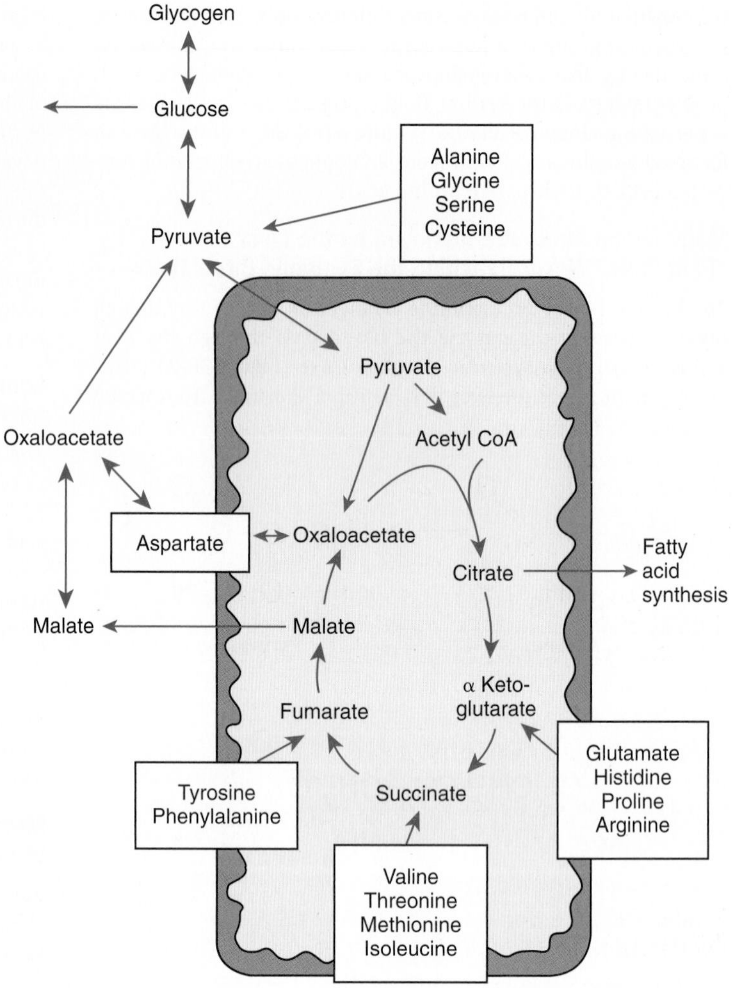

Glycogen

Glucose

Pyruvate ← Alanine / Glycine / Serine / Cysteine

Pyruvate

Acetyl CoA

Oxaloacetate

Aspartate ↔ **Oxaloacetate**

Citrate → Fatty acid synthesis

Malate ← **Malate**

Fumarate

α Keto-glutarate ← Glutamate / Histidine / Proline / Arginine

Tyrosine / Phenylalanine

Succinate ← Valine / Threonine / Methionine / Isoleucine

FIGURE 32-8 Sites of entry of various amino acids into the scheme of carbohydrate metabolism. This figure illustrates the means by which glucose can be synthesized from amino acids in the process of gluconeogenesis. In the case of the dispensable amino acids, the reactions are reversible, allowing amino acid production from carbohydrate.

acids is important for homeostasis of glucose and other fuels. For example, the natural diets of the true carnivores (e.g., cats, mink) contain a large portion of protein and little carbohydrate, but their glucose needs are no less than those of other animals, so it is extremely important that they synthesize glucose from amino acids. Ruminants are in a similar situation because most of the carbohydrates they consume undergo fermentative digestion and are absorbed as volatile fatty acids rather than glucose. As with carnivores, ruminants depend on amino acids for some of their glucose needs, although a large portion of ruminant glucose requirements may be met through conversion of propionate.

To allow carbohydrate production and the deamination of excess amino acids, the endocrine reactions to high-protein meals are somewhat different from those to meals containing substantial amounts of carbohydrate. During the digestion of high-protein meals, insulin and glucagon secretion does not occur in its usual reciprocal pattern. Insulin secretion is stimulated by amino acids as well as by glucose. Glucagon secretion, which is inhibited by glucose, is stimulated by amino acids as long as glucose concentrations are moderately low. This relationship means that during the digestion of a high-protein, low-carbohydrate meal, there is simultaneous secretion of insulin and glucagon. One of the effects of insulin is the greater cellular uptake of amino acids as well as glucose. Thus the effect of insulin in this situation is to increase transport of amino acids into tissues.

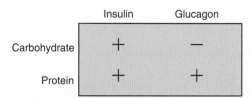

	Insulin	Glucagon
Carbohydrate	+	−
Protein	+	+

FIGURE 32-9 Influence of dietary carbohydrate and protein on insulin and glucagon secretion.

If insulin secretion were the only action stimulated by amino acid absorption, however, the animal would risk insulin-stimulated hypoglycemia when it consumed a high-protein, low-carbohydrate diet. An important action of glucagon is to stimulate gluconeogenesis through the deamination of amino acids in the liver. This process ensures that adequate glucose will be available to counterbalance the effects of amino acid–stimulated insulin secretion. Figure 32-9 illustrates the relationship between insulin secretion and glucagon secretion during the absorption of diets with different carbohydrate and protein concentrations.

Not All Amino Acids Are Subject to Hepatic Destruction

During the absorptive period, amino acids for peripheral (nonhepatic) protein synthesis must come from that portion of amino acids that escape hepatic destruction. As seen from Figure 32-7, this portion amounts to only about 23% of the amino acids absorbed from the gut. Although this may seem like a meager portion of amino acids to be allocated for protein synthesis by all body tissues except liver, two considerations make it more appropriate. First, amino acids are selectively taken up by the liver, so the distribution of individual amino acids in blood leaving the liver is not the same as that in blood reaching the liver. The indispensable amino acids, especially the BCAAs, are not avidly extracted by the liver, whereas some of the dispensable amino acids (e.g., alanine) are extensively taken up by hepatic tissue. The dispensable amino acids can be synthesized by protein-producing tissues; thus the relatively low concentration of serum amino acids resulting from hepatic amino acid removal is not rate limiting for tissue protein synthesis. Second, the proportion of amino acids taken up by the liver, as well as the fate of the amino acids that are taken up, is not constant and can be adjusted according to the body's protein needs. Low-protein diets lead to reductions in hepatic amino acid uptake, protein synthesis, and amino acid destruction by the liver.

Metabolism at the Tissue Level Is Coordinated with Hepatic Metabolism and Results in the Deposition of Fuel into Storage Tissues During the Absorptive Period

The overall effects of hepatic metabolism during the absorption of a meal are the removal of glucose and amino acids and the synthesis of protein and fat. Complementary changes occur in peripheral tissues, so additional glucose and amino acids are removed by skeletal muscle and adipose tissue. In addition, fatty acids secreted by the liver as VLDL triglycerides are deposited in adipose tissue, as are the triglycerides of chylomicrons.

Insulin Promotes the Synthesis of Protein and the Deposition of Glycogen in Muscle

The absorptive period is dominated by the effects of insulin. In skeletal muscle, the largest tissue mass of the body, insulin promotes the uptake of glucose and amino acids and thus tends to moderate the increase in blood concentration of these nutrients during absorption of a meal. The uptake of glucose by muscle is associated with glycogen synthesis, just as in the liver. Muscle glycogen, in contrast to liver glycogen, cannot be made directly available to augment blood glucose concentrations during periods of low glucose availability. Muscle glycogen is primarily for metabolism in the muscle.

Insulin-Stimulated Uptake of Amino Acids by Muscle Results in a Net Increase in Muscle Protein Synthesis

The term *net increase* is used in reference to muscle protein synthesis because muscle protein is in a state of dynamic equilibrium, that is, a constant state of flux. Protein molecules are continuously being broken down and their amino acids added to an intracellular amino acid pool. Simultaneously, new proteins are constantly being made, deriving their amino acids from the same pool (Figure 32-10). The size of the amino acid pool depends on the relative rates of entry and exit of amino acids. Amino acids enter the pool from the blood during the absorptive phase and at all times from the breakdown of body protein. Exit of amino acids from the pool results from protein synthesis and oxidative catabolism. In the absorptive phase of digestion, the amino acid pool is large because amino acids are being taken up from the blood. In addition, few of the amino acids leaving the pool are directed toward oxidative catabolism because sufficient glucose is available for oxidation and energy generation. Therefore the amino acid

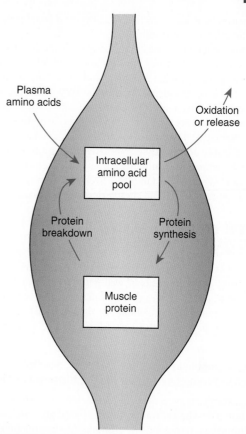

FIGURE 32-10 Intracellular amino acid pool. The size of the pool depends on the rates of amino acid uptake from plasma and muscle protein relative to the rates of amino acid loss resulting from oxidation, export to plasma, and protein synthesis.

pool is large, and a high proportion of amino acids is directed to protein synthesis. When the rate of protein synthesis exceeds the rate of protein breakdown, there is a net increase in the amount of muscle protein. Thus, during the absorptive phase, amino acids are stored in muscle protein, protein that has a functional role not only for locomotion and posture, but also for amino acid storage.

During the Absorptive Phase, Triglyceride Accumulation in Adipose Tissue Occurs by Two Mechanisms: Uptake from Very-Low-Density Lipoproteins and Direct Lipid Synthesis from Glucose

Triglyceride fatty acids are transferred from chylomicrons and VLDLs to adipose tissue by the action of *lipoprotein lipase* (LPL). This enzyme resides on endothelial surfaces of capillaries and, when activated, binds to chylomicrons and VLDLs, catalyzing the hydrolysis of fatty acids from their core triglycerides and allowing the transfer of those fatty acids to the surrounding tissues. The sensitivity of LPL to specific hormones varies in different tissues. Adipose tissue LPL is stimulated by insulin; thus, during the absorptive phase, fatty acids from chylomicrons and VLDLs are selectively transferred to adipose tissue. Therefore, under the influence of insulin, excess carbohydrate and amino acids are converted to fatty acids in the liver, and those fatty acids are subsequently transported, via VLDLs, to the adipose tissue. Similarly, chylomicron triglyceride arising from intestinal fatty acid absorption is also selectively transported to adipose tissue, under the influence of insulin.

Adipose tissue fatty acids may also arise from direct synthesis in addition to uptake from chylomicrons and VLDLs. Adipose tissue cells are metabolically active, and under the influence of insulin, they take up glucose. Within the adipocytes, glucose can be converted to fatty acids by the same metabolic mechanisms by which fatty acids were synthesized in the liver. In addition, acetate from fermentative digestion also can serve as a substrate for fatty acid synthesis in adipose tissue (see later discussion of the special fuel considerations of ruminants). Thus there are two major sites of fatty acid synthesis in the body: liver and adipose tissue. The relative importance of these sites varies with species.

NUTRIENT UTILIZATION DURING THE POSTABSORPTIVE PHASE

The *postabsorptive phase* is the relatively brief period (usually a few hours) between meals in well-fed animals. It is characterized by short-term changes that mobilize nutrients from storage pools to maintain fuel availability for metabolically active tissue. Figure 32-11 illustrates the general scheme of postabsorptive metabolism.

Hepatic Metabolism Switches from Glucose Utilization to Glucose Production During the Postabsorptive Phase

As the absorption of a meal is completed, the rate of glucose absorption from the gut wanes, and the blood glucose concentration diminishes, removing the stimulus for insulin production. As blood glucose concentrations decline, glucagon secretion is stimulated. The primary target organ of glucagon is the liver, in which glucagon creates marked metabolic changes. Through stimulation of specific cell surface receptors on hepatocytes, glucagon activates adenyl cyclase, leading to the phosphorylation of numerous cellular enzymes (see Chapter 1). Some enzymes are activated by phosphorylation, whereas others are inactivated, and unless the overall scheme of substrate flow is considered, the whole phosphorylation-dephosphorylation system appears to be quite random and to make little sense. Considering the actions of the individual enzymes in light of their effect on the flow of energy substrate through the liver, however, reveals that the system is an elegant and incredibly well-orchestrated mechanism for the maintenance of fuel homeostasis.

The enzymes that stimulate mobilization and utilization of fuels are activated by phosphorylation, whereas those stimulating storage of fuels are inactivated by phosphorylation. It must be understood that many enzymes of intermediary metabolism serve a passive role, catalyzing reactions that can go in either direction, depending on substrate concentrations. A relatively small number of regulatory enzymes usually stand at the head of metabolic pathways and determine the substrate concentrations to which the other, unregulated enzymes are exposed. Through its effect on several key regulatory enzymes, glucagon (a stimulator of phosphorylation) places the liver in a fuel-mobilization state. In contrast, insulin (an inhibitor of phosphorylation) promotes a hepatic metabolic pattern that favors fuel storage, as previously discussed.

The opposing actions of insulin and glucagon on hepatic metabolism are evident from their actions on two key regulatory enzyme pairs: *glycogen synthase* and *glycogen phosphatase,* and *phosphofructokinase* and *fructose-1,6-bisphosphatase.* The first of these pairs regulates glycogen synthesis and breakdown, whereas the second regulates glycolysis and gluconeogenesis, respectively. Figure 32-12 illustrates the actions of these enzymes and their regulatory effects. Glycogen synthase and phosphofructokinase are inhibited by phosphorylation and thus are stimulated by insulin. Glycogen phosphatase and fructose-1,6-bisphosphatase are stimulated by phosphorylation and thus stimulated by glucagon. The actions of insulin and glucagon on these antagonistic enzyme pairs emphasize the importance of the insulin/glucagon ratio to which the liver is exposed. Neither hormone elicits an "all-or-none" reaction, but rather alters the balance of opposing reactions by influencing the relative activity of antagonistic enzymes. Thus the fuel-mobilizing or fuel-storing activity of the liver depends on which hormone is most dominant. For this reason, the insulin/glucagon ratio appears to be more important to liver metabolism than the absolute concentration of either hormone.

Under the influence of glucagon, glycogen phosphatase is activated by phosphorylation, promoting glycogenolysis and the elevation of intracellular glucose concentrations. As glucose accumulates, it is prevented from cycling back into glycogen because the major enzyme catalyzing that reaction, glycogen synthase, is blocked by phosphorylation. In addition, the flow of glucose into glycolysis is also blocked by phosphorylation inhibition of phosphofructokinase (see Figure 32-12). Thus the normal pathways

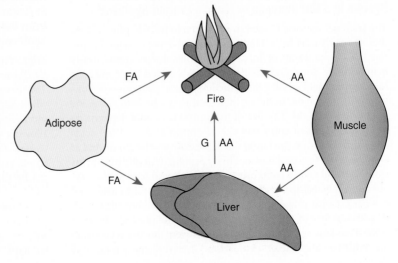

FIGURE 32-11 Postabsorptive metabolism is characterized by movement of fuels out of depot sites for immediate use. Glucose *(G)* arising from glycogenolysis or gluconeogenesis is a major fuel, although some fatty acid *(FA)* is consumed as well. Amino acid *(AA)* forms the substrate for gluconeogenesis.

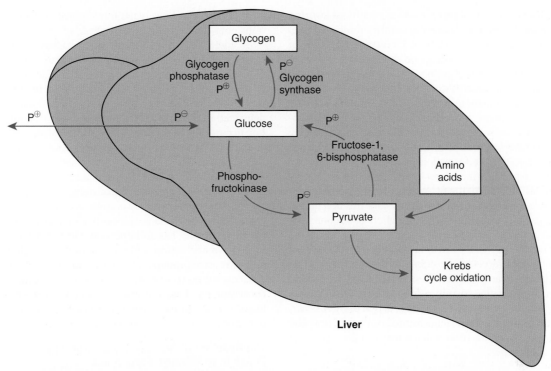

FIGURE 32-12 Effects of phosphorylation on four key enzymes of glucose production and utilization. All four enzymes are phosphorylated under the influence of cyclic adenosine monophosphate *(cAMP)*. Note, however, that the enzymes that favor glucose formation are stimulated by phosphorylation *(P⁺)*, whereas those that favor glucose utilization and storage are inhibited by phosphorylation *(P⁻)*.

for glucose utilization within the hepatocyte are all inhibited by glucagon, allowing glucose from glycogen breakdown to accumulate in the cells. Eventually, intracellular glucose escapes into the extracellular fluid and on into the blood. In this manner, hepatic glycogen is mobilized to elevate and maintain blood glucose concentrations when they begin to decline.

The liver stores of glycogen are relatively limited and cannot maintain blood glucose concentrations for a long period. Estimates in humans are that hepatic glycogen will serve blood glucose needs for 6 to 12 hours under conditions of light exertion and for only about 20 minutes under conditions of heavy exertion. Values for animals are probably similar. Therefore, in addition to glycogen mobilization, some other means must exist for maintaining the body's glucose supply during periods of exertion and prolonged periods between meals. Under these conditions of greater demand, glucose is provided by gluconeogenesis. Gluconeogenesis is promoted by the phosphorylation-stimulated enzyme fructose-1,6-bisphosphatase. This enzyme essentially puts the glycolytic pathway into reverse, leading to glucose production from the same molecules that are intermediates in its oxidative destruction. Important substrates are pyruvate and all the intermediates of the Krebs cycle.

At this point, it is important to remember that most of the Krebs cycle intermediates or pyruvate can be supplied by the deamination of amino acids. The entry point of the various amino acids into the scheme of carbohydrate metabolism is illustrated in Figure 32-8. Pyruvate and all the Krebs cycle intermediates can flow backward through the oxidative pathway (not all the reactions of gluconeogenesis are the exact reverse of the corresponding reactions in glycolysis, but the net result of gluconeogenesis

is the reverse of glycolysis), resulting in the production of glucose. Thus, amino acids provide a large store of precursors for glucose formation. The end result of glucagon stimulation is to promote the production of glucose through glycogenolysis and gluconeogenesis, turning the liver into a glucose-synthesizing organ.

Fuel Mobilization in Peripheral Tissues Occurs When the Blood Insulin Concentration Declines

The pattern of metabolism in the peripheral tissues changes in the postabsorptive phase to support the liver's capacity to maintain fuel supplies.

Muscle Reacts to a Metabolic Demand for Glucose by Mobilizing Amino Acids to Support Hepatic Gluconeogenesis

Mobilization of amino acid from muscle appears to be stimulated largely by a relative lack of insulin; thus mobilization occurs when blood glucose concentrations are low. Amino acids mobilized from skeletal muscle come from the intracellular amino acid pool cited earlier (see Figure 32-10). However, the mobilizing reactions are complex, and the distribution of amino acids leaving the muscle does not reflect the distribution of amino acids in the intracellular pool, as explained later.

Muscle Release of Amino Acids Is Related to Reduced Glucose and Amino Acid Uptake

The postabsorptive decline in the serum insulin concentration has a twofold effect on muscle: the entry of amino acids from the serum into the intracellular amino acid pool is diminished, and the entry of glucose into muscle cells for energy production declines. Reduced amino acid entry results in conditions favoring net protein degradation to maintain the cellular amino acid pool size. Reduced glucose entry results in increased utilization of amino acids from the pool for energy production.

The pattern of utilization of amino acids for energy by muscle may at first seem unnecessarily complex, involving selective use and extensive transformation of amino acids. BCAAs serve as primary sources of energy in muscle cells during the postabsorptive phase because these amino acids account for approximately one third of all muscle amino acid. Catabolism of BCAAs begins with deamination and the formation of the α-keto-acid of the BCAA. The α-keto-acids then enter the Krebs cycle for energy production. Deamination of the BCAA requires that some acceptor be available to receive the amino group, and this acceptor is ultimately pyruvate, resulting in the formation of alanine. The source of pyruvate can be muscle glycogen, blood glucose, or the metabolic products of BCAA α-keto-acids. When metabolism of BCAA α-keto-acids serves as the supply of pyruvate for alanine synthesis, the net reaction is conversion of BCAA to alanine (Figure 32-13). Thus the overall metabolic activity in muscle during the postabsorptive phase is the destruction of BCAAs and the formation of alanine. The alanine formed is released from the muscle cells into the blood, from which it may be taken up by the liver for gluconeogenesis.

The Complex Pattern of Muscle Amino Acid Catabolism and Release Is Necessary to Accommodate the Liver's Limited Capacity for Uptake of Branch-Chain Amino Acids and to Facilitate the Removal of Amino Nitrogen from the Muscle

It might appear that a simpler system of amino acid transfer to the liver would suffice. Why are amino acids not just released from muscle cell amino acid pools into the blood and transported to the liver for glucose synthesis? The answer lies in the limited uptake capacity of the liver for BCAAs and the need to transport amino nitrogen out of the muscle. BCAAs, the predominant amino acids of skeletal muscle, are not taken up readily by the

liver; thus, if BCAAs were not transformed to alanine, amino acid transfer to the liver would be limited.

In addition, alanine is a convenient means by which nitrogen from the deamination of muscle amino acid can be transported to the liver. This is important because free amino groups liberated by the catabolism of amino acids in muscle, if not removed, could lead to the formation of toxic levels of ammonia. Ammonia is detoxified in the body by the formation of urea, but urea formation occurs only in the liver. Thus, alanine forms a gluconeogenic precursor that also transports nitrogen to the liver for urea synthesis. Figures 32-13 and 32-14 illustrate the role of alanine in the transport of amino acid nitrogen and carbon to the liver for synthesis of urea and glucose, respectively.

The regulation of muscle protein mobilization is influenced to a large extent by the lack of insulin. However, the adrenocortical hormone cortisol has an important effect of stimulating protein breakdown and amino acid mobilization. Through the mobilization of muscle protein and stimulation of hepatic gluconeogenesis, cortisol exerts one of its major effects, raising blood glucose concentration. Under normal conditions, glucagon, the other major gluconeogenic hormone, exerts its effects on the liver and does not appear to have a direct effect on muscle.

The Reaction of Adipose Tissue During the Postabsorptive Phase Is to Mobilize Fatty Acids

Fatty acids are released from adipose tissue because of the action of the phosphorylation-stimulated enzyme *hormone-sensitive lipase* (HSL). This enzyme is stimulated by the relative lack of insulin in the postabsorptive period; insulin suppresses the action of HSL by promoting its dephosphorylation. Glucagon may have some adipose tissue activity in promoting triglyceride breakdown by stimulating the phosphorylation and activation of HSL. More likely, however, glucagon's effects are restricted to the liver, and the normal stimulation of HSL comes from epinephrine or norepinephrine; norepinephrine originates from sympathetic nerves in the adipose tissue. The exact means by which sympathetic nerve activity in adipose tissue is coordinated with body fuel availability is not well established, but the catecholamine

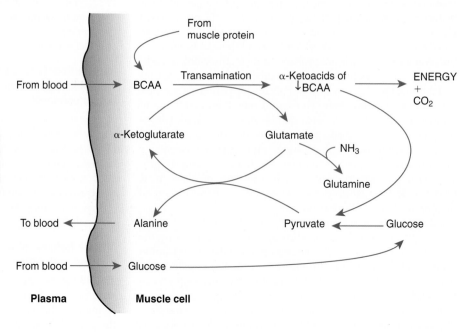

FIGURE 32-13 Catabolism of branch-chain amino acids *(BCAAs)* by muscle cells. The pyruvate for export of amino groups may be derived from glucose or the amino acids themselves.

hormones and neuroregulators appear to be the primary positive stimulus for breakdown of adipose triglyceride. However, the negative stimulus provided by the absence of insulin may be the most important regulator of adipose fat mobilization.

Stimulation of HSL in the postabsorptive state leads to the release of fatty acids from adipose tissue into the blood. Fatty acids in blood are reversibly bound to albumin because they are not otherwise soluble in water. Albumin-bound fatty acids in blood are usually referred to as *nonesterified fatty acids* (NEFAs) to distinguish them from triglyceride fatty acids in chylomicrons and lipoproteins. NEFAs in blood may be used directly for energy

by many tissues. However, many NEFAs are taken up by the liver and used for either ketone body production or VLDL synthesis, as discussed in the next section.

NUTRIENT UTILIZATION DURING PROLONGED ENERGY MALNUTRITION OR COMPLETE FOOD DEPRIVATION

During Prolonged Periods of Fasting or Undernutrition, Glucose and Amino Acids Are Conserved by Extensive Utilization of Fats and Ketone Bodies for Energy Production

From the previous discussion of postabsorptive metabolism, you can appreciate that amino acids form an important depot for glucose precursors and energy-producing substrate. During prolonged fasting or undernutrition, however, it would not be advantageous for animals to rely heavily on their skeletal muscle for energy and glucose production; doing so would soon lead to severe weakness as the skeletal muscle protein was consumed. Thus, protective mechanisms have developed by which skeletal muscle is preserved during periods of insufficient energy intake. In utilization of stored fuels, shifts away from glucose and toward adipose fat stores are necessary for protein sparing. Figure 32-15 illustrates the general scheme of metabolism during prolonged catabolic periods.

A Large Portion of the Fatty Acids Released from Adipose Tissue Is Taken up Directly by the Liver

During prolonged periods of undernutrition, low glucose availability leads to rapid mobilization of adipose fatty acids in the form of NEFAs. Although NEFAs are metabolized by various tissues, many are extracted from the blood by the liver, which receives much of the total blood flow and has an efficient hepatic NEFA extraction mechanism. When the NEFAs are in the hepatocytes, they may follow any of three potential metabolic paths. The first is complete oxidation for energy production; however, the hepatic requirements for energy are such that only a small amount of the total fatty acid supply during adipose mobilization needs to be used for complete oxidation. The second pathway is esterification leading to triglyceride formation, and the third is production of ketone bodies. Triglyceride synthesis is discussed later; the focus here is ketone body production.

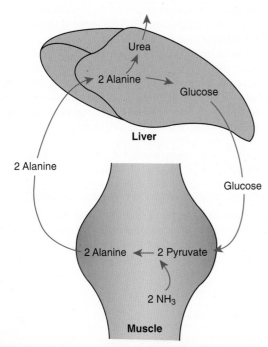

FIGURE 32-14 Alanine arising from BCAA catabolism in muscle is converted to glucose and urea in the liver. The glucose produced can potentially return to the muscle for alanine production. Thus the cycle of alanine to glucose forms a shuttle to transport nitrogen from the muscle to the liver for urea synthesis. *NH₃*, Ammonia.

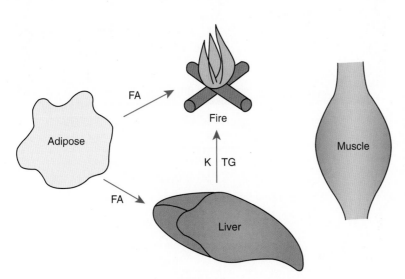

FIGURE 32-15 During prolonged periods of food deprivation or energy deficiency, the ketone bodies *(K)*, fatty acids *(FA)*, and triglycerides *(TG)* become the major fuels. Glucose oxidation becomes minor, thus sparing muscle protein that otherwise would be needed for gluconeogenesis.

Hepatic Ketone Body Formation Is Promoted by Low Glucose Availability, a High Glucagon/Insulin Ratio, and a Ready Supply of Fatty Acids

Ketone body formation occurs within the hepatic mitochondria, and the rate of ketone body synthesis is controlled by the regulated transport of fatty acids across the mitochondrial membrane (Figure 32-16). Fatty acids enter mitochondria in combination with a molecule known as *carnitine,* and transport depends on an enzyme known as *carnitine palmitoyltransferase I* (CPT-I). The activity of this enzyme, along with the availability of fatty acid, is the primary determinant of the rate of ketone body formation. CPT-I activity is regulated in an interesting manner, being inhibited by an intermediate of the fatty acid synthesis pathway, *malonyl CoA.* Malonyl CoA concentrations are high when the liver is responding to insulin and glucose is being used for fatty acid synthesis. When glucagon concentrations are high relative to insulin, little fatty acid is synthesized in the liver. Thus, malonyl CoA concentrations are low, and CPT-I is fully active when the insulin/glucagon ratio is low. Ketone body synthesis is stimulated under these hormonal conditions.

Under conditions when CPT-I is active, most available fatty acid is transported into the mitochondria for ketone body synthesis. This well-orchestrated but somewhat complex regulatory system is important because the liver can both produce and consume fatty acids. If there were not a way of "turning off" fatty acid destruction during periods of synthesis, a futile cycle of synthesis and destruction would occur. The inhibition of CPT-I by malonyl CoA provides a system that blocks the metabolic destruction of newly synthesized fatty acid while still providing a mechanism for the utilization of fatty acids derived from adipose tissue. The overall pattern of metabolism results in a reciprocal relationship between glucose availability and ketone body production. Although ketone bodies are produced in the liver, they cannot be used there for energy production. Therefore, all ketone bodies are transported to peripheral tissues for utilization. When the concentration of ketone bodies in the blood becomes abnormally high, some are excreted in urine.

Glucagon Plays an Important Role in the Excessive Production of Ketone Bodies in Diabetes Mellitus

If untreated, diabetes mellitus in animals, especially dogs, leads to high concentrations of ketone bodies in the blood. Diabetes mellitus occurs because of a lack of insulin, but the hepatic production of ketone bodies results from the unrestrained action of glucagon. Even though serum concentrations of glucose are high in diabetes mellitus, the inability of the pancreas to secrete insulin leads to a low insulin/glucagon ratio; thus the liver is functioning solely under the direction of glucagon. Glucagon inhibits fatty acid production from glucose, so malonyl CoA concentrations are low and CPT-I activity is high. Because of the lack of insulin to suppress adipose HSL, blood NEFA concentrations are high. The combination of high NEFA availability and unrestrained CPT-I activity results in rapid transport of fatty acids into the mitochondria with extensive ketone body production, even though blood glucose concentrations are high.

Fatty Acids Cannot Be Used for Glucose Synthesis

It is important to understand that the metabolism of fat within the mitochondria cannot contribute directly to gluconeogenesis. When they cross the mitochondrial membrane, fatty acids undergo β-oxidation, which leads to the successive removal of

FIGURE 32-16 The liver is a site of both destruction and synthesis of fatty acids. To keep both processes from occurring simultaneously, fatty acid destruction is inhibited during periods of fatty acid synthesis. *Solid lines,* pathway of fatty acid synthesis; *irregular broken line,* fatty acid destruction. Oxidative destruction is suppressed by the action of malonyl CoA, an intermediate in the synthesis of fatty acid. Malonyl CoA blocks the transport of fatty acids into the mitochondria at the translocation enzyme carnitine palmitoyltransferase I *(CPT I)*.

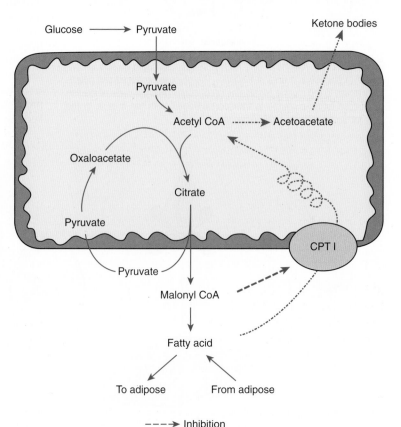

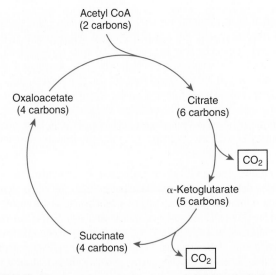

FIGURE 32-17 Oxidation of acetyl CoA (from acetate) by the Krebs cycle. The two carbons of acetyl CoA result in the formation of carbon dioxide; there is no net synthesis of oxaloacetate. Because oxaloacetate forms the precursor for glucose synthesis, acetyl CoA (and thus acetate) cannot lead to glucose formation.

two-carbon acetyl CoA units from the carbon chains of the fatty acids. The resulting acetyl CoA can enter the Krebs cycle through condensation with oxaloacetate. Because any of the Krebs cycle intermediates can lead to glucose production, it may first appear that acetyl CoA from fatty acid β-oxidation could lead to the production of glucose. However, this is not the case; there is no *net* production of oxaloacetate associated with the consumption of acetyl CoA by the Krebs cycle (Figure 32-17). Existing oxaloacetate combines with acetyl CoA to form citrate in the initial step of the cycle. At the end of the cycle, the original oxaloacetate is re-formed as the two carbons from the acetyl CoA are converted to carbon dioxide. No new oxaloacetate can be produced by this process.

Ketone Bodies Are Formed in the Mitochondria from Acetyl Coenzyme A

Not all mitochondrial acetyl CoA must enter the Krebs cycle. In fact, when fatty acids are rapidly entering the mitochondria, there is much more acetyl CoA available than necessary for Krebs cycle activity. It is this excess acetyl CoA, originating from fatty acids, from which the ketone bodies are synthesized (see Figure 32-16). Ketone bodies are able to leave the mitochondria freely.

Ketone bodies affect fuel homeostasis in peripheral tissues, where they may serve as a substitute for glucose. In this way, they conserve available glucose and reduce the need for gluconeogenesis.

Hepatic Very-Low-Density Lipoproteins May Be Synthesized from Adipose-Derived Fatty Acid as Well as from Newly Synthesized Fatty Acid

The section on absorptive-phase metabolism discusses the hepatic production of VLDL. During the absorptive phase, triglyceride for VLDL synthesis comes from fatty acids synthesized from glucose. During catabolic periods, VLDLs may continue to be produced, but fatty acids derived from serum NEFAs are used for VLDL synthesis (see Figure 32-5). This may initially appear to be an unnecessary and inefficient metabolic step. Why should fatty

acids from adipose tissue be transported to the liver for VLDL formation when they can be directly metabolized for energy by the tissues? The need for VLDL synthesis occurs because of the need for a better transport system. The capacity of the serum to transport NEFA is limited because NEFA must circulate bound to albumin. The NEFA-binding capacity of albumin is finite and may become almost saturated during periods of rapid adipose mobilization. VLDLs provide a transport system for fatty acids that is independent of serum albumin.

Hormonal Conditions Direct the Distribution of Very-Low-Density Lipoprotein Fatty Acids in the Body

During the absorptive phase, VLDLs are directed to adipose tissue by the action of adipose tissue LPL, an insulin-stimulated enzyme. LPL also exists in muscle tissue, but does not depend on insulin stimulation for activity. Thus, during periods of low glucose availability, adipose tissue LPL is inhibited because of a lack of insulin, but muscle tissue LPL is fully active. This situation leads to the selective direction of VLDL fatty acids to muscle tissue during times of adipose mobilization.

Changes in Growth Hormone Concentrations May Aid in Shifting Peripheral Fuel Utilization from Glucose and Amino Acids to Ketone Bodies and Fatty Acids

The fat mobilization–induced changes in hepatic metabolism are effective in conserving protein only because of changes that occur in glucose and amino acid utilization in peripheral tissues. As ketone bodies, NEFAs, and VLDL triglycerides become the major energy supplies, there is less tissue demand for glucose or amino acids as energy substrates. Endocrine alterations, in addition to low insulin concentrations, may aid in promoting this switch in peripheral fuel utilization. In several species, growth hormone concentrations rise during a prolonged period of energy deprivation. Growth hormone is antagonistic to insulin, thus promoting an increase in the serum glucose concentration even in the presence of normal or near-normal serum insulin levels. In addition, growth hormone may have some direct effect on conserving protein and mobilizing lipid.

SPECIAL FUEL CONSIDERATIONS OF RUMINANTS

Ruminants Exist in a Perpetual State of Gluconeogenesis Because of Their Unique Digestive Process

Most carbohydrate digestion in ruminants occurs in the forestomach through fermentative digestion. The result is that almost no digestible carbohydrate enters the intestine for glandular digestion and absorption as glucose. Therefore, ruminants exist in a constant state of potential glucose deficiency. To cope with this situation, ruminants have developed efficient systems of both production and conservation of glucose.

Essentially, all the glucose available to ruminants with typical diets originates from gluconeogenesis. Quantitatively, the most important glucose precursor is the volatile fatty acid (VFA) propionate. Propionate contributes to glucose synthesis after entering the Krebs cycle at the level of succinate (Figure 32-18). Note that succinate is a four-carbon Krebs cycle intermediate that can lead to net formation of oxaloacetate, the entry metabolite for gluconeogenesis. The other VFAs, acetate and butyrate, also enter the Krebs cycle, although they enter as acetyl CoA. As previously discussed, acetyl CoA cannot lead to the net production of oxaloacetate or glucose. Therefore, of the ruminant's major energy sources—acetate, propionate, and butyrate—only propionate can

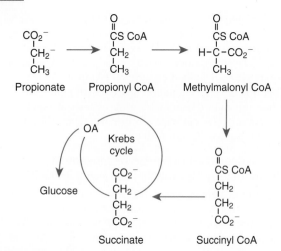

FIGURE 32-18 Gluconeogenesis from propionate involves its initial conversion to succinate. Succinate is a four-carbon krebs cycle intermediate that can lead to net glucose synthesis.

support glucose production. Almost all propionate absorbed from the rumen is extracted from the portal blood by the liver, never entering the systemic circulation.

In addition to constant gluconeogenesis, ruminants also support their glucose needs by efficiently conserving glucose. Fatty acids are synthesized in the liver of some animals (e.g., primates, rats, dogs) but only in the adipose tissue of ruminants. Furthermore, glucose is essentially not used for fatty acid synthesis. Rather, fatty acids are synthesized from acetate, which is the most abundant energy source in ruminants. The only glucose used by adipose tissue is for the synthesis of the glycerol backbone for triglycerides. In lactating animals, fatty acids produced in the udder for milk fat are synthesized from either acetate or ketone bodies, never from glucose.

Some important metabolic diseases of ruminants occur during periods when their system of glucose homeostasis is stressed. Dairy cows are especially vulnerable in early lactation because the synthesis of lactose (milk sugar) requires glucose. In high-producing cows, nearly all the glucose they produce goes to lactose synthesis, whereas the remaining tissues function on alternative fuels. Sheep experience a similar stress on glucose synthesis in late gestation. The energy needs of the fetus and placenta can be met only by glucose (or glucose-derived lactate) and amino acids. Compared with many other animals, sheep have a high ratio of fetal mass to body size; thus their fuel homeostatic mechanisms are particularly stressed by pregnancy. Failure of the glucose homeostatic mechanism frequently occurs under these circumstances, resulting in conditions known as *lactational ketosis* in dairy cows and *pregnancy toxemia* in ewes.

CLINICAL CORRELATIONS

HEPATIC LIPIDOSIS IN A CAT

History. You are asked to examine a 3-year-old intact female cat. She apparently was normal, even fat and happy, until 2 weeks ago, when she disappeared from her owner's apartment for 4 days. When she returned, the cat seemed depressed and would not eat. Over the next few days she became progressively more listless, almost somnolent.

Clinical Examination. The cat has a normal pulse, temperature, and respiratory rate, but she is depressed and responds little to handling. The ocular sclerae (whites of the eyes) appear icteric, or jaundiced. The latter physical sign leads you to suspect liver disease, so you submit blood samples for biochemical analysis. Analysis of blood taken from the jugular vein reveals a higher-than-normal concentration of bile acids and bilirubin, confirming a diagnosis of liver disease. A needle aspiration biopsy of the liver reveals hepatocytes that are distended with large droplets of nonstaining material, probably fat.

Comment. The presence of significant concentrations of bile acids in blood, other than in the hepatic-portal circulation, is evidence of reduced liver function. Recall that bile acids are absorbed from the ileum into the portal vein, in which they return to the liver. The normal liver extracts bile acids from portal blood efficiently, allowing only small amounts to escape into the systemic circulation; thus, elevated concentrations of bile acids in jugular blood indicate liver disease.

Hepatic lipidosis, or "fatty liver," is a common disease of cats, initiated by a period of stress combined with either an unwillingness to eat or a lack of available food. In either situation the cat begins to mobilize large quantities of fat to support metabolic energy needs. Normally, much of the mobilized NEFA would be expected to be taken up by the liver and converted to VLDL for export to energy-using tissues. In cats that experience fatty liver, the hepatic influx of NEFA appears to overwhelm the liver's capacity to synthesize and secrete VLDL, so fat accumulates in the liver. When the fat accumulation becomes severe, hepatic function is compromised, and the cat becomes systemically ill. Appetite becomes severely depressed, leading to a downward spiral of events in which the hepatic lipidosis becomes more and more severe.

Treatment. Treatment consists of reversing the state of negative energy balance by force-feeding. Various methods of force-feeding exist; the most practical approach is placement of an indwelling gastric tube. The tube is often passed through the nostrils but may be placed by a number of different techniques, including direct intubation through the wall of the abdomen. The latter technique is facilitated by the use of a fiberoptic gastroscope. When the cat is in positive energy balance, adipose mobilization ceases, and the liver eventually clears of fat. Tube feeding may need to continue for several days before the cat begins to eat on its own. Tube feeding has greatly improved the prognosis for hepatic lipidosis, although it is still a life-threatening condition.

HYPERLIPEMIA IN A HORSE

History. A client calls you concerned about his 25-year-old Morgan mare that is depressed, and has not been eating or drinking well for the past few days. It is the middle of the winter. The mare has poor teeth and she has been losing weight this winter, but the clients think the weight loss has been more dramatic in the last few weeks.

Clinical Examination. The mare's temperature, pulse, and respiratory rate are normal. She appears mentally dull, and she is dehydrated. The feces look somewhat dry. Her mucous membranes are yellow (icteric). She has decreased gastrointestinal borborygmi in all quadrants. On palpation per rectum, she has some dry feces, but no other abnormalities are detected. On nasogastric intubation, she does not have any reflux. Based on her age, inappetance, and weight loss, you are concerned that she might be hyperlipidemic/hyperlipemic. You submit blood work for complete blood count (CBC) and biochemical profile including triglycerides. You give her some water via the nasogastric tube, and you float her remaining teeth. You recommend that they feed her an equine senior diet (which is a highly digestible feed).

Laboratory Results. Her clinical chemistry demonstrates increased glucose (170 mg/dL), triglycerides (TG) (550 mg/dL), and bilirubin (2.5 mg/dL) concentrations. A CBC reveals an increased white blood cell count (leukocytosis) characterized by increased neutrophils (neutrophilia), monocytosis (increased monocytes), and decreased lymphocytes (lymphopenia).

Comment. Negative energy balance due to decreased intake with current or increased calorie demands, results in increased lipolysis of the adipose tissue. This results in the mobilization of adipose fat in the form of nonesterified fatty acids (NEFA). Circulating NEFA may be used for energy by a wide variety of tissues, but a large proportion is extracted from serum by the liver. In the liver, NEFA can potentially be utilized for complete oxidization, ketone body synthesis, or reesterification to triglycerides. In horses, a large portion of NEFA arriving at the liver are reesterified. The resulting TG are either stored in the liver or released to the circulation as components of very-low-density lipoproteins (VLDL). Removal of VLDL from the blood is regulated by lipoprotein lipase, an enzyme that, especially in adipose tissue, is insulin dependent. When the rate of hepatic VLDL secretion exceeds their removal, TG accumulates in the blood serum. Various terms including *hyperlipidemia, hypertriglyceridemia,* and *hyperlipemia* are used to describe this condition. The use of the specific terms is usually dependent on the severity of the serum lipid accumulation.

Treatment. If there is a primary cause of the inappetance (i.e., colic, neoplasia), which can create a catabolic state, it needs to be identified and treated first. For this horse, it was likely the poor teeth, which decreased the ability of the horse to chew hay, and thus the horse was not eating sufficient calories to equal its metabolic needs. Additionally, during the winter, many horses will drink less; the horse may have more easily become dehydrated. This could lead to an impaction colic, which would be an additional reason why the horse was not eating sufficient calories. Basal metabolism may also be increased as it is winter. Thus, all of these factors (i.e., teeth, decreased drinking, colic) are likely causes of the decreased intake and increased caloric needs. It is also possible that the mare has neoplasia. Regardless of the primary cause, because of the decreased intake, it led to the catabolic state, thus precipitating the hyperlipidemia/hyperlipemia. Treatment is aimed at treating both the primary cause as well as the hyperlipidemia/hyperlipemia. The horse can be given good quality grass when available and the senior diet. Based on her blood work, there are no overt signs of neoplasia. She could be treated based on the possible issues of teeth, decreased intake, and increased metabolic demands for thermoregulation as the primary causes, and her progress should be monitored. For the hyperlipidemia/hyperlipemia, she can be given insulin and maybe glucose. Insulin increases gluconeogenesis, both by inhibiting hormone-sensitive lipase, which causes lipolysis of adipose tissue, and increasing lipoprotein lipase. Thus adipose storage in the liver will be decreased. Depending on the severity of disease and initial causes, this treatment may be sufficient. Many horses require in-clinic care with intravenous fluids, as well as heparin, to promote insulin sensitivity through

increased activity of lipoprotein lipase, while decreasing activity of hormone-sensitive lipase. Overall, these horses need careful monitoring, whether on the farm or in the clinic, as it can take some period of time to correct hyperlipidemia/hyperlipemia, including addressing the caloric/nutritional needs and addressing the primary cause.

PRACTICE QUESTIONS

1. All the following are metabolites that can be oxidized for fuel in the animal body. Which one is *not* important in the transport of energy between organs and organ systems?
   a. Triglyceride
   b. Ketone bodies
   c. Oxaloacetic acid
   d. Nonesterified fatty acids
   e. Amino acids

2. Which of the following reactions is not characteristic of the absorptive phase of digestion?
   a. Hepatic synthesis of glycogen
   b. Hepatic uptake of glucose
   c. Destruction of dietary amino acid
   d. Utilization of muscle-derived amino acid for gluconeogenesis
   e. Hepatic synthesis of triglyceride from glucose

3. Which of the following reactions in the liver could be expected to occur during both the digestive phase and a prolonged fast?
   a. Glycogen synthesis
   b. Fatty acid synthesis
   c. Ketone body synthesis
   d. Ketone body oxidation
   e. Triglyceride synthesis from fatty acids

4. Which of the following statements is true of both ketone bodies and nonesterified fatty acids?
   a. They are water soluble.
   b. They provide energy for muscle metabolism.
   c. They circulate in blood bound to albumin.
   d. They can provide energy to the brain.
   e. They are formed exclusively in the liver.

5. Which of the following amino acids is not extensively catabolized by the liver?
   a. Valine
   b. Alanine
   c. Glutamine
   d. Asparagine
   e. Glycine

BIBLIOGRAPHY

Aschenbach JR, Kristensen NB, Donkin SS, et al: Gluconeogenesis in dairy cows: the secret of making sweet milk from sour dough, *IUBMB Life* 62(12):869–877, 2010.

Barton MH: Disorders of the liver. In Reed SM, Bayly WM, Sellon DC, editors: *Equine internal medicine,* ed 2, St Louis, 2004, Saunders.

Bauman DE, Currie WB: Partitioning of nutrients during pregnancy and lactation: a review of mechanisms involving homeostasis and homeorrhesis, *J Dairy Sci* 63(9):1514–1529, 1980.

Bender DA: *Introduction to nutrition and metabolism*, ed 2, Bristol, Pa, 1997, Taylor & Francis.

Brody T: *Nutritional biochemistry*, ed 2, San Diego, 1999, Academic Press.

Cheeke PR, Dierenfeld ES: *Comparative animal nutrition and metabolism*, Cambridge, Mass, 2010, CABI.

Gillham B, Papachristodoulou DK, Thomas JH: *Will's biochemical basis of medicine*, ed 3, Boston, 1996, Butterworth-Heinemann.

Hand MS, Thatcher CD, Remillard RL, Roudebush P: *Small animal clinical nutrition*, Topeka, Kan, 2010, Mark Morris Institute.

Herdt TH: Fuel homeostasis in the ruminant, *Vet Clin North Am Food Anim Pract* 4(2):213–231, 1988.

Kaneko JJ, Harvey JW, Bruss ML: *Clinical biochemistry of domestic animals*, ed 5, San Diego, 1997, Academic Press.

McCue MD: Starvation physiology: reviewing the different strategies animals use to survive a common challenge, *Comp Biochem Physiol A Mol Integr Physiol* 156(1):1–18, 2010.

McKenzie HC III: Equine hyperlipidemias, *Vet Clin North Am Equine Pract* 27(1):59–72, 2011.

Nordlie RC, Foster JD, Lange AJ: Regulation of glucose production by the liver, *Annu Rev Nutr* 19:379–406, 1999.

Pearson EG: Diseases of the hepatobiliary system. In Smith BP, editor: *Large animal internal medicine*, ed 4, St Louis, 2009, Mosby.

Storey KB, editor: *Functional metabolism: regulation and adaptation*, Ottawa, 2004, John Wiley & Sons.

VanItallie TB, Nufert TH: Ketones: metabolism's ugly duckling, *Nutr Rev* 61(10):327–341, 2003.

Wang T, Hung CC, Randall DJ: The comparative physiology of food deprivation: from feast to famine, *Annu Rev Physiol* 68:223–251, 2006.

CHAPTER 33
The Endocrine System

KEY POINTS

General concepts

1. Hormones are chemicals produced by specific tissues that are transported by the vascular system to affect other tissues at low concentrations.
2. The endocrine and nervous systems are integrated in their control of physiological processes.

Synthesis of hormones

1. Protein hormones are initially synthesized as preprohormones and then cleaved in the rough endoplasmic reticulum to form prohormones and in the Golgi apparatus to form the active hormones, which are stored in granules before being released by exocytosis.
2. Steroids are synthesized from cholesterol, which is synthesized by the liver; steroids are not stored but are released as they are synthesized.

Transport of hormones in the blood

1. Protein hormones are hydrophilic and carried in the plasma in dissolved form.
2. Steroids and thyroid hormones are lipophilic and carried in plasma in association with both specific and nonspecific binding proteins; the amount of unbound, active hormone is relatively small.

Hormone-cell interaction

1. Protein hormones have specific receptors on target tissue plasma membranes, whereas steroids have specific receptors within the cytoplasm or nucleus.

Postreceptor cell responses

1. Steroids interact directly with the cell nucleus through the formation of a complex with its cytosolic receptor, whereas protein hormones need a messenger because they cannot enter the cell.

Metabolism of hormones

1. Steroid hormones are metabolized by conjugation with sulfates and glucuronides, which makes steroids water soluble.

Feedback control mechanisms

1. The most important feedback control for hormones is the negative-feedback system, in which increased hormone concentrations result in less production of the hormone, usually through an interaction with the hypothalamus or pituitary gland.
2. Endocrine secretory patterns can be influenced by factors such as sleep or light and can produce circadian rhythms.

The hypothalamus

1. The hypothalamus coordinates the activity of the pituitary gland through the secretion of peptides and amines.

The pituitary gland

1. The neurohypophysis has cell bodies that originate in the hypothalamus, with cell endings that secrete oxytocin and vasopressin.
2. Oxytocin and vasopressin are synthesized in cell bodies within the hypothalamus and are carried by axon flow to the posterior lobe, where they are released.
3. The main effects of oxytocin are on the contraction of smooth muscle (mammary gland and uterus); the effects of vasopressin are primarily on the conservation of water (antidiuresis) and secondarily on blood pressure.
4. Plasma osmolality controls the secretion of vasopressin.
5. The anterior pituitary produces growth hormone, prolactin, thyroid-stimulating hormone, follicle-stimulating hormone, luteinizing hormone, and corticotropin.
6. Adenohypophyseal activity is controlled by hypothalamic releasing hormones, which are released into the portal system, which in turn connects the median eminence of the hypothalamus and the anterior pituitary gland.

GENERAL CONCEPTS

Hormones Are Chemicals Produced by Specific Tissues That Are Transported by the Vascular System to Affect Other Tissues at Low Concentrations

The endocrine system has evolved to allow physiological processes to be coordinated and regulated. The system uses chemical messengers called *hormones.* Hormones have traditionally been defined as "chemicals that are produced by specific endocrine organs, are transported by the vascular system, and are able to affect distant target organs in low concentration." Although this definition is useful from a veterinary medical point of view, it should be recognized that some substances, such as prostaglandins and somatomedins, are produced by many other tissues and are still considered hormones.

Other types of control systems use chemical substances that are not transported in the vascular system to influence distant cell activity. These systems serve as means of local integration among or between cells, as follows:

- *Paracrine effectors,* in which the messenger diffuses through the interstitial fluids, usually to influence adjacent cells; if the messenger acts on the cell of its origin, the substance is called an *autocrine effector* (Figure 33-1).

- *Neurotransmitters,* which affect communication between neurons, or between neurons and target cells; the substances are limited in the distance traveled and the area of the cell influenced (Figure 33-2).
- *Exocrine effectors,* such as hormones produced by the pancreas, are released into the gastrointestinal tract.

The Endocrine and Nervous Systems Are Integrated in Their Control of Physiological Processes

The endocrine system interacts with the other main regulatory system, the *nervous system,* which coordinates activities that require rapid control. An example of the close interaction of the two systems is the reflex in which suckling causes the release of milk. Suckling initiates the transmission of nerve impulses from the mammary gland to the hypothalamus (by way of the spinal tract). Neurosecretory neurons within the supraoptic and paraventricular nuclei are stimulated to synthesize *oxytocin.* Oxytocin is transported along axons of these nerves and is released from nerve endings in the posterior pituitary into the blood vascular system. Oxytocin is then carried to the mammary gland, where it causes contraction of myoepithelial cells. These cells surround the smallest unit of milk-secreting cells, called an *alveolus.* This results in the movement of milk into the large cisternae adjacent to the teat and subsequently into the teat.

The interaction between the nervous and endocrine systems can be even more direct. For example, endocrine cells of the adrenal medulla are directly controlled by preganglionic neurons of the adrenal medulla, and the medullary hormones are released immediately in response to stressful stimuli. The endocrine and nervous systems also share transmitters; substances such as epinephrine, dopamine, histamine, and somatostatin are found in both endocrine and neural tissues.

The endocrine system is involved in control of physiological functions, including metabolism, growth, and reproduction. *Metabolism* can be divided into two forms: energy and mineral. The hormones that control *energy metabolism* include insulin, glucagon, cortisol, epinephrine, thyroid hormone, and growth hormone. The hormones that control *mineral metabolism* include parathyroid hormone, calcitonin, angiotensin, and renin. The hormones that control *growth* include growth hormone, thyroid hormone, insulin, estrogen and androgen (both reproductive hormones), and a large number of growth factors. The hormones that control *reproduction* include estrogen, androgen, progesterone, luteinizing hormone (LH), follicle-stimulating hormone (FSH), prolactin (PRL), and oxytocin.

One of the important characteristics of the endocrine system is the *amplification* of the signal. The action of one steroid molecule to activate a gene can result in the formation of many messenger ribonucleic acid (mRNA) molecules, and each of these can induce the formation of many enzyme molecules. Also, one protein molecule can influence the formation of many cyclic adenosine 3′,5′-monophosphate (cAMP) molecules, and each of these can activate many enzymes. Amplification is the basis for the sensitivity of the endocrine system, which allows small amounts of hormones in plasma (10^{-11} to 10^{-12} mol) to produce significant biological effects. Hormone action also influences rates of existing enzyme reactions, but not the initiation of new reactions. This implies that there are certain basal levels of enzyme activities even in the absence of hormones. Hormone action is relatively slow and prolonged, with the effects of hormones lasting minutes to days. This contrasts with the nervous system, in which the response is rapid and short (milliseconds to seconds).

SYNTHESIS OF HORMONES

Protein Hormones Are Initially Synthesized as Preprohormones and Then Cleaved in the Rough Endoplasmic Reticulum to Form Prohormones and in the Golgi Apparatus to Form the Active Hormones, Which Are Stored in Granules Before Being Released by Exocytosis

The major classes of hormones include proteins (e.g., growth hormone, insulin, corticotropin [previously called adrenocorticotropic hormone, or ACTH]); peptides (e.g., oxytocin and vasopressin); amines (e.g., dopamine, melatonin, epinephrine); and steroids (e.g., cortisol, progesterone, vitamin D). The protein and peptide hormones are initially synthesized on ribosomes as larger precursor proteins, which are referred to as *preprohormones* (Figure 33-3). Synthesis of protein hormones begins in ribosomes, with the "pre" portion immediately attaching to the rough endoplasmic reticulum (RER), which pulls the ribosomes into close apposition with the RER. During synthesis, the preprohormone is secreted into the interior of the RER. The presence of a peptidase within the wall of the RER allows the "pre" portion of the molecule to be rapidly removed and the prohormone to leave the RER in vesicles that have been pinched off from the RER. These vesicles then move to the Golgi apparatus, where they coalesce with Golgi membranes to form secretory granules. The prohormone is cleaved during this process, so most of the hormone is in its final form within the Golgi apparatus, although some prohormone can also be found.

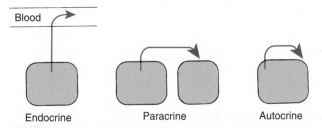

FIGURE 33-1 Types of cell communication via chemical mediators. (From Hedge GA, Colby HD, Goodman RL: *Clinical endocrine physiology,* Philadelphia, 1987, Saunders.)

FIGURE 33-2 Comparison of functional arrangements of an ordinary neuron releasing its neurotransmitter *(NT)* into a synapse and a neurosecretory neuron releasing its neurohormone *(NH)* into a blood vessel. (From Hedge GA, Colby HD, Goodman RL: *Clinical endocrine physiology,* Philadelphia, 1987, Saunders.)

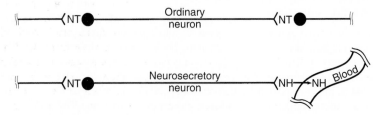

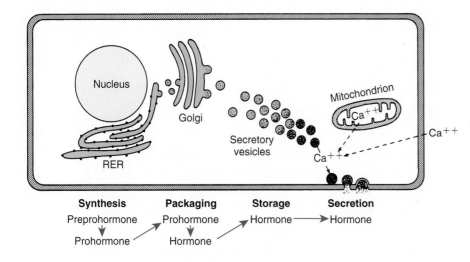

FIGURE 33-3 Subcellular components of peptide hormone synthesis and secretion. *RER*, Rough endoplasmic reticulum. (From Hedge GA, Colby HD, Goodman RL: *Clinical endocrine physiology*, Philadelphia, 1987, Saunders.)

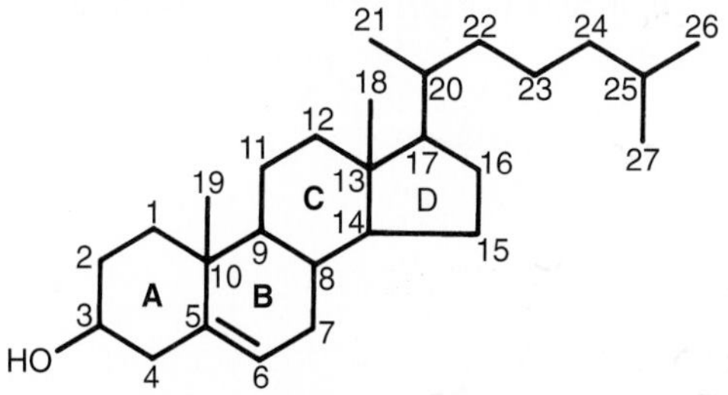

FIGURE 33-4 The ring structure and numbering system of the carbon atoms in steroid hormones, illustrated for the cholesterol molecule. (From Hedge GA, Colby HD, Goodman RL: *Clinical endocrine physiology*, Philadelphia, 1987, Saunders.)

Protein hormones are stored in granules within the gland until needed for release. Although some of the hormone is secreted on a continuous basis, most is secreted through the process of *exocytosis* of granules in response to a specific signal. The process of exocytosis requires adenosine triphosphate (ATP) and calcium (Ca^{2+}). Increased cytoplasmic calcium results from intracellular release of Ca^{2+} from mitochondria, or endoplasmic reticulum, or from the influx of extracellular Ca^{2+}.

Steroids Are Synthesized from Cholesterol, Which Is Synthesized by the Liver; Steroids Are Not Stored but Are Released as They Are Synthesized

Steroids represent a class of hormones that, unlike protein hormones, are lipophilic. In general, they belong to one of two categories: *adrenocortical hormones* (glucocorticoids, mineralocorticoids) and *sex hormones* (estrogens, progesterone, androgens). They have a common four-ring, 17-carbon skeleton that is derived from *cholesterol* (Figure 33-4). Although the steroids can be synthesized *de novo* within the cell from the two-carbon molecule acetate, the majority of steroids are formed from cholesterol, which is synthesized by the liver (Figure 33-5). Low-density lipoproteins (LDLs) enter steroid-producing cells through interaction with a membrane receptor. Cholesterol is released through the degradation of LDLs by lysosomal enzymes. Cholesterol is either used immediately for steroid synthesis or stored in granules in an ester form within the cell. The first step in the synthesis of all steroid hormones from cholesterol involves cleavage of the side chain of cholesterol to form *pregnenolone;* this step occurs within the mitochondrion. Subsequent modifications of the steroid molecule may occur within the mitochondrion or may involve movement to other compartments of the cell (Figure 33-6). The control of movement of steroids among cell compartments during the synthesis process is not well understood.

The type of steroid hormone that is eventually synthesized depends on the presence of specific enzymes within the particular cell. For example, only cells of the adrenal cortex contain enzymes (hydroxylases) that result in hydroxylation of the eleventh and twenty-first carbon molecules, a process that is essential for the production of glucocorticoids and mineralocorticoids. The pattern for sex steroid biosynthesis is for pregnenolone to be modified in a sequence that involves progesterone, androgens, and finally estrogens. Cells that synthesize androgens (e.g., Leydig cells of the testis) have the enzymes required for the formation of pregnenolone and progesterone, as well as for the modification of progesterone to androgen, but lack the enzymes necessary to modify androgens into estrogens. Although the sex steroid–forming cells do not have enzymes that allow the formation of adrenocortical hormones, the adrenal cortex contains the enzyme systems necessary for the formation of both adrenocortical hormones and sex hormones, although the former are emphasized. As a result, the adrenal cortex normally produces small amounts of sex steroids and produces larger amounts in certain pathophysiological conditions.

There is no provision for the storage of steroid hormones within the cell; they are secreted immediately after formation by simple diffusion across the cell membrane because of their lipophilic structure. Thus, synthesis and secretion of steroid hormones occur in a tightly coupled manner, whereby the rate of hormone secretion is controlled by the rate of synthesis. The only storage form of steroids within these cells involves that of the precursor molecule, cholesterol, as an ester.

TRANSPORT OF HORMONES IN THE BLOOD

Protein Hormones Are Hydrophilic and Carried in the Plasma in Dissolved Form

This chapter focuses mainly on hormones that are transported to target tissues in the vascular system. The means by which hormones are transported in the blood varies according to the

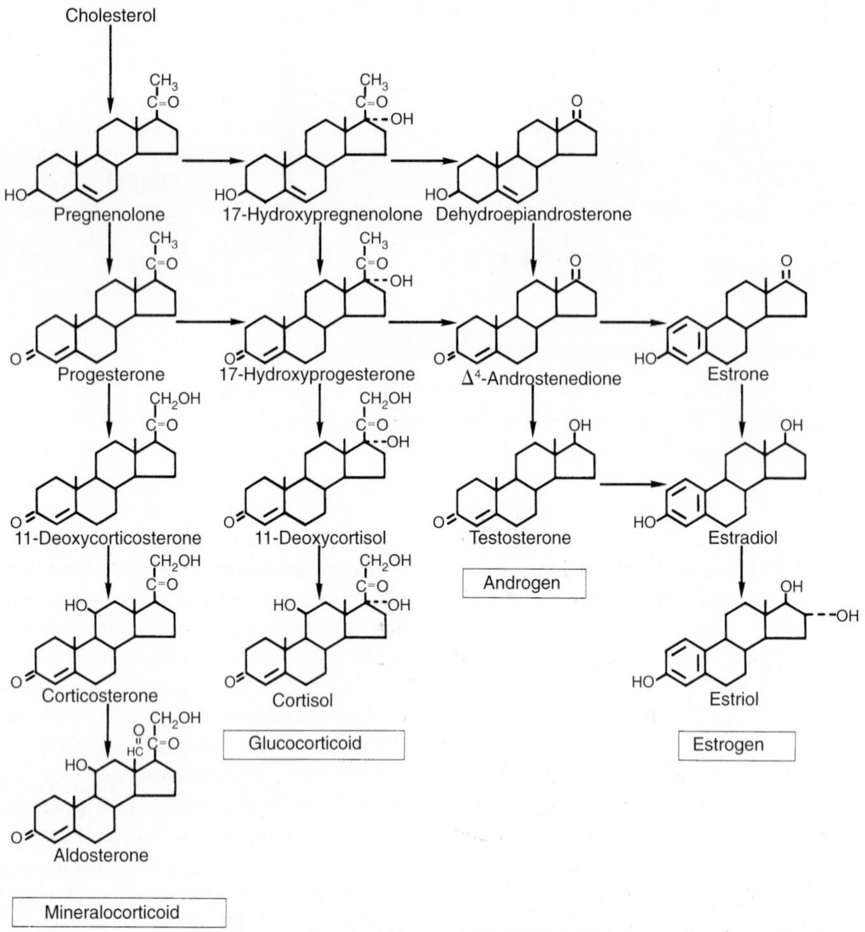

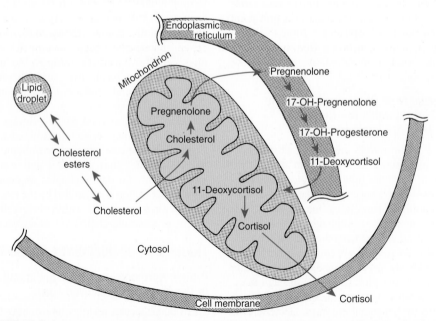

FIGURE 33-5 Pathways involved in the production of the major steroid hormones. (From Hedge GA, Colby HD, Goodman RL: *Clinical endocrine physiology,* Philadelphia, 1987, Saunders.)

FIGURE 33-6 Subcellular compartmentalization of cortisol biosynthesis. (From Hedge GA, Colby HD, Goodman RL: *Clinical endocrine physiology*, Philadelphia, 1987, Saunders.)

solubility of the hormone. Protein and peptide hormones are hydrophilic and are carried in the plasma in dissolved form. The protein hormones may circulate in *monomeric* (single-unit) or *polymeric* (multiple-unit) form (e.g., insulin). Hormones that have subunits can appear in the circulation in subunit form, although this reduces the biological potency of the molecule.

Steroids and Thyroid Hormones Are Lipophilic and Carried in Plasma in Association with Both Specific and Nonspecific Binding Proteins; the Amount of Unbound, Active Hormone Is Relatively Small

The transport of steroid and thyroid hormones is more complicated than that of protein hormones, because the steroid and thyroid hormones are lipophilic and thus have limited solubility in aqueous solutions. These hormones are transported in the blood through association with various types of proteins. Some of the proteins that bind steroids have a high affinity for a particular steroid; for example, a globulin, *transcortin,* has a high affinity for cortisol and corticosterone but also serves as an important transport vehicle for progesterone, even though it has a lower affinity for this hormone. The carrier proteins that have high affinities have low capacity because of their low plasma concentration. In contrast, the general class of plasma proteins called *albumins* have low affinities for steroid hormones but have a high capacity for steroid transport because of their high concentration in plasma.

A hormone must be in the *free,* or unbound, form before it can penetrate a target cell and elicit biological activity. This is accomplished by the establishment of equilibrium between bound and free hormone levels in the plasma. The free form usually represents only about 1% of the total amount of hormone in the plasma (up to 10% of cortisol may be in the free form). The system is responsive to use of the free form, and the free form is replenished quickly by dissociation of bound hormone from the protein. The *total* amount of the hormone is usually measured, with the exception of thyroid hormone, for which attempts are usually made to estimate the amounts of bound and free. As indicated for steroid hormones, synthesis and release are tightly linked, and because metabolic clearance rates are usually constant, concentrations of steroids in plasma are usually a good reflection of the secretion rate. Under certain physiological conditions, such as pregnancy in humans, metabolism of estrogens can change because of the increased production of estrogen-binding proteins.

HORMONE-CELL INTERACTION

Protein Hormones Have Specific Receptors on Target Tissue Plasma Membranes, Whereas Steroids Have Specific Receptors Within the Cytoplasm or Nucleus

A central question in endocrinology is how hormones and target cells of a particular tissue interact in a specific manner. The problem seems almost overwhelming for steroids because they are lipid soluble and able to permeate all cells of the body. The solution is that target cells have receptors that are *specific* for a particular hormone. For steroids, the receptors are located in the cytoplasm or nucleus of the target cells, whereas receptors for protein and peptide hormones are located on the plasma membrane of the cell. In addition to specificity, receptors have a high *affinity* for their respective hormone. These characteristics of the receptor allow hormones to be in low concentration in the blood but effective in producing significant tissue response.

The greater the affinity of the receptor for the hormone, the longer is the biological response. Termination of the action of a hormone usually requires *dissociation* of the hormone from the receptor. This occurs most often as a result of a decrease in plasma concentrations of the hormone; the binding of receptor and hormone is noncovalent, and declining hormone concentrations favor a chemical equilibrium of dissociation over association. Termination of hormone action can also result from *internalization* of the receptor-hormone complex through the process of endocytosis. The hormone is degraded by lysosomal enzymes, whereas the receptor, protected because of its association with the vesicle membrane, can be recycled to the plasma membrane.

Receptors are present on cells in much greater numbers than required for the elicitation of a biological response. Occupancy by a hormone of considerably less than 50% of the receptors usually elicits a maximal biological response. Even so, changes in receptor numbers that affect the sensitivity of the cell, although not its maximal responsiveness, can occur. Changes in receptor number affect the probability that an interaction will occur between receptor and hormone. Receptor synthesis can be stimulated by a hormone that is different from the hormone that interacts with the receptor. For example, predominant gonadotropin receptors on ovarian granulosa cells change from FSH to LH receptors late in the ovarian follicle phase because of the influence of FSH. This allows the control of the ovarian follicle to pass from FSH to LH, which facilitates ovulation and the formation of a corpus luteum. Conversely, receptor numbers can decrease in conjunction with continued interaction of receptor and hormone. This often occurs when an agonist that has great affinity for the receptor is administered or when amounts of hormone are pathologically elevated. The receptor numbers are downregulated in this situation. The end result is that the animal becomes resistant to continued therapy with the hormone in question.

POSTRECEPTOR CELL RESPONSES

Steroids Interact Directly with the Cell Nucleus Through the Formation of a Complex with Its Cytosolic Receptor, Whereas Protein Hormones Need a Messenger Because They Cannot Enter the Cell

The events that follow binding of the hormone and receptor depend on whether a steroid, protein, or peptide hormone is involved. With steroids, the hormone is able to interact within the cell because of its ability to penetrate the lipoprotein plasma membrane (Figure 33-7). The interaction of receptor and steroid hormone results in activation of the subsequent complex translocation to the nucleus, where it interacts with specific sites on the chromatin. The result is the production of mRNA, which, when translocated to the ribosomes, directs synthesis of proteins that produce the desired biological result.

Protein or peptide hormones require an intermediary to act in their behalf because they are not able to penetrate the plasma membrane of the cell; the intermediary substance is known as a *second messenger* (Figure 33-8). The best-documented second messenger is cAMP, which is produced by the activation of an enzyme, adenyl cyclase, through interaction of the hormone and receptor in the plasma membrane. The activation of adenyl cyclase and the production of cAMP result in the phosphorylation of protein kinases, which are responsible for the biological response. Other second messengers include cytosolic calcium and its associated phosphodiesterase, calmodulin, as well as inositol triphosphate (IP_3) and diacylglycerol, both of which are products

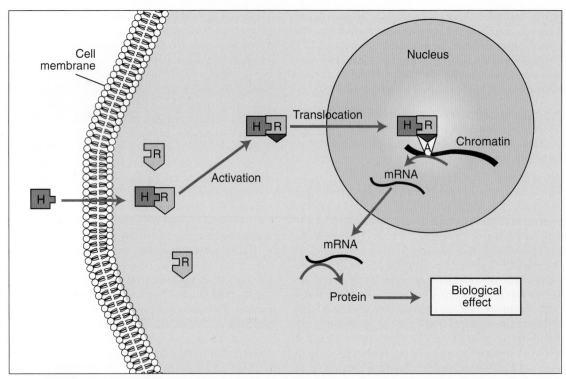

FIGURE 33-7 Subcellular mechanism of action of a lipophilic hormone *(H)* via an intracellular receptor *(R)*. The H-R complex induces messenger ribonucleic acid *(mRNA)* synthesis by binding to an acceptor site *(A)* on the chromatin. (From Hedge GA, Colby HD, Goodman RL: *Clinical endocrine physiology,* Philadelphia, 1987, Saunders.)

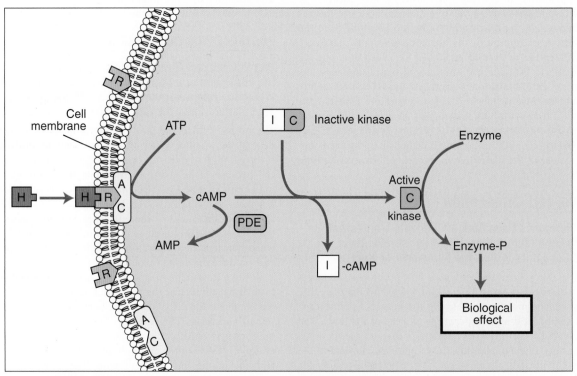

FIGURE 33-8 Subcellular mechanism of action of a hydrophilic hormone *(H)* via a membrane receptor *(R)*, adenyl cyclase *(AC)*, and cyclic adenosine monophosphate *(cAMP)*. *ATP,* Adenosine triphosphate; *I* and *C,* inhibitory and catalytic subunits of the kinase, respectively; *PDE,* phosphodiesterase. (From Hedge GA, Colby HD, Goodman RL: *Clinical endocrine physiology,* Philadelphia, 1987, Saunders.)

of phosphatidylinositol metabolism. An important action of IP_3 is the stimulation of intracellular calcium release. One important response to diacylglycerol is the activation of phospholipase A and the formation of arachidonic acid, which leads to formation of members of the prostaglandin family of molecules. The biological response to a protein or peptide hormone–receptor interaction is more rapid than that to steroids; preexisting enzymes are activated, whereas the biological response to steroid requires the synthesis of enzyme protein.

METABOLISM OF HORMONES

Steroid Hormones Are Metabolized by Conjugation with Sulfates and Glucuronides, Which Makes Steroids Water Soluble

Hormone activity is limited by the metabolism of hormones. The metabolism of steroids usually involves reduction of the molecule, followed by conjugation with sulfates and glucuronides, which increases the water solubility of the steroids, allowing them to be excreted in urine. The liver is the main organ responsible for this process. Iodine molecules are removed from thyroid hormones during metabolism. Protein hormones are cleaved by peptidases; this is preceded by reduction of disulfide bonds if this is a characteristic of the molecule. Although a metabolite is usually less biologically potent than the original molecule, some evidence suggests that conjugates of steroids can have significant biological activity. This raises the question of whether the conversion of hormones intracellularly, such as testosterone to dihydrotestosterone, represents metabolism, because dihydrotestosterone is more potent biologically than testosterone. Another example, the conversion of estradiol-17β to estrone by peripheral tissues, including adipose cells, is described as a form of metabolism; however, estrone is a natural, and relatively potent, estrogen.

Although in some situations the *rate of clearance* of a hormone can change (e.g., decrease as a result of increased hormone-binding plasma proteins during pregnancy, or increase as the result of decreased hormone-binding plasma proteins in conjunction with liver disease), *metabolism* of hormones is relatively constant, and the concentration of a hormone usually reflects the other determinant of hormone activity: the *rate of synthesis* of the hormone.

FEEDBACK CONTROL MECHANISMS

The Most Important Feedback Control for Hormones Is the Negative-Feedback System, in Which Increased Hormone Concentrations Result in Less Production of the Hormone, Usually Through an Interaction with the Hypothalamus or Pituitary Gland

The effects of hormones are proportional to their concentrations in blood, and therefore control of these concentrations is an important aspect in ensuring that physiological function is normal. As indicated previously, the primary factor affecting hormone concentrations in blood is the secretion rate by a particular organ. Feedback-loop control systems have evolved in which concentrations of hormones are monitored at the controlling point either to increase or to decrease secretion of a hormone by an endocrine organ. The most common feedback system is *negative feedback,* in which continuous monitoring allows the system to counteract changes in hormone secretion or to maintain a relatively constant environment.

An example of systems in which negative-feedback control involves both the endocrine and the nervous system is shown in Figure 33-9. The hypothalamus, which controls secretion of tropic hormones in the anterior pituitary through the secretion of peptide-releasing hormones, has cells with a certain set point by which they compare concentrations of hormone in the blood with the output of releasing hormones. If blood concentrations fall below the physiological set point, releasing-hormone output increases; this in turn increases production of tropic hormones by the anterior pituitary and subsequently the secretion of the hormone by the target organ. Conversely, if the hormone concentration increases above acceptable physiological limits, a shutdown of releasing-hormone production occurs within the hypothalamus, tropic hormone secretion by the anterior pituitary decreases, and production of the hormone by the target organ decreases. This type of control system is not an "all-or-none" arrangement because changes and adjustments are being continuously made to maintain an optimal concentration of hormone.

In the negative-feedback system an increase in secretion of hormone results in a decrease in tropic hormone secretion. It is also possible to have a negative-feedback system in which an increase in a physiological substance, such as glucose, causes an increase in a hormone, in this case insulin, which plays an

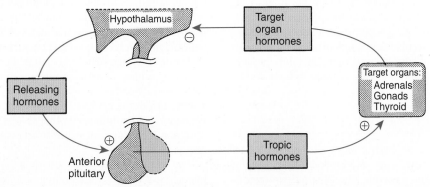

FIGURE 33-9 Negative feedback of tropic and releasing hormones by target organ hormones. The *plus signs* indicate stimulation, and the *minus sign* indicates inhibition. In some cases, such inhibition occurs at the pituitary gland. (From Hedge GA, Colby HD, Goodman RL: *Clinical endocrine physiology,* Philadelphia, 1987, Saunders.)

important role in glucose metabolism. This is considered to be a negative-feedback system because blood glucose concentrations are being "dampened," or returned toward normal levels, through the action of insulin.

Positive-feedback systems also exist, although they are much less common than negative-feedback systems. One example is the preovulatory release of LH, in which the pulsatile rate of LH secretion greatly increases during the late stages of ovarian follicular development because of increased estrogen production by the follicle. In this situation, there is a definitive end point: ovulation results in a decline in the stimulus, estrogen, although the duration of the LH surge is probably determined within the hypothalamus, and therefore the LH response to estrogen is modulated.

Endocrine Secretory Patterns Can Be Influenced by Factors Such as Sleep or Light and Can Produce Circadian Rhythms

Endocrine secretion patterns can occur outside the control of negative-feedback inhibition. Hormone patterns can change on an approximately 24-hour basis, a process referred to as a *diurnal rhythm,* or *circadian rhythm. Circadian* is the preferred term because *diurnal* refers to activity in the daytime; *nocturnal* should be used for the rhythms that are active at night. Most of the daily rhythms have some aspects of light, or lack of light, as a major influence in the rhythm. Rhythmic changes in hormone patterns that occur at shorter intervals, often in the range of an hour, are called *ultradian rhythms.*

THE HYPOTHALAMUS

The Hypothalamus Coordinates the Activity of the Pituitary Gland Through the Secretion of Peptides and Amines

As indicated previously, the two major controlling systems are the nervous and the endocrine systems. The interface between these systems occurs, for the most part, in the hypothalamus. The hypothalamus is an area of the diencephalon that forms the floor of the third ventricle and includes the optic chiasma, tuber cinereum, mammillary bodies, and the median eminence. Often not included in this classification are the infundibulum and the neurohypophysis (stalk of the posterior lobe and the posterior lobe, respectively), although both tissues represent extensions of the hypothalamus into the pituitary gland.

The hypothalamus produces peptides and amines that influence the pituitary gland to produce (1) tropic hormones (e.g., corticotropin), which in turn influence the production of hormones (e.g., cortisol) by peripheral target endocrine tissues, or (2) hormones that directly cause a biological effect in tissues (e.g., PRL). The hypothalamus is also the center for the control of a large number of autonomic nervous system control pathways.

THE PITUITARY GLAND

The pituitary gland, or hypophysis cerebri, is composed of the *adenohypophysis* (pars distalis, or anterior lobe), the *neurohypophysis* (pars nervosa, or posterior lobe), the *pars intermedia* (intermediate lobe), and the *pars tuberalis* (Figure 33-10). The adenohypophysis is formed from an area of the roof of the embryonic oral ectoderm called *Rathke's pouch,* which extends upward to meet the neurohypophysis, which extends downward as an

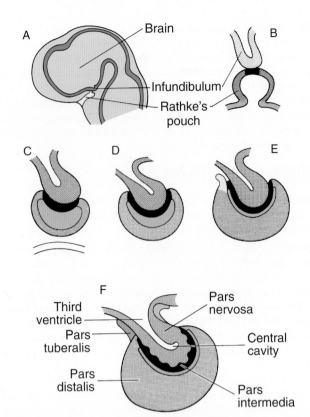

FIGURE 33-10 Diagrams showing progressive stages in the embryonic development of the pituitary gland. Rathke's pouch becomes detached from the oral epithelium at stage C. (From Villee CA, Walker WF Jr, Smith FE: *General zoology,* ed 2, Philadelphia, 1963, Saunders; Turner CD, Bagnara JT: *General endocrinology,* ed 6, Philadelphia, 1976, Saunders.)

outpouching of neural ectoderm from the floor of the third ventricle.

The Neurohypophysis Has Cell Bodies That Originate in the Hypothalamus, with Cell Endings That Secrete Oxytocin and Vasopressin

The neurohypophysis is composed of axons whose neural origin is largely within the supraoptic and paraventricular nuclei of the hypothalamus. The neurohypophysis is an extension of the hypothalamus into the pituitary; that is, the cell bodies are in the hypothalamus. The axons form the stalk of the posterior lobe, and the nerve endings are in the lobe proper (Figure 33-11).

The endocrine-secretory neurons that constitute the neurohypophysis differ from neurons involved in the transmission of neural signals in several ways: (1) neurosecretory neurons do not innervate other neurons, even though they are innervated; (2) the secretory product of neurosecretory neurons is secreted into the blood; and (3) the secretory product can act at distances greatly removed from the neuron. Also, in contrast to anterior pituitary hormones, which influence other tissues to produce hormones, posterior lobe hormones can directly cause the desired tissue response.

The first indication of the physiological activity of the neurohypophyseal lobe was the finding of Oliver and Schafer in 1895 that the injection of whole pituitary extracts caused a rise in blood pressure. This effect was soon found to be associated with the *pars nervosa.* This action represents the effects of one of the main neurohypophyseal hormones, *vasopressin.* The existence of the other main neurohypophyseal hormone, *oxytocin,* was first indicated in 1915, when Gaines showed that the injection of posterior pituitary gland extracts caused milk ejection. In 1941, Ely and Peterson showed that a denervated mammary gland could eject milk if the gland was perfused with blood that had been enriched with posterior pituitary extract. Both neurohypophyseal hormones were isolated and sequenced by du Vigneaud in 1954. These were some of the first proteins whose amino acid sequences were elucidated.

Oxytocin and Vasopressin Are Synthesized in Cell Bodies Within the Hypothalamus and Are Carried by Axon Flow to the Posterior Lobe, Where They Are Released

As indicated, the two important hormones produced by the neurohypophysis are vasopressin and oxytocin. Although it was previously thought that the two hormones were produced in separate nuclei, evidence now indicates that both hormones are produced in both the supraoptic and the paraventricular nucleus. The cell bodies that synthesize the hormones are large and thus the neurons are called *magnocellular neurons.* The synthesis of vasopressin and oxytocin, as described previously for protein and peptide hormones, involves first the production of a preprohormone, prepropressophysin for vasopressin and prepro-oxyphysin

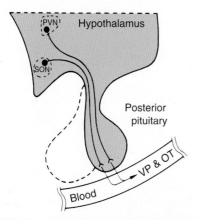

FIGURE 33-11 The hypothalamoneurohypophyseal system, which secretes vasopressin *(VP)* and oxytocin *(OT)*. *PVN,* Paraventricular nucleus; *SON,* supraoptic nucleus. (From Hedge GA, Colby HD, Goodman RL: *Clinical endocrine physiology,* Philadelphia, 1987, Saunders.)

for oxytocin, at the level of the cell body within the hypothalamus (Figure 33-12). The "pre" portion of the molecule is cleaved before the molecules are packaged into granules. During passage of the granules down the axon, the prohormone is cleaved to produce either oxytocin or vasopressin; the remaining peptide fragments are called neurophysin I or neurophysin II, respectively. Neurophysin I, which is released into the vascular system along with oxytocin, has been quantified as an alternative means of following the release of oxytocin. At present, the physiological function of the neurophysins is not known.

The release of the posterior lobe peptide hormones is initiated in the hypothalamus as a result of depolarization of the cell body because of stimulation by neural afferents. The action potential generated extends down the axon to the nerve terminal, where the secretory granules containing the hormone are stored. The depolarization of the nerve cell membrane allows the influx of calcium ions, which initiates the release of hormone through the process of exocytosis.

The Main Effects of Oxytocin Are on the Contraction of Smooth Muscle (Mammary Gland and Uterus); the Effects of Vasopressin Are Primarily on the Conservation of Water (Antidiuresis) and Secondarily on Blood Pressure

The main effects of oxytocin involve the contraction of the myoepithelial cells, which surround the alveoli in the mammary gland and the myometrium of the uterus (see Chapters 38 and 39).

The main activity of vasopressin belies its name because its main effect is antidiuretic, the enhancement of water retention by the kidney. As a consequence, the hormone is often called *antidiuretic hormone* (ADH) (Figure 33-13). Vasopressin is the most important hormone for the control of water balance. Vasopressin also has a pressor effect, which involves the contraction of smooth muscle of the vascular system and therefore has an effect on blood pressure. The main form of vasopressin in most species is arginine vasopressin, whereas in pigs it is lysine vasopressin, and in birds arginine vasotocin.

Plasma Osmolality Controls the Secretion of Vasopressin

The control of vasopressin secretion as a result of changes in plasma osmolality is through *osmoreceptors* located in the hypothalamus as well as through receptors located in the esophagus and stomach that immediately sense water intake (Figure 33-14). An increase in osmolality of body fluids increases the rate of

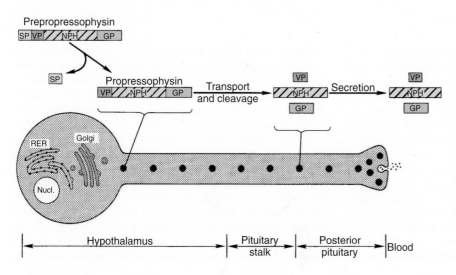

FIGURE 33-12 Diagram of a vasopressin-secreting neuron illustrating the subcellular components involved in synthesis and secretion. This process begins with the synthesis of prepropressophysin, which consists of (1) a signal peptide *(SP)*, (2) vasopressin *(VP)*, (3) neurophysin *(NPH)*, and (4) a glycoprotein *(GP)*. The production and release of oxytocin is identical except that no glycoprotein is involved. *RER,* Rough endoplasmic reticulum; *Nucl.,* nucleus. (From Hedge GA, Colby HD, Goodman RL: *Clinical endocrine physiology,* Philadelphia, 1987, Saunders.)

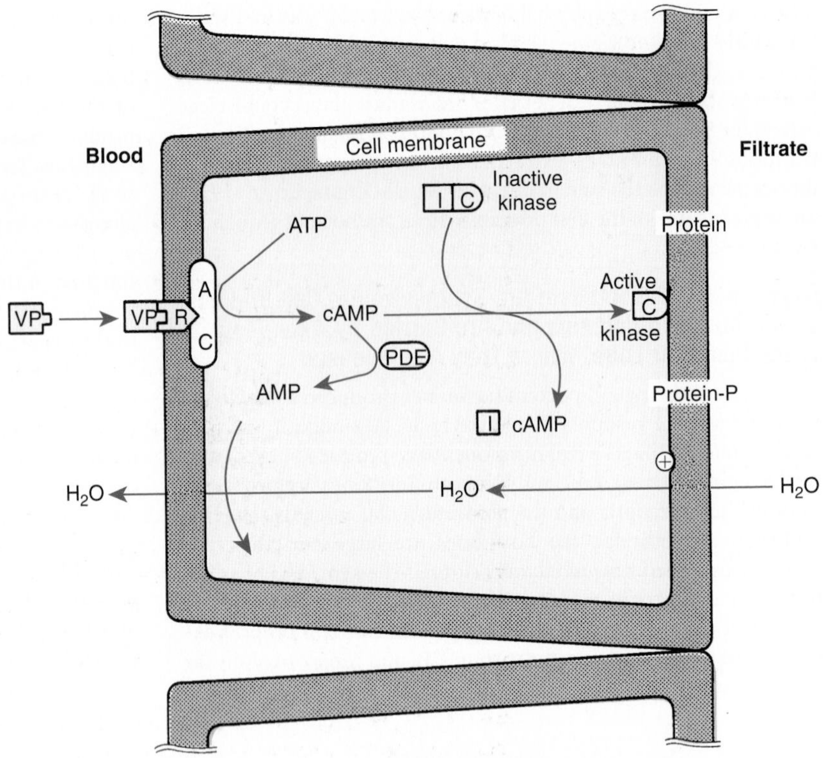

FIGURE 33-13 Antidiuretic mechanism of action of vasopressin *(VP)* on cells of the distal tubule and collecting ducts. *AC,* Adenyl cyclase; *AMP,* adenosine monophosphate; *ATP,* adenosine triphosphate; *cAMP,* cyclic AMP; *I* and *C,* inhibitory and catalytic subunits of the kinase, respectively; *PDE,* phosphodiesterase; *R,* receptor. (From Hedge GA, Colby HD, Goodman RL: *Clinical endocrine physiology,* Philadelphia, 1987, Saunders.)

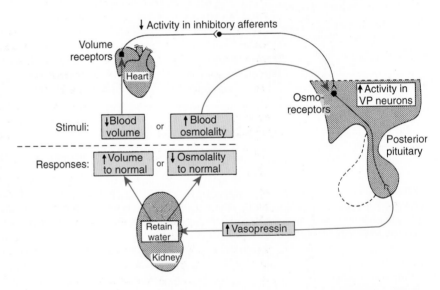

FIGURE 33-14 Major mechanisms regulating vasopressin *(VP)* secretion. A perturbation in either blood volume or osmolality modifies vasopressin secretion to restore these parameters to their normal values. However, this restoration requires appropriate water intake adjustments by thirst as well as by the modulation of water retention depicted. Also, the two responses indicated may be affected by simultaneous changes in sodium balance. (From Hedge GA, Colby HD, Goodman RL: *Clinical endocrine physiology,* Philadelphia, 1987, Saunders.)

action potential firing in the osmoreceptors, which in turn activates hypothalamic cells that synthesize vasopressin. This negative-feedback system is sensitive to changes in osmolality, and the solute-to-water ratio is maintained within 1% to 2% of the normal values. The regulation of the pressor effect of vasopressin—that is, through blood volume—is achieved by increasing the number of action potentials in stretch receptors located in the atria. A decrease in blood volume activates the stretch receptors, which inhibit activity of neurons, vagal in origin, that inhibit the osmoreceptor cells. Blood volume changes that decrease blood pressure also affect vasopressin release through activation of *baroreceptors* in the carotid sinus and aortic arch.

Diabetes insipidus (DI) is a disorder of water metabolism characterized by polyuria, urine of low specific gravity or osmolality, and polydipsia. It is caused by defective secretion of ADH (central

DI) or by the inability of the renal tubule to respond to ADH (nephrogenic DI). Deficiency of ADH can be partial or complete. *Central* DI is characterized by an absolute or relative lack of circulating ADH and is classified as *primary* (idiopathic and congenital) or *secondary.* Secondary central DI usually results from head trauma or neoplasia.

Central DI may appear at any age, in any breed of dog or cat, and in either gender; however, young adults (6 months of age) are most often affected. The major clinical signs of DI are profound polyuria and polydipsia (>100 mL/kg/day; normal range, 40 to 70 mL/kg/day), nocturia, and incontinence, usually of several months' duration. The severity of the clinical signs varies because DI may result from a partial or complete defect in ADH secretion or action. Other, less consistent signs include weight loss (because these animals are constantly seeking water) and dehydration.

Routine complete blood cell count and serum biochemical and electrolyte profiles are usually normal in animals with DI. Plasma osmolality is often high (>310 mOsm/L) in central or nephrogenic DI as a result of *dehydration*. Animals with primary polydipsia often exhibit low plasma osmolality (<290 mOsm/L) as a result of *overhydration*. When present on initial evaluation, abnormalities (e.g., slightly increased hematocrit, hypernatremia) are usually secondary to dehydration from water restriction by the pet owner. In DI the urinalysis is unremarkable except for the finding of a persistently dilute urine (urine specific gravity, 1.004 to 1.012).

Diagnostic tests to confirm and differentiate central DI, nephrogenic DI, and psychogenic polydipsia include the *modified water deprivation test* or response to ADH supplementation. The modified water deprivation test is designed to determine whether endogenous ADH is released in response to dehydration and whether the kidneys can respond to ADH. The more common causes of polyuria and polydipsia should be ruled out before this procedure is performed. Failure to recognize renal failure before water deprivation may lead to an incorrect or inconclusive diagnosis or may cause significant morbidity in the patient.

Hypersecretion of vasopressin in the absence of osmotic or volumetric stimulation is called the *syndrome of inappropriate antidiuretic hormone secretion* (SIADH). Neoplastic processes are often involved in SIADH; ectopic tumors, often located in the lung, are the neoplasms most frequently involved.

The Anterior Pituitary Produces Growth Hormone, Prolactin, Thyroid-Stimulating Hormone, Follicle-Stimulating Hormone, Luteinizing Hormone, and Corticotropin

The adenohypophysis comprises the pars distalis and the pars intermedia. The major hormones produced by the anterior pituitary are growth hormone (GH, also called *somatotropin*), PRL, thyroid-stimulating hormone (TSH), FSH, LH, and corticotropin (Table 33-1). GH is produced by acidophilic somatotropes, and PRL is produced by lactotropes; both are classified as *somatomammotropins*. GH and PRL are single-chain proteins that contain two and three disulfide bonds, respectively. There is overlap of activity between GH and PRL; this overlap is based on the approximately 50% homology of their amino acid sequences. Of these two major somatomammotropins, GH is uniquely species specific as to its activity.

TSH, produced by thyrotropes, and FSH and LH, produced by gonadotropes, are classified as *glycoproteins* because all three

molecules have carbohydrate moieties. These hormones have α and β subunits that are linked by noncovalent binding. The α subunits are identical (and interchangeable) among the three glycoproteins. The β subunits, unique for each hormone, impart the specific action of each hormone. Other members of this family of hormones that are not of anterior pituitary origin include *equine chorionic gonadotropin* (also called *pregnant mare's serum gonadotropin*) and *primate chorionic gonadotropin*, which are produced by cells of the placental chorion.

Corticotropin and β-lipotropin belong to the *pro-opiomelanocortin* family in that they originate from a common prohormone (Figure 33-15). Cells in both the *pars distalis* and the *pars intermedia* synthesize pro-opiomelanocortin molecules. The emphasis on the type of hormone produced is different in the end product; corticotropin is produced by *pars distalis* corticotropes. In the *pars intermedia*, corticotropin is cleaved by corticotropes to form *α-melanocyte–stimulating hormone* (α-MSH), the predominant hormone of this lobe. The remaining peptide fragment is known as *corticotropin-like intermediate lobe peptide*; the physiological activity of this peptide fragment is not known. In both the *pars distalis* and the *pars intermedia*, β-lipotropin is cleaved

TABLE 33-1 Six Major Hormones Secreted by the Anterior Pituitary Gland

Hormone	Abbreviations
Glycoproteins	
Follicle-stimulating hormone	FSH
Luteinizing hormone (interstitial cell–stimulating hormone)	LH (ICSH)
Thyroid-stimulating hormone (thyrotropin)	TSH
Somatotropins	
Growth hormone (somatotropin)	GH
Prolactin	PRL
Pro-opiomelanocortins	
β-Lipotropin	
Corticotropin (adrenocorticotropic hormone)	ACTH

Modified from Hedge GA, Colby HD, Goodman RL: *Clinical endocrine physiology,* Philadelphia, 1987, Saunders.

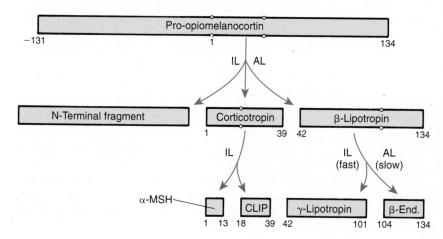

FIGURE 33-15 Cleavage of pro-opiomelanocortin to yield corticotropin and related peptides. By convention, the numbering of the amino acids begins with the first one of corticotropin and then increases positively toward the carboxy terminal and negatively toward the amino terminal. Cleavage occurs at pairs of basic amino acids indicated by the circles. *AL,* Anterior lobe; *α-MSH,* alpha-melanocyte–stimulating hormone; *β-End,* beta-endorphin; *CLIP,* corticotropin-like intermediate lobe peptide; *IL,* intermediate lobe. (From Hedge GA, Colby HD, Goodman RL: *Clinical endocrine physiology,* Philadelphia, 1987, Saunders.)

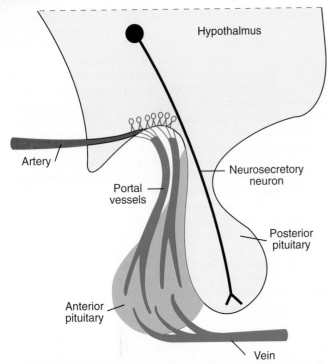

FIGURE 33-16 Diagram of the hypothalamopituitary unit, contrasting the vascular connection between the brain and the anterior pituitary gland with the neuronal connection between the brain and the posterior pituitary gland. (From Hedge GA, Colby HD, Goodman RL: *Clinical endocrine physiology,* Philadelphia, 1987, Saunders.)

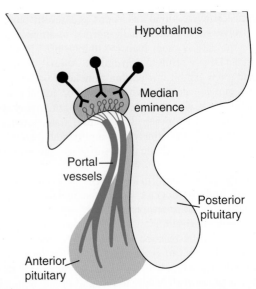

FIGURE 33-17 Hypothalamic neurosecretory neurons and hypothalamohypophyseal portal vessels. (From Hedge GA, Colby HD, Goodman RL: *Clinical endocrine physiology,* Philadelphia, 1987, Saunders.)

to form β-endorphins and γ-lipotropin. Endorphins have opioid activity and appear to modulate gonadotropin secretion.

Control of adenohypophyseal activity was not understood for many years, primarily because the functional connection between the brain and the anterior pituitary gland was not understood. In the 1930s, Popa and Fielding (Budapest medical student and university professor, respectively) described the vascular system that connects the hypothalamus with the pituitary gland but were unable to determine the direction in which blood flowed. In about 1950, Geoffrey Harris drew the important conclusion that the linkage involved blood passage from the hypothalamus to the anterior pituitary gland through the portal blood system previously described by Popa and Fielding (Figure 33-16). The dorsal hypophyseal artery, which supplies nutrients and oxygen to the adenohypophysis (the ventral hypophyseal artery supplies the neurohypophysis), terminates in the median eminence as a capillary plexus. Blood from this plexus is drained by two veins that empty into sinusoidal capillaries of the *pars distalis,* completing the portal venous system (one vein supplies the ventral, central part of the *pars distalis;* the other supplies the dorsal, peripheral areas).

Adenohypophyseal Activity Is Controlled by Hypothalamic Releasing Hormones, Which Are Released into the Portal System, Which in Turn Connects the Median Eminence of the Hypothalamus and the Anterior Pituitary Gland

Whereas neurons that compose the neurohypophysis are influenced directly by neural input within the hypothalamus, the imposition of a vascular system between the hypothalamus and the adenohypophysis requires a different type of control system. The hypothalamus produces regulatory or *hypophysiotropic*

hormones, which are transported to and released within the median eminence (comparable to posterior lobe hormones) (Figure 33-17). These regulatory hormones then pass via the portal venous system to the adenohypophysis, where they stimulate the release of the various anterior pituitary hormones. The synthesis of adenohypophyseal regulatory hormones is controlled by both neural and hormonal inputs at the level of the hypothalamus. Some of the hypophyseal hormones have been found in other areas of the brain and extraneural sites, including the gastrointestinal tract and the pancreas.

The initial isolation and identification of the hypothalamic hormones required large amounts of tissue as well as expertise in biochemistry. The first identified hypothalamic hormone, which controls corticotropin release, was originally called *corticotropin-releasing factor* (now changed from *factor* to *hormone*). The initial work, done by Guillemin's group at the University of Houston in the early 1960s, required the collection, freezing, and transport of several hundred thousand sheep brains from abattoirs located in the western United States, as well as the subsequent dissection of the hypothalami. The hypothalamic hormones that have been characterized and the hormones they release include the following (Table 33-2):

- *Corticotropin-releasing hormone* (CRH). A 41–amino acid polypeptide that stimulates corticotropes to release all components of the pro-opiomelanocortin family of molecules.
- *Gonadotropin-releasing hormone* (GnRH). A decapeptide that stimulates gonadotrope secretion of both FSH and LH.
- *Thyrotropin-releasing hormone* (TRH). A tripeptide that stimulates thyrotrope secretion of TSH.
- *Dopamine.* A catecholamine precursor of norepinephrine that inhibits lactotrope secretion of PRL and thyrotrope secretion of TSH.
- *Somatostatin.* A tetradecapeptide that inhibits somatotrope secretion of GH.
- *Growth hormone–releasing hormone* (GHRH). A 44–amino acid polypeptide that stimulates somatotrope secretion of GH.

Except for dopamine, all these hypophysiotropic hormones are peptides.

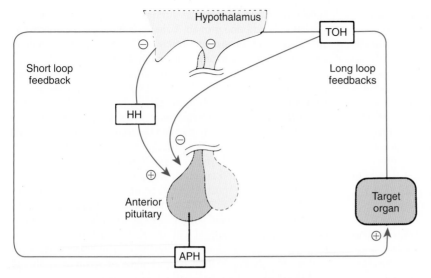

FIGURE 33-18 Regulation of anterior pituitary hormone *(APH)* secretion by hypophysiotropic hormones *(HH)*, short-loop negative feedback, and long-loop negative feedback by target organ hormones *(TOH)*. Plus signs indicate stimulation, and minus signs indicate inhibition. (From Hedge GA, Colby HD, Goodman RL: *Clinical endocrine physiology*, Philadelphia, 1987, Saunders.)

TABLE 33-2 Major Hypophysiotrophic Hormones

Hormone	Abbreviation	Site of Origin
Thyrotropin-releasing hormone	TRH	Paraventricular nucleus
Gonadotropin-releasing hormone	GnRH	Preoptic area of hypothalamus
Growth hormone–inhibiting hormone (somatostatin)	GHIH	Anterior hypothalamic area
Growth hormone–releasing hormone	GHRH	Arcuate nucleus
Corticotropin-releasing hormone	CRH	Paraventricular nucleus
Prolactin-releasing factor	PRF	?
Prolactin-inhibiting hormone (or dopamine)	PIH	Arcuate nucleus

Modified from Hedge GA, Colby HD, Goodman RL: *Clinical endocrine physiology*, Philadelphia, 1987, Saunders.

Previously, only four of the anterior pituitary hormones (FSH, LH, TSH, and corticotropin) were considered to be *tropic*; that is, their main effect was stimulation of hormone secretion by specific endocrine organs located peripheral to the pituitary gland. More recently, GH has been added to this list because GH stimulates the liver to produce *somatomedins,* which have a negative-feedback effect on GH secretion. PRL remains as the only *pars distalis* hormone for which negative-feedback inhibition has not been demonstrated through hormones produced by PRL target tissues.

The most important regulation of secretion of the protein hormones by the *pars distalis* is by feedback inhibition. One feedback system involves negative-feedback inhibition of the tropic pituitary hormone by interaction of the target organ hormone with the hypothalamus, as well as with the pituitary gland; this system is called a *long-loop feedback system* (Figure 33-18). For example, cortisol is produced by the adrenal cortex as a result of corticotropin stimulation, and cortisol in turn has a negative-feedback effect on corticotropin production at the level of the hypothalamus and the anterior pituitary gland. *Short-loop feedback systems* have also been described; an anterior pituitary hormone such as corticotropin has a direct negative-feedback inhibition of hormone secretion, in this case CRH, within the hypothalamus.

Even under conditions of negative-feedback inhibition, the secretion of anterior pituitary hormones is not constant. For example, even though estrogens exert a continuous, potent negative-feedback inhibition on gonadotropin secretion, gonadotropin secretion alternates between secretion and no secretion, with pulses of gonadotropins released into the vascular system. In the case of gonadotropins, the ovarian endocrine status influences the pulse rate and the amplitude of each pulse. Progesterone domination is associated with a decreased pulse rate and an increased pulse amplitude, whereas estrogen causes the opposite effect. The work of Irvine and Alexander has provided the best documentation of the precise relationship between secretory activity of hypothalamic regulatory and anterior pituitary hormones. Their data were obtained through analysis of hormones obtained from the intercavernal sinus, which collects venous blood from the pituitary gland of the horse.

Clinical syndromes of somatotropin deficiency and excess include pituitary dwarfism in the dog and acromegaly in the cat, respectively. Pituitary dwarfism results from destruction of the pituitary gland through a neoplastic, degenerative, or anomalous process. It may be associated with decreased production of other pituitary hormones, including TSH, ACTH, LH, FSH, and GH. *Pituitary dwarfism* is most common in German shepherd dogs aged 2 to 6 months. Other affected breeds include Carnelian bear dogs, Spitz-type dogs, toy pinschers, and Weimaraners. In German shepherd dogs the disease is inherited as a simple autosomal recessive trait and occurs as a result of cystic Rathke's pouch. The first observable clinical signs of pituitary dwarfism are slow growth, noticed in the first 2 to 3 months of life, and mental retardation, usually manifested as difficulty in house training. Physical examination findings may include proportionate dwarfism, retained puppy hair coat, hypotonic skin, truncal alopecia, cutaneous hyperpigmentation, infantile genitalia, and delayed dental eruption. Clinicopathological features include eosinophilia, lymphocytosis, mild normocytic-normochromic anemia, hypophosphatemia, and occasionally hypoglycemia resulting from secondary adrenal insufficiency. Differential diagnoses include other causes of stunted growth, such as hypothyroid dwarfism, portosystemic shunt, diabetes mellitus, hyperadrenocorticism, malnutrition, and parasitism. Diagnosis is made by measuring serum growth hormone concentrations (assay no longer commercially available) or serum somatomedin C (insulin-like growth factor 1 [IGF-1]). The advantage of IGF-1 is that it is not species specific. There is usually a subnormal response to exogenous TSH and ACTH stimulation tests; furthermore, endogenous TSH and ACTH are decreased in affected dogs as a result of panhypopituitarism.

Acromegaly, or *hypersomatotropism,* is the condition resulting from chronic excessive GH secretion in the adult animal. Canine acromegaly is an extremely rare disorder observed after the administration of progestational compounds for suppression of estrus in intact female dogs. The disease is caused by excessive secretion of GH from mammary cells under the influence of exogenous progesterone. Acromegaly in cats, as in humans, is caused by a GH-secreting tumor of the anterior pituitary gland. Such tumors in cats grow slowly and may be present for a long time before the onset of clinical signs. Feline acromegaly occurs in older (8- to 14-year-old) cats and occurs more frequently in males. Canine acromegaly occurs in intact female dogs given progestational compounds for estrus prevention.

Clinical signs of uncontrolled diabetes mellitus (DM) are often observed as the first manifestations of acromegaly; therefore polydipsia, polyuria, and polyphagia are the most common presenting signs. Net weight gain of lean body mass in animals with uncontrolled DM is a key sign of acromegaly. Organomegaly, including renomegaly (observed in both cats and humans with acromegaly), hepatomegaly, and enlargement of endocrine organs, is also observed. Some dogs and cats show the classic enlargement of extremities, body size, jaw, tongue, and forehead that is characteristic of acromegaly in humans. Some of the most striking manifestations of acromegaly occur in the musculoskeletal system, such as an increase in muscle mass and growth of the acral segments of the body, including the paws, chin, and skull. Cardiovascular abnormalities, such as cardiomegaly (as determined radiographically and echocardiographically), systolic murmurs, and congestive heart failure, develop late in the course of the disease. Azotemia develops late in the disease in approximately 50% of acromegalic cats. Neurological signs of acromegaly in humans, such as peripheral neuropathies (paresthesias, carpal tunnel syndrome, sensory and motor defects), and parasellar manifestations, such as headache and visual field defects, are not generally detected in acromegalic small animals.

Impairments in glucose tolerance and insulin resistance that result in DM are observed in all cats and most dogs with acromegaly. Measurement of endogenous insulin reveals dramatically increased serum insulin concentrations. Despite severe insulin resistance and hyperglycemia, ketosis is rare in acromegalic animals. Feline acromegaly should be suspected in any diabetic cat (especially males) that has severe insulin resistance (insulin requirement >20 U/cat/day). Hypercholesterolemia and mild increases in serum activities of liver enzymes are attributed to the diabetic state. Hyperphosphatemia without azotemia is also a

common clinicopathological finding, perhaps as a result of GH-stimulated bone growth. Urinalysis findings are unremarkable except for persistent proteinuria, probably as a result of systemic hypertension and glomerulosclerosis.

A definitive diagnosis of acromegaly requires documentation of increased plasma G or somatomedin C concentrations. Unfortunately, feline and canine GH assays are no longer commercially available. However, insulin-like growth factor 1 is a non-species–specific assay that can be used to identify suspected cases of acromegaly. In cats, it is estimated that almost 30% of cats with diabetes who do not go into remission on an ultra low carbohydrate diet and insulin therapy are acromegalic.

At this time the most definitive test for the diagnosis of acromegaly in cats is computed tomography (CT) or MRI of the pituitary region coupled with increased serum IGF-1 concentrations. CT findings, coupled with the exclusion of other disorders that cause insulin resistance (hyperthyroidism, hyperadrenocorticism), in cats that exhibit clinical signs of acromegaly should lead the clinician to a diagnosis of acromegaly.

CLINICAL CORRELATIONS

EQUINE CUSHING'S DISEASE

History. You are called to examine a 15-year-old mare whose owner complains that the mare has had stiffness in her legs for the past 9 months. The mare has been used as a broodmare and delivered a foal the past spring (and for the previous seven years). She failed to conceive last spring, and now, in the early summer of the next year, she has yet to exhibit normal estrous cycles.

Clinical Examination. As you gain a general perspective on the mare, you notice that she appears to have been clipped recently. She is not a show mare, and because it is early summer, you inquire why she has been clipped. The owner indicates that the mare has been slow to shed this spring, and she is tired of seeing the mare with a rough hair coat. The finding of a long hair coat out of season prompts you to ask about the water consumption of the mare; the owner indicates that the mare drank more water (and urinated accordingly) than would be expected. You examine the feet and find that the soles appear slightly "dropped"; you find a small abscess in the sole of one of the feet.

Comment. The main clue regarding the nature of the disease is the presence of a long hair coat out of season; this is the *sine qua non* of the disease. The usual complaints of owners of horses with Cushing's disease are related to chronic processes, such as pneumonia, laminitis, or weight loss, the latter often associated with parasitism and an inability to masticate properly because of tooth problems. Broodmares progressing into Cushing's disease often have a recent history of infertility after a successful broodmare career. Although the cause of infertility is not known, a disturbance of gonadotropin secretion is likely, along with a perturbation of the pro-opiomelanocortin system.

The disease represents a classic case of loss of control of the intermediate lobe of the pituitary gland by the hypothalamus, in this case the loss of dopaminergic control. Under normal conditions, melanotropes of the intermediate lobe process pro-opiomelanocortin to α-MSH and acetylated β-endorphin, residues 1 to 31, and nonopiate active carboxy-terminally shortened 1 to 26, or 1 to 27, endorphin. In the absence of dopamine, the melanotropes produce α-MSH, as well as β-endorphin, 1 to 31 (the active form), and small amounts of corticotropin; the latter stimulates glucocorticoid production by the adrenal cortex. The negative-feedback control system fails in this situation because the melanotropes do not have glucocorticoid receptors, even under normal conditions. The result is unchecked synthesis and secretion of melanotrope products, including corticotropin, and unchecked glucocorticoid secretion. Activity of the corticotropes in the *pars distalis* is decreased because of negative-feedback inhibition by the glucocorticoids. One of the long-term effects of excess glucocorticoid secretion is muscle wasting, a common finding in these animals. Also, typical manifestations of the disease include polydipsia and polyuria, which result from compression of the *pars nervosa* by the enlarging pars intermedia and reduction in ADH synthesis.

Although there is hyperplasia of the intermediate lobe in Cushing's disease, it has not been established whether this disease occurs because of autonomous hyperplasia of the intermediate lobe or, conversely, whether the hyperplasia occurs because of gradual loss of dopaminergic control by the hypothalamus. One theory is that chronic stress, such as that occurring with laminitis, could affect dopamine secretion by the hypothalamus, leading to loss of control of the intermediate lobe and the development of hyperplasia.

Treatment. At present the only proven treatment is to provide the best possible husbandry for animals with Cushing's disease. This care includes parasite control, floating of teeth, providing good nutrition, and taking proper care of the feet.

AGALACTIC MARE

History. A client calls you with a mare that has just foaled, and the mare does not appear to have any milk.

Clinical Examination. The mare and foal otherwise appear to be normal. However, the mare has little milk for the foal. On examining the placenta, the placenta appears to be a little bit thickened.

Comment. This mare likely has agalactia due to ingestion of fescue, likely contaminated with the fungus *Claviceps* sp, contained within the hay. The fungus produces an ergot alkaloid that is a dopamine agonist, and thus inhibits prolactin secretion. Ergot alkaloids can also produce thickened fetal membranes. Domperidone can be given to inhibit dopamine, which will block the inhibition of prolactin. The increase in prolactin should increase milk production. Additionally, milk production could be increased by giving oxytocin several times daily. If the foal is nursing, this will stimulate oxytocin release which should stimulate milk let down.

Treatment. The mare can be given a combination of domperidone as well as oxytocin to stimulate milk production. Depending on when the domperidone is started, it can take up to 10 to 14 days to see the full effects. The foal may likely have to be supplemented with a milk replacement as well to be sure the foal is getting sufficient calories.

PRACTICE QUESTIONS

1. In general, hormones are classified as proteins, peptides, and steroids. Which one of the following hormones is a peptide?
   a. Growth hormone
   b. Insulin
   c. Vasopressin
   d. Dopamine
   e. Epinephrine
   f. Melatonin

2. In general, steroid hormones are classified as mineralocorticoid, glucocorticoid, and sex steroids. Which one of the following hormones is a glucocorticoid?
   a. Aldosterone
   b. Corticosterone
   c. Cortisol
   d. Testosterone
   e. Estrone

3. Direct feedback control of corticotropin-releasing hormone by corticotropin is termed:
   a. Negative feedback.
   b. Positive feedback.
   c. Short-loop feedback.
   d. Long-loop feedback.

4. Hormones from the pro-opiomelanocortin family are synthesized from precursor hormones produced in either the *pars distalis* or the *pars intermedia*. The two main hormones produced by these two lobes (in respective order) are:
   a. α-MSH and endorphin.
   b. Corticotropin and endorphin.
   c. α-MSH and corticotropin.
   d. Corticotropin and α-MSH.
   e. Corticotropin and α-lipotropin.

5. Increased hormonal activity that occurs during daylight hours is termed _____ rhythm.
   a. Circadian
   b. Diurnal
   c. Nocturnal
   d. Ultradian

BIBLIOGRAPHY

Eiler H: Endocrine glands. In Reece WO, editor: *Dukes' physiology of domestic animals*, ed 12, Ithaca, NY, 2004, Comstock Publishing.

Feldman EC, Nelson RW, editors: *Canine and feline endocrinology and reproduction*, ed 3, Philadelphia, 2004, Saunders.

Frazer GS: The pregnant mare. In Reed SM, Bayly WM, Sellon DC, editor: *Equine internal medicine*, ed 2, St Louis, 2004, Elsevier Saunders.

Hedge GA, Colby HD, Goodman RL: *Clinical endocrine physiology*, Philadelphia, 1987, Saunders.

Martin CR: *Endocrine physiology*, New York, 1985, Oxford University Press.

Melmed S, Polonsky KS, Larsen PR, Kronenberg HM: *Williams textbook of endocrinology*, ed 12, Philadelphia, 2012, Elsevier Saunders.

Pineda MH, Dooley MP, editors: *McDonald's veterinary endocrinology and reproduction*, ed 5, Ames, Iowa, 2003, Iowa State University Press.

Tepperman J, Tepperman HM: *Metabolic and endocrine physiology*, ed 5, Chicago, 1987, Year Book Medical Publishers.

Troedsson MG, Christensen BW: Alerations in sexual function. In Smith BP, editor: *Large animal internal medicine*, ed 4, St Louis, 2009, Mosby Elsevier.

CHAPTER 34
Endocrine Glands and Their Function

KEY POINTS

The thyroid gland

1. The thyroid hormones are synthesized from two connected tyrosine molecules that contain three or four iodine molecules.
2. Thyroid hormones are stored outside the cell and attached to thyroglobulin in the form of colloid.
3. The release of thyroid hormones involves transport of thyroglobulin with attached thyroid hormones into the cell, cleavage of the thyroid hormones from thyroxine-binding globulin, and release into the interstitial tissues.
4. Thyroid hormones are transported in the plasma attached to plasma proteins.
5. The main routes of metabolism of thyroid hormones are through deiodination or the formation of glucuronides and sulfates via hepatic mechanisms.
6. Thyroid hormones are the primary factors for the control of basal metabolism.
7. The ingestion of compounds that inhibit the uptake or organic binding of iodine blocks the thyroid's ability to secrete thyroid hormones and causes goiter.

The adrenal glands

1. The adrenal glands are composed of two organs: the outer gland (cortex) and the inner gland (medulla).

The adrenal cortex

1. The adrenal cortex has three zones: the zona glomerulosa, which secretes mineralocorticoids, and the zona fasciculata and the zona reticularis, which secrete glucocorticoids and sex steroids.
2. Adrenal corticoids are synthesized from cholesterol; the critical difference in the activity of these corticoids is related to the hydroxyl group on C-17 of glucocorticoids.
3. Adrenocortical hormones are carried in plasma in association with specific binding globulins (corticosteroid-binding globulin).
4. The metabolism of adrenocortical hormones involves the reduction of double bonds and conjugation of the steroids to glucuronides and sulfates.
5. One of the most important functions of glucocorticoids is control of metabolism, in particular the stimulation of hepatic gluconeogenesis.
6. Corticotropin is the pituitary hormone that regulates glucocorticoid synthesis by the adrenal cortex.

7. One of the most important clinical uses of glucocorticoids is the suppression of the inflammatory response.

The adrenal medulla

1. The synthesis of catecholamines is from tyrosine; the main catecholamine synthesized by the adrenal medulla is epinephrine.
2. The primary actions of catecholamines are on metabolism, especially effects that increase the concentration of glucose.
3. The main factors that stimulate catecholamine secretion are hypoglycemia and conditions that produce stress.

Hormones of the pancreas

1. The synthesis of insulin is biphasic: an acute phase involves the release of preformed insulin, and a chronic phase involves the synthesis of protein.
2. The metabolism of insulin involves splitting the A and B chains and reducing the chains to amino acids and peptides.
3. The main metabolic functions of insulin are anabolic.
4. Insulin deficiency produces diabetes mellitus, which can culminate in diabetic ketoacidosis.
5. Dietary management is an important consideration in therapy for feline type 2 diabetes.
6. The most important functions of glucagon are to decrease glycogen synthesis, increase glycogenolysis, and increase gluconeogenesis.
7. Glucagon synthesis is stimulated by decreased glucose concentrations in the blood.
8. The main functions of somatostatin are to inhibit the secretion of hormones produced by the pancreas (insulin, glucagon, pancreatic polypeptide).

Calcium and phosphate metabolism

1. Calcium is important for many intracellular reactions, including muscle contraction, nerve cell activity, release of hormones through exocytosis, and activation of enzymes.
2. Phosphate is important for the structure of bone and teeth, and organic phosphate serves as part of the cell membrane and several intracellular components.
3. The most important body pool of calcium involved in homeostasis is the extracellular fluid component.

THE THYROID GLAND

In most mammals the thyroid gland is located caudal to the trachea at the level of the first or second tracheal ring. The thyroid gland is composed of two lobes lying on either side of the trachea and connected by a narrow piece of tissue called the *isthmus*.

The thyroid gland is the most important endocrine gland for metabolic regulation. The glandular tissue has cells formed in a circular arrangement called a *follicle* (Figure 34-1). The follicles are filled with a homogeneous-staining substance called *colloid*, which is the main storage form of the thyroid hormones. The follicular cells are cuboidal when the secretion is basal and are elongated when the cells are stimulated to release hormone. Another important endocrine cell, the *parafollicular cell,* or *C cell,* is located outside the follicles. This cell secretes *calcitonin,* a hormone important for the regulation of calcium. The activity of this hormone is discussed in the section on calcium metabolism.

The Thyroid Hormones Are Synthesized from Two Connected Tyrosine Molecules That Contain Three or Four Iodine Molecules

The synthesis of thyroid hormone is unusual because a large amount of the active hormone is stored as a colloid outside the follicle cells, within the lumen (or acinus) created by the circular arrangement of glandular cells. Two molecules are important for thyroid hormone synthesis: tyrosine and iodine. *Tyrosine* is a part of a large molecule (molecular weight, 660,000 D) called *thyroglobulin* that is formed within the follicle cell and secreted into the lumen of the follicle. *Iodine* is converted to iodide in the intestinal tract and then is transported to the thyroid, where the follicle cells effectively trap the iodide through an active transport process. This allows intracellular iodide concentrations to be 25 to 200 times higher than extracellular concentrations.

As iodide passes through the apical wall of the cell, it attaches to the ring structures of the tyrosine molecules, which are part of the thyroglobulin amino acid sequence. The tyrosyl ring can accommodate two iodide molecules; if one iodide molecule attaches, it is called *monoiodotyrosine,* and if two attach, it is called *diiodotyrosine.* The coupling of two iodinated tyrosine molecules results in the formation of the main thyroid hormones; two diiodotyrosine molecules form *tetraiodothyronine,* or *thyronine* (T_4), and one monoiodotyrosine and one diiodotyrosine molecule form *triiodothyronine* (T_3) (Figure 34-2). A key enzyme in the biosynthesis of thyroid hormones is *thyroperoxidase* (which works in concert with an oxidant, hydrogen peroxide). Thyroperoxidase catalyzes the iodination of the tyrosyl residues of *thyroxine-binding globulin* (TBG) and the formation of T_3 and T_4. In addition to the unusual molecular storage form of the hormone, thyroid hormones are also unique in that they are the only hormones that contain a halide (i.e., iodine).

Thyroid Hormones Are Stored Outside the Cell and Attached to Thyroglobulin in the Form of Colloid

When thyroid hormones are synthesized, they remain in the extracellular acinar lumen until release. This extracellular storage of hormone within an endocrine gland is a unique storage arrangement. It allows the thyroid gland to have a large reserve of hormone. From a teleologic standpoint, thyroid hormone is the most important hormone of metabolism; it allows mammals to withstand periods of iodine deprivation without an immediate effect on the production of thyroid hormones.

The Release of Thyroid Hormones Involves Transport of Thyroglobulin with Attached Thyroid Hormones into the Cell, Cleavage of the Thyroid Hormones from Thyroxine-Binding Globulin, and Release into the Interstitial Tissues

For thyroid hormones to be released from the thyroid gland, thyroglobulin with its attached monoiodotyrosine, diiodotyrosine, T_3, and T_4 molecules must be translocated into the follicle cell, and the hormones must be cleaved from thyroglobulin (Figure 34-3). Key enzymes in this transfer are found in the lysosomes. On entering the cell, the TBG molecules fuse with lysosomes, and lysosomal enzymes cleave both the iodinated tyrosine molecules and the iodinated thyronines from the thyroglobulin molecule. The thyronines are released through the basal cell membrane (they freely pass through the cell membrane); monoiodotyrosine and diiodotyrosine are deiodinated by an enzyme called *iodotyrosine dehalogenase;* and both the iodide and the remaining tyrosine molecules are recycled to form new hormone in association with thyroglobulin.

The majority of T_3 formation occurs outside the thyroid gland by deiodination of T_4. Tissues that have the highest concentration of deiodinating enzymes are those of the liver and kidneys, although muscle tissue produces more T_3 on the basis of relative size. The enzyme that is involved in the removal of iodide from

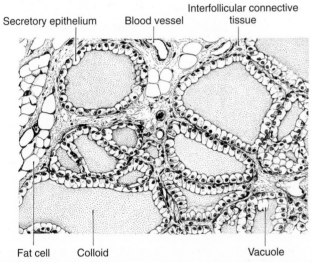

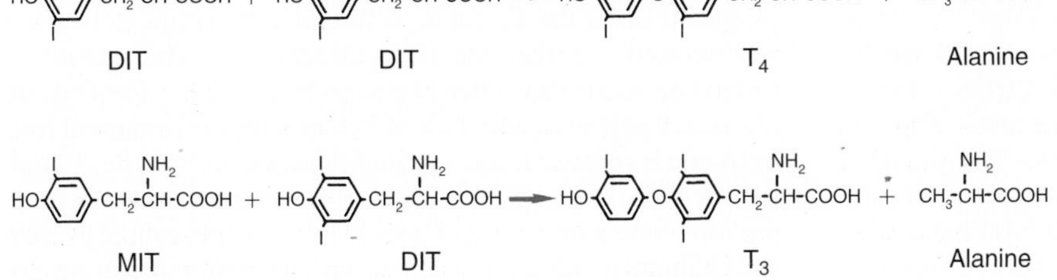

Secretory epithelium   Blood vessel   Interfollicular connective tissue

Fat cell   Colloid   Vacuole

FIGURE 34-1 Histological features of the normal thyroid gland of the rat. All normal thyroid glands are structurally similar, although slight variations occur with age, diet, habitation, and sexual status (neutered or intact). The normal animals of the colony to which this rat belonged were maintained on a high-protein ration, which probably accounts for the slight hypertrophic condition of the secretory epithelium. (From Turner CD, Bagnara JT: *General endocrinology,* ed 6, Philadelphia, 1976, Saunders.)

DIT   DIT   T4   Alanine

MIT   DIT   T3   Alanine

FIGURE 34-2 Production of tetraiodothyronine (thyronine, *T4*) and triiodothyronine (*T3*) by the coupling of iodinated tyrosyl residues with thyroglobulin molecule. *DIT,* Diiodotyrosine; *MIT,* monoiodotyrosine. (From Hedge GA, Colby HD, Goodman RL: *Clinical endocrine physiology,* Philadelphia, 1987, Saunders.)

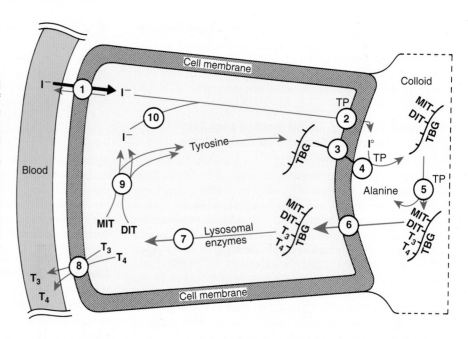

FIGURE 34-3 Depiction of follicular cell showing steps in the synthesis and release of triiodothyronine *(T₃)* and thyronine *(T₄)*. The numbers identify the major steps: *1,* trapping of iodide; *2,* oxidation of iodide; *3,* exocytosis of thyroglobulin; *4,* iodination of thyroglobulin; *5,* coupling of iodotyrosines; *6,* endocytosis of thyroglobulin; *7,* hydrolysis of thyroglobulin; *8,* release of T₃ and T₄; *9,* deiodination of monoiodotyrosine *(MIT)* and diiodotyrosine *(DIT);* and 10, recycling of iodide. *TBG,* Thyroxine-binding globulin; *TP,* thyroperoxidase. (From Hedge GA, Colby HD, Goodman RL: *Clinical endocrine physiology,* Philadelphia, 1987, Saunders.)

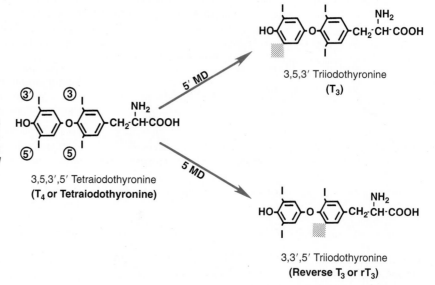

FIGURE 34-4 Structure and nomenclature of thyroxine and its conversion to the two triiodothyronines by 5′-monodeiodinase and 5-monodeiodinase *(MD)*. *Shaded squares* indicate the sites of deiodination. (From Hedge GA, Colby HD, Goodman RL: *Clinical endocrine physiology,* Philadelphia, 1987, Saunders.)

the outer phenolic ring of T₄ in the formation of T₃ is called *5′-monodeiodinase* (Figure 34-4). Another type of T₃ in which an iodide molecule is removed from the inner phenolic ring of T₄, a compound called *reverse T₃,* is also formed. Reverse T₃ has little of the biological effects of thyroid hormones and is formed only by the action of extrathyroidal deiodinating enzymes and not by activity of the thyroid gland.

Thyroid Hormones Are Transported in the Plasma Attached to Plasma Proteins

As indicated in Chapter 33, lipid-soluble hormones are transported in the vascular system through association with specific binding plasma proteins. There is considerable species variation in the proteins that bind thyroid hormones. The most important carrier protein is TBG, which has high affinity for T₄, although it also has low capacity because of its low concentration. TBG also is an important carrier protein for T₃. TBG has been reported in all domestic animals except the cat. *Albumin* is also involved in

the transport of thyroid hormones; however, albumin has low affinity for T₃ and T₄ but high capacity because of its high concentration in plasma. In the absence of TBG, albumin is the most important carrier of thyroid hormones. All species have a third plasma protein, thyroxine-binding prealbumin, which is specific for T₄ and has a specificity and capacity that are intermediate between those of TBG and albumin. The term *prealbumin* refers to the migration of the protein during electrophoresis, not to synthesis of the molecule.

As with all lipid-soluble hormones that are transported in plasma, most of the T₃ and T₄ is bound; little is free to interact with receptors on the cells of the target tissues. The amount of thyroid hormone that is free in plasma is remarkably low (e.g., in humans, 0.03% of T₄ and 0.3% of T₃). In dogs the amount of free hormone is somewhat greater (slightly less than 1.0% for T₄ and slightly more than 1.0% for T₃) because of less affinity between plasma-binding proteins and thyroid hormones in canine plasma than in human plasma. The equilibrium between free and bound

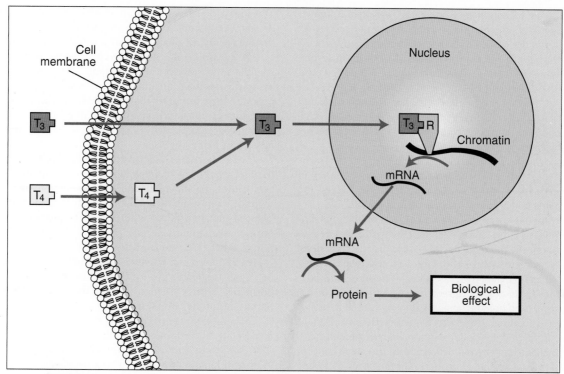

FIGURE 34-5 Proposed subcellular mechanism of thyroid hormone action. *mRNA,* Messenger ribonucleic acid; *R,* receptor. (From Hedge GA, Colby HD, Goodman RL: *Clinical endocrine physiology,* Philadelphia, 1987, Saunders.)

hormone is easily shifted because of physiological or pharmacological situations, such as the increase in estrogen concentrations that occurs during pregnancy. Estrogens cause increased synthesis of TBG by the liver, resulting in a shift toward the bound form. Adjustments to maintain a normal amount of free hormone occur rapidly, with a decline in the rate of metabolism or with stimulation of thyroid hormone production through the release of *thyroid-stimulating hormone* (TSH).

The Main Routes of Metabolism of Thyroid Hormones Are Through Deiodination or the Formation of Glucuronides and Sulfates via Hepatic Mechanisms

The main form of metabolism of thyroid hormones involves the removal of iodide molecules. Except for the T_3 formed from T_4, none of the deiodinated thyronine derivatives has any significant metabolic activity. The two enzymes involved in T_3 and reverse T_3 synthesis, 5′-deiodinase and 5-deiodinase, are also involved in the catabolism of thyroid hormones. Only these two enzymes are needed for catabolism because they do not differentiate between the 3 and 5 positions of the phenolic rings of the thyronines. Skeletal muscle, liver, and kidney tissues are important tissues involved in the catabolism of thyroid hormones through deiodination. The formation of thyroid hormone conjugates represents another form of inactivation; sulfates and glucuronides are formed mainly in the liver and kidneys. Conjugation is less common than deiodination as a means of metabolism of thyroid hormones. Another form of metabolism involves modification of the alanine moiety of the thyronines by either transamination or decarboxylation. The deiodinated and conjugated forms of the thyronines are eliminated primarily in the urine; unmetabolized thyronines are excreted with feces through bile secretion.

Degradation of the conjugate forms in the feces results in the production of iodide molecules, which are reabsorbed as part of the *enterohepatic cycle.* Humans are more efficient than dogs in recovery of iodide both intrathyroidally and enterohepatically.

One of the striking aspects of thyroid hormones is their long half-lives in humans; T_3 has a half-life of 1 day and T_4 of 6 to 7 days, whereas most other hormones have half-lives of seconds or minutes. One reason for these long half-lives is the large percentage of the circulating thyronines that are bound to the plasma proteins, which protects them from degradation. The difference in half-lives between T_3 and T_4 results from the tighter T_4 protein binding compared with T_3 and the resultant reduction in free circulating hormone. In contrast, the half-life for T_4 is relatively short in certain domestic species; dogs and cats exhibit a T_4 half-life of less than 24 hours.

Thyroid Hormones Are the Primary Factors for the Control of Basal Metabolism

The mechanism of action of thyroid hormones at the cellular level is based on their ability to penetrate the cell membrane even though they are amino acids; in essence, they are lipophilic. Although it is thought that thyroid hormones interact directly with the nucleus to initiate the transcription of *messenger ribonucleic acid* (mRNA) (Figure 34-5), the presence of T_3 receptors has been reported on mitochondria.

Thyroid hormones are likely the primary determinants of basal metabolism. It is difficult to define their precise physiological effects, however, because many of the effects of thyroid hormones have been demonstrated through the creation of hypothyroid or hyperthyroid states. Nevertheless, it has long been recognized that thyroid hormones increase oxygen consumption of tissues and, as a result, heat production. This effect is known as the calorigenic effect. One site of action of the *calorigenic effect* of thyroid hormones is within the mitochondrion.

Thyroid hormones affect carbohydrate metabolism in several ways, including increasing intestinal glucose absorption and facilitating the movement of glucose into both fat and muscle. Furthermore, thyroid hormones facilitate insulin-mediated glucose uptake by cells. Glycogen formation is facilitated by small amounts of thyroid hormones; however, glycogenolysis occurs after larger dosages.

Thyroid hormones in concert with growth hormone are essential for normal growth and development. This is accomplished in part by the enhancement of amino acid uptake by tissues and enzyme systems that are involved in protein synthesis.

Whereas thyroid hormones affect all aspects of lipid metabolism, the emphasis is placed on *lipolysis*. One particular effect of thyroid hormones is the tendency to reduce plasma cholesterol levels. This appears to involve both increased cell uptake of *low-density lipoproteins* (LDLs) with associated cholesterol molecules and a tendency for increased degradation of both cholesterol and LDL. These effects on lipid metabolism are usually seen in pathophysiological situations involving hypersecretion of thyroid hormone or in thyroid deficiency states in which hypercholesterolemia is a hallmark of thyroid deficiency. In this same context, the effects of thyroid hormones on metabolic processes, including carbohydrate, protein, and lipid metabolism, are often described as *catabolic*.

Thyroid hormones have noteworthy effects on the nervous and cardiovascular systems. The effects of the sympathetic nervous system are enhanced by the presence of thyroid hormones. This is thought to occur through thyroid stimulation of β-adrenergic receptors in tissues that are targets for the catecholamines, such as epinephrine and norepinephrine. In the central nervous system (CNS), thyroid hormones are important for normal development of tissues in the fetus and neonate; inhibition of mental activity occurs when thyroid hormone exposure is inadequate. In humans, persons with hypothyroid activity are mentally dull and lethargic, which suggests that normal CNS function in the adult depends on the presence of adequate amounts of thyroid hormone.

Thyroid hormones increase the heart rate and force of contraction, probably through their interaction with the catecholamines.

This interaction is caused by an increase in tissue responsiveness through the induction of catecholaminergic β receptors by thyroid hormones. Blood pressure is elevated because of increased systolic pressure, with no change in diastolic pressure; the end result is an increase in cardiac output. These responses are most easily observed in situations of increased thyroid activity. In regard to the effect of thyroid hormones on cardiovascular activity, it may be concluded that they are important for maintaining normal contractile activity of cardiac muscle, including the transmission of nerve impulses.

Thyroid hormone was used in classic experiments involving the metamorphosis of amphibian larvae. Thyroxine administration causes the differentiation of tadpoles into frogs, whereas thyroidectomy results in development into large tadpoles. Thyroid-induced metamorphosis is limited to amphibians, but thyroid hormones are important for many (subtle) aspects of differentiation in other classes of animals.

Thyroid hormone activity is usually defined in terms of tissue or organ responses to inadequate or excessive amounts of hormone. A more balanced view is that thyroid hormones are important for the *normal* metabolic activity of all tissues.

TSH, or *thyrotropin*, is the most important regulator of thyroid activity. It acts through the initiation of cyclic adenosine 3′,5′-monophosphate (cAMP) formation and the phosphorylation of protein kinases. Thyrotropin secretion is regulated by thyroid hormones through negative-feedback inhibition of the synthesis of *thyrotropin-releasing hormone* (TRH) at the level of the hypothalamus and by inhibition of TSH activity at the level of the pituitary gland (Figure 34-6).

The Ingestion of Compounds That Inhibit the Uptake or Organic Binding of Iodine Blocks the Thyroid's Ability to Secrete Thyroid Hormones and Causes Goiter

An inability to secrete adequate amounts of thyroid hormone often leads to the enlargement of the thyroid gland, a condition known as *goiter*. In many places in the world, this condition is, or has been, caused by a deficiency of iodine in the diet. This has largely been corrected through the use of iodized salt. Certain plants, such as cruciferous plants (e.g., cabbage, kale, rutabaga, turnip, rapeseed), contain a potent antithyroid compound called *progoitrin*, which is converted into goitrin within the digestive tract. *Goitrin* interferes with the organic binding of iodine. Many

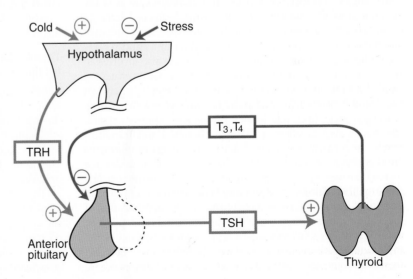

FIGURE 34-6 Hypothalamopituitary-thyroid axis. *Plus signs* indicate stimulation; *minus signs* indicate inhibition. T_3, Triiodothyronine; T_4, thyronine; *TRH,* thyrotropin-releasing hormone; *TSH,* thyroid-stimulating hormone. (From Hedge GA, Colby HD, Goodman RL: *Clinical endocrine physiology,* Philadelphia, 1987, Saunders.)

of the goitrogenic feeds also contain thiocyanates, which interfere with the trapping of iodine by the thyroid gland. The feeding of excess iodine can sometimes overcome the effects of thiocyanate but has less influence on overcoming the effects of goitrin. Studies of these phenomena have led to the development of compounds for the treatment of hyperthyroidism, the most potent being the thiocarbamides, *thiourea* and *thiouracil*. Other antithyroid drugs include sulfonamides, *p*-aminosalicylic acid, phenylbutazone, and chlorpromazine.

Hypothyroidism in Dogs

Hypothyroidism is most common in the dog, and the usual etiology of primary hypothyroidism is lymphocytic thyroiditis. Congenital hypothyroidism may be caused by thyroid dysgenesis, dyshormonogenesis, T_4 transport defects, goitrogens, or in rare cases, iodine deficiency. Secondary hypothyroidism may be a secondary effect of pituitary tumors, radiation therapy, or ingestion of endogenous or exogenous glucocorticoids. Tertiary hypothyroidism can be acquired, as in the case of hypothalamic tumors, or can be congenital as a result of defective TRH or TRH receptor defects.

The signalment of hypothyroid dogs carries a distinct breed predisposition; high-risk breeds manifest symptoms as early as 2 to 3 years of age, and low-risk breeds manifest symptoms at a slightly older age (4 to 6 years of age). Breeds predisposed to hypothyroidism include golden retrievers, Doberman pinschers, dachshunds, Irish setters, miniature schnauzers, Great Danes, miniature poodles, boxers, Shetland sheepdogs, Newfoundlands, chow chows, English bulldogs, Airedale terriers, cocker spaniels, Irish wolfhounds, giant schnauzers, Scottish deerhounds, and Afghan hounds.

Clinical signs of hypothyroidism are gradual and subtle in onset; lethargy and obesity are most common. Dermatological evidence of hypothyroidism is the next most common clinical finding. Symmetric truncal or tail head alopecia is a classic finding in hypothyroid dogs. The skin is often thickened because of myxedematous accumulations in the dermis. Common hair coat changes seen in the hypothyroid dog include dull dry hair, poor hair regrowth after clipping, and presence or retention of puppy hair.

Cardiovascular signs of hypothyroidism include bradycardia, decreased cardiac contractility, and atherosclerosis, but these are uncommon presenting complaints. Neuromuscular signs such as myopathies and megaesophagus are also uncommon manifestations of canine hypothyroidism. Neuropathies, including bilateral or unilateral facial nerve paralysis, vestibular disease, and lower motor neuron disorders, are occasionally seen in hypothyroid dogs. Myxedema coma is an unusual finding in hypothyroid dogs and is secondary to myxedematous fluid accumulations in the brain and severe hyponatremia. Less common signs of hypothyroidism include reproductive disorders in female dogs, such as prolonged interestrous intervals, silent heat, and delivery of weak or stillborn puppies. Corneal lipid deposits and gastrointestinal problems such as constipation are occasionally observed in hypothyroid dogs.

Clinicopathological findings, such as anemia resulting from erythropoietin deficiency, decreased bone marrow activity, and decreased serum iron and iron-binding capacity, are observed in about 25% to 30% of hypothyroid dogs. Hypercholesterolemia is seen in approximately 75% of hypothyroid dogs because of altered lipid metabolism, decreased fecal excretion of cholesterol, and decreased conversion of lipids to bile acids. Hyponatremia, a common finding in humans with hypothyroidism, is observed as a mild decrease in serum sodium in about 30% of hypothyroid dogs in one study. Hyponatremia is caused by an increase in total body water as a result of impaired renal excretion of water and by retention of water by hydrophilic deposits in tissues. An unusual clinicopathological feature of hypothyroidism is increased serum creatine phosphokinase levels, possibly as a result of hypothyroid myopathy.

Diagnosis is based on measurement of serum basal total thyroxine (T_4) and triiodothyronine (T_3) concentrations, serum free T_4 and T_3 concentrations, and endogenous canine serum thyrotropin (TSH) levels (Table 34-1) and/or results of dynamic thyroid function tests, including the TRH and TSH stimulation tests. The many variables that affect T_4 include age, breed, environmental and body temperature, diurnal rhythm, obesity, and malnutrition. Specifically, affected greyhounds have approximately half the normal total thyroxine (TT_4) and free thyroxine (unbound) (FT_4) concentrations of normal dogs. Obese dogs have mild increases in serum TT_4 concentrations. In puppies the serum TT_4 concentration is two to five times higher than in adult dogs. Furthermore, there is an age-related decline in serum TT_4 concentrations and response to TSH stimulation in dogs. *Euthyroid sick*

TABLE 34-1 Serum T_4 and T_3 Values by Radioimmunoassay

Species*	T_4 (mg/dL)	T_3 (ng/dL)
Equine		
M ± SD	1.63 ± 0.51	77.1 ± 45.75
Range	0.95-2.38	31-153
Bovine		
M ± SD	6.22 ± 2.03	92.50 ± 53.61
Range	3.60-8.9	41-170
Caprine		
M ± SD	3.45 ± 0.47	145.9 ± 29.32
Range	3.0-4.23	88-190
Ovine		
M ± SD	4.41 ± 1.13	99.6 ± 27.34
Range	2.95-6.15	63-150
Porcine		
M ± SD	3.32 ± 0.80	89.8 ± 36.7
Range	1.70-4.68	43-140
Canine		
M ± SD	1.15 ± 0.38	96.2 ± 21.39
Range	0.70-2.18	63-130
Feline		
M ± SD	2.02 ± 0.61	64.7 ± 20.62
Range	1.18-2.95	39-112

From McDonald LE: *Veterinary endocrinology and reproduction*, ed 4, Philadelphia, 1989, Lea & Febiger.

T_3, Triiodothyronines; T_4, thyronine; *M ± SD*, median plus/minus standard deviation.

*N = 10, for all species listed.

syndrome is characterized by a decrease in serum TT_4 and increase in reverse T_3. Concurrent illnesses such as diabetes mellitus, chronic renal failure, hepatic insufficiency, and infections can cause euthyroid sick syndrome, resulting in decreases in serum TT_4 concentrations. Drugs such as anesthetics, phenobarbital, primidone, diazepam, trimethoprim-sulfa, quinidine, phenylbutazone, salicylates, and glucocorticoids can also decrease serum basal TT_4 concentrations.

Free thyroid hormone concentrations, or unbound T_4 and T_3, are used in human medicine to differentiate between euthyroid sick syndrome and true hypothyroidism. In humans the diagnostic accuracy of a single FT_4 measurement is approximately 90%. Measurement of FT_4 concentrations is achieved by equilibrium dialysis (*gold standard*) or analogue immunoassays. Theoretically, FT_4 is not subject to spontaneous or drug-induced changes that occur with TT_4. Results of early studies, classifying dogs as hypothyroid on the basis of TSH stimulation tests, indicated that FT_4 measurements by equilibrium dialysis were 90% accurate, whereas other FT_4 assays (analogue assays) were no better than TT_4. Glucocorticoids decrease both FT_4 fraction and TT_4 in dogs.

With the advent of the endogenous canine TSH assay, veterinarians now have a method of assessing the thyroid-pituitary axis in dogs without dynamic testing. With thyroid gland failure, decreases in serum FT_4 and TT_4 are sensed by the pituitary gland, resulting in an increase in serum endogenous TSH concentration. Initial studies in dogs with experimentally induced hypothyroidism have been encouraging. In humans, when endogenous TSH concentrations are increased and FT_4 concentrations are decreased, diagnostic accuracy for primary hypothyroidism approaches 100%. As FT_4 concentration falls, there is a logarithmic increase in serum endogenous TSH concentration, which makes the TSH assay the most sensitive test for the detection of early hypothyroidism. The use of endogenous TSH *alone* is not recommended as a method of assessing thyroid function.

The antithyroglobulin autoantibody test (ATAA) appears promising on the basis of initial study results. The presence of antithyroglobulin antibodies theoretically presages the onset of hypothyroidism in dogs with autoimmune thyroiditis. It is hoped that this test will identify dogs with hereditary thyroid disease before breeding. However, no large studies of dogs with naturally occurring thyroid disease have been performed to evaluate this assay.

For many years the TSH stimulation test was considered the gold standard for diagnosis of hypothyroidism in dogs. Unfortunately, this test does not differentiate between early hypothyroidism and euthyroid sick syndrome and does not identify dogs with secondary or tertiary hypothyroidism. Furthermore, exogenous bovine TSH is no longer commercially available. Other thyroid function tests include the TRH stimulation test, thyroid scan, and thyroid biopsy. However, each test has drawbacks (expense, inaccuracy, or invasiveness).

In summary, diagnosis of canine hypothyroidism is based on signalment, historical findings, physical examination findings, clinicopathological features, and confirmation with a battery of thyroid function tests. The author uses TT_4 and endogenous TSH (eTSH) initially, followed by FT_4 by dialysis. If all measurements are abnormal, the dog is hypothyroid. If two of the three are abnormal, secondary hypothyroidism (low FT_4, low TSH) or early primary hypothyroidism (high TSH, low FT_4) is possible. If only one of the three thyroid measurements is abnormal, the dog should be reevaluated in 3 to 6 months.

Hyperthyroidism in Cats

Hyperthyroidism is the most common endocrinopathy of cats and is caused by adenomatous hyperplasia of the thyroid gland. Middle-aged to older cats are typically affected, and there is no predilection for breed or gender.

Balanced pet foods normally provide sufficient iodine but vary widely in iodine content. The effects of this feed variation have been theorized to be important in cats, but there is no data to support or refute the theory. Although acute changes in dietary iodine have been associated with changes in FT_4 in cats, most chronic changes in dietary iodine are associated with "adaptation" of the thyroid gland and therefore are unlikely to be the cause of feline hyperthyroidism.

As noted earlier, goitrogens can result in hypothyroidism. However, some have theorized that chronic exposure to goitrogens can lead to toxic nodular goiter resulting in hyperthyroidism. Flavinoids from soy proteins have been suggested to play a role in the pathogenesis of hyperthyroidism in cats. Polyphenolic soy isoflavones, such as genistein and daidzein, were identified in almost 60% of dry cat foods tested. This contradicts the epidemiologic data which shows that hyperthyroidism is less common in cats fed dry foods. Some dry foods contain isoflavone contents consistent with levels shown to interfere with thyroid function by inhibiting thyroperoxidase in rats and 5'-deiodinase activity in cats. In a prospective study of 18 clinically normal cats eating a soy diet (400 mg isoflavones/kg diet), total T_4 and FT_4 concentrations were modestly, but significantly, increased while T_3 concentrations were unchanged. However, many studies in humans have shown no detrimental effect of soy isoflavones on thyroid function particularly when incorporated into a balanced diet with adequate iodine intake.

Canned cat food has been implicated as a cause of feline hyperthyroidism in multiple epidemiological studies. The suspected goitrogen is bisphenol-A-diglycidyl ether (BADGE), a substance used in making the liner of easy-open "pop-top" cans. It is suspected that this compound can leach into the foods and be consumed by cats. Although this BADGE-based lining is generally considered safe and is used for foods for human consumption, cats may be more susceptible to toxic effects of this compound because they have a greatly reduced ability to detoxify it via hepatic glucuronidation. Bisphenol A also reduces triiodothyronine binding and causes increased TSH secretion resulting in hyperthyroidism and goiter in rats and some humans. While cat studies may not be available, rodent studies show a very high safety margin. It should be noted that epidemiological studies showing associations are not the same as cause and effect. More than 90% of cats in the United States consume commercial pet foods as their primary nutritional source, and relatively few develop hyperthyroidism.

More recently, investigators have honed in on the molecular aspects of feline hyperthyroidism. The disease in cats is more similar to toxic nodular goiter in humans and is characterized by autonomous growth of thyroid follicles. The pathogenesis of toxic nodular goiter is an abnormality in the signal transduction of the thyroid cell. The TSH receptor on the thyroid cells activates receptor-coupled guanosine triphosphate-binding proteins (G proteins; see Chapter 1). Uniquely, the thyroid cell proliferation and hormone production are both controlled by the TSH receptor-G-protein-cAMP signaling. Overexpression of stimulatory G proteins and underexpression of inhibitory G proteins have been demonstrated in some humans with toxic nodular goiter. Mutations of the TSH receptor that result in the receptor remaining activated without ligand (i.e., TSH) have also been reported in humans with toxic nodular goiter.

In hyperthyroid cats, the same abnormalities have been investigated and it appears that activation mutation (activation without ligand) of the TSH receptor may be part of the pathogenesis of feline hyperthyroidism in some cats. Furthermore, abnormalities of G proteins, specifically significantly decreased G inhibitory protein expression, have been described in tissues from hyperthyroid cats.

Although cat litter was associated with an increased risk of hyperthyroidism, the use of litter may simply be a marker of cats that are kept indoors. Indoor cats are likely to live longer and hence have a higher risk of developing hyperthyroidism. Exposure to pesticides and herbicides has been associated with thyroid abnormalities in other species. In particular, the use of flea control products was associated with an increased risk of developing hyperthyroidism; however, no specific product or ingredient could be identified.

One recent report implicated brominated flame retardants (BFRs) as carcinogens/goitrogens possibly associated with feline hyperthyroidism. Coincidently BFRs were introduced 30 years ago at the same time that feline hyperthyroidism emerged. Bromide, a halide, is an intriguing agent to implicate in feline hyperthyroidism because of the unique composition of thyroid hormones which contain the halide iodide. In this report, serum levels of lipid-adjusted serum polybrominated diphenyl ethers (PBDE) were ten- to four-hundred-fold higher than those found in humans. It has been theorized that findings of higher than human polybrominated diphenyl ether (PBDE) serum levels in cats is in accord with the most consistently identified risk factor, which is indoor living. The authors also propose that cats are at increased risk because of meticulous grooming behavior and increased exposure to flame retardants in furniture and carpets. The smaller size of cats, relative to humans, is also a possible risk factor for increased serum levels of PBDEs.

Hyperthyroidism is characterized by hypermetabolism; therefore, polyphagia, weight loss, polydipsia, and polyuria are the most prominent features of the disease. Activation of the sympathetic nervous system is also seen; hyperactivity, tachycardia, pupillary dilation, and behavioral changes are characteristic of the disease in cats. Long-standing hyperthyroidism leads to hypertrophic cardiomyopathy, high-output heart failure, and cachexia, which may lead to death.

Clinicopathological features of hyperthyroidism include erythrocytosis and an excitement leukogram (neutrophilia, lymphocytosis) caused by increased circulating catecholamine concentrations. Increased catabolism of muscle tissue in hyperthyroid cats may result in increased levels of blood urea nitrogen (BUN) but not creatinine. In fact, glomerular filtration rate (GFR) is increased in hyperthyroid cats, and this increase may mask underlying renal insufficiency. Although hyperthyroidism increases GFR, the effect of thyroid hormone excess on the urinalysis is variable. Most cats, however, have decreased urine specific gravity, particularly if they are exhibiting polyuria as a clinical sign. Increased metabolic rate results in liver hypermetabolism; therefore, serum activities of liver enzymes (alanine aminotransferase, aspartate aminotransferase) increase in 80% to 90% of hyperthyroid cats. Serum cholesterol decreases, not because of decreased synthesis, but rather because of increased hepatic clearance mediated by thyroid hormone excess.

Feline hyperthyroidism is diagnosed through measurement of TT_4; TT_3 measurement is generally noncontributory to a diagnosis. Because the disease has become more common and recognized in its early stages, FT_4 concentrations have been shown to be more diagnostic of early or "occult" hyperthyroidism. However, FT_4 concentrations should be interpreted in light of the TT_4 because nonthyroidal illness (chronic renal failure) can result in spurious elevations of FT_4 as well. Free triiodothyronine (FT_3) concentrations do not provide any further advantage over FT_4.

THE ADRENAL GLANDS

The Adrenal Glands Are Composed of Two Organs: the Outer Gland (Cortex) and the Inner Gland (Medulla)

The adrenal glands are two bilaterally symmetric endocrine organs located just anterior to the kidneys. Each gland is divided into two separate entities, a medulla and a cortex (Figure 34-7), each of which produces different types of hormones. These adrenal tissues have different embryonic origins. The *medulla* arises from the neuroectoderm and produces amines such as norepinephrine and epinephrine. The *cortex* arises from the mesodermal coelomic epithelium and produces steroid hormones such as cortisol, corticosterone, sex steroids, and aldosterone. The utility of placing two such disparate tissues together is not apparent. The one common factor is that both sets of hormones are important for adaptation to adverse environmental conditions (i.e., stress).

Interest in the function of the adrenal cortex was heightened in the 1930s because of the research of Hans Selye. He published a series of papers on the effects of adrenalectomy and the ability of the surgically treated animal to defend itself against injury. Selye's hypothesis was termed the *general adaptation syndrome,* which he divided into three parts: the alarm reaction, the stage of resistance, and the stage of exhaustion. The critical aspect of this theory was that in addition to specific responses to injury, animals responded in *nonspecific* ways to combat injury, and the adrenal cortex was the most important organ in leading the nonspecific response. One example of the beneficial effects of glucocorticoids in a situation of injury is the mobilization of glucose, a readily usable source of energy for running away or healing injury. The adaptation of animals to stressful environments is often accompanied by enlargement of the adrenal cortex, such as in domestic chickens raised in crowded conditions and wild animals living in relatively high density.

THE ADRENAL CORTEX

The Adrenal Cortex Has Three Zones: the Zona Glomerulosa, Which Secretes Mineralocorticoids, and the Zona Fasciculata and the Zona Reticularis, Which Secrete Glucocorticoids and Sex Steroids

The adrenal cortex is organized into three zones in mammals (see Figure 34-7). The outer zone, the *zona glomerulosa,* is relatively narrow, and its cells are organized in a whorl-type arrangement. The middle zone, the *zona fasciculata,* is relatively wide, and its cells are organized in columns. In the cow and sheep, the zona fasciculata is further divided into inner and outer layers. The inner zone of the adrenal cortex, the *zona reticularis,* which is adjacent to the adrenal medulla, is intermediate in size, and cells are more randomly organized.

All the cells of the adrenal cortex have intracellular features characteristic of steroid hormone synthesis: an abundance of lipid droplets (containing cholesterol esters), mitochondria, and smooth endoplasmic reticulum. Human adrenal glands have an

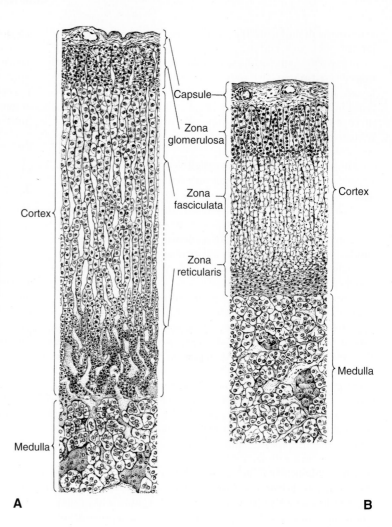

FIGURE 34-7 Depiction of comparable sections through the adrenal glands of **A,** normal rats, and **B,** hypophysectomized rats. Because the functional capacity of the adrenal cortex is conditioned by the release of corticotropin, hypophysectomy results in tremendous shrinkage of the cortex. The medulla is not influenced by hypophysectomy. Both sections are drawn to scale. (From Turner CD, Bagnara JT: *General endocrinology,* ed 6, Philadelphia, 1976, Saunders.)

additional zone, the fetal zone, that is present during fetal life and for the first year of life. The fetal zone participates with the placenta in the production of estrogen during gestation. Immature mice and rabbits have an inner X zone that becomes the zona reticularis at puberty.

The adrenal cortex produces two major types of steroid hormones: the mineralocorticoids and the glucocorticoids. These hormones have distinctly different functions. The *mineralocorticoids,* produced by the zona glomerulosa, play an important role in electrolyte balance and therefore are important in the regulation of blood pressure (see later discussion). The major mineralocorticoid is *aldosterone.* The *glucocorticoids,* produced by the zona fasciculata (which accounts for the majority of glucocorticoid production) and zona reticularis, are important in the regulation of all aspects of metabolism, either directly or through an interaction with other hormones. The major glucocorticoid is *cortisol.*

Adrenal Corticoids Are Synthesized from Cholesterol; the Critical Difference in the Activity of These Corticoids Is Related to the Hydroxyl Group on C-17 of Glucocorticoids

The synthesis of adrenal steroids involves the classic pathways for steroid biosynthesis. As indicated previously, cholesterol is the major starting material for the synthesis of steroid hormones. Cholesterol is readily available to the steroid-synthesizing cells because it is stored in large quantities in ester form within lipid droplets in these cells. One of the initial steps in steroid formation

is the hydrolysis of the ester. The first step in steroid synthesis involves an enzyme that cleaves the carbon side chain from the steroid molecule, leaving a C-21 steroid known as *pregnenolone.* This step occurs within the mitochondrion (Figure 34-8). The synthesis of all steroid hormones, regardless of their form, utilizes pregnenolone in the synthetic pathway (see Figure 33-5).

The critical aspect of adrenal corticoid synthesis, which differentiates adrenal corticoids from the progesterone family of steroids, is a hydroxylation step at C-21 (directed by a C-21 hydroxylase). The difference between the mineralocorticoids (aldosterone) and the glucocorticoids (cortisol) is a hydroxyl group on C-17, which is part of the glucocorticoid molecule. As expected, cells of the zona fasciculata and zona reticularis have the hydroxylating enzyme for C-17 (17α-hydroxylase), whereas cells of the zona glomerulosa do not have this enzyme. Both aldosterone and cortisol have hydroxyl groups on C-11. Because of the marked difference in biological activity of the mineralocorticoids and glucocorticoids, it is useful to view the zona glomerulosa as an endocrine organ that is distinct from the zona fasciculata and zona reticularis.

Two intermediate compounds in the synthesis of aldosterone have significant adrenocortical activity. *11-Deoxycorticosterone* has significant mineralocorticoid activity, although it is secreted in relatively small amounts. *Corticosterone,* the immediate precursor to aldosterone, is a relatively important glucocorticoid in animals, although its potency is less than that of cortisol.

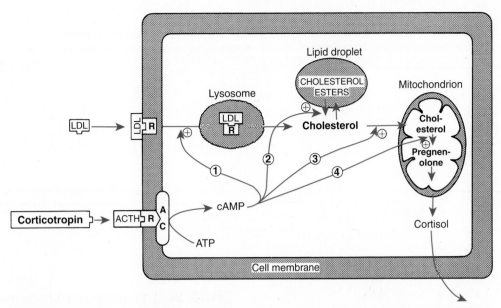

FIGURE 34-8 Mechanism of action of corticotropin (adrenocorticotropic hormone, *ACTH*) on adrenocortical steroidogenesis. The numbers indicate the processes stimulated (indicated by *plus signs*) by corticotropin as follows: *1*, stimulation of the uptake of low-density lipoproteins *(LDL)*, which are further processed to free cholesterol; *2*, stimulation of the hydrolysis of stored cholesterol esters to generate free cholesterol; *3*, stimulation of the transport of cholesterol into mitochondria, where cleavage of the cholesterol side chain occurs; and *4*, promotion of the binding of cholesterol to the enzyme. *AC*, Adenyl cyclase; *ATP*, adenosine triphosphate; *cAMP*, cyclic adenosine monophosphate; *R*, receptor. (From Hedge GA, Colby HD, Goodman RL: *Clinical endocrine physiology*, Philadelphia, 1987, Saunders.)

In adrenal cortical cells, biosynthetic pathways allow some synthesis of androgens and estrogens. Although the amount of sex steroids produced by the adrenal cortex under normal conditions is low, significant amounts can be synthesized under pathological conditions.

Adrenocortical Hormones Are Carried in Plasma in Association with Specific Binding Globulins (Corticosteroid-Binding Globulin)

Steroid hormones, as indicated previously, are lipids and depend on binding to plasma proteins for transport in the blood. A specific globulin that has a high affinity for cortisol has been identified: *corticosteroid-binding globulin,* or *transcortin.* Of the cortisol carried in plasma, 75% is bound to transcortin and 15% to albumin, leaving 10% in the unbound, or free, state. This amount of free hormone is large compared with thyroid hormones: less than 0.1% of T_4 is free. The transport of aldosterone is mainly associated with albumin (50%), and only 10% is associated with transcortin, leaving a very large amount (40%) in the free state.

Changes in physiological or pathophysiological states can influence the amount of binding proteins present in plasma. Estrogen produced in increasing amounts by the fetoplacental unit during pregnancy results in an increase in hepatic synthesis of transcortin, whereas liver dysfunction can result in lower concentrations of transcortin. The large pool of hormone present in the bound state during pregnancy gives animals a good reserve from which to make appropriate adjustments in the amount of free hormone available for influencing biological activity. Because the total amount of glucocorticoid is determined in the assay of plasma concentrations, the veterinary clinician needs to be aware

that total concentrations not only reflect secretion rate, but also can be influenced by the amount of glucocorticoid-binding plasma proteins.

The Metabolism of Adrenocortical Hormones Involves the Reduction of Double Bonds and Conjugation of the Steroids to Glucuronides and Sulfates

The clearance half-life of cortisol is about 60 minutes, and that of aldosterone is about 20 minutes. This difference is attributable to the observed difference in protein binding of these hormones within the plasma. In general, metabolism of mineralocorticoid and glucocorticoid hormones involves the reduction of double bonds and ketone configurations, which reduces the biological activity of the molecules. The liver, an organ important for modification of these hormones, is also an important site for the conjugation of these steroids with sulfates and glucuronides; this reduces their biological potency and renders them water soluble for passage in the urine.

One of the Most Important Functions of Glucocorticoids Is Control of Metabolism, in Particular the Stimulation of Hepatic Gluconeogenesis

The mechanism of action of adrenal hormones is similar to that of other lipophilic hormones: they are able to penetrate the cell membrane and interact in the cytoplasm with specific cytosolic receptors. This complex is transferred to the nucleus, resulting in transcription of certain genes and the synthesis of specific proteins that affect the biological action of the adrenal hormones.

As emphasized previously, adrenocortical hormones are classified as either glucocorticoid or mineralocorticoid in their

TABLE 34-2 Relative Glucocorticoid and Mineralocorticoid Potencies of Various Steroids

Steroid	Glucocorticoid Potency (Relative to Cortisol)	Mineralocorticoid Potency
Cortisol	1	1
Aldosterone	0.1	400
Corticosterone	0.2	2
11-Deoxycorticosterone	<0.1	20
Dexamethasone	30	2
Fludrocortisone	10	400
Prednisone	4	0.7
Triamcinolone	5	<0.1

From Hedge GA, Colby HD, Goodman RL: *Clinical endocrine physiology,* Philadelphia, 1987, Saunders.

activity. Before the biological actions of each class are discussed, it is important to realize that there is overlap of activity (Table 34-2). For example, whereas cortisol is the dominant glucocorticoid hormone, it also has mineralocorticoid effects, although at a reduced potency.

The glucocorticoid hormones are important mediators of intermediary metabolism. One of the important specific effects of glucocorticoids is the stimulation of hepatic gluconeogenesis, which involves the conversion of amino acids to carbohydrates. The net result is an increase in hepatic glycogen and a tendency to increase blood glucose levels. These effects on glycogen metabolism are observed mainly in animals that have excessive glucocorticoid secretion (hyperadrenocorticism) or an insulin deficiency. The effect of glucocorticoids on carbohydrate metabolism is "permissive"; that is, their presence is required for the gluconeogenic and glycogenolytic actions of glucagon and epinephrine, respectively.

Whereas glucocorticoids and insulin have similar effects on liver glycogen metabolism, their effects on the peripheral use of glucose are different. Glucocorticoids inhibit glucose uptake and metabolism in the peripheral tissues, particularly in muscle and adipose cells. This effect has been termed the *anti-insulin effect.* The chronic administration of glucocorticoids can lead to the development of a syndrome called *steroid diabetes* because of the hyperglycemic effect produced at the level of the liver; use of glucose decreases in the peripheral tissues because of insulin antagonism.

Whereas the actions of glucocorticoids on fat metabolism tend to be complex, the direct effect on adipose tissue is to increase the rate of lipolysis and to redistribute fat into the liver and abdomen. This fat redistribution leads to the classic "potbelly" appearance of animals and humans with hyperadrenocorticism.

Protein synthesis is inhibited by glucocorticoids; in fact, protein catabolism is enhanced, with an accompanying release of amino acids. This process supports hepatic gluconeogenesis. Two tissues, cardiac and brain, are spared from the effect of glucocorticoids on protein catabolism. Chronic administration of glucocorticoids results in muscle wasting and the weakening of bone. The mobilization and incorporation of amino acids into glycogen result in an increase in urinary excretion of nitrogen and a negative nitrogen balance.

Glucocorticoids play a role in water diuresis (i.e., the enhancement of water excretion). Whereas glucocorticoids inhibit vasopressin activity in the distal tubule, the most important effect

TABLE 34-3 Glucocorticoid Effects and Target Tissues

Effect	Site of Action
Stimulates gluconeogenesis	Liver
Increases hepatic glycogen	Liver
Increases blood glucose	Liver
Facilitates lipolysis	Adipose tissue
Is catabolic (negative nitrogen balance)	Muscle, liver
Inhibits corticotropin secretion	Hypothalamus, anterior pituitary gland
Facilitates water excretion	Kidney
Blocks inflammatory response	Multiple sites
Suppresses immune system	Macrophages, lymphocytes
Stimulates gastric acid secretion	Stomach

From Hedge GA, Colby HD, Goodman RL: *Clinical endocrine physiology,* Philadelphia, 1987, Saunders.

is to increase the GFR. Table 34-3 summarizes the effects of glucocorticoids.

Corticotropin Is the Pituitary Hormone that Regulates Glucocorticoid Synthesis by the Adrenal Cortex

The control of the secretion of the glucocorticoids by the zona fasciculata and zona reticularis is by the tropic hormone (corticotropin) (Figure 34-9). A negative-feedback system exists, whereby glucocorticoids inhibit the release of hypothalamic corticotropin–releasing hormone, which in turn results in decreased corticotropin secretion by the pituitary gland. Some evidence indicates that glucocorticoids also have a negative-feedback effect at the level of the pituitary gland. The potency of a glucocorticoid in negative-feedback inhibition of corticotropin is directly related to its glucocorticoid potency; for example, cortisol has more potent negative-feedback effects than corticosterone and has more potent glucocorticoid effects.

The negative-feedback control system that exists for the secretion of glucocorticoids does not result in the maintenance of uniform hormone concentrations in blood throughout the day. Sleep and activity patterns are superimposed on the negative-feedback system, so a predictable circadian rhythm occurs in

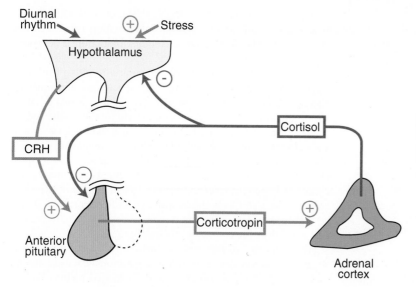

FIGURE 34-9 Regulation of cortisol secretion by the hypothalamopituitary axis. *Plus signs* indicate stimulation; *minus signs* indicate inhibition. *CRH,* Corticotropin-releasing hormone. (From Hedge GA, Colby HD, Goodman RL: *Clinical endocrine physiology,* Philadelphia, 1987, Saunders.)

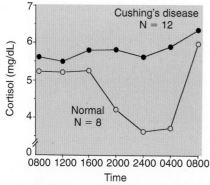

FIGURE 34-10 Circadian changes in cortisol secretion in normal horses *(open circles),* in comparison with no circadian change in horses with equine Cushing's disease *(solid circles).* (From Dybdal N: The pathophysiology of pituitary pars intermedia dysfunction in the horse, Davis, 1989, University of California–Davis [PhD thesis].)

which concentrations of glucocorticoids are lowest late at night and highest in the early-morning hours (Figure 34-10).

Another factor that can modify the negative-feedback control of glucocorticoids is stress. Stress can result from physical or psychological stimuli that are harmful to the individual. The effects of stress, as with the factors that influence circadian rhythms of glucocorticoid secretion, are mediated through the CNS. The glucocorticoid response to stress is immediate: concentrations of cortisol increase rapidly to reach, within minutes, values that are several-fold higher than normal. The glucocorticoid response is proportional to the severity of the stress; that is, lower levels of stress result in less cortisol production than do higher levels of stress.

One of the Most Important Clinical Uses of Glucocorticoids Is the Suppression of the Inflammatory Response

Glucocorticoids have valuable clinical effects, particularly the inhibition of the inflammatory response, including the prevention of capillary dilation, extravasation of fluid into tissue spaces, leukocyte migration, fibrin deposition, and connective tissue

synthesis. Whereas the process of inflammation is important for the walling off and destruction of systemic noxious agents, the end response is often the replacement of functional tissue with fibrous connective tissue, with a resultant loss of function. For example, inflammatory processes in the mammary gland often result in the isolation of the injurious agent by the laying down of connective tissue as a part of the defense mechanism; however, the gland may lose much of its functional capacity as a result. Administration of glucocorticoids, in conjunction with antibiotic therapy, can help reduce the loss of functional tissue by inhibiting the development of connective tissue. Figure 34-11 shows the chemical structures of some of the synthetic glucocorticoids used in clinical practice.

One of the ways in which glucocorticoids inhibit the inflammatory response is through the inhibition of the formation of substances that promote inflammation. Glucocorticoids inhibit the synthesis of inflammatory mediators, such as prostaglandins, thromboxanes, and leukotrienes, that arise as a result of arachidonic acid metabolism. This effect is mediated through the stabilization of lysosomal membranes and the prevention of phospholipase A_2 activation. Glucocorticoids are also used to inhibit allergic reactions. This action occurs through the inhibition of the release of certain biogenic amines, such as histamine, from the granules of mast cells.

Hyperadrenocorticism

Hyperadrenocorticism (Cushing's syndrome) in the dog may be caused by a pituitary tumor, pituitary hyperplasia, adrenal tumors, adrenal hyperplasia, or nonendocrine tumors (usually of the lung), or it may be iatrogenic. Approximately 85% of dogs with hyperadrenocorticism have pituitary gland–dependent disease, whereas 15% exhibit adrenal tumors. Hyperadrenocorticism is a disease of middle-aged and older dogs (7 to 12 years of age). Breeds typically affected by pituitary-dependent hyperadrenocorticism include miniature poodles, dachshunds, boxers, Boston terriers, and beagles. Adrenal tumors are seen more frequently in large-breed dogs, and there is a predilection for females (3 : 1 ratio with males). Hyperadrenocorticism is a rare endocrine disorder of cats and is usually pituitary in origin in that species.

The most common clinical signs associated with canine hyperadrenocorticism are polydipsia, polyuria, polyphagia, heat

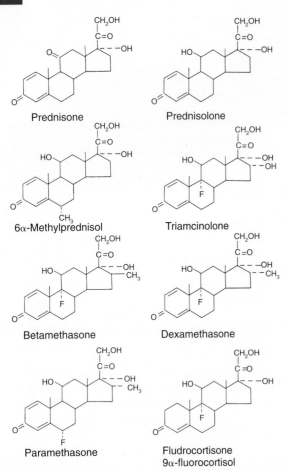

FIGURE 34-11 Chemical structures of some clinically useful glucocorticoid analogues. (From Martin CR: *Endocrine physiology,* New York, 1985, Oxford University Press.)

intolerance, lethargy, abdominal enlargement or "potbelly," panting, obesity, muscle weakness, and recurrent urinary tract infections (UTIs). Dermatological manifestations of canine hyperadrenocorticism can include alopecia (especially truncal), thin skin, phlebectasias, comedones, bruising, cutaneous hyperpigmentation, calcinosis cutis, pyoderma, dermal atrophy (especially around scars), seborrhea, and secondary demodicosis. Thin skin is the hallmark of feline hyperadrenocorticism. Cats with Cushing's syndrome develop such severe thinning of the epidermis that they may incur open wounds just by grooming themselves.

Attempts to diagnose hyperadrenocorticism can be challenging. Uncommon clinical manifestations of hyperadrenocorticism in dogs can include signs such as hypertension, congestive heart failure, bronchial calcification, pulmonary thromboembolism, polyneuropathy, polymyopathy, pseudomyotonia, behavioral changes, and blindness. Evidence of increased collagenase activity caused by hypercortisolemia may result in nonhealing corneal ulceration and bilateral cranial cruciate rupture (in small dogs). Unusual reproductive signs may include testicular atrophy, prostatomegaly in castrated male dogs, clitoral hypertrophy, and perianal adenoma in females or castrated males.

Serum chemistry abnormalities associated with hypercortisolemia in dogs include increased serum activities of alkaline phosphatase and alanine aminotransferase, hypercholesterolemia,

hyperglycemia, and decreased BUN. The hemogram is often characterized by evidence of erythroid regeneration (nucleated red blood cells) and a classic *stress leukogram.* Basophilia is occasionally observed. Many dogs with hyperadrenocorticism have evidence of UTI without pyuria. Proteinuria resulting from glomerulosclerosis is also common. Urine specific gravity is usually decreased and may be hyposthenuric. Thyroid status is often affected in animals with hyperadrenocorticism, as evidenced by (1) decreases in TT_4 and TT_3 caused by euthyroid sick syndrome and (2) a response to TSH stimulation that is attenuated as a result of overcrowding of pituitary thyrotrophs by adrenocorticotrophs. Overt diabetes mellitus may result from the insulin antagonism caused by hypercortisolemia in about 15% of dogs with hyperadrenocorticism and 85% of cats with hyperadrenocorticism. Conversely, hyperadrenocorticism can be a cause of insulin resistance and poor glycemic control in diabetic animals.

The diagnosis of hyperadrenocorticism should be based on suggestive clinical signs and supporting minimal database abnormalities (e.g., high serum cholesterol, increased serum alkaline phosphatase activity) and confirmed by an appropriate screening test. If screening test results are inconclusive, the dog should be retested at a later date (3 to 6 months) rather than be subjected to treatment without a definitive diagnosis.

Screening tests for hyperadrenocorticism, such as the low-dose dexamethasone suppression (LDDS) test and the corticotropin stimulation test, work on the principle of suppression or stimulation of the pituitary-adrenal axis. In the case of the LDDS test, dexamethasone is administered at a low dosage to cause negative feedback to the pituitary gland. In a normal animal, this negative feedback results in a decrease in endogenous corticotropin secretion and a resultant decrease in circulating cortisol concentrations. Dexamethasone is the only synthetic corticosteroid that does not cross-react with the cortisol assay. The corticotropin stimulation is used to determine the extent of adrenal enlargement. Adrenal glands that are enlarged because of chronic pituitary stimulation by corticotropin or that are neoplastic show an exaggerated response to exogenous corticotropin.

The LDDS test has traditionally been the screening test of choice for canine hyperadrenocorticism. It is sensitive (92% to 95%); only 5% to 8% of dogs with pituitary-dependent hyperadrenocorticism exhibit suppressed cortisol concentrations at 8 hours (i.e., 5% to 10% false-negative results). In addition, 30% of dogs with pituitary-dependent hyperadrenocorticism exhibit suppression at 3 or 4 hours, followed by "escape" of suppression at 8 hours; this pattern is diagnostic for pituitary-dependent disease and makes further testing unnecessary. The major disadvantage of the LDDS test is the lack of specificity in dogs with nonadrenal illness. It is recommended that a dog be allowed to recover from the nonadrenal illness before being assessed for hyperadrenocorticism with the LDDS test.

The urine cortisol-to-creatinine ratio (UC:CR) is sensitive (useful for its negative predictive value, i.e. if a normal UC:CR is obtained, hyperadrenocorticism is unlikely), inexpensive, and easy to perform and interpret. Home collection (non-stressed) of urine is preferred. An at-home LDDS test using the UC:CR is an extremely sensitive and simple test to perform. Morning urine samples are collected for 3 days. After the second urine collection on day 2, three doses of oral dexamethasone (0.1 mg/kg each) are given 6 hours apart. Urine is then obtained the following morning (day 3) after dexamethasone administration. Failure to suppress UC:CR on day 3 compared with day 1 and 2 is consistent with feline hyperadrenocorticism.

Mineralocorticoids

The mineralocorticoids, produced in the outer zone (zona glomerulosa) of the adrenal cortex, have surprisingly different functions compared with glucocorticoids; the functions are surprising because both types of hormones are produced by tissues that are part of the same gland. As indicated previously, electrolyte balance and blood pressure homeostasis represent the principal physiological effects of mineralocorticoids (Table 34-4). These actions are carried out at the level of the distal tubules in the kidney. The effect of the mineralocorticoids is to promote retention of sodium and secretion of potassium and hydrogen. The cellular response to mineralocorticoids is to synthesize a protein that increases the permeability of the luminal cell surface to sodium influx from the renal filtrate and increases sodium/potassium-adenosinetriphosphatase (Na^+,K^+-ATPase) activity in the contraluminal cell surface, which allows movement of Na^+ out of the cell into the interstitial tissue (Figure 34-12).

The control of secretion of K^+ by mineralocorticoids is passive in the sense that K^+ is retained in the renal filtrate to maintain the osmolality of urine. However, evidence suggests that mineralocorticoids have an effect on Na^+ secretion that is independent of Na^+ retention. The secretion of K^+ continues to be influenced by mineralocorticoids after mineralocorticoid administration, whereas Na^+ retention decreases within a few days.

In situations of excessive mineralocorticoid production, the effects of increased Na^+ retention are to increase the extracellular fluid volume and to cause hypertension; conversely, low blood pressure (hypotension) occurs as a result of inadequate secretion of mineralocorticoids. Hypersecretion of mineralocorticoids can also lead to excessive hydrogen ion (H^+) loss and metabolic alkalosis, whereas hyposecretion can result in increased retention of H^+ and metabolic acidosis.

The regulation of mineralocorticoid secretion, in contrast to glucocorticoid secretion, is not controlled by tropic hormones from the pituitary gland (Figure 34-13). In the case of mineralocorticoids, the main controlling factors are produced in the target organ, the kidney. Cells in the juxtaglomerular apparatus of the kidney produce an enzyme, *renin*, in response to decreases in blood pressure. Renin acts on *angiotensinogen*, an α_2 globulin produced by the liver and present in the circulation, and this results in the production of *angiotensin I*, a decapeptide. Angiotensin I is further hydrolyzed to *angiotensin II*, an octapeptide, by angiotensin-converting enzyme. Angiotensin II stimulates the zona glomerulosa to produce mineralocorticoids. Angiotensin II also increases peripheral resistance of the blood vascular system by causing vasoconstriction of smooth muscle of the blood

vessels. Angiotensin II, if present on a long-term basis, also increases the size of the zona glomerulosa.

Evidence indicates that cells of the macula densa, groups of specialized cells located at the origin of the kidney's distal tubule (Figure 34-14), exert control on the *renin-angiotensin system*. This is done through the sensing of changes in Na^+ concentrations in

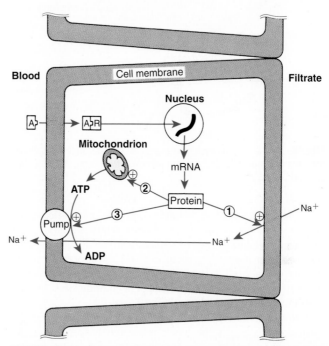

FIGURE 34-12 Mechanisms of action of aldosterone on sodium transport in the renal tubular cell. The *numbered arrows* indicate the three putative sites of action of aldosterone: *1,* increasing the permeability of the luminal membrane to sodium; *2,* increasing mitochondrial adenosine triphosphate *(ATP)* production; *3,* increasing Na^+,K^+-ATPase activity in the contraluminal membrane. *Plus signs* indicate stimulation. *A,* Aldosterone; *ADP,* adenosine diphosphate; *mRNA,* messenger ribonucleic acid; *R,* receptor. (From Hedge GA, Colby HD, Goodman RL: *Clinical endocrine physiology,* Philadelphia, 1987, Saunders.)

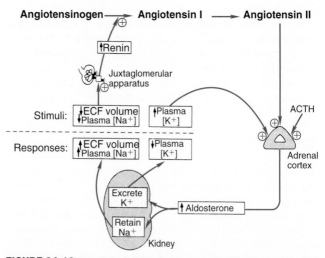

FIGURE 34-13 Regulation of aldosterone secretion by the zona glomerulosa of the adrenal cortex. *Plus signs* indicate stimulation. *ACTH,* Corticotropin (adrenocorticotropic hormone); *ECF,* extracellular fluid. (From Hedge GA, Colby HD, Goodman RL: *Clinical endocrine physiology,* Philadelphia, 1987, Saunders.)

TABLE 34-4 Mineralocorticoid Effects and Target Tissues

Effect	Site of Action
Stimulates Na^+ reabsorption	Kidney, salivary glands, sweat glands
Stimulates K^+ excretion	Kidney, salivary glands, sweat glands
Stimulates H^+ excretion	Kidney

From Hedge GA, Colby HD, Goodman RL: *Clinical endocrine physiology,* Philadelphia, 1987, Saunders.

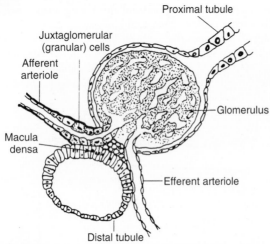

FIGURE 34-14 Diagrammatic representation of juxtaglomerular apparatus. (From Martin CR: *Endocrine physiology*, New York, 1985, Oxford University Press.)

tissue fluids; increased Na⁺ results in decreased renin release, and decreased Na⁺ results in increased renin release. In either case, the change produced tends to restore the mineralocorticoid concentrations to normal. In addition to the effect of sodium, the macula densa may control changes in the renin-angiotensin system through the sensing of changes in chloride ion (Cl^-) concentrations in tissue fluids.

Another major regulatory factor in the control of mineralocorticoid secretion is the blood potassium concentration. An increase in K⁺ concentration stimulates the zona glomerulosa to secrete mineralocorticoids, whereas a decline in K⁺ has the opposite effect. This stimulation is independent of the renin-angiotensin system.

It has been thought that corticotropin has minimal effect on control of the zona glomerulosa, because experimental studies showed that hypophysectomy has little effect on the zona glomerulosa. More recent studies have shown that cells of the zona glomerulosa have receptors for corticotropin, and corticotropin may play some role, although minor, in the control of mineralocorticoid secretion.

In contrast to the sodium-conserving effect of mineralocorticoids, the 28–amino acid *atrial natriuretic peptide* (ANP) reduces Na⁺ retention by the kidneys. ANP also causes peripheral vasodilation and thus a lowering of blood pressure. ANP may inhibit the production of mineralocorticoids and renin as well. ANP is produced by cells of the cardiac atria, but it is also produced in other sites, including the brain.

Hypoadrenocorticism

Hypoadrenocorticism, caused by lack of mineralocorticoids and glucocorticoids, is most often diagnosed in young female dogs and usually has an immune-mediated etiology. Certain breeds, such as Leonbergers, standard poodles, and Portuguese water dogs, are at increased risk for the disease; however, hypoadrenocorticism may be diagnosed in any breed. Addison's disease is a rare condition of young to middle-aged cats. Historical findings compatible with hypoadrenocorticism include intermittent vomiting, diarrhea, weight loss, lethargy, anorexia, and weakness. These symptoms often resolve with fluid therapy and corticosteroid treatment. Physical examination of animals in an acute hypoadrenal crisis reveals weak pulse, bradycardia, prolonged capillary refill time, severe mental slowness, and profound muscle

weakness. Clinical features of hypoadrenocorticism that should raise suspicion include a normal or slow heart rate in the presence of circulatory shock and the "waxing and waning" course of disease before collapse. Cats with hypoadrenocorticism may exhibit similar clinical signs; however, bradycardia is much less common.

Electrolyte abnormalities consisting of severe hyponatremia and hypochloremia associated with hyperkalemia are the hallmarks of hypoadrenocorticism. Azotemia and hyperphosphatemia also accompany primary hypoadrenocorticism, which makes it difficult to differentiate it from acute renal failure. Azotemia may be prerenal as a result of dehydration and hypovolemia, or increase in BUN may be caused by gastrointestinal hemorrhage. Hematological abnormalities consist of eosinophilia and lymphocytosis, or eosinophil and lymphocyte counts may be normal in the presence of severe metabolic stress. The anemia of hypoadrenocorticism has classically been attributed to lack of glucocorticoid effects on the bone marrow. However, more recent studies have suggested that hemorrhagic gastroenteritis contributes significantly to the anemia. Although hypoglycemia is more common with secondary or atypical hypoadrenocorticism, it is rarely seen with typical hypoadrenocorticism.

Urine specific gravity is frequently low, attributable to medullary washout (inadequate medullary gradient caused by sodium depletion) and decreased medullary blood flow. Dilute urine in the presence of azotemia and hyperkalemia may easily be mistaken for acute renal failure. Hormonal assays are necessary to confirm the presence or absence of adrenal disease and to differentiate between hypoadrenocorticism and renal failure.

Diagnosis of primary hypoadrenocorticism is based on clinical signs, classic electrolyte imbalances, and confirmation with a corticotropin response test. The baseline cortisol sample should be collected with the initial blood work, and synthetic corticotropin (cosyntropin [Cortrosyn], 0.25 mg) should be administered intravenously during the initial fluid therapy. A 1-hour, postcorticotropin sample may then be drawn, and glucocorticoids may be administered after the 1-hour sample is taken. Intramuscular injection of corticotropin (gel or synthetic) may not be absorbed in animals in circulatory shock; therefore, intravenous administration of synthetic corticotropin is preferred. If glucocorticoids must be administered before the measurement of cortisol, dexamethasone sodium phosphate is preferred because it does not interfere with the cortisol assay. Endogenous plasma corticotropin may be measured to determine whether the hypoadrenocorticism is primary or secondary.

Dogs and cats with primary hypoadrenocorticism exhibit a subnormal response to corticotropin administration. Both the baseline and the postcorticotropin cortisol concentrations are usually low or undetectable. Endogenous plasma corticotropin concentrations are dramatically increased in animals with primary hypoadrenocorticism as a result of loss of negative feedback to the pituitary gland, caused by decreased serum cortisol concentrations. In the case of secondary hypoadrenocorticism, caused by a pituitary deficiency of corticotropin, the endogenous corticotropin concentrations are typically decreased (<20 pg/mL). The response to exogenous corticotropin is diminished, but not as dramatically as for primary hypoadrenocorticism. Baseline and postcorticotropin cortisol concentrations may be in the normal range.

Hyperaldosteronism (Conn's Syndrome)

Hyperaldosteronism is caused by either an adrenal tumor hypersecreting aldosterone or bilateral adrenal hyperplasia; the condition is usually diagnosed in older cats and occasionally dogs. Oversecretion of aldosterone results in the classic electrolyte changes of hypokalemia (increased plasma K⁺), hypernatremia (elevated plasma Na⁺), and metabolic alkalosis (increased pH; opposite of Addison's disease). Tumors of the adrenal gland are usually benign. Clinical signs consist of muscle weakness and cervical ventroflexion in cats with aldosterone-secreting adrenal tumors. Less commonly, hypertension and blindness occur. In cats with bilateral adrenal hyperplasia, hypertension, blindness, and renal failure are more common than signs of hypokalemia (i.e., muscle weakness). Laboratory signs include hypokalemia, elevated creatine kinase (CK), and metabolic alkalosis in all adrenal tumors and less commonly with bilateral adrenal hyperplasia. Hypernatremia is seen in less than 30% of cases. Diagnosis is achieved by documentation of increased plasma aldosterone (N = 150 to 430 pmol/L), low to undetectable plasma renin, and/or increased plasma aldosterone concentration-to-plasma renin activity ratios (PAC:PRA; normal = 0.3 to 3.8) and visualization of bilateral adrenal hyperplasia or unilateral enlargement of the adrenal gland on ultrasound. Treatment of hyperaldosteronism consists of potassium supplementation (oral and intravenous), spironolactone, and calcium channel blockers for hypertension. Surgical removal of the adrenal tumor is usually curative.

THE ADRENAL MEDULLA

The adrenal medulla, as its name indicates, occupies the central portion of the adrenal gland (see Figure 34-7). A stimulatory effect of adrenal medullary extracts on cardiac activity was first recognized by Oliver and Schafer in 1894. Thereafter, the main hormone of the adrenal medulla, epinephrine, became the first hormone to be isolated (by Abel in 1898), crystallized (by Takamine and Aldrich in 1901), and synthesized (by Stolz in 1904). Theories on the importance of the adrenal medulla include that of Cannon, who in 1932 proposed the "fight or flight" hypothesis, in which the adrenal medulla is activated to aid in combating situations of extreme stress. Others advocated the "tonus" theory, which stated that cells of the adrenal medulla are constantly in a state of readiness. In fact, the adrenal medulla has a constant output of catecholamines that can be accentuated dramatically if the need arises.

It was recognized early in this research that cells of the adrenal medulla are the equivalent of postganglionic cells of the sympathetic nervous system. Therefore, it was assumed that *epinephrine* was the mediator of postganglionic activity of the sympathetic nervous system. It was later recognized that another catecholamine, *norepinephrine,* is the neurotransmitter of the sympathetic nervous system. Both epinephrine and norepinephrine are released when preganglionic nerve fibers to the adrenal medulla are stimulated; in fact, most of the norepinephrine found in plasma originates from the adrenal medulla. However, epinephrine is the major catecholamine secreted by the adrenal medulla of most mammals. Exceptions to this generalization include the dominance of norepinephrine over epinephrine in whales and chickens and in the fetal tissues of all species.

The Synthesis of Catecholamines Is from Tyrosine; the Main Catecholamine Synthesized by the Adrenal Medulla Is Epinephrine

The cells of the adrenal medulla that synthesize catecholamines are classified as *chromaffin cells.* This classification is based on the histochemical reaction of the cells when exposed to potassium dichromate, that is, a darkening of the cells as a result of the

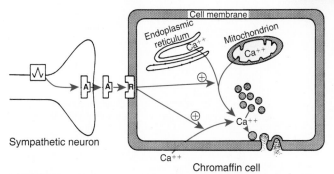

FIGURE 34-15 Stimulus-secretion coupling in the adrenal chromaffin cell. Note that cytosolic calcium may be derived from intracellular or extracellular sources. *Circled plus signs* indicate stimulation. *A,* Acetylcholine; *R,* receptor. (From Hedge GA, Colby HD, Goodman RL: *Clinical endocrine physiology,* Philadelphia, 1987, Saunders.)

formation of colored pigments in conjunction with the oxidation of the catecholamines. The cells that produce epinephrine are different from those that synthesize norepinephrine; accordingly, the type of chromaffin granule present is different for each cell type. In cattle the epinephrine-secreting cells tend to be on the outer edge of the medulla. *Acetylcholine* release from the preganglionic nerve fibers initiates the synthesis of the catecholamines by the medullary cells (Figure 34-15). Acetylcholine also stimulates the release of catecholamines from chromaffin granules, a phenomenon called *stimulus-secretion coupling.*

The synthesis of the catecholamines begins with either of the amino acids phenylalanine or *tyrosine.* However, tyrosine is a naturally occurring amino acid, and most synthesis of catecholamines begins with it (Figure 34-16). The initial step in the biosynthetic pathway begins with the conversion of tyrosine to 3,4-dihydroxyphenylalanine, or *DOPA.* Tyrosine hydroxylase, the enzyme responsible for the conversion of tyrosine, is the rate-limiting enzyme in the formation of catecholamines. The end products of tyrosine metabolism, including DOPA, dopamine, norepinephrine, and epinephrine, inhibit the activity of tyrosine hydroxylase. DOPA is converted to dopamine through the enzymatic activity of aromatic-L-amino acid decarboxylase (DOPA decarboxylase). To this point, the biochemical transformations have occurred in the cytosol. The conversion of dopamine to norepinephrine occurs within the chromaffin granule because the key enzyme, dopamine-β-hydroxylase, is localized within the granule (Figure 34-17).

If the cell secretes norepinephrine, the biochemical pathway is ended, and the hormone remains in the norepinephrine granule, ready for secretion. If the cell secretes epinephrine, norepinephrine moves back into the cytosol, where it is converted to epinephrine through the activity of phenylethanolamine-*N*-methyltransferase (PMNT). Epinephrine then moves into an epinephrine granule for storage before its release. The metabolism of catecholamines is rapid (2 minutes for norepinephrine, less for epinephrine), and is accomplished mainly by the liver and kidneys.

The importance of the anatomical association of the adrenal cortex and medulla may be related to the fact that cortisol is important for the activity of the enzyme PMNT. The chromaffin cells are located close to the venous sinuses that drain the adrenal cortex and therefore are exposed to venous effluent that contains high concentrations of cortisol.

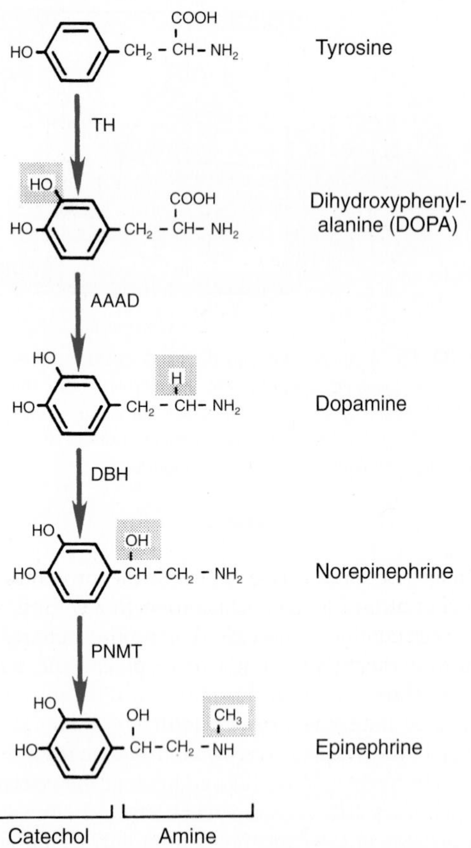

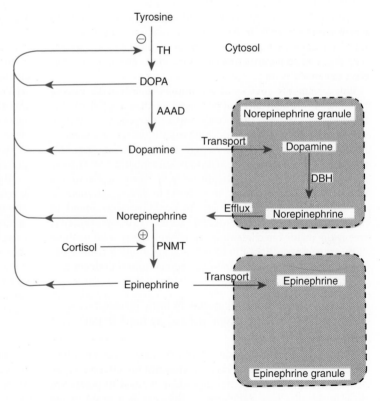

FIGURE 34-16 Pathway of catecholamine synthesis in the adrenal medulla. *Shaded areas* denote the structural changes occurring at each step. *AAAD,* Aromatic-L-amino acid decarboxylase; *DBH,* dopamine-β-hydroxylase; *PNMT,* phenylethanolamine-*N*-methyltransferase; *TH,* tyrosine hydroxylase. (From Hedge GA, Colby HD, Goodman RL: *Clinical endocrine physiology,* Philadelphia, 1987, Saunders.)

The Primary Actions of Catecholamines Are on Metabolism, Especially Effects that Increase the Concentration of Glucose

The actions of the catecholamines involve the regulation of intermediary metabolism, as well as responses that allow animals to adjust to situations involving acute stress. The actions of catecholamines are mediated through adrenergic receptors located on target tissues (Figure 34-18). There are two major types of adrenergic receptors, alpha (α) and beta (β), which are subdivided into α_1, α_2, β_1, and β_2. The α-adrenergic receptors control catecholamine release from sympathetic nerve endings, with α_1 affecting postsynaptic nerve endings and α_2 affecting presynaptic terminals. The β_1 receptors affect mainly the heart, and β_2 receptors affect smooth muscle contraction and intermediary metabolism. Whereas all adrenergic receptors are responsive to both epinephrine and norepinephrine, the responses to the two catecholamines are different. In addition, the receptor types on various tissues vary in number, which, together with the different responses of adrenergic receptors on tissues, results in variable adrenergic responses being produced by a particular catecholamine.

The metabolic effects of catecholamines are mediated mainly by β_2 receptors. Because epinephrine is 10 times more potent than norepinephrine with β_2 receptors, epinephrine plays a much more important role in the control of intermediary metabolism than does norepinephrine. The effects of epinephrine on glucose metabolism are similar to those of glucagon and opposite to those of insulin. Epinephrine increases blood glucose concentrations, with the effect mainly in the liver; that is, epinephrine promotes both hepatic glycogenolysis and gluconeogenesis. Epinephrine also stimulates glycogenolysis in skeletal muscle, which in this situation is in contrast with the action of glucagon. Because glucose-6-phosphatase is not present in skeletal muscle, lactate is produced instead of glucose; the liver takes up lactate and

FIGURE 34-17 Regulation of catecholamine biosynthesis in the adrenal medulla. *Plus sign* indicates stimulation; minus sign indicates inhibition. *AAAD,* Aromatic-L-amino acid decarboxylase; *DBH,* dopamine-β-hydroxylase; *DOPA,* dihydroxyphenylalanine; *PNMT,* phenylethanolamine-*N*-methyltransferase; *TH,* tyrosine hydroxylase. (From Hedge GA, Colby HD, Goodman RL: *Clinical endocrine physiology,* Philadelphia, 1987, Saunders.)

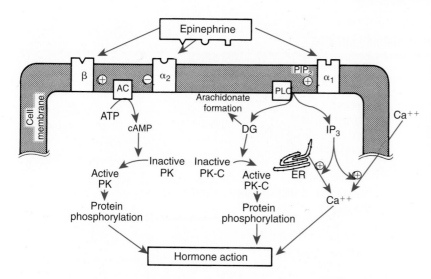

FIGURE 34-18 Mechanisms of action of epinephrine in target cells mediated by β-, α_2-, and α_1-adrenergic receptors. *Plus signs* indicate stimulation; *minus sign* indicates inhibition. *AC,* Adenyl cyclase; *ATP,* adenosine triphosphate; *cAMP,* cyclic adenosine monophosphate; *DG,* diacylglycerol; *ER,* endoplasmic reticulum; *IP₃,* inositol 1,4,5-triphosphate; *PIP₂,* phosphatidylinositol 4,5-bisphosphate; *PK,* protein kinase; *PK-C,* protein kinase C; *PLC,* phospholipase C. (From Hedge GA, Colby HD, Goodman RL: *Clinical endocrine physiology,* Philadelphia, 1987, Saunders.)

converts it to glucose. Additional effects on glucose metabolism include the inhibition of insulin secretion (through α receptors) and stimulation of glucagon secretion by the pancreas; both actions increase blood glucose concentrations.

Epinephrine promotes lipolysis through interaction with two receptors on adipose cells. Activation of a lipase enzyme results in an increase in free fatty acids in the blood. Glucocorticoids potentiate the effect of epinephrine on lipolysis.

Catecholamines stimulate cardiac function. Both epinephrine and norepinephrine interact with β_1 receptors to increase both the force of contraction and the heart rate, the latter resulting from the promotion of a shorter period of diastolic depolarization. Whereas both catecholamines promote arteriolar constriction through interaction with α receptors, epinephrine, through its high affinity for β_2 receptors, causes the dilation of blood vessels both in the heart and in skeletal muscle. The end result is that total peripheral resistance is decreased by the action of epinephrine, with a concomitant decline in diastolic pressure; however, blood pressure is minimally changed, and cardiac output increases because of the increase in heart rate. The action of epinephrine to increase cardiac output is an obvious beneficial effect in situations that are described as "fight or flight."

Catecholamines affect smooth muscle. Epinephrine causes relaxation of bronchial smooth muscle, particularly when the muscle is in a contracted state. Because the action is mediated through β_2 receptors, norepinephrine has little effect on bronchial smooth muscle. Epinephrine causes relaxation of the smooth muscle of the gastrointestinal (GI) tract through interaction with β_2 receptors. Catecholamine stimulation of β-adrenergic receptors results in contraction of uterine smooth muscle, and stimulation of β_2 receptors results in relaxation. Because of its dominant effect on β_2 receptors, epinephrine causes relaxation of the uterus, whereas both epinephrine and norepinephrine interact with α receptors to cause contraction.

The effects of the catecholamines on bladder smooth muscle depend on different locations of α and β receptors; α-adrenergic receptors are located within the neck of the bladder, and β-adrenergic receptors are located within the body of the bladder. Epinephrine relaxes the body and contracts the neck of the bladder; norepinephrine contracts the neck of the bladder. The net effect is retention of urine.

Although the parasympathetic nervous system is the principal system involved in penile erection, the sympathetic nervous system may also play a role. Epinephrine promotes erection through vasodilation of the vasculature mediated by β receptors. Higher concentrations of epinephrine (and norepinephrine) can cause ejaculation through α-receptor interaction and vasoconstriction.

In the eye, epinephrine causes relaxation of the lens through stimulation of β receptors on the ciliary muscles. It causes dilation of the pupil through stimulation of α receptors, with resultant contraction of the radial muscle of the iris.

The effects of epinephrine on the CNS are excitatory. Drugs that affect the CNS probably do so by modulation of catecholamine concentrations, whereby sedation is associated with lower values of epinephrine. Other effects of catecholamine include the promotion of sweating and piloerection. Epinephrine also increases renin production by the renal juxtaglomerular cells. Table 34-5 summarizes the effects of catecholamines.

The Main Factors That Stimulate Catecholamine Secretion Are Hypoglycemia and Conditions That Produce Stress

Any factor that increases sympathetic nervous system stimulation of the adrenal medulla results in the immediate secretion of catecholamines. The main physiological factor that influences catecholamine secretion is hypoglycemia. In this situation, epinephrine secretion is stimulated by decreases in blood glucose concentrations that are within normal physiological limits. In contrast, other parts of the sympathetic nervous system are depressed by decreases in blood glucose levels. Factors that elicit a massive release of catecholamines are categorized as "stressful," particularly those that are acute. Catecholamines are especially important for the maintenance of blood pressure in conjunction with severe blood loss; decreased blood pressure stimulates epinephrine secretion. Catecholamines are also important for adaptation to cold exposure in terms of increased heat production; decreased temperature increases epinephrine secretion. The response to acute stress can be particularly marked, because each preganglionic sympathetic neuron that supplies the adrenal medulla affects a number of chromaffin cells; that is, the signal is greatly amplified.

HORMONES OF THE PANCREAS

The pancreas has important endocrine and nonendocrine functions. The nonendocrine functions result from activity of the

TABLE 34-5 Responses of Target Tissues to Catecholamines

Target Tissue	Receptor Type	Responses
Liver	β_2	Glycogenolysis, lipolysis, gluconeogenesis
Adipose tissue	β_2	Lipolysis
Skeletal muscle	β_2	Glycogenolysis
Pancreas	α_2	Decreased insulin secretion
	β_2	Increased insulin secretion
Cardiovascular system	β_1	Increased heart rate, increased contractility, increased conduction velocity
	α_2	Vasoconstriction
	β_2	Vasodilation in skeletal muscle arterioles, coronary arteries, and all veins
Bronchial muscle	β_2	Relaxation
Gastrointestinal tract	β_2	Decreased contractility
Urinary bladder	α_2	Sphincter contraction
	β_2	Detrusor relaxation
Uterus	α_2	Contraction
	β_2	Relaxation
Male sex organs	α_2	Ejaculation, detumescence
	β_2	Erection?
Eye	α_1	Radial muscle contraction
	β_2	Ciliary muscle relaxation
Central nervous system	α_2	Stimulation
Skin	α_2	Piloerection, sweat production
Renin secretion	β_1	Stimulation

From Hedge GA, Colby HD, Goodman RL: *Clinical endocrine physiology,* Philadelphia, 1987, Saunders.

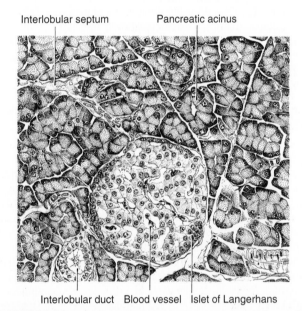

FIGURE 34-19 Depiction of section through the pancreas of the rat. The islet of Langerhans is a gland of internal secretion, whereas the surrounding acinar tissue forms an exocrine gland. (From Turner CD, Bagnara JT: *General endocrinology,* ed 6, Philadelphia, 1976, Saunders.)

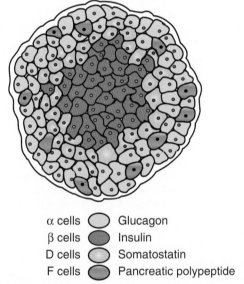

α cells	Glucagon
β cells	Insulin
D cells	Somatostatin
F cells	Pancreatic polypeptide

FIGURE 34-20 Depiction of the pancreatic islet. (From McDonald LE: *Veterinary endocrinology and reproduction,* ed 4, Philadelphia, 1989, Lea & Febiger.)

exocrine part of the pancreas and are involved in GI function. The endocrine portion of the pancreas is organized as discrete islets (islets of Langerhans) that contain four cell types, each of which produces a different hormone (Figure 34-19). The most numerous of the islet cells are β cells, which produce insulin; α cells produce glucagon; D cells produce somatostatin; and F or PP cells produce pancreatic polypeptide (Figure 34-20). Although these hormones have different functions, all are involved in the control of metabolism and, more specifically, in glucose homeostasis.

Insulin

The first studies that associated the pancreas with carbohydrate metabolism were done by von Mering and Minkowski in 1889,

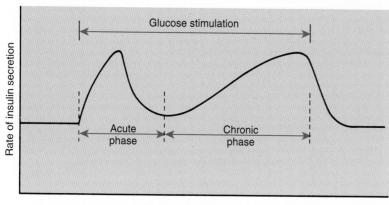

FIGURE 34-21 Kinetics of insulin secretion by the β cell in response to a continued glucose stimulus. (From Hedge GA, Colby HD, Goodman RL: *Clinical endocrine physiology,* Philadelphia, 1987, Saunders.)

when they showed that pancreatectomy of dogs resulted in signs similar to those characteristic of diabetes mellitus. Later, Banting and Best were able to show that injection of pancreatic extracts could alleviate the signs of diabetes mellitus in dogs and humans. Able was the first to crystallize insulin, and its structure was elucidated by Sanger in 1960.

Insulin is a protein consisting of two chains, designated A (21 amino acids) and B (30 amino acids), that are connected by two disulfide bridges. The monomer form of the hormone is thought to be the active form; insulin also exists in dimer and hexamer forms, the latter complexed with two zinc molecules. Although there are some differences in amino acid composition among species, the differences are small; for example, cattle, sheep, horses, dogs, and whales differ only in positions 8, 9, and 10 of the A chain. As a result, the biological activities of insulin are not highly species specific. Of the domestic species, feline insulin is most similar to bovine insulin, and canine insulin is identical to porcine insulin in its amino acid structure.

The Synthesis of Insulin Is Biphasic: an Acute Phase Involves the Release of Preformed Insulin, and a Chronic Phase Involves the Synthesis of Protein

The synthesis of insulin, similar to that of other peptide hormones, begins with the formation of a linear polypeptide preproinsulin within the rough endoplasmic reticulum. A small peptide fragment is removed to form proinsulin. Proinsulin is coiled, and the end fragments are joined by disulfide bonds. Proinsulin is transferred to the Golgi apparatus, where it is further processed and packaged into granules that contain both insulin and the connecting or C peptide (33 amino acids in length).

The secretion of insulin follows biphasic kinetics in response to appropriate stimuli (Figure 34-21). The initial, acute release of insulin involves the exocytosis of preformed insulin from secretion granules. After the acute phase, a chronic phase of secretion occurs that involves the synthesis of protein and thus probably the synthesis of insulin.

The Metabolism of Insulin Involves Splitting the A and B Chains and Reducing the Chains to Amino Acids and Peptides

Insulin is metabolized mainly by the liver and kidneys. Enzymes that are present reduce the disulfide bonds that link the A and B chains, and the chains are then subjected to protease activity, which reduces them to peptides and amino acids. The half-life of insulin is about 10 minutes.

The Main Metabolic Functions of Insulin Are Anabolic

Insulin acts at a number of sites within the metabolic pathways of carbohydrates, fats, and proteins (Figure 34-22). It is important to realize that the liver is an especially important target organ, in part because the pancreatic venous effluent passes directly to the liver. The net effect of the actions of insulin is to lower blood concentrations of glucose, fatty acids, and amino acids and to promote intracellular conversion of these compounds to their storage forms: glycogen, triglycerides, and protein, respectively (Table 34-6). Glucose does not readily penetrate cell membranes except in a few tissues, such as brain, liver, and red and white blood cells, all of which must have continual access to glucose. The presence of insulin is critical to the movement of glucose through the plasma membrane into the cell.

Insulin has profound effects on carbohydrate metabolism. Insulin facilitates the use of glucose: namely, glycolysis, which involves the oxidation of glucose to pyruvate and lactate through the induction of enzymes, such as glucokinase, phosphofructokinase, and pyruvate kinase. Insulin promotes glycogen production in the liver, in adipose tissue, and in skeletal muscle by increasing glycogen synthetase activity with a concomitant decrease in glycogen phosphorylase activity. Gluconeogenesis is decreased by insulin because of the promotion of protein synthesis in peripheral tissues, thereby decreasing the amount of amino acids available for gluconeogenesis. In addition, insulin decreases the activities of hepatic enzymes (fructose 1,6-bisphosphate aldolase, pyruvate carboxylase, phosphoenolpyruvate carboxylase, and glucose-6-phosphatase) that are involved in the conversion of amino acids to glucose.

In adipose tissue, insulin promotes the synthesis of triglycerides. Insulin facilitates the intracellular use of glucose, which results in increased levels of pyruvate, a precursor of acetyl-coenzyme A (acetyl-CoA) (in turn, a precursor of fatty acids) and increased glycerol-3-phosphate for the esterification of fatty acids. Insulin activates the enzymes pyruvate dehydrogenase and acetyl-CoA carboxylase, which promote the synthesis of fatty acids from acetyl-CoA. Insulin also increases the activity of lipoprotein lipase located in the endothelium of capillaries of extrahepatic tissues, which promotes the movement of fatty acids into adipose tissue. Finally, insulin decreases lipolysis in adipose tissue.

With protein metabolism, insulin promotes uptake of amino acids by most tissues, including skeletal muscle, but not liver. Insulin promotes protein synthesis and inhibits protein degradation. Therefore, insulin promotes the maintenance of a positive

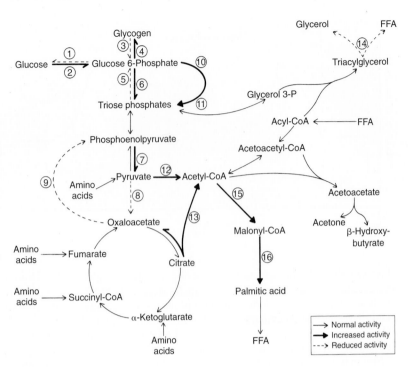

FIGURE 34-22 Metabolic pathways affected by insulin. The numbers correspond to each of the following enzymes: *1,* glucose-6-phosphatase; *2,* glucokinase; *3,* phosphorylase; *4,* glycogen synthase; *5,* fructose-1,6-bisphosphate aldolase; *6,* 6-phosphofructokinase; *7,* pyruvate kinase; *8,* pyruvate carboxylase; *9,* phosphoenolpyruvate carboxykinase; *10,* glucose-6-phosphate-dehydrogenase; *11,* 6-phosphogluconate dehydrogenase; *12,* pyruvate dehydrogenase; *13,* adenosine triphosphate (ATP)–citrate lyase; *14,* hormone-sensitive lipase; *15,* acetyl–coenzyme A (CoA) carboxylase; *16,* fatty-acid synthase. *FFA,* Free fatty acid. (From Hedge GA, Colby HD, Goodman RL: *Clinical endocrine physiology,* Philadelphia, 1987, Saunders.)

TABLE 34-6 Sites of Action and Effects of Insulin on Carbohydrate, Lipid, and Protein Metabolism

	Site of Action		
Process Affected	**Liver**	**Muscle**	**Adipose**
Carbohydrate Metabolism			
↑Glucose transport		X	X
↑Glycogen synthesis	X	X	X
↓Glycogenolysis	X	X	X
↓Gluconeogenesis	X		
Lipid Metabolism			
↑Lipogenesis	X		X
↓Lipolysis	X		X
Protein Metabolism			
↑Amino acid uptake		X	
↑Protein synthesis		X	
↓Protein degradation		X	
↓Gluconeogenesis	X		

From Hedge GA, Colby HD, Goodman RL: *Clinical endocrine physiology,* Philadelphia, 1987, Saunders.

nitrogen balance. With insulin deficiency, protein catabolism increases, with increased amounts of amino acids available for hepatic gluconeogenesis and a resultant increase in the blood glucose concentrations.

The most important factor in the control of insulin secretion is the concentration of blood glucose. Increased concentrations of blood glucose initiate the synthesis and release of insulin by the β cells of the pancreatic islets (Figure 34-23). Two theories explain the mechanism of cellular induction of insulin synthesis and release. In the first, insulin exists within the plasma membrane, whereby glucose interacts with a membrane receptor protein that directs intracellular events toward the synthesis and release of insulin. In the second theory, insulin occurs at the intracellular level, whereby the metabolism of glucose produces the signal for insulin synthesis and release. Glucose control of insulin secretion is a positive-feedback system in which increased concentrations of glucose lead to increased concentrations of insulin.

Because the oral administration of glucose produces a greater insulin response than systemic administration, factors from the intestinal tract were thought to affect insulin secretion. It is now known that a number of GI hormones stimulate insulin secretion, including gastrin, cholecystokinin, secretin, and gastric inhibitory peptide. The presence of amino acids and fatty acids in the intestinal tract also stimulates the release of insulin, although with less potency than that of glucose (Box 34-1).

Hormones other than those from the GI tract are important for the control of insulin secretion. Glucagon from the α cells of the pancreas has a direct stimulatory effect on the β cells to secrete insulin. Conversely, somatostatin inhibits the secretion of insulin. Both hormones work through the adenyl cyclase system, glucagon being stimulatory and somatostatin being inhibitory. Catecholamines tend to decrease insulin secretion through an interaction with the α-adrenergic receptors on the β cells. Whereas epinephrine is the main circulating catecholamine that affects insulin secretion, norepinephrine also influences insulin secretion because the pancreas has adrenergic innervation by the autonomic nervous system. The pancreas also has cholinergic innervation by the autonomic nervous system, and in contrast to adrenergic stimulation, cholinergic activity increases insulin secretion through the release of acetylcholine.

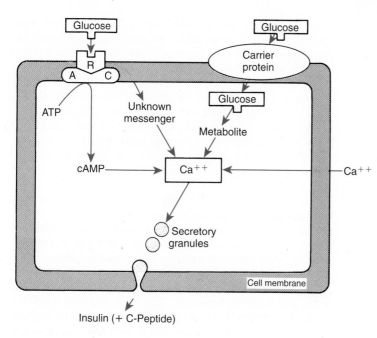

FIGURE 34-23 Proposed mechanisms of action of glucose on insulin secretion by the β cell. *AC,* Adenyl cyclase; *ATP,* adenosine triphosphate; *R,* receptor; *cAMP,* cyclic adenosine monophosphate. (From Hedge GA, Colby HD, Goodman RL: *Clinical endocrine physiology,* Philadelphia, 1987, Saunders.)

Insulin Deficiency Produces Diabetes Mellitus, Which Can Culminate in Diabetic Ketoacidosis

A lack or deficiency of insulin produces a syndrome called *diabetes mellitus* (DM). DM may be *type 1,* which is most common in dogs, or *type 2,* which is most common in cats. Type 1 DM is caused by an autoimmune destruction of the β cells of the pancreas; it leads to absolute insulin deficiency and a propensity to develop ketosis. *Diabetic ketoacidosis* (DKA) is the culmination of DM that results in unrestrained ketone body formation in the liver, metabolic acidosis, severe dehydration, shock, and possibly death. Hepatic lipid metabolism becomes deranged with insulin deficiency, and nonesterified fatty acids are converted to acetyl-CoA rather than incorporated into triglycerides. Acetyl-CoA accumulates in the liver and is converted into acetoacetyl-CoA, then ultimately to ketones, including acetoacetic acid, β-hydroxybutyrate (primary ketone in dogs and cats), and acetone.

As insulin deficiency culminates in DKA, accumulation of ketones and lactic acid in the blood and loss of electrolytes and water in the urine result in profound dehydration, hypovolemia, metabolic acidosis, and shock. Ketonuria and osmotic diuresis, resulting from glycosuria, cause sodium and potassium loss in the urine, exacerbating hypovolemia and dehydration. Nausea, anorexia, and vomiting, caused by stimulation of the chemoreceptor trigger zone through ketonemia and hyperglycemia, contribute to the dehydration caused by osmotic diuresis. Dehydration leads to further accumulation of glucose and ketones in the blood. Stress hormones such as cortisol and epinephrine contribute to the hyperglycemia in a vicious cycle. Eventually, severe dehydration may result in hyperviscosity, thromboembolism, severe metabolic acidosis, renal failure, and finally death.

Historical Findings. Most dogs and cats with DKA present with a previous history of uncomplicated diabetes, including polyuria, polydipsia, and dramatic rapid weight loss in the presence of a good or even ravenous appetite. More recent historical findings include anorexia, weakness, depression, vomiting, and diarrhea. Occasionally, owners fail to notice the significance of the classic signs of DM, and the animals are presented solely with an acute history of DKA. DKA may also develop in previously well-controlled, treated diabetic patients.

Physical Examination Findings. The most common examination findings in DKA are lethargy and depression, dehydration, unkempt hair coat, and muscle wasting. Hepatomegaly is common in both diabetic cats and diabetic dogs. Cataracts are often observed in diabetic dogs. A plantigrade rear limb stance resulting from diabetic neuropathy is often observed in diabetic cats. Other findings include tachypnea, dehydration, weakness, vomiting, and occasionally a strong acetone breath odor. Cats may present recumbent or comatose, which may be a manifestation of mixed ketotic-hyperosmolar syndrome. Icterus can develop from the complicating factors of hemolysis, hepatic lipidosis, and acute pancreatitis.

Laboratory Findings. Glucose level is greatly elevated. The average blood glucose concentration in patients with DKA is 25 mmol/L. Values can range from 10 mmol/L to greater than 50 mmol/L, but the latter is more characteristic of hyperosmolar coma. Although portable glucose meters are typically used to monitor glucose concentrations in DKA, caution is advised in relying on these monitors for baseline glucose concentrations because of inaccuracies in animals with severe hyperglycemia. All DKA patients have a relative or absolute deficiency of insulin and excessive hepatic production of glucose, resulting in hyperglycemia. Hyperglycemia is further exacerbated by dehydration and the corresponding reduction in GFR, and these factors are important determinants of its severity. This is supported by the findings that (1) glucose concentrations should exceed 25 mmol/L only when dehydration is severe enough to reduce GFR, and thus the ability of the kidneys to excrete glucose, and (2) fluid administration alone can significantly reduce blood glucose concentrations.

Osmolality usually is mildly to extremely increased in the DKA patient as a result of hyperglycemia, but this may not be detected, in part because of concurrent hyponatremia. Sodium (and to a lesser extent potassium), glucose, and urea concentrations are the determinants of the calculated serum osmolality. Reference values for serum osmolality in dogs and cats are approximately 290 to 310 mOsm/kg. Hyperosmolality is generally mild enough to resolve with intravenous fluid and insulin therapies.

Nonketotic hyperosmolar diabetes is defined by extreme hyperglycemia (>30 mmol/L), hyperosmolality (>350 mOsm/L), severe dehydration, and CNS depression, without ketone formation and with absent or mild metabolic acidosis. Affected patients are more likely to have underlying renal or cardiovascular disease and to be non–insulin dependent. Although this specific syndrome, as defined in humans, is infrequently encountered in veterinary medicine, ketotic or nonketotic diabetic cats may be seen, with significant hyperosmolality and CNS alterations.

Most patients with DKA have a total body K$^+$ deficit caused by urinary (osmotic diuresis), anorexia, and GI losses (vomiting, anorexia). The metabolic acidosis, relative or absolute insulin deficiency, and serum hypertonicity combine to cause a K$^+$ shift from the intracellular to the extracellular compartment. This is capable of masking the severity of total-body hypokalemia when plasma concentrations are measured. Insulin therapy, as well as correction of the acid-base disturbance with fluids and bicarbonate, will drive serum K$^+$ intracellularly, potentially causing marked circulating hypokalemia. Polyuric patients are predisposed to severe hypokalemia, whereas oliguric or anuric patients are predisposed to severe hyperkalemia.

In general, DKA causes significant total-body Na$^+$ deficits. Excessive urinary loss of Na$^+$ results from the osmotic diuresis induced by high glucose and ketone concentrations and the lack of insulin, which usually aids in reabsorption of Na$^+$ from the distal nephron. Hyperglucagonemia, vomiting, and diarrhea also contribute to the total-body Na$^+$ loss. Hyperosmolality may contribute to a low Na$^+$ concentration because as osmolality increases, water is drawn from the interstitium into the vascular space, thus diluting plasma Na$^+$ and Cl$^-$.

Phosphorus is the major intracellular anion and is important for energy production and for maintenance of cell membranes. Concentrations are regulated by dietary intake, renal elimination, factors promoting its movement into and out of cells, and vitamin D and parathyroid interactions. In DKA, circulating concentrations are usually within reference range or increased initially because of dehydration and renal disease. Phosphorus may also be low at presentation because of urinary loss from osmotic diuresis. As long as renal function is not compromised, a significant decrease in phosphorus should be anticipated with therapy. After insulin administration, phosphorus shifts to the intracellular compartment with glucose. Clinical signs of hypophosphatemia, such as hemolytic anemia (also seen with Heinz bodies in DKA), lethargy, depression, and diarrhea, may develop once concentrations reach 0.32 mmol/L. Oversupplementation of phosphorus should be avoided because hypocalcemia or metastatic calcification may result.

Magnesium (total serum) is not usually measured routinely, but concentrations may be abnormal in DKA. A recent study in cats demonstrated high total serum magnesium concentrations at presentation in those with DKA; after 48 hours of therapy, however, total serum magnesium concentrations were significantly decreased. Magnesium deficiency may be caused by poor oral intake, decreased intestinal absorption, increased renal loss, or changes in distribution because it is the second most abundant intracellular cation. Clinical signs of hypomagnesemia include neuromuscular weakness and cardiac arrhythmias, signs that can be seen with other electrolyte alterations. Hypomagnesemia can also cause decreases in other electrolytes, such as potassium and calcium. Correction of deficits may resolve electrolyte disturbances and may improve clinical outcome in the severely deficient patient.

Liver enzyme elevations are common in DM patients. Further increases potentially occur in DKA. Alanine aminotransferase and aspartate aminotransferase are most often affected, increasing secondary to hypovolemia and poor hepatic blood flow, with subsequent hepatocellular damage. Further increases in serum alkaline phosphatase concentration may occur if pancreatitis and secondary cholestasis ensue. Cholesterol and triglycerides may be elevated secondary to derangements of lipid metabolism resulting from decreased insulin.

Metabolic acidosis is one of the most prominent features of DKA. As ketone bodies accumulate in the blood and overwhelm the body's buffering capabilities, there is an increase in hydrogen ions and a decrease in bicarbonate. As dehydration worsens, blood flow to peripheral tissues decreases, and the resulting lactic acidosis may contribute to the acid-base disturbance. Acidosis may manifest as lethargy, vomiting, hyperventilation, decreased myocardial contractility, peripheral vasodilation, stupor, and coma. Initiation of insulin therapy (to stop ketogenesis) and fluid therapy (to correct dehydration) will help improve the metabolic acidosis in most patients. Bicarbonate supplementation should be pursued with caution and is generally not recommended unless the patient's blood pH is less than 7.1 or serum bicarbonate is less than 12 mmol/L.

Anion gap may be normal or elevated. An elevated value further characterizes the metabolic acidosis caused by DKA. The anion gap is a representation of the circulating anions not routinely measured on biochemical analyses. The normal anion gap ranges from 10 to 20 and is calculated by the following equation:

$$Osmolality\ (mOsm) = 2(Na^+ + K^+\ [mEq/L]) + Glucose\ (mmol/L) + BUN\ (mmol/L)$$

In DKA the ketones become unmeasured anions as they dissociate from ketoacids. However, if significant dehydration is present secondary to the osmotic diuresis and vomiting, lactic acidosis secondary to tissue hypoxia may contribute to the unmeasured anions, thus increasing the anion gap.

Circulating urea and creatinine concentrations may be within reference range or high. These values are high in most patients because of severe dehydration, but renal insufficiency or failure is also a possible cause. Increases in urea and creatinine must be evaluated in light of the urine specific gravity. A low urine specific gravity at presentation does not always guarantee a diagnosis of renal insufficiency or failure, because osmotic diuresis and chronic hypokalemia can contribute to low specific gravities in DM patients. Therefore, reevaluation of urea, creatinine, and urine specific gravity must be done after treatment of the crisis. If urea and creatinine are initially elevated and remain static or increase with appropriate therapy, concurrent renal disease is strongly suspected.

The most important part of urinalysis is measurement of glucose and ketones. A strongly positive glucose result confirms DM, and a positive result for ketones confirms DKA. However, a negative ketone result does not definitively rule out ketosis. The nitroprusside reagent used in urine sticks detects only acetoacetate and acetone. It is not as sensitive for β-hydroxybutyrate, the most prevalent ketone body, and therefore may be negative in the presence of ketosis. A recent study reported that β-hydroxybutyrate concentrations greater than 1.9 mmol/L were the most sensitive indicator of DKA, and values greater than 4.8 mmol/L were highly specific for its diagnosis. Using a cutoff value of 3.8 mmol/L was associated with the best combination of specificity (95%) and sensitivity (72%) for DKA.

The presence of pyuria and hematuria on urinalysis, along with confirmation by examination of urine sediment, supports the presence of UTI. However, urine culture should be performed regardless of urine sediment activity.

The hemogram may be normal at presentation but usually reveals a leukocytosis with a mature neutrophilia (common in cats) or a stress leukogram. There may be a regenerative or degenerative left shift suggestive of a severe inflammatory and infectious process. The red blood cell count and hematocrit may be elevated as a result of dehydration. Heinz bodies, with or without anemia, may be noted in cats because feline hemoglobin is uniquely susceptible to oxidative damage.

Concurrent Disease. Frequently, an underlying stressful event precipitates the shift from DM to DKA or nonketotic hyperosmolar DM. Impaired immune function secondary to DM increases the risk of infections. The precipitating event may be a UTI or other viral or bacterial infection or inflammatory disorder, such as pancreatitis, pyelonephritis, cholangiohepatitis, inflammatory bowel disease (IBD), eosinophilic granuloma complex, prostatitis, pyometra, upper respiratory infection, or pneumonia. Other concurrent diseases may include renal insufficiency or failure, hepatic lipidosis, neoplasia, and congestive heart failure. Recent drug therapy may also precipitate a crisis, especially administration of corticosteroids or progestagens. Therefore, further diagnostic testing of the diabetic patient that presents in a crisis is essential, particularly abdominal radiography or ultrasonography, as well as thoracic radiography and echocardiography if indicated. Additional testing for concurrent endocrine diseases, such as hyperthyroidism in cats and hypothyroidism and hyperadrenocorticism in dogs, may also be indicated but should be postponed until some control of the DM is achieved, because uncontrolled disease may affect the results of the tests.

Ancillary tests for pancreatitis include abdominocentesis or diagnostic peritoneal lavage if pancreatitis is suspected. Serum amylase and lipase, if determined on presentation, may be elevated in the absence of pancreatitis, secondary to severe dehydration or renal insufficiency, and demonstration of an elevated circulating concentration of trypsin-like immunoreactivity (TLI) may be preferable. Cats and dogs with acute necrotizing pancreatitis usually present with vomiting, abdominal pain, and concurrent DKA. Physical examination findings include icterus, cranial abdominal pain, and abdominal effusion. Radiographs may reveal a "ground glass" appearance of the abdomen, and abdominal ultrasound usually shows enlargement and hypoechogenicity of the pancreas. Concurrent hepatopathies are often present in patients with DKA, but evaluation is complicated by the effect of both DM and DKA on liver enzymes and liver function tests. Ultrasonography may be more useful in these cases. Diagnostic peritoneal lavage is usually necessary to demonstrate inflammatory, nonseptic peritonitis, and abdominal lipase is usually increased dramatically in affected cats and dogs.

Dietary Management Is an Important Consideration in Therapy for Feline Type 2 Diabetes

Type 2 DM is caused by insulin resistance and secondary β-cell failure. Type 2 DM may be managed using oral hypoglycemic agents, diet, or insulin. DM is one of the most common feline endocrinopathies, affecting 1 in 300 cats. The pathogenesis of type 2 DM in cats is reviewed earlier. Diagnosis of DM can be challenging, particularly in the early stages when the cats are non–insulin dependent. However, when clinical signs of diabetes are observed (polyuria, polydipsia, neuropathy), many cats may still benefit from alternatives to insulin therapy. In general, the primary abnormalities associated with type 2 DM, such as obesity and insulin resistance, are reversible. Insulin secretory ability, however, may be reversible (glucose toxicity) or irreversible (pancreatic amyloid deposition). In cats the differentiation of insulin-dependent (type 1) DM and non–insulin-dependent (type 2) DM is virtually impossible before treatment; therefore the clinician may have to rely on the response to oral hypoglycemic agents as a guide to whether the cat has sufficient β-cell function to be managed with oral hypoglycemic agents.

Goals of therapy for DM include restoration of normal fasting serum glucose concentrations, normalization of serum fructosamine, and reversal or attenuation of chronic complications, such as diabetic neuropathy and nephropathy. As in human patients with type 2 DM, the best approach to cats is a stepwise progression from dietary management to oral hypoglycemics and finally to insulin therapy when "islet burnout" occurs.

Exercise and diet is the cornerstone of therapy in human patients with type 2 DM. In most diabetic cats, exercise is not a reasonable option. One mechanism by which cats may be encouraged to exercise is by feeding the cat multiple small meals hidden in various places within the house. For example, an obese diabetic cat might be encouraged to jump up on the refrigerator or counter to find small amounts of food and then have to hunt for the rest of the food at the opposite end of the house.

In human diabetic patients, fiber supplementation is beneficial in the management of the disease. In humans and dogs, increased amounts of fiber slow the rate of glucose absorption from the intestine and minimize the postprandial fluctuations in blood glucose. This allows better glycemic control and correction of obesity; however, the data in cats are less compelling. In the only study of high-fiber diets in cats, 9 of 13 diabetic cats showed significant improvement in glycemic control with consumption of a high-fiber diet. Examples of high-fiber diets include prescription diet w/d and r/d, Science Diet Maintenance Light, Purina OM, and Iams Less Active. Because many cats find high-fiber diets unpalatable, soluble fiber such as psyllium can be mixed into the cat's regular food, and glycemic control may still be enhanced. If the cat's weight is normal at the start of therapy, the diet should be fed at a maintenance level of 60 to 70 kcal/kg/day. If the patient is obese, caloric intake should be limited to 70% to 75% of the energy needs for the cat's optimal weight.

The cat is an obligate carnivore and as such is unique among mammals in its insulin response to dietary carbohydrates, protein, and fat. The feline liver exhibits normal hexokinase activity, but glucokinase activity is virtually absent. *Glucokinase* converts glucose to glycogen for storage in the liver and is important in "mopping up" excess postprandial glucose. Normal cats are similar to diabetic humans because glucokinase levels drop precipitously with persistent hyperglycemia in humans with type 2 DM. Amino acids, rather than glucose, are the signal for insulin release in cats. In fact, a recent study demonstrated more effective assessment of insulin reserve in cats using the arginine response test rather than a glucose tolerance test. Another unusual aspect of feline metabolism is the increase in hepatic gluconeogenesis seen after a normal meal. Normal cats maintain essential glucose requirements from gluconeogenic precursors (i.e., amino acids) rather than from dietary carbohydrates. As a result, cats can maintain normal blood glucose concentrations even when deprived of food for more than 72 hours; furthermore, feeding has negligible effect on blood glucose concentrations in normal cats. In summary, the cat is uniquely adapted to a carnivorous diet (mice) and is not metabolically adapted to ingestion of excess carbohydrate.

When type 2 DM occurs in cats, the metabolic adaptations to a carnivorous diet become even more deleterious, leading to severe protein catabolism; feeding a diet rich in carbohydrates may exacerbate hyperglycemia and protein wasting in these diabetic cats. In humans with type 2 DM, the first recommendation is to restrict excess dietary carbohydrates such as potatoes and bread and to control obesity by caloric restriction. Furthermore, human patients with type 2 DM have improved glycemic control and nitrogen turnover during weight loss when a low-energy diet (high protein) is combined with oral hypoglycemic therapy.

High-protein, low-carbohydrate diets have been found to be beneficial in increasing lean body mass and reducing postprandial hyperglycemia. Caution should be used when high-protein, low-carbohydrate diets are used in cats also treated with insulin because the insulin requirement may decrease. Usually the insulin dose is decreased by 25% in cats given high-protein diets and insulin. On the other hand, high-protein diets and oral hypoglycemic agents appear to be complementary treatments in cats that are underweight. In recent studies, 60% to 90% of diabetic cats discontinued insulin injections after 4 to 8 weeks on an ultra low carbohydrate (< 5% dry matter), high-protein diet.

Glucagon

Glucagon is a protein hormone produced by the α cells of the islets of Langerhans. It has a close relationship with insulin in the control of glucose metabolism.

Glucagon is a polypeptide consisting of a single chain composed of 29 amino acids. There is considerable homology in amino acid composition among species. Glucagon is produced in other sites besides the pancreas; the stomach produces a molecule called *gut glucagon* that is identical to the pancreatic glucagon molecule, and the small intestine produces an immunologically similar molecule called *glicentin*. As with other polypeptide

hormones, glucagon is first synthesized in the endoplasmic reticulum as part of a precursor molecule, packaged in the Golgi apparatus, and final processing occurs in the secretory granules. Glucagon is released by exocytosis. Glucagon is metabolized mainly by the liver and kidneys. It has a half-life in plasma of about 5 minutes.

The Most Important Functions of Glucagon Are to Decrease Glycogen Synthesis, Increase Glycogenolysis, and Increase Gluconeogenesis

The physiological actions of glucagon are the opposite of those of insulin; the main effect of glucagon is centered in the liver. Glucagon increases cAMP production in the liver, which leads to decreased glycogen synthesis, increased glycogenolysis, and increased gluconeogenesis, the last related to the effects of glucagon on protein metabolism (Figure 34-24). The net result is an increase in glucose concentrations in the blood.

Changes in glucagon secretion counterbalance the effects of insulin in association with the daily ingestion of food and the intervals between food intake periods. After the consumption of food, the initial response of the metabolic system is increased insulin secretion, which results in conservation of energy through the formation of storage forms of carbohydrates, fats, and proteins. Glucagon secretion, which begins with the ingestion of food, increases as the interval from food ingestion lengthens and blood glucose concentrations begin to decline. This secretion allows the individual to mobilize energy stores for the maintenance of glucose homeostasis (i.e., to prevent postprandial hypoglycemia) (Figure 34-25).

Glucagon Synthesis Is Stimulated by Decreased Glucose Concentrations in the Blood

The main factor that regulates glucagon secretion is plasma glucose concentration. In contrast to insulin synthesis, decreased glucose concentrations stimulate glucagon synthesis and release, a relationship that represents a negative-feedback system. It must be remembered that glucagon regulation works in tandem with insulin regulation to maintain glucose concentrations within the physiological range. In fact, if glucagon were not secreted to maintain blood glucose concentrations, the individual would die of hypoglycemic shock. Because the α cells require insulin for glucose entry into the cells (as do most cells), in clinical syndromes involving insulin insufficiency (diabetes mellitus), glucose entry into the α cells is reduced and plasma glucagon concentrations are paradoxically elevated. Glucagon promotes lipolysis and an increase in fatty acids, which has a negative-feedback effect on glucagon secretion.

Protein ingestion represents an exception to the rule of opposite responses of glucagon and insulin. The release of both insulin and glucagon in response to protein ingestion appears logical; increased insulin secretion, in response to increased plasma amino acid levels, leads to lower glucose concentrations, and increased glucagon would counteract this through increased hepatic gluconeogenesis, resulting in maintenance of blood glucose within normal limits. The complementary responses of insulin and glucagon allow growth to occur in animals fed a diet only of protein and fat.

Intestinal hormones, with the exception of secretin, stimulate both glucagon and insulin secretion. A similar (inhibitory) response to somatostatin is observed for both glucagon and insulin. Both sympathetic and parasympathetic stimulation of the autonomic nervous system induce secretion of glucagon (Figure 34-26).

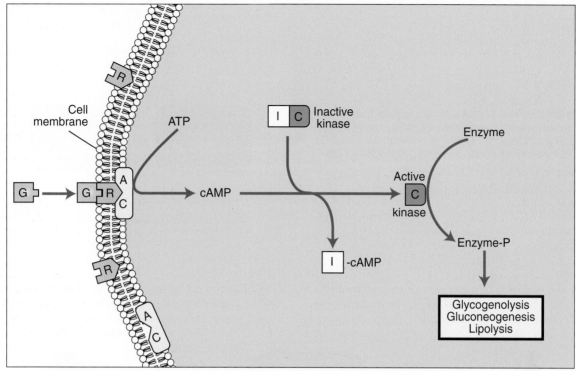

FIGURE 34-24 Mechanism of action of glucagon *(G)* on its target cells. *AC,* Adenyl cyclase; *ATP,* adenosine triphosphate; *cAMP,* cyclic adenosine monophosphate; *I* and *C,* inhibitory and catalytic subunits of the kinase, respectively; *R,* receptor. (From Hedge GA, Colby HD, Goodman RL: *Clinical endocrine physiology,* Philadelphia, 1987, Saunders.)

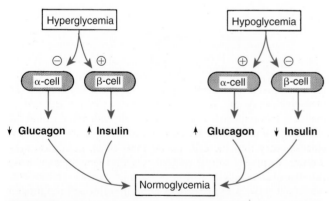

FIGURE 34-25 Effects of hyperglycemia and hypoglycemia on the secretion of insulin and glucagon by the pancreatic β cells and α cells, respectively. *Plus signs* indicate stimulation; *minus signs* indicate inhibition. (From Hedge GA, Colby HD, Goodman RL: *Clinical endocrine physiology,* Philadelphia, 1987, Saunders.)

Some birds have a predominance of glucagon in the pancreas, which suggests that glucagon may have a more important role in carbohydrate metabolism of avian species than in mammals.

Somatostatin

As indicated in Chapter 33, somatostatin was first described in the brain as a 14–amino acid peptide that inhibits growth hormone secretion by the pars distalis. The molecule has since been identified in a number of tissues, including other areas of the brain, the GI tract, and the D cells of the pancreatic islets. Its synthesis and secretion are similar to those observed for other

protein hormones. The metabolism of somatostatin is rapid (about 5 minutes) and occurs mainly in the liver and kidneys.

The Main Functions of Somatostatin Are to Inhibit the Secretion of Hormones Produced by the Pancreas (Insulin, Glucagon, Pancreatic Polypeptide)

The actions of somatostatin can be classified as inhibitory. Pancreatic somatostatin inhibits the digestive processes by decreasing nutritive absorption and digestion. The motility and secretory activity of the GI tract are decreased by somatostatin. One of the most important physiological functions of pancreatic somatostatin is the regulation of the endocrine cells of the pancreas (Figure 34-27). Somatostatin inhibits secretion of all endocrine cell types of the islets of Langerhans, including the D cells. The α cells are more affected by the inhibitory action of somatostatin than are β cells; therefore, glucagon secretion is more affected by somatostatin than is insulin secretion.

Somatostatin secretion is increased by nutrients (e.g., glucose, amino acids) and by the neurotransmitters of the autonomic nervous system (epinephrine, norepinephrine, acetylcholine). Of the hormones produced by the pancreas, only glucagon stimulates somatostatin secretion.

Pancreatic Polypeptide

Pancreatic polypeptide, a 36–amino acid polypeptide, is produced by the F cells of the pancreas (see Figure 34-20). In contrast to somatostatin secretion, pancreatic polypeptide secretion is limited to the pancreas.

The effects of pancreatic polypeptide are directed toward the GI tract. The secretion of pancreatic enzymes and the contraction of the gallbladder are inhibited by the actions of this hormone.

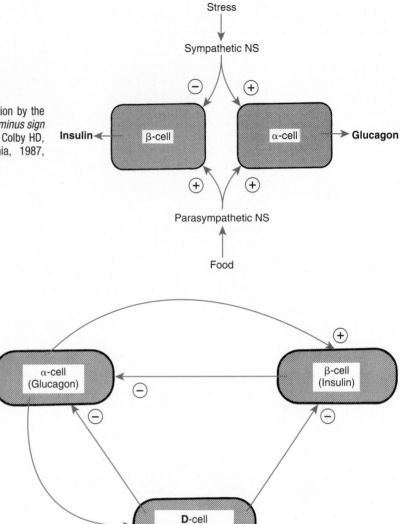

FIGURE 34-26 Regulation of insulin and glucagon secretion by the autonomic nervous system. *Plus signs* indicate stimulation; *minus sign* indicates inhibition. *NS,* Nervous system. (From Hedge GA, Colby HD, Goodman RL: *Clinical endocrine physiology,* Philadelphia, 1987, Saunders.)

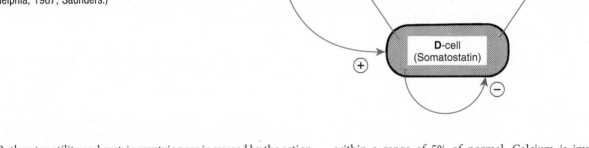

FIGURE 34-27 Possible cell-to-cell interactions in the pancreatic islets. *Plus signs* indicate stimulation; *minus signs* indicate inhibition. (From Hedge GA, Colby HD, Goodman RL: *Clinical endocrine physiology,* Philadelphia, 1987, Saunders.)

Both gut motility and gastric emptying are increased by the action of pancreatic polypeptide.

The secretion of pancreatic polypeptide is stimulated by intestinal hormones, including cholecystokinin, secretin, and gastrin. Stimulation of the vagus nerve also promotes pancreatic polypeptide secretion. The ingestion of protein is stimulatory for secretion, whereas carbohydrates and fats have little effect. As indicated previously, somatostatin inhibits pancreatic polypeptide secretion.

CALCIUM AND PHOSPHATE METABOLISM

Calcium Is Important for Many Intracellular Reactions, Including Muscle Contraction, Nerve Cell Activity, Release of Hormones Through Exocytosis, and Activation of Enzymes

The control of calcium and phosphate metabolism is important because these ions play a major role in physiological processes. Calcium homeostasis is tightly controlled; adjustments are made within a range of 5% of normal. Calcium is important for a number of intracellular reactions, including muscle contraction, nerve cell activity, the release of hormones through the process of exocytosis, and the activation of several enzymes. Calcium is important for coagulation of blood and for maintaining the stability of cell membranes and the linkage between cells. On a less acute basis, calcium is important for the structural integrity of bone and teeth.

Phosphate Is Important for the Structure of Bone and Teeth, and Organic Phosphate Serves as Part of the Cell Membrane and Several Intracellular Components

Phosphate concentrations are controlled by the same systems that control calcium concentrations. *Inorganic phosphate* in blood serves as the source of phosphate, which is important for the structure of bone and teeth. Inorganic phosphate also functions as an important H^+ buffering system in blood. *Organic phosphate* is an important part of the cell, including the plasma membrane and intracellular components, such as nucleic acids, adenosine triphosphate, and adenosine monophosphate.

The Most Important Body Pool of Calcium Involved in Homeostasis Is the Extracellular Fluid Component

Almost all calcium (99%) in the body is in bone in the form of *hydroxyapatite* crystals, which contain calcium, phosphate, and water. The next largest pool of calcium is intracellular calcium. As stated previously, calcium is important for the response of cells in carrying out their physiological activities, including the secretion of hormones. In the inactive cell state, calcium concentrations are relatively low in the cytosol; calcium is bound to proteins or contained within the mitochondria or granules of the endoplasmic reticulum. Increased intracellular calcium concentrations are indicative of increased cell activity.

The smallest pool of calcium, which resides in the extracellular fluid (ECF), is the most important pool for physiological control of calcium concentrations in the blood. This component comprises interstitial calcium, blood calcium, and a small (0.5%) but important part of the bone calcium pool, which exists as amorphous crystals or in solution. The soluble bone calcium pool allows access to the large reserve of calcium that resides in bone.

The regulation of calcium levels involves control of the movement of calcium between the ECF and three body organs: bone, GI tract, and kidneys. The exchange of calcium ions between the ECF and intracellular fluid occurs in conjunction with the control of intracellular metabolism, with little effect on plasma concentrations of calcium.

The absorption of calcium from the GI tract is by passive diffusion and active transport. The *passive diffusion* of calcium across the intestinal mucosa occurs in the presence of high concentrations and, as such, is not an important aspect of calcium absorption. *Active transport* involves the movement of calcium into the intestinal cell down a concentration gradient, which is facilitated by carrier proteins located on the luminal side of the mucosal cell. Calcium is moved through the serosal side of the mucosal cell into the interstitial fluid through a calcium pump system. The active transport system adjusts according to the amount of calcium in the diet, becoming more active when calcium concentrations in the diet are lower and less active when calcium concentrations are higher. Calcium excretion into the GI tract is not affected by calcium uptake, and this can exacerbate conditions involving hypocalcemia. The GI tract serves as the source of calcium for the body, even though both absorption and excretion of calcium occur through the tract. As discussed later, vitamin D plays an important role in the absorption of calcium from the GI tract.

The kidneys serve as the route of excretion of calcium. Most of the calcium that passes into the kidneys is reabsorbed, with a net loss of only about 2%. This amount is matched by net absorption of calcium by the GI tract. Most of the calcium filtered by the kidneys is reabsorbed in the proximal tubules; the next largest amount is absorbed by the distal tubules, and a lesser amount, by the ascending loop of Henle. The distal tubules are under hormonal control and therefore are the sites of regulation of calcium in the kidneys.

The most important regulation of calcium metabolism between bone and ECF involves the soluble portion of bone. Amorphous crystals and soluble calcium, which form the source of ready exchange of ions with the blood, are located between the *osteoblasts,* which line the blood vessel channels, and the *osteocytes,* which are deeper in the bone (Figure 34-28). These two cell types have cytoplasmic projections that interact intimately through the presence of tight cell junctions. For labile bone calcium to reach the blood, calcium must cross the membrane barrier created by the osteoblasts and osteocytes. Movement of calcium from stable bone into the ECF also occurs but has little impact on the acute regulation of calcium concentrations. The process of remodeling bone, which occurs on a continuous basis, involves the breakdown of hydroxyapatite crystals by osteoclasts, a laying down of organic matrix by osteoblasts in the tunnels made by the osteoclasts, and finally the mineralization of the organic matrix by hydroxyapatite crystals. If an animal is subjected to prolonged changes involving calcium metabolism, the slowness of bone calcium exchange can have a significant impact on calcium metabolism.

Parathyroid Hormone

The main organ involved in the control of calcium and phosphate metabolism is the parathyroid gland (Figure 34-29). Most domestic animals have four pairs of parathyroid glands that are generally located at the poles of the two lobes of the thyroid gland; the pig has only one pair of parathyroid glands, which lie anterior to the thyroid. The cranial pair of parathyroid glands in dogs and cats is at the craniolateral poles of the thyroid, and the pair of ruminants and horses is anterior to the thyroid. The caudal pair of parathyroid glands in dogs, cats, and ruminants is located within the medial surface of the thyroid, whereas in the horse it is near the bifurcation of the carotid trunk. The parathyroid cells that are in the active process of hormone secretion are called *chief cells,* whereas inactive, or degenerate, cells are called *oxyphil cells.*

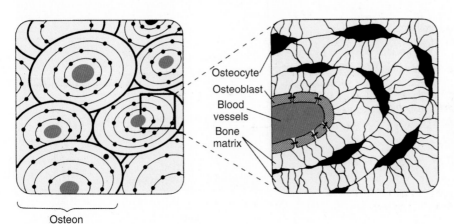

FIGURE 34-28 Structure of the osteon, the functional unit of bone, depicted in cross section at two magnifications. (From Hedge GA, Colby HD, Goodman RL: *Clinical endocrine physiology,* Philadelphia, 1987, Saunders.).

The synthesis of parathyroid hormone (PTH) is similar to the synthesis of other protein hormones; a prepro-PTH of 115 amino acids is synthesized in the rough endoplasmic reticulum and then cleaved by 25 amino acids to form pro-PTH. A 6–amino acid "pro" portion is removed by the Golgi apparatus; the resulting PTH has 84 amino acids. PTH is secreted by the process of exocytosis. PTH is rapidly metabolized by the liver and kidneys and has a relatively short half-life (5 to 10 minutes) in blood.

The effect of PTH is to increase calcium and decrease phosphate concentrations in ECFs. PTH has direct effects on bone and kidney metabolism of calcium and indirect effects on GI metabolism of calcium. The initial effect of PTH on bone is to promote the transfer of calcium across the osteoblast-osteocyte membrane. This level of action occurs without the movement of

phosphate and therefore has no effect on phosphate concentrations in blood. PTH has additional effects on stable bone, which results in the resorption of the bone. This effect involves increased osteoclast activity and an inhibition of osteoblast activity. The effect of PTH on stable bone results in the release of both calcium and phosphate.

PTH acts on the distal convoluted tubules of the kidneys to increase absorption of calcium and decrease renal phosphate reabsorption through an effect on the proximal tubules. PTH is involved also in the activation of vitamin D at the kidney level. PTH mediates the absorption of calcium from the gut indirectly through its effect on vitamin D.

PTH secretion is controlled by free (ionized) calcium concentrations in blood; decreases in calcium levels stimulate PTH secretion, and increases in calcium turn off secretion (Figure 34-30). Both actions are mediated by an effect on cAMP metabolism. Epinephrine stimulates PTH secretion through stimulation of β-adrenergic receptors. Magnesium affects PTH secretion in the same manner as calcium, but its physiological impact is much less. Sleep affects the secretion of PTH; values are highest immediately after waking.

Calcitonin

Calcitonin, a hormone produced by cells in the thyroid gland, also affects calcium metabolism. Cells of the type involved in the synthesis of calcitonin—parafollicular, or C, cells—are scattered throughout the thyroid gland and are distinctly different from the cells that synthesize thyroid hormones. During the early studies of calcitonin in animal classes such as fish, amphibians, reptiles, and birds, which have separate thyroid and ultimobranchial glands, it was found that all the calcitonin activity was in the ultimobranchial glands. Therefore the calcitonin cells represent ultimobranchial gland tissue that has been incorporated into the thyroid during embryonic development.

Calcitonin, synthesized as a preprohormone, has 32 amino acids; a ring structure at the amino terminus contains a disulfide link that bridges between amino acids 1 and 7. The processing of the molecule is interesting because calcitonin is located in the middle of procalcitonin, so an additional enzyme cleavage is

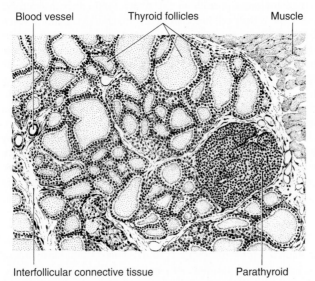

Blood vessel   Thyroid follicles   Muscle

Interfollicular connective tissue   Parathyroid

FIGURE 34-29 Depiction of a section of the thyroid and parathyroid glands of the rat as seen under low power of the microscope. Notice that the parathyroid gland lies near the surface of the thyroid gland and is surrounded on three sides by the thyroid follicles. (From Turner CD, Bagnara JT: *General endocrinology*, ed 6, Philadelphia, 1976, Saunders.)

FIGURE 34-30 Changes in plasma immunoreactive parathyroid hormone *(PTH)* levels in response to hypercalcemia induced by calcium infusion; in response to hypocalcemia produced by ethylenediaminetetraacetic acid *(EDTA)* infusion; and in response to hyperphosphatemia with normocalcemia in a cow. (From Capen CC: The calcium regulating hormones: parathyroid hormone, calcitonin, and cholecalciferol. In McDonald LE: *Veterinary endocrinology and reproduction*, ed 4, Philadelphia, 1989, Lea & Febiger.)

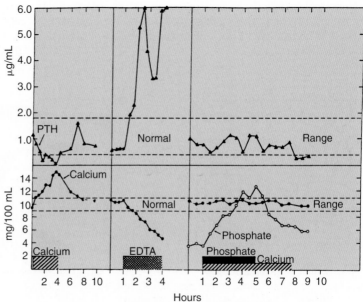

required for the formation of the active molecule. The secretion of calcitonin is by exocytosis from granules.

Calcitonin acts as a counterbalance to PTH because it causes hypocalcemia and hypophosphatemia. The effect of calcitonin on mineral metabolism is mainly on bone (Figure 34-31). Calcitonin decreases the movement of calcium from the labile bone calcium pool (behind the osteoblast-osteocyte barrier) to the ECF and decreases bone resorption through an inhibitory effect on osteoclasts. Whereas the inhibition of bone resorption explains one aspect of the hypophosphatemic effects of calcitonin, calcitonin also increases movement of phosphate from the ECF into bone. Calcitonin decreases GI activity directly by inhibiting gastric acid secretion and indirectly by inhibiting gastrin secretion. The physiological importance of this is not known. Calcitonin also increases renal excretion of calcium and phosphate.

The control of calcitonin secretion is by calcium; increased calcium concentrations cause increased secretion of calcitonin. The physiological control of calcium metabolism by calcitonin operates in situations of hypercalcemia with increased secretion of calcitonin and concomitant inhibition of PTH secretion. During hypocalcemic conditions (see Figure 34-31), calcitonin synthesis is inhibited, and PTH becomes responsible for reestablishing normal calcium concentrations in the ECFs. GI hormones, including gastrin, cholecystokinin, secretin, and glucagon, stimulate the secretion of calcitonin, with gastrin the most potent. These hormones limit postprandial hypercalcemia.

Vitamin D

Vitamin D is important for the absorption of calcium from the gut. It is a steroidlike molecule, and because it is produced in one tissue and transported by the blood to a distant site of action, it should probably be called a hormone instead of a vitamin. All the vitamin D produced by the body is produced in the skin. Epithelial cells of the skin synthesize the immediate precursor of vitamin D, 7-dehydrocholesterol, from acetate. Exposure of the skin to ultraviolet light results in cleavage of the C-9 and C-10 bonds of 7-dehydrocholesterol, which results in the formation of vitamin D (Figure 34-32). The vitamin D molecule, as such, is inactive

FIGURE 34-31 Negative-feedback loops controlling parathyroid hormone *(PTH)* and calcitonin *(CT)* secretion. *Plus signs* indicate stimulation; *minus signs* indicate inhibition. (From Hedge GA, Colby HD, Goodman RL: *Clinical endocrine physiology,* Philadelphia, 1987, Saunders.)

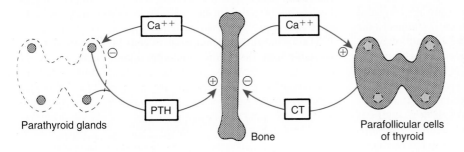

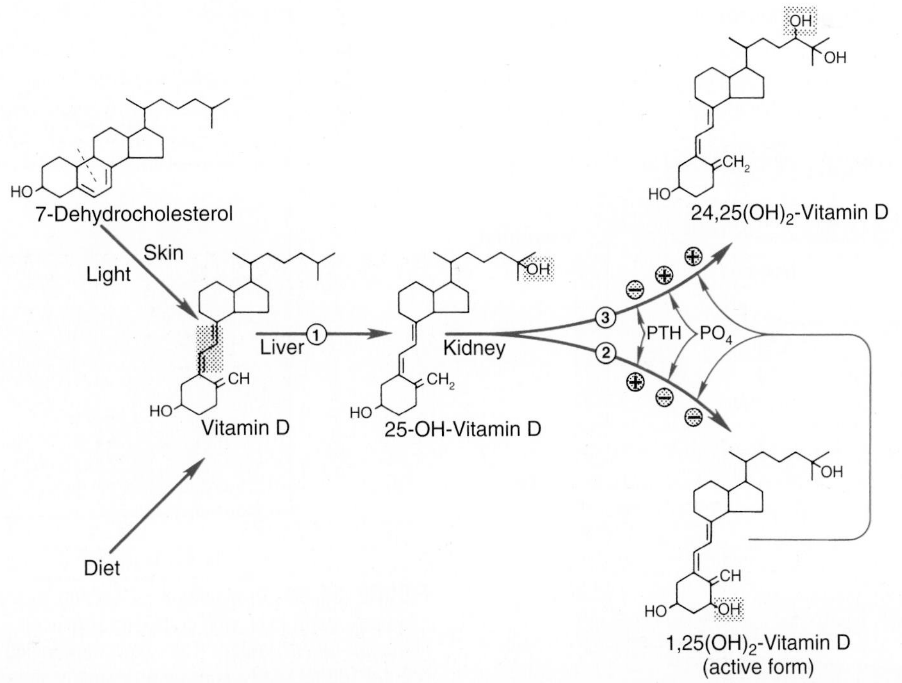

FIGURE 34-32 Synthesis and metabolism of vitamin D. The position of hydroxylation of 25-OH-vitamin D in the kidney is controlled by parathyroid hormone *(PTH)*, phosphate *(PO₄)*, and 1,25-(OH)₂-vitamin D. *Shading* indicates structural change at each step; *dashed line* indicates the position of cleavage of 7-dehydrocholesterol to produce vitamin D. Enzymes: *(1)* 25-hydroxylase, *(2)* 1α-hydroxylase, *(3)* 24-hydroxylase. *Plus signs* indicate stimulation; *minus signs* indicate inhibition. (From Hedge GA, Colby HD, Goodman RL: *Clinical endocrine physiology,* Philadelphia, 1987, Saunders.)

and must be transformed by both the liver and the kidney before the molecule is biologically activated. The liver first hydroxylates the molecule at the C-25 position, and the kidney subsequently hydroxylates the molecule at C-1 to produce the active compound, 1,25-(OH)$_2$-vitamin D (1,25-vitamin D).

Control of the C-1 hydroxylase in the kidney by PTH is the most important control linkage for the synthesis of 1,25-vitamin D. Decreases in calcium concentrations stimulate PTH secretion, which in turn favors the synthesis of active vitamin D and increased intestinal absorption of calcium. Phosphate also regulates vitamin D metabolism. Increased serum phosphate concentrations stimulate an enzyme that promotes hydroxylation of C-24 (instead of C-1) by the kidney, which leads to the formation of 24,25-(OH)$_2$-vitamin D, an inactive molecule. The active molecule, 1,25-vitamin D, also regulates itself by decreasing C-1 hydroxylase and increasing C-24 hydroxylase activity; decreased amounts of active vitamin D is the result.

Because of its lipid nature, 1,25-vitamin D is transported by binding to proteins in the plasma. Most of vitamin D is carried in association with a specific α globulin called *transcalciferin,* a molecule synthesized by the liver.

The most important effects of vitamin D involve increased absorption of calcium by the GI tract. Vitamin D stimulates the synthesis of protein within the mucosal cells, which aids the rate-limiting step in calcium absorption: movement of calcium into the mucosal cell (Figure 34-33). Because the intestinal effect of vitamin D depends on the activation of protein synthesis by mucosal cells, the effect on calcium absorption usually requires several hours. Although the stimulation of protein synthesis relates mostly to active transport of calcium, vitamin D also stimulates passive transfer of calcium. Vitamin D also has effects on bone, promoting the movement of calcium ions from the labile pool into ECFs and the resorption of bone, as well as enhancing the effects of PTH on bone metabolism of calcium.

The control of 1,25-vitamin D synthesis is by PTH and phosphate. A decrease in calcium concentrations results in increased PTH secretion and increased formation of 1,25-vitamin D through enhancement of C-1 hydroxylation (Figure 34-34). This action leads to the correction of hypocalcemia by increasing absorption of calcium by the gut. A decline in phosphate concentrations results in decreased inhibition of the C-1 hydroxylation, which indirectly results in increased 1,25-vitamin D production and increased absorption of phosphate. Some evidence suggests that hormones associated with pregnancy, such as growth hormone and prolactin, increase 1,25-vitamin D production by stimulating C-1 hydroxylation.

In the overall control of calcium metabolism, PTH is primarily responsible for the maintenance of calcium homeostasis. The primary target tissue for PTH in calcium homeostasis is the labile pool in bone; changes in renal absorption of calcium are also important. In the case of long-term calcium deficit in the diet, both PTH and 1,25-vitamin D are important for correction of the deficit. Decreased dietary calcium leads to decreased concentrations of calcium in the ECFs and the release of PTH. PTH affects resorption of calcium by the kidneys, but most importantly for long-term correction of the problem, it causes increased 1,25-vitamin D secretion with increased absorption of dietary calcium. PTH also contributes to the overall calcium pool through its effect on stable bone, that is, the promotion of resorption.

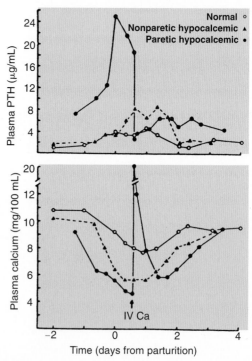

FIGURE 34-34 Development of varying degrees of hypocalcemia in cows near parturition, with corresponding increases in plasma parathyroid hormone *(PTH)* levels. The cow developing severe hypocalcemia (<5 mg/100 mL) had a considerably greater increase in plasma PTH levels than the moderate rise detected in the nonparetic hypocalcemic and the normal cow. Note that PTH levels declined rapidly after treatment of the paretic cow with intravenous calcium *(IV Ca)*. (From Mayer CP: The roles of parathyroid hormone and thyrocalcitonin in parturient paresis. In Anderson JJB, editor: *Parturient hypocalcemia,* New York, 1970, Academic Press.)

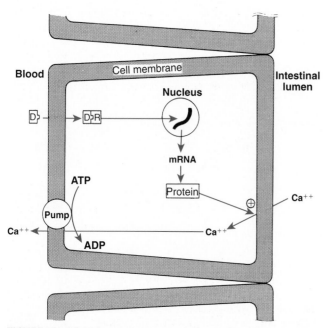

FIGURE 34-33 Mechanism of action of 1,25-(OH)$_2$-vitamin D *(D)* to increase calcium absorption in the intestine. *Plus sign* indicates stimulation. *R,* Receptor. (From Hedge GA, Colby HD, Goodman RL: *Clinical endocrine physiology,* Philadelphia, 1987, Saunders.)

Hypercalcemia has a variety of causes, including malignancy, hyperparathyroidism, fungal disease, osteoporosis, hypoadrenocorticism, chronic renal disease, and hypervitaminosis D. The initial signs of hypercalcemia are polydipsia and polyuria resulting from impaired response of distal renal tubules to antidiuretic hormone. Listlessness, depression, and muscle weakness result from depressed excitability of neuromuscular tissue. Mild GI signs of hypercalcemia include inappetence, vomiting, and constipation. Persistent mild elevations in serum calcium (12 to 14 mg/dL) can cause uroliths and signs of urinary tract disease such as hematuria and stranguria. On the other hand, severe hypercalcemia (>14 mg/dL) can progress rapidly to acute renal failure when the calcium-phosphorus product ($Ca \times PO_4$) exceeds 60 to 80 mg/dL because of mineralization of renal tissue.

The diagnostic approach to hypercalcemia consists of ruling out the most common cause: hypercalcemia of malignancy. A thorough history and physical examination, including lymph node and rectal examination (for anal sac adenocarcinoma), complete blood cell count, urinalysis, serum chemistry profile, and chest and abdominal radiographs, are necessary to search for underlying neoplastic processes. If lymphoma is not detected on the minimum database, a bone marrow examination and survey skeletal radiographs may be necessary. When a diagnosis of neoplasia has been excluded, the next primary differential for hypercalcemia is chronic renal failure. This is the most difficult differential to exclude because other causes of hypercalcemia may result in renal damage because of soft tissue mineralization of the kidneys. Therefore an animal with hypercalcemia, azotemia, and hyperphosphatemia could have primary hyperparathyroidism, primary renal failure with secondary renal hyperparathyroidism, or vitamin D intoxication. Furthermore, patients with hypercalcemia secondary to renal disease may also exhibit elevations in intact PTH. Diagnosis of primary hyperparathyroidism is based on the findings of hypercalcemia (preferably ionized), hypophosphatemia (unless azotemic), high-normal to elevated serum PTH concentrations, and a mass in the cervical region. Intact PTH, demonstrated by a "sandwich" assay validated for use in the dog and cat, should be measured. A normal PTH concentration in the presence of elevated total and/or ionized calcium is considered inappropriate for the calcium level and would be considered diagnostic for primary hyperparathyroidism. For suspected cases of hypercalcemia of malignancy in which the diagnostic approach has failed to identify a neoplastic process, PTH-related protein (PTH-rp) concentrations may be measured.

The classic biochemical findings in animals with hypoparathyroidism are *hypocalcemia* (both total and ionized) and *hyperphosphatemia*. Other causes of hypocalcemia include iatrogenic (post-thyroidectomy) hypoparathyroidism, chronic and acute renal failure, acute pancreatitis, hypoalbuminemia, puerperal tetany (eclampsia), ethylene glycol intoxication, intestinal malabsorption, and nutritional secondary hyperparathyroidism. Early signs of hypocalcemia are nonspecific and include anorexia, facial rubbing, nervousness, and a stiff, stilted gait. Later signs progress to paresthesias, hyperventilation, and finally generalized tetany and seizures.

Primary hypoparathyroidism is diagnosed by means of an intact PTH assay. Serum or plasma PTH concentrations should be measured on a freshly drawn morning sample in a fasting animal. Handling of the sample is crucial to appropriate diagnosis because PTH may degrade if subjected to warm temperatures. *Intact PTH* refers to the entire 85–amino acid sequence of PTH; this is measured in a double-antibody "sandwich" assay in most endocrine laboratories that perform PTH measurement. For the diagnosis of primary hypoparathyroidism, the sample should be analyzed for both ionized calcium and intact PTH. Low ionized calcium and undetectable intact PTH concentrations are diagnostic for hypoparathyroidism.

CLINICAL CORRELATIONS

DIABETES MELLITUS

History. You are presented with a 10-year-old, intact, female poodle whose owner is upset because the dog urinates in the house. In addition, the owner has noticed that the animal now drinks larger amounts of water than in the past. Although the owner indicates the dog has a good appetite, it appears to have lost weight over the past few months.

Clinical Examination. During the examination you check the dog's breath and detect a sweet odor. Among the organ systems you check are the eyes, and you find developing cataract formation. Because you have seen this dog many times, you check its weight and find that it has lost 2 pounds since its last admittance a year ago. You are able to run a blood glucose determination in your hospital and tell the owner that the glucose concentration is 278 mg/dL.

Comment. The findings in diabetes mellitus (DM) are all attributable to inadequate availability of insulin. Glycogen synthesis decreases in tissues, whereas glycogenolysis and gluconeogenesis increase, contributing to the high concentrations of glucose found in blood. When glucose concentrations exceed the reabsorption capacity in the tubular cells of the kidney, glucose appears in the urine. The loss of glucose in urine causes an osmotic diuresis (polyuria), and the dog compensates for this by drinking additional amounts of water. The sweetness of the breath is caused by the presence of ketone bodies. These form as the result of decreased triglyceride synthesis in adipose tissue, which stimulates lipase activity and the release of free fatty acids. These fatty acids are metabolized to ketone bodies (acetoacetate, acetone, β-hydroxybutyrate) by the liver in a situation of excess fatty acids. The end result is both a ketonemia and a ketonuria. Protein metabolism shifts toward catabolism during DM, with decreased protein synthesis and increased protein degradation by muscle cells. This process increases the circulating concentrations of amino acids available to the liver for gluconeogenesis. The end result is nitrogen loss and a decrease in the muscle mass of the animal. The changes noted in the lenses of the eyes represent only one of a number of changes that occur in the presence of DM as a result of glycosylation of proteins, including lens proteins and hemoglobin.

Treatment. Insulin administration is essential in the treatment of insulin-dependent (type 1) DM. During the initial stages of treatment, considerable care must be taken to ensure that the dosage is correct. The goal of treatment is to maintain glucose concentrations between a low of 80 mg/dL and a high of 200 mg/dL, with a serum fructosamine less than 400 μmol/L and one or two insulin injections every 24 hours. Too much insulin has the potential for producing a hypoglycemic coma. Two other important aspects of treatment include feeding the animal a diet high in soluble fiber in conjunction with insulin administration and adequate exercise. Finally, the owner needs to be educated and prepared for the necessity of intensive involvement in the management of the disease.

PANCREATIC TUMOR IN A GERMAN SHEPHERD

History. A 10-year-old female, spayed, overweight German shepherd presents for a progressive history of collapse and weakness over the last few weeks. The owners noticed that she did not want to walk as far, that she seemed worse in her back legs, and had less energy. She also seemed slightly dull and disoriented recently, particularly after exercise. They also thought she had been eating, drinking, and urinating more frequently. They wondered if she had gained weight. Today, a few hours prior to presentation, she had what appeared to be one or two seizures.

Clinical Examination. On exam, she was ataxic (delayed conscious proprioception/ability to know where her legs are) more so in her hind end than in her front legs. She also appeared to be weak in all four limbs, with her hind legs being more affected than her front end. The rest of the physical and neurologic exam was normal.

Comment. Routine blood work demonstrated hypoglycemia. Based on the concern for pancreatic and insulin function, insulin levels were submitted. Abdominal radiographs were normal. Abdominal ultrasound revealed a mass in the pancreas. No evidence of metastatic lesions was found in the abdomen. Computed tomography (CT) could be used to further delineate the insulinoma. Insulin levels are increased.

When function is normal, glucose is metabolized to ATP within the pancreatic β cells. This results in closure of the K^+-ATP-sensitive channels. There is a decrease in K^+ efflux, which then depolarizes the β cells and opens the voltage-sensitive calcium channels. The increase in Ca^{2+} causes the exocytosis of insulin.

With abnormal function (neoplasia), the neoplastic cells secrete insulin independent of blood glucose. In some cases, localized growth hormone levels are increased in dogs with insulinoma. It has been proposed that growth hormone may increase through paracrine or autocrine mechanisms.

With hypoglycemia, there is an increase in glucagon, catecholamines, growth hormones, and glucocorticoids. Glucagon and catecholamines are most important in regulation of blood glucose.

Clinical signs are associated with hypoglycemia. Decreased glucose concentrations in the central nervous system result in decreased cerebral oxygenation and can cause lethargy, weakness, and seizures. Clinical signs can be episodic due to the counter-regulatory mechanisms described.

Treatment. Immediate treatment includes intravenous dextrose. Long-term management includes surgical removal of the mass(es) if possible, based on size and extent of tumor(s). Some dogs will develop diabetes. Diet recommendations include small, more frequent feedings of high protein, fat, and complex carbohydrates with decreased simple sugars. Medical treatment includes streptozocin, which destroys the β cells; treatment of the hypoglycemia with prednisone, which increases gluconeogenesis, or with dexamethasone; diazoxide, which decreases insulin secretion through inhibiting closure of ATP-dependent K^+ channels of β cells; and octreotide, which inhibits insulin secretion. Median survival time for dogs with partial pancreatectomy was 12 to 14 months. Prognosis is better in dogs with stage I versus stage II or III (50% vs. 20% normothermic at 12 to 14 months). Stage I was defined as primary tumor with no evidence of regional lymph nodes or metastasis; stage II was primary tumor with regional lymph node metastasis; and stage III was primary tumor, no regional lymph node metastasis, but liver involvement. Most dogs are reported as stage II or III involvement.

PRACTICE QUESTIONS

1. The other main hormone secreted by the thyroid gland, in addition to tetraiodothyronine and triiodothyronine, is:
   a. Calcitonin.
   b. Insulin.
   c. Parathyroid hormone.
   d. Glucagon.
   e. Somatostatin.

2. The most important function of mineralocorticoids is control of:
   a. Carbohydrate metabolism.
   b. Glucose metabolism.
   c. Electrolyte metabolism.
   d. Protein metabolism.

3. The pancreas has four types of cells, each of which produces a specific hormone. For example, the α cells of the pancreas produce:
   a. Insulin.
   b. Glucagon.
   c. Somatostatin.
   d. Pancreatic polypeptide.

4. Two hormones play an important role in calcium homeostasis. The two hormones, _____ and _____, cause an increase and a decrease in calcium concentrations, respectively:
   a. Calcitonin; glucagon
   b. Somatostatin; calcitonin
   c. Calcitonin; parathyroid hormone
   d. Parathyroid hormone; calcitonin
   e. Parathyroid hormone; glucagon

5. The main functions of the catecholamines are to allow rapid body responses to acute stimuli, which include the mobilization of glucose. The catecholamines are secreted by the sympathetic portion of the autonomic nervous system. The _____ hormone is the main neurotransmitter of the sympathetic nervous system, whereas _____ is the main hormone produced by the postganglionic fibers of the adrenal medulla.
   a. Serotonin; epinephrine
   b. Epinephrine; serotonin
   c. Epinephrine; norepinephrine
   d. Norepinephrine; epinephrine
   e. Serotonin; melatonin

BIBLIOGRAPHY

Court MH, Freeman LM: Identification and concentration of soy isoflavones in commercial cat foods, *Am J Vet Res* 63(2):181–185, 2002.

Doerge DR, Sheehan DM: Goitrogenic and estrogenic activity of soy isoflavones, *Environ Health Perspect* 110(suppl 3):349–353, 2002.

Dye JA, Venier M, Ward CA: Brominated-flame retardants (BFRs) in cats—possible linkage to feline hyperthyroidism (abstract), *J Vet Intern Med*, May: 595, 2007.

Dye JA, Venier M, Zhu L, et al: Elevated PBDE levels in pet cats: sentinels for humans? *Environ Sci Technol* 41(18):6350–6356, 2007.

Edinboro CH, Scott-Moncrieff JC, Janovitz E, et al: Epidemiologic study of relationship between consumption of commercial canned food and risk of hyperthyroidism in cats, *J Am Vet Med Assoc* 224(6):879–886, 2004.

Eiler H: Endocrine glands. In Reece WO, editor: *Dukes' physiology of domestic animals*, ed 12, Ithaca, NY, 2004, Comstock Publishing.

Engelking LR: *Metabolic and endocrine physiology*, Jackson, Wyo, 2000, Teton New Media.

Feldman EC, Nelson RW, editors: *Canine and feline endocrinology and reproduction*, ed 3, Philadelphia, 2004, Saunders.

Fernandez NJ, Barton J, Spotswood T: Hypoglycemia in a dog, *Can Vet J* 50(4):423–426, 2009.

Hess RS: Insulin secreting islet cell neoplasia. In Ettinger SJ, Feldman EC, editors: *Textbook of veterinary internal medicine*, ed 6, St Louis, 2005, Elsevier Saunders.

Kass PH, Peterson ME, Levy J, et al: Evaluation of environmental, nutritional, and host factors for feline hyperthyroidism, *J Vet Intern Med* 13(4):323–329, 1999.

Martin KM, Rossing MA, Ryland LM: Evaluation of dietary and environmental risk factors for feline hyperthyroidism, *J Am Vet Med Assoc* 217(6): 853–856, 2000.

Melmed S, Polonsky KS, Reed PR, et al: *Williams textbook of endocrinology*, ed 12, Philadelphia, 2012, Saunders Elsevier.

Molina P: *Endocrine physiology*, ed 3, New York, 2010, McGraw-Hill Medical.

Mooney CT: Pathogenesis of feline hyperthyroidism, *J Feline Med Surg* 4(3):167–169, 2002.

Peterson ME, Kintzer PP, Cavanaugh PG, et al: Feline hyperthyroidism: pretreatment clinical and laboratory evaluation of 131 cases, *J Am Vet Med Assoc* 183(1):103–110, 1983.

Pineda MH, Dooley MP, editors: *McDonald's veterinary endocrinology and reproduction*, ed 5, Ames, Iowa, 2003, Iowa State University Press.

Wakeling J, Everard A, Brodbelt D, et al: Risk factors for feline hyperthyroidism in the UK, *J Small Anim Pract* 50(8):406–414, 2009.

CHAPTER 35
Control of Gonadal and Gamete Development

KEY POINTS

Development of the reproductive system
1. Organization of the gonads is under genetic control (genetic sexual differentiation).
2. Sexual organization of the genitalia and brain depends on the presence or absence of testosterone.

Hypothalamopituitary control of reproduction
1. The hypothalamus and anterior pituitary (adenohypophysis) secrete protein and peptide hormones, which control gonadal activity.
2. The adenohypophysis *(pars distalis)* produces follicle-stimulating hormone, luteinizing hormone, and prolactin, all of which control reproductive processes.

Modification of gonadotropin release
1. The pulsatile release of gonadotropin releasing hormone (GnRH) induces the critical pulsatile production of the gonadotropins, follicle stimulating hormone (FSH) and luteinizing hormone (LH).

2. Gonadotropin release is then modulated by the process of negative feedback from estrogen and progesterone.

Ovarian follicle development
1. Gamete development occurs initially without gonadotropin support and subsequently with pulsatile gonadotropin secretion.
2. In the preantral follicle, gonadotropin receptors for luteinizing hormone develop on the theca, which results in androgen synthesis; follicle-stimulating hormone directs the granulosa to transform the androgens to estrogens.
3. Late in the ovarian follicular phase, luteinizing hormone receptors develop on the granulosa, which permits the preovulatory surge of luteinizing hormone to cause ovulation.

DEVELOPMENT OF THE REPRODUCTIVE SYSTEM

Organization of the Gonads Is Under Genetic Control (Genetic Sexual Differentiation)

The initial development of the embryonic ovary involves the migration of germ cells into the genital ridge from the yolk sac. These primordial germ cells populate sex cords that have formed in the cortical region of the embryonic gonad from the proliferation of cells from the *coelomic epithelium* (so-called germinal epithelium) of the genital ridge. The sex cords contribute cells, known initially as *follicle cells* and subsequently as *granulosa cells*, which immediately surround the oocyte. The mesenchyme of the genital ridge contributes cells that will become the theca. The entire structure is called a *follicle*, which includes oocyte, granulosa, and theca cells.

No direct connections are formed between the oocytes and the tubes destined to become the oviducts, which are derived from *müllerian ducts*. The final result is that oocytes are released through the surface of the ovary by rupture of tissue elements that surround the ovary; this process is called *ovulation*. A specialized end of the oviduct, the *fimbria*, develops to enable the oocyte to be removed efficiently from the surface of the ovary. In some animals, oocytes are funneled to the fimbria through the use of a bursa, which tends to encompass the ovary; oocytes are directed to a relatively small opening in the bursa.

The development of the embryonic testis is similar to that of the ovary: germ cells migrate into the genital ridge and populate sex cords that have formed from an invagination of the surface (coelomic) epithelium (Figure 35-1). *Sertoli cells* (male counterparts of granulosa cells) develop from the sex cords, and *Leydig cells* (male counterparts of thecal cells) develop from the mesenchyme of the genital ridge. One fundamental difference from ovarian development is that the invagination of the sex cords in the male continues into the medulla of the embryonic gonad, where connections are made with medullary cords from the mesonephros (primitive kidney). The duct of the mesonephros *(wolffian duct)* becomes the epididymis, vas deferens, and urethra, which has a direct connection to the seminiferous tubules. Thus, male germ cells pass to the exterior of the animal through a closed tubular system.

Sexual Orientation of the Genitalia and Brain Depends on the Presence or Absence of Testosterone

The development of the genital tubular system and the external genitalia *(genital sexual differentiation)* is under the control of the developing gonad. If the individual is female—that is, the developing gonad is an ovary—the müllerian duct develops into oviduct, uterus, cervix, and vagina, whereas the wolffian duct regresses; the absence of testosterone is important for both changes (Figure 35-2). If the individual is male, the rete testis produces müllerian-inhibiting factor, which causes regression of the müllerian ducts. The *wolffian duct* is maintained in the male because of the influence of androgens produced by the testis. To

†Deceased

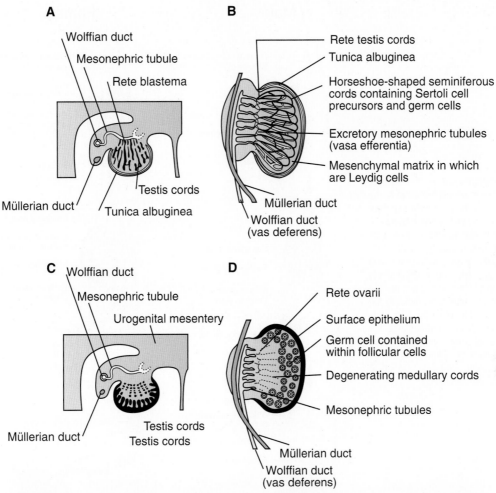

FIGURE 35-1 Testicular development during the eigth week **(A)** and the sixteenth to twentieth weeks **(B)** of human fetal life. **A,** The primitive sex cords proliferate in the medulla and establish contact with the rete testis. The tunica albuginea (fibrous connective tissue) separates the testis cords from the coelomic epithelium and eventually forms the capsule of the testis. **B,** Note the horseshoe shape of the seminiferous cords and their continuity with the rete testis cords. The vasa efferentia, derived from the excretory mesonephric tubules, connect the seminiferous cords with the wolffian duct (see text). Comparable diagrams of ovarian development around the seventh week **(C)** and the twentieth to twenty-fourth weeks **(D)** of development. **C,** Any primitive medullary sex cords degenerate and are replaced by the well-vascularized ovarian stroma. The cortex proliferates, and mesenchymal condensations later develop around the arriving primordial germ cells. **D,** In the absence of medullary cords and a true persistent rete ovarii, no communication is established with the mesonephric tubules. Therefore, in the adult, ova are shed from the surface of the ovary and are not transported by tubules to the oviduct. (From Johnson M, Everitt B, editors: *Essential reproduction,* ed 3, London, 1988, Blackwell Scientific.)

summarize, the müllerian ducts are permanent structures, and the wolffian ducts are temporary structures unless acted on by the presence of male hormones. The presence of an enzyme, *5α-reductase,* is important for the effect of the androgens because testosterone must be converted intracellularly into dihydrotestosterone for masculinization of the tissues to occur. The use of synthetic 5α-reductase inhibitors for the treatment of benign prostatic disease in humans is contraindicated without concurrent birth control measures, because drug levels in semen deposited in the female can lead to disorders of sexual development in male fetuses.

Development of the external genitalia follows the development and direction of the gonads. If the individual's genotype is female, folds of tissue called *labia* form the *vulva,* and a *clitoris* develops. If the individual is male, androgens from the testis

direct formation of the *penis* (male counterpart of the clitoris) and the *scrotum* (male counterpart of the labia). Again, the absence or presence of androgens is an important factor influencing the formation of external genitalia.

The final organization of the individual with regard to gender comes with sexual differentiation of the hypothalamus. Exposure of the hypothalamus to androgens at about the time of birth causes the hypothalamus to be organized as male. A paradoxical finding is that conversion *(aromatization)* of androgens to estrogens is essential for maleness, mediated by enzymes in the neural tissue. In the absence of androgens, the *hypothalamus* is organized as female.

The fundamental concept of organization of the reproductive system with regard to genotype is that the female system is organized in the absence of testes. If the individual is to be male, there

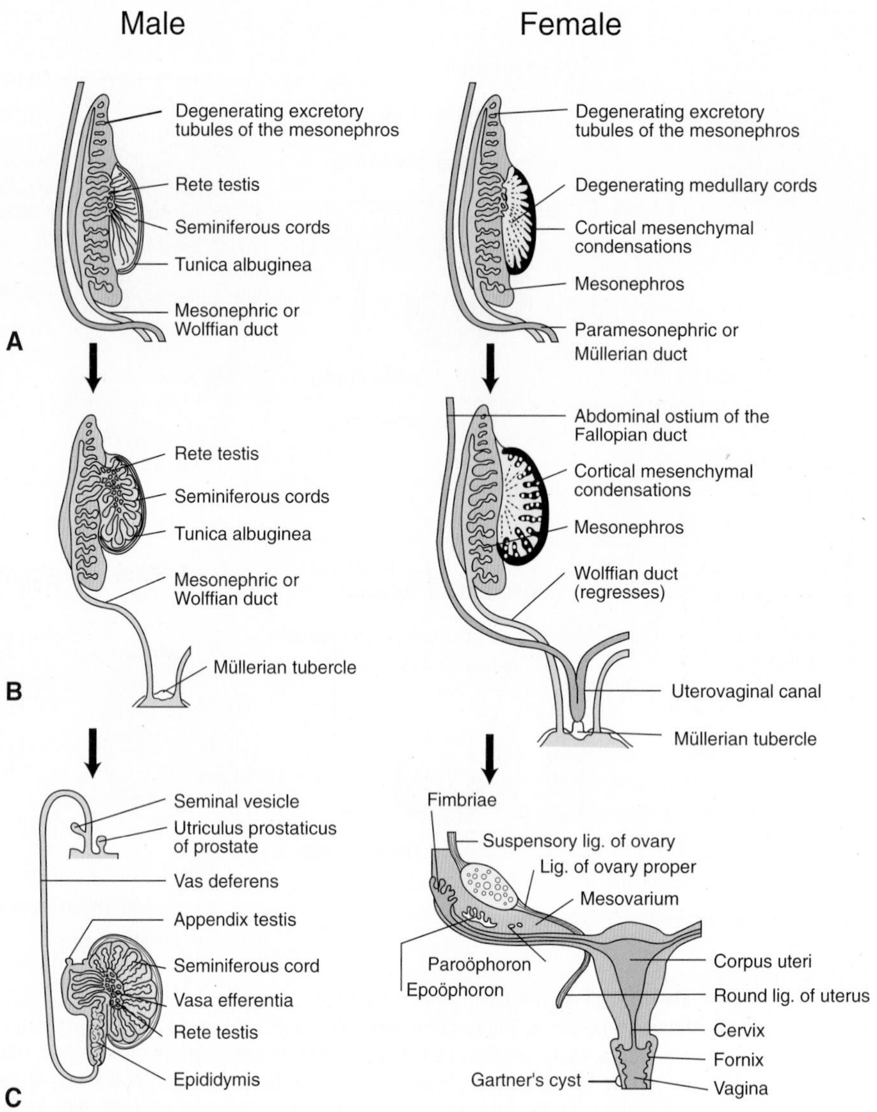

Male   Female

FIGURE 35-2 Differentiation of the internal genitalia in the human male and female at **A,** the sixth week of gestation, **B,** the fourth month of gestation, and **C,** the time of descent of testis and ovary. Note that the müllerian and wolffian ducts are present in both genders early on; the müllerian ducts eventually regress in the male and persist in the female, and the wolffian ducts regress in the female and persist in the male. The appendix testis and utriculus prostaticus in the male and epoöphoron, paroöphoron, and Gartner's cyst in the female are remnants of the degenerated müllerian and wolffian ducts, respectively. *Lig,* Ligament. (From Johnson M, Everitt B, editors: *Essential reproduction,* ed 3, London, 1988, Blackwell Scientific.)

must be active intervention by the testes through the production of androgens and appropriate tissue enzymes in two circumstances: (1) within the internal genitalia for conversion to more potent androgens, and (2) within the hypothalamus for conversion to estrogens.

HYPOTHALAMOPITUITARY CONTROL OF REPRODUCTION

The Hypothalamus and Anterior Pituitary (Adenohypophysis) Secrete Protein and Peptide Hormones, Which Control Gonadal Activity

Gonadal activity is under the control of both the *hypothalamus* and the *anterior pituitary gland* (Figure 35-3). The hypothalamus lies near the ventral midline of the diencephalon. It is divided into halves by the third ventricle and actually forms the ventral and lateral walls of the third ventricle. The hypothalamus has clusters of neurons, collectively called *nuclei,* which secrete peptide hormones important for controlling pituitary activity. As described in more detail later, these peptides move to the pituitary either directly by passage through the axons of neurons or by a vascular portal system. The pituitary responds to the

hypothalamic peptides to produce hormones that are important for the control of the gonads.

The Adenohypophysis *(Pars Distalis)* Produces Follicle-Stimulating Hormone, Luteinizing Hormone, and Prolactin, All of Which Control Reproductive Processes

The pituitary gland is composed of three parts: an anterior lobe called the *adenohypophysis,* or *pars distalis;* an intermediate lobe called the *pars intermedia;* and a posterior lobe called the *neurohypophysis,* or *pars nervosa.* The lobes are of different embryological origins; the *pars distalis* is derived from the endoectoderm (derived in turn from a small diverticulum off the dorsal pharynx, called *Rathke's pouch*), and the *pars intermedia* and *pars nervosa* are derived from neuroectoderm. The adenohypophysis produces protein hormones that are important for the control of reproduction: two *gonadotropins* (follicle-stimulating hormone [FSH] and *luteinizing hormone* [LH]) and a third hormone called *prolactin;* other pituitary hormones include *growth hormone* (GH), *corticotropin* (adrenocorticotropic hormone, ACTH), and *thyroid-stimulating hormone* (TSH). FSH and LH are synergistic in *folliculogenesis* and ovulation in the ovary. FSH plays a more

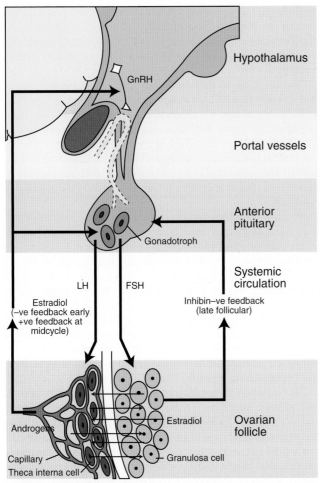

FIGURE 35-3 Summary of hypothalamic-pituitary-ovarian interactions during the follicular phase of the cycle. *FSH,* Follicle-stimulating hormone; *GnRH,* gonadotropin-releasing hormone; *LH,* luteinizing hormone; *-ve,* negative; *+ve,* positive. (From Johnson M, Everitt B, editors: *Essential reproduction,* ed 3, London, 1988, Blackwell Scientific.)

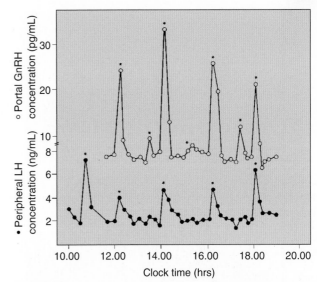

FIGURE 35-4 Concentrations of gonadotropin-releasing hormone *(GnRH)* in portal plasma *(open circles)* and luteinizing hormone *(LH)* in jugular venous plasma *(solid circles)* of four ovariectomized ewes. Asterisks indicate secretory episodes (pulses) of GnRH and LH. (From Johnson M, Everitt B, editors: *Essential reproduction,* ed 3, London, 1988, Blackwell Scientific.)

dominant role during the growth of follicles, and LH plays a more dominant role during the final stages of follicle maturation through ovulation. The *gonadotropins,* as well as TSH, are called *glycoproteins* because their molecules contain carbohydrate moieties that contribute to their function. *Oxytocin,* which is released by the neurohypophysis, is a hormone of importance in reproduction.

Besides being an important center for the control of reproduction, the *hypothalamus* regulates appetite and temperature and integrates the activity of the autonomic nervous system. Because of a common embryological origin, the *hypothalamus* has a direct connection to the neurohypophysis. This connection is through the neural stalk, which contains axons that originate from neuronal cell bodies located in the hypothalamus. Two sets of neurons within the hypothalamus, the *supraoptic* and *paraventricular* nuclei, are responsible for the synthesis of vasopressin and oxytocin, respectively. These small peptide hormones are coupled to larger peptide molecules, called *neurophysins,* and are transported from the site of synthesis in the hypothalamus (neuronal cell bodies) through axons to the site of storage and eventual release, the neurohypophysis.

The connection of the hypothalamus to the adenohypophysis does not involve the direct passage of axons through the *neural*

stalk. A *venous portal system* connects the median eminence within the hypothalamus to the adenohypophysis. Hypothalamic substances that control the adenohypophysis are carried from the median eminence of the hypothalamus to the pituitary by a venous portal system. For example, *gonadotropin-releasing hormone* (GnRH), a peptide, is produced in the medial preoptic nucleus, and *dopamine,* an amino acid, is produced in the arcuate nucleus. Axons transport both substances from the hypothalamus to the *median eminence,* where they are released into the venous portal system. The synthesis of GnRH, as with oxytocin and vasopressin, involves the production of a larger precursor molecule, with a C-terminal region of 56 amino acids, called *GnRH-associated peptide* (GAP). Although GAP can stimulate the release of FSH and LH, GnRH is still thought to be the critical hormone for gonadotropin release. An even more important function of GAP may be its ability to inhibit prolactin secretion.

MODIFICATION OF GONADOTROPIN RELEASE

The Pulsatile Release of Gonadotropin Releasing Hormone (GnRH) Induces the Critical Pulsatile Production of the Gonadotropins, Follicle Stimulating Hormone (FSH) and Luteinizing Hormone (LH)

The main secretory pattern of gonadotropins is *pulsatile;* the pattern is driven by pulsatile secretion of GnRH from the hypothalamus (Figure 35-4). The pulsatile release of gonadotropin-releasing hormone (GnRH) induces the critical pulsatile production of the gonadotropins, follicle-stimulating hormone (FSH) and luteinizing hormone (LH).

Gonadotropin Release Is then Modulated by the Process of Negative Feedback from Estrogen and Progesterone

Gonadotropin release is then modulated by the process of negative feedback from estrogen and progesterone. The importance of this mode of delivery is shown by the fact that if GnRH is

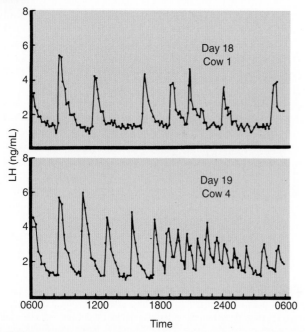

FIGURE 35-5 Pattern of plasma luteinizing hormone (LH) concentration on day 18 or 19 of the estrous cycle in two cows. (From Rahe CH, Owens RE, Fleeger JL, et al: Pattern of plasma luteinizing hormone in the cyclic cow: dependence upon the period of the cycle, *Endocrinology* 107(2):498–503, 1980.)

administered in a continuous (pharmacological) manner, the system can be downregulated. Continual occupancy of GnRH receptors on gonadotrophs by GnRH interrupts the intracellular signal for the synthesis and release of gonadotropins. Successful induction of a fertile estrus in bitches can be performed by administering canine analogue GnRH; however, the dose must be diminished as ovulation approaches, or downregulation will occur.

In general, *the pulse generator system* for gonadotropin secretion is increased in the *follicular phase* and decreased in the *luteal phase* of the estrous cycle (Figure 35-5). Estrogen decreases the pulse amplitude, and progesterone decreases the pulse frequency of *gonadotropin* secretion. This means that during the follicular phase, pulse frequency increases because of the absence of progesterone, and pulse amplitude decreases because of the presence of estrogen. This combination of increased pulse frequency and decreased pulse amplitude is important for nurturing the final growth phase of the developing antral follicle.

The hypothalamus and adenohypophysis are capable of responding to a sustained increase in estrogen secretion by increased secretion of gonadotropins, a relationship that is termed *positive feedback*. The sudden sustained increase in estrogen levels, which occurs over one to several days during final antral follicle development, causes an increase in gonadotropin secretion by increasing the frequency of pulsatile release of GnRH and, as a result, gonadotropin secretion. In essence, the frequency of pulsatile release of gonadotropins overcomes the metabolic clearance rate. The purpose of the gonadotropin surge is to induce changes within the follicle that lead to its rupture (ovulation). The duration of the gonadotropin surge is relatively short, usually 12 to 24 hours, possibly because the main factor driving the response, estrogen, declines in concentration as the follicles respond to the preovulatory gonadotropin surge. This particular physiological

mechanism for initiating the onset of ovulation is effective because the follicle is able to signal its stage of maturity to the hypothalamus and adenohypophysis by a product (estrogen) that is produced in increasing amounts with increasing follicle maturity.

The secretion of gonadotropins is modified by the ovarian steroid hormones *estrogen* and *progesterone*. With time, the effect of these hormones is suppressive for gonadotropin secretion. Estrogens, in particular, cause *negative-feedback inhibition* of gonadotropin secretion, which is characterized by its sensitivity (effective at low concentrations) and its rapid onset (within a few hours). The substantial increase in gonadotropin concentrations that occurs after ovariectomy is caused largely by the removal of estrogens.

Because progesterone affects gonadotropin pulse frequency, it is thought that its modulatory effect is at the level of the hypothalamus. Estrogens are thought to affect gonadotropin secretion through an effect on both the pituitary gland and the hypothalamus. Although there are differences in the site of action among species, it appears that the hypothalamic site for negative-feedback inhibition of gonadotropins by both progesterone and estrogen is in an area immediately above the median eminence, known as the *arcuate nucleus*. The hypothalamic site for positive-feedback stimulation of gonadotropin release by estrogen is probably further anterior, that is, in the preoptic anterior hypothalamic region.

The secretion of gonadotropins can be modified by peptide and protein hormones produced by both the hypothalamus and the ovary. β-Endorphin, an opioid peptide produced from the hypothalamic precursor molecule pro-opiomelanocortin, can inhibit LH secretion when pharmacologically administered systemically. Its role in the physiological modulation of gonadotropin secretion, however, remains to be identified. Another hormone, inhibin, a protein produced by the granulosa cells of the developing follicle, also inhibits gonadotropin secretion, particularly FSH, during the final stages of follicle development. As described in the section on *folliculogenesis,* this depression of FSH secretion may be important to the animal for controlling the number of follicles that are brought to final maturation.

Control of gonadotropin secretion in the male is similar to that in the female; pulses of GnRH, arising in the hypothalamus, affect pulsatile secretion of the gonadotropins. This in turn causes the secretion of testosterone, also in pulsatile form, from the testes. One major difference between the genders is that the need for positive-feedback release of gonadotropins in males does not exist; gametes are produced and released on a continuous basis within a tubular system that opens to the exterior. This negates any need for a surge release of gonadotropins, as is required in the female to rupture the ovarian surface for the release of oocytes.

Prolactin is the third adenohypophysis-produced hormone that is important in the reproductive process, mainly because of its effect on the mammary gland and lactation in mammals. Although the secretion of prolactin is pulsatile, the control of secretion has more emphasis on inhibition than does stimulation of secretion. This concept is supported by the finding that prolactin secretion increases if the pituitary gland is disconnected from the hypothalamus by either cutting the pituitary stalk or transplanting the pituitary gland to another site (e.g., kidney capsule). Thus, most attention has focused on factors that inhibit prolactin secretion. The catecholamine dopamine, which is produced by neurons in the ventral hypothalamus (arcuate nucleus), is a potent inhibitor of prolactin secretion (Figure 35-6). Other

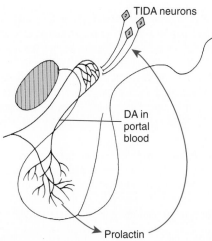

TIDA neurons

DA in portal blood

Prolactin

FIGURE 35-6 Diagrammatic summary of the proposed negative-feedback relationship between prolactin and dopamine *(DA)*. Prolactin is believed to accelerate dopamine turnover in the arcuate nucleus neurons (tuberoinfundibular dopamine *[TIDA]* neurons), and the amine is then released into the portal capillaries to gain access to the lactotropes. Hyperprolactinemia could be caused by either a failure of prolactin inhibitory factor activity at the dopamine receptor level in the anterior pituitary or a reduction of TIDA neuron activity in the hypothalamus. (From Johnson M, Everitt B, editors: *Essential reproduction,* ed 3, London, 1988, Blackwell Scientific.)

factors that inhibit prolactin secretion are γ-aminobutyric acid (GABA) and GAP. Dopamine agonists, such as the ergot-type compounds *bromocriptine* and *cabergoline*, can be used to suppress prolactin secretion in cases of hyperprolactinemia. Cabergoline, a potent prolactin inhibitor, can be used to shorten interestrous intervals in female dogs and promote luteolysis in female dogs and female cats during the latter half of pregnancy (prolactin is a luteotropin). The negative-feedback control of prolactin is shown in Figure 35-6.

One of the first known prolactin-releasing factors was *thyrotropin-releasing hormone* (TRH). The physiological relevance of TRH in prolactin secretion is still unknown despite that receptors for TRH have been identified on lactotropes within the adenohypophysis. *Vasoactive intestinal peptide* (VIP), a potent stimulator of prolactin secretion, may play a physiological role in prolactin secretion through inhibition of dopamine synthesis within the hypothalamus. Estrogens can increase prolactin secretion by lactotropes by decreasing lactotrope sensitivity to dopamine and increasing the number of TRH receptors. Interestingly, female dogs undergoing ovariohysterectomy with a cesarean section usually maintain the ability to lactate effectively afterward, but this should always be evaluated before ovariohysterectomy or ovariectomy is performed. Removal of the ovary, the primary source of estrogen, could be detrimental if lactation is marginal.

OVARIAN FOLLICLE DEVELOPMENT

Gamete Development Occurs Initially Without Gonadotropin Support and Subsequently with Pulsatile Gonadotropin Secretion

Oocyte proliferation, which occurs by *mitotic division* during fetal development, ends at about the time of birth in most mammalian species. Oocytes begin the process of reduction of chromosome numbers to the haploid state by *meiosis* shortly after birth under the influence of *meiosis-initiating factor,* thought to be produced by the *rete ovarii.* The process is soon interrupted at the *diplotene,* or *dictyate,* stage of meiosis I by the meiosis-inhibiting factor, which is probably produced by the developing follicle cells. Oocytes remain in this stage until the follicle begins its final development, an interval that can be as long as 50 years or more in humans. The *follicle,* at this point, is delineated by an outer basement membrane *(membrana propria),* which is secreted by the follicle cells.

The initial development of the follicle involves growth of the oocyte. This growth is accompanied by intense synthetic activity; a large amount of ribonucleic acid (RNA) is synthesized. At the same time, follicle cells begin to divide and form a *granulosa* that is several cells thick. The granulosa cells then secrete another boundary substance, the *zona pellucida,* that lies within the granulosa and that immediately surrounds the oocyte. Granulosa cells maintain contact with the oocyte through the zona pellucida by means of the development of cytoplasmic processes. Interaction among granulosa cells is facilitated by the development of gap junctions. This form of communication is important because the granulosa has no blood supply; blood vessels are excluded at the level of the membrana propria. The *thecal layer* of the follicle forms around the membrana propria to complete the layers of the follicle. Follicles at this stage are called *primary,* or *preantral, follicles.*

Factors that control initial follicle growth are not known. External factors, such as gonadotropins, are not required because preantral follicles can develop in hypophysectomized animals. In species such as cattle and horses (perhaps sheep and goats as well), in which several dominant follicles develop during the estrous cycle, it is likely that a few follicles begin to develop each day. In animals in which a cohort of follicles develops synchronously (pigs, cats, dogs), there appears to be less tendency to have competing follicle growth waves during the luteal phase (pig) and a tendency to have only one cohort of follicles during the preovulatory period (cat and dog). Thus the development of a cohort of follicles may limit follicle development from the primordial state, at least during the period of active follicle development leading to ovulation. Initial follicle growth is under genetic control, and the pattern reflects the needs of the particular species.

In the Preantral Follicle, Gonadotropin Receptors for Luteinizing Hormone Develop on the Theca, Which Results in Androgen Synthesis; Follicle-Stimulating Hormone Directs the Granulosa to Transform the Androgens to Estrogens

For follicles to progress beyond the preantral stage, the granulosa and theca need to develop *receptors* for gonadotropins. FSH and LH receptors develop on the granulosa and theca, respectively. The onset of the antral follicle is marked by the appearance of fluid that begins to divide the granulosa. The follicular fluid, a secretory product of the granulosa, coalesces to form an increasingly larger fluid cavity *(antrum)* within the granulosa. In later development of the antral follicle, the oocyte remains surrounded by a layer of granulosa cells called the *cumulus oophorus,* which are attached to the wall of the follicle by a small stalk of granulosa cells.

The proximity of the granulosa and theca cells allows cooperative estrogen synthesis. The theca produces *androgens* (testosterone and androstenedione) under the influence of LH, which diffuses across the membrana propria into the granulosa, where the androgens are transformed into *estrogen* (estradiol-17). At this time of development, the granulosa is incapable of forming androgens, the precursors of estrogen biosynthesis, and the theca has limited capacity for producing estrogens. This concept of cooperative effort, called the *two-cell mechanism* for estrogen secretion, is generally accepted as being the way most follicular estrogen is produced. These estrogens have a positive-feedback effect on the granulosa; they stimulate the cells to undergo mitotic division, and thus the follicle grows in size as the granulosa proliferates in response to its own secretory product (estrogen).

One effect of estrogen is the formation of additional receptors for FSH as follicle development proceeds. In this situation the antral follicle becomes increasingly sensitive to FSH as it develops and is able to grow under a relatively steady state of FSH secretion.

Late in the Ovarian Follicular Phase, Luteinizing Hormone Receptors Develop on the Granulosa, Which Permits the Preovulatory Surge of Luteinizing Hormone to Cause Ovulation

Late in antral follicle development, FSH and estrogens initiate the formation of LH receptors on the granulosa, whereas FSH receptors begin to diminish. Increasing secretion of estrogen by the antral follicle finally results in the initiation of the *preovulatory surge of gonadotropins.* Thus, in the last stages of development, the follicle falls progressively under the control of LH as it makes its last growth spurt to the point of ovulation.

CLINICAL CORRELATIONS

ANDROGEN INSENSITIVITY

History. You are called to examine a mare that has recently been brought to a broodmare farm after a successful racing career. It is late spring, but the mare has shown estrous behavior only on an intermittent basis.

Clinical Examination. As you approach the mare, you notice that she is large. The genital examination reveals a normal vulva, but when you introduce the speculum, it can be inserted only about 5 to 6 inches. Digital examination of the genital tract through the vulva results in a finding of complete blockage at the level of the vestibulovaginal conjunction, with no evidence of the external os of the cervix. On examination per rectum, you find the vagina, cervix, uterus, and oviducts to be absent; the gonads are symmetric in shape without the usual indentation caused by the ovulation fossa that is characteristic of equine ovaries.

Comment. You tell the shocked owner that you are suspicious that the animal is not really a mare, but a male masquerading as a female. One of the easiest ways to confirm the diagnosis is to have a testosterone analysis done on plasma. If the gonads are testes, they still retain the ability to secrete significant amounts of testosterone, even though they are retained (cryptorchid, in a sense) within the abdominal cavity. You could also have a chromosomal analysis to verify that the animal has an XY sex chromosome complement. In this case, it is likely that the testes were able to secrete the müllerian-inhibiting factor, which resulted in regression of the tubular system of the genital tract that forms the female system (oviducts, uterus, cervix, vagina). But why, asks the owner, did the external genitalia not turn out to be

male? There is evidence, in cases such as this, that the tissues of the external genitalia lacked critical receptors for androgens; thus the external genitalia were female in type. The rule of sexual development is that the female state develops in the absence of testicular input, the latter including müllerian-inhibiting factor and testosterone. In this case the lack of sexual differentiation also appeared to involve the hypothalamus, because the "mare" did not exhibit male behavior despite relatively high testosterone concentrations.

Treatment. There is obviously no treatment for this syndrome. It would be unethical to take her back to the track and race her again as a female, when the owner knows that "she" is a male. The horse could be used as a performance horse (i.e., hunter/jumper, dressage, eventing) or for pleasure riding.

PRACTICE QUESTIONS

1. Which of the following statements is true?
   a. Müllerian ducts develop in the female because of the presence of estrogen.
   b. Müllerian ducts develop in the female because of a müllerian-stimulating factor.
   c. Wolffian ducts develop in the male because of a wolffian-stimulating factor.
   d. Wolffian ducts develop in the male because of the presence of androgen.

2. The most potent factor involved in the organization of the internal and external parts of the genital tract is:
   a. Müllerian-inhibiting factor.
   b. Müllerian-stimulating factor.
   c. Estrogen.
   d. Androgen.

3. Which of the following groups of hormones is transported to the anterior pituitary by the hypothalamohypophyseal portal system?
   a. Oxytocin, GnRH, and dopamine
   b. GnRH, dopamine, and vasopressin
   c. Dopamine, vasopressin, and oxytocin
   d. Dopamine and GnRH

4. Which of the following groups of hormones controls the synthesis and release of hypophyseal hormones involved in reproductive processes?
   a. Oxytocin, GnRH, VIP, and dopamine
   b. GnRH, dopamine, VIP, and vasopressin
   c. Dopamine, vasopressin, VIP, and oxytocin
   d. GAP, dopamine, VIP, and GnRH
   e. GAP, GnRH, VIP, and oxytocin

5. Which of the following factors is responsible for causing oocytes to remain in a diplotene or dictyate state?
   a. Müllerian-inhibiting factor
   b. Müllerian-stimulating factor
   c. Meiosis-inhibiting factor
   d. Meiosis-stimulating factor
   e. Wolffian-inhibiting factor
   f. Wolffian-stimulating factor

BIBLIOGRAPHY

Austin CR, Short RV, editors: *Reproduction in mammals*, vols 1-6, Cambridge, UK, 1986, Cambridge University Press.

Cain JL, Lasley BL, Cain GR, et al: Induction of ovulation in bitches with pulsatile or continuous infusion of GnRH, *J Reprod Fertil Suppl* 39:143–147, 1989.

Concannon PW, Morton DB, Weir BJ, editors: Dog and cat reproduction, contraception and artificial insemination, *J Reprod Fertil Suppl* 39, 1989.

Cupps PT, editor: *Reproduction in domestic animals*, ed 4, New York, 1991, Academic Press.

Feldman EC, Nelson RW, editors: *Canine and feline endocrinology and reproduction*, ed 4, Philadelphia, 2009, Saunders.

Hafez ESE, Hafez B, editors: *Reproduction in farm animals*, ed 7, Baltimore, 2000, Lippincott Williams & Wilkins.

Jöchle W, Arbeiter K, Post K, et al: Effects on pseudopregnancy, pregnancy and interoestrous intervals of pharmacological suppression of prolactin secretion in female dogs and cats, *J Reprod Fertil Suppl* 39:199–207, 1989.

Johnson MH, Everitt BJ, editors: *Essential reproduction*, ed 5, London, 2000, Blackwell Scientific.

Neill JD, editor: *Knobil and Neill's physiology of reproduction*, vols 1 and 2, ed 3, Philadelphia, 2005, Elsevier.

Pineda MH, Dooley MP, editors: *McDonald's veterinary endocrinology and reproduction*, ed 5, Ames, 2003, Iowa State University Press.

Romagnoli S, Schlafer DH: Disorders of sexual differentiation in puppies and kittens: a diagnostic and clinical approach, *Vet Clin North Am Small Anim Pract* 36(3):573–606, 2006.

CHAPTER 36
Control of Ovulation and the Corpus Luteum

KEY POINTS

Ovulation
1. Ovulatory follicles are selected at the onset of luteolysis (in large domestic animals).
2. Ovulation is caused by an estrogen-induced preovulatory surge of gonadotropins.

Corpus luteum
1. The corpus luteum secretes progesterone, which is essential for pregnancy.
2. Luteinizing hormone is important for the maintenance of the corpus luteum.

3. Regression of the corpus luteum in nonpregnant large domestic animals is controlled by uterine secretion of prostaglandin $F_{2\alpha}$.
4. Changes in luteal life span in large domestic animals occur because of changes in prostaglandin $F_{2\alpha}$ synthesis by the uterus.

Ovarian cycles
1. In spontaneously ovulating animals, ovarian cycles have two phases: follicular and luteal; animals that require copulation for ovulation can have only a follicular phase.
2. The luteal phase is modified by copulation in some species.

OVULATION

Ovulatory Follicles Are Selected at the Onset of Luteolysis (in Large Domestic Animals)

Until the advent of ultrasonography, it was difficult to identify growth patterns of follicles in domestic animals, especially those of follicles that develop during the luteal phase of the cycle. The concept that follicles do develop during the luteal phase was emphasized by the earlier work of Rajakowski, who described the midcycle follicle in the cow. With ultrasonography, it has been possible to define follicular growth and regression during the luteal phase of the cycle in the cow and mare. In cattle the predominant pattern is for several dominant (large) antral follicles to develop sequentially during the cycle (Figure 36-1). The follicular cycles are distinct to the extent that follicle regression usually begins (as indicated by follicle size) before the onset of the growth of the next follicle. The first dominant follicle regresses about midluteal phase, with a second dominant follicle beginning growth immediately. Whether the second dominant follicle is the ovulatory follicle, or whether a third develops, depends on the stage of the follicle at the time of regression of the *corpus luteum* (CL). If the second dominant follicle has begun to regress at the time of CL regression, a third follicle develops. Thus the selected ovulatory follicle is, by chance, the dominant follicle that is still in a developmental stage at the time that regression of the CL is initiated. The duration required for the development of the antral follicle to the point of ovulation has been estimated by various techniques to be about 10 days in domestic animals, perhaps slightly longer in some primates.

From ultrasonographical and endocrinological studies, two different phases in final antral follicle development apparently occur in large domestic animals: a relatively slow phase that lasts 4 to 5 days, followed by a second phase of accelerated growth, again lasting 4 to 5 days, that terminates in ovulation

(Figure 36-2). Because the final growth phase of follicle development can be initiated during the luteal phase, the initiation of this phase can occur under the influence of a relatively slow pulse rate of gonadotropin release that occurs during the luteal phase. The rapidly growing follicle requires exposure to a faster gonadotropin pulse rate by the third, or fourth, day in order for the follicle(s) to complete the normal growth pattern through ovulation. This situation usually occurs in conjunction with the onset of CL regression, which passively allows an increase in pulsatile rate of gonadotropin secretion (see Figure 35-4).

One of the ways the *dominant follicle* maintains its status is to produce substances that inhibit the development of other antral follicles. One of the substances is *inhibin,* a peptide hormone produced by the granulosa, which inhibits the secretion of follicle-stimulating hormone (FSH). The dominant follicle is able to compensate for the lower FSH concentrations and continue to grow because of the numbers of FSH receptors it has compared with competitor follicles. Follicle development is dynamic once the rapid growth phase is achieved; the follicle(s) must be acted on through proper gonadotropin stimulation within a few days, or the result is death of the follicle. If the rapidly growing antral follicle is not exposed to the proper gonadotropin environment, *atresia* (regression) of the follicle begins almost immediately. Follicles that regress are invaded by inflammatory cells, and the area previously occupied by the antral follicle is eventually filled by connective tissue; that is, the follicle is replaced by an ovarian scar.

Ovulation Is Caused by an Estrogen-Induced Preovulatory Surge of Gonadotropins

The preovulatory surge of luteinizing hormone (LH), which begins about 24 hours before ovulation in most domestic species, including the cow, dog, goat, pig, and sheep, initiates the critical changes in the follicle that affect its endocrine organ status and

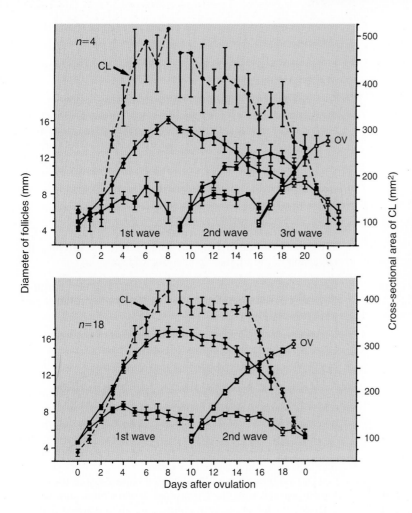

FIGURE 36-1 Mean (± standard error of the mean) profiles of diameters of dominant follicles and the largest subordinate follicle and the cross-sectional luteinized area of the corpus luteum *(CL)* for the interovulatory intervals with three and two follicular waves in cattle. Regression (P <0.05) of the CL began between days 18 and 20 for three-wave intervals and between days 15 and 16 for two-wave intervals. *OV,* Ovulation. (From Ginther OJ, Knopf L, Kastelic JP: Temporal associations among ovarian events in cattle during oestrous cycles with two and three follicular waves, *J Reprod Fertil* 87(1): 223–30, 1989.)

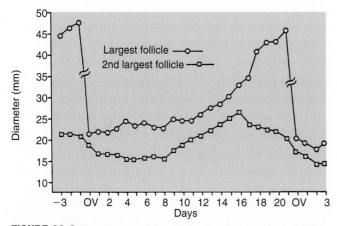

FIGURE 36-2 Development of the dominant and second-largest follicle during the estrous cycle of the mare. Note the divergence in diameter between the largest and second-largest follicles 1 day after ovulation. (From Pierson RA, Ginther OJ: Follicular population dynamics during the estrous cycle of the mare, *Anim Reprod Sci* 14:219, 1987.)

result in release of the oocyte (Figure 36-3). Two important tissues, the oocyte and the granulosa, have been kept under control by the production of inhibitory substances that are probably of granulosa origin. An *oocyte-inhibiting factor* prevents the oocyte from resuming meiosis, and a *luteinizing-inhibiting factor*

prevents the granulosa from prematurely being changed into luteal tissue. The impact of the LH surge blocks the production of both these factors. In most animals the resumption of meiosis results in the first division of meiosis (meiosis I), or formation of the *first polar body,* which is complete before ovulation. In animals with the potential for reasonably long reproductive longevity (e.g., cattle), the initiation of the meiotic process could have begun as many as 10 years or more before its completion.

The effect of the LH surge on the granulosa is to allow initiation of the process of *luteinization,* which transforms the cells from estrogen to progesterone secretion. This process is underway before ovulation occurs. With the advent of the LH surge, estrogen secretion declines concomitantly with the onset of progesterone secretion.

Another function of the preovulatory surge release of LH is to cause the granulosa to produce substances, such as relaxin and *prostaglandin* $F_{2\alpha}$ (PGF$_{2\alpha}$), that affect the continuity of the connective tissue of the thecal layers of the follicle. These and other unknown substances disrupt the theca through the development of vesicles (within fibrocytes) that contain hydrolytic enzymes capable of breaking down the collagen matrix of connective tissue. The rupture of the follicle is caused by the disintegration of the connective tissue.

In summary, estrogen is used by the follicle(s) (1) to stimulate the growth and development of the granulosa and (2) to signal the hypothalamus and anterior pituitary as to the readiness of the follicle(s) for ovulation.

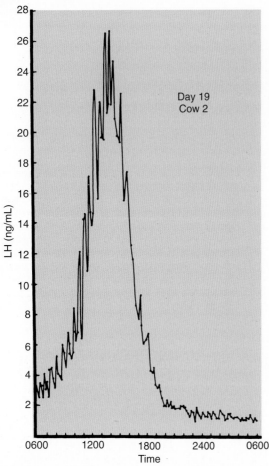

FIGURE 36-3 Preovulatory surge of luteinizing hormone *(LH)* on day 19 of the estrous cycle in a cow. (From Rahe CH, Owens RE, Fleeger JL, et al: Pattern of plasma luteinizing hormone in the cyclic cow: dependence upon the period of the cycle, *Endocrinology* 107(2):498–503, 1980.)

CORPUS LUTEUM

The Corpus Luteum Secretes Progesterone, Which Is Essential for Pregnancy

The main function of the CL is the secretion of progesterone, which prepares the uterus for the initiation and maintenance of pregnancy. The CL forms from the wall of the follicle, which is collapsed and folded after ovulation. With rupture of the follicle, there is a breakdown of the tissues that surround the granulosa, particularly the membrana propria, and hemorrhage into the cavity can occur from vessels in the theca. The folds of tissue that protrude inward into the cavity contain granulosa and theca cells and, importantly, the vascular system that will support cell growth and differentiation. Although the granulosa cell is the dominant cell of the CL, theca cells also contribute significantly to the composition of the structure. The process that granulosa cells undergo during the change from estrogen to progesterone secretion, *luteinization,* begins with the onset of the preovulatory LH surge and accelerates with ovulation.

In most domestic species, significant production of progesterone by the CL begins within 24 hours of ovulation. In some species, including the dog and primates, small amounts of progesterone are produced during the preovulatory LH surge; in the dog, this is important for the expression of sexual receptivity,

which occurs as estrogen levels decline while progesterone levels increase.

Luteinizing Hormone Is Important for the Maintenance of the Corpus Luteum

For most domestic animals, LH is the important *luteotropin,* with the CL maintained in either nonpregnant or pregnant animals by a relatively slow pulsatile pattern of LH release (one pulse every 2 to 3 hours). In rodents, prolactin is the important luteotropin; daily biphasic release of prolactin is initiated by copulation, which is essential for the maintenance of the CL. Of the domestic species, prolactin has been implicated as a luteotropin in sheep and dogs.

Normal folliculogenesis, a prerequisite for ovulation, sets the stage for the subsequent development of the postovulatory CL. Thus, more clinical attention is paid to factors controlling the regression of the CL than to luteotropic factors.

Regression of the Corpus Luteum in Nonpregnant Large Domestic Animals Is Controlled by Uterine Secretion of Prostaglandin F$_{2\alpha}$

Regression of the CL is important in large domestic nonpregnant animals so that animals reenter a potentially fertile state as soon as possible. The CL life span after ovulation must be of sufficient duration to allow a newly developing conceptus to synthesize and release factors that allow the CL to be maintained, but it must be relatively short so that a nonpregnant animal can return to a potentially fertile state. In large domestic animals the duration of the luteal phase is about 14 days in the absence of pregnancy. This allows large domestic animals to recycle at relatively frequent intervals, approximately every 3 weeks.

Leo Loeb first showed (in 1923) the importance of the uterus for the regression of the CL through hysterectomy studies that extended the luteal phase in guinea pigs. He concluded that the uterus must produce a substance that terminated luteal activity. This information lay dormant for many years, until hysterectomy studies in cattle, pigs, and sheep in the 1950s produced similar results, that is, a prolongation of the luteal phase of the estrous cycle. Through these studies the concept developed that the uterus is responsible for control of the duration of the life span of the CL, at least in large domestic species (and guinea pigs).

It is now accepted that PGF$_{2\alpha}$, a 20-carbon unsaturated fatty acid, is the uterine substance that causes regression of the CL in large domestic animals, including cattle, goats, horses, pigs, and sheep; PGF$_{2\alpha}$ has no known natural role in CL regression in cats and dogs or in primates. Prostaglandin (PGF$_{2\alpha}$ and PGE) therapy has been used clinically to cause luteolysis in the bitch and queen, for the treatment of pyometra, or to induce abortion. In large domestic species, regression of the CL is initiated by uterine synthesis and release of PGF$_{2\alpha}$ (likely of endometrial origin) at about 14 days postovulation. The mode of transfer of PGF$_{2\alpha}$ from the uterus to the ovary is thought to occur either by *local countercurrent transfer* or *general systemic transfer.* Countercurrent transfer involves the movement of molecules across the blood vascular system from higher concentrations in the venous effluent (utero-ovarian vein) to an area of lower concentration (ovarian artery) (Figure 36-4). Systemic transfer involves passage of the molecules through the general circulatory system. In some species (cow and ewe), PGF$_{2\alpha}$ synthesis from a uterine horn only influences the life span of the CL in the ipsilateral ovary. In other species (sow and perhaps mare), PGF$_{2\alpha}$ synthesis from one horn is sufficient to cause regression of CL in both ovaries. This effect likely occurs

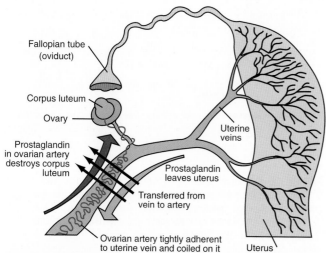

FIGURE 36-4 Postulated route by which prostaglandin secreted by the progesterone-primed uterus is able to enter the ovarian artery and destroy the corpus luteum in sheep. (From Baird DT: The ovary. In Austin CR, Short RV, editors: *Reproduction in mammals*, vol 3, Cambridge, UK, 1986, Cambridge University Press.)

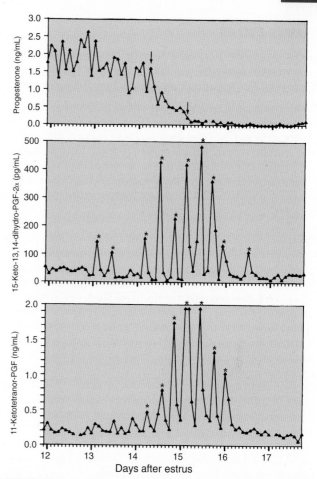

FIGURE 36-5 Concentrations of progesterone, 15-keto-13,14-dihydro-PGF$_{2\alpha}$, and 11-ketotetranor-PGF metabolites in a nonpregnant ewe. Values identified as significant pulses of either PGF$_{2\alpha}$ metabolite are indicated by asterisks. The times of initiation and completion of functional luteolysis are indicated by arrows. *PGF*, Prostaglandin F. (From Zarco L, Stabenfeldt GH, Basu S, et al: Modification of prostaglandin F-2 alpha synthesis and release in the ewe during the initial establishment of pregnancy, *J Reprod Fertil* 83(2):527–36, 1988.)

because of greater production of PGF$_{2\alpha}$ by uterine tissue, as well as a difference in the rate of metabolism of PGF$_{2\alpha}$. PGF$_{2\alpha}$ is rapidly metabolized systemically, with more than 90% changed by one passage through the lungs. Thus the system involving the use of PGF$_{2\alpha}$ as the luteolytic agent in large domestic species requires that PGF$_{2\alpha}$ be conserved through a special transfer system, or that it be produced in relatively large amounts.

The pattern of synthesis and release of PGF$_{2\alpha}$ is essential to its luteolytic effect. For example, PGF$_{2\alpha}$ synthesis and release must be pulsatile, with pulses occurring at about 6-hour intervals, in order for *luteolysis* to be affected (Figure 36-5). The concept has developed that a minimum of four to five pulses within 24 hours is required to cause complete *luteolysis*. If pulse intervals increase significantly before complete luteolysis (e.g., to 12 hours), the CL can recover and continue to function, even if at a lower level of steroid synthetic activity. The uterus must be exposed to estrogen and progesterone to synthesize and release PGF$_{2\alpha}$. Although the initiation of PGF$_{2\alpha}$ synthesis that leads to *luteolysis* is not completely understood, one possible explanation is that estrogen (from an antral follicle) causes the initial synthesis and release of PGF$_{2\alpha}$. In sheep it is thought that interplay occurs between the uterus and ovary after the initial PGF$_{2\alpha}$ pulse. PGF$_{2\alpha}$ affects the CL to cause both a reduction in progesterone production and the release of *luteal oxytocin*. Oxytocin then interacts with receptors within the uterus to initiate another round of PGF$_{2\alpha}$ synthesis. PGF$_{2\alpha}$ synthesis ceases 6 to 12 hours after progesterone concentrations have become basal, that is, with the completion of *luteolysis*. A system for early recycling is not present in nonpregnant dogs and cats as far as regression of CL; the luteal phase is about 70 and 35 days, respectively. Bitches experiencing infertility as a result of frequent estrous cycles may have pathologically shortened diestrus or anestrus.

Changes in Luteal Life Span in Large Domestic Animals Occur Because of Changes in Prostaglandin F$_{2\alpha}$ Synthesis by the Uterus

Significant changes in the length of the life span of the CL in nonpregnant large domestic species occur only because of changes

within the uterus. As discussed in Chapter 38, the presence of an embryo results in the blockage of PGF$_{2\alpha}$ synthesis and a continuance in luteal activity. Prolonged luteal phases also typically occur in mares in the absence of uterine infection. This deficit in mares appears to be a genetic propensity toward inadequate synthesis and release of PGF$_{2\alpha}$. The absence of a uterine horn can also result in a lengthened luteal phase in animals in which the ipsilateral horn controls the CL (local control). In this situation (e.g., in the cow), if ovulation occurs in the ovary ipsilateral to the missing horn, the luteal phase is prolonged because of the need for the ipsilateral uterine horn to control the life span of the CL.

In nonpregnant large domestic animals, inflammatory responses of the endometrium caused by bacterial contamination can result in significant synthesis and release of PGF$_{2\alpha}$, leading to premature luteolysis and a shortening of the estrous cycle. It should be emphasized that luteal activity is almost always normal in the absence of uterine abnormality in large domestic species. Thus, short estrous cycles in large domestic animals are pathognomonic for uterine infection.

OVARIAN CYCLES

In Spontaneously Ovulating Animals, Ovarian Cycles Have Two Phases: Follicular and Luteal; Animals That Require Copulation for Ovulation Can Have Only a Follicular Phase

An *ovarian cycle* in a nonpregnant animal is defined as the interval between successive ovulations. The cycle is composed of two phases, an initial *follicular phase* and a subsequent *luteal phase*, with ovulation separating the phases. In most domestic animals and primates, the ovulatory process is governed by internal mechanisms; estrogen from the antral follicle initiates the ovulatory release of gonadotropins. These animals are called *spontaneous ovulators.*

Fundamental differences exist among animals regarding the relationship of the *follicular* and *luteal phases* of the cycle. In higher primates, there is complete separation of follicular and luteal phases, with no significant follicle growth occurring until luteolysis is complete. In large domestic animals, significant follicle growth does occur during the luteal phase of the cycle. For example, in the cow a large antral follicle is present at the onset of *luteolysis,* and in the mare, follicle growth can even result in ovulation of follicles during the luteal phase (about 5% of cycles). Thus, in large domestic animals, much of the follicle growth is telescoped into the luteal phase. This situation results in shorter cycles in large domestic animals versus primates (17 to 21 days versus 28 days); the interval of *luteolysis* to ovulation is shorter in large domestic animals (5 to 10 days) than in primates (12 to 13 days). The period of antral follicle growth leading to ovulation is not appreciably different, however, with the final progression of antral follicle growth requiring about 10 days in large domestic animals and about 12 to 13 days in primates.

Animals that require copulation for ovulation are known as *induced ovulators.* They include cats, rabbits, ferrets, mink, camels, llamas, and alpacas. Copulation replaces estrogen as the stimulus that induces the ovulatory release of gonadotropins. However, these animals require exposure to elevated estrogen concentrations before they can respond to copulation by the release of gonadotropins.

Induced ovulators have follicle growth patterns (in the absence of coitus) in which cohorts of follicles develop, are maintained in a mature state for a few days, and then regress. Follicle growth patterns can be distinctly separated, as in the cat, in which follicles develop and regress over 6 to 7 days, with a minimum of 8 to 9 days between follicle growth waves. Follicle waves can also have some overlap, as in llamas and alpacas (Figure 36-6), or can closely overlap, as in the rabbit.

The Luteal Phase Is Modified by Copulation in Some Species

In rodent species the luteal phase of the ovarian cycle is extended by copulation. The life span of CL is only 1 to 2 days in the absence of copulation. Copulation initiates the release of prolactin, which results in prolongation of luteal activity for up to 10 or 11 days in the absence of pregnancy. This phenomenon is often called *pseudopregnancy.* In the canine, spontaneous regression of the CL marking the end of diestrus occurs in association with increased levels of prolactin, causing clinical pseudopregnancy. Nonpregnant bitches can nest, lactate, and nurture objects during this time. The queen can exhibit pseudopregnancy if copulation occurred with an infertile tom.

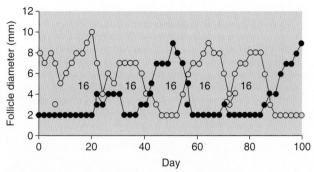

FIGURE 36-6 Ovarian follicular activity over a period of 100 days in a llama, indicating follicle growth alternating between the left *(open circles)* and the right *(solid circles)* ovaries. (From Vaughan JL, Macmillan KL, D'Occhio MJ: Ovarian follicular wave characteristics in alpacas, *Anim Reprod Sci* 80:353–361, 2004.)

CLINICAL CORRELATIONS

INABILITY TO IMPREGNATE A MARE

History. A 14-year-old American Saddlebred mare has been bred two times this season and still is not pregnant. The mare has had three prior foals without any difficulty. This season the owners have had the mare bred by artificial insemination (AI) at the barn where the stallion is kept. The trainer wanted more control over the situation, and she is now going to have the mare kept here. The semen will be shipped here for AI breeding. The trainer has had the semen measured to ensure that the motility is good, which it is. The mare has had a uterine culture and cytology performed, which are within normal limits. On previous ultrasound examinations the mare had no fluid in her uterus and no other abnormalities (e.g., cysts). The stallion is only collected on certain days of the week, so the mare's cycle must be timed so that the semen will arrive before the mare ovulates.

Clinical Examination. The mare is in good body condition. Based on her previous history and diagnostics, it appears that she has a cycle that is difficult to follow. Most mares will ovulate a follicle that is at least 35 mm. Additional parameters to assess when she will ovulate include the following: her cervix will be very relaxed, her edema will maximize and then start to regress, and her progesterone level should be 0 ng/mL. On palpation, the mare has a large corpus luteum (CL) present on one ovary, and she appears to be in diestrus. Because it is desirable to get her back in heat as soon as possible, the mare is given PGF$_{2\alpha}$. This will cause regression of the CL, and the mare should be in heat in 5 to 7 days.

Comment. It is not clear why the mare has not yet become pregnant. The semen appears to be of good quality, and the mare does not appear to have any preexisting conditions that decrease her fertility. The mare will be followed closely to optimize her potential for a pregnancy.

Treatment. The mare is rechecked 4 days after the administration of PGF$_{2\alpha}$. She has a 30-mm follicle on the right, multiple small follicles (MSFs) on the left, but no edema, and the cervix is toned. The mare is rechecked 2 days later, and she has a 35-mm follicle on the right, a 25-mm follicle on the left, edema is 2 (of 3), and cervix is starting to relax. To be sure that she is not missed, progesterone is checked and it is 1 to 2.5 ng/mL. She will be ready to breed soon. The stallion trainer is called because it is anticipated that semen will be needed the following day. The recheck of the mare on the next day shows a 38-mm follicle on the right, MSFs on the left, and edema of 3, with a relaxing cervix (2). Semen is ordered for the next day. The next morning the mare has a greater than 40-mm follicle on the right, MSFs on the left, 3+ edema, and cervix is a 3. Her progesterone is 0 ng/mL. When the semen arrives, the motility, morphology, and numbers are good, and the mare is bred. She has a 42-mm follicle on the right, MSFs on the left, edema of 3, and cervix is a 3. Although it is anticipated, based on her cycle, that she will ovulate that night, she is given one dose of human chorionic gonadotropin (hCG). This will stimulate FSH and LH to help induce ovulation. When the mare is checked the next morning, she has ovulated. The mare is checked again at 14 days and found to be pregnant. She is rechecked at 24 days, and she is still pregnant. The fetus is growing, and a fetal heartbeat is detected.

PERSISTENT LUTEAL PHASE IN THE MARE

History. You have been called to examine a mare that foaled this spring but was not bred at the foal "heat" because of a retained placenta. It has been 40 days since the foal "heat," and the owner wants to know why the mare has not returned to estrus.

Clinical Examination. The main clinical findings are a cervix that is found (through speculum examination) to be relatively small and tightly constricted and (through palpation per rectum) to have considerable tone. Rectal palpation also reveals a uterus that has considerable tone. The ovaries are normal in size; in fact, one ovary has a 35-mm follicle. This prompts you to ask the owner whether the mare has been vigorously teased by a stallion for the detection of estrus. The owner brings the teasing stallion to the mare to demonstrate the farm's teasing technique, and as predicted, the mare vigorously rejects the stallion.

Comment. A history of a mare that has been previously in estrus and has not returned to estrus within 30 days usually indicates the presence of a persistent corpus luteum (CL). The CL persists because of inadequate PGF$_{2\alpha}$ synthesis and release, which normally occurs approximately 14 days after ovulation and causes regression of the CL in the absence of pregnancy. The incidence of the syndrome may be as high as 15% to 20%. The CL can remain active for as long as 3 months before the mare is able to synthesize and release PGF$_{2\alpha}$ in amounts sufficient to cause regression of the CL. It is difficult to palpate a persistent CL per rectum because it tends to shrink into the interior of the ovary. The structure may be visualized by ultrasonography, but this is not always possible. The appearance of the cervix and the tone of the cervix and uterus suggest that the genital tubular system is under the influence of progesterone; these findings, together with the history, support a tentative diagnosis. A tentative diagnosis can also be made if the mare returns to estrus within a few days after the administration of PGF$_{2\alpha}$. A definitive diagnosis can be made by progesterone analysis of blood; values are often 1 to 2 ng/mL in this syndrome, versus 3 ng/mL or more in mares with normal–estrous-cycle CLs. Additional supportive diagnostics would be to repeat the palpation and ultrasound examination in several days. If the mare maintains her uterine tone, does not have edema, and maintains cervical tone, these findings would also support a persistent CL.

The clinical finding that can be confusing in this syndrome is the presence of a large follicle in the absence of estrus. Ovarian follicles develop in this syndrome, and sometimes ovulation even occurs. However, mares do not show sexual receptivity in the presence of large follicles if luteal-phase concentrations of progesterone are present. Additionally, they do not develop marked uterine edema or cervical relaxation if progesterone is still present. One possibility that should be considered in a differential diagnosis is that ovarian activity has stopped (i.e., the mare has become anestrous). Although this does not occur often in foaling mares, mares that foal early can be adversely affected by the relatively short photoperiod that is present. In this case the clinical signs do not support the diagnosis of anestrus.

Treatment. The administration of PGF$_{2\alpha}$ (or one of its analogues) usually initiates regression of the persistent CL and results in the appearance of estrus within 5 to 7 days. The early return to estrus is based on the fact that ovarian follicles tend to develop on a continuous basis throughout the persistent luteal-phase syndrome. Regression of the CL allows the current dominant follicle to continue to develop and produce estrogen, which brings the mare into estrus. One caveat: If a large follicle (e.g., 40 to 45 mm) is present at treatment, the follicle may ovulate before the mare manifests estrus, and the treatment will be judged as failing. In this case the animal needs to be monitored daily; if ovulation occurs within a few days of treatment, the animal may need to be inseminated artificially if breed rules allow.

PRACTICE QUESTIONS

1. The main hormone secreted by the dominant follicle that allows the follicle to maintain its dominant state is:
   a. Estrogen.
   b. Inhibin.
   c. Oocyte-inhibiting factor.
   d. Progesterone.

2. The factor that is most important in deciding whether a luteal-phase dominant follicle will go on to ovulation is:
   a. Inadequate pituitary stimulation.
   b. Regression of the CL.
   c. Atresia of the follicle.

3. The initiation of the preovulatory LH surge that leads to ovulation in spontaneous ovulators results from:
   a. Estrogen.
   b. Inhibin.
   c. Progesterone.
   d. FSH.
   e. Prolactin.

4. The substance responsible for the regression of the CL in large domestic animals is:
   a. Estrogen.
   b. Inhibin.
   c. Oxytocin.
   d. Prolactin.
   e. PGF$_{2\alpha}$.

5. Ovarian follicle patterns in animals that are induced ovulators—that is, those that require copulation for the induction of ovulation—are as follows:
   a. Ovarian follicle waves greatly overlap
   b. Ovarian follicle waves slightly overlap
   c. Ovarian follicle waves are distinctly separated
   d. All the above

BIBLIOGRAPHY

Austin CR, Short RV, editors: *Reproduction in mammals*, vols 1-6, Cambridge, UK, 1986, Cambridge University Press.

Bocci F, Di Salvo P, Zelli R, et al: *Ovarian ultrasonography and progesterone concentration during the periovulatory period in bitches.* Presented at 5th Biannual Congress, European Veterinary Society for Small Animal Reproduction (EVSSAR), Budapest, Hungary, 2005.

Concannon PW, Morton DB, Weir BJ, editors: Dog and cat reproduction, contraception and artificial insemination, *J Reprod Fertil Suppl* 39, 1989.

Cupps PT, editor: *Reproduction in domestic animals*, ed 4, New York, 1991, Academic Press.

Feldman EC, Nelson RW, editors: *Canine and feline endocrinology and reproduction*, ed 4, Philadelphia, 2009, Saunders.

Hafez ESE, Hafez B, editors: *Reproduction in farm animals*, ed 7, Baltimore, 2000, Lippincott Williams & Wilkins.

Johnson MH, Everitt BJ, editors: *Essential reproduction*, ed 5, London, 2000, Blackwell Scientific.

Neill JD, editor: *Knobil and Neill's physiology of reproduction*, vols 1 and 2, ed 3, Philadelphia, 2005, Elsevier.

Pineda MH, Dooley MP, editors: *McDonald's veterinary endocrinology and reproduction*, ed 5, Ames, 2003, Iowa State University Press.

CHAPTER 37

Reproductive Cycles

KEY POINTS

Reproductive cycles

1. The two types of reproductive cycles are estrual and menstrual.

Puberty and reproductive senescence

1. Puberty is the time when animals initially release mature germ cells.
2. Reproductive senescence in primates occurs because of ovarian inadequacy, not inadequacy of gonadotropin secretion.

Sexual behavior

1. Sexual receptivity is keyed by the interaction of the hormones estrogen and progesterone, via gonadotropin-releasing hormone in the female and testosterone in the male.

External factors controlling reproductive cycles

1. Photoperiod, lactation, nutrition, and animal interaction are important factors that affect reproduction.
2. Inadequate nutrition results in ovarian inactivity, especially in cattle.

REPRODUCTIVE CYCLES

The Two Types of Reproductive Cycles Are Estrual and Menstrual

Two types of reproductive cycles are recognized, *estrual* and *menstrual,* with the term *ovarian cycle* representing the interval between two successive ovulations. These terminologies have developed in order to use certain external characteristics for accurately identifying a particular stage of the reproductive cycle and, most importantly, relating it to the time of ovulation.

Domestic animals have limited periods of *estrus* (or *sexual receptivity*); the term *estrous cycle* is used, and the onset of *proestrus* defines the start of the cycle (Figure 37-1). Primates are sexually receptive during most of the reproductive cycle; the term *menstrual cycle* is used, with the onset of *menstruation* (vaginal discharge of blood-tinged fluids and tissues) designated as the start of the cycle (Figure 37-2). The first day of the cycle for both estrual and menstrual cycles in many species begins shortly after the end of the *luteal phase*. In the dog a normal *anestrous* period separates *diestrus* and *proestrus* (the stages of the cycle are described later).

In domestic animals, proestrus usually begins within 48 hours after the end of the luteal phase; the dog and pig are exceptions, with proestrus in the dog delayed by the anestrus phase (2 to 3 months) and proestrus in the pig not occurring for 5 to 6 days. In primates, menstruation usually begins within 24 hours of the end of the luteal phase. Even though both cycles begin at the same time in relation to the luteal phase (shortly after), the time of ovulation differs. This is because, as previously discussed, luteal and follicular phases are separated in primates, with ovulation occurring at a minimum of 12 to 13 days after the onset of menses. In most domestic animals the *follicular phase* overlaps the luteal phase, and therefore ovulation occurs relatively earlier in the estrous cycle. Ovulation is easier to predict in domestic animals (versus primates) because estrus is usually tightly coupled to the preovulatory release of *gonadotropins* and ovulation. The

onset of follicular development in primates can be delayed for a variety of reasons (e.g., stress), making the time of ovulation less predictable for primates than for domestic animals.

The estrous cycle has been classically divided into stages that represent either behavioral or gonadal events (see Figure 37-1). The terminology, originally developed for the guinea pig, rat, and mouse, is as follows:

- *Proestrus.* Period of follicle development, occurring subsequent to luteal regression and ending at estrus.
- *Estrus.* Period of sexual receptivity.
- *Metestrus.* Period of initial development of the corpus luteum (CL).
- *Diestrus.* Period of mature phase of the CL.

The classic terminology is not particularly useful for domestic animals. The common terminologies used for domestic animals involve either *behavioral* or *gonadal* activity. The cycle can be described in a behavioral manner by indicating whether animals are in *estrus* (sexually receptive) or not, including the stages of proestrus, metestrus, and diestrus. The cycle can also be described with reference to the activity of the gonads if differentiation of follicles and the CL is possible. Animals can be in the *follicular phase* (proestrus and estrus) or the *luteal phase* (metestrus and diestrus).

Because the equine CL is relatively difficult to identify by palpation per rectum, horses are usually classified by sexual behavior: estrus or nonestrus. The behavioral classification is also used in other domestic species, including the goat, pig, and sheep, because of the difficulty of determining their ovarian status. The ovarian status of cattle can be determined accurately by palpation per rectum, and cows are usually classified by ovarian status: follicular or luteal. The ovarian status of the dog and cat can be determined by performing vaginal cytology (estrogen effect) and measuring serum progesterone levels. If a CL can be identified, the judgment can be made that ovarian activity is normal in the particular animal, because the CL represents the culmination of follicle growth and ovulation.

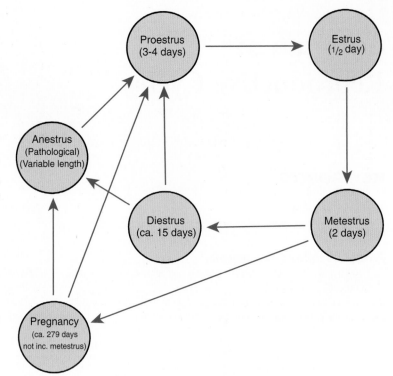

FIGURE 37-1 Various stages of the ovarian cycle of the cow. (From McDonald LE: *Veterinary endocrinology and reproduction,* ed 4, Philadelphia, 1989, Lea & Febiger.)

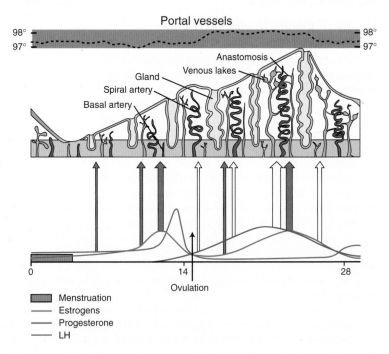

FIGURE 37-2 Changes in human endometrium during the menstrual cycle. Underlying steroid changes are indicated below, and basal body temperature is indicated above. Thickness of *arrows* (estrogens, *shaded*; progestogens, *white*) indicates strength of action. *LH,* Luteinizing hormone. (From Johnson M, Everitt B, editors: *Essential reproduction,* ed 3, London, 1988, Blackwell Scientific.)

PUBERTY AND REPRODUCTIVE SENESCENCE

Puberty Is the Time When Animals Initially Release Mature Germ Cells

For females to begin reproductive cycles, they must undergo a process called *puberty.* The term *puberty* is used to define the onset of reproductive life. For the female, although the onset of sexual activity (in domestic animals) or first menstrual bleeding (in primates) is often used as the onset of puberty, the most precise definition is the time of first ovulation. For all species, there is a critical requirement for the attainment of a certain size in order for puberty to be initiated, in cattle about 275 kg, for example, and in sheep about 40 kg (Figure 37-3). If this critical requirement is not met because of inadequate nutrition, puberty is delayed. The age at puberty for domestic animals is as follows: cats, 6 to 12 months; cows, 8 to 12 months; dogs, 6 to 12 months; goats, 7 to 8 months; horses, 12 to 18 months; and sheep, 7 to 8 months. Classically, bitches have attained 75% of their adult size before puberty occurs.

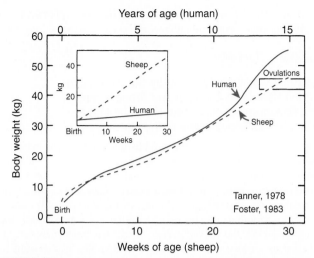

FIGURE 37-3 Body weight from birth through the initiation of ovulation for sheep (mean) and humans (50th percentile). *Inset* shows absolute growth during the first 30 weeks. (From Foster DL, Karsch FJ, Olster DH, et al: Determinants of puberty in a seasonal breeder, *Recent Prog Horm Res* 42:331–84, 1986.)

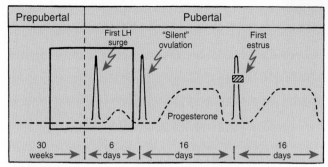

FIGURE 37-4 Schematic overview of major events during the transition into adulthood in the female sheep. *LH,* Luteinizing hormone. (From Foster DL, Ryan KD: Mechanisms governing onset of ovarian cyclicity at puberty in the lamb, *Ann Biol Anim Biochim Biophys* 19:1369, 1979.)

The physiological mechanisms involving control of puberty in domestic animals are best known in sheep. One of the fundamental concepts of the onset of puberty involves an increase in the synthesis and release of *gonadotropin-releasing hormone* (GnRH) from the hypothalamus, which drives *gonadotropin* secretion (in pulsatile form) and follicle growth. Before puberty, GnRH and gonadotropin secretion are kept in check because the hypothalamus is highly sensitive to *negative-feedback inhibition by estrogens.* One of the keys to puberty in lambs is a maturation of the hypothalamus, which results in reduced sensitivity to negative feedback by estrogen. Puberty onset is not held back because of lack of responsiveness of the prepubertal gonads, because ovarian follicle development can be elicited by gonadotropin administration.

Changes in *photoperiod* are important for allowing lambs to enter puberty. It has been shown that lambs must have some exposure to a long photoperiod during their prepubertal development; the period can be as short as 1 to 2 weeks (under experimental conditions). Termination of the long photoperiod, which occurs with the summer solstice, allows the sensitivity of the hypothalamus to decrease in response to negative estrogen feedback. The minimal interval from the end of the long photoperiod exposure to the onset of puberty is 10 weeks under experimental conditions. This aspect agrees well with the timing of spontaneous puberty, in which the first ovulation often occurs in the latter part of September (in the Northern hemisphere), or about 13 weeks from the occurrence of the summer solstice. Note that this concept of the initiation of puberty does not involve decreasing photoperiod; the emphasis is on a turning point that involves the cessation of exposure to a long photoperiod.

With appropriate growth and photoperiod exposure, the secretion of gonadotropins in lambs causes significant follicle growth. This growth is maintained because of decreased sensitivity of the hypothalamus to estrogens produced by growing follicles. The first endocrine event of puberty in the ewe lamb is the appearance of a preovulatory-type surge of gonadotropins, presumably induced by estrogens produced by developing follicles (Figure 37-4). The gonadotropin surge results in the production

of a luteal structure, through luteinization of a follicle(s), which has a short life span, 3 to 4 days. After the demise of the initial luteal structure, another gonadotropin surge occurs, leading to ovulation and the formation of a CL, usually of a normal life span. At this time, cyclical ovarian activity is finally initiated in the ewe lamb.

Photoperiod can have a suppressive effect on the timing of puberty in animals whose ovarian cyclicity is controlled by light. Kittens born in the spring may be large enough to enter puberty by late autumn, but puberty could be delayed a few months if the kittens are under the natural photoperiod.

Photoperiod influences the timing of puberty onset in macaque monkeys, depending on the physiological maturity of the individual. The first ovulation, or puberty onset, can occur during the late autumn or early winter, at about 30 months of age (20% of animals) or 12 months later at about 42 months of age (80% of animals). The animals undergoing puberty at about 30 months of age have an earlier maturation of the neuroendocrine system, in which significant gonadotropin secretion begins during the previous spring. Thus, there is a window of opportunity for the onset of puberty in macaques that must be entered within the favorable photoperiod of decreasing light if puberty is to occur at an earlier time; nutrition and growth are likely determinants of the earlier time for onset of puberty.

The onset of puberty usually results in the establishment of cyclical ovarian activity within a relatively short period (i.e., within a few weeks to a month in lambs). Ewe lambs can initiate normal ovarian activity at the onset of puberty, which can lead to pregnancy (if mated) at the first estrus, or they can have false starts with the establishment of limited luteal phases and cessation of ovarian activity for several weeks to a month before they resume ovarian activity. In general, the onset of ovarian cyclicity starts later and ends earlier for ewe lambs compared with adults of the same breed. The earlier cessation of ovarian activity results from an earlier response to negative estrogen feedback.

The initiation of cyclical ovarian activity in pubertal primates takes longer; the first significant follicle growth usually ends in ovulatory failure. In macaque monkeys, 3 to 6 months is usually required after the onset of menarche, or first vaginal bleeding, before the occurrence of the first ovulation of puberty. In humans, follicle growth without ovulation can occur for up to a year before the establishment of normal ovarian cyclicity, including ovulation and CL formation.

For male lambs, the onset of puberty is first keyed when lambs begin to lose their sensitivity to estrogen feedback inhibition, usually by about 15 weeks of age. For many males, this occurs during the period of increasing, or long, photoperiod, which is in contrast to the ewe lamb. Spermatogenesis (process of sperm production resulting in the presence of mature sperm) usually begins at this time, but because of the length of the process, lambs are usually not capable of successful breeding until about 30 weeks of age or more, or in concert with the onset of puberty in ewe lambs. Thus, puberty is a relatively gradual phenomenon in male sheep compared with the abrupt process in females.

Because adult ewes experience the same double gonadotropin surge at the onset of the breeding season, it has been suggested that adult animals recapitulate puberty each year as they enter the breeding season. Recent studies in adult ewes, however, indicate that *refractoriness* to the long photoperiod experienced by animals during the spring and summer is the most critical aspect for the establishment of ovarian activity. Thus the concept that the renewal of ovarian activity in sheep recapitulates puberty appears not to be accurate, at least in some aspects.

Reproductive Senescence in Primates Occurs Because of Ovarian Inadequacy, Not Inadequacy of Gonadotropin Secretion

The end to ovarian activity that occurs in primates is called *menopause.* In humans, for example, it usually occurs between 45 and 50 years of age. Menopause results from the depletion of oocytes, which has occurred throughout the reproductive life of the individual; in essence, it represents ovarian failure. It is not clear whether follicles fail to develop from their primordial state because of an absolute, or relative, reduction in follicle numbers, or whether the absence of gonadotropin receptors prohibits follicles from entering the gonadotropin-dependent stage of growth. The initiation of menopause often involves cyclical irregularity caused by failure of follicle development and ovulation. Gonadotropin secretion can be increased, or can be normal, because of the lack of estrogen and therefore lack of negative feedback on gonadotropin secretion. In the end, ovarian follicle activity ceases, estrogen concentrations decline, and in the absence of negative-feedback inhibition, gonadotropin concentrations increase dramatically.

Reproductive senescence is not recognized in domestic animals. This is partly because some domestic species have lives that are shortened for economic or humane reasons. Nevertheless, a phenomenon such as menopause clearly does not occur in domestic animals. One effect of age can be noted in the dog: estrous-cycle intervals gradually increase from the norm of 7.5 months to 12 to 15 months toward the end of the life span. Also, litter size diminishes, and increased neonatal mortality, probably associated with dystocia, occurs with increasing age of the dam.

Reproductive senescence in the cheetah has been reported to be a consequence of uterine rather than ovarian changes.

SEXUAL BEHAVIOR

Sexual Receptivity Is Keyed by the Interaction of the Hormones Estrogen and Progesterone via Gonadotropin-Releasing Hormone in the Female and Testosterone in the Male

As indicated previously, the establishment of sexual behavior depends on exposure, or lack of exposure, of the hypothalamus to testosterone during the early neonatal period. In essence, testosterone (aromatized to estrogen) causes masculinization of the sexual centers in the hypothalamus; in the absence of testosterone, the hypothalamus becomes feminized. An area within the hypothalamus, the *medial preoptic area,* has been identified in the rat as an area that is modified structurally by exposure to testosterone.

Several principles exist regarding the effects of hormones on sexual behavior of domestic animals. First, the magnitude of change in hormone concentration that affects sexual behavior is small; in the cat, for example, an increase in estradiol-17 concentration from 10 to 20 pg/mL of plasma results in signs of proestrus. Second, synergism between hormones is often important for sexual receptiveness; in the dog, for example, estrogen priming followed by progesterone is important. Third, the sequence of exposure to hormones can be important; in the ewe, for example, progesterone priming is required before estrogen exposure for manifestation of estrus.

Estrogen, from the developing antral follicle, is the one hormone required for sexual receptivity in all domestic animals. *Progesterone,* derived from either the granulosa of the preovulatory follicle or the CL, is also important for estrus in some animals.

In sheep and goats, estrus occurs in response to estrogen only if the animal has been exposed previously to progesterone (through the presence of a previous CL). Estrus usually begins within a short period after the end of the luteal phase (i.e., 24 to 36 hours) because of the presence of large antral follicles at luteolysis; thus the period from last exposure to progesterone and the onset of estrus is short (Figure 37-5). The requirement of progesterone for sexual receptivity means that the first follicular phase of the breeding season, which leads to ovulation in the ewe, is not accompanied by estrus. Most adult ewes show estrus after the first luteal phase. Ewe lambs often require the exposure of two or more luteal phases before they express estrus.

Of the domestic species, dogs are unusual in that sexual receptivity is keyed by progesterone, produced initially by the

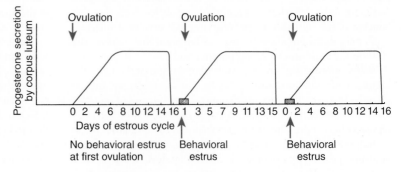

FIGURE 37-5 Estrous cycle of the ewe, showing how the first ovulation of the season is unaccompanied by estrus. Note the short interval between regression of the corpus luteum and the next ovulation. (From Short RV: Oestrous and menstrual cycles. In Austin CR, Short RV, editors: *Reproduction in mammals,* vols 1-6, Cambridge, UK, 1986, Cambridge University Press.)

granulosa during the preovulatory luteinizing hormone (LH) surge and subsequently by the developing CL. Prior exposure to estrogen makes the female attractive to males but does not produce sexual receptivity; estrus requires the additional exposure to progesterone. Estrus is often maintained for up to a week in the presence of a developing luteal phase. In other domestic species, progesterone is inhibitory for estrous activity.

The importance of prior progesterone priming for estrus manifestation has been suggested for dairy cattle by the finding of a reduced incidence of estrus at the first postpartum ovulation (days 15 to 20). Complete progesterone withdrawal occurs in the cow immediately before delivery, and animals would not have been exposed to progesterone for 2 to 3 weeks in this situation. Sows also have a reduced incidence of estrus at the first ovulation, which usually does not occur until after weaning, usually not until at least 45 days after parturition. Other domestic species (i.e., cats, goats, horses) all show estrus with the first ovulation of the season with no apparent requirement for progesterone priming.

Testosterone is important for *libido* in female primates. The theca layer from degenerating follicles forms an active interstitium that secretes the androgens androstenedione and testosterone. Androgens are also essential for the maintenance of libido in males. Occasionally, castrated males, particularly horses, are able to maintain libido despite the lower concentrations of androgens (of adrenal origin) that are present after castration. These animals can sometimes be differentiated from those with retained testicles (*cryptorchid* animals) by testosterone analysis of plasma; however, serum testosterone levels in intact males vary by the minute. A GnRH stimulation test more accurately identifies remaining testicular tissues (2.2 μg/kg intravenously, sampling before and 1 to 3 hours later). When commercially available, serum LH levels are better for differentiating bilaterally cryptorchid individuals (LH <1 ng/mL) from castrated animals (LH >1 ng/mL).

Both experimental and circumstantial evidence indicates that GnRH plays a role in sexual receptivity. The administration of GnRH to ovariectomized rats produced sexual (lordotic) responses, and in prepubertal gilts, GnRH administration resulted in the occurrence of estrus within 24 hours. The circumstantial evidence is that the onset of sexual receptivity in animals is tightly coupled to the onset of the preovulatory gonadotropin surge. Because the preovulatory gonadotropin surge is the result of an increased rate of pulsatile release of gonadotropins driven by increased GnRH synthesis and release, it is likely that this increased GnRH secretory activity affects sexual centers within the hypothalamus for the promotion of sexual receptivity. This allows the onset of the ovulatory process, triggered by the gonadotropin surge, to be tightly coupled with sexual receptivity.

EXTERNAL FACTORS CONTROLLING REPRODUCTIVE CYCLES

Photoperiod, Lactation, Nutrition, and Animal Interaction Are Important Factors That Affect Reproduction

Photoperiod

Photoperiod controls the occurrence of reproductive cycles in a number of domestic species, including cats, goats, horses, and sheep. The result is that these animals have an annual period in which they have continuous (cyclical) ovarian activity, as well as another period of no ovarian activity, termed *anestrus*. The

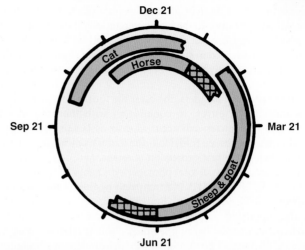

FIGURE 37-6 Diagrammatic representation of the effect of photoperiod on ovarian activity in the typical cat, horse, sheep, and goat. The *bars* represent periods of ovarian inactivity (anestrum). The transitional periods for the horse, sheep, and goat are shown by the *hatched portions* of the bars. (From Stabenfeldt GH, Edqvist LE: Female reproductive processes. In Swenson MJ, editor: *Dukes' physiology of domestic animals,* ed 10, Ithaca, NY, 1984, Cornell University Press.)

response to photoperiod is different among these species; cats and horses are positively affected by increasing light, and goats and sheep are positively affected by decreasing photoperiod (Figure 37-6).

A positive response to a change in the photoperiod usually occurs relatively soon after the occurrence of the summer or winter solstice (i.e., within 1 to 2 months). A negative response to a change in photoperiod usually requires a longer duration for an effect (i.e., 2 to 4 months to suppress ovarian activity after the occurrence of the particular solstice). The net result is that in the absence of pregnancy, cyclical ovarian activity usually occupies more than half the year for these four seasonally breeding species.

In cats, cyclical ovarian activity can range from late January through October (in the Northern Hemisphere). In horses, the usual range of ovarian activity is from March through October. Conversely, sheep and goats have ovarian activity from late July through February or March (depending on the breed). As indicated previously, progesterone priming immediately before follicle development is required for sexual receptivity in sheep. The full length of the reproductive season of sheep is not manifested externally because (1) the first ovulation is not preceded by the presence of a CL, and (2) the last follicle phase may be delayed because of a negative photoperiod, with the priming effects of progesterone lost before follicle growth.

The main translator of photoperiod is the *pineal gland*, which produces *melatonin* in response to darkness. The central nervous system pathway involved with the translation of light includes the retina, suprachiasmatic nucleus, superior cervical ganglion, and pineal gland. Whereas melatonin has been previously described as *antigonadal,* this is obviously not true, because both short and long phases of darkness, with resultant short and long duration of melatonin secretion, can have a positive effect on reproductive cycles. In sheep, however, exposure to increasing darkness may be important only for maintaining ovarian activity. The onset of ovarian activity is thought to occur in response to the development of refractoriness to the long photoperiod. The development of *photorefractoriness* to a long photoperiod as a requisite to ovarian cyclicity is consonant with the fact that sheep can begin cyclical ovarian activity even before the onset of the summer solstice.

Of the seasonal breeders, the cat is the most sensitive to photoperiod change; estrus, in conjunction with the presence of mature antral follicles, can occur as early as January 15 (in the Northern hemisphere). Initial follicle activity likely begins at least 10 days before the first expression of estrus, or 15 days after the winter solstice. Thus a total photoperiod change as brief as 15 minutes can be perceived and translated by the cat into ovarian activity.

The suppressive effects of photoperiod can be overcome by exposure to artificial lighting regimens. This is relatively easy in the case of cats and horses, in which environments with photoperiods are compatible with ovarian activity (i.e., at least 12 hours of light per day). If the photoperiod is established before the end of ovarian activity in the autumn, cyclical ovarian activity continues through the time associated with anestrus. If mares are allowed to become anestrous in the autumn, it can take a minimum of 2 months of exposure of mares to increased light to reestablish ovarian activity. The usual time for placing mares under lights is December 1 (in the Northern Hemisphere), with cyclical ovarian activity expected by early February.

It is usually not possible to place sheep and goats in light-tight barns to increase their exposure to dark in order to overcome the suppressive effects of increasing light. One recent development in this regard has been the oral or systemic (implant) administration of melatonin to sheep during the spring. This exposure to melatonin has resulted in an early onset of ovarian activity and increased the number of multiple ovulations above that normally observed at the beginning of the breeding season.

Lactation

Lactation can have suppressive effects on ovarian activity. In pigs, suppression of ovarian activity is complete; sows do not come into estrus until after piglets are weaned. Cats can have ovarian activity suppressed throughout lactation, although they occasionally come into estrus during the latter part of lactation. Ovarian activity tends to be suppressed in lactating beef cows, with the first estrus and ovulation not occurring before day 45 postpartum. The suckling process appears important to ovarian suppression; dairy cows are not suppressed by lactation unless it involves a large nutritional deficit.

Goats and sheep usually begin lactation during a photoperiod that is increasingly suppressive for ovarian activity, and therefore the reestablishment of ovarian activity in these species is confounded by the photoperiod. Ewes delivering in the autumn ovulated as early as postpartum day 12 (average, postpartum day 23), indicating that lactation has little suppressive effect on ovarian activity in sheep. Mares usually ovulate by postpartum days 10 to 15, with lactation having no suppressive effect on ovarian activity regarding this ovulatory interval.

One of the concepts of *lactational suppression of ovarian activity* involves the importance of suckling with its related stimulation of prolactin synthesis. Inhibiting factors for prolactin synthesis, including dopamine and the GnRH-associated peptide, need to be suppressed in order for prolactin synthesis to proceed. The sensory input from suckling suppresses the production of these prolactin-inhibiting factors. Because both dopamine and GnRH-associated peptide are essential links in the synthesis of gonadotropins, their reduced output results in reduced ovarian activity through decreased gonadotropin synthesis and release.

Pheromones

Pheromones are chemical compounds that allow communication among animals through the olfactory system. When sexual behavior is affected, the compounds are called *sex pheromones.* Pheromones arise from several tissue sources; the most prominent sources for animals are sebaceous glands, the reproductive tract, and the urinary tract.

Some of the first experiments that demonstrated the potency of male odors to influence reproductive behavior were done in mice. One syndrome, called the *Whitten effect,* involves the synchronization of estrus in female mice through the sudden introduction of a male (or male odor through bedding), with a large number of animals cycling within 3 days of introduction of the male. The effect of the pheromones in this case is to stimulate the synthesis and release of gonadotropins. Another syndrome, called the *Bruce effect,* involves the blockage of pregnancy development by the introduction of a different (strange) male in proximity to a recently bred female. The effect of the odor of the strange male is to block the release of prolactin, the hormone responsible for the maintenance of the CL in association with pregnancy in rodents. Regression of the CL in this case produces fetal loss. Thus, pheromones can strongly affect reproductive cycles.

Pheromones are important for the attraction of the male to the female at the time of sexual receptivity. Sexual attractiveness of the female evolves from the pheromones that she elicits on a limited, cyclical basis in association with estrus. For example, methyl-p-hydroxybenzoate, isolated from the vaginal secretions of dogs in proestrus and estrus, has produced intense anogenital interest by males when applied to anestrous females. Females are also influenced by male odors; sows in estrus assume a breeding (rigidity) stance when exposed to the urine of males. Androgens can serve as pheromones, or they can influence the production of substances within the kidney that influence female sexual behavior. The attractiveness of the female to the male involves a change in perception of the male by the female resulting from a changing physiological state within the female, not because of changes that are occurring in the male.

The classic way for males to delineate their territory has been for them to mark the area with urine. In general, pheromones that affect sexual behavior tend to have a musk type of odor. The classic pheromone used by humans is perfume, which is derived from civetone, a cyclical 17-carbon compound obtained from the civet cat.

The Whitten effect has been used to manipulate the estrous cycles of animals. In sheep, males are introduced into a flock of ewes before the breeding season to advance, or ensure, ovarian cyclicity at the beginning of the breeding season. Whereas it was previously thought the effect of the introduction of a male was short-lived (i.e., a gonadotropin response could only be obtained within the first few days from ewes that had antral follicles), it is now clear that the interaction of rams with ewes over extended periods of the anestrus results in earlier ovarian activity.

As discussed, pheromones can account for some of the effect of the male. More recent studies, however, have shown that *sight* of the male by the female, as well as *physical contact,* are important factors that influence gonadotropin secretion and thus ovarian activity.

The Whitten effect has also been used to influence the onset of puberty in pigs. The introduction of males into groups of gilts beginning several weeks before the expected time of puberty (180 to 200 days) has been used to ensure, or advance, the onset of puberty. The *dormitory effect,* the well-recognized synchronization of menstrual cycles in roommate women, occurs in bitches kenneled together as well.

Inadequate Nutrition Results in Ovarian Inactivity, Especially in Cattle

In dairy cattle, genetically selected for high productivity, the ability to produce up to 100 pounds of milk per day is a remarkable achievement. It is almost impossible for dairy cows to consume enough feed during the first part of the lactation cycle to maintain their body weight, and they are often in a negative nutritional balance for up to 100 days postpartum. Animals must have an adequate level of nutrition to initiate ovarian activity, so ovarian activity is suppressed until a positive energy balance is established. If an owner wants a dairy cow to produce large quantities of milk, the owner must be willing to wait for nutrition to "catch up" with milk production.

Inadequate nutrition can affect ovarian activity in the postpartum period. A management practice sometimes used to enhance production efficiency is to maintain beef cows on a marginal plane of nutrition during the winter. This approach forces animals to use fat that has been developed and stored during the grazing season. If pregnant beef cows are not returned to a positive nutritional balance by the last month of gestation, the reestablishment of ovarian cyclicity, which usually occurs between days 45 and 60 postpartum, will be delayed. Another situation that can affect ovarian activity involves pregnant beef heifers. These animals often need extra nutrition in the postpartum period to reestablish ovarian activity because they have requirements for growth as well as for lactation.

CLINICAL CORRELATIONS

SEXUAL ATTRACTIVENESS IN THE SPAYED BITCH

History. You are called by a veterinary colleague who has seen a bitch owned by one of her important clients. The client is upset because the dog is attracting males despite recently having undergone an ovariohysterectomy. You inquire whether the dog allows intromission by males. Although the answer is "no," the owner is sure that a portion of an ovary was left *in situ.* Your colleague is sure she removed the ovaries during the surgical procedure. You are asked to examine the dog as a favor to your colleague.

Clinical Examination. The dog has a vulva that is slightly swollen with a small amount of creamy discharge present. An examination of a vaginal mucosal smear reveals noncornified epithelial cells and an increased number of neutrophils. You indicate to the owner that you believe the (nondiscriminatory) male dogs are being attracted by the presence of an infection in the urogenital tract; the owner needs more convincing. You decide to obtain a reproductive endocrine panel (progesterone level and an LH test) and a urinalysis from the dog. The values for progesterone are low (<1.0 ng/mL) and the LH is positive (indicating lack of feedback) and thus do not support the active presence of ovarian tissue. The presence of white blood cells and bacteria in the urine suggests a urinary tract infection. A culture and sensitivity can be submitted to determine the specific bacteria and its antibiotic sensitivity.

Comment. It is common for bitches with genitourinary infections to attract male dogs, presumably because of the odors generated by the infection. One of the most important points of differentiation as to cause (i.e., bladder infection versus presence of ovarian remnant) is to know about the sexual behavior of the animal. The bitch normally allows intromission by a male only if she has been exposed to progesterone after priming with estrogen. This situation occurs only if an ovarian follicle is present and has begun to luteinize after the preovulatory luteinizing hormone surge. If the animal in question had allowed intromission, the presence of an ovarian remnant would be more likely. Because of the failure of the bitch to allow intromission, you can conclude that the animal almost certainly lacks ovarian tissue. With regard to the endocrine analysis, if the animal was completely ovariectomized, the LH level will be high, indicating a lack of negative feedback from either estrogen (not seen in the vaginal cytology) or progesterone (< 1.0 ng/mL). Nonestrogenized vaginal cytology and a low progesterone level do not rule out the presence of ovarian tissue, but if the sample is obtained when the animal is showing the sexual attractiveness, it can be stated with assurance that the behavior is not caused by hormones or, by extension, activity of ovarian tissue.

Treatment. The bladder infection is treated, and the owner is instructed to keep the female away from males until the infection has cleared.

TRYING TO GET A MARE PREGNANT

History. You work in Minnesota. Your clients have a 4-year-old Thoroughbred mare that they would like to breed early in the season, so that they will have as old of foal as possible, when it is old enough to race.

Clinical Examination. The mare has never been bred before. The breeding soundness exam (which assesses conformation, ultrasonography of her reproductive tract, cytology, and culture of her uterus) is normal.

Comment. If the mare can be bred as early in the year as possible, the owner will hopefully have a foal early in January (in the Northern Hemisphere). This will hopefully result in the foal being at its maximal development to race. The photoperiod is regulated by the pineal gland, which produces melatonin. Processing of light signals through the central nervous system (CNS) is regulated by the retina, suprachiasmatic nucleus, superior cervical ganglion, and the pineal gland. Ovarian activity begins in response to refractoriness of the photoperiod. There are two major methods for stimulating ovulatory activity in mares. One is to increase the total light per day. The other involves pulsatile amounts of light. Alternatively, drugs can be used to alter the cycle.

Treatment. The typical method to stimulate ovulation involves mimicking the photoperiod for 60 days prior to breeding. For this mare, 16 hours of day light should be started in November. In other cases, short periods of "flashes" of light (i.e., 1 hour of light 9.5 hours after onset of darkness) during the photosensitive period (10 hours after onset of darkness) can be used to stimulate ovulatory activity. An alternative option is to stimulate the mare with dopamine antagonists (i.e., domperidone) while increasing the photoperiod (i.e., increase photoperiod for 2 weeks, and then add dopamine antagonist until mare starts to cycle). Using one of these methods, the mare should begin ovulatory activity early in January, and hopefully will be bred and become pregnant for an early January foal.

PRACTICE QUESTIONS

1. The first estrous cycle of the cow subsequent to parturition follows which sequence?
   a. Anestrus, diestrus, estrus, metestrus, proestrus
   b. Anestrus, estrus, diestrus, metestrus, proestrus
   c. Anestrus, metestrus, diestrus, estrus, proestrus
   d. Anestrus, proestrus, estrus, diestrus, proestrus
   e. Anestrus, proestrus, estrus, metestrus, diestrus

2. The usual situation in large domestic animals is for a dominant follicle or dominant follicles to be present at the time of luteal regression, with sexual receptivity manifested within 1 to 2 days after luteal regression; the one large animal species that is the exception to this generalization is the:
   a. Cow.
   b. Doe.
   c. Ewe.
   d. Mare.
   e. Sow.

3. The hormones that form the foundation for sexual receptivity are:
   a. Estrogen and $PGF_{2\alpha}$.
   b. Progesterone and estrogen.
   c. Estrogen and GnRH.
   d. Progesterone and $PGF_{2\alpha}$.
   e. $PGF_{2\alpha}$ and GnRH.

4. Decreasing light turns off cyclical ovarian activity after a number of months, whereas increasing light reverses the process after a number of months, including the development of a transitional period. This description fits which domestic species?
   a. Cat
   b. Cow
   c. Dog
   d. Goat
   e. Horse
   f. Pig
   g. Sheep

5. What response results from the Whitten effect, in which the introduction of a male into a group of noncyclical animals results in the reestablishment of ovarian activity?
   a. Increased estrogen secretion
   b. Increased progesterone secretion
   c. Increased prolactin secretion
   d. Increased follicle-stimulating hormone secretion
   e. Increased luteinizing hormone secretion
   f. Increased follicle-stimulating hormone and luteinizing hormone secretion

6. Which one of the following domestic species requires progesterone priming, in addition to estrogen, to manifest estrus (therefore not manifesting estrus with the first ovarian cycle in the postpartum period)?
   a. Cat
   b. Dog
   c. Goat
   d. Horse
   e. Pig
   f. Sheep

BIBLIOGRAPHY

Austin CR, Short RV, editors: *Reproduction in mammals*, vols 1-6, Cambridge, UK, 1986, Cambridge University Press.

Beach FA: Coital behavior in dogs, *Behavior* 36:544, 1970.

Breen KM, Billings HJ, Wagenmaker ER, et al: Endocrine basis for disruptive effects of cortisol on preovulatory events, *Endocrinology* 146(4):2107–2115, 2005.

Card C: Hormone therapy in the mare. In Samper JC, editor: *Equine breeding management and artificial insemination*, ed 2, St Louis, 2009, Saunders.

Concannon PW, Morton DB, Weir BJ, editors: Dog and cat reproduction, contraception and artificial insemination, *J Reprod Fertil Suppl* 39, 1989.

Cupps PT, editor: *Reproduction in domestic animals*, ed 4, New York, 1991, Academic Press.

Davidson AP, Stabenfelt GH: Reproductive cycles. In Cunningham JG, Klein BG, editors: *Textbook of veterinary physiology*, ed 4, St Louis, 2007, Saunders.

Feldman EC, Nelson RW, editors: *Canine and feline endocrinology and reproduction*, ed 4, Philadelphia, 2009, Saunders.

Hafez ESE, Hafez B, editors: *Reproduction in farm animals*, ed 7, Baltimore, 2000, Lippincott Williams & Wilkins.

Johnson MH, Everitt BJ, editors: *Essential reproduction*, ed 5, London, 2000, Blackwell Scientific.

National Research Council: *Nutrient requirements of dogs and cats*, Washington, DC, 2005, National Academies Press.

Neill JD, editor: Knobil and Neill's physiology of reproduction, vols 1 and 2, ed 3, Philadelphia, 2005, Elsevier.

Pineda MH, Dooley MP, editors: *McDonald's veterinary endocrinology and reproduction*, ed 5, Ames, 2003, Iowa State University Press.

Simpson GM, England GCW, Harvey MJ, editors: *BSAVA manual of small animal reproduction and neonatology*, Gloucester, UK, 2010, BSAVA.

CHAPTER 38

Pregnancy and Parturition

KEY POINTS

Pregnancy
1. The development of an embryo involves fusion of an oocyte and spermatozoon within the oviduct.
2. Extension of the life span of the corpus luteum in large domestic species and cats is essential for pregnancy maintenance.
3. The placenta acts as an endocrine organ.

Parturition
1. Fetal cortisol initiates delivery through increased secretion of estrogen and thus prostaglandin $F_{2\alpha}$.

PREGNANCY

The Development of an Embryo Involves Fusion of an Oocyte and Spermatozoon Within the Oviduct

The development of a new individual requires the transfer of male gametes to the female genital tract for fertilization of the female gamete(s). *Spermatozoa,* which have been concentrated and stored in the epididymis, gradually change from *oxidative* (aerobic) to *glycolytic* (anaerobic) *metabolism* as they progress through the epididymis. In this situation, spermatozoa are in a state of reduced metabolism. Mature sperm are only able to metabolize a special sugar, *fructose,* within the reproductive tract. Lactose, glucose, dextrose, and fructose have all been used in commercially available semen extenders.

Sperm are ejaculated usually into the vagina, although some domestic species (dog, horse, and pig) ejaculate directly into the cervix and uterus. The movement of sperm through the cervix is aided by estrogen-induced changes in cervical mucus, which result in the formation of channels that facilitate movement of sperm. This has been particularly emphasized in primates, in which the thinning of mucus occurs just before ovulation, a factor that can be used to predict the time of ovulation.

The environment of the female genital system is generally inhospitable to the survival of sperm; for example, white blood cells are quickly attracted to the uterine lumen because sperm cells are foreign to the female genital tract. Special reservoirs have evolved in the female tract to aid in the survival of sperm during transport; these include the cervix and oviduct, the latter involving areas at the uterotubule junction and within the ampulla. The reservoirs are progressively filled (from caudal to cranial in the tract), requiring hours before the *oviductal reservoirs* are full. Finally, the reservoir within the ampulla is able to release a few sperm on a continuous basis, so that *fertilization* can occur shortly after the arrival of oocytes within the oviduct.

The first studies in *sperm transport* emphasized the rapidity of the process, with sperm reported passing from the vagina to the fimbriated end of the oviduct within minutes. It is now known that sperm undergoing so-called fast transport are not involved in *fertilization;* in fact, they are damaged by the rapid transport.

Sperm need to undergo changes within the female genital tract that are a prerequisite for fertilization; the process is called *capacitation.* One of the effects of *capacitation* is the removal of glycoproteins from the sperm cell surface.

The glycoproteins, perhaps added for protective purposes, interfere with *fertilization.* This change allows sperm to undergo the *acrosome reaction* when they come in contact with oocytes. The *acrosome reaction* involves the release of hydrolytic enzymes from the acrosomal cap; this may be important for penetration of the sperm through the granulosa and zona pellucida to the oocyte plasma membrane. *Hyaluronidase* causes breakdown of hyaluronic acid, an important component of the intercellular matrix of granulosa cells that surround the oocyte. *Acrosin,* a proteolytic enzyme, digests the acellular coating around the oocyte. Both enzymatic events allow the sperm to penetrate to the oocyte. The *acrosome reaction* also changes the surface of the sperm, which allows it to fuse with the oocyte. The *acrosome reaction* results in tail movements that feature a flagellar beat that tends to drive sperm in a forward direction.

Because of the changes that spermatozoa must undergo within the female reproductive tract before *fertilization,* the deposition of sperm before ovulation is the preferred timing for producing maximal fertility. An exception to this takes place when sperm with reduced longevity are used, such as the case with chilled-extended semen or frozen semen. In these cases, deposition of semen into the female reproductive tract should occur close to the time of ova maturation associated with fertilization. Females are usually sexually receptive for at least 24 hours before ovulation and, in the natural setting (free interaction between genders), insemination usually occurs a number of hours before the occurrence of ovulation. Even with induced ovulators, such as cats, the interval from copulation to ovulation is usually 24 hours or more. In essence, the system has evolved to have ready-to-fertilize sperm at the fertilization site when oocytes arrive. This concurs with the finding that the life span of male gametes tends to be twice that of female gametes.

The presentation of male gametes before female gametes in the oviduct implies that oocytes are ready for fertilization on arrival in the ampulla; this is likely true for a majority of animals. A prerequisite for fertilization of the oocyte is that it must undergo the first meiotic division before fertilization. Although this occurs in a number of species before ovulation, in the horse and dog the first meiotic division does not occur until after ovulation (in the dog, not for at least 48 hours). In this situation, spermatozoa often wait for oocytes to mature in the oviduct before *fertilization* can occur. One means of adaptation to delayed completion of meiosis is that spermatozoa have a longer life span in the dog (6 to 11 days) and horse compared with other domestic species.

After *fertilization* has occurred, the *embryo* usually develops to the *morula,* or early *blastocyst* stage, within the oviduct before moving into the uterus. This period, lasting usually 4 to 5 days, affords the uterus time to finish its inflammatory response involving the removal of spermatozoa. This period also allows the endometrial glands time to secrete nutrients under the influence of progesterone from the developing corpus luteum (CL); the nutrients are essential for the development of embryos during their preimplantation stage.

An interesting finding in the mare is her ability to distinguish fertilized from unfertilized oocytes; unfertilized oocytes from previous cycles are retained within the oviduct, whereas recently fertilized oocytes (embryos) move through the oviduct to the uterus. It is likely that all animals recognize pregnancy by the presence of an embryo(s) at the early oviductal stage. However, this recognition does not necessarily result in prolongation of the CL and the continued production of progesterone, which is essential for the maintenance of pregnancy. In the bitch, despite ovulation and ova maturation spanning several hours, embryonic ages are synchronized by some mechanism inherent to the bitch's reproductive tract.

Extension of the Life Span of the Corpus Luteum in Large Domestic Species and Cats Is Essential for Pregnancy Maintenance

For those domestic animals (cattle, goats, horses, pigs, sheep) whose luteal activity is controlled by the uterus, modification of *uterine prostaglandin $F_{2\alpha}$* (PGF$_{2\alpha}$) synthesis and release is critical for the establishment of pregnancy. The embryo apparently produces substances that modify uterine production of PGF$_{2\alpha}$. *Estrogen synthesis* by the embryo is one way the endometrium may be informed regarding the presence of an embryo. A specific protein of embryonic origin called *trophoblastin,* produced before day 14

of pregnancy (or postovulation) in both sheep and cattle, is of immunological interest for the establishment of pregnancy; it has a close structural relationship to the molecule *interferon.* Movement of the embryo(s) in the tract is also important for pregnancy recognition. In the mare the embryo moves throughout both horns before being fixed at day 16. In pigs a minimal number of embryos need to be present (about four), presumably to occupy a sufficiently large area of the endometrium. Litter-bearing animals also use transuterine migration to maximize the opportunity for fetal development, a procedure that aids the recognition of pregnancy process. The end result is either suppression of PGF$_{2\alpha}$ synthesis, as seen in the cow (Figure 38-1), or modification of the secretion mode (*continuous* instead of *pulsatile*), as seen in sheep. The absence of *pulsatile secretion* of PGF$_{2\alpha}$ seems to be critical for the extension of the life span of the CL and the establishment of pregnancy in large domestic species.

In the cat the CL lasts for 35 to 40 days after ovulation regardless of the presence of pregnancy, and thus early modification of luteal activity is not essential for the establishment of pregnancy. Implantation occurs at about day 13, which allows the fetoplacental unit to influence and extend luteal activity that is compatible with pregnancy maintenance. The luteotropic hormone that is responsible for luteal maintenance in the cat is not known. One hormone that likely synergizes with progesterone for the support of pregnancy is relaxin, a placental hormone produced in the cat beginning at about day 20 of gestation (see later discussion).

The dog does not extend its luteal phase during pregnancy; the luteal phase in the nonpregnant animal is often slightly longer (70 days) than in pregnant animals. Nevertheless, enhancement of luteal activity occurs through a placental *luteotropin,* likely *relaxin,* with progesterone secretion enhanced beginning at about day 20 of gestation or a few days after implantation. Early in the *luteal phase,* luteal function in the bitch is likely autonomous. During the second half of the *luteal phase,* luteinizing hormone (LH) and prolactin are likely *luteotrophs* (Figure 38-2).

The rescue of the CL at the onset of pregnancy in primates involves the production of a *luteotropin* called *chorionic gonadotropin* (CG; for humans, hCG), which is produced by trophoblastic cells (*syncytiotrophoblasts*) of the embryo (Figure 38-3). For trophoblast tissue to produce CG, it must have intimate contact with the interstitium of the endometrium. This contact occurs by a type of implantation called *interstitial,* in which the embryo

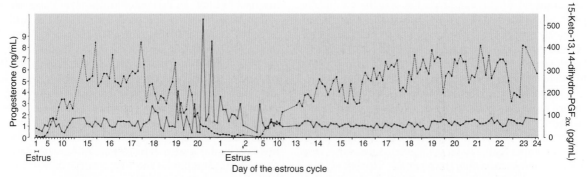

FIGURE 38-1 Relationship between prostaglandin release, as indicated by the measurement of 15-keto-13,14-dihydroprostaglandin F$_{2\alpha}$, and progesterone production by the corpus luteum during a nonfertile cycle and after a conception in the same cow. (From Kindahl H, Edquist LE, Bane A: Blood levels of progesterone and 15-keto-13,14-dihydro-prostaglandin F2alpha during the normal oestrous cycle and early pregnancy of heifers, *Acta Endocrinol (Copenh)* 82(1):134–49, 1976.)

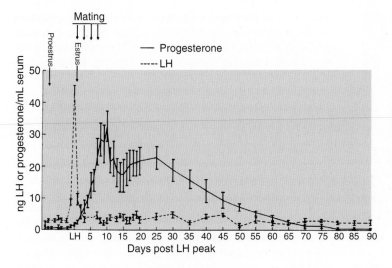

FIGURE 38-2 Luteinizing hormone *(LH)* and progesterone concentrations during pregnancy in nine dogs. *Vertical bars* represent the standard error of the mean. (From Smith MS, McDonald LE: Serum levels of luteinizing hormone and progesterone during the estrous cycle, pseudopregnancy and pregnancy in the dog, *Endocrinology* 94(2):404–12, 1974. Copyright © by The Endocrine Society.)

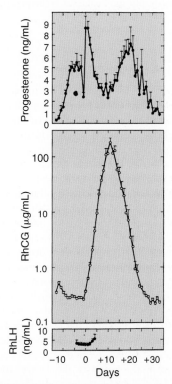

FIGURE 38-3 Summarization of 15 early pregnancies in normal rhesus monkeys normalized to the day of corpus luteum rescue (day 0). Points are means plus or minus standard error. Note the temporal relationship between luteal progesterone production (before day +10) and chorionic gonadotropin output. *RhCG,* Rhesus chorionic gonadotropin; *RhLH,* rhesus luteinizing hormone. (From Knobil E: On the regulation of the primate corpus luteum, *Biol Reprod* 8:246, 1973.)

penetrates the endometrium at about 8 to 9 days after fertilization in humans and nonhuman primates. Secretion of CG begins 24 to 48 hours after implantation, with immediate enhancement of luteal progesterone production. Rescue of the CL in human pregnancy occurs as late as 4 to 5 days before the end of the luteal phase.

As indicated, interstitial implantation is essential to the development of pregnancy in primates. *Implantation* is less invasive in the dog and cat, with the type termed *eccentric.* In the large

domestic species, "invasion" of the endometrium is minimal; implantation occurs within special endometrial protrusions called *caruncles* in ruminants and by relatively minor *villus* invasion of the endometrium in horses and pigs. Domestic animals depend more on uterine secretions for the support of pregnancy than do primates. For cattle and horses the first indications of implantation begin about days 25 to 30, and another 7 to 10 days likely passes before a significant amount of embryonic nutrition is obtained through the implantation site. Subclinical uterine infections, or an inadequate number of endometrial glands, can interfere with the establishment of pregnancy in the species in which a long interval exists from fertilization to implantation. The cervix forms an important barrier to contamination of the uterine lumen in both the nonpregnant and the pregnant animal; in the latter the cervix becomes sealed.

The Placenta Acts as an Endocrine Organ

Besides the essential role of providing nutrients and oxygen for embryonic metabolism, the *placenta* functions as an endocrine organ. One of the most important functions of the placenta is the *production of progesterone.* In primates this function is established early in gestation, and the placenta likely can maintain pregnancy within 2 to 3 weeks after implantation in primates. Placental production of sufficient progesterone to maintain pregnancy occurs later in domestic animals (sheep, day 50 of 150-day gestation; horse, day 70 of 340-day gestation; cat, day 45 of 65-day gestation); in some species the placenta never produces enough progesterone to support pregnancy (cattle, goats, pigs, dogs).

The *production of estrogen,* in contrast to that of progesterone, requires interaction between the fetus and the placenta. This interaction has been best described in primates, in particular by the experiments of the Hungarian immigrant to Sweden Egon Dicfaluszy. He and his co-workers found that the primate placenta is unable to produce estrogen from progesterone even though the steroids are only separated by androgens in the steroid biochemical synthetic pathway. The placenta simply does not possess the enzymes necessary for the conversion of progesterone to androgens. Therefore a system has evolved in which the placenta supplies *pregnenolone,* the immediate precursor of progesterone, to the fetus, and the *fetal zone of the adrenal cortex* transforms pregnenolone to a C-19 androgen, *dehydroepiandrosterone.* This is returned to the placenta, which is able to convert dehydroepiandrosterone to an estrogen. In humans the primary

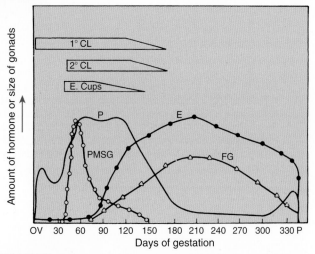

FIGURE 38-4 Summary of the temporal relationships among changes in hormonal concentrations and morphological changes throughout the gestational period of the mare. *1° CL,* Primary corpus luteum; *2° CL,* secondary corpora lutea; *E,* estrogens; *E. Cups,* endometrial cups; *FG,* fetal gonads; *P,* progesterone; *PMSG,* pregnant mares' serum gonadotropin (equine chorionic gonadotropin). (From Daels PF, Hughes JP, Stabenfeldt GH: Reproduction in horses. In Cupps PT, editor: *Reproduction in domestic animals,* ed 4, New York, 1991, Academic Press.)

estrogen of pregnancy is *estriol.* Because the fetus is involved in the production of estriol, the well-being of the fetus can be judged by determining estriol concentrations in the plasma of the mother.

The production of estrogen in the mare also involves an interaction between the placenta and fetus (Figure 38-4). From the work of Pashen and Allen, we know that the fetal gonads replace the fetal adrenals in primates as the key fetal endocrine organ involved in the cooperative synthesis of estrogen. The interstitial cells of the gonads appear to be the interactive cells, with fetal gonads enlarging to a size greater than the maternal gonads during the latter part of gestation. The production of estrogens during pregnancy in other domestic species, occurring relatively late in gestation, may involve the development of placental enzymes that allow progesterone to be metabolized to estrogens without the direct intervention of a fetal endocrine organ. (Fetal cortisol, however, is important for the induction of these placental enzymes, particularly in sheep; see next section.)

The protein hormones that are produced during pregnancy tend to be of placental origin. For example, *relaxin* is a hormone produced by the placenta in the cat, dog, and horse beginning at about days 20, 20, and 70, respectively. Besides its importance for preparing the soft tissues of the pelvic canal for passage of the fetus at birth (see the discussion on parturition), *relaxin* may be important for the support of pregnancy through a synergistic action with progesterone. In exception to the general rule of protein hormone production by the placenta, *relaxin* is produced by the CL in the pig, cow, and primates during pregnancy, with prepartum release occurring in conjunction with *luteolysis.*

The only CG identified in domestic animals to date is *equine CG* (eCG, formerly called *pregnant mares' serum gonadotropin* by its discoverer, Harold Cole) (see Figure 38-4). The eCG is produced by trophoblast cells that initially form as a band on the chorion *(chorionic girdle),* detach themselves around day 35 of pregnancy, penetrate the endometrium, and form associations of cells called *endometrial cups.* The eCG enhances progesterone

production by the primary CL of pregnancy and aids in the formation of additional (secondary) CL through the *luteinization,* or ovulation, of preformed follicles. The essentiality of eCG for pregnancy maintenance is not known, because the primary CL is adequate for maintaining pregnancy.

Placental lactogen is another placental protein hormone. Its production increases in primates as CG secretion wanes during pregnancy. Placental lactogen has been reported in goats and sheep, with secretion increasing during the latter part of gestation. The hormone appears to have both *somatotropic* and *lactogenic effects* on the basis of growth hormone–like and prolactin-like properties. In dairy cattle, for example, placental lactogen may be important for mammary gland alveolar development, setting the stage for the next lactation. Another hormone whose production is increased during pregnancy, *prolactin,* also is important for alveolar development during the prepartum period. Prolactin is not a hormone of placental origin; prolactin increases during the latter part of gestation due to the effect of estrogen on its release from the adenohypophysis. Prolactin is luteotrophic in the dog.

PARTURITION

Fetal Cortisol Initiates Delivery Through Increased Secretion of Estrogen and Thus Prostaglandin F$_{2\alpha}$

During pregnancy the uterus progressively enlarges and stretches because of the growing fetus. Progesterone plays an important role in maintaining the quiescence of the myometrium as well as promoting a tightly contracted cervix. During the latter part of gestation, estrogen begins to influence uterine muscle by stimulating the production of *contractile protein* and the formation of *gap junctions;* the former increases the contractile potential of the uterus, and the latter facilitates the contractile process through increased communication among smooth muscle cells. Thus, important changes that set the stage for parturition begin weeks before the actual process begins. In the end, the uterus is converted from a quiescent to a contractile organ, and importantly, the cervix relaxes and opens to allow the fetus to be delivered.

The most important question about parturition concerns what initiates the process. In domestic animals, maturation of the fetus eventually brings about changes that initiate the delivery process. The key organ system of the fetus responsible for initiating the process is the *fetal adrenal cortex,* with the hypothalamus and adenohypophysis playing important supporting roles. This concept came from the work at the University of California (UC)–Davis by Liggins and Kennedy, who showed that destruction of the anterior pituitary of the sheep fetus resulted in prolongation of gestation; Drost subsequently found the same results after fetal adrenalectomy. Critical changes in *cortisol secretion* by the fetus eventually result in the synthesis and release of PGF$_{2\alpha}$ from the uterus, which produces muscle contraction and relaxation of the cervix. The following details of the initiation of parturition emphasize ruminants. It is postulated that elevated cortisol levels also contribute to the initiation of parturition in the dog.

The maturation of the fetal adrenal cortex is of critical importance in the initiation of parturition. The adrenal cortex likely becomes progressively sensitive to fetal adrenocorticotropic hormone (ACTH, corticotropin) (Figure 38-5). The time of adrenal maturation is under fetal genetic control, as shown by studies conducted on fetal lambs of different breeds in the same uterus (produced by embryo transfer) in which the prepartum initiation of cortisol production occurred at times that were

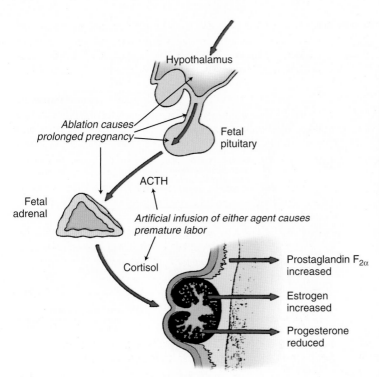

FIGURE 38-5 Diagrammatic summary explaining how the fetal lamb controls the onset of labor. Experimental procedures that lengthen or shorten pregnancy are shown. *ACTH,* Adrenocorticotropic hormone (corticotropin). (Redrawn from Liggins CG: The foetal role in the initiation of parturition in the ewe. In Wolstenholme GEW, O'Connor M, editors: *Foetal autonomy,* London, 1969, J & A Churchill.)

characteristic (and different) for the breed. Fetal cortisol induces placental enzymes (*17-hydroxylase* and *C17-20 lyase*) that direct steroid synthesis away from progesterone to estrogen. This process occurs at different times prepartum in domestic species, beginning at prepartum days 25 to 30 in cattle, 7 to 10 in pigs, and 2 to 3 in sheep. The end result of increased estrogen secretion is the secretion of *prostaglandins,* particularly $PGF_{2\alpha}$. $PGF_{2\alpha}$ is the pivotal hormone for the initiation of parturition; once its secretion begins, the acute phase of delivery is activated. The role of oxytocin in the initiation of delivery is not certain; it likely complements $PGF_{2\alpha}$ when the delivery process has started.

The synthesis of $PGF_{2\alpha}$ is thought to come about through increased availability of the substrate *arachidonic acid,* which is the main rate-limiting step in the synthesis of $PGF_{2\alpha}$. Estrogens are proposed to influence the system by making available the enzyme *phospholipase A,* a membrane-bound lysosomal enzyme that initiates the subsequent hydrolysis of phospholipids and release of arachidonic acid. This likely results from an increasing estrogen/progesterone ratio, with progesterone initially stabilizing, then estrogens destabilizing, lysosomal membranes. The end result is increased availability of arachidonic acid for the synthesis of $PGF_{2\alpha}$. The onset of $PGF_{2\alpha}$ synthesis results in the immediate release of the hormone because $PGF_{2\alpha}$ is not synthesized and stored. The critical effect of $PGF_{2\alpha}$ on the myometrium is to release intracellular calcium ion, which binds to *actin* and *myosin* to initiate the contractile process. Prostaglandins, both PGE and $PGF_{2\alpha}$, also have important effects on the *cervix,* which allow it to relax and dilate, permitting the passage of the fetus. The end result is a direct effect of $PGF_{2\alpha}$ on the intracellular matrix of the cervix in which there is a loss of collagen with a concomitant increase in *glycosaminoglycans,* the latter affecting the aggregation of collagen fibers.

In some animals, such as the cow, goat, dog, and cat, $PGF_{2\alpha}$ synthesis and release initiate regression of the CL beginning 24 to 36 hours before delivery, with complete withdrawal of progesterone occurring 12 to 24 hours before delivery. Although

essential for delivery in these species, progesterone withdrawal does not initiate delivery; it is the release of $PGF_{2\alpha}$ that both causes *luteolysis* and drives myometrial contractions.

In the mare, as in primates, delivery occurs even though progesterone concentrations remain elevated during the process. In this situation, $PGF_{2\alpha}$ is able to overcome the suppressive effects of progesterone on myometrial activity. For animals dependent on placental production of progesterone for pregnancy maintenance, it is not possible to turn off one function (i.e., steroid synthesis) and still continue with other functions that are necessary for the support of the fetus through the time of delivery.

Oxytocin is also important to the delivery process (Figure 38-6). Estrogen induces *oxytocin receptor* formation in the myometrium. Recent information indicates that significant amounts of oxytocin are released only with the entry of the fetus into the birth canal. Oxytocin release occurs through the *Ferguson reflex.* The afferent arm of the reflex involves passage of impulses through sensory nerves in the spinal cord to the appropriate nuclei in the hypothalamus; the efferent arm involves transport of oxytocin from the neurohypophysis by the vascular system. Oxytocin is synergistic with $PGF_{2\alpha}$ in promoting contraction of the uterus.

As noted earlier, a hormone important for the preparation of parturition is *relaxin.* This hormone was first identified as being responsible for the separation of the pubic symphysis through relaxation of the interpubic ligament. Relaxin causes the ligaments and associated muscles surrounding the pelvic canal to relax, which allows the fetus to expand the pelvic canal to its fullest potential. In the mare, a well-defined area of muscle softening can be discerned on the midline from the top of the croup through the ventral commissure of the vulva. In the cow, muscles posterior to the hip become relaxed to the point that they undulate as the animal walks in the final 24 hours before parturition. In the cow and pig, the CL is the source of relaxin. In both these species the prepartum release of $PGF_{2\alpha}$ causes luteolysis, with a concomitant decline in progesterone production and the release of preformed relaxin. In other domestic species, such as cats,

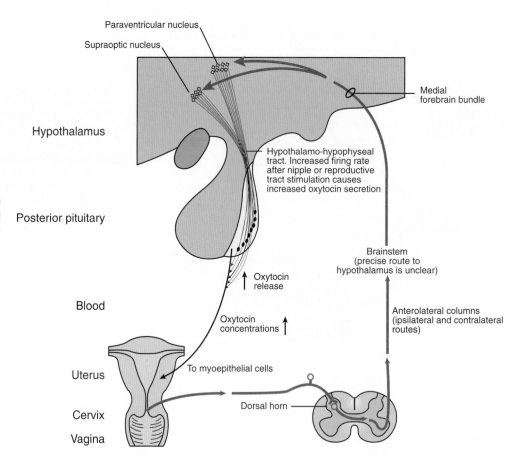

FIGURE 38-6 The neuroendocrine reflex (Ferguson reflex) underlying oxytocin synthesis and secretion. (From Johnson M, Everitt B, editors: *Essential reproduction,* ed 3, London, 1988, Blackwell Scientific.)

dogs, and horses, the source of relaxin is the placenta. In these species, significant relaxin production begins during the first part of gestation, with values sustained through parturition. A relaxin assay has been developed for the diagnosis of pregnancy in the dog, with good accuracy after 25 days of gestation. Relaxin may be important in these species for the maintenance of pregnancy in synergism with progesterone (see Figure 38-2).

The *first stage of parturition* involves presentation of the fetus at the internal os of the cervix. This likely results from increased myometrial activity caused by $PGF_{2\alpha}$ release. When the cervix opens and the fetus passes into the pelvic canal, myometrial contractions become less important for delivery of the fetus; *abdominal press,* accomplished by closure of the epiglottis and contraction of maternal abdominal muscles, becomes the main force involved in the delivery process. The actual delivery process is called the *second stage of parturition.*

The *third stage of parturition* involves the delivery of the fetal membranes. In litter-bearing animals, such as the cat, dog, and pig, the placental membranes are delivered often with, or immediately after, the appearance of each fetus. In single-bearing species, the placenta may be delivered immediately or within a few hours. From studies done on the mare at UC–Davis, we know that major, sustained surges of $PGF_{2\alpha}$ occur in the immediate postpartum period and are important for expulsion of placental membranes and reduction of uterine size through myometrial contraction. $PGF_{2\alpha}$ is likely the most important component of uterine size reduction in the immediate postpartum period for all domestic species. This can be inferred from the episodes of discomfort that parturient animals undergo during the hours immediately after delivery.

The neonate must make a major physiological adjustment to life on the outside. The major change involves the vascular system, in particular the respiratory system. During fetal life, blood bypasses the lungs (except for the perfusion of lung tissue in support of development) by two routes: through the ventricles by way of the *foramen ovale,* and from the pulmonary artery to the aorta by the *ductus arteriosus.* The foramen ovale is closed functionally at birth by a flap of tissue in the left ventricle through the development of higher pressures within the left versus the right ventricle. Although the ductus arteriosus immediately constricts at birth, it requires months before it is completely closed. This course of closure is also true for the *ductus venosus,* which serves as a hepatic shunt during fetal life. The rapid conversion from a fluid to a gaseous environment, as occurs at birth, is a truly remarkable adaptation.

CLINICAL CORRELATIONS

PROLONGED GESTATION

History. You are called to examine a purebred Holstein cow that is 12 days overdue compared with the herd gestation average of 280 days. She was artificially inseminated, was diagnosed pregnant 35 days later, and has not been observed in estrus since insemination. You inquire about the presence of bulls on the dairy farm, but there are none.

Clinical Examination. The cow has a greatly enlarged abdomen. On palpation of the uterus per rectum, you find the presence of a large calf. The cow certainly appears to be term as far as the size of the calf. You are puzzled, however, by the lack of colostrum in the udder.

Comment. The history and physical examination findings are compatible with an animal that has a fetus that is defective in terms of the initiation of parturition. A normal fetal hypothalamic-pituitary-adrenocortical system is essential for the production of cortisol, which initiates the delivery process. In the cow, this can begin 3 to 4 weeks prepartum, with fetal cortisol directing the increased production of estrogen; this in turn eventually initiates PGF$_{2\alpha}$ synthesis and release. The deficit could be caused by a malformed adrenal gland, pituitary, or hypothalamus. In one syndrome described for Holsteins, the critical defect was a lack of corticotropin-producing cells in the pituitary, which led to inadequate stimulation of the adrenal cortex and inadequate fetal cortisol production. The lack of lactogenesis reflects that the endocrine changes beginning 3 to 4 weeks prepartum as a prelude to delivery are also important for lactogenesis, and in their absence, colostral formation is delayed.

Treatment. The animal can respond to glucocorticoids, with delivery usually occurring 2 to 3 days later. The placenta is normal in this situation, and the systemic administration of glucocorticoids substitutes for fetal cortisol in initiating the endocrine events that lead to parturition. Lactogenesis is usually initiated by glucocorticoid treatment, although the process is usually less advanced than that expected at normal delivery. Because the calf continues to grow in utero in this syndrome, it is often too large to be delivered *per vaginam,* and a cesarean section may have to be performed 2 to 3 days after treatment in concert with dilation of the cervix.

You need to tell the owner that the calf will likely not survive because of inadequate adrenal secretion. If the calf were an extremely valuable bull prospect, one could administer both glucocorticoids and mineralocorticoids for a number of months with the hope the animal would eventually be able to take over its own adrenal support (this actually occurred in one case at UC–Davis). It would be questionable, however, to initiate treatment of the calf on the basis that the disease is an autosomal recessive inherited condition.

EARLY EMBRYONIC DEATH IN A MARE

History. A new client calls; they have a 10-year-old Quarter Horse mare they would like to breed. The mare has previously had a few foals. Last year, she was bred, and determined to be pregnant by ultrasound exam at day 24 post-ovulation, but was not pregnant at day 60.

Clinical Examination. You perform a breeding soundness on the exam and everything appears to be normal. You recommend uterine cytology, culture, and biopsy to determine if there is an apparent cause of the pregnancy loss. The cytology and culture are normal. The biopsy detects some inflammation and fibrosis (category 2b). The inflammation is around the endometrial glands, and it can limit motility and clearance. These changes may be reversible, but a mare with a category 2b uterus has a decreased pregnancy rate (30% to 70%) depending on the severity of inflammation.

Comment. The normal cytology and culture at this time does not rule out that the mare did not have an infection (endometritis) at the time of her pregnancy last year. The biopsy indicates some inflammation, which could limit the ability of the endometrial cups to form and/or placenta to provide sufficient nutrition, oxygen and/or hormones (progesterone). Normally, the corpus luteum (CL) on the ovary will provide sufficient progesterone to maintain the pregnancy. If there is inflammation (i.e., endometritis, colic) present to stimulate release of PGF$_{2\alpha}$, this can cause lysis of the CL and loss of pregnancy. Mares can be checked to determine if they are producing sufficient levels of progesterone. If not, progesterone can be supplemented. The fetoplacental unit takes over production of progesterone at 90 days.

Treatment. The cause of the early embryonic death (EED) is not clear. It is possible that the fibrotic changes in the uterus could limit nutritional support of the fetus. It is also possible that the mare had endometritis last year, and/or the mare did not produce sufficient progesterone to maintain the pregnancy. To increase the chances the most, the mare can be flushed after breeding to decrease inflammation, administer oxytocin to decrease fluid accumulation, and supplement with progesterone.

PRACTICE QUESTIONS

1. Active rescue of luteal activity through suppression of pulsatile prostaglandin synthesis and release by the production of embryonic signals must occur in which of the following species in order for a developing pregnancy to have the early progestational support essential for pregnancy maintenance? (Select all that apply.)
   a. Cattle
   b. Dog
   c. Goat
   d. Horse
   e. Pig
   f. Sheep

2. In primates it has been established that estrogen production during much of pregnancy is a cooperative venture between fetal adrenals and the placenta. The domestic species most extensively studied in this regard is the horse. In this species the main two interactive organs involved in the synthesis of estrogen during pregnancy are the placenta and the:
   a. Fetal adrenals.
   b. Fetal gonads.
   c. Fetal liver.
   d. Fetal hypothalamus.
   e. Fetal pituitary.

3. Which of the following hormones initiates the final process that eventually leads to parturition?
   a. Maternal estrogen
   b. Maternal progesterone
   c. Fetal cortisol
   d. Maternal relaxin
   e. Maternal prostaglandin
   f. Maternal oxytocin

4. The hormone that initiates the myometrial contractile process that acutely initiates parturition is:
   a. Maternal estrogen.
   b. Maternal progesterone.
   c. Fetal cortisol.
   d. Maternal relaxin.
   e. Maternal prostaglandin.
   f. Maternal oxytocin.

5. The hormone released by the passage of the fetus into the pelvic canal through the cervix is:
   a. Maternal estrogen.
   b. Maternal progesterone.
   c. Fetal cortisol.
   d. Maternal relaxin.
   e. Maternal prostaglandin.
   f. Maternal oxytocin.

BIBLIOGRAPHY

Austin CR, Short RV, editors: *Reproduction in mammals*, vols 1-6, Cambridge, UK, 1986, Cambridge University Press.

Concannon PW, Morton DB, Weir BJ, editors: Dog and cat reproduction, contraception and artificial insemination, *J Reprod Fertil Suppl* 39, 1989.

Cupps PT, editor: *Reproduction in domestic animals*, ed 4, New York, 1991, Academic Press.

Feldman EC, Nelson RW, editors: *Canine and feline endocrinology and reproduction*, ed 4, Philadelphia, 2009, Saunders.

Hafez ESE, Hafez B, editors: *Reproduction in farm animals*, ed 7, Baltimore, 2000, Lippincott Williams & Wilkins.

Jackson PGG: *Handbook of veterinary obstetrics*, Philadelphia, 2004, Saunders.

Johnson MH, Everitt BJ, editors: *Essential reproduction*, ed 5, London, 2000, Blackwell Scientific.

LeBlanc MM, Lopate C, Knottenbelt DC, Pascoe RR: The mare. In Knottenbelt DC, Pascoe RR, Lopate C, LeBlanc MM, editors: *Equine stud farm medicine and surgery*, ed 2, Edinburgh, 2003, Saunders.

Lennoz-Roland M: *Practical uses of aglepristone: review of a recent expert meeting*. Presented at 5th Biannual Congress, *European Veterinary Society for Small Animal Reproduction (EVSSAR)*, Budapest, Hungary, 2006.

Neill JD, editor: *Knobil and Neill's physiology of reproduction*, vols 1 and 2, ed 3, Philadelphia, 2005, Elsevier.

Olson PN, Nett TM, Bowen RA, et al: Endocrine regulation of the corpus luteum of the bitch as a potential target for altering fertility, *J Reprod Fertil Suppl* 39:27–40, 1989.

Pineda MH, Dooley MP, editors: *McDonald's veterinary endocrinology and reproduction*, ed 5, Ames, 2003, Iowa State University Press.

Silva LD, Verstegen JP: Comparisons between three different extenders for canine intrauterine insemination with frozen-thawed spermatozoa, *Theriogenology* 44(4):571–579, 1995.

Simpson GM, England GC, Harvey MJ, editors: *BSAVA manual of small animal reproduction and neonatology*, Gloucester, UK, 2010, BSAVA.

Stout TA: The early pregnancy. In Samper JC, editor: *Equine breeding management and artificial insemination*, ed 2, St Louis, 2009, Saunders.

Van der Weyden GC, Taverne MA, Dieleman SJ, et al: Physiological aspects of pregnancy and parturition in dogs, *J Reprod Fertil Suppl* 39:211–214, 1989.

CHAPTER 39
The Mammary Gland

KEY POINTS

Anatomical aspects of the mammary gland

1. The milk-secreting cells of the mammary gland develop through the proliferation of epithelium into hollow structures called alveoli.
2. Most of the milk that accumulates before suckling or milking is stored in the alveoli, even though animals have enlarged milk-storage areas called cisterns.
3. A suspensory system involving the udder of the cow allows the animal to carry a large amount of milk.

Control of mammogenesis

1. Initial development of the mammary gland is programmed by embryonic mesenchyme.
2. Proliferation of the mammary duct system begins at puberty, with ducts under the control of estrogens, growth hormone, and adrenal steroids, and alveoli under the control of progesterone and prolactin.

Colostrum

1. Prepartum milk secretion (without removal) results in the formation of colostrum.
2. The ingestion of colostrum is important because of the passive immunity it confers through the presence of high concentrations of immunoglobulins.
3. The time immunoglobulins can be absorbed through the neonatal gut is limited to the first 24 to 36 hours of life.
4. Lipids (particularly vitamin A) and proteins (caseins and albumins) are high in concentration in colostrum; carbohydrates (lactose) are low.

Lactogenesis

1. Prolactin, inhibited by dopamine and stimulated by vasoactive intestinal peptide, is the most important hormone involved in the process of milk synthesis, or lactogenesis; growth hormone is also important for lactogenesis.
2. The release of fat into milk from the alveolar cell involves constriction of the plasma membrane around the fat droplet; fats are dispersed in milk in droplet form.

3. Milk proteins and lactose are released from alveolar cells by the process of exocytosis.

Milk removal

1. Efficient milk removal requires the release of oxytocin, which causes contraction of muscle cells that surround the alveoli (myoepithelial cells), and movement of milk into the ducts and cisterns.

First nursing

1. Carbohydrate stores are good in neonates born as singles or twins, whereas carbohydrate stores are low in neonates born in litters; consequently the former can stand a longer interval to first suckling than can the latter.

Composition of milk

1. Fats are the most important energy source in milk.
2. Lactose, composed of glucose and galactose, is the main carbohydrate of mammalian milk.
3. The main proteins in milk are called *caseins* and are found in curd.

The lactation cycle

1. Milk production peaks at 1 month postpartum in dairy cattle, followed by a slow decline in production; milking usually stops at 305 days of lactation so that the animal can prepare the mammary gland for the next lactation.
2. Lactation can be induced by hormone administration (estrogen and progesterone) and enhanced by growth hormone and increased photoperiod exposure.

Diseases associated with the mammary gland

1. The main diseases that affect the mammary gland directly are mastitis (prevalent in dairy cattle and dogs) and neoplasia (prevalent in intact dogs and cats).
2. The main conditions that involve the mammary gland indirectly are passive transfer of red blood cell agglutinating antibodies by the ingestion of colostrum (mare, queen) and hypocalcemia caused by the transient drain of calcium that occurs with initiation of lactation (dairy cattle) or during the perinatal period (dog).

A nimals that belong to the class *Mammalia* are characterized as having bodies that are basically covered with hair, delivering live young instead of eggs (the monotremes are an exception), and, pertinent to this chapter, nurturing their young through the use of structures called *mammary glands*. The ability of mammals to nurture their young through milk secretion by mammary glands during the early part of post-fetal life has given these animals survival advantages. Because the reproductive strategy of mammals involves the production of far fewer young, compared with reptiles, amphibians,

and birds, mammary glands have allowed mammals to be much more efficient in the nurture of their young. Egg-laying classes of animals, such as fish, reptiles, and amphibians, depend on favorable environmental factors for the nurture of their young; the offspring are often vulnerable to the vagaries of nature. Mammalian young do not require teeth for the suckling process and thus can be delivered with immature maxillae and mandibles, which facilitates the delivery of the head. The development of teeth coincides with the need to consume food other than milk.

ANATOMICAL ASPECTS OF THE MAMMARY GLAND

The Milk-Secreting Cells of the Mammary Gland Develop Through the Proliferation of Epithelium into Hollow Structures Called Alveoli

Embryonic ectoderm is the source of the mammary glands. The mammary ectoderm is first represented by parallel linear thickenings on the ventral belly wall. The continuity of the ridge that is formed is broken into the appropriate number of *mammary buds,* from which the functional part of the mammary gland will be derived.

The *parenchyma,* or milk-secreting cells, of the mammary gland develops through the proliferation of epithelial cells that arise from the primary mammary cord. The epithelial cells eventually form hollow, circular structures called *alveoli,* which are the fundamental milk-secreting units of the mammary gland (Figure 39-1). In concert with this development, an enlarged area of epithelium, the *nipple,* which is the external connection to the internal milk-secreting system, develops on the surface. In males, although nipples often develop, the underlying primary mammary cord does not develop into substantial glandular tissue.

Most of the Milk That Accumulates Before Suckling or Milking Is Stored in the Alveoli, Even Though Animals Have Enlarged Milk-Storage Areas Called Cisterns

Duct systems connect alveoli with the nipple, or teat, enabling milk to pass from the area of formation to the area of delivery (nipple). The ducts may come together so that there is only one final duct per gland, which has one opening through the nipple, or teat, such as occurs in cattle, goats, and sheep. Two main ducts and associated openings occur in the mare and sow, whereas the cat and dog can have 10 or more openings in the nipple, with each opening representing separate glands (Figure 39-2). Both the cow

and the doe (goat) have specialized areas for holding milk, called *cisterns,* which are located in the ventral part of the gland and into which all main ducts empty (Figure 39-3). This has enabled the cow, for example, to synthesize and store larger amounts of milk than would otherwise be possible. Despite this adaptation, it is important to realize that a majority of the milk present at the time of milking is stored in the duct system of the mammary glands.

Mammary glands develop typically as paired structures. The number of pairs in domestic animals varies from one in goats, horses, and sheep; two in cattle; to seven to nine in the sow and seven to ten in the bitch and queen. The position of mammary glands varies in animals, being thoracic in primates; extending the length of the thorax and abdomen in cats, dogs, and pigs; and being inguinal in cattle, goats, and horses. In domestic species, such as cattle, goats, horses, and sheep, pairs of mammary glands are closely apposed to each other; the resulting structure is called an *udder.* In the cow, for example, two pairs of glands (four quarters) compose the udder.

A Suspensory System Involving the Udder of the Cow Allows the Animal to Carry a Large Amount of Milk

One of the important anatomical adaptations of the udder that allows dairy cows to carry large amounts of milk is the development of a suspension system for the udder. This system is formed by the median suspensory ligament (formed between pairs of mammary glands) composed of elastic connective tissue that originates from the abdominal tunic. The lateral (nonelastic) suspensory ligament, which originates from prepubic and subpubic ligaments, enters the glands laterally at various levels to become part of the interstitial connective tissue framework of the udder. It is not unusual for heavy-producing dairy cows to have 25 kg (55 lb) of milk in their udder immediately before milking. If the suspensory support system were not in place, the mammary gland system would soon break down from the weight of the milk.

CONTROL OF MAMMOGENESIS

Initial Development of the Mammary Gland Is Programmed by Embryonic Mesenchyme

The fetal development of the mammary gland is under both genetic and endocrine control. The initial development of the mammary bud is under control of embryonic *mesenchyme* (connective tissue). If mammary mesenchyme is transplanted to another area, mammary bud formation will occur at the site of transplantation. Although little is known about fetal mammary development, it is not thought to be driven by hormones. However, actively secreting mammary glands may be present at birth as a result of exogenous administration of certain hormones to the mother.

Proliferation of the Mammary Duct System Begins at Puberty, with Ducts Under the Control of Estrogens, Growth Hormone, and Adrenal Steroids, and Alveoli Under the Control of Progesterone and Prolactin

Development of the mammary gland in post-fetal life usually starts in concert with puberty. Cyclical ovarian activity results in the production of estrogen and progesterone. Estrogen, with growth hormone and adrenal steroids, is responsible for

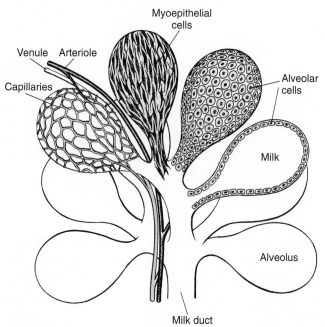

FIGURE 39-1 Diagram of a cluster of alveoli in the mammary gland of a goat. (From Cowie AT: Lactation. In Austin CR, Short RV, editors: *Reproduction in mammals,* ed 2, vol 3, Hormonal control of reproduction, Cambridge, UK, 1984, Cambridge University Press.)

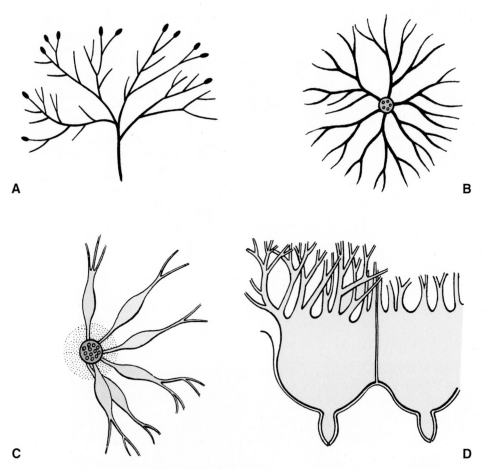

A

B

C

D

FIGURE 39-2 Diagram showing different arrangements of the mammary duct system. **A,** Cow, goat, sheep. **B,** Horse, pig. **C,** Cat, dog. **D,** Cow, goat cistern. (From Cowie AT: Lactation. In Austin CR, Short RV, editors: *Reproduction in mammals,* ed 2, vol 3, Hormonal control of reproduction, Cambridge, UK, 1984, Cambridge University Press.)

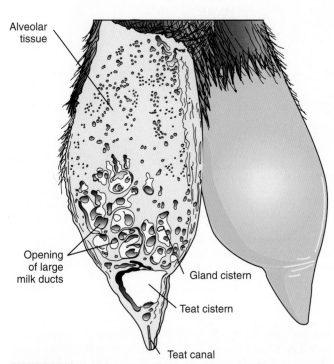

Alveolar tissue

Opening of large milk ducts

Gland cistern

Teat cistern

Teat canal

FIGURE 39-3 Depiction of the udder of a goat in which a section of the left mammary gland shows the dense alveolar tissues, the gland cistern with the large ducts opening into it, the teat cistern, and the teat canal. (From Cowie AT: Lactation. In Austin CR, Short RV, editors: *Reproduction in mammals,* ed 2, vol 3, Hormonal control of reproduction, Cambridge, UK, 1984, Cambridge University Press.)

proliferation of the duct system. The development of alveoli from the terminal ends of the ducts requires the addition of progesterone and *prolactin* (Figure 39-4).

Although the development of the mammary gland begins with the onset of puberty, the gland remains relatively undeveloped until the occurrence of pregnancy. In most domestic animals, udder development usually becomes evident by the middle of gestation; the secretion of milk often begins during the latter part of gestation (mainly from increasing *prolactin* secretion) and results in the formation of colostrum, as discussed later. By the end of pregnancy, the mammary gland has been transformed from a structure involving mostly stromal (connective tissue) elements to a structure that is filled with alveolar cells that are actively synthesizing and secreting milk. Groups of adjacent alveoli form *lobules* that further combine into larger structures called *lobes.* Connective tissue bands delineate the lobules and the lobes (Figure 39-5).

COLOSTRUM

Prepartum Milk Secretion (Without Removal) Results in the Formation of Colostrum

The milk formed before parturition is called *colostrum.* Its formation represents a secretory process in which lactogenesis occurs in the absence of milk removal. *Lactation* cannot fully blossom until pregnancy is terminated, however, because of the inhibitory effects of progesterone and estrogen on milk secretion, inhibitory factors that are removed at or just before delivery.

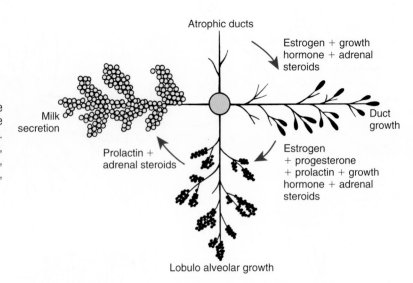

FIGURE 39-4 Hormones involved in the growth of the mammary gland and in the initiation of milk secretion in the hypophysectomized-ovariectomized-adrenalectomized rat. (From Lyons WR: *Proc R Soc B* 149:303, 1958. In Austin CR, Short RV, editors: *Reproduction in mammals,* ed 2, vol 3, Hormonal control of reproduction, Cambridge, UK, 1984, Cambridge University Press.)

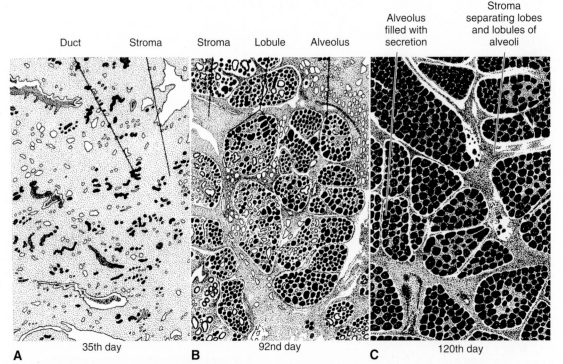

FIGURE 39-5 Drawings of sections of the mammary gland of the goat at three different times during pregnancy (which lasts approximately 150 days). **A,** Note the small collections of ducts scattered throughout the stroma on the 35th day. **B,** On the 92nd day the lobules of alveoli are forming in groups known as lobes; secretion is present in some of the alveolar lumina, and there is still considerable stromal tissue. **C,** On the 120th day the lobules of alveoli are almost fully developed; the alveoli are full of secretion, and the stromal tissue is reduced to thin bands separating lobules and thicker strands between lobes. (From Falconer IR, editor: *Lactation,* London, 1970, Butterworths.)

The Ingestion of Colostrum Is Important Because of the Passive Immunity It Confers Through the Presence of High Concentrations of Immunoglobulins

When colostrum is formed before parturition, certain substances are concentrated in the process. Ingestion of colostrum is important for the well-being of the neonate. In addition to nutrition, colostrum has an important function in temporary, or passive, protection against infectious agents. *Immunoglobulins* (e.g., immunoglobulin A, or IgA) are produced in the mammary gland by plasma cells (derived from B lymphocytes originating in the gut) as a result of exposure of the mother to certain microorganisms. The immunoglobulins gain access to the milk system through the migration of the plasma cells from adjacent tissue sites. The immunoglobulins are highly concentrated in colostrum, and through the consumption of colostrum, the neonate can receive passive immunity against pathogens experienced by the mother. This allows the young to receive immediate protection from environmental organisms. The neonates of all domestic animals acquire antibodies through the ingestion of colostrum. The absorption of antibodies through milk in domestic animals contrasts with the situation in other species, including humans, rabbits, and guinea pigs, in which a more substantial amount of antibody is passed to the fetus through the placenta.

The Time Immunoglobulins Can Be Absorbed Through the Neonatal Gut Is Limited to the First 24 to 36 Hours of Life

Neonates usually have a limited time (24 to 36 hours) in which immunoglobulins (proteins) can be absorbed through the gut. Thus the feeding of colostrum within this period is important to ensure the presence of immunoglobulins in the newborn. Other antimicrobial factors found in milk that are important for protection against the development of pathogenic enteric bacterial flora include lysozymes, lactoferrin, and the lactoperoxidase system.

Lipids (Particularly Vitamin A) and Proteins (Caseins and Albumins) Are High in Concentration in Colostrum; Carbohydrates (Lactose) Are Low

Colostrum is a rich source of nutrients, especially vitamin A, in addition to immunoglobulins. Placental transfer of vitamin A is limited in domestic animals, with calves and piglets being particularly low in vitamin A at birth. This deficiency is corrected by the ingestion of colostrum. Lipids and proteins, including caseins and albumins, are also present in relatively high concentration in colostrum. One exception is lactose; its synthesis is significantly inhibited by progesterone until about the time of delivery. Nevertheless, at the moment of delivery, the newborn's milk supply is nutritive (high protein, fat, and vitamin A content) and protective (immunoglobulins) (Table 39-1).

TABLE 39-1 Amounts of Selected Components of Bovine Colostrum as Percentage of Level in Normal Milk

Constituent	Day(s) After Parturition		
	0	3	4
Dry matter	220	100	100
Lactose	45	90	100
Lipids	150	90	100
Minerals	120	100	100
Proteins			
Casein	210	110	110
Albumin	500	120	105
Globulin	3500	300	200
Vitamins			
A	600	120	100
Carotene	1200	250	125
E	500	200	125
Thiamine	150	150	150
Riboflavin	320	130	110
Pantothenic acid	45	110	105

From Jacobson NL, McGilland AD: The mammary gland and lactation. In Swenson MJ, editor: *Dukes' physiology of domestic animals*, ed 10, Ithaca, NY, 1984, Cornell University Press.

LACTOGENESIS

Prolactin, Inhibited by Dopamine and Stimulated by Vasoactive Intestinal Peptide, Is the Most Important Hormone Involved in the Process of Milk Synthesis, or Lactogenesis; Growth Hormone Is Also Important for Lactogenesis

Prolactin plays an important role in the secretion of milk, or *lactogenesis*. Prolactin is released in conjunction with manipulation of the teat through either the suckling or the milking process. Sensory stimuli are carried into the hypothalamus, and the synthesis and release of *dopamine,* a major inhibitor of prolactin secretion, is blocked while neurons in the *paraventricular nucleus* are stimulated to produce and release *vasoactive intestinal peptide,* a stimulator of prolactin release (Figure 39-6). A short-lived surge of prolactin secretion occurs immediately after the onset of milk removal; peak values are usually reached within 30 minutes after the initial stimulus. Major surges of prolactin apparently do not need to be elicited on an hourly basis to maintain lactation because 12-hour release intervals, as occur in association with the milking of dairy cows, are sufficient to maintain lactogenesis. Prolactin responses, as judged by the amount of hormone release after mammary gland stimulation, decrease as the lactation period progresses.

Another major hormone required for milk production in ruminants is *growth hormone* (GH). There is now considerable interest in the use of GH to promote additional milk production from cows through exogenous administration of the hormone.

The Release of Fat into Milk from the Alveolar Cell Involves Constriction of the Plasma Membrane Around the Fat Droplet; Fats Are Dispersed in Milk in Droplet Form

The synthesis and release of milk by alveolar epithelial cells is a remarkable physiological process (Figure 39-7). Alveolar cells synthesize fats, proteins, and carbohydrates and extrude the products into the lumen of the alveolus. Fat droplets first accumulate in the basal cytoplasm of the cell and then move to the apex, where the droplet protrudes into the alveolar lumen. The cell membrane constricts about the base of the fat droplet, so fat is dispersed in milk in small droplets, surrounded by cell membranes; the droplet often contains portions of cell cytoplasm.

Milk Proteins and Lactose Are Released from Alveolar Cells by the Process of Exocytosis

Milk proteins are synthesized on the endoplasmic reticulum; the casein molecules pass to the Golgi apparatus, where they are phosphorylated and formed into micelles within the Golgi vesicles. Lactose is also synthesized within the Golgi vesicles and is released in conjunction with milk proteins. The process of extrusion of proteins and carbohydrates is different from that of fat; the Golgi vesicles fuse with the cell membrane, and the release of proteins and carbohydrates occurs by *exocytosis*. Although it is not certain how often cells go through a synthesis and extrusion cycle, it may occur twice daily, particularly in dairy cows that are milked two times per day.

MILK REMOVAL

For lactogenesis to be maintained, milk must be removed from the mammary gland by suckling or milking. If milk is not removed within about 16 hours in dairy cows, the synthesis of milk begins to be suppressed. As indicated previously, most of the milk in the

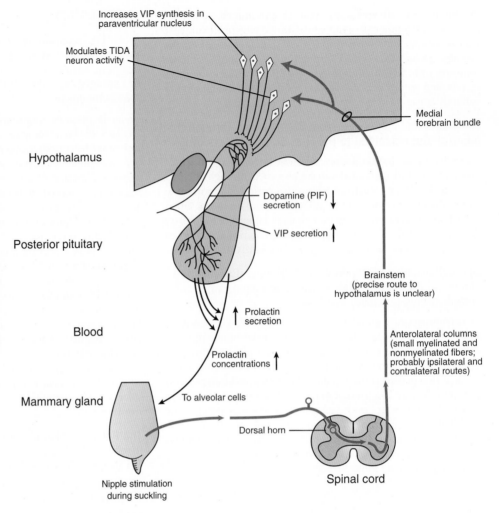

FIGURE 39-6 Somatosensory pathways in the suckling-induced reflex release of prolactin. The exact route taken by sensory information between brainstem and hypothalamus is speculative. Although tuberoinfundibular *(TIDA)* dopamine neuron activity is modulated as a result of the arrival of this somatosensory-derived input (prolactin inhibiting factor, *PIF*), the increased secretory activity of neurons containing vasoactive intestinal peptide *(VIP)* in the paraventricular nucleus is probably also crucial in driving prolactin secretion during suckling. (Modified from Johnson M, Everitt B: *Essential reproduction,* ed 3, London, 1988, Blackwell Scientific.)

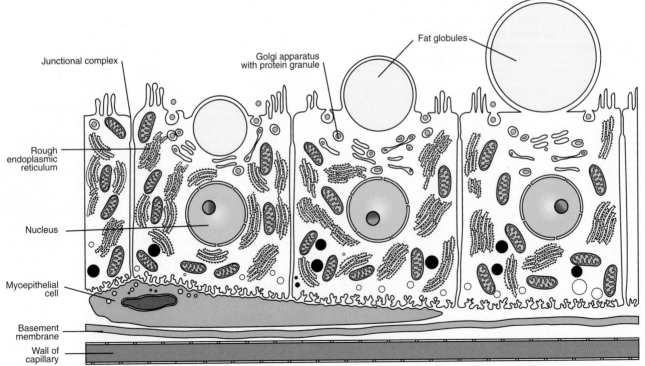

FIGURE 39-7 Diagram of the ultrastructure of three alveolar cells and a myoepithelial cell. (From Cowie AT: Lactation. In Austin CR, Short RV, editors: *Reproduction in mammals,* ed 2, vol 3, *Hormonal control of reproduction,* Cambridge, UK, 1984, Cambridge University Press.)

udder of a dairy cow at the time of milking is located in the ducts and alveoli. The movement of milk into the gland cistern at suckling or milking would be slow, and less milk would be obtained during the milking of a cow, if the drainage of milk were a passive process.

Efficient Milk Removal Requires the Release of Oxytocin, Which Causes Contraction of Muscle Cells That Surround the Alveoli (Myoepithelial Cells), and Movement of Milk into the Ducts and Cisterns

To facilitate the process of milk removal, *myoepithelial cells* surround the alveoli and ducts (see Figures 39-1 and 39-7). The myoepithelial cells are particularly responsive to oxytocin and, in fact, contract when exposed to the hormone. The synthesis and release of oxytocin from the posterior pituitary is elicited by a neuroendocrine reflex involving tactile stimulation of the udder by suckling by the young, or the manual stimulation of washing before milking. The sensory stimuli from the udder are carried through the spinal cord into the hypothalamus. Neurons in the paraventricular and supraoptic nuclei are stimulated to synthesize oxytocin and release it from nerve terminals that impinge on the median eminence (Figure 39-8). Other sensory stimuli that elicit oxytocin release include auditory, visual, and olfactory stimuli that occur near or within the kennel, cattery, or milking parlor. Past societies used various deceptions to have earlier breeds of cattle release their milk. They often allowed the calf to suckle one teat while they milked the other glands. They also knew about the

Ferguson reflex, if not in name, in which stimulation of the cervix (and release of oxytocin) was elicited by blowing air into the vagina using hollow tubes.

The release of oxytocin occurs within seconds after the stimulus arrives in the hypothalamus; increased pressure within the mammary gland is evident within a minute of stimulation as milk is forced out of the alveoli and ducts because of contraction of the myoepithelial cells. The term used in mammals to describe this phenomenon is *milk letdown.* Increased pressure within the udder is often obvious within a minute of the stimulation. The release of oxytocin lasts only a few minutes, and it is important that the milking process begin soon after milk letdown is complete (Figure 39-9). The milking process, as done by machine or by hand in earlier times, is often completed within 4 to 5 minutes.

It is interesting to compare stimuli that release oxytocin, which initiates the passive part of lactogenesis, with stimuli that release prolactin, which directly influences lactogenesis. Any sensory stimulus that a cow associates with milking has the potential for releasing oxytocin. The neuroendocrine reflex is elicited in the expectation of milk removal because of the environment (kennel, cattery, or milking parlor) to which the animal is exposed. Prolactin, on the other hand, is released only by tactile stimulation of the udder. The latter makes sense, because there is no need to stimulate milk synthesis and release unless the evidence for milk removal (udder stimulation) is strong. Milk removed during hand milking is trapped in the teat and forced out, whereas milk removed by milking machines moves by suction.

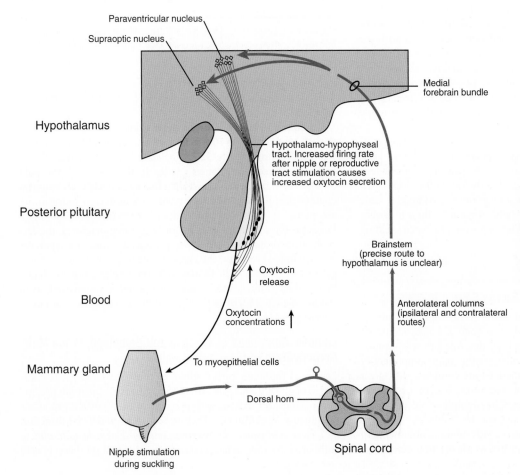

FIGURE 39-8 Somatosensory pathways in the suckling-induced reflex release of oxytocin. The actual pathway of sensory input in the hypothalamus is unknown, but it probably involves the medial forebrain bundle. (Modified from Johnson M, Everitt B: *Essential reproduction,* ed 3, London, 1988, Blackwell Scientific.)

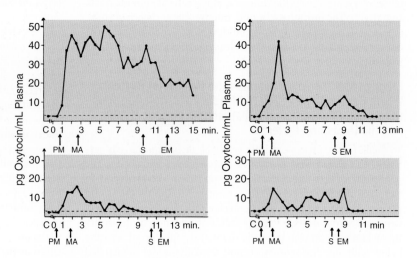

FIGURE 39-9 Oxytocin in the blood of cows before, during, and after milking. *Abscissae* show time in minutes. *C,* Control level; *EM,* end of machine milking; *PM,* preparation for milking; *MA,* application of teat cups; *S,* stripping. (From Schams et al: *Acta Endocrinologica* 92:258–270, 1979.)

FIRST NURSING

Carbohydrate Stores Are Good in Neonates Born as Singles or Twins, Whereas Carbohydrate Stores Are Low in Neonates Born in Litters; the Former Can Stand a Longer Interval to First Suckling Than Can the Latter

In domestic animals that have one or two offspring, such as cattle, horses, sheep, and goats, the young have to be able to stand in order to suckle. In this situation, neonates have reasonably good carbohydrate stores, and suckling may not occur for 1 to 2 hours without adverse effect as the young gain the ability to stand and locate the mammary gland. Young that are part of litters (cats, dogs, and pigs) are usually immediately nestled toward the mammary glands and often will be sucking in less than 30 minutes. This is important for animals born in litters because they tend to be immature at birth and susceptible to hypoglycemia, and suckling delays are often detrimental to their survival. Hypoglycemia results in stasis of the bowel (ileus) and can promote neonatal sepsis (overwhelming infection).

The suckling interval during the neonatal period varies considerably among domestic animals. Species nursing litters, such as cats, dogs, and pigs, often nurse at intervals of 1 hour or less. Goats, horses, and sheep nurse at slightly longer intervals, often up to 2 hours. Rabbits are an exception regarding the time between suckling periods; their young nurse at 24-hour intervals. As can be imagined, baby rabbits are engorged after each suckling period.

COMPOSITION OF MILK

Fats Are the Most Important Energy Source in Milk

Of the components of milk, fat is the most important energy source. Milk fat is composed of a number of lipids, including monoglycerides, diglycerides, triglycerides, free fatty acids, phospholipids, and steroids. Triglycerides are the main component of milk fat. The types of lipid synthesized are complex, with great variations in both chain length and saturation of fatty acids observed on the basis of species. The amount of fat produced varies greatly both within and among species (Table 39-2). Marine mammal milk has a high fat content, with values of about 40% to 50% in seals, 40% in dolphins, and 30% in whales. In these species

TABLE 39-2 Composition of Milk from Various Species (Percentage)

Species	Fat	Protein	Lactose	Ash
Cat	7.1	10.1	4.2	0.5
Cow	3.5	3.1	4.9	0.7
Dog	9.5	9.3	3.1	1.2
Goat	3.5	3.2	4.6	0.8
Horse	1.6	2.4	6.1	0.5

Modified from Jacobson NL, McGilland AD: The mammary gland and lactation. In Swenson MJ, editor: *Dukes' physiology of domestic animals,* ed 10, Ithaca, NY, 1984, Cornell University Press.

the high energy content of the milk through fat helps offset the heat loss of the young.

In domestic animals, sheep, swine, dogs, and cats have milk that ranges from 7% to 10% in fat content. Dairy cattle have values that range from 3.5% to 5.5%; goats are similar to cows (3.5%); and mares have lower values (1.6%). In the past, milk was sold on a butterfat basis, and breeds that had a relatively high butterfat content of milk (e.g., the Jersey with 5% butterfat) found more acceptance in dairy operations than is currently the case. Small farms produced mainly cream (for butter manufacture); the fat-concentrated portion of milk was produced by use of a separator that separated cream on the basis of specific gravity and centrifugal force. Because milk is now sold on a solids, not fat, basis, breeds that produce more milk (and protein) are favored, even though the fat content of the favored breed, Holstein-Friesian, is lower (3.5%).

Lactose, Composed of Glucose and Galactose, Is the Main Carbohydrate of Mammalian Milk

Lactose is the main carbohydrate of most mammals. It is composed of glucose and galactose. Blood glucose is the main precursor molecule for lactose, with propionate an important precursor for glucose in ruminants. Lactose is formed under the direction of *lactose synthetase,* an enzyme composed of α-*lactalbumin* (a milk protein) and *galactosyl transferase.* Lactose synthesis is held in abeyance until immediately before term because progesterone is inhibitory for the formation of α-lactalbumin. Prolactin, on the other hand, is stimulatory for the formation of lactose synthetase. Animals must have the enzyme *lactase* present in the jejunum for lactose to be cleaved (to glucose and galactose) and used. Lactase is present in most mammalian young but is sometimes not present in adult animals, including humans. In the absence of lactase, lactose can have an osmotic effect in the gastrointestinal tract, which can lead to diarrhea.

The Main Proteins in Milk Are Called *Caseins* and Are Found in Curd

The main proteins produced by the alveolar cells are called *caseins.* Caseins can be removed (as a curd) from milk through a process called *curdling* or *coagulation,* with other milk proteins, such as albumins and globulins, remaining in the fluid part of the milk (whey).

THE LACTATION CYCLE

The time required for changeover from colostrum to normal milk secretion varies with each species. In cattle, colostral milk tends to be stringy and yellow for several days postpartum. The complex bovine udder needs time for all areas to be flushed of colostrum. The milk of cattle is withheld from the milk supply for several days because of its unacceptable aesthetic quality, not because of the basic quality of the milk.

Milk Production Peaks at 1 Month Postpartum in Dairy Cattle, Followed by a Slow Decline in Production; Milking Usually Stops at 305 Days of Lactation So That the Animal Can Prepare the Mammary Gland for the Next Lactation

Milk production tends to increase for the first 3 to 4 weeks of lactation and then begins to slowly decline through the end of lactation (Figure 39-10). Cows are usually "dried up" after 305-day lactational periods; pounds of milk and butterfat production rates are calculated on this basis. Dairy animals are forced to stop lactating in order to prepare for the next lactation. The usual procedure is to stop milking. The back pressure of milk within the alveoli gradually inhibits the secretion of milk by the alveolar epithelial cells, with a resultant regression of the alveolar cells and small ducts. The process, called *involution,* often requires at least a month, with a 6-week period usually desired as the minimal interval from drying off to the onset of the next lactational period. Within 1 to 2 months, the secretory (alveoli) and excretory (duct) systems regress and are once again replaced. The process by which epithelial structures regress, yet retain coding for the renewal of duct and alveolar systems, is truly remarkable.

Lactation Can Be Induced by Hormone Administration (Estrogen and Progesterone) and Enhanced by Growth Hormone and Increased Photoperiod Exposure

The *induction of lactation* by hormone treatment is sometimes desired, especially in dairy animals with high-lactation records but poor reproductive performance. The use of a combined treatment of estrogen and progesterone over a relatively short period (1 week) has induced alveolar development sufficiently to result in milk production. Although the amount of milk produced is less than normal, the cows can be maintained in the milking string while efforts to impregnate them continue. To induce lactogenesis by hormonal means, animals should not be

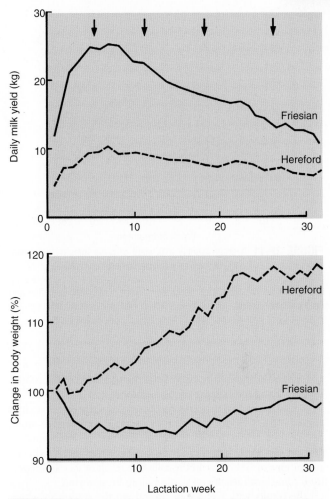

FIGURE 39-10 Average daily milk yield *(top)* and average percentage change in body weight *(bottom)* in seven low-yielding cows *(broken line)* and eight high-yielding cows *(solid line). Arrows* indicate times of blood sampling. (Courtesy Dr IC Hart. From Cowie AT: Lactation. In Austin CR, Short RV, editors: *Reproduction in mammals,* ed 2, vol 3, *Hormonal control of reproduction,* Cambridge, UK, 1984, Cambridge University Press.)

lactating at treatment and should have mammary glands free of infection.

Growth hormone, which is important to the normal lactational process, can be used for the enhancement of lactation when administered over a rather wide range of concentrations (Figure 39-11). The ability to synthesize GH is relatively recent; its availability has expanded interest in its use for increasing the amount of milk produced by dairy cows. In general, GH acts on the postabsorptive use of nutrients so that protein, fat, and carbohydrate metabolism in the whole body are changed, and the nutrients are directed toward milk synthesis. If cows are in early lactation and in a negative energy balance, GH administration results in the mobilization of body fats that are used for milk formation. If cows are in positive energy balance, GH has no effect on the metabolism of body fat. Initially, GH treatment decreases the energy balance of cows; however, this is adjusted by a voluntary increase in feed consumption. Despite the increased feed consumption, GH administration increases the gross efficiency of lactation by as much as 19%. In essence, the effects of exogenous GH do not depend on gross alterations in nutrient

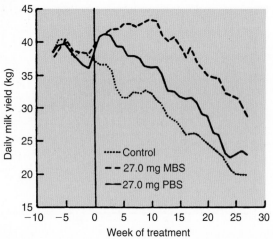

FIGURE 39-11 Average weekly milk yield of cows injected daily with diluent (control), 27 mg of methionyl bovine somatotropin *(MBS)*, or 27 mg of pituitary bovine somatotropin *(PBS)*. Treatments began at week 0 at an average of 84 ±10 days after parturition. (From Tucker HA: Lactation and its hormonal control. In Knobil E, Neill J, Ewing LL, et al, editors: *The physiology of reproduction,* vol 2, New York, 1988, Raven Press.)

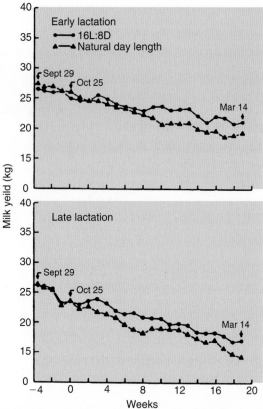

FIGURE 39-12 Influence of day length on milk production of Holstein cows. Between September 29 and October 24, cows at 37 to 74 days (early lactation) or 94 to 204 days (late lactation) after parturition were exposed to natural photoperiods of 12 hours of light per day and standardized diets. Between October 25 and March 14, cows were exposed to natural photoperiod (9 to 12 hours of light daily) or to 16 hours of fluorescent lighting superimposed on the natural photoperiod. *L,* Light; *D,* dark. (From Tucker HA: Lactation and its hormonal control. In Knobil E, Neill J, Ewing LL, et al, editors: *The physiology of reproduction,* vol 2, New York, 1988, Raven Press.)

digestibility or on body maintenance requirements. The use of GH may be economically viable, with the increased milk production justifying the expense of the hormone.

An interesting controversy has arisen from the fact that cows treated with GH do not produce "organically" derived milk, despite that synthetic GH is almost identical to endogenously derived GH. Although there is no evidence that increased concentrations of GH occur in the milk as a result of its administration, some consider the resultant milk to be abnormal.

The results with GH are in contrast to the studies in which thyroid hormone administration, in the form of *iodinated casein* (thyroprotein), was used to increase lactation in cows. Although the administration of thyroprotein increased lactation, extra feed was necessary to prevent excessive body weight loss, and milk production declined abruptly when thyroprotein was removed from the diet. In essence, the use of thyroprotein does not affect the efficiency of the lactational process as GH does. In dogs, one differential for gynecomastia (mammary enlargement) is profound hypothyroidism, causing elevated thyrotropin-releasing hormone (TRH) levels, which in turn stimulate prolactin secretion.

Another interesting finding concerning the manipulation of lactation has been that the milk yield in cows can be increased by exposing them to increased light (called a *photoperiod*). Cows under a photoperiod regimen of 16 hours of light (8 hours of dark) produced 6% to 10% more milk than animals under the reverse photoperiod (8 hours of light and 16 hours of dark) (Figure 39-12). Although the mechanism by which light affects lactation is not known, it likely involves prolactin secretion, at least to some extent, in that increased light exposure results in increased prolactin secretion. Similarly, the queen's estrous cycle is affected by photoperiod, mediated by melatonin and prolactin levels. Melatonin and prolactin secretion may play a role in ovarian function in the cat, with lower levels of both hormones present during estrus than during the interestrous period. Protocols exist for inducing improved lactation in postpartum bitches using low-dose oxytocin and metoclopramide (a dopamine D-2 receptor antagonist).

DISEASES ASSOCIATED WITH THE MAMMARY GLAND

The Main Diseases That Affect the Mammary Gland Directly Are Mastitis (Prevalent in Dairy Cattle and Dogs) and Neoplasia (Prevalent in Intact Dogs and Cats)

The most important problems involved in the production of milk are those caused by inflammation of the gland *(mastitis)*. One fundamental cause of mastitis is injury to the teat canal from the repeated stretching that occurs with the milking process. Organisms that ordinarily would be excluded from the gland are able to make their way past the barrier located within the teat canal; with repeated microorganism exposure, an infection is established.

One of the adverse consequences of mastitis is the formation of connective tissue within the udder as a result of the attempt of the gland to wall off the infection. The presence of connective tissue limits the area into which ducts and alveoli can proliferate, thus reducing the milk-producing potential of the gland. The mammary gland is an example of an organ (the eye is another example) in which the elicitation of an inflammatory response is often detrimental to the function of the organ. Thus, therapies directed toward the treatment of mastitis often combine antiinflammatory and antibacterial agents.

Another process that disturbs the structure of the mammary gland is *neoplasia*. In domestic animals, the dog is most susceptible to the occurrence of mammary tumors. The exposure of the mammae to the ovarian hormones estrogen and progesterone greatly increases the chance of neoplasia. The incidence of mammary tumors is relatively low if the dog is ovariectomized before the first estrous cycle, but it increases progressively through exposure to two ovarian cycles; ovariectomy has little effect on neoplasia if done after the third or fourth cycle. Some owners want their dogs to have one or two cycles before they are ovariectomized. It is important for veterinarians to point out the beneficial aspects of ovariectomy before the onset of puberty because of the incidence of mammary neoplasia, as well as the usual benefits of fertility and behavioral control.

The Main Conditions That Involve the Mammary Gland Indirectly Are Passive Transfer of Red Blood Cell Agglutinating Antibodies by the Ingestion of Colostrum (Mare, Queen) and Hypocalcemia Caused by the Transient Drain of Calcium That Occurs with Initiation of Lactation (Dairy Cattle) or During the Perinatal Period (Dog)

An immunological disease associated with the mammary gland involves the transfer of red blood cell agglutinating antibodies to the neonate through the milk. The situation is most common in the horse, in which fetal red blood cells (RBCs) pass into the maternal system and elicit antibody formation against the fetal RBCs. These antibodies tend to be concentrated in the colostrum along with other immunoglobulins. At birth the foal is able to absorb the RBC agglutinating antibodies (as well as other beneficial immunoglobulins) for up to 48 hours. Foals often go into a hemolytic crisis between 24 and 48 hours after delivery and can die unless given vigorous therapy, including blood transfusions. If fetal RBC antibody formation is suspected in a mare, the disease can be handled by muzzling the foal at birth through 48 hours and feeding with colostrum saved (frozen) from other preparturient mares. A similar condition has been reported in group A blood type kittens (usually purebred) born to group B blood type queens bred to toms with type A blood type. Unfortunately, no feline colostrum is commercially available, but kittens can be given serum or plasma from another blood type A queen for immunoglobulin transfer, while being prevented from nursing from their dam.

Diseases associated with the mammary gland and life threatening to the dam are *hypocalcemia, puerperal tetany,* or *eclampsia.* At parturition the acceleration of lactogenesis causes a great increase in the movement of calcium from the blood into the milk. Both cows and dogs are particularly susceptible, with some dams unable to respond immediately to the calcium drain from the blood by the mobilization of calcium. As a result, the animals lose their ability to maintain normal muscle activity; cows are often unable to stand, and become prostrate with the appearance of being comatose. Bitches develop tremors progressing to seizures. The syndrome occurs in cows at parturition and in dogs during the last weeks of pregnancy or the first few weeks postpartum, when lactation reaches its peak. Inappropriate prenatal nutrition, often with calcium supplementation, sets bitches up for this condition by inhibiting normal parathyroid gland development, necessary to meet the demands for mobilization of calcium by lactation. The systemic administration of calcium to hypocalcemic cows or bitches often produces a dramatic recovery in 10 to 20 minutes.

CLINICAL CORRELATIONS

PREGNANT MARE THAT DOES NOT HAVE SUFFICIENT MILK OR UDDER DEVELOPMENT

History. A 13-year-old pregnant Arabian mare is due to foal in the next week, based on breeding dates. This is her second foal; the first foal did well. She has had limited udder development. The mare is current on vaccinations and deworming; she has no previous medical problems. She has been on pasture with all the other horses. She is supplemented with 2 pounds of 14% mare and foal feed per day. She is given grass hay, and she is in good body condition. The farm is located in eastern Tennessee.

Clinical Examination. The mare is pregnant. The foal is viable based on movement and heartbeat. The foal is in the pelvic inlet, indicating that the mare will foal soon. All other parameters of the examination are normal. The mare is in good body condition.

Comment. With a mare close to parturition that has had limited udder development, one concern is whether the mare has been fed fescue. The owners are asked about this and say that she has been receiving a grass hay with fescue in it. They did not know that fescue could cause problems. The clients are informed that fescue can contain an endophytic fungus, *Neotyphodium coemophialum,* which produces alkaloid toxins. These toxins are dopaminergic and inhibit prolactin. Additionally, the increase in dopamine activity directly decreases prolactin. Normally, neurons in the proventricular nucleus would release prolactin, which would stimulate lactogenesis. In some animals, progesterone levels are also decreased.

Treatment. Domperidone can be given because it inhibits the dopaminergic effects. If domperidone is started 5 to 10 days before parturition, this is often sufficient time for the mare to develop adequate milk for the foal. If domperidone is not started until up to 24 hours after foaling, it must be given for 10 to 14 days. Some mares will respond and will increase the milk production, whereas some mares will not respond. Although this treatment is often useful in stimulating milk production by the mare, it does not necessarily reverse other complications associated with fescue. Mares that have been given fescue may have foals that appear dysmature, are weak, or have prolonged gestation. The placenta from these affected mares is often thickened. To prevent these effects of fescue, clients are encouraged to keep the mares off fescue-containing feeds for at least 30 to 60 days before foaling. In addition, endophyte-free fescue grasses are available, but expensive.

NEONATAL ISOERYTHROLYSIS

History. You are called to examine a mare, 7 months pregnant, that has a previous history of having conceived and delivered a normal foal after her first pregnancy; the foal was subsequently suckled and was sold as a weanling. The mare had no trouble conceiving and carrying the next two pregnancies, but the foals died within 2 to 4 days of birth, even though they were healthy and vigorous at birth and the mare had colostrum and milk. The previous owner became discouraged because of these deaths and sold the mare to the current owner at a bargain price.

Clinical Examination. You perform a general physical examination of the mare and find all organ systems to be normal. Palpation of the uterus per rectum reveals the presence of a viable fetus that appears to be of the correct size for a pregnancy of the purported duration. Both the external genitalia and the mammary glands are normal in appearance.

Comment. From the history, and because the mare appears to be undergoing a normal pregnancy, you conclude that there is nothing wrong with the reproductive process. The fact that the previous two foals were healthy at birth and yet weakened rapidly and died within 4 days indicates that something likely happened to them after delivery. If the deaths were caused by an issue associated with the mare, the most likely cause of these deaths would be *neonatal isoerythrolysis.* In this situation the mare becomes exposed to the red blood cells (RBCs, erythrocytes) of the fetus during pregnancy, or the mare could have been exposed to RBCs from a stallion, whose erythrocytes are recognized as foreign. If the mare is exposed to the RBCs from the stallion or the fetus, those RBCs enter the circulation of the dam. She responds by making antibodies to the RBCs because of the presence of foreign antigen on the fetal erythrocytes that were inherited from the sire. In the mare, these antibodies do not pass through the placental barrier, so the fetus is protected from these antibodies during pregnancy. The antibodies do pass into the colostrum and are concentrated during the process of colostrum formation. Therefore, when the foal suckles the colostrum, it acquires the antibodies that will react to its own RBCs. The foal develops a type II hypersensitivity reaction in which the antibodies destroy the foal's RBCs through different mechanisms.

Treatment. The foal needs to be prevented from suckling the mare for the first 2 to 3 days of life. During the first 1 to 2 days, the foal is able to absorb large protein molecules, including the important immunoglobulins that enable the foal to ward off infections, as well as, in this case, antibodies against fetal RBC antigens. The gut epithelium closes to the passage of large protein molecules by 36 to 48 hours of life; at this time, or shortly thereafter, the foal can be allowed to suckle without risk of absorbing the antibodies. The key is to prevent the foal from suckling during the first 2 to 3 days of life to prevent absorption of the antibodies that will react to its own RBCs. The mare needs to be monitored closely before parturition so that the foal can be muzzled shortly after delivery. The foal does need nourishment during the first 2 to 3 days of life; thus it is important that the foal be fed colostrum obtained from other mares (usually maintained frozen). If the foal does receive the mare's colostrum containing antibodies that will react to its own RBCs, the foal can still be treated. The foal should not nurse the mare for the first 3 to 5 days of life, and the foal can be given packed RBCs from a donor if necessary. To anticipate the potential risk, blood typing of stallions and mares is now available.

PRACTICE QUESTIONS

1. The development of the duct system in the mammary gland is under the control of estrogens, growth hormone, and adrenal steroids. If the duct system is to develop functional milk-secreting units, called *alveoli,* which of the following hormone(s) are essential to this development?
   a. Progesterone
   b. Prolactin
   c. Relaxin
   d. Prolactin and progesterone
   e. Prolactin and relaxin
   f. Progesterone and relaxin

2. The hormone that is most important for the maintenance of lactation (lactogenesis) is:
   a. Estrogen.
   b. Oxytocin.
   c. Progesterone.
   d. Prolactin.
   e. Relaxin.

3. Sensory inputs (including sound, sight, and smell, but not necessarily touch) elicit the release of what important hormone required for the lactation process in the cow?
   a. Estrogen
   b. Oxytocin
   c. Progesterone
   d. Prolactin
   e. Relaxin

4. The contraction of what anatomical structure is of fundamental importance for the release of milk from the udder of the cow?
   a. Alveoli
   b. Duct
   c. Myoepithelial cell
   d. Duct cistern
   e. Teat cistern

5. The most important energy source in milk is:
   a. Carbohydrates.
   b. Lactose.
   c. Lipids.
   d. Proteins.

BIBLIOGRAPHY

Bogaerts P: *Clinical approach to genital and mammary pathologies in cats.* Presented at 5th Biannual Congress, *European Veterinary Society for Small Animal Reproduction (EVSSAR),* Budapest, Hungary, 2006.

Cowie T: Lactation. In Austin CR, Short RV, editors: *Reproduction in mammals,* vols 1-6, Cambridge, UK, 1986, Cambridge University Press.

Feldman EC, Nelson RW, editors: *Canine and feline endocrinology and reproduction,* ed 4, Philadelphia, 2009, Saunders.

Leyva H, Madley T, Stabenfeldt GH: Effect of light manipulation on ovarian activity and melatonin and prolactin secretion in the domestic cat, *J Reprod Fertil Suppl* 39:125-133, 1989.

Neill JD, editor: Knobil and Neill's physiology of reproduction, vols 1 and 2, ed 3, Philadelphia, 2005, Elsevier.

Park CS, Lindberg GL: The mammary gland and lactation. In Reece WO, editor: *Dukes' physiology of domestic animals,* ed 12, Ithaca, NY, 2004, Comstock Publishing.

Peterson ME, Kutzler MI, editors: *Small animal pediatrics: the first 12 months of life,* Philadelphia, 2011, Saunders.

CHAPTER 40
Reproductive Physiology of the Male

KEY POINTS

Functional anatomy
1. The male reproductive system consists of many individual organs acting in concert to produce spermatozoa and deliver them to the female's reproductive tract.
2. Normal spermatogenesis requires maintenance of uniform testicular temperature 2° to 6° C lower than core body temperature.
3. Emission is the release of spermatozoa and accessory gland fluids into the pelvic urethra, whereas ejaculation is the forceful expulsion of semen from the urethra.

Spermatogenesis
1. Spermatogenesis is a lengthy orchestrated process in which diploid stem cells divide by mitosis to maintain their own numbers and cyclically produce progeny that undergo meiotic division and differentiation into haploid germ cells.
2. Testicular size can predict daily sperm production.

Hypothalamic-pituitary-testicular axis
1. The reproductive system of the male is regulated by the hypothalamus, which is hormonally linked to the anterior pituitary and testes by luteinizing hormone and follicle-stimulating hormone.

Puberty
1. Puberty is not synonymous with sexual maturity.
2. Puberty results from a continuous process of endocrine changes that are initiated shortly after birth.

Anabolic steroids
1. Anabolic steroids are androgen derivatives that exert negative feedback on the hypothalamic-pituitary-testicular axis.

FUNCTIONAL ANATOMY

The Male Reproductive System Consists of Many Individual Organs Acting in Concert to Produce Spermatozoa and Deliver Them to the Female's Reproductive Tract

The male reproductive system is made up of a number of individual organs acting in concert to produce spermatozoa and deliver them to the reproductive tract of the female. This concerted effort involves both the neuroendocrine (hypothalamus and anterior pituitary glands) and the genital system. The genital organs consist of two testes, each suspended within the scrotum by a spermatic cord and external cremaster muscle; two epididymides; two deferent ducts; accessory sex glands; and the penis. The accessory sex glands include paired ampullae, paired seminal vesicles (vesicular glands), a prostate gland, and paired bulbourethral glands (Cowper glands). The presence of individual accessory glands, the testicular orientation, the type of penis, and the site of semen deposition in the female are dependent on the species (Table 40-1).

Normal Spermatogenesis Requires Maintenance of Uniform Testicular Temperature 2° to 6° C Lower Than Core Body Temperature

Normal *spermatogenesis* in most mammals is dependent upon maintenance of uniform testicular temperature between 2° to 6° C lower than core body temperature. Elevated testicular temperature reduces the numbers of live, normal spermatozoa. Thermoregulation of the testes in domestic animals is maintained by the pendulous scrotal sac, the testicular vasculature, the dartos and cremaster muscles, and the scrotal skin. A pendulous scrotum facilitates thermoregulation by using several mechanisms such as conduction, convection, and evaporation. The internal spermatic artery of many mammals is highly convoluted and in farm animals the coiling is so extensive that the artery forms a vascular cone on the dorsal pole of the testis. The testicular vascular cone is composed of a venous pampiniform plexus network surrounding the highly coiled testicular artery. This ramification reduces the mean blood pressure and permits transfer of heat from the testicular arteries (high temperature) to the veins (low temperature) by a counter-current heat-exchange system. This mechanism of heat exchange is possible because the spermatic artery is extensively coiled and in close proximity to the venous pampiniform plexus. In addition, there are periarterial veins and arteriovenous shunts that facilitate heat transfer as well as the transfer of hormones such as testosterone from the veins to the arteries. The dartos and cremaster muscles can increase or reduce the exposure surface area of the scrotum and move the testes closer to or farther from the abdomen, depending on their state of contracture. The scrotal skin is usually thin, generally lacks subcutaneous fat, has relatively little hair or wool, and contains numerous sebaceous and sweat glands. The blood and lymphatic system in the scrotal skin is very extensive, with blood vessels near the skin surface, facilitating radiation of heat. In hot environments the blood flow in the scrotal skin increases and the evaporation per unit area of scrotal skin is greater than the evaporation from the general body surface. In the scrotum, the number and volume of the sweat glands per unit skin surface is greater than

TABLE 40-1 Male Reproductive Parameters

	Bull, Buck, and Ram	Stallion	Boar	Dog	Tom	Llama/Alpaca
Testis orientation	Vertical cauda down	Horizontal	Perineal cauda up	Horizontal	Perineal cauda up	Perineal cauda up
Ampullae	+	+	−	+	−	+
Seminal vesicle	+	+	+	−	−	−
Bulbourethra	+	+	++	−	+	+
Prostate	+	+	+	+	+	+
Penis type	Fibroelastic sigmoid	Vascular	Fibroelastic sigmoid	Vascular	Vascular	Fibroelastic sigmoid
Semen deposition	Vagina	Uterus	Cervix/uterus	Vagina	Vagina	Uterus

other body regions. In addition, the scrotal skin has thermoreceptors that trigger a local and a systemic response in the presence of an increase in local temperature. Locally the blood flow and scrotal sweating will increase. The systemic response will increase the number of breaths per minute (polypnea).

As previously mentioned, in domestic mammals, normal testicular function, especially normal spermatogenesis, is temperature dependent and requires an environment that is lower than core body temperature. Therefore, in normal domestic males, the testes are located outside the abdominal cavity, in the scrotum. Failure of one or both of the testes to descend into the scrotum is known as *cryptorchidism*. Although the cryptorchid testis is still capable of producing *androgens*, it is incapable of producing normal spermatozoa. Consequently, a bilaterally cryptorchid male would be sterile. The cryptorchid testis is more prone to torsion of the spermatic cord and 10 times more likely to be neoplastic. Cryptorchidism appears to be genetic, although the exact mechanism is not completely understood and may vary among species. It is most common in boars, dogs, and stallions and least common in bulls, rams, and bucks. Descent of the testes into the scrotum normally occurs in domestic animals during the following time periods:

- *Horse.* 9 to 11 months of gestation
- *Cattle.* 3.5 to 4 months of gestation
- *Sheep.* 80 days of gestation
- *Pig.* 90 days of gestation
- *Dog.* 5 days after birth
- *Cat.* 2 to 5 days after birth
- *Llama/alpaca.* Usually present at birth

For the majority of domestic species, passage of the testes through the internal rings by 2 weeks after birth is necessary for a final scrotal position to occur. Many animals may have testes in the inguinal region at birth, and the testes may remain there for weeks or months before descending into the scrotum. In the dog, testicular descent is uncommon after 14 weeks of age and does not occur after 6 months of age. In the stallion, although it is considered abnormal, descent of inguinally retained testes has been known to occur as late as 2 to 3 years of age.

The testis is the pivotal organ of the male reproductive system. It must be remembered, however, that all testicular functions are profoundly influenced by the neuroendocrine system. The testis is responsible for steroidogenesis, primarily the production of androgens, as well as the generation of haploid germ cells by spermatogenesis. These two functions occur in the Leydig cells and the seminiferous tubules, respectively.

Functionally, the testis is considered to have three compartments. The interstitial tissue compartment, containing the Leydig cells, surrounds the seminiferous tubules and bathes them with testosterone-rich fluid. The other two compartments reside within the seminiferous tubules. The basal compartment contains spermatogonia, which divide through mitosis, whereas the adluminal compartment represents a special environment where spermatocytes undergo meiosis and continue their meiotic divisions to differentiate into spermatids and finally into spermatozoa. Within the seminiferous tubules, the Sertoli cells, which provide support and nourishment to the developing germ cells, extend from the basal compartment into the adluminal compartment. Tight-junctional complexes between the Sertoli cells separate the basal and adluminal compartments and form the major component of the blood-testis barrier, which functionally prevents many compounds found in the blood and interstitial fluid from entering the adluminal compartment.

The seminiferous tubules empty their contents into the rete testis, which subsequently transports the spermatozoa and seminiferous tubular fluid into the epididymis. The epididymis is a single tortuous duct of considerable length (from 2 m in the cat to 80 m in the stallion) that is anatomically divided into three segments: head, or caput; body, or corpus; and tail, or cauda. The epididymis not only is a conduit for spermatozoa but also provides a special environment in which spermatozoa are concentrated, undergo maturation, and acquire fertilizing capacity. Spermatozoa that enter the caput from the rete testis are immotile and incapable of fertilization. Only after they undergo migration and maturation through the caput and corpus are both motility and the capacity for fertilization achieved. The cauda epididymis and the deferent duct, into which the cauda empties, serve as a storage depot for mature spermatozoa; together, these are known as the extragonadal sperm reserves. The spermatozoal transit time through the caput and corpus epididymis is not altered by *ejaculation* and is similar (2 to 5 days) for domestic species. Storage time in the cauda epididymis is more variable among species (3 to 13 days) and can be reduced by several days in sexually active males. Animals that rest sexually for 7 to 10 days have a maximum number of spermatozoa in the cauda epididymis, and this reserve is reduced by at least 25% with daily or every-other-day ejaculation.

The deferent ducts, or *vasa deferentia,* pass through the inguinal rings into the abdomen and connect the cauda epididymis with the pelvic urethra. In most species the terminal portion of the deferent ducts enlarges to form prominent ampullae such as those found in ruminants and the stallion. In other species the ampullae either are absent or are anatomically indistinct from the vasa deferentia. The ampullae serve as an additional storage depot for spermatozoa, and in some species, such as the bull, stallion,

TABLE 40-2 Seminal Characteristics from Domestic Animals

Parameter	Bull	Ram	Buck	Boar	Stallion	Alpaca/Llama	Dog*	Tom
Ejaculate volume (mL)	5-8	0.7-1.3	0.7-1.4	150-250	50-100	0.7-3.0	2.0-25	0.03-0.3
Spermatozoa concentration (millions/mL)	800-2,000	2,000-3,500	2,000-4,500	200-300	150-300	80-250	60-500	1,700-2,900
Motile spermatozoa (%)	40-75	60-80	60-85	50-80	40-75	40-70	50-90	40-90
Normal spermatozoa (%)	65-95	80-95	75-95	70-90	60-90	55-85	50-90	50-90

*The ejaculate of the dog consists of three fractions.

and dog, ampullary glands add to the ejaculate. Along with spermatozoa, ejaculated semen is composed primarily of accessory gland secretions that add volume, nutrients, buffers, and a number of other substances whose exact functions are unknown. The contribution to the ejaculate by each of the accessory glands varies with the species and is responsible for the variation in concentration, volume, and character between ejaculates. The seminal vesicles lie lateral to the ampullae near the neck of the bladder. In the bull, ram, and buck, these organs are firm and lobulated with a narrow lumen, whereas in the stallion and boar, they are more saclike. The dog and tom lack seminal vesicles but have relatively prominent prostate glands, especially the dog. The prostate gland is present in all domestic males and is intimately associated with the pelvic urethra, but it varies in size and appearance among species. The bulbourethral glands of the tom are almost as large as the prostate, but these glands are absent in the dog. In the stallion and bull, the bulbourethral glands are small, round to ovoid structures that lie adjacent to the pelvic urethra near the ischial arch, whereas those of the boar are large and cylindrical. The male llama/alpaca lacks seminal vesicles, and the bulbourethral and prostate glands are present.

The copulatory organ of the male is the penis. It is more or less cylindrical in all species and extends from the ischial arch to near the umbilicus on the ventral abdominal wall, except in the tom and the llama/alpaca, in which the penis points posteriorly in the relaxed state. The body of the penis is surrounded by a thick fibrous capsule (the tunica albuginea) that encloses numerous cavernous spaces (the corpus cavernosum penis) as well as the corpus spongiosum penis, which immediately surrounds the urethra. Erection is a psychosomatic event that involves mutually occurring actions of the vascular, neurological, and endocrine systems. Contraction of the ischiocavernosus muscle during erection results in occlusion of venous outflow. At the same time, the parasympathetically mediated relaxation of corpus cavernosum and corpus spongiosum results in these cavernous spaces becoming engorged with blood, and the penis becomes elongated and turgid.

Emission Is the Release of Spermatozoa and Accessory Gland Fluids into the Pelvic Urethra, Whereas Ejaculation Is the Forceful Expulsion of Semen from the Urethra

Emission is the release of spermatozoa and accessory gland fluids into the pelvic urethra as a result of sympathetically mediated thoracolumbar reflex contraction of the smooth muscle in the ductus deferens and accessory glands. Ejaculation is the forceful expulsion of semen from the urethra and is prompted by a parasympathetically mediated sacral reflex that induces rhythmic contractions of the bulbospongiosus, ischiocavernosus, and

urethralis muscles. After ejaculation, a sacral sympathetically mediated increase in the smooth muscle tone of the cavernous spaces increases the outflow of blood, and contraction of the retractor penis muscle withdraws the penis into the prepuce. The seminal characteristics of the different species are listed in Table 40-2.

SPERMATOGENESIS

Spermatogenesis Is a Lengthy Orchestrated Process in Which Diploid Stem Cells Divide by Mitosis to Maintain Their Own Numbers and Cyclically Produce Progeny That Undergo Meiotic Division and Differentiation into Haploid Germ Cells

Spermatogenesis is a lengthy orchestrated process in which diploid stem cells at the base of the seminiferous tubules (spermatogonia) divide through mitosis to maintain their own numbers. These cells also cyclically produce progeny that undergo further meiotic division and differentiation into haploid spermatids, which are released as spermatozoa (Figure 40-1). Spermatogenesis is generally divided into three major events: spermatocytogenesis, meiosis, and spermiogenesis. Spermatocytogenesis accomplishes two important functions. First, the mitotic divisions of type A spermatogonia produce other spermatogonia that are not yet committed to the immediate spermatozoal production process, thus maintaining a population of stem cells. These stem cell divisions are responsible for the ability of the male to continuously produce spermatozoa throughout his adult life. Second, type A spermatogonia become type B spermatogonia, which further divide through mitosis to produce primary spermatocytes. The primary spermatocytes enter into the pool of meiotically dividing cells and ultimately produce spermatozoa.

Meiosis occurs only during the processes of oogenesis and spermatogenesis, in which the haploid condition results after two cell divisions with only one chromosomal duplication. During meiosis, homologous chromosomes pair up, and this facilitates the exchange of genetic material between chromosomes. At the first meiotic division, the homologous chromosomes segregate into the two resulting cells, creating a haploid condition. In the male the resultant haploid cells are the secondary spermatocytes with duplicated chromatids. In less than 1 day after their formation, secondary spermatocytes divide to form spermatids that contain one chromatid from each of the haploid chromosomes.

The newly formed spermatids continue to differentiate without dividing to form mature spermatids through the process of spermiogenesis. Spermiogenesis occurs just before spermatids are released as spermatozoa at the luminal surface of the seminiferous tubule (spermiation). The major features of spermiogenesis

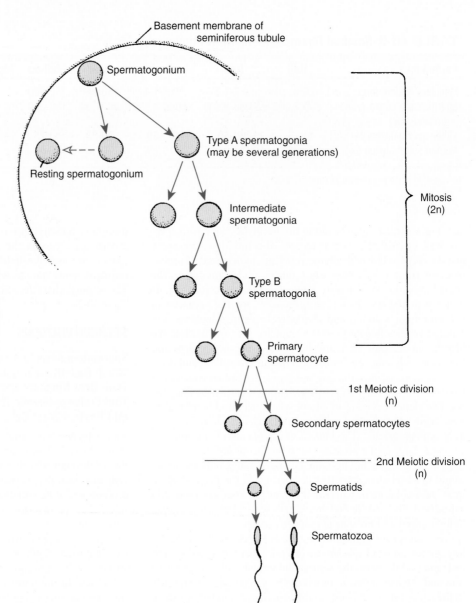

FIGURE 40-1 Diagram of spermatogenesis. (From McDonald LE, Pineda MH, editors: *Veterinary endocrinology and reproduction,* Philadelphia, 1989, Lea & Febiger.)

include formation of the acrosome from the Golgi apparatus, condensation and elongation of the nucleus, formation of the flagellum, and extensive shedding of cytoplasm. The spermiated *spermatozoon* consists of a head, middle piece, and tail (Figure 40-2). The head contains the genetic material to be combined with that of the oocyte during fertilization. Overlying the head is the acrosome, which contains hydrolytic enzymes necessary for penetration of the oocyte. The middle piece contains mitochondria, which provide the energy for microtubules extending into the tail to slide back and forth, past each other, thus producing tail movement.

Taking epididymal transit time into account, the interval from type A spermatogonia to ejaculated spermatozoa is approximately 60 to 70 days for the ram and the bull and 50 to 60 days for the boar, the dog, and the stallion. Therefore the interval from an event that may adversely affect the testis or epididymis to a decline in seminal quality may be as short as a few days to as long as 2 months. Similarly, at least 60 days would likely be required for an ejaculate to return to normal after a toxic insult to the testis.

In theory, 16 primary spermatocytes and 64 spermatozoa develop from one type A spermatogonium in the bull and the ram. However, a percentage of potential sperm production is lost to degeneration during the normal course of spermatogenesis. In humans, approximately 40% of the sperm production potential is lost during the latter stages of meiosis. Daily sperm production is the number of spermatozoa produced per day by the testes. It is highly correlated with testicular size and is not affected by frequency of use for breeding.

Testicular Size Can Predict Daily Sperm Production

Testicular size is an important trait of medium to high heritability that provides an accurate estimate of the amount of sperm-producing parenchyma in the testis. Because of the influence of testicular size, there is a wide range in daily sperm production among domestic species. For example, daily sperm production has been calculated to be 0.37×10^9 in the dog and 16.2×10^9 in the boar. Within a species, both individual and breed variation in testicular size can also influence daily sperm production.

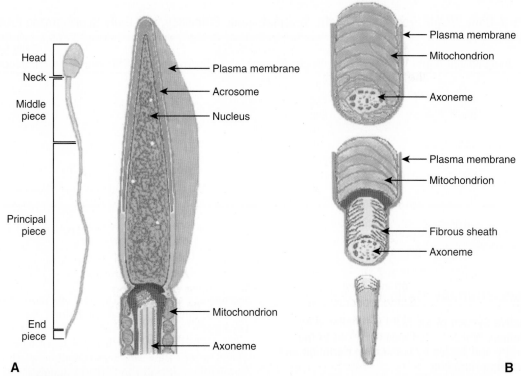

Head
Neck
Middle piece
Principal piece
End piece

Plasma membrane
Acrosome
Nucleus
Mitochondrion
Axoneme

Plasma membrane
Mitochondrion
Axoneme

Plasma membrane
Mitochondrion
Fibrous sheath
Axoneme

A

B

FIGURE 40-2 A, Major elements of the mammalian spermatozoa. **B,** Middle piece *(top),* principal *(middle),* and end piece *(bottom)* of a spermatozoon viewed in cross section. (From Robaire B, Pryor JL, Trasler JM: *Handbook of andrology,* Lawrence, Kan, 1995, Allen Press.)

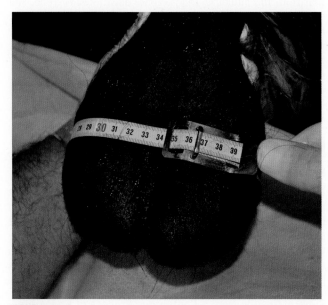

FIGURE 40-3 Measurement of scrotal circumference in a bull by using a scrotal tape.

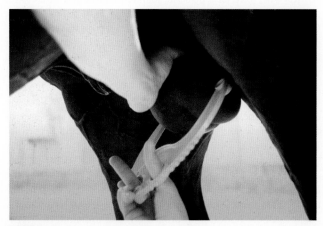

FIGURE 40-4 Measurement of total scrotal width in the stallion using calipers. (From Brinsko SP, Blanchard TL, Varner DD, et al: *Manual of equine reproduction,* ed 3, St Louis, 2010, Mosby.)

Testicular size cannot be measured directly; therefore, an indirect measure commonly used in ruminants is *scrotal circumference* (Figure 40-3). In other species with more horizontally oriented testes, total scrotal width (Figure 40-4) or testicular volume as determined by ultrasonographic measurements is used. Testicular size is influenced by species, breed, age, and body condition score. Each gram of normal testicular parenchyma produces the same quantity of spermatozoa according to the species but differs among species (Table 40-3). Therefore, males with larger testes will produce more spermatozoa than males with smaller testes for the same age and species. In ruminants, scrotal circumference is also an accurate predictor of the age of puberty onset and of the percentage of normal seminiferous tubules. In cattle, there is a negative correlation between scrotal circumferences and age of puberty in the female offspring; this means, bulls with larger scrotal circumferences will produce females that attain puberty at an earlier age.

TABLE 40-3 Body Weight, Testicular Weight, Spermatogenic Efficiency, and Daily Spermatozoa Production

	Body Weight (kg)	Pair Testes Weight (Grams)	Spermatogenic Efficiency[a]	Daily Spermatozoa Production ($\times 10^9$)[b]
Alpaca	65	20	NA	NA
Boar	150	750	23	17.3
Bulls	600	600	11	6.6
Dog	15	30	17	0.5
Lama	115	30	NA	NA
Ram	100	550	21	11.6
Stallion	500	350	16	5.6
Tom	5	20	16	0.3

NA, Not available.
[a]Spermatozoa produced per gram of testicular parenchyma ($\times 10^6$).
[b]Spermatozoa produced daily by the two testes.

HYPOTHALAMIC-PITUITARY-TESTICULAR AXIS

The Reproductive System of the Male Is Regulated by the Hypothalamus, Which Is Hormonally Linked to the Anterior Pituitary and Testes by Luteinizing Hormone and Follicle-Stimulating Hormone

The reproductive system of male mammals is regulated by intricate feedback mechanisms involving the hypothalamus, anterior pituitary, and testes (Figure 40-5). The hypothalamus synthesizes and secretes the *decapeptide gonadotropin-releasing hormone* (GnRH). Secreted in a pulsatile manner, GnRH acts directly on gonadotropic cells in the anterior pituitary. On stimulation by GnRH, these gonadotropes synthesize and secrete the gonadotropins follicle-stimulating hormone (FSH) and luteinizing hormone (LH). Both FSH and LH are heterodimeric glycoproteins made up of two noncovalently linked polypeptides. The alpha (α) subunit protein is common to both FSH and LH, whereas the beta (β) subunit is specific for each. Individual gonadotropes have the ability to synthesize and secrete FSH, LH, or both. The release of FSH and LH depends on the pulsatile pattern of GnRH secretion. Irregular, low-amplitude GnRH pulses result in FSH release, whereas high-frequency GnRH pulses induce the release of LH.

Within the testis, LH binds to membrane receptors on the Leydig cells and stimulates them to convert cholesterol to *testosterone*. Synthesized androgens diffuse into blood and lymph, where they are bound to androgen-binding protein (ABP) produced by the Sertoli cells. High local concentrations of androgens within the testis are considered essential for normal spermatogenesis to occur. ABP enhances the accumulation of testosterone and dihydrotestosterone in high concentrations within the seminiferous tubules and the interstitium of the testis. Within the testis, the target cells for testosterone are the peritubular myoid cells and the Sertoli cells, which envelop and support the developing sperm cells. ABP also facilitates the transport of androgens from the testis to the epididymis, where these hormones influence epididymal transit and the further maturation of spermatozoa.

Studies have demonstrated that FSH specifically targets receptors on the Sertoli cells within the seminiferous tubules. FSH and testosterone stimulate a variety of Sertoli cell functions, including the synthesis and secretion of ABP, inhibin, activin, estrogen, and several products (e.g., transferrin) that are involved in the transfer of nutrients to germ cells; meiosis; spermatocyte maturation;

spermiation; and Leydig cell function. Sertoli and Leydig cells appear to interact in a paracrine fashion. Steroid production of Leydig cells can be stimulated by a product released by Sertoli cells, the secretion of which is enhanced by FSH. A potential candidate for such a substance is inhibin, which is produced by Sertoli cells in response to FSH and stimulates steroidogenesis in Leydig cells. Inhibin, a glycoprotein hormone, along with testosterone, is involved in the complex feedback regulation of pituitary function. Gonadal steroids are known to suppress FSH release, but inhibin appears to be the most potent inhibitor of FSH secretion from the pituitary. Testosterone, dihydrotestosterone, and estrogen regulate LH synthesis and secretion through negative feedback exerted at the level of the hypothalamus or the anterior pituitary gland. Because FSH and LH are necessary for high testicular concentrations of substances responsible for normal spermatogenesis, exogenous administration of testosterone or inhibin to enhance fertility would be contraindicated since they would impede the secretion of those factors responsible for maintaining an optimal spermatogenic environment.

PUBERTY

Puberty Is Not Synonymous with Sexual Maturity

Puberty in the male is when he is first able to produce sufficient numbers of sperm to impregnate a female. For practical reasons, for bulls, boars, rams, and stallions, this could be defined as the age when the ejaculate contains 50×10^6 spermatozoa, of which 10% or more are motile. It must be remembered that puberty is not synonymous with sexual maturity, which can occur months to years later, depending on the species.

Puberty Results from a Continuous Process of Endocrine Changes That Are Initiated Shortly After Birth

The pituitary gland, gonads, and steroid-dependent target tissues are capable of responding to stimulatory hormones before puberty; therefore the hypothalamus is considered to play a pivotal role in the initiation of puberty. Puberty appears to be the end result of a continuous process of endocrine changes that are initiated shortly after birth. Some investigators theorize that puberty occurs when the animal's hypothalamic-pituitary complex becomes desensitized to the feedback inhibition of gonadal steroids. This desensitization would apparently allow

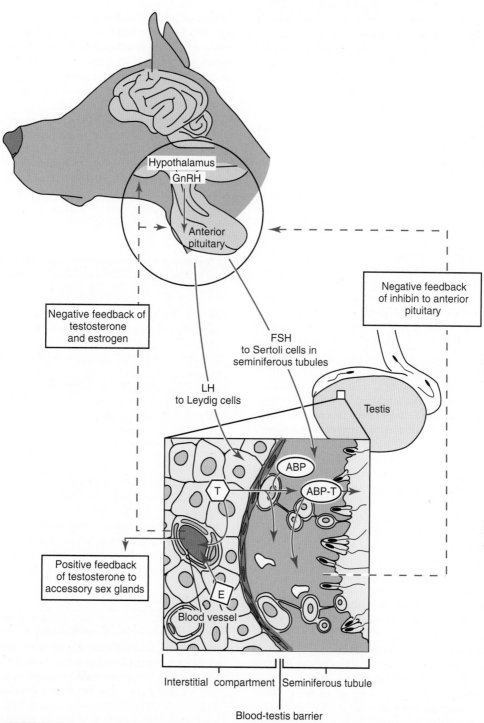

FIGURE 40-5 The reproductive system of male mammals is regulated by intricate feedback mechanisms that involve the hypothalamus, anterior pituitary, and testes. *GnRH,* Gonadotropin-releasing hormone; *FSH,* follicle-stimulating hormone; *LH,* luteinizing hormone; *ABP,* androgen-binding protein; *ABP-T,* androgen-binding protein–testosterone; *E,* estrogen; *T,* testosterone.

increased discharge of GnRH from the hypothalamus and a greater response of the pituitary to GnRH. Although numerous factors can influence the modulation by the central nervous system of the endocrine system, the major factors that affect age at puberty in domestic animals are breed, energy intake, and season of birth.

The hypothalamic-pituitary-gonadal system in humans differentiates and functions during fetal life and briefly during infancy; it then is suppressed during childhood and is reactivated during puberty after almost a decade of low activity. Inhibition of the hypothalamic-pituitary-gonadal system in prepubertal children is mediated through the suppression of GnRH synthesis and pulsatile secretion. Progressive pulsatile stimulation of the pituitary by GnRH and the gonads by LH and FSH is required for the initiation and progression of puberty. Prepubertal children secrete small amounts of FSH and LH from the pituitary, indicating that the hypothalamic-pituitary-gonadal axis is functional, but at a low level. This low level of gonadotropin secretion rapidly decreases when sex steroids are administered. Therefore, a highly sensitive negative-feedback mechanism appears to exist in young prepubertal children, and a similar mechanism is likely to exist in prepubertal domestic animals.

ANABOLIC STEROIDS

Anabolic Steroids Are Androgen Derivatives That Exert Negative Feedback on the Hypothalamic-Pituitary-Testicular Axis

The use of *anabolic* steroids has become widespread in human and animal athletes as many attempt to increase performance. Testimonials from veterinarians, physicians, human athletes, and trainers indicate that improvements in the athlete's mental attitude, stamina, and physical strength are attained after anabolic steroids are administered. The major concern is that many individuals receiving anabolic steroids are peripubescent or prepubescent. Anabolic steroids are androgen derivatives that have been altered to maximize their anabolic action and to minimize their androgenic side effects. It is not yet possible, however, to produce anabolic steroids that are devoid of androgenic activity, and many of the undesirable side effects of these drugs are caused by their androgenic activity. The adverse reproductive side effects observed with anabolic steroid use are similar to those associated with testosterone administration. Sustained testosterone or anabolic steroid administration affects pituitary function and leads to long-lasting impairment of testicular endocrine function. Potential side effects of the use of anabolic steroids in young animals may lead to incomplete development of the hypothalamic-pituitary-gonadal axis. The long-term side effects of anabolic steroid use on reproductive parameters in sexually immature animals are not yet known.

A high percentage of colts and stallions in training or racing receive androgenic drugs, including anabolic steroids, and these horses have smaller testicles than similar horses not receiving such drugs. Only two anabolic steroids, stanozolol and boldenone undecylenate, are approved by the U.S. Food and Drug Administration (FDA) for use in horses. Neither of these is approved for use in stallions. The administration of anabolic steroids to stallions has been shown to reduce seminal quality, daily sperm output, daily sperm production, and testicular size. These effects most likely result from a negative-feedback mechanism on gonadotropin release from the pituitary. Alterations in seminal parameters are also observed, including depression of sperm concentration, sperm motility, and total number of sperm per ejaculate. Histological examination of the testes demonstrates a reduction in the number of developing germ cells other than type A spermatogonia. In addition, the mean diameter of Leydig cells is decreased, and changes indicative of testicular degeneration (including marked cytoplasmic vacuolization, shrunken tubules, and Leydig cells) and phagocytosis of spermatids by multinucleated giant cells have been observed. These adverse effects on the testes tend to be more severe in younger stallions. Repeated implantation of anabolic steroids in prepubertal bulls also results in decreased testicular size. Effects on testicular growth depend on the type of anabolic steroid administered, the age of the patient, and the dosage and duration of therapy.

Human studies, which did not directly investigate the effects of anabolic steroids on spermatogenesis, also found reduced levels of circulating gonadotropins, testosterone, or both.

Individuals using high doses of testosterone and anabolic steroids for only 3 months still had hypogonadotropic hypogonadism 3 weeks after the cessation of drug use. The presence of atrophic testicles and low LH, FSH, and testosterone levels after drug withdrawal indicates that long-term androgenic or anabolic steroid use affects pituitary function and leads to long-lasting impairment of testicular endocrine function.

Questions regarding the possibility of permanent sterility or testicular atrophy with long-term anabolic steroid use have not been answered for adults, and even less is known about the effects in prepubertal or peripubertal individuals. Indirect evidence suggests that prepubertal individuals may be at a higher risk for permanent derangements from anabolic steroid use than adults. Therefore the indiscriminant use of anabolic steroids in males intended for breeding should be strongly discouraged.

CLINICAL CORRELATIONS

INFERTILITY IN A STALLION

History. You are asked to perform a "breeding soundness" examination on a 3-year-old Quarter Horse stallion that was mated with 10 mares last year and impregnated only one mare. The stallion is in demand because of his bloodlines and because his muscular and mature appearance contributed to winning a number of shows as a yearling. All the mares mated to this young stallion have been shown to be free of reproductive abnormalities. You ask whether the horse has had any illness or febrile episodes or has received any medication recently. The answer to all these queries is "no."

Clinical Examination. The stallion demonstrates normal *libido* when exposed to a mare in estrus, and two ejaculates are obtained 1 hour apart by means of an artificial vagina. Examination of both semen samples reveals poor spermatozoal concentration, low sperm numbers, and a high percentage of morphologically abnormal spermatozoa and immature germ cells. The stallion has a normal penis and prepuce, but his testes are small and soft. You ask if the stallion has ever received anabolic steroids, and with some reluctance the owner admits that the trainer did give anabolic steroids to the horse in preparation for the yearling futurity and for shows thereafter.

Comment. The use of anabolic steroids in performance animals is not uncommon. Even so, many owners and trainers are reluctant to admit to their use. Many colts are administered these drugs to give them a competitive edge in the show ring or on the racetrack so that they will later be in demand as sires. Unfortunately, because they are testosterone derivatives, the negative-feedback effects of anabolic steroids adversely affect the fertility of these animals, sometimes permanently. It is not known how severe or long-standing the adverse effects will be if anabolic steroids are given in the peripubertal period. Because this animal's testes are so small and soft, he apparently received high doses of anabolic steroids for a prolonged period during the development of the hypothalamic-pituitary-testicular axis, and the effects are most likely irreversible. It must be noted that as a 3-year-old, the horse is not yet sexually mature, and in the future he may still be able to produce sufficient numbers of normal spermatozoa to impregnate a small number of mares per season, but certainly not a "full book."

Treatment. Other than time, no known treatment will reverse the detrimental side effects caused by anabolic steroid use in adult males. Even less is known about the long-term effects in young animals. Depending on the percentage of normal, progressively motile sperm, this animal may be able to breed a limited number of mares, most likely through artificial insemination. The owners could also have the stallion reexamined in several months or longer to see if there is any improvement in sperm morphology.

INFERTILITY IN A BULL

History. You are asked to perform a "breeding soundness" examination at your veterinary clinic on a 5-year-old Brangus bull before the breeding season that will start in 1 month. This bull was used in a single sire mating system in the last breeding season with 20 females (75 days exposure) producing 90% of calf crop. The bull was vaccinated against *Clostridium* and respiratory virus with killed products and dewormed 3 months ago. Forty days ago this bull had a short but intense febrile respiratory illness, which resulted in recumbency and lasted 3 days. The bull was treated with antibiotics and antiinflammatory drugs for 5 days and the problem resolved promptly.

Clinical Examination. This bull is in good body condition score (6; scale between 1 and 9) without foot/leg problems detectable when walking and the general physical examination was unremarkable. The accessory sexual organs examined by palpation per rectum were normal. The scrotal contents were within normal limits and the scrotal circumference was 42 cm. Semen was collected via *electroejaculation* and normal penile protrusion and erection was observed. No abnormalities in the penis were detected. Semen evaluation revealed 20% of the spermatozoa to be motile with 50% of the spermatozoa having abnormal morphology. Most of the morphologic abnormalities consisted of detached heads, bent tails, and distal and proximal droplets among other defects.

Comment. Testicular function requires a low testicular temperature compared to systemic temperature in order to allow normal spermatogenesis. This bull had two instances that affected the testicular thermoregulatory function: fever and recumbency. The abnormalities noted in the semen are in agreement with the process of testicular degeneration. The spermatogenesis requires approximately 60 days. The degree of testicular compromise depends on the degree and duration of the insult as well as the inherent natural susceptibility of the male. Remember every ejaculate that you collect today is a snapshot of a process that began at least 60 days ago. Therefore the recommendation would be to re-evaluate this animal at least 60 days from the last day of the illness. It is also important to remark that there is variability among males in the degree of response to this insult.

Treatment. No known treatment, other than time, will reverse the detrimental effects caused by the fever. Due to the fact that spermatogenesis will require approximately 60 days in bulls (54 days plus epididymus transit time), the recommendation would be to not use this bull for breeding until the next evaluation is performed. Moreover, because this bull is used in single sire breeding season, the owner needs to find a new satisfactory potential breeder for this upcoming breeding season. Based on your recommendation you can educate your client that the best time to perform a breeding soundness examination is at least 2 months before the breeding season.

PRACTICE QUESTIONS

1. For most domestic species, the duration of spermatogenesis is approximately:
   a. 120 days.
   b. 10 days.
   c. 60 days.
   d. 6 months.
   e. 21 days.

2. Normal spermatogenesis in domestic mammals requires a testicular temperature that is:
   a. Higher than core body temperature.
   b. Lower than core body temperature.
   c. The same as core body temperature.
   d. Above freezing but below boiling.
   e. Conducive to testosterone metabolism.

3. Normal spermatogenesis requires an intratesticular testosterone concentration that is:
   a. The same as circulating levels.
   b. Lower than circulating levels.
   c. Static and unchanging.
   d. Much higher than circulating levels.
   e. Able to change rapidly with the maturational stage of the spermatozoon.

4. Puberty in the male:
   a. Occurs at about the same time for all species.
   b. Is influenced only by the age of the animal.
   c. Is synonymous with sexual maturity.
   d. Is defined as when he is first able to produce sufficient numbers of sperm to impregnate a female.
   e. Is independent of GnRH secretion.

5. Anabolic steroids are testosterone derivatives and therefore:
   a. Should be helpful in treating infertile males.
   b. Have no effect on male fertility.
   c. Enhance testicular function.
   d. Are only approved for use in stallions.
   e. Should not be used in males intended for breeding because of negative-feedback effects.

BIBLIOGRAPHY

Amann RP, Schanbacher BD: Physiology of male reproduction, *J Anim Sci* 57(suppl 2):380–403, 1983.

Coulter GH, Kastelic JP: Testicular thermoregulation in bulls, *Proc 15th Conf AI Reproduction N.A.A.B.* 28–34, 1994.

Neill JD, editor: *Knobil and Neill's physiology of reproduction,* vols 1 and 2, ed 3, Philadelphia, 2005, Elsevier.

Robaire B, Chan P: *Handbook of andrology,* ed 2, Lawrence, Kan, 2010, Allen Press.

Roberts SJ: Veterinary obstetrics and genital diseases. In *Theriogenology,* ed 3, Woodstock, Vt, 1986, David & Charles.

Strauss JF, Barbieri RL: *Yen and Jaffe's reproductive endocrinology: physiology, pathophysiology, and clinical management,* ed 6, Philadelphia, 2010, Saunders.

CHAPTER 41
Glomerular Filtration

KEY POINTS

1. Introduction to the physiology of the kidney.
2. The glomerulus filters the blood.
3. The structure of the glomerulus allows efficient, selective filtration.
4. Glomerular filtration rate is determined by the mean net filtration pressure, permeability of the filtration barrier, and area available for filtration.

5. The filtration barrier is selectively permeable.
6. Glomerular filtration rate is regulated by systemic and intrinsic factors.
7. Glomerular filtration rate is measured by determining the plasma clearance rate of a substance.

Introduction to the Physiology of the Kidney

The kidney has diverse roles in maintaining homeostasis. In mammals the two kidneys normally receive approximately 25% of the cardiac output. The kidneys filter the blood and thereby excrete metabolic waste, while retrieving filtered substances that are needed by the body, including water, glucose, electrolytes, and low–molecular-weight proteins. The kidneys respond to water, electrolyte, and acid-base disturbances by specifically altering the rate of reabsorption or secretion of these substances. The kidneys also produce hormones that regulate systemic blood pressure and red blood cell production.

These myriad functions are accomplished by an extensive variety of cell types, each with specific responses to direct and indirect signals, arranged in a particular pattern to form the functional unit of the kidney, the *nephron*. The nephron is composed of the *glomerulus*, where the blood is filtered, and its associated renal tubule segments, where filtered substances are absorbed from, and plasma components are secreted into, the tubule fluid. In the renal cortex the nephrons merge into the collecting duct system, which traverses the kidney and empties into the renal pelvis. Figure 41-1 provides an overview of the anatomical arrangement of nephrons within the kidney and the major functions of the nephron and collecting duct segments.

Most of our knowledge of renal physiology comes from experimental evidence from the mouse, rat, and rabbit. Our understanding of renal physiology continually evolves as more information is gathered.

The Glomerulus Filters the Blood

The first step in renal function is filtration of the blood by the glomerulus. The glomerulus is a compact network of capillaries that retains cellular components and medium– to high–molecular-weight proteins within the vessels while extruding a fluid nearly identical to plasma in its electrolyte and water composition. This fluid is the *glomerular filtrate;* the process of its formation is glomerular filtration.

The rate of glomerular filtration is a clinically useful measure of renal function. The *glomerular filtration rate* (GFR) is expressed as milliliters of glomerular filtrate formed per minute per kilogram of body weight (mL/min/kg). To understand GFR, it may help to think of these numbers in more tangible terms. An average-size beagle of 10-kg body weight with a typical GFR of 3.7 mL/min/kg would produce approximately 37 mL of glomerular filtrate per minute, or 53.3 L (~14 gallons) of glomerular filtrate per day, almost 27 times the beagle's extracellular fluid volume.

The Structure of the Glomerulus Allows Efficient, Selective Filtration

The *glomerular tuft* is composed of a network of capillaries (Figure 41-2). In mammals, renal arterial blood flows to the afferent arteriole, which divides into numerous glomerular capillaries. The capillaries anastomose to form the efferent arteriole, which conducts the filtered blood away from the glomerulus (Figure 41-3). Avian kidneys contain both mammalian-type and reptilian-type nephrons; in glomeruli of reptilian-type nephrons, the capillaries have few branches.

The glomerular tuft is encased by *Bowman's capsule,* which is lined with a single layer of cells, the parietal epithelium. The area between the glomerular tuft and Bowman's capsule is *Bowman's space.* This is where the glomerular filtrate first appears. From here, the glomerular filtrate enters the lumen of the first segment of the proximal tubule.

The structure of the glomerular capillaries is important in determining the rate and selectivity of glomerular filtration. The wall of the capillary consists of three layers: the capillary endothelium, the basement membrane, and the visceral epithelium (Figure 41-4). The *capillary endothelium* is a single layer of very thin cells that faces the blood in the capillary lumen. Endothelial fenestrae ("windows") are transcellular pores that conduct water and noncellular components in the blood to the second layer of the glomerular capillary wall, the *glomerular basement membrane* (GBM). The GBM is acellular and composed of various glycoproteins, primarily laminins, type IV collagens, nidogens, and the heparin sulfate proteoglycans, agrin in mature animals and perlecan in developing glomeruli. Compared to other basement membranes, the GBM is thicker and contains distinct glycoprotein isoforms. The GBM has three layers, created during

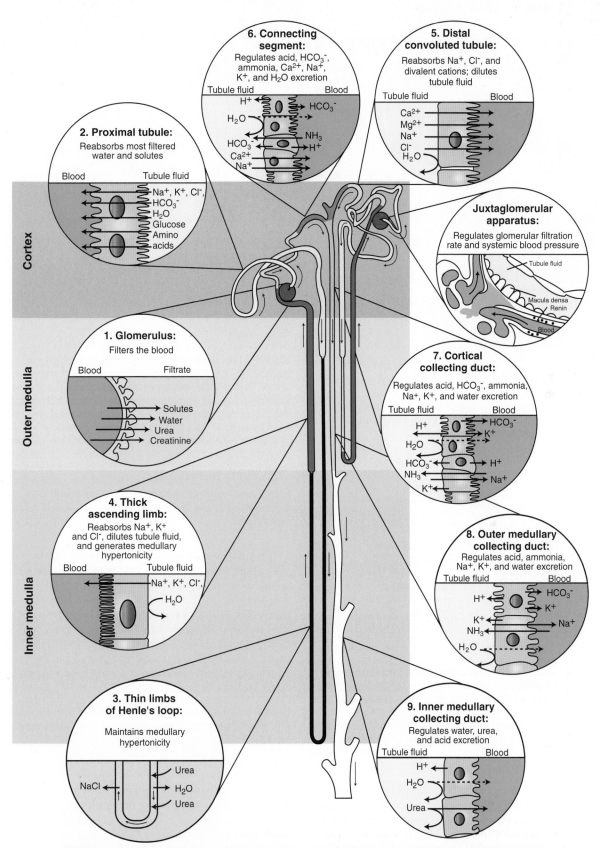

FIGURE 41-1 Schematic illustration of juxtamedullary and superficial nephrons, listing functions of the segments of nephron and collecting duct. The glomerulus of a juxtamedullary nephron is located deep in the cortex near the corticomedullary junction. The thin limb of Henle's loop extends deep into the inner medulla. The glomerulus of a superficial nephron is located in the outer cortex, and Henle's loop extends only into the outer medulla. *Arrows* indicate the direction of tubule fluid flow. Segments are numbered in sequential order of modification of the tubule fluid, beginning with the glomerulus. (Modified from Madsen KM, Verlander JW: Anatomy of the kidney. In Tisher CC, Wilcox CS, editors: *Nephrology for the house officer,* Baltimore, 2006, Williams & Wilkins.)

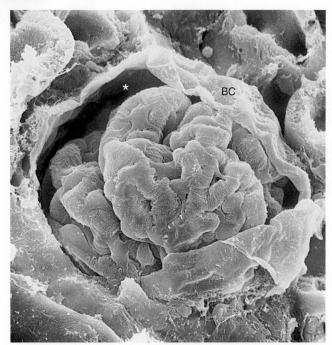

FIGURE 41-2 Scanning electron micrograph of rat glomerulus. The glomerular tuft is a complex network of capillaries that is encased in visceral epithelial cells and Bowman's capsule *(BC)*. Between the visceral epithelial cells and BC is Bowman's space *(asterisk),* where the glomerular filtrate is collected and delivered to the proximal tubule.

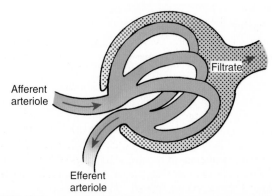

FIGURE 41-3 Schematic illustration of glomerulus. The afferent arteriole carries blood to the glomerulus and subdivides into numerous glomerular capillaries. Water and solutes cross the glomerular capillary wall into Bowman's space, forming the glomerular filtrate *(stippled area),* which flows into the proximal tubule. The glomerular capillaries coalesce, and the filtered blood leaves the glomerulus through the efferent arteriole.

development by the fusion of the basement membranes of the endothelial and epithelial cell layers. The three layers are named according to their density and relative position. As shown in Figure 41-4, the *lamina densa* (dense layer) is relatively dark because it is relatively resistant to the passage of electrons when viewed with a transmission electron microscope. The lamina densa is composed of tightly packed glycoprotein fibrils. It is sandwiched between the *lamina rara interna* (inside thin layer) on the endothelial side of the GBM and the *lamina rara externa* (outside thin layer) on the epithelial side of the GBM. The laminae rarae are composed of a loose network of glycoprotein fibrils.

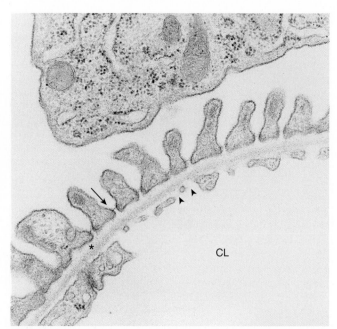

FIGURE 41-4 Transmission electron micrograph of rat glomerular capillary wall. The three main layers of the capillary wall are viewed in cross section. A single layer of glomerular capillary endothelial cells lines the capillary lumen *(CL).* Numerous fenestrae *(arrowheads)* pierce the endothelial cells. On the outside of the capillary is a single layer of visceral epithelial cells. At the top of the micrograph is a portion of the cell body of a visceral epithelial cell. The secondary foot processes are aligned along the capillary wall, and the spaces between them are spanned by the slit diaphragm *(arrow).* Between the endothelial and epithelial cell layers is the glomerular basement membrane, consisting of the electron-lucent lamina rara interna adjacent to the endothelial cells, the lamina densa *(asterisk),* and the lamina rara externa adjacent to the visceral epithelial cells.

The third compartment of the glomerular capillary wall is the *visceral epithelium,* which is a layer of intricate, interlocking cells called *podocytes.* Numerous long, narrow extensions, the *primary* and *secondary foot processes,* interdigitate with foot processes from other podocytes and wrap around the individual capillaries (Figure 41-5). The *epithelial slit diaphragm* spans between adjacent foot processes (see Figure 41-4). The transmembrane protein, nephrin, is a critical component of this structure; the extracellular domain of nephrin molecules extending from adjacent foot processes interacts to form the slit diaphragm.

Glomerular Filtration Rate Is Determined by the Mean Net Filtration Pressure, Permeability of the Filtration Barrier, and Area Available for Filtration

The glomerular capillary wall creates a barrier to the forces favoring and opposing filtration of the blood. The forces favoring filtration—that is, movement of water and solutes across the glomerular capillary wall—are the hydrostatic pressure of the blood within the capillary and the oncotic pressure of the fluid in Bowman's space (the ultrafiltrate). Normally, the oncotic pressure of the ultrafiltrate is inconsequential because medium– to high–molecular-weight proteins are not filtered. Therefore the main driving force for filtration is the glomerular capillary hydrostatic pressure. Forces opposing filtration are the plasma oncotic pressure within the glomerular capillary and the hydrostatic pressure in Bowman's space. Figure 41-6 illustrates the direction and magnitude of these forces under normal conditions.

The net filtration pressure (P_f) at any point along the glomerular capillary is the difference between the capillary hydrostatic pressure (P_{gc}) favoring filtration and the capillary oncotic pressure (π_b) plus the hydrostatic pressure of the ultrafiltrate (P_t) opposing filtration. This relationship is expressed mathematically as follows:

$$P_f = P_{gc} - (\pi_b + P_t)$$

As blood travels through the glomerular capillary, a large proportion of the fluid component of the plasma is forced across the capillary wall, whereas the plasma proteins are retained in the capillary lumen. Therefore the plasma oncotic pressure increases significantly along the capillary bed. At the same time, the loss of plasma volume along the capillary bed causes a decrease in the hydrostatic pressure in the capillary, although this change is small because of resistance in the efferent arteriole. The result is that the net filtration pressure tends to decrease along the capillary bed. However, during conditions that increase blood flow through the glomerular capillaries, the increase in capillary oncotic pressure is blunted and filtration in the distal portions of the glomerular capillaries is consequently increased.

The GFR is the product of the mean net filtration pressure ($\overline{P}_f$), the permeability of the filtration barrier, and the surface area available for filtration. The permeability of the filtration barrier is determined by the structural and chemical characteristics of the glomerular capillary wall. The product of the filtration barrier permeability and its surface area is the ultrafiltration coefficient (K_f). Thus the combined effects of the determinants of GFR are mathematically represented by the following equation:

$$GFR = \overline{P}_f \times K_f$$

The Filtration Barrier Is Selectively Permeable

In addition to determining the hydraulic permeability of the filtration barrier, the structural and chemical characteristics of the glomerular capillary wall establish the selective permeability (*permselectivity*) of the filtration barrier. The permselectivity of the filtration barrier is responsible for differences in the rate of filtration of blood components. Normally, essentially all cellular components and plasma proteins the size of albumin molecules or larger are retained in the bloodstream, whereas water and solutes are freely filtered. In general, substances with a molecular radius of 4 nm or more are not filtered, whereas molecules with a radius of 2 nm or less are filtered without restriction.

However, characteristics other than size affect the ability of blood components to cross the filtration barrier. The net electrical charge of a molecule has a dramatic effect on its rate of filtration. The *cationic* (positively charged) form of many substances is more freely filtered than the neutral form, which is more freely filtered than the *anionic* (negatively charged) form of the same molecule. For example, the cationic form of albumin is excreted at a rate approximately 300 times that of native albumin, which has a net negative charge. These differences are caused by a charge-selective barrier in the glomerular capillary wall that is created by negatively charged residues of glycoproteins incorporated in the glomerular basement membrane and coating the endothelial and epithelial cells. These fixed negative charges repel negatively charged plasma proteins and thus inhibit their passage across the filtration barrier. The shape and deformability of the molecule also affect its ability to cross the filtration barrier. Neutral dextran, a long, flexible molecule, crosses the filtration barrier approximately seven times as easily as horseradish peroxidase, a globular protein with a similar molecular radius and net charge.

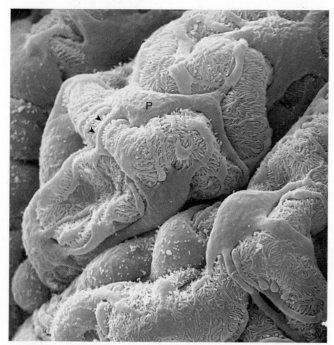

FIGURE 41-5 Scanning electron micrograph of the surface of rat glomerular capillaries viewed from Bowman's space. The cell bodies *(P)* of visceral epithelial cells, or podocytes, nestle between the capillary loops. The primary foot processes *(arrowheads)* radiate outward and wrap around the capillaries. Secondary foot processes extend from the primary foot processes and interdigitate with secondary foot processes from other podocytes.

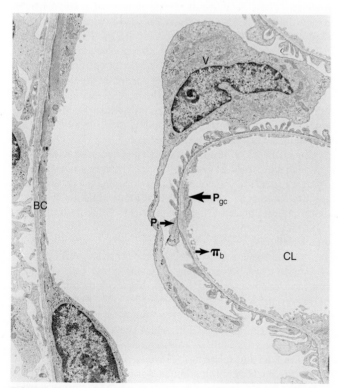

FIGURE 41-6 Transmission electron micrograph of rat glomerular capillary and Bowman's capsule *(BC)* illustrating the forces favoring and opposing filtration. The main force favoring filtration is the hydrostatic pressure of the glomerular capillary (P_{gc}). The forces opposing filtration are the hydrostatic pressure of Bowman's space (P_t) and the oncotic pressure of the blood (π_b). *CL*, Capillary lumen; *V*, visceral epithelial cell.

Glomerular Filtration Rate Is Regulated by Systemic and Intrinsic Factors

The kidney normally maintains the GFR at a relatively constant level despite changes in systemic blood pressure and renal blood flow. The GFR is kept within the physiological range by renal modulation of systemic blood pressure and intravascular volume and by intrinsic control of renal blood flow, glomerular capillary pressure, and K_f. Renal effects on systemic blood pressure and volume are mediated primarily through humoral factors, particularly the renin-angiotensin-aldosterone system. Intrinsic control of glomerular capillary perfusion is mediated by two autoregulatory systems that control the resistance to flow in the afferent and efferent arterioles: the myogenic reflex and tubuloglomerular feedback.

The *renin-angiotensin-aldosterone* system is an important regulator of GFR and renal blood flow. *Renin* is a hormone produced primarily by cells located in the wall of the afferent arteriole, the *granular extraglomerular mesangial cells,* which are specialized *juxtaglomerular cells.* Renin release is stimulated by a decrease in renal perfusion pressure, most often caused by systemic hypotension. Renin catalyzes the transformation of *angiotensinogen,* which is produced by the liver, to *angiotensin I.* Angiotensin I is converted to the more active *angiotensin II* by *angiotensin-converting enzyme* (ACE), which is located primarily in the vascular endothelium of the lung. ACE is also present in other organs, including the kidney, where it is largely in interstitial capillary endothelium and the proximal tubule. Local conversion of angiotensin I to angiotensin II in the kidney may regulate renal blood flow and transport processes independent of systemic effects.

Angiotensin II is a potent vasoconstrictor and thus directly increases systemic blood pressure and renal perfusion pressure. Angiotensin II activates sodium uptake in several renal tubules, including the proximal tubule, distal convoluted tubule, and collecting duct, and it stimulates the release of *aldosterone* from the adrenal gland and *vasopressin* from the pituitary, other hormones that enhance renal sodium and water reabsorption. Thus, angiotensin II increases salt and water retention, intravascular volume, and vascular resistance, all of which contribute to increased systemic blood pressure and renal perfusion pressure. Renin release is suppressed by both the improved renal perfusion and the elevated plasma angiotensin II, creating a negative-feedback system that maintains renal perfusion and GFR within the physiological range (Figure 41-7).

Within the kidney, there is direct control of glomerular capillary perfusion by two systems previously mentioned: the *myogenic reflex* and *tubuloglomerular feedback.* The myogenic reflex is an autoregulatory mechanism triggered by changes in glomerular perfusion, whereas tubuloglomerular feedback is an autoregulatory mechanism triggered by changes in tubule fluid delivery. The myogenic reflex regulates renal blood flow and GFR by almost immediate afferent arteriolar constriction after an increase in arteriolar wall tension, thus increasing resistance to blood flow in response to increased perfusion pressure. Conversely, arteriolar dilation occurs almost immediately after a decrease in arteriolar wall tension, thus reducing resistance to flow when vascular perfusion pressure decreases. Arcuate and interlobular arteries respond similarly. These changes in vascular resistance contribute to maintenance of GFR and renal blood flow at a constant level, despite marked alterations in the blood pressure in the renal artery. The vasoconstrictive arm of this reflex is associated with

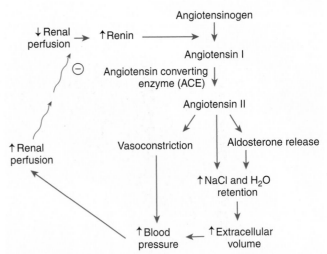

FIGURE 41-7 Schematic illustration of renin-angiotensin-aldosterone system. *Circled minus sign* represents inhibition.

depolarization of vascular smooth muscle cells in pre-glomerular arteries and arterioles and rapid entry of calcium through voltage-gated calcium channels, which stimulates smooth muscle cell contraction. The myogenic response is independent of renal innervation but may be influenced by chemical mediators, such as nitric oxide.

The second intrinsic control mechanism is *tubuloglomerular feedback* (TGF). To understand this concept, it is important to review the anatomical arrangement of an individual nephron (see Figure 41-1 and Figure 41-8). Specifically, recall that the distal nephron is closely associated with the glomerulus of the same nephron. An anatomically distinct cluster of epithelial cells, the *macula densa,* is located in the distal portion of the thick ascending limb of the loop of Henle. The macula densa is situated between the afferent and efferent arterioles, adjacent to the extraglomerular mesangial region. These four structures together are known as the *juxtaglomerular apparatus.*

The elements of tubuloglomerular feedback are summarized here and illustrated in Figure 41-8. An increase in glomerular filtration in a single nephron increases tubule fluid flow and sodium chloride concentration in the tubule fluid at the macula densa. Apical uptake of NaCl via the Na^+, K^+, $2Cl^-$ co-transporter (NKCC2) in macula densa cells leads to depolarization of the cells and basolateral release of adenosine triphosphate (ATP). By various intermediate steps, not entirely defined as yet, ATP release suppresses renin release from juxtaglomerular cells, increases resistance in the afferent arteriole, decreases glomerular capillary perfusion pressure, triggers mesangial cell contraction, and reduces K_f. These responses lead to reduced GFR in the individual nephron (single-nephron GFR), which prevents tubule fluid flow rates that exceed the tubule's transport capacity and thus prevents excessive fluid and solute loss. Conversely, increased NaCl delivery to the distal nephron stimulates production of vasodilatory agents by macula densa cells; nitric oxide (NO) via nitric oxide synthase and prostaglandin E_2 (PGE_2) via cyclooxygenase-2 (COX-2). NO and PGE_2 release modulates arteriolar and mesangial constriction and blunts the TGF response, serving as a brake to prevent excessive reductions in single-nephron GFR. In addition, the endothelium itself contributes to local control of renal

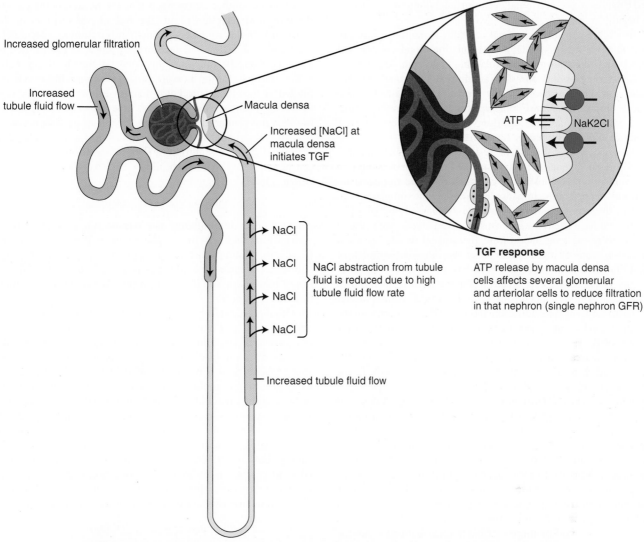

FIGURE 41-8 Schematic illustration of tubuloglomerular feedback mechanism and juxtaglomerular apparatus. Increased GFR increases tubule fluid flow rate; increased flow in the thick ascending limb (TAL) increases NaCl delivery to the macula densa (MD); increased NaCl uptake at the MD causes basal ATP release; ATP release suppresses renin release from juxtaglomerular (JG) cells in the afferent arteriole, causes afferent arteriolar constriction, mesangial cell contraction and thereby decreased K_f. The result is decreased single-nephron GFR.

vascular tone by producing potent vasoconstrictors and vasodilators. Endothelium-derived constricting factors include the vasoconstrictors, endothelin, thromboxane A_2 (a metabolite of arachidonic acid), and angiotensin II. Endothelin isoforms activate specific endothelin receptors in vascular smooth muscle cells of afferent and efferent arterioles in vitro and in general, cause vasoconstriction and thereby regulate glomerular perfusion pressure. Angiotensin II activates specific receptors and induces vasoconstriction, mediated by increased production of reactive oxygen species in vascular smooth muscle cells.

Endothelium-derived relaxing factors include nitric oxide (NO), prostacyclin (prostaglandin I_2), and PGE_2. NO is produced in the kidney by oxidation of L-arginine, catalyzed by isoforms of nitric oxide synthase, and has important protective effects on the kidney. NO prevents renal damage by quenching reactive oxygen species, thus inhibiting intrarenal vasoconstriction, glomerular hypertension, mesangial cell proliferation, and mesangial matrix production. Cyclooxygenase in renal vasculature and tubules

mediates PGE_2 production which generally acts to dilate the glomerular and medullary microcirculation and increase glomerular perfusion. Clinical use of nonsteroidal anti-inflammatory drugs (NSAIDs), which are cyclooxygenase inhibitors, commonly causes significant reductions in GFR and even renal failure, particularly in volume-contracted patients.

The intrarenal regulation of vascular tone and glomerular filtration is subject to complex interactions among the various regulatory mechanisms. For example, angiotensin II can stimulate endothelin release; endothelin can stimulate release of the vasodilators, NO and PGE_2; NO modulates renal COX-2 expression and PGE_2 production. Additional complications arise from counterregulatory effects of the same agent on specific receptor subtypes; for example, angiotensin II has been shown both to inhibit and to enhance macula densa COX-2 expression and PGE_2 production depending on which angiotensin receptor subtype is activated. These complicated interactions remain to be fully deciphered, but undoubtedly provide a refined system of checks and balances to preserve renal perfusion and glomerular function in healthy animals.

In addition to intrinsic renal controls, systemic factors can contribute to changes in GFR by regulating blood volume and vessel tone. Many hormones regulate blood volume. Angiotensin II, aldosterone, and vasopressin (antidiuretic hormone) enhance water and solute reabsorption by the kidney and thus increase blood volume. *Atrial natriuretic peptides,* produced in the cardiac atria, cause both natriuresis (sodium wasting) and *diuresis* (water wasting) and thereby reduce blood volume.

Systemic factors that affect vessel tone also affect systemic blood pressure, renal perfusion, and ultrafiltration. Vasopressin and circulating catecholamines can cause systemic vasoconstriction and increase blood pressure. Beta-adrenergic stimulation can activate the renin-angiotensin system, and alpha-adrenergic stimulation can cause renal vasoconstriction, which can both reduce and redistribute renal blood flow. In addition to altering renal perfusion, vasoconstrictors can affect the other determinant of GFR, the ultrafiltration coefficient K_f. Vasoconstrictors may cause contraction of the mesangial cells within the glomerulus and thus reduce the area available for filtration. Because K_f is the product of the area available for filtration and the hydraulic permeability, mesangial cell contraction in vivo would reduce K_f and thus reduce GFR.

Other factors that increase GFR include insulin-like growth factor and high dietary protein. Insulin-like growth factor increases GFR in normal and ischemic kidneys. A single high-protein meal causes transient elevations in renal blood flow and GFR; chronically high dietary protein intake causes sustained increases in renal blood flow and GFR. These observations are clinically relevant in the management of chronic renal insufficiency and renal failure. Although it may seem desirable to increase GFR by any means in patients with chronic renal disease, in fact the increase in GFR resulting from some high-protein diets can cause more rapid progression of glomerular injury and renal failure in animals and in humans.

In birds the GFR is more variable than in mammals, but the regulatory mechanisms are not well understood. Birds, unlike mammals, exhibit intermittent filtration in reptilian-type glomeruli; this occurs during dehydration and decreases the GFR. This may result from the release of arginine vasotocin, the avian analogue of mammalian arginine vasopressin, which decreases GFR in birds by causing constriction of the afferent arteriole of reptilian-type nephrons. Although some authors report that a juxtaglomerular apparatus is present in avian kidneys, the macula densa is either absent or rudimentary, and tubuloglomerular feedback has not yet been demonstrated.

Glomerular Filtration Rate Is Measured by Determining the Plasma Clearance Rate of a Substance

In experimental settings and in clinical practice, GFR is one of the most important parameters of renal function. Determination of GFR relies on the concept of clearance, that is, the rate the plasma is cleared of a substance. The rate of clearance is measured by the rate of elimination of a substance divided by its plasma concentration, mathematically expressed as follows:

$$C_X = (U_X V)/P_X$$

where C_X is the volume of plasma cleared of substance X per unit time, U_X is the urine concentration of substance X, V is the volume of urine collected divided by the time period of the collection, and P_X is the plasma concentration of substance X.

The net clearance rate of a substance is the sum of the rates of filtration and secretion minus the rate of reabsorption of the substance. To determine the glomerular filtration rate accurately, the rates of secretion and reabsorption must be determined or excluded from the equation. This is neatly done by using inulin as the substance for the measurement of clearance. Inulin is freely filtered by the glomerulus but is neither reabsorbed nor secreted by the renal tubule cells. Because of these properties, and because inulin is not produced by the body, the rate of its disappearance from the blood after intravascular injection is strictly related to the rate of glomerular filtration. Therefore, measurement of GFR can be expressed mathematically by the clearance equation, in which substance X is inulin:

$$GFR = C_{inulin} = (U_{inulin} V)/P_{inulin}$$

where GFR is in milliliters per minute, C_{inulin} is the rate of clearance of inulin from the plasma in milliliters per minute, U_{inulin} is the inulin concentration in a urine sample collected over a time T, V is the volume of the urine in milliliters collected over time T in minutes, and P_{inulin} is the mean plasma inulin concentration during time T.

Although the standard method of determining GFR is by the rate of clearance of inulin from the blood, GFR can be measured in a variety of ways. In clinical situations the most widely used measure of glomerular filtration is endogenous creatinine clearance. *Creatinine* is a byproduct of muscle metabolism that is handled similar to inulin by the kidney. It is freely filtered, is not reabsorbed by the tubule, and, at least in the dog, is not secreted by the tubule. In some species, however, approximately 10% of the excreted creatinine is secreted by the tubule. Nevertheless, depending on the accuracy of the assay used for creatinine, the endogenous creatinine clearance test provides a good estimate of GFR. In practice, a 24-hour urine collection is done and urine volume and mean urine and plasma creatinine are measured. These values are used in the clearance equation as follows:

$$C_{creatinine} = U_{creatinine} V/P_{creatinine}$$

This results in an approximation of GFR in milliliters per minute. In veterinary medicine the GFR is better expressed on the basis of body weight or body surface area—that is, as milliliters per minute per kilogram or milliliters per minute per square meter—because of the large variation in size within individual species.

In birds, creatinine clearance cannot be used for determination of GFR because avian renal tubules can secrete creatinine when the plasma level is elevated and can reabsorb creatinine when the plasma level is normal.

In clinical practice, the serum creatinine level alone is frequently used to assess renal function. It must be remembered that a very small increase in serum creatinine correlates with a large reduction in glomerular filtration rate and conversely, that a normal serum creatinine does not necessarily reflect normal renal function.

CLINICAL CORRELATIONS

CHRONIC RENAL FAILURE

History. You examine a 15-year-old male Siamese cat. The owner reports that her cat is listless, inappetent, and thin. The cat has been drinking more water than usual lately, urinating large volumes, and vomiting frequently.

Clinical Examination. The cat is very thin and moderately dehydrated. The mucous membranes are pale. Both kidneys are easily palpable and feel small, firm, and slightly irregular. The hematocrit is 22% (normal, 30% to 42%), serum creatinine level is 8.7 mg/dL (normal, 0.5 to 1.2 mg/dL), and urine specific gravity is 1.012. The urine sediment is unremarkable.

Comment. The cat has *chronic renal failure,* which is seen frequently in geriatric patients in small animal practice. The serum creatinine level is elevated because progressive loss of glomerular function has severely reduced the GFR, and creatinine is not cleared from the plasma normally. The urine is not concentrated in response to dehydration because tubular function is also compromised. The small kidney size is an indication of chronicity and is a result of gradual nephron loss and scarring. Anemia is common in chronic renal failure and results from many factors, including decreased production of erythropoietin by the kidney.

Treatment. In veterinary medicine the treatment of chronic renal failure is usually supportive and symptomatic. This cat would probably benefit initially from rehydration with intravenous fluids and correction of electrolyte and acid-base disturbances as dictated by the serum chemistry profile. Chronic support may greatly improve the cat's quality of life and slow the progression of disease. This should include a diet containing low total protein that is high in bioavailability, low sodium, and low phosphorus. Supplementing with the water-soluble vitamins may be beneficial. Anabolic steroids may help improve the anemia, although exogenous erythropoietin has become standard treatment in humans with anemia caused by chronic renal failure and is now being used in veterinary medicine as well.

GLOMERULONEPHRITIS

History. A client presents his 3-year-old, spayed female springer spaniel. He reports that the dog has not been eating well for several days and seems to tire easily.

Clinical Examination. The dog seems bright and alert and is in good flesh. The only abnormality detected by physical examination is slight pitting edema in the distal extremities. The left kidney is palpable, and feels smooth and of normal size. A urinalysis yields normal results except for 3+ protein (normal, negative to trace amounts) and the presence of a few red blood cell casts. A complete blood cell count is normal, and the only abnormality on a serum chemistry profile is a serum albumin level of 1.5 g/dL (normal, 2.3 to 4.3 g/dL).

Comment. This dog has *acute glomerulonephritis.* Proteinuria is indicative of glomerular disease because normally the filtration barrier established by the glomerular capillary wall prevents the passage of proteins into the tubular fluid. When the glomerulus is damaged, it becomes leaky and protein appears in the urine. The loss of albumin in this case appears to be marked because the serum albumin level has dropped below normal levels. The peripheral edema is probably caused by the hypoalbuminemia, and thus lowered intracapillary oncotic pressure and leakage of fluid into the extravascular space.

In this case, acute glomerulonephritis is likely because of the recent onset of clinical signs, the absence of renal failure, and the presence of red blood cell casts in the urine. Additional tests that are helpful in assessing the patient and guiding therapy include a 24-hour urine collection to measure the severity of the protein loss and an endogenous creatinine clearance test done at the same time to determine whether the GFR has been altered. A renal biopsy is necessary to determine the type and severity of glomerular injury. Potential causes of acute glomerulonephritis, such as recent or concurrent bacterial or viral infections or autoimmune diseases, should be explored. Renal ultrasound may provide additional information on the condition of the kidneys.

Treatment. The treatment of glomerulonephritis varies. Occasionally, the initiating cause can be determined and removed. Some cases resolve spontaneously; at other times, various combinations of immunosuppressive and antiinflammatory agents are used to combat ongoing damage from immune complex deposition and glomerular inflammation. If pulmonary edema secondary to hypoalbuminemia is present, the hypoalbuminemia must be treated with plasma or other colloids to sustain the animal until the glomerular lesion is resolved or controlled. Frequent assessment of urine protein/creatinine ratios as well as serum creatinine is warranted to monitor disease progression.

PRACTICE QUESTIONS

1. The major force favoring filtration across the glomerular capillary wall is the:
   a. Oncotic pressure of the plasma.
   b. Oncotic pressure of the glomerular filtrate.
   c. Hydrostatic pressure of the blood.
   d. Hydrostatic pressure of the glomerular filtrate.
   e. Ultrafiltration coefficient.

2. The glomerular filtration rate (GFR) is the:
   a. Volume of blood filtered by the kidneys per minute per kilogram of body weight.
   b. Volume of plasma filtered by the kidneys per minute per kilogram of body weight.
   c. Volume of urine produced by the kidneys per minute per kilogram of body weight.
   d. Volume of glomerular filtrate formed by the kidneys per minute per kilogram of body weight.
   e. Volume of blood cleared of creatinine by the kidneys per minute per kilogram of body weight.

3. In clinical practice the GFR is often estimated by determining the rate of creatinine clearance. The rate of creatinine clearance is the:
   a. Volume of plasma cleared of creatinine per minute per kilogram of body weight.
   b. Volume of glomerular filtrate formed per minute per kilogram of body weight.
   c. Weight of creatinine filtered from the blood per minute per kilogram of body weight.
   d. Weight of creatinine per volume of urine formed per minute per kilogram of body weight.
   e. Difference between the rate of plasma flow in the afferent and efferent arterioles.

4. The two major characteristics that determine whether a blood component is filtered or retained in the capillary lumen are its:
   a. Molecular radius and molecular weight.
   b. Molecular radius and lipid solubility.
   c. Molecular radius and plasma concentration.
   d. Molecular radius and electrical charge.
   e. Molecular weight and length.

5. The GFR is increased by:
   a. A low-protein meal.
   b. Afferent arteriolar constriction.
   c. Tubuloglomerular feedback.
   d. Release of atrial natriuretic peptide.
   e. Activation of the renin-angiotensin-aldosterone system.

BIBLIOGRAPHY

Bell PD, Komlosi P, Zhang ZR: ATP as a mediator of macula densa cell signaling, *Purinergic Signal* 5(4):461–471, 2009.

Castrop H, Höcherl K, Kurtz A, et al: Physiology of kidney renin, *Physiol Rev* 90(2):607–673, 2010.

Dantzler WH: Challenges and intriguing problems in comparative renal physiology, *J Exp Biol* 208(Pt 4):587–594, 2005.

Harris RC: An update on cyclooxygenase-2 expression and metabolites in the kidney, *Curr Opin Nephrol Hypertens* 17(1):649, 2008.

Kone BC: Nitric oxide synthesis in the kidney: isoforms, biosynthesis, and functions in health, *Semin Nephrol* 24(4):299–315, 2004.

Miner JH: Glomerular basement membrane composition and the filtration barrier, *Pediatr Nephrol* 26(9):1413–1417, 2011.

Munger KA, Kost CK Jr, Brenner BM, Maddox DA: The renal circulations and glomerular ultrafiltration. In Taal MW, Chertow GM, Marsden PA, et al, editors: *Brenner & Rector's the kidney*, ed 9, Philadelphia, 2012, Saunders.

CHAPTER 42
Solute Reabsorption

KEY POINTS

1. The renal tubule reabsorbs filtered substances.
2. Renal tubule function may be assessed by determining fractional excretion rate.
3. The proximal tubule reabsorbs the bulk of filtered solutes.
4. The proximal tubule secretes organic ions.
5. The thick ascending limb and distal convoluted tubule reabsorb salts and dilute the tubule fluid.
6. The collecting duct reabsorbs sodium chloride and can secrete or reabsorb potassium.
7. Solute transport is regulated by systemic and intrarenal signals.

8. Angiotensin II stimulates sodium uptake in proximal tubule, distal nephron, and collecting duct.
9. Aldosterone enhances sodium reabsorption and potassium secretion.
10. Other hormones and ligands that regulate sodium transport include antidiuretic hormone, nitric oxide, endothelin-1, and atrial natriuretic peptide.
11. Phosphate uptake in the proximal tubule is decreased by parathyroid hormone.
12. Calcium reabsorption in the distal nephron and connecting segment is enhanced by parathyroid hormone, vitamin D_3, and calcitonin.

The Renal Tubule Reabsorbs Filtered Substances

The bulk of the ultrafiltrate formed in the glomerulus must be reabsorbed by the renal tubules rather than excreted in the urine. To understand the importance of tubule reabsorption of filtered substances, consider the 10-kg beagle that forms 53.3 L of glomerular filtrate each day. The ultrafiltrate contains virtually the same concentration of salts and glucose as plasma; without tubular reabsorption, the urinary loss of sodium, chloride, potassium, bicarbonate, and glucose alone would total more than 500 g of solute. Without tubular reabsorption, the beagle would need to replace these losses constantly throughout the day by eating more than a pound of salts and drinking more than 50 L of water at the same rate as the urinary loss to maintain fluid and salt balance.

Fortunately, the renal tubule efficiently retrieves these and other constituents of the ultrafiltrate. Figure 42-1 illustrates the percentages of various filtered substances that remain in the tubule fluid at different points along the tubule. One hundred percent of the filtered glucose is reabsorbed by the proximal tubule; by the time the final urine is formed in the terminal collecting duct, approximately 99% of the filtered water and sodium has been retrieved.

Renal Tubule Function May Be Assessed by Determining Fractional Excretion Rate

The net rate of tubular reabsorption and secretion of a filtered substance is expressed as the *fractional excretion rate*. The fractional excretion rate of a substance X is the ratio of the urinary concentration of X (U_X) to the plasma concentration of X (P_X) divided by the urinary/plasma (U/P) ratio of a reference substance that is neither secreted nor reabsorbed. Relating U_X/P_X to the U/P ratio of a reference substance eliminates the confounding effect of water reabsorption on the urinary concentration of X. In experimental settings the urinary and plasma concentrations of

inulin during a constant inulin infusion may be used for reference. However, it is more practical in clinical situations to use creatinine as the reference substance. Therefore the fractional excretion rate of X (FE_X) is determined by the following equation:

$$FE_X = U_X/P_X \div U_{creatinine}/P_{creatinine}$$

where $U_{creatinine}$ and $P_{creatinine}$ are the urinary and plasma concentrations of creatinine. By multiplying FE_X by 100, the fractional excretion rate is expressed as the percentage of filtered X that is excreted. The fractional excretion rate, typically of sodium, can be used to assess the functional integrity of the renal tubules in clinical cases of acute renal failure.

The Proximal Tubule Reabsorbs the Bulk of Filtered Solutes

The rate of reabsorption and secretion of filtered substances varies among segments of the renal tubule. In general, the proximal tubule reabsorbs more of the ultrafiltrate than the other tubule segments combined, at least 60% of most filtered substances.

The structure of the proximal tubule and its proximity to the peritubular capillary facilitate the movement of tubule fluid components into the blood through two pathways: the *transcellular pathway* and the *paracellular pathway*. The tubule fluid flows over the apical surface of the proximal tubule epithelial cell. Substances transported through the transcellular pathway cross the apical plasma membrane, cytoplasm, and the basolateral plasma membrane into the interstitial fluid. Movement across the apical and basolateral plasma membranes occurs largely by carrier-mediated transport. The vast plasma membrane surface area of the proximal tubule contributes to transcellular transport. The apical plasma membrane has extensive microprojections, called *microvilli*, which collectively create the *brush border* (Figures 42-2 and 42-3). On the blood side of the cell, the basolateral plasma

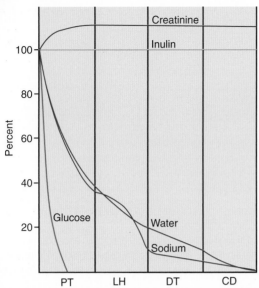

FIGURE 42-1 Illustration of the percentage of filtered substances $[(U_X/P_X) \times 100/(U_{inulin}/P_{inulin})]$ remaining in the tubule fluid in various tubule segments. In some species, creatinine is secreted by the proximal tubule and is excreted at a greater rate than the reference substance, inulin. *CD,* Collecting duct; *DT,* distal tubule; *LH,* loop of Henle; *PT,* proximal tubule. (Modified from Sullivan LP, Grantham JJ, editors: *Physiology of the kidney,* ed 2, Philadelphia, 1982, Lea & Febiger.)

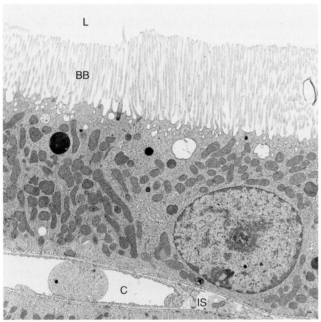

FIGURE 42-2 Transmission electron micrograph of cross section of rat proximal tubule. The brush border *(BB)* of the apical plasma membrane extends from the epithelial cells into the tubule lumen *(L),* where it is bathed by the tubule fluid. On the basal side of the cell is the interstitial space *(IS)* and the peritubular capillary *(C).*

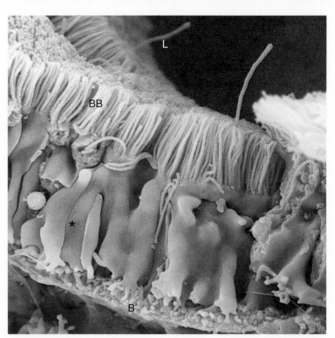

FIGURE 42-3 Scanning electron micrograph of rat proximal tubule, viewed from the lateral intercellular space. The lush brush border *(BB)* carpets the luminal aspect *(L).* Lateral cellular processes *(asterisk)* interdigitate with those of neighboring cells. The surface of the basal plasma membrane *(B)* is amplified by extensive membrane infoldings, creating numerous processes called *micropedici* ("tiny feet").

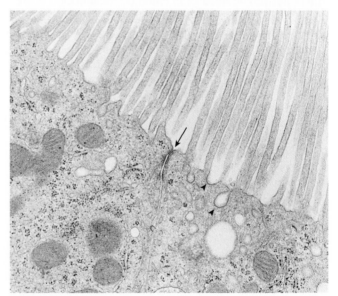

FIGURE 42-4 Transmission electron micrograph of apical region of rat proximal tubule viewed in cross section. The zonula occludens *(arrow)* joins adjacent proximal tubule cells. The zonula occludens divides the apical plasma membrane from the basolateral plasma membrane and separates the tubule fluid from the fluid of the lateral intercellular space. Also seen are coated pits *(arrowheads)* that contain the binding sites for substances reabsorbed by receptor-mediated endocytosis.

membrane has complex infoldings that enhance the surface area; the basolateral surface area equals that of the apical surface area in portions of the proximal tubule. The benefits of the enhanced plasma membrane surface area include increased capacity for the multitude of solute transporters and increased exposure to the luminal and interstitial fluids.

The second route of transport in the proximal tubule is the *paracellular pathway.* Substances pass through the paracellular pathway from the tubule fluid across the *zonula occludens,* a permeable structure that attaches the proximal tubule cells to each other at the junction of the apical and basolateral plasma membrane domains (Figure 42-4). Paracellular transport occurs by passive diffusion or by *solvent drag,* which is the entrainment of solute by the flow of water. Substances crossing the zonula occludens enter the lateral intercellular space, which is thought to communicate freely with the interstitial fluid; from there, reabsorbed substances can be taken up by the peritubular capillary.

Movement of water and solute from the interstitial fluid into the bloodstream is driven by Starling's forces (see Chapter 23) and aided by the proximity of the *peritubular capillary*. In mammals

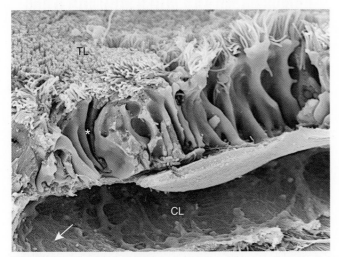

FIGURE 42-5 Scanning electron micrograph of rat proximal tubule and peritubular capillary. The peritubular capillary wraps around the basal aspect of the proximal tubule cells. Substances retrieved from the tubule lumen *(TL)* are delivered through either the transcellular pathway or the paracellular pathway into the fluid bathing the basolateral aspect of the epithelial cells. Water and solutes enter the interstitial space and diffuse into the peritubular capillary lumen *(CL)*. *Asterisk* represents lateral intercellular space; *arrow* represents fenestrae of peritubular capillary endothelium.

the peritubular capillary originates at the glomerular efferent arteriole, subdivides, and wraps closely around the basal aspect of the proximal tubule (Figure 42-5). The plasma leaving the glomerulus has a high oncotic pressure because water and salts are filtered, but proteins are retained in the capillary. The peritubular capillary has low resistance, and thus the hydrostatic pressure in the capillary is low. Both these conditions—high peritubular plasma oncotic pressure and low peritubular capillary hydrostatic pressure—favor fluid and solute uptake from the interstitium into the bloodstream.

In birds the effect of the peritubular blood supply on tubular reabsorption and secretion is complicated by the presence of a renal portal circulation. Renal portal veins anastomose with the efferent glomerular arterioles and supply peritubular blood to the reptilian-type nephrons and the proximal and distal tubules of mammalian-type nephrons; thus these tubules, but not the loops of Henle of the mammalian-type nephrons, are supplied with a mixture of portal venous and arterial blood. The rate of flow to the renal portal supply varies and is controlled by a smooth muscle valve.

Reabsorption of solutes takes place by a number of mechanisms, including primary active transport, carrier-mediated secondary active transport, solvent drag, and passive diffusion. (Transport mechanisms are described in Chapter 1.) In the proximal tubule, most solute reabsorption is driven by the active transport of sodium ions (Na^+) by the sodium-potassium–adenosinetriphosphatase (Na^+,K^+-ATPase) pump, which is located in the basolateral plasma membrane. The Na^+,K^+-ATPase extrudes 3 Na^+ ions and takes up 2 K^+ ions on each turnover of the pump (Figure 42-6).

Na^+,K^+-ATPase activity reduces the intracellular Na^+ concentration and increases the intracellular K^+ concentration. Outward

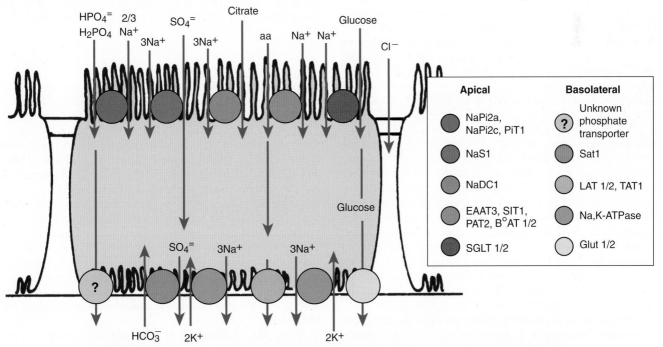

FIGURE 42-6 Schematic illustration of transport processes in the proximal tubule epithelial cell. Virtually all transport is believed to be driven by active reabsorption of Na^+ by the Na^+,K^+-ATPase located in the basolateral plasma membrane. Glucose, phosphate, sulfate, citrate, and amino acids *(aa)*, and other solutes enter the cell by Na^+-coupled secondary active transport on solute specific transporters, driven by the low intracellular Na^+ concentration resulting from the active transport of Na^+ out of the cell. Cl^- diffuses across the zonula occludens into the lateral intercellular spaces down its electrochemical gradient.

diffusion of K^+ down its chemical gradient through K^+ channels makes the cell interior electrically negative relative to the exterior. These two factors create an electrochemical gradient for Na^+ across the apical plasma membrane, favoring Na^+ uptake from the tubule fluid into the cell. Na^+ uptake across the apical plasma membrane is facilitated by specific transporters in the membrane that couple the movement of other solutes either in the same direction as Na^+ *(co-transport)* or in the opposite direction *(counter-transport)*. Specific Na^+-dependent transporters for glucose (SGLT1, SGLT2), amino acids (EAAT3, SIT1, and more), phosphate (NaPi2a, NaPi2c, PiT-1), sulfate (NaS1), and citrate (NaDC1, NaDC3) mediate their uptake from the proximal tubule fluid by this mechanism of *secondary active transport*. The uptake of these substances increases their intracellular concentration, and they move across the basolateral plasma membrane and into the blood down their electrical or chemical gradient, facilitated by solute specific transporters and partly by passive diffusion. The list of solute transporters in the apical and basolateral plasma membranes continues to grow as more are discovered by researchers. Several of the apical Na^+-coupled solute co-transporters and corresponding basolateral exit mechanisms are illustrated in Figure 42-6.

Bicarbonate (HCO_3^-) reabsorption in the proximal tubule is also driven by the Na^+ gradient, although indirectly. The chemical gradient for Na^+ drives Na^+ and proton (hydrogen ion, H^+) counter-transport across the apical plasma membrane through a Na^+/H^+ exchanger (NHE3). Secreted H^+ combines with filtered HCO_3^- in the tubule fluid to form water (H_2O) and carbon dioxide (CO_2), catalyzed by the enzyme carbonic anhydrase in the apical plasma membrane of proximal tubule cells. CO_2 enters the cell across the apical plasma membrane, in part facilitated by the integral membrane protein, aquaporin 1 (AQP1). Cytoplasmic carbonic anhydrase catalyzes the hydroxylation of CO_2 with OH^- donated from H_2O, forming H^+ and HCO_3^- in the cell. HCO_3^- crosses the basolateral plasma membrane through a $Na^+,3\text{-}(HCO_3^-)$ co-transporter (NBCe1) and a Na^+-dependent HCO_3^-/Cl^- exchanger. The majority of H^+ is transported into the tubule fluid through the Na^+/H^+ antiporter (NHE3); the electrogenic proton pump, H^+ATPase, also contributes to proton secretion. By this complex mechanism, illustrated in Figure 42-7, the proximal tubule reabsorbs 60% to 85% of filtered HCO_3^-.

Chloride ion (Cl^-) reabsorption in the proximal tubule is also indirectly powered by the Na^+,K^+-ATPase pump and occurs through both paracellular and transcellular routes. As Na^+, HCO_3^-, glucose, amino acids, and other solutes are selectively reabsorbed and water is taken up along with these solutes, the concentration of Cl^- in the tubule fluid rises, establishing a chemical gradient for Cl^- movement toward the blood side of the epithelium. In addition, in the early proximal tubule, the selective uptake of Na^+ exceeds that of anions, resulting in a net positive charge on the blood side. This creates a small electrical gradient favoring anion reabsorption. Thus, in the early proximal tubule, the chemical and electrical gradients favor Cl^- reabsorption. The zonula occludens is highly permeable to Cl^-, thus passive, paracellular transfer of Cl^- from the tubule lumen to the interstitial fluid occurs. Transcellular Cl^- absorption also occurs in the proximal tubule. Cl^--coupled transporters in both the apical and basolateral plasma membranes and Cl^- channels in the basolateral plasma membrane facilitate transmembrane Cl^- transport, which is also driven by electrical and chemical gradients established by Na^+,K^+-ATPase activity.

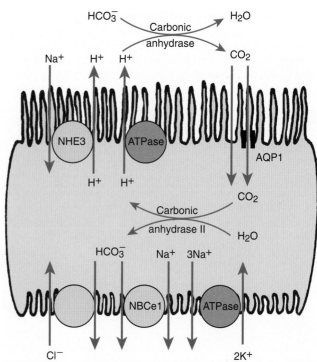

FIGURE 42-7 Schematic illustration of bicarbonate (HCO_3^-) reabsorption and acid secretion in the proximal tubule. The active reabsorption of Na^+ by the basolateral Na^+,K^+-ATPase pump drives the secretion of H^+ through the Na^+/H^+ exchanger (NHE3) in the apical plasma membrane; apical H^+ATPase also contributes to proximal tubule proton secretion. In the lumen the secreted H^+ and filtered HCO_3^- form H_2O and CO_2, catalyzed by apical membrane–associated carbonic anhydrase. The CO_2 crosses the apical plasma membrane into the cell, facilitated by AQP1 channels. Intracellular CO_2 combines with intracellular H_2O to form H^+ and HCO_3^-, catalyzed by cytoplasmic carbonic anhydrase II. The H^+ is secreted into the tubule fluid, and the HCO_3^- is transported to the blood side of the cell through co-transport with Na^+ (NBCe1) or counter-transport with Cl^-.

In distal portions of the proximal tubule, the tubule fluid becomes depleted of many of the substances necessary for Na^+ reabsorption by co-transport. There, Na^+,K^+-ATPase continues to move Na^+ from the cell into the interstitial fluid; Na^+ uptake from the lumen occurs predominantly by electrically neutral sodium chloride (NaCl) uptake facilitated by coordinated Na^+- and Cl^--coupled transporters and by passive reabsorption of Na^+ through the paracellular pathway. Paracellular transport of Na^+ is made possible here by the chemical gradient for Cl^- established by the selective reabsorption of other solutes in the early proximal tubule. As Cl^- moves down its chemical gradient from the tubule lumen to the blood side, it carries Na^+ along with it by electrostatic attraction. The passage of Cl^- down its chemical gradient also abolishes the small, lumen-negative charge and in fact establishes a small, lumen-positive charge in the late proximal tubule, which further favors the passive transfer of Na^+ to the blood side.

Other filtered solutes, such as potassium (K^+) and calcium (Ca^{2+}) ions, are present in the tubule fluid in low concentrations and are reabsorbed by the proximal tubule. Approximately 65% of filtered Ca^{2+} is reabsorbed in the proximal tubule. About 90% of the Ca^{2+} uptake in the proximal tubule is paracellular because of a favorable electrochemical gradient in the late proximal tubule

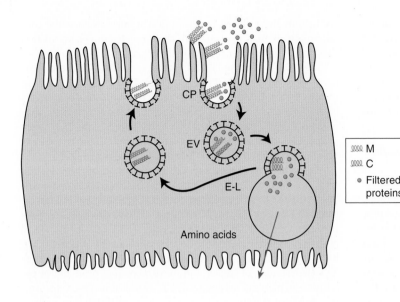

FIGURE 42-8 Schematic illustration of receptor-mediated endocytosis of filtered proteins in the proximal tubule. Filtered proteins bind with receptors, megalin *(M)* and cubilin *(C)*, in the membrane of coated pits *(CP)* in the apical plasma membrane. The coated pits invaginate and form endocytic vesicles *(EV)* that transport the proteins to the endosomal-lysosomal system *(E-L)*. The proteins are degraded and the amino acids transported to the interstitium; megalin and cubilin are recycled to the apical plasma membrane.

and solvent drag. The majority of K^+ reabsorption in the proximal tubule also occurs by passive mechanisms, primarily through the paracellular route.

The proximal tubule also reabsorbs filtered peptides and low–molecular-weight proteins. A large proportion of filtered peptides are degraded to amino acids by peptidases in the proximal tubule brush border and are reabsorbed by co-transport with Na^+ across the apical plasma membrane. Short-chain peptides are themselves transported through co-transport with H^+ on specific transporters (PEPT1 and PEPT2) in the proximal tubule brush border, driven by the proton gradient between the tubule fluid and cytoplasm. Most of these dipeptides and tripeptides are degraded by intracellular peptidases, although some may exit intact to the blood side through another peptide transporter.

Low–molecular-weight proteins are avidly reabsorbed by the proximal tubule, but by a different mechanism. Filtered proteins such as insulin, glucagon, parathyroid hormone, and many more are taken up at the apical plasma membrane by receptor-mediated endocytosis (see Figure 42-4). The proteins bind receptors (megalin and cubilin) in the plasma membrane, are endocytosed, and delivered by the endocytic vesicles to intracellular organelles called *lysosomes* while the receptors are recycled to the apical plasma membrane (Figure 42-8). Proteolytic enzymes in the lysosomes degrade the reabsorbed proteins; the amino acids that are the end products are transported into the interstitial fluid and returned to the blood. Diseased glomeruli often leak protein into the filtrate; in these instances, the proximal tubule endocytic machinery is upregulated and the lysosomal compartment is expanded, often to the extent that the increased number and size of lysosomes in proximal tubules are appreciable in histologic sections.

The Proximal Tubule Secretes Organic Ions

The proximal tubule secretes a wide variety of organic ions into the tubule fluid. Many organic ions, including both endogenous waste products and exogenous drugs or toxins, are protein bound in the plasma and thus are poorly filtered by the glomerulus. However, the proximal tubule clears these substances from the blood by basolateral uptake and apical secretion into the tubule fluid by carrier-mediated processes; transporters involved include

organic anion transporters (basolateral, OAT1 and OAT3; apical, OAT4), organic cation transporters (basolateral OCT1-3), apical P-glycoprotein (Pgp), which mediates secretion of organic cations, basolateral Na^+-dicarboxylate co-transporter, and several multidrug resistance transporters (MRP) including apical MRP2, which mediates primary active luminal secretion of organic anions. Endogenous organic compounds secreted by the proximal tubule include bile salts, oxalate, urate, creatinine, prostaglandins, epinephrine, and hippurates. Drugs and toxins secreted by the proximal tubule include antibiotics (e.g., penicillin G, trimethoprim), diuretics (e.g., chlorothiazide, furosemide), antiviral agents (e.g., acyclovir, ganciclovir), the analgesic morphine and many of its derivatives, the potent herbicide paraquat, and many more.

This aspect of proximal tubule function has broad practical applications. Tubule secretion of endogenous organic ions, drugs, and toxins provides the basis for urine testing for hormones and foreign substances as a reflection of blood levels that may be only transiently elevated. Tubule secretion of exogenous *p*-aminohippurate is used to estimate renal plasma flow. Tubule secretion of certain antibiotics is important in choosing antibiotics that reach high concentrations in the urine for more effective treatment of urinary tract infections. Similarly, secretion of diuretics enhances delivery of these drugs to their site of action, such as furosemide to the thick ascending limb of Henle's loop and thiazides to the distal convoluted tubule. Tubule secretion of certain drugs determines in part their excretion rate and affects appropriate dosing, which can be particularly important in patients with compromised renal function. Finally, competitive inhibitors of organic ion secretion raise blood levels and prolong the activity of other drugs administered simultaneously that are excreted by this route, which can create unintended drug toxicities or can be used for therapeutic advantage. For example, penicillins are normally excreted rapidly by the kidney, in large part due to proximal tubule secretion. Probenecid, which inhibits secretion of organic anion drugs via OATs, is often administered with penicillin to prolong its half-life and reduce the frequency of dosing needed to maintain therapeutic levels.

Tubule secretion plays a larger role in birds than in mammals. The end product of protein metabolism in mammals is *urea*, which is excreted primarily through glomerular filtration. In birds the end product of protein metabolism is *uric acid*. Uric acid is produced by the liver and the kidney in birds and is excreted primarily by tubule secretion. In fact, in starlings the total amount of uric acid excreted by the kidney is more than five times the amount filtered. The principal site of uric acid secretion in the avian kidney is believed to be the proximal portion of reptilian-type nephrons.

The Thick Ascending Limb and Distal Convoluted Tubule Reabsorb Salts and Dilute the Tubule Fluid

The structure of the tubule epithelium changes abruptly and dramatically at the end of the proximal tubule. The proximal tubule, with its abundant mitochondria, luxuriant brush border, and pronounced basolateral plasma membrane infoldings, is suited for high-volume transport of a large variety of substances by both active and passive mechanisms. The segments that follow the proximal tubule each have a unique structure, in keeping with their specialized functions. Immediately downstream from the straight portion of the proximal tubule is the thin limb of Henle's loop, which is a low epithelium with few mitochondria and few membranous infoldings (Figure 42-9). As might be expected, physiological studies indicate that active transport of solutes in this segment is virtually nonexistent. The function of the thin limb is determined by the segmental distribution of specific solute and water transporters and passive permeability properties and its spatial orientation in the medulla. These characteristics are essential to its role in the urine concentrating mechanism and are discussed in Chapter 43.

In the ascending limb of Henle's loop, the low epithelium of the thin limb abruptly changes to the relatively tall epithelium of the thick ascending limb. The thick ascending limb has many mitochondria and basolateral plasma membrane infoldings, reflecting its high capacity for active solute transport (Figure 42-10). The distal convoluted tubule follows with an even taller epithelium and a dense array of mitochondria. Next is the connecting segment, a segment with a heterogeneous cell population that connects the nephrons to the collecting duct system.

The thick ascending limb of Henle's loop (TAL) and the distal convoluted tubule (DCT) reabsorb Na^+, Cl^-, and the divalent cations Ca^{2+} and Mg^{2+}. These segments reabsorb solutes against a high gradient. By the time the tubule fluid leaves the distal convoluted tubule, more than 90% of the filtered salts have been reabsorbed, and the osmolality of the tubule fluid is typically reduced from approximately 300 to 100 mOsm/kg H_2O.

As in the proximal tubule, salt reabsorption in the TAL and DCT is driven by Na^+,K^+-ATPase in the basolateral plasma membrane. In the TAL, the electrochemical gradient for Na^+ established by basolateral Na^+,K^+-ATPase activity drives ion uptake through the $Na^+,K^+,2Cl^-$ co-transporter (NKCC2) in the apical plasma membrane (Figure 42-11). Intracellular Cl^- diffuses down its chemical gradient into the interstitial fluid through Cl^- channels (heteromers of ClC-K and barttin channel proteins) in the basolateral plasma membrane. The K^+ moves down its concentration gradient through apical K^+ channels (ROMK), thus is recycled to the lumen. The Cl^- absorption and K^+ secretion cause a lumen-positive voltage relative to the interstitium. The lumen-to-blood electrical gradient drives diffusion of the divalent cations, Ca^{2+} and Mg^{2+}, as well as Na^+ through cation-selective paracellular channels formed by tight junction proteins known as *claudins*. The apical $Na^+,K^+,2Cl^-$ co-transporter in the thick ascending limb is inhibited by the *loop* diuretics (named for Henle's loop), such as bumetanide and furosemide, which are often used in clinical veterinary medicine.

The distal convoluted tubule contains an apical NaCl co-transporter (NCC) that mediates Na^+ movement from the tubule fluid down the chemical gradient for Na^+ generated by the

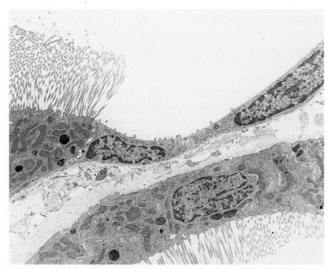

FIGURE 42-9 Transmission electron micrograph of rat kidney illustrating the transition from the proximal tubule to the thin descending limb of Henle's loop. The tall epithelium of the proximal tubule with the extensive brush border and abundant mitochondria abruptly changes to the low epithelium of the thin limb of Henle's loop. Epithelial cells of the thin limb have a smooth, simple plasma membrane surface and few mitochondria, which is consistent with the apparent absence of significant active transport.

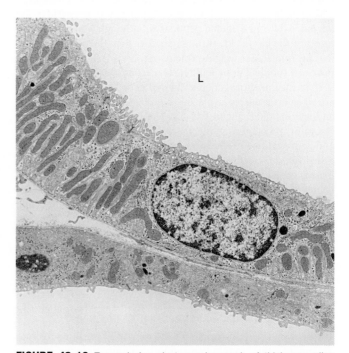

FIGURE 42-10 Transmission electron micrograph of thick ascending limb of Henle's loop in the rat. In accordance with its important role in active Na^+ reabsorption, the thick ascending limb is a tall epithelium, with extensive basolateral plasma membrane infoldings and numerous mitochondria. A collecting duct is adjacent to the basolateral aspect of the thick limb. *L,* Tubule lumen.

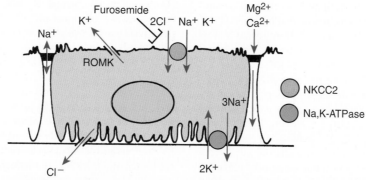

FIGURE 42-11 Schematic illustration of transport functions of the thick ascending limb of Henle's loop. Na$^+$ is actively reabsorbed through the basolateral Na$^+$,K$^+$-ATPase pump. Na$^+$, K$^+$, and Cl$^-$ enter the cell from the luminal fluid through secondary active co-transport via the Na$^+$, K$^+$, 2 Cl$^-$ co-transporter, NKCC2. Cl$^-$ exits through basolateral Cl$^-$ channels formed from ClC-K and barttin subunits. K$^+$ leaves the cell down its concentration gradient through apical K$^+$ channels (ROMK). A lumen-to-blood gradient for cations is established and drives reabsorption of Ca^{2+} and Mg^{2+} through cation-selective paracellular channels in the tight junction formed by claudins. Na$^+$ also crosses paracellular channels, initially from lumen to blood, but as the tubule fluid becomes more dilute, paracellular Na$^+$ back-leak occurs. Loop diuretics, such as furosemide, inhibit NKCC2.

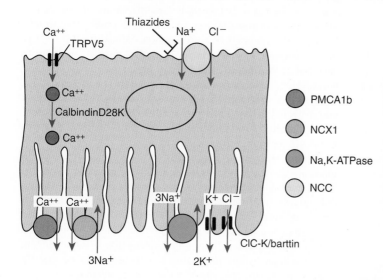

FIGURE 42-12 Schematic illustration of transport functions of the distal convoluted tubule. Na$^+$ is actively reabsorbed by the basolateral Na$^+$,K$^+$-ATPase pump. Na$^+$ and Cl$^-$ enter the cell from the luminal fluid through secondary active co-transport via the thiazide-sensitive Na$^+$, Cl$^-$ co-transporter, NCC. Cl$^-$ exits through basolateral ClC-K/barttin Cl$^-$ channels. K$^+$ is recycled to the interstitium through basolateral K$^+$ channels. Calcium uptake is driven by basolateral Ca^{2+}ATPase (PMCA1b) and Na$^+$,K$^+$-ATPase, which drive Ca^{2+} uptake through the basolateral Na$^+$/Ca^{2+} exchanger (NCX1) and apical Ca^{2+} channel (TRPV5). Calbindin 28k facilitates diffusion of Ca^{2+} from the apical to the basolateral cytoplasm.

basolateral Na$^+$,K$^+$-ATPase (Figure 42-12). Cl$^-$ exits through basolateral ClC-K/barttin Cl$^-$ channels, driven by the electrical gradient. The apical NaCl co-transporter is inhibited by thiazide diuretics.

The thick ascending limb and the distal convoluted tubule are impermeable to water. The avid reabsorption of salts without water produces a hypotonic tubule fluid; thus these segments are sometimes called the *diluting segments*. Dilution of the tubule fluid takes place regardless of the volume status of the animal. It is an important component of fluid volume regulation, allowing the kidney to excrete excess water without salt, thereby preventing water overload and plasma hypotonicity, and also generates a hypertonic medullary interstitium which is necessary for urine concentration and water conservation. The roles of the thick ascending limb and the distal convoluted tubule in water balance are discussed further in Chapter 43.

The Collecting Duct Reabsorbs Sodium Chloride and Can Secrete or Reabsorb Potassium

The collecting duct system begins with the connecting segment, which follows the distal convoluted tubule. The tubules of individual nephrons begin merging in the connecting segment and the downstream initial collecting tubule. Depending on the species, the connecting segment contains several distinct epithelial cell types, including distal convoluted tubule cells, connecting segment cells, intercalated cells, and principal cells. Each of these structurally distinct cell types has specific physiological functions.

The initial collecting tubules merge into the collecting duct, which traverses the cortex and medulla to the papillary tip, where the tubule fluid (urine) discharges into the renal pelvis. In most of the collecting duct system, two main cell types exist: the *intercalated cell*, which has many intracytoplasmic vesicles and mitochondria, and the *principal cell*, which has fewer intracytoplasmic vesicles and mitochondria but more extensive basolateral plasma membrane infoldings (Figure 42-13). The principal cell is the major cell type in the initial collecting duct, the cortical collecting duct, and the outer medullary collecting duct, accounting for approximately two thirds of the cells in most regions. Intercalated cells account for the remainder of the cortical and outer medullary collecting duct cells, and in some species (rat, mouse, and human, at least) persist even in the inner medullary collecting duct.

NaCl reabsorption in the collecting duct is primarily a function of principal cells and is driven by basolateral Na$^+$,K$^+$-ATPase. As in other tubule segments, Na$^+$ is actively transported by this pump into the interstitial fluid, establishing an electrochemical gradient that promotes Na$^+$ uptake through apical *epithelial Na$^+$ channels* (ENaC). The resulting lumen-negative electrical potential drives Cl$^-$ absorption through the paracellular pathway. Intercalated cells also contribute to NaCl reabsorption in the collecting duct. A subpopulation of intercalated cells contributes to Cl$^-$ reabsorption via an apical Cl$^-$/HCO$_3^-$ exchanger, *pendrin*, and basolateral Cl$^-$ channels. In addition to mediating Cl$^-$ uptake from the lumen, pendrin activity in intercalated cells enhances ENaC activity in principal cells, thus promoting both Cl$^-$ and Na$^+$ reabsorption.

Control of net renal K$^+$ excretion is another function of the collecting duct. K$^+$ is pumped actively into the cell by Na$^+$,K$^+$-ATPase, raising the intracellular K$^+$ concentration above that of the interstitial and tubule fluid. Intracellular K$^+$ exits the cell down the chemical gradient through K$^+$ channels present in the apical (ROMK, BK) and basolateral plasma membranes. Under normal circumstances, however, net K$^+$ secretion occurs for two reasons:

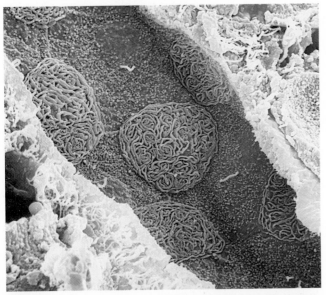

FIGURE 42-13 Scanning electron micrograph of outer medullary collecting duct in the rat, viewed from the luminal surface. Two cell types are evident: the principal cell, with short, small projections over the apical surface and a single central cilium; and the intercalated cell, with extensive, complex membrane folds (microplicae) over the apical surface.

(1) the apical K$^+$ channel, ROMK, is more permeable than the basolateral K$^+$ channel, and (2) the lumen-negative electrical potential favors K$^+$ secretion (Figure 42-14).

The collecting duct can also reabsorb K$^+$. Intracellular potassium is actively transported in exchange for hydrogen ions in the tubule fluid by apical H$^+$,K$^+$-ATPases similar to that in the gastric parietal cell. H$^+$,K$^+$-ATPases are most abundant in intercalated cells, but are also present in principal cells. When dietary potassium is restricted, H$^+$,K$^+$-ATPase activity and expression in the collecting duct is upregulated and apical K$^+$ channel (ROMK and BK) activity is inhibited; these effects enhance net K$^+$ uptake from the lumen and favor K$^+$ exit through basolateral K$^+$ channels, thus promoting K$^+$ reabsorption.

Solute Transport Is Regulated by Systemic and Intrarenal Signals

In the proximal tubule, most filtered solutes and water are reabsorbed regardless of the animal's physiological state, but the rate of reabsorption of sodium, chloride, phosphate, and other solutes is regulated by specific hormones. The distal tubule and collecting duct control the ultimate rate of excretion of electrolytes and water to maintain homeostasis despite variations in dietary intake and extrarenal losses of salts and water. The specific homeostatic responses of these segments are controlled in large part by several hormones, including angiotensin II, aldosterone, antidiuretic hormone, endothelin-1, atrial natriuretic peptide, parathyroid hormone, 1α,25-(OH)$_2$-vitamin D$_3$, and calcitonin. Many of these hormones are produced exclusively by other organs and delivered to the kidney through the circulation. Others, such as angiotensin II and endothelin-1, are produced at least partly in the kidney and exert local effects on renal transport.

In birds the relative importance of the reptilian-type and the mammalian-type nephrons in regulation of salt balance has not been established. Furthermore, in many species of birds, particularly marine and desert species, sodium balance is regulated largely by secretion of NaCl by the nasal (supraorbital) gland, rather than by regulation of renal excretion. Finally, ureteral urine delivered to the cloaca moves in a retrograde manner into the digestive tract, where additional salt reabsorption occurs; the importance of this mechanism varies among avian species.

Angiotensin II Stimulates Sodium Uptake in Proximal Tubule, Distal Nephron, and Collecting Duct

Angiotensin II directly enhances sodium reabsorption in the proximal tubule, thick ascending limb of Henle's loop, distal convoluted tubule, and the collecting duct. These segments contain specific angiotensin II receptors (AT$_1$ receptors) that, when activated, increase Na$^+$ transport. In the proximal tubule, angiotensin

FIGURE 42-14 Schematic illustration of transport in the principal cell of the collecting duct. Basolateral Na$^+$,K$^+$-ATPase actively transports Na$^+$ and drives passive diffusion of Na$^+$ from the tubule lumen into the cell through a Na$^+$-selective channel, ENaC, in the apical plasma membrane. K$^+$-selective channels (ROMK, BK) in the apical plasma membrane enable K$^+$ secretion into the tubule fluid. The hormone aldosterone enhances Na$^+$,K$^+$-ATPase and ENaC channel activity and increases K$^+$ permeability of the apical plasma membrane, thus enhancing Na$^+$ reabsorption and K$^+$ secretion.

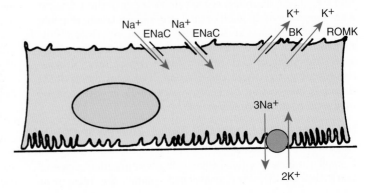

II stimulates Na^+ uptake through the apical Na^+/H^+ exchanger and the basolateral $Na^+(HCO_3^-)_3$ co-transporter and Na^+,K^+-ATPase. Angiotensin II also increases expression of the apical Na^+/H^+ exchanger and the $Na^+,K^+,2Cl^-$ transporter in the thick ascending limb. In the distal convoluted tubule, it increases the apical expression of the NaCl co-transporter, NCC. In the collecting duct, angiotensin II enhances Na^+ transport via ENaC in principal cells and apical Cl^-/HCO_3^- exchange via pendrin in intercalated cells.

By contrast, activation of angiotensin type 2 receptors (AT_2) enhances renal sodium excretion. The sodium transport mechanisms regulated by AT_2 and the interplay between AT_2 activation and the sodium-retaining effects of AT_1 receptors are the subject of many current investigations.

Aldosterone Enhances Sodium Reabsorption and Potassium Secretion

Aldosterone is a mineralocorticoid hormone that is secreted by the adrenal cortex. Aldosterone release is stimulated by systemic hypotension through the renin-angiotensin system. Aldosterone acts on connecting segment cells and the principal cells of the collecting duct to enhance Na^+ reabsorption, which in turn enhances water reabsorption to increase fluid volume. At the cellular level, aldosterone stimulates Na^+,K^+-ATPase activity and increases the *open probability* of the apical plasma membrane Na^+ channels (ENaC), thereby enhancing Na^+ reabsorption. Chronic aldosterone stimulation causes proliferation of the basolateral plasma membrane and increased Na^+,K^+-ATPase abundance. In addition, chronic aldosterone stimulation increases the apical plasma membrane expression of the apical NaCl co-transporter (NCC) in the distal convoluted tubule, the epithelial Na^+ channel (ENaC) in collecting duct principal cells, and the Cl^-/HCO_3^- exchanger, pendrin, in collecting duct intercalated cell subtypes, all of which contribute to enhanced NaCl reabsorption.

Aldosterone release is also stimulated by hyperkalemia (elevated plasma K^+ level) and has an important role in regulating K^+ homeostasis. Aldosterone increases basolateral K^+ entry into principal cells by stimulating Na^+,K^+-ATPase activity. Enhanced apical ENaC activity and luminal Na^+ uptake create a favorable electrical gradient for K^+ secretion through apical K^+ channels and thereby enhances urinary K^+ excretion. Aldosterone may also directly or indirectly increase the activity of the apical K^+ channel, ROMK.

Other Hormones and Ligands That Regulate Sodium Transport Include Antidiuretic Hormone, Nitric Oxide, Endothelin-1, and Atrial Natriuretic Peptide

In some species, *antidiuretic hormone* (ADH, vasopressin), which is released when an animal is volume depleted, dehydrated, or hypotensive, enhances salt reabsorption from the thick ascending limb and the collecting duct. The increased salt transport partly results from vasopressin-stimulated increases in the activity of the apical $Na^+,K^+,2Cl^-$ co-transporter (NKCC2) in the thick ascending limb and ENaC in the collecting duct. Although ADH stimulation of salt reabsorption in the thick ascending limb has the seemingly paradoxical effect of enhancing the dilution of the tubule fluid, this in fact allows maximal salt and water conservation because the increased salt uptake contributes to the interstitial osmolarity and enables enhanced water reabsorption in the collecting ducts (see Chapter 43).

Nitric oxide (NO) is a gas produced by the catabolism of L-arginine, catalyzed by nitric oxide synthase (NOS) in renal endothelial and epithelial cells. Nitric oxide increases renal Na^+ and water excretion by inhibiting Na^+ uptake mechanisms in several renal tubule segments. In the thick ascending limb, NO production inhibits apical Na^+ uptake by inhibiting the apical Na^+ transporters, NKCC2 and NHE3; in the collecting duct, NO production inhibits Na^+ uptake via ENaC. NO-mediated inhibition of Na^+ reabsorption in these segments, and probably also in the proximal tubule, plays an important role in regulating systemic extracellular fluid volume and blood pressure.

Endothelin-1 is a peptide hormone produced in the kidney in the collecting duct, endothelial cells, and the thick ascending limb of Henle's loop. Endothelin-1 binding to ET-B receptors in the proximal tubule, collecting duct, and thick ascending limb increases renal NaCl and water excretion by effects on epithelial transport and renal microcirculation, mediated by nitric oxide and prostaglandins. The transport mechanisms that are inhibited include the apical Na^+/H^+ exchanger (NHE3) and Na^+,K^+-ATPase in the proximal tubule, the $Na^+,K^+,2Cl^-$ co-transporter (NKCC2) in the thick ascending limb, and the epithelial sodium channel (ENaC) and Na^+,K^+-ATPase in the collecting duct.

Atrial natriuretic peptide (ANP) is produced in the cardiac atria. ANP release is stimulated by atrial distention in healthy subjects and plasma ANP levels are elevated in patients with congestive heart failure and other conditions causing extracellular fluid retention. ANP inhibits aldosterone and renin release and increases renal Na^+ excretion but the precise mechanisms causing the natriuresis have not been defined.

Phosphate Uptake in the Proximal Tubule Is Decreased by Parathyroid Hormone

The majority of filtered phosphate is reabsorbed in the proximal tubule, but the rate of reabsorption is regulated by several factors. Filtered phosphate is reabsorbed via Na-coupled phosphate transporters (NaPi2a, NaPi2c, PiT2) located in the proximal tubule brush border; the mechanisms of basolateral transport have not been determined. Regulation of phosphate uptake is mediated largely by changes in the apical abundance of these transporters. Parathyroid hormone (PTH) decreases brush border NaPi2a, NaPi2c, and PiT2, thereby decreasing phosphate uptake and increasing urinary phosphate excretion. The acute response to PTH is removal of NaPi2a and PiT2 from the brush border; in fact, NaPi2a removal occurs within minutes after PTH administration. Regulation of NaPi2c contributes to the chronic response to PTH.

Several other factors regulate phosphate uptake in the proximal tubule. In addition to PTH, factors that downregulate proximal tubule phosphate uptake include dietary potassium deficiency, metabolic acidosis, high phosphate diet, estrogen, glucocorticoids, and circulating peptides collectively known as phosphatonins. Factors that upregulate proximal tubule phosphate uptake include dietary phosphorus deficiency, thyroid hormone, insulin-like growth factor, and possibly vitamin D_3.

Calcium Reabsorption in the Distal Nephron and Connecting Segment Is Enhanced by Parathyroid Hormone, Vitamin D_3, and Calcitonin

The kidney reabsorbs the majority of filtered calcium (Ca^{2+}) and contributes significantly to the regulation of systemic Ca^{2+} balance. Approximately 65% of filtered Ca^{2+} is absorbed in the proximal tubule; the majority of Ca^{2+} reabsorption in the proximal tubule is paracellular and passive, driven by electrical and chemical gradients. Approximately 20% of filtered Ca^{2+} is reabsorbed in the thick ascending limb of Henle's loop. Ca^{2+} reabsorption in this segment occurs primarily by passive, paracellular means, driven by electrochemical gradients (see Figure 42-11); TAL Mg^{2+} uptake is by the same mechanism and reclaims approximately 50% to 60% of filtered Mg^{2+}. A small percentage of Ca^{2+} reabsorption in the TAL occurs by transcellular transport, at least partly mediated by a basolateral Ca^{2+}ATPase. Ca^{2+} transport in the thick ascending limb is suppressed when serum Ca^{2+} is elevated, through activation of the basolateral calcium-sensing receptor (CaSR), which inhibits sodium chloride uptake in the TAL and reduces the electrical gradient driving paracellular Ca^{2+} uptake.

The distal convoluted tubule and the connecting segment reabsorb an additional 10% of the filtered Ca^{2+}, primarily by active transcellular transport (see Figure 42-12). The basolateral plasma membrane of distal convoluted tubule and connecting segment cells contains a Ca^{2+}-ATPase (PMCA1b) that actively pumps intracellular Ca^{2+} into the interstitial fluid. Ca^{2+} is also transported across the basolateral plasma membrane by a Na^+/Ca^{2+} antiporter (NCX1) that exchanges extracellular Na^+ for intracellular Ca^{2+}. Ca^{2+} in the tubule fluid enters the cell across the apical plasma membrane through a Ca^{2+} channel (TRPV5), and diffusion to the basolateral side of the cell is facilitated by the cytoplasmic Ca^{2+}-binding protein, calbindin 28k. Only 1% to 2% of the filtered Ca^{2+} is reabsorbed in the collecting ducts, by mechanisms that have not been identified.

Regulation of Ca^{2+} transport occurs in the distal convoluted tubule, the connecting segment, and the cortical thick ascending limb of Henle's loop. Parathyroid hormone, $1\alpha,25\text{-}(OH)_2$–vitamin D_3, and calcitonin have important roles in controlling renal Ca^{2+} excretion.

Hypocalcemia (low plasma Ca^{2+} level) stimulates parathyroid hormone release, which affects bone, the intestines, and the kidneys to raise the plasma Ca^{2+} level. The renal response occurs in the cortical thick ascending limb, the distal convoluted tubule, and the connecting segment. *Parathyroid hormone* (PTH) is believed to increase apical uptake of Ca^{2+} in these segments by increasing the activity of the apical Ca^{2+} channel. Furthermore, at least in the distal convoluted tubule, PTH increases the Cl^- conductance at the basolateral plasma membrane, which hyperpolarizes the cells (the interior becomes more electrically negative) and thus increases the driving force for Ca^{2+} entry. The hormone, vitamin D, is converted to its active form in the proximal convoluted tubules; this process is stimulated by PTH. Receptors for vitamin D_3 are located predominantly in the distal convoluted tubule and connecting segment, where vitamin D_3, $1\alpha,25\text{-}(OH)_2$–vitamin D_3, increases the cellular content of the Ca^{2+}-binding protein, calbindin 28k, and thus contributes to enhanced Ca^{2+} reabsorption.

Calcitonin reduces the serum Ca^{2+} concentration, largely by decreasing osteoclast-mediated bone resorption and thus increasing net Ca^{2+} deposition in bone. Calcitonin reduces renal Ca^{2+} excretion by enhancing Ca^{2+} reabsorption in the thick ascending limb and the distal convoluted tubule via mechanisms that are not fully characterized.

CLINICAL CORRELATIONS

GLUCOSURIA

History. A client presents her 10-year-old female miniature schnauzer with the complaint of a dramatic increase in water consumption and urine volume over the previous 2 weeks.

Clinical Examination. No major abnormalities are found on physical examination. The dog appears alert and is moderately overweight. The urinalysis reveals 4+ glucose (normally negative) and urine specific gravity of 1.030. The plasma glucose level is tested immediately and is 275 mg/dL (normal, 80 to 120 mg/dL).

Comment. The dog has *diabetes mellitus,* which results from a relative or absolute deficiency of insulin secreted from the β cells of the pancreas, similar to Type 1 diabetes mellitus in humans, or by a state of insulin resistance, similar to Type 2 diabetes mellitus in humans. Regardless of the cause, the effective insulin deficiency results in elevated plasma glucose levels. Glucose is freely filtered by the glomerulus and normally is entirely reabsorbed by the proximal tubule, via Na^+-coupled apical uptake by SGLT1/2 glucose transporters, and basolateral facilitated diffusion via GLUT1/2 glucose carriers. As the plasma glucose level rises, the glucose concentration in the glomerular filtrate rises. When it exceeds the reabsorptive capacity of the proximal tubule (the renal threshold) of approximately 180 mg/dL, glucose appears in the urine *(glucosuria).* The glucose acts as an osmotic agent and increases the volume of urine excreted. The dog then drinks more water to replace the excessive fluid loss.

Treatment. Treatment of diabetes mellitus in veterinary patients usually involves the administration of insulin injections two to three times each day, with adjustments of the dose in accordance with frequent evaluations of the plasma or urine glucose values. When the insulin dosage is appropriate, the plasma glucose level is normalized, the glucosuria disappears, and the urine volume and water consumption decrease. In some cases, oral hypoglycemic drugs, such as glipizide, may also be used to help normalize serum glucose.

HYPOADRENOCORTICISM

History. A concerned client presents her 1-year-old spayed female Samoyed with the complaint of severe weakness, inappetence, and vomiting since the previous day.

Clinical Examination. The dog is lethargic, weak, and extremely dehydrated. The heart rate is normal, but pulses are weak. No other abnormalities are detected on physical examination. Samples of blood and urine are collected immediately for a complete blood count, serum chemistry profile, and urinalysis, and then an intravenous catheter is placed to start volume replacement therapy with a balanced electrolyte solution. The urinalysis is normal, with a specific gravity of 1.025. Abdominal radiographs are normal, but the thoracic radiographs demonstrate a small cardiac silhouette and small thoracic vessels. The serum creatinine level is 2.5 mg/dL (normal, 0.6 to 1.2 mg/dL), serum K^+ level is 6.5 mEq/L (normal, 3.6 to 5.6 mEq/L), serum Na^+ is 129 mEq/L (normal, 141 to 155 mEq/L), serum Cl^- is 97 mEq/L (normal, 103 to 115 mEq/L), and serum HCO_3^- is 12 mEq/L (normal, 18 to 24 mEq/L).

Comment. The dog has *hypoadrenocorticism.* The metabolic disturbances result from a deficiency of the mineralocorticoid hormone aldosterone. In a normal animal, aldosterone stimulates connecting segment and collecting duct Na^+,K^+-ATPase activity and enhances apical Na^+ uptake by increasing apical ENaC open probability and abundance in principal cells; these effects on Na^+ reabsorption promote K^+ secretion by increasing transport of K^+ into the cell from the interstitium and by creating a favorable electrical gradient for apical K^+ exit. Aldosterone may also directly or indirectly enhance apical K^+ channel activity. When aldosterone is deficient, Na$^+$ conservation and K$^+$ secretion in these segments are impaired and hyponatremia and hyperkalemia can occur. Cl$^-$ and water follow the path of Na$^+$ and also are excreted excessively by the kidney. *Hyperkalemia* (high serum K$^+$ level) has profound effects on excitable tissue, including nerve and muscle cells, and results in muscle weakness, decreased cardiac output, hypotension, and cardiac arrhythmias. The loss of Na$^+$ and water results in volume depletion and decreased size of the heart and thoracic blood vessels and exacerbates the hypotension and poor tissue perfusion.

Poor perfusion of the kidneys is probably the major cause of the elevated serum creatinine level *(azotemia)* because inadequate renal blood flow and reduced glomerular capillary hydrostatic pressure prevent adequate glomerular filtration. This is called prerenal azotemia. In most cases of *prerenal azotemia* the urine is maximally concentrated in an attempt to retain fluid and restore blood volume, but in hypoadrenocorticism, this response is often blunted, possibly by the *hyponatremia* (reduced serum Na$^+$ level) or by the absence of glucocorticoids, which have been shown to have a permissive effect on maximal urine concentration (see Chapter 43). The decreased serum bicarbonate level indicates metabolic acidosis, which is the result of both the diminished renal ability to secrete H$^+$ and reabsorb HCO$_3^-$ (see Chapter 44) and the increased production of acid from poorly perfused tissue.

Treatment. Prompt treatment is important for the animal's survival because the hyperkalemia and acidosis can cause fatal cardiac arrhythmias. Volume repletion with normal saline and correction of the *base deficit* (low serum HCO$_3^-$ level) often stabilizes the animal. Replacement therapy with mineralocorticoid hormones (e.g., desoxycorticosterone acetate, desoxycorticosterone pivalate, fludrocortisone acetate) restores apical Na$^+$ channel and basolateral Na$^+$,K$^+$-ATPase activity and should be started as soon as possible. Frequently, glucocorticoid hormones are given early to treat shock even before the electrolyte status is known; these hormones are beneficial for two reasons. First, hypoadrenocorticism usually results in glucocorticoid deficiency, sometimes manifested by hypoglycemia, and replacement therapy is indicated. Second, the mineralocorticoid activity in many glucocorticoid preparations may be beneficial in correcting the hyperkalemia and hyponatremia.

A definitive diagnosis may be obtained by an adrenocorticotropic hormone (ACTH, corticotropin) challenge test, which maximally stimulates the release of cortisol from the adrenal gland and shows little or no response in animals with hypoadrenocorticism.

Chronic maintenance usually involves oral therapy with fludrocortisone acetate; the proper dosage is determined by periodic evaluations of the serum K$^+$ and Na$^+$ levels. Chronic replacement of glucocorticoids is also recommended.

PRACTICE QUESTIONS

1. Which segment of the renal tubule is responsible for the reabsorption of the bulk of filtered solutes?
   a. Proximal tubule
   b. Thin limbs of Henle's loop
   c. Thick ascending limb of Henle's loop
   d. Distal convoluted tubule
   e. Collecting duct

2. The main driving force for the reabsorption of solutes from the tubule fluid is:
   a. Active transport of solutes across the apical plasma membrane.
   b. Secondary active transport of solutes across the apical plasma membrane.
   c. Active transport of Na$^+$ from the tubule epithelial cell across the basolateral plasma membrane by the electrogenic Na$^+$ channel.
   d. Active transport of Na$^+$ from the tubule epithelial cell across the basolateral plasma membrane by the Na$^+$,K$^+$-ATPase pump.
   e. Passive diffusion of solutes through the paracellular pathway.

3. Glucose is found in the urine of an animal when:
   a. Glucose transporters in the proximal tubule are inhibited by furosemide.
   b. Glucose secretion in the proximal tubule is stimulated by angiotensin II.
   c. Glomerular filtration barrier is defective causing increased glucose in the tubule fluid.
   d. Plasma glucose is elevated, increasing glucose concentration in the tubule fluid above the proximal tubule transport capacity.
   e. Elevated plasma glucose stimulates proximal tubule glucose secretion.

4. The ultimate rate of excretion of K$^+$ in the urine is determined by the:
   a. Concentration of K$^+$ in the glomerular filtrate.
   b. Proximal tubule, which reabsorbs or secretes K$^+$ to meet the physiological requirements of the animals.
   c. Thick ascending limb, where K$^+$ secretion is enhanced by high plasma K$^+$ concentrations.
   d. Distal convoluted tubule, which has K$^+$ pumps that are inserted in the apical or basolateral plasma membranes, depending on the need for reabsorption or secretion of K$^+$.
   e. Collecting duct, where the principal cells are capable of K$^+$ secretion, and the intercalated cells are capable of K$^+$ reabsorption.

5. Which of the following are effects of aldosterone on Na$^+$ transport in the connecting segment and collecting duct?
   a. Enhances the permeability of Na$^+$ channels in the apical plasma membrane, thereby enhancing Na$^+$ reabsorption
   b. Stimulates Na$^+$,K$^+$-ATPase activity in the basolateral plasma membrane, thereby enhancing Na$^+$ reabsorption
   c. Reduces the Na$^+$ permeability of the apical plasma membrane, thereby inhibiting Na$^+$ reabsorption
   d. Reduces Na$^+$,K$^+$-ATPase activity in the basolateral plasma membrane, thereby inhibiting Na$^+$ reabsorption
   e. Reduces the K$^+$ permeability of the apical plasma membrane, thereby inhibiting K$^+$ reabsorption

BIBLIOGRAPHY

Arroyo JP, Ronzaud C, Lagnaz D, et al: Aldosterone paradox: differential regulation of ion transport in distal nephron, *Physiology (Bethesda)* 26(2):115–123, 2011.

Biber J, Hernando N, Forster I, et al: Regulation of phosphate transport in proximal tubules, *Pflugers Arch* 458(1):39–52, 2009.

Christensen EI, Verroust PJ, Nielsen R: Receptor-mediated endocytosis in renal proximal tubule, *Pflugers Arch* 458(6):1039–1048, 2009.

Garvin JL, Herrera M, Ortiz PA: Regulation of renal NaCl transport by nitric oxide, endothelin, and ATP: clinical implications, *Annu Rev Physiol* 73:359–376, 2011.

Launay-Vacher V, Izzedine H, Karie S, et al: Renal tubular drug transporters, *Nephron Physiol* 103(3):97–106, 2006.

Mather A, Pollock C: Glucose handling by the kidney, *Kidney Int* 79(Suppl 120): S1–S6, 2011.

McDonough AA: Mechanisms of proximal tubule sodium transport regulation that link extracellular fluid volume and blood pressure, *Am J Physiol Regul Integr Comp Physiol* 298(4): R851–R861, 2010.

Planelles G: Chloride transport in the renal proximal tubule, *Pflugers Arch* 448(6):561–570, 2004.

Taal MW, Chertow GM, Marsden PA, et al, editors: *Brenner & Rector's the kidney*, ed 9, Philadelphia, 2012, Saunders.

Unwin RJ, Capasso G, Shirley DG: An overview of divalent cation and citrate handling by the kidney, *Nephron Physiol* 98(2):1520, 2004.

Wand WH, Giebisch G: Regulation of potassium (K) handling in the renal collecting duct, *Pflugers Arch* 458(1):157–168, 2009.

CHAPTER 43
Water Balance

KEY POINTS

1. The kidney maintains water balance.
2. The proximal tubule reabsorbs more than 60% of filtered water.
3. The kidney can produce either concentrated or diluted urine.
4. A hypertonic medullary interstitium is needed to form concentrated urine.
5. Short-loop and long-loop nephrons have different roles in urine concentration.
6. Sodium chloride reabsorption by the medullary thick ascending limb generates medullary hypertonicity.
7. Urea reabsorption by the inner medullary collecting duct and urea recycling enhance medullary hypertonicity.

8. The countercurrent mechanism increases medullary interstitial osmolality with minimal energy expenditure.
9. Countercurrent exchange in the vasa recta removes water from the medullary interstitium without reducing medullary interstitial hypertonicity.
10. Active sodium chloride reabsorption in the thick ascending limb and the distal convoluted tubule dilutes the tubule fluid.
11. Antidiuretic hormone regulates collecting duct water permeability to determine the final urine osmolality.
12. Cells in the inner medulla adapt to interstitial hyperosmolality by accumulation of organic osmolytes.

The Kidney Maintains Water Balance

One of the most important functions of the kidney is maintaining the water content of the body and the tonicity of the plasma. Terrestrial animals must constantly guard against desiccation, thus their kidneys evolved to reabsorb most of the water in the glomerular filtrate. Under normal conditions, a 10-kg beagle that produces 53.3 L of glomerular filtrate every day may reabsorb more than 99% of the water contained in the glomerular filtrate, excreting only 0.2 to 0.25 L of urine. A water-deprived dog with normal renal function can produce urine that is seven to eight times more concentrated than the osmolality of plasma, significantly higher than 2000 milliosmoles per kilogram of water ($mOsm/kg\ H_2O$). However, the kidney also can produce hypotonic urine in response to a water overload. After a water load, the same dog can excrete urine with an osmolality as low as 100 $mOsm/kg\ H_2O$, approximately one third that of plasma. This chapter discusses how the kidney accomplishes these feats.

The Proximal Tubule Reabsorbs More Than 60% of Filtered Water

The proximal tubule reabsorbs the majority of the glomerular filtrate. It takes up solutes from the tubule fluid by both active and passive means. The sodium-potassium-adenosine triphosphatase (Na^+,K^+-ATPase) pump in the basolateral plasma membrane actively transports Na^+ and drives carrier-mediated secondary active transport and passive uptake of solutes. Removal of solute from the tubule fluid creates a slight gradient favoring the movement of water into the cells and the intercellular spaces. The complex apical brush border and basolateral plasma membrane infoldings create large surface areas that are highly permeable to water primarily because of the water channel, aquaporin-1 (AQP1), in the apical and basolateral plasma membranes throughout the proximal tubule. Thus, the small chemical gradient results

in rapid movement of water from the tubule fluid to the interstitial fluid. The high oncotic pressure and low hydrostatic pressure in the peritubular capillaries favor the movement of reabsorbed water and solute from the interstitial fluid to the blood.

The proximal tubules in the kidneys of our 10-kg beagle reabsorb 32 to 37 L of water per day. However, because the water is reabsorbed nearly isotonically with salt, the osmolality of the tubule fluid remains similar from Bowman's space to the beginning of the thin descending limb of Henle's loop.

The Kidney Can Produce Either Concentrated or Diluted Urine

An elegant system has evolved in the mammalian kidney that allows excretion of either concentrated or diluted urine as needed. This system has three main components: (1) generation of a hypertonic medullary interstitium, which allows excretion of concentrated urine; (2) dilution of the tubule fluid by the thick ascending limb and the distal convoluted tubule, which allows excretion of dilute urine; and (3) variability in the water permeability of the collecting duct in response to antidiuretic hormone (ADH, vasopressin), which determines the final urine concentration. The beauty of this system is that all the factors necessary for urine concentration and dilution are operative at any given time, so the kidney can respond immediately to changes in ADH levels with corresponding changes in urine osmolality and water excretion.

A Hypertonic Medullary Interstitium Is Needed to Form Concentrated Urine

Terrestrial animals usually produce urine that is concentrated well above the plasma osmolality. Excretion of concentrated wastes conserves water and thus reduces the volume of water that must be consumed to prevent dehydration. Two of the three factors just mentioned are responsible for the formation of concentrated urine: (1) generation of a hypertonic medullary interstitium and (2) enhanced water permeability in the collecting duct in the presence of ADH.

The hypertonicity of the medullary interstitium is produced and maintained primarily by (1) the reabsorption of osmotically active substances by tubules in the medulla and (2) the removal of water from the medullary interstitium by the vasa recta.

Short-Loop and Long-Loop Nephrons Have Different Roles in Urine Concentration

The anatomical arrangement of the renal tubules in the medulla is a crucial element of the urine-concentrating mechanism. The nephrons of the mammalian kidney are subdivided into superficial and juxtamedullary nephrons based on the location of their respective glomeruli (see Figure 41-1). The majority are *superficial nephrons,* which have short loops of Henle that extend only into the inner stripe of the outer medulla. These *short-loop nephrons* have a descending thin limb that parallels the thick ascending limb, but they do not have an ascending thin limb; the thin descending limb merges with the thick ascending limb near the hairpin turn (Figure 43-1).

Juxtamedullary nephrons have long loops of Henle that extend deep into the inner medulla. These *long-loop nephrons* have several segments of descending and ascending thin limbs with specific urea and water transporter expression that contribute to their role in maintaining the medullary hypertonicity and urine concentrating ability. The juxtamedullary nephrons are particularly responsible for the kidney's ability to concentrate urine at a much higher level than the osmolality of plasma.

In birds, the reptilian-type nephrons have glomeruli that are near the surface in the renal cortex and have no loops of Henle. The mammalian-type nephrons have glomeruli that are deeper in the cortex and have either short or long loops of Henle that extend into the medullary cone. The mammalian-type nephrons have a countercurrent arrangement and are thought to be largely responsible for the ability of birds to excrete hypertonic urine.

Sodium Chloride Reabsorption by the Medullary Thick Ascending Limb Generates Medullary Hypertonicity

The thick ascending limb of Henle's loop actively reabsorbs sodium chloride (NaCl) but is impermeable to water. Therefore, this segment raises the osmolality of the interstitial fluid, thus generating medullary interstitial hypertonicity and a lumen-to-interstitium osmotic gradient. This process occurs in both short-loop and long-loop nephrons. The hypertonic interstitium allows water to be abstracted from water-permeable descending thin limbs and returned to the circulation.

Urea Reabsorption by the Inner Medullary Collecting Duct and Urea Recycling Enhance Medullary Hypertonicity

The *inner medullary collecting duct* (IMCD) also actively reabsorbs NaCl, but its more important contribution to the medullary hypertonicity is the reabsorption of urea (see Figure 43-1). Although the cortical and outer medullary collecting ducts are impermeable to urea, the terminal IMCD is highly permeable to urea via specific urea transporters (UT-A1, UT-A3). Thus, urea remains in the tubule fluid until it reaches the terminal IMCD deep in the medulla. Because urea reabsorption by the IMCD is enhanced by ADH, when conditions demand water conservation and ADH is released, urea reabsorption is enhanced and the osmotic gradient for water uptake increases. Because the thin limbs of Henle's loop are permeable to urea, the high interstitial urea concentration drives urea into the thin limb luminal fluid. The tubule segments that intervene between the thin ascending limb and the terminal IMCD are impermeable to urea, thus urea reabsorbed from the terminal IMCD and taken up by the thin limbs is recycled back to the IMCD. In mammals this system of *urea recycling* enhances the efficiency of the urine-concentrating mechanism. In birds, however, urea is nearly absent in the medullary interstitium; urates do not contribute appreciably to osmotic pressure because they have low water solubility. Thus, medullary hypertonicity in birds appears to depend on single-solute (NaCl) recycling.

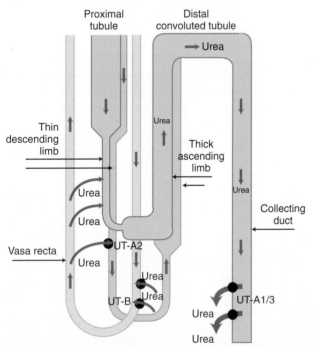

FIGURE 43-1 Urea recycling in the kidney. Filtered urea is reabsorbed in the IMCD by carrier-mediated, facilitated transport (UT-A1, UT-A3) and diffuses down its concentration gradient into the vasa recta. Urea diffuses out of the fenestrated ascending vasa recta down its concentration gradient and returns to the tubule lumen by transport into the thin limbs of Henle's loop. Urea uptake in the descending thin limbs and descending vasa recta is enhanced by the urea transporters, UT-A2 and UT-B, respectively. Because the thick ascending limb, distal convoluted tubule, and cortical and outer medullary collecting ducts are impermeable to urea, urea in the thin limb luminal fluid is recycled to the IMCD. Urea reabsorption in the IMCD is enhanced by ADH. The result is enhanced accumulation of urea in the medullary interstitium, which contributes to the medullary interstitial osmotic pressure and promotes water reabsorption.

The Countercurrent Mechanism Increases Medullary Interstitial Osmolality with Minimal Energy Expenditure

The prevailing hypothesis for decades has been that a countercurrent mechanism in the thin limbs of Henle's loop is responsible for the progressive amplification of the medullary hypertonicity initiated by the active reabsorption of salt by the thick ascending limb of Henle's loop (Figure 43-2). This may be accomplished with minimal energy expenditure because of two characteristics: (1) the anatomical arrangement of the thin limbs of Henle's loop and (2) the differential water and salt permeabilities of the descending and ascending thin limbs. Although recent data on the specific distribution of water and solute permeabilities and

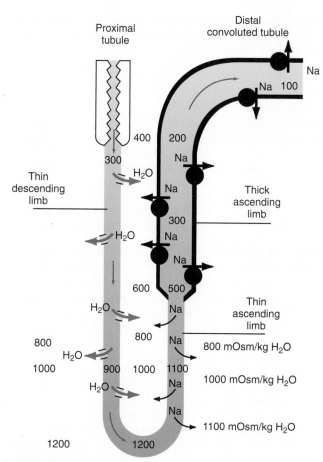

FIGURE 43-2 Generation of medullary hypertonicity and a dilute tubule fluid in the distal nephron and preservation of medullary hypertonicity by the thin limbs of Henle's loop. The thick ascending limb of Henle's loop actively transports NaCl into the interstitium without water, thus diluting the tubule fluid and raising the medullary interstitial tonicity. The proximal tubule luminal fluid osmolality is approximately 300 mOsm/kg H2O when it enters the progressively more concentrated medullary interstitium. Because portions of the thin descending limbs are impermeable to sodium (Na) but are permeable to water (H2O), at least in part due to AQP1, water diffuses into the interstitium and the tubule fluid concentrates. After the hairpin turn deep in the inner medulla, the concentrated tubule fluid crosses regions of progressively lower interstitial osmolality as it flows through the ascending thin limb of Henle's loop. Because this segment is impermeable to water but is permeable to sodium, the gradient draws luminal sodium into the interstitium. The differential permeabilities of the descending and ascending thin limbs and the countercurrent arrangement preserve the medullary interstitial concentration gradient. The distal convoluted tubule continues NaCl reabsorption without water, so that the osmolality of the tubule fluid delivered to the collecting duct system is approximately 100 mOsm/kg H2O, much less than that of plasma (295-300 mOsm/kg H2O).

the complex anatomical associations of tubules and vessels in the medulla have raised doubts about the countercurrent multiplier hypothesis, the fundamentals of the concept remain the basis of understanding the mechanisms maintaining medullary hypertonicity.

The thin limbs of Henle's loop in juxtamedullary nephrons extend deep into the inner medulla. The descending and ascending thin limbs are joined by a sharp, hairpin turn. Thus the descending and ascending thin limbs are parallel and juxtaposed, with the tubule fluid flow in opposite directions.

The descending thin limb originates from the straight portion of the proximal tubule and runs parallel to the thick ascending limb of Henle's loop. The tubule fluid entering the thin limb is essentially isosmotic to plasma, whereas the surrounding interstitial fluid in the outer medulla is hyperosmotic because of active Na$^+$ reabsorption by the water-impermeable thick ascending limb. The descending thin limb, at least in long-loop nephrons, contains AQP1 water channels and is highly permeable to water. However, the descending thin limb, at least in the outer medulla, is not permeable to salt. Thus, the tubule fluid equilibrates with the hypertonic interstitial fluid by the movement of water into the interstitium and the tubule fluid osmolality rises.

The osmolality of the medullary interstitial fluid is progressively higher in the deeper regions of the medulla, and the tubule fluid osmolality also progressively rises until it reaches its maximal concentration at the hairpin turn. Formerly, this was believed to result from continued equilibration by diffusion of water without salt into the interstitium. However, new evidence shows that descending thin limbs in the inner medulla are salt permeable; with this knowledge the precise explanation for how the tubule fluid osmolality continues to increase to the hairpin turn is in question.

As the thin limb ascends through regions of progressively lower interstitial osmolality, the concentrated luminal fluid flows through lower ambient osmolalities, and once again the tubule fluid equilibrates with the interstitial fluid. However, the ascending thin limb is impermeable to water and permeable to NaCl, so the equilibration occurs not by movement of water into the tubule fluid, but by diffusion of NaCl from the tubule fluid into the interstitial fluid. Thus the tubule fluid osmolality decreases and solute is added to the interstitium, contributing to the elevated interstitial osmolality. This process continues until the ascending thin limb merges with the thick ascending limb in the outer medulla. At the transition to the thick ascending limb, the tubule fluid osmolality is only moderately hypertonic.

At this point, what has been accomplished? By passive means, the thin limbs have reabsorbed both water and salt. Water was reabsorbed from the descending thin limb, and salt was reabsorbed from the ascending thin limb. At the same time, the countercurrent flow in these two segments and variable water and salt permeabilities have helped to maintain the medullary hypertonicity.

Countercurrent Exchange in the Vasa Recta Removes Water from the Medullary Interstitium Without Reducing Medullary Interstitial Hypertonicity

The diffusion of water from the descending thin limb into the interstitium would dilute the effect of salt and urea transport into the interstitium and cause swelling of the inner medulla if it were not for the ability of the vasa recta to remove the reabsorbed fluid. The vasa recta are permeable to water, salts, and urea. The relatively high plasma oncotic pressure in the vasa recta entering the medulla favors the movement of water into the capillary lumen, and luminal NaCl and urea concentrations equilibrate with the interstitial concentration. Thus, as the vessels descend in the inner medulla, the plasma osmolality and urea concentration rise at the vasa recta near the hairpin turn, then fall as the vessels ascend out of the medulla (Figure 43-3). What is the net effect of passive equilibration of the interstitial fluid with the plasma in the vasa recta? Two observations indicate that by the time the ascending vasa recta leave the medulla, there has been net movement of fluid into the capillary: (1) the plasma oncotic pressure has fallen, and (2) the blood flow in the ascending vasa recta is approximately double that in the descending vasa recta. Thus the relatively high initial plasma oncotic pressure, the countercurrent arrangement of the vasa recta, and the passive equilibration of the plasma with the changing interstitial osmolalities in different

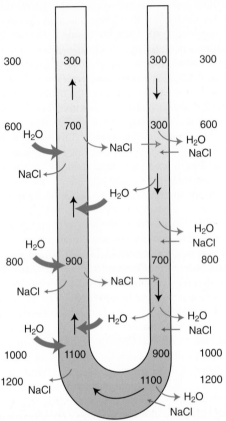

FIGURE 43-3 Countercurrent exchange in the vasa recta. The walls of the vasa recta are permeable to water and salt (NaCl). Plasma entering the medulla in the descending vasa recta has an osmolality of approximately 300 mOsm/kg H₂O, and progressively increases by equilibration with the progressively higher interstitial osmolality of the inner medulla. Similarly, the plasma osmolality progressively decreases as the vessel passes through regions of progressively lower interstitial osmolality. In both arms of the vasa recta, the gradient between the plasma and interstitial osmolality is reduced by movement of water and solute in opposite directions. This system prevents the dissipation of the medullary concentration gradient. In addition, there is net removal of water from the interstitium because of the relatively low hydrostatic pressure and relatively high oncotic pressure in the vasa recta.

regions of the medulla allow the removal of both water and solute from the medullary interstitium, without dissipating the medullary hypertonicity.

Active Sodium Chloride Reabsorption in the Thick Ascending Limb and the Distal Convoluted Tubule Dilutes the Tubule Fluid

The thick ascending limb and the distal convoluted tubule actively reabsorb Na⁺, which drives Cl⁻ reabsorption, via mechanisms described in detail in Chapter 42. Because these segments are impermeable to water, active solute reabsorption causes a progressive decline in the tubule fluid osmolality. Thus, the thick ascending limb and distal convoluted tubule are often called the *diluting segments*. The result is that the tubule fluid delivered to the collecting duct is hypotonic, even in a dehydrated animal.

Antidiuretic Hormone Regulates Collecting Duct Water Permeability to Determine the Final Urine Osmolality

The generation of medullary hypertonicity and dilution of the tubule fluid in the distal nephron segments set the stage for the elimination of either concentrated or dilute urine, as warranted by the fluid volume status, plasma tonicity, and blood pressure of the animal. The water permeability of the collecting duct, which is regulated by ADH (arginine vasotocin in birds), determines the osmolality of the excreted urine.

During water overload, ADH is absent, and the collecting duct is relatively impermeable to water. The tubule fluid delivered by the distal convoluted tubule remains hypotonic because the water is retained in the collecting duct lumen. Thus, in the absence of ADH, dilute urine is formed, and excess water is excreted (Figure 43-4).

During dehydration, hypotension or volume depletion, ADH is released from the pituitary. ADH release is triggered by a rise in plasma osmolality of as little as 3 to 5 mOsm/kg H₂O resulting from dehydration or salt overload and by decreased blood pressure as a result of systemic vasodilation, heart failure, or isosmotic volume depletion from vomiting, diarrhea, or hemorrhage. In these circumstances, the animal needs to reduce the plasma osmolality to normal or to restore fluid volume or blood pressure.

When ADH is present, water flows from the dilute tubule fluid into the cell and then the interstitium down the concentration gradient, producing structural alterations that include cell swelling and dilation of the intercellular spaces (Figure 43-5). As the now water-permeable collecting duct traverses the inner medulla through regions of progressively higher interstitial fluid osmolality, the tubule fluid equilibrates by diffusion of water into the interstitium, and highly concentrated urine is eliminated.

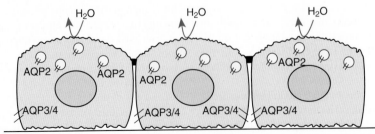

FIGURE 43-4 Collecting duct epithelium in the absence of antidiuretic hormone (ADH). When ADH is absent, the apical plasma membrane is impermeable to water, and dilute urine is excreted.

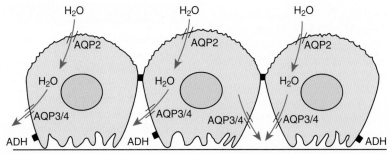

FIGURE 43-5 Water permeability of apical plasma membrane of collecting duct epithelium in the presence of antidiuretic hormone (ADH). ADH stimulates the insertion of aquaporin-2 *(AQP2)* water channels into the apical plasma membrane, which enhances its water permeability. Water rushes into the cells and across the basolateral plasma membrane via aquaporin-3 and -4 *(AQP3, AQP4)* into the lateral intercellular spaces. Concurrent morphological changes include translocation of membrane containing AQP2 from intracytoplasmic vesicles to the apical plasma membrane, cell swelling into the tubule lumen, and dilation of the lateral intercellular spaces.

ADH acutely regulates the water permeability of the collecting duct by regulating the location of the water-channel protein *aquaporin-2* (AQP2) in collecting duct cells. When ADH is absent, AQP2 is contained in cytoplasmic vesicles in principal cells and IMCD cells (see Figure 43-4). ADH secretion stimulates the insertion of AQP2 into the apical plasma membrane of these cells, and water freely passes through these channels (see Figure 43-5). Chronic ADH stimulation leads to an overall increase in the amount of AQP2 in the collecting duct; conversely, chronically low ADH leads to decreased AQP2 expression. As already mentioned, ADH also upregulates urea transporters and enhances urea reabsorption by the IMCD, enabling increased urea contribution to the medullary tonicity. The basolateral water channels, aquaporin-3 and aquaporin-4, are present in the basolateral plasma membrane of collecting duct cells regardless of ADH status, and allow the movement of water from inside the cell to the hypertonic interstitial space. In birds, AQP2 homologues are present in collecting ducts of mammalian-type nephrons and are stimulated by arginine vasotocin to enhance water permeability; an avian AQP4 homologue has been identified in the basolateral plasma membrane of collecting duct cells. Forms of the clinical condition known as *nephrogenic diabetes insipidus,* which is characterized by renal unresponsiveness to ADH, are caused by congenital or acquired abnormalities or deficiency of AQP2 proteins, often accompanied by decreased expression of other aquaporins.

In birds, salt and water reabsorption also occurs distal to the collecting ducts. Birds lack a urinary bladder; urine travels from the kidneys via the ureters to the cloaca, where both salt and water are reabsorbed. Furthermore, cloacal urine passes retrograde into the digestive tract, where additional salt and water are reabsorbed. The importance of this process with respect to both salt and water recovery varies among bird species.

Cells in the Inner Medulla Adapt to Interstitial Hyperosmolality by Accumulation of Organic Osmolytes

Cells in the inner medulla not only exist in a hypertonic environment, but also regulate cell volume during changes in ambient osmolality. These cells accomplish this by accumulating organic *osmolytes* that maintain the intracellular osmotic pressure and prevent cell shrinkage without marked increases in the concentration of intracellular electrolytes. These substances include sorbitol, betaine, myoinositol, amino acids, and glycerophosphorylcholine (GPC). The intracellular concentrations of these osmolytes vary with the diuretic state of the animal, increasing during periods of urine concentration, when the medullary interstitial osmolality is maximized, and decreasing during diuresis, when medullary interstitial osmolality decreases. Changes in the intracellular content of organic osmolytes in response to changes in ambient osmolality occur by parallel changes in either the production (e.g., sorbitol, GPC) or transmembrane transport (e.g., betaine, myoinositol, amino acids) of the osmolytes, or by counter-regulation of degradation of osmolytes (e.g., GPC).

CLINICAL CORRELATIONS

DIABETES INSIPIDUS

History. A client presents her 6-month-old female Boston terrier with the complaint of excessive water consumption and urination.

Clinical Examination. The physical examination reveals no abnormalities. The dog is alert and active. A urinalysis is normal, and the urine specific gravity is 1.002 (osmolality, 152 mOsm/kg H_2O). The serum chemistry profile and a complete blood cell count (CBC) are normal.

You admit the dog to your clinic for a modified water deprivation test. The urine fails to become concentrated despite a 5% loss of body weight. You administer vasopressin (ADH), and the urine specific gravity is 1.029 (osmolality, 852 mOsm/kg H_2O) 1 hour later.

Comment. The dog has *central diabetes insipidus* (DI), which is a deficiency of ADH. The urine is diluted by the thick ascending limb of Henle's loop and the distal convoluted tubule. Solute-free water absorption in the collecting duct depends on the action of ADH. In the absence of ADH, excessive volumes of water are excreted, and the dog drinks voraciously to prevent dehydration.

Other causes of excretion of dilute urine (urine osmolality much lower than serum osmolality) are psychogenic polydipsia, hyperadrenocorticism, glucocorticoid therapy, hypercalcemia, hypokalemia, and nephrogenic DI. Most of these can be detected from a thorough history, physical examination, CBC, and serum chemistry profile. When only psychogenic polydipsia, central DI, and nephrogenic DI remain in the differential diagnosis, the diagnosis usually can be made using the modified water deprivation test. Animals with psychogenic polydipsia can secrete ADH and have normal kidneys; therefore they concentrate their urine after water deprivation. Dogs with DI can concentrate their urine minimally or not at all after water deprivation. If the problem is insufficient ADH release (central DI), the urine concentration increases in response to exogenous ADH. If the kidney is unresponsive to ADH (nephrogenic DI), the urine concentration does not increase further in response to additional ADH.

Treatment. Treatment of central DI includes free access to water and daily administration of a vasopressin analogue, such as desmopressin (DDAVP), by parenteral or intranasal route.

CHRONIC RENAL INSUFFICIENCY

History. You recommend routine dentistry for a 15-year-old male miniature schnauzer that appears to be in good health. Before administering general anesthetic to this aged animal, you obtain a CBC, serum chemistry profile, and urinalysis to detect any subclinical organ dysfunction.

Clinical Examination. The CBC and serum chemistry profile are normal. The urinalysis is normal with a specific gravity of 1.010 (osmolality, 352 mOsm/kg H_2O). You ask the owner to submit a sample of the dog's urine from the first void of the day. The specific gravity of this sample is 1.012 (osmolality, 401 mOsm/kg H_2O).

Comment. Chronic renal insufficiency is common in geriatric patients and is probably responsible for the two urine specific gravity values in the "fixed range" of 1.008 to 1.012. These values correspond to osmolalities similar to or slightly higher than normal plasma osmolality. Additional evaluation would have to be performed to verify that this animal could neither dilute nor concentrate his urine significantly; however, in an animal of advanced age and in the absence of other clinical or laboratory abnormalities, further evaluation is probably not indicated.

In chronic renal insufficiency the loss of functional nephrons is first manifested by the inability to alter significantly the urine concentration in response to a water load or water deprivation. The residual nephrons are able initially to sustain adequate filtration rates to prevent azotemia (elevated serum creatinine and urea nitrogen levels), but the compensatory increase in flow rates in individual nephrons probably exceeds the capacity of the thick ascending limb and distal convoluted tubule to dilute the tubule fluid significantly or to generate a steep medullary concentration gradient. Thus the tubule fluid cannot be concentrated greatly above or diluted below the level of the plasma osmolality. If there is progressive nephron loss, the glomerular filtration rate will continue to decline, and renal failure will ensue.

Treatment. It is important to be aware that your patient has chronic renal insufficiency and is unable to respond efficiently to changes in fluid and salt intake. Water should be withheld only briefly, and caution should be exercised in supporting the animal with intravenous fluids during anesthesia while avoiding fluid overload.

A highly bioavailable, low-protein diet that is also low in sodium and phosphorus may slow the progression of chronic renal disease and delay the onset of renal failure, at least in some species.

PRACTICE QUESTIONS

1. The bulk of filtered water is reabsorbed by which renal tubule segment?
   a. Proximal tubule
   b. Thin limbs of Henle's loop
   c. Thick ascending limb of Henle's loop
   d. Cortical collecting duct
   e. Inner medullary collecting duct

2. The kidney responds rapidly to changing water requirements. The ability to alter quickly the rate of water excretion by greatly concentrating or diluting the urine is the result of several factors. Which of the following does not contribute to this ability?
   a. Generation of hypertonic medullary interstitium
   b. Countercurrent flow and differential salt and water permeabilities in the thin limbs of Henle's loop
   c. Dilution of the tubule fluid by the thick ascending limb and the distal convoluted tubule
   d. Responsiveness of the collecting duct to antidiuretic hormone (ADH)
   e. ADH-regulated countercurrent flow and enhanced water permeability in the vasa recta

3. The hypertonic medullary interstitium is generated in large part by:
   a. Active transport of Na^+ by the straight portion of the proximal tubule.
   b. Active reabsorption of Na^+ by the water-impermeable, ascending thin limb of Henle's loop.
   c. Active reabsorption of Na^+ by the water-impermeable, thick ascending limb of Henle's loop.
   d. Increase in water channels in the apical plasma membrane of collecting duct cells under the influence of vasopressin.
   e. Enhanced urea permeability of the thick ascending limb of Henle's loop under the influence of vasopressin.

4. In dehydration, ADH is released, which reduces water excretion by:
   a. Enhancing water reabsorption in the proximal tubules by stimulating Na^+,K^+-ATPase.
   b. Enhancing water reabsorption in the thick ascending limb by stimulating the insertion of aquaporin-2 water channels into the apical plasma membrane.
   c. Enhancing water reabsorption in the collecting duct by stimulating Na^+,K^+-ATPase activity.
   d. Enhancing water permeability in the collecting duct by stimulating the insertion of aquaporin-2 water channels into the apical plasma membrane.
   e. Reducing the glomerular filtration rate by activation of tubuloglomerular feedback.

5. In clinical situations the excretion of dilute urine may be caused by all the following *except*:
   a. Chronic renal disease.
   b. Glucocorticoid administration.
   c. ADH deficiency.
   d. Hypoadrenocorticism.
   e. Acute renal hypoperfusion.

BIBLIOGRAPHY

Laverty G, Skadhauge E: Adaptive strategies for post-renal handling of urine in birds, *Comp Biochem Physiol A Mol Integr Physiol* 149(3):246–254, 2008.

Nielsen S, Kwon TH, Frøkiær J, et al: Regulation and dysregulation of aquaporins in water balance disorders, *J Intern Med* 261(1):53–64, 2007.

Nishimura H: Urine concentration and avian aquaporin water channels, *Pflugers Arch* 456(4):755–768, 2008.

Pallone TL, Zhang Z, Rhinehart K: Physiology of the renal medullary microcirculation, *Am J Physiol Renal Physiol* 284(2):F253–F266, 2003.

Pannabecker TL, Dantzler WH, Layton HE, Layton AT: Role of three-dimensional architecture in the urine concentrating mechanism of the rat renal inner medulla, *Am J Physiol Renal Physiol* 295(5): F1271–F1285, 2008.

Sands JM, Layton HE, Fenton RA: Urine concentration and dilution. In Taal MW, Chertow GM, Marsden PA, et al, editors: *Brenner & Rector's the kidney*, ed 9, Philadelphia, 2012, Saunders.

CHAPTER 44
Acid-Base Balance

KEY POINTS

1. Buffers, lungs, and kidneys together maintain acid-base balance.
2. Acid excretion is achieved by proton secretion by tubule epithelial cells, buffering in the tubule fluid, and bicarbonate absorption.
3. Renal ammonia metabolism generates new bicarbonate and promotes acid excretion.
4. The proximal tubule has a high capacity for H^+ secretion and bicarbonate reabsorption.

5. The thick ascending limb of Henle's loop absorbs filtered bicarbonate.
6. The collecting duct determines the final urine pH.
7. The collecting duct can secrete protons, reabsorb bicarbonate, and generate acidic urine.
8. The collecting duct can secrete bicarbonate and generate alkaline urine.

Buffers, Lungs, and Kidneys Together Maintain Acid-Base Balance

Normal blood pH is approximately 7.4; normal cellular function requires a pH close to this value. Three systems maintain acid-base homeostasis: (1) intracellular and extracellular buffers, (2) the lungs, and (3) the kidneys. The first two make rapid corrections of blood pH, whereas the kidneys more slowly control acid-base homeostasis and excrete excess hydrogen ion (H^+).

Maintaining acid-base balance usually requires preventing excess acid in the body. Acid is constantly produced in the body as a byproduct of metabolism. The amount of acid produced varies depending on changes in diet, exercise, other organ functions, and in birds the phases of the egg-laying cycle. Therefore the systems that maintain acid-base homeostasis must adapt to changes in the acid load. Less often there is an excess base load that must be eliminated.

Several intracellular and extracellular buffers titrate H^+ to maintain a physiological pH. These include hemoglobin and other proteins, carbonate in bone, phosphate, and bicarbonate (HCO_3^-). These buffers rapidly normalize the pH after acute changes in the acid load, unless the buffering capacity is exceeded. In addition, during chronic metabolic acidosis, bone provides a reservoir of buffer that is mobilized to help normalize systemic pH. Excess H^+ and low HCO_3^- in the extracellular fluid promote physicochemical as well as osteoclast-mediated dissolution of bone, releasing carbonate, which buffers H^+. In chronic acidosis, this can lead to abnormally low bone mineral density.

The respiratory system also responds rapidly to maintain normal blood pH by altering the rate of removal of carbon dioxide (CO_2) from the blood. The enzyme carbonic anhydrase (CA), present in red blood cells and many other cells, catalyzes the following reaction:

$$CO_2 + H_2O \xleftrightarrow{\text{CA}} HCO_3^- + H^+$$

Removal of CO_2 from the blood by respiration shifts this reaction to the left, and the concentration of H^+ is consequently reduced (pH is raised). Thus the lung is important for stabilizing blood pH, particularly in response to rapid changes in the acid load.

The kidney is the third line of defense of acid-base balance. Although buffering and respiration are able to stabilize blood pH, the kidneys are responsible for the actual excretion of most excess H^+.

Acid Excretion Is Achieved by Proton Secretion by Tubule Epithelial Cells, Buffering in the Tubule Fluid, and Bicarbonate Absorption

The kidney excretes acid efficiently by the combined effects of (1) carbonic anhydrases, which make protons and bicarbonate readily available for transport; (2) transporters that move H^+ from the epithelial cells into the tubule fluid and bicarbonate into the interstitial fluid; and (3) buffers that minimize increases in H^+ concentration in the tubule fluid.

The kidneys excrete acid by secretion of H^+, primarily in the proximal tubule, the thick ascending limb of Henle's loop, and the collecting duct. These segments use different mechanisms to excrete excess acid and to control blood pH precisely. The proximal tubule secretes the majority of acid, whereas the collecting duct controls net acid excretion and the final urine pH.

Most secreted H^+ is transported across the apical plasma membrane by the following three transporters: (1) a sodium ion (Na^+)/H^+ exchanger, (2) an H^+-adenosine triphosphatase (ATPase) pump, and (3) an H^+,K^+-ATPase pump. The Na^+/H^+ exchanger secretes acid by electrically neutral exchange of luminal Na^+ for intracellular H^+. The Na^+ gradient generated by basolateral Na^+,K^+-ATPase drives apical Na^+/H^+ exchange (secondary active transport). Na^+/H^+ exchange is the main route of H^+ secretion in the proximal tubule and the thick ascending limb.

The electrogenic H^+-ATPase pump actively transports intracellular H^+ across the apical plasma membrane and contributes a net positive charge to the tubule fluid. The collecting duct H^+,K^+-ATPase pumps, which are similar to gastric and colonic proton pumps, actively secrete acid by electrically neutral exchange of intracellular H^+ for K^+ in the tubule fluid. Although the H^+-ATPase pump is responsible for most H^+ secretion by the collecting duct, H^+,K^+-ATPases may equal or exceed the acid secretion rate of the H^+-ATPase pump under some conditions.

Buffering of the tubule fluid is necessary for efficient acid excretion. Buffers accept secreted H^+ and minimize the decrease in tubule fluid pH that would otherwise follow rapid H^+ secretion by the epithelial cells. In mammals the most important buffers are bicarbonate, phosphate, and ammonia (NH_3); to a lesser extent, creatinine and citrate serve as luminal buffers. In birds, urates significantly contribute to titration of secreted acid. Figure 44-1 illustrates the removal of acid by intraluminal buffers.

In the proximal tubule, HCO_3^- is the most important intraluminal buffer, for two main reasons. First, the concentration of HCO_3^- in the tubule fluid is high. Although large amounts of HCO_3^- are reabsorbed in the proximal tubule, roughly proportional amounts of H_2O are reabsorbed, and the HCO_3^- concentration remains similar to that of the glomerular filtrate. Second, secreted H^+ combines with luminal HCO_3^- to form H_2O and CO_2; this reaction is catalyzed by carbonic anhydrase associated with the apical plasma membrane. The CO_2 crosses the plasma membrane, partly by diffusion and partly facilitated by membrane proteins serving as gas channels, such as the water channel, aquaporin-1, which has been shown to function as a CO_2 channel in proximal tubule cells. Intracellular carbonic anhydrase catalyzes CO_2 hydration to form H^+ and HCO_3^-, which are transported across the apical and basolateral plasma membranes respectively, resulting in acid secretion and bicarbonate reabsorption.

Filtered phosphate also buffers the tubule fluid. Secreted H^+ titrates HPO_4^{2-} to form $H_2PO_4^-$. The monovalent phosphate ion ($H_2PO_4^-$) is lipid insoluble and is transported only at very low rates on the apical Na^+-inorganic phosphate (P_i) co-transporters. Thus the secreted protons bound to $H_2PO_4^-$ are retained in the tubule fluid. In birds, titration of luminal urate forms uric acid. Besides being lipid insoluble, uric acid also has a low aqueous solubility, and thus a significant portion of acid is removed as uric acid precipitates. The role of NH_3 in acid excretion is discussed in the following sections.

Apical acid secretion is coordinated with basolateral bicarbonate transport. In the proximal tubule bicarbonate reabsorption is mediated primarily by the sodium bicarbonate co-transporter, NBCe1. In the collecting duct, the basolateral anion exchanger, kAE1, is a chloride/bicarbonate exchanger that is responsible for the majority of bicarbonate uptake by acid-secreting cells.

Renal Ammonia Metabolism Generates New Bicarbonate and Promotes Acid Excretion

Renal ammonia metabolism is a major component in the maintenance of acid-base balance and is illustrated in Figure 44-2. In proximal tubule cells the amino acid *glutamine* is metabolized to produce NH_4^+. This process is called *ammoniagenesis*. The intracellular NH_4^+ enters the tubule fluid through secondary active transport by substitution for H^+ on the Na^+/H^+ exchanger. Glutamine metabolism also produces new bicarbonate anions, which are transported across the basolateral plasma membrane. Thus proximal tubule ammoniagenesis enables bicarbonate production and absorption and distal delivery of ammonia. Renal ammoniagenesis is enhanced by acidosis and is an important renal response to an increase in the acid load.

In the thick ascending limb of Henle's loop, luminal NH_4^+ is reabsorbed by substitution for K^+ on the apical $Na^+,K^+,2Cl^-$ co-transporter. NH_4^+ reabsorption in this segment reduces the amount of ammonia species delivered to the late distal tubule and increases ammonia (NH_3) in the medullary interstitium.

High NH_3/NH_4^+ concentrations are enhanced and maintained in the medullary interstitium by a countercurrent multiplication system in the loops of Henle, similar to that described in Chapter 43. This creates a steep concentration gradient for NH_3, which favors its movement into the medullary collecting duct. Until recently, the prevailing model for NH_4^+ excretion in the collecting duct was NH_3 *diffusion and trapping*. The belief was that ammonia freely diffused across plasma membranes and into the luminal fluid where it bound protons, rendering it impermeant across plasma membranes and trapped in the luminal fluid. However, NH_3, although not a charged molecule *is* a polar molecule, much like water, and it is now known that the lipid bilayer is relatively impermeable to NH_3. In fact, specific ammonia transporters, the Rh glycoproteins, Rhcg and Rhbg, are present in plasma membranes of the majority of cell types in the collecting duct and facilitate transepithelial ammonia transport. These transporters are required for normal collecting duct ammonia transport and renal ammonia excretion and their abundance and subcellular distribution are regulated in accordance with physiologic conditions that increase renal ammonia excretion, such as acidosis. In addition, in the terminal inner medullary collecting duct, NH_4^+ is transported by substitution for K^+ on the basolateral Na^+,K^+-ATPase.

The majority of secreted NH_3 is titrated by secreted H^+ to form NH_4^+ in the tubule luminal fluid. The formation of NH_4^+ from intraluminal NH_3 and H^+ lowers the concentration of both NH_3 and H^+ in the tubule fluid. This contributes to the maintenance of a favorable gradient for the transport of NH_3 into the tubule fluid and reduces the electrochemical gradient for H^+ that is created by active proton secretion in the collecting duct.

Finally, the comparative aspects of ammonia excretion are intriguing. Ammoniagenesis and ammonia excretion are

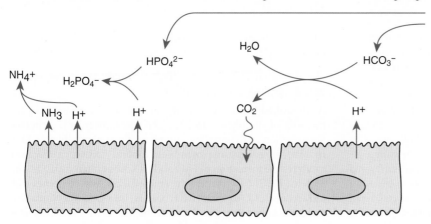

FIGURE 44-1 Schematic illustration of buffer mechanisms at work in tubule fluid. In the proximal tubule, buffering by filtered bicarbonate (HCO_3^-) predominates because of the relatively high concentration of HCO_3^-. In the cortical collecting duct, buffering by filtered, nonbicarbonate buffers, such as HPO_4^{2-}, predominates. NH_3 secretion in the collecting duct, in basal conditions and particularly in response to acidosis, increases luminal buffering in the collecting duct, which enhances acid secretion.

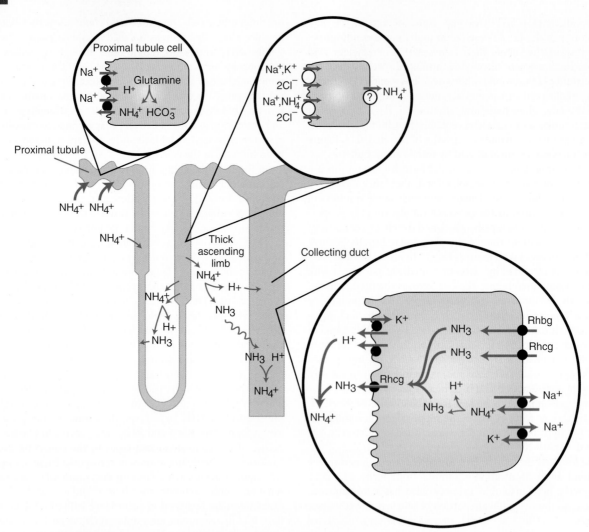

FIGURE 44-2 Schematic illustration of the roles of various nephron segments in ammonium excretion. In the proximal tubule, glutamine is catabolized to generate ammonium ion (NH$_4^+$) and bicarbonate (HCO$_3^-$). NH$_4^+$ is secreted into the lumen by substitution for H$^+$ on the Na$^+$/H$^+$ exchanger in the apical plasma membrane. Ammonium ion recycles in the loop of Henle by reabsorption by the thick ascending limb, where NH$_4^+$ is reabsorbed by substitution for K$^+$ on the Na$^+$/K$^+$,2Cl$^-$ co-transporter in the apical plasma membrane, followed by some form of facilitated transport across the basolateral plasma membrane. The elevation of the interstitial NH$_3$ and NH$_4^+$ concentration results in movement into the descending thin limbs of Henle's loop and subsequent return to the thick ascending limb. This medullary recycling results in a high concentration of ammonia (NH$_3$) and NH$_4^+$ in the medullary interstitium and prevents its return to the cortex, where it would be reabsorbed into the blood. Ammonia or NH$_4^+$ is transported by specific ammonia transporters (the Rh glycoproteins, Rhbg and Rhcg) in the collecting duct and by substitution of NH$_4^+$ for K$^+$ on Na$^+$,K$^+$-ATPase in the inner medullary collecting duct, and is excreted in the urine.

important mechanisms controlling acid-base homeostasis in mice, rats, dogs, chickens, and humans. In these species, ammonia excretion accounts for up to 60% of net acid excretion in basal conditions and can increase to 90% of net acid excretion in models of metabolic acidosis. However, these findings cannot be applied generally to other species. Rabbits have low basal urinary ammonia excretion rates and do not increase ammonia excretion during metabolic acidosis. In one model of metabolic acidosis, domestic cats acidified the urine but apparently did not increase renal ammoniagenesis and only increased urinary ammonia excretion to a level comparable to basal excretion in mice. In humans and rats, dietary potassium restriction increases renal ammonia excretion despite concurrent development of metabolic

alkalosis, but potassium restriction causes metabolic acidosis in dogs and cats and reduces renal ammonia excretion in dogs.

The Proximal Tubule Has a High Capacity for H$^+$ Secretion and Bicarbonate Reabsorption

As described in Chapter 42, the proximal tubule reabsorbs the majority of the filtered HCO$_3^-$. The mechanism of bicarbonate reabsorption in the proximal tubule is illustrated in Figure 42-7. In brief, apical plasma membrane-bound carbonic anhydrase catalyzes the formation of H$_2$O and CO$_2$ from filtered HCO$_3^-$ and secreted H$^+$. The CO$_2$ enters the epithelial cell and combines with intracellular H$_2$O to form HCO$_3^-$ and H$^+$ catalyzed by cytoplasmic carbonic anhydrase. HCO$_3^-$ is transported to the blood side of the tubule primarily by the basolateral sodium bicarbonate co-transporter, NBCe1, driven by the electrical gradient for anions. Concurrently, H^+ is transported into the lumen, primarily by the Na^+/H^+ antiporter, but also by the H^+-ATPase pump, which may transport up to 35% of the total H^+ secreted by the proximal tubule. Bicarbonate reabsorption/acid secretion in the proximal tubule is increased during chronic metabolic acidosis. Several hormones regulate proximal tubule bicarbonate reabsorption and acid secretion: angiotensin II stimulates transport by the basolateral sodium bicarbonate co-transporter, the apical Na^+/H^+ exchanger, and the apical vacuolar H^+-ATPase; glucocorticoid receptor activation and endothelin enhance the Na^+/H^+ exchanger; parathyroid hormone suppresses the Na^+/H^+ exchanger and basolateral sodium bicarbonate transport.

Although the proximal tubule has a large capacity for H^+ secretion and reabsorbs 80% or more of the filtered HCO_3^-, it cannot maintain a large pH gradient across the apical plasma membrane. Net H^+ secretion in this segment is particularly dependent on the intraluminal buffers discussed earlier, which combine with secreted H^+ and prevent the H^+ concentration in the tubule fluid from rising significantly. As a result, although the majority of renal acid secretion occurs in the proximal tubule, the pH of the tubule fluid when it leaves this segment is similar to that of the glomerular filtrate.

The Thick Ascending Limb of Henle's Loop Absorbs Filtered Bicarbonate

Bicarbonate reabsorption continues in the thick ascending limb of Henle's loop, which reabsorbs approximately 15% of filtered bicarbonate. Carbonic anhydrase generates protons and bicarbonate for transport as in the proximal tubule. In the thick ascending limb, protons are secreted primarily by apical Na^+/H^+ exchange, also similar to the proximal tubule. Bicarbonate uptake is mediated by the basolateral anion exchanger, AE2, and by anion channels.

The Collecting Duct Determines the Final Urine pH

The rate of acid secretion by the collecting duct determines the final urine pH and renal net acid excretion. Despite robust acid secretion in the proximal tubule and the additional contribution by the thick ascending limb, because of luminal buffering the pH of the tubule fluid that reaches the connecting segment is still similar to that of the glomerular filtrate, pH approximately 7.4. However, the normal urine pH of carnivores ranges from 5.5 to 7.5, that of ruminants ranges from 6 to 9, and even greater extremes of pH occur in response to acidosis and alkalosis. The collecting duct is responsible for this ability to excrete urine with a pH extremely different from that of plasma.

The Collecting Duct Can Secrete Protons, Reabsorb Bicarbonate, and Generate Acidic Urine

In contrast to the proximal tubule, which is a high-capacity, low-gradient system of H^+ secretion, the collecting duct has a lower capacity for H^+ secretion but can generate a steep H^+ concentration gradient.

Acid secretion in most of the collecting duct system is primarily a function of specialized epithelial cells, the *intercalated cells* (see Figure 42-13). Intercalated cells comprise approximately 40% of cells in the connecting segment, cortical collecting duct, and outer medullary collecting duct in most species examined, diminishing and ultimately disappearing in the inner medulllary collecting duct. Intercalated cells contain abundant cytoplasmic

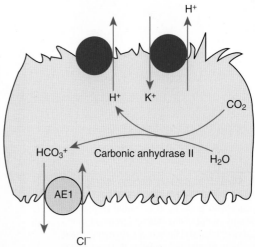

FIGURE 44-3 Schematic illustration of the mechanisms of H^+ secretion and HCO_3^- reabsorption in the acid-secreting intercalated cells of the collecting duct. Two means of active transport of H^+ across the apical plasma membrane are present: the electrogenic proton pump, H^+-ATPase, and the electrically neutral H^+,K^+-ATPase pump. The intracellular formation of H^+ and HCO_3^- from CO_2 and H_2O is catalyzed by cytoplasmic carbonic anhydrase. The basolateral plasma membrane contains a Cl^-/HCO_3^- exchanger (AE1) that allows HCO_3^- reabsorption.

carbonic anhydrase, which catalyzes the formation of intracellular H^+ and HCO_3^- from intracellular H_2O and CO_2. The collecting duct contains specific intercalated cell subtypes that are structurally and functionally distinct; approximately half of the intercalated cells in the renal cortex and virtually all in the renal medulla are an acid-secreting subtype (type A or α). In these cells, H^+ is secreted into the tubule fluid by the apical electrogenic proton pump, H^+-ATPase, or by electrically neutral H^+,K^+-ATPase pumps. HCO_3^- is transported to the blood side of the cell by a basolateral Cl^-/HCO_3^- exchanger (kidney anion exchanger 1, kAE1) similar to the Cl^-/HCO_3^- exchanger in red blood cell membranes (Figure 44-3). Acid-secreting intercalated cells alter the rate of H^+ secretion by altering the number of proton pumps in the apical plasma membrane. The insertion or removal of proton pump–containing membrane vesicles causes structural changes that reflect the physiological response (Figure 44-4). In rabbits, the Cl^-/HCO_3^- exchanger also is translocated from intracellular compartments to the basolateral plasma membrane in acidosis. In this way, the acid-secreting intercalated cells respond to physiological conditions and alter acid secretion accordingly. Less is known about the roles and response mechanisms of the renal H^+,K^+-ATPases in acidosis, but metabolic acidosis and hypokalemia enhance renal H^+,K^+-ATPase activity.

The terminal segments of the inner medullary collecting duct, where there are few or no intercalated cells, also can secrete acid. A Na^+/H^+ exchanger, an electrogenic proton pump, a H^+,K^+-ATPase pump, and substitution of NH_4^+ for K^+ on the basolateral Na^+,K^+-ATPase all participate in acid secretion in this segment, but the relative importance of these mechanisms is currently unclear.

Acid secretion in the collecting duct is generally enhanced by acidosis and suppressed by alkalosis. The hormones angiotensin II, aldosterone, and endothelin stimulate H^+-ATPase in acid-secreting intercalated cells in the collecting duct, but the roles of

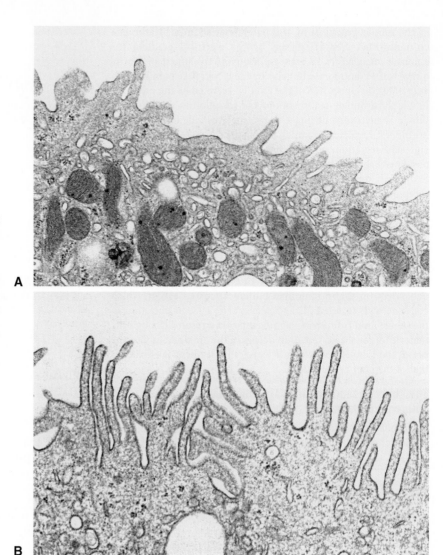

FIGURE 44-4 Transmission electron micrographs of an acid-secreting (type A) intercalated cell from rat cortical collecting duct. **A,** In a control animal, the apical plasma membrane contains few small membranous projections, and the apical cytoplasm is filled with numerous membrane vesicles. **B,** In a rat with acute respiratory acidosis, the apical surface is covered with numerous long, membranous projections, and the number of apical cytoplasmic vesicular profiles is greatly reduced. This is the result of the insertion of membrane vesicles containing H$^+$ transporters into the apical plasma membrane in response to acidosis, thus enhancing the acid-secreting capacity of the cell. (Magnification × 11,300.)

these hormones in systemic acid-base homeostasis is not fully understood.

The Collecting Duct Can Secrete Bicarbonate and Generate Alkaline Urine

The proximal tubule reabsorbs HCO$_3^-$ and secretes H$^+$, regardless of the plasma HCO$_3^-$ concentration and the blood pH. In fact, as the plasma HCO$_3^-$ concentration increases, the concentration of HCO$_3^-$ in the glomerular filtrate increases, and the amount of HCO$_3^-$ reabsorption by the proximal tubule epithelium also increases. However, the collecting duct is capable of net HCO$_3^-$ secretion in response to alkalosis, but this only occurs in the connecting segment and the cortical collecting duct. In addition to acid-secreting intercalated cells (type A or α) similar to those in the medulla, two additional intercalated cell subtypes (type B or β, and non A, non B, or type C) that can secrete bicarbonate ion are present in these segments (Figure 44-5). These cells are rich in carbonic anhydrase and secrete HCO$_3^-$ by an apical Cl$^-$/HCO$_3^-$ exchanger, pendrin, which is distinct from the basolateral Cl$^-$/HCO$_3^-$ exchanger in acid-secreting intercalated cells. Type B intercalated cells have a basolateral proton pump and functionally represent a mirror image of acid-secreting cells, with active H$^+$

reabsorption and exchange of Cl$^-$ in the tubule fluid for intracellular HCO$_3^-$ (Figure 44-6). Type C (non A, non B) intercalated cells have the apical anion exchanger, pendrin, as well as apical H$^+$-ATPase. These intercalated cells secrete bicarbonate, but the apical proton pump suggests they may not contribute to net bicarbonate excretion; their role may be more important in chloride reabsorption.

Alkalosis stimulates and acidosis suppresses bicarbonate secretion. Bicarbonate secretion is also stimulated by dietary restriction of NaCl or Cl$^-$ alone, and by aldosterone analogues and angiotensin II. These hormones also enhance apical proton transport by acid-secreting intercalated cells, which seems counterproductive. However, the stimulation of both proton secretion and apical chloride/bicarbonate exchange by these hormones enhances Cl$^-$ and Na$^+$ uptake, and is an additional mechanism supporting the NaCl retention stimulated by aldosterone and angiotensin II. The role of intercalated cells in NaCl uptake in the collecting duct is discussed in Chapter 42.

In Cl$^-$ depletion, the amount of Cl$^-$ delivered to the collecting duct may fall so low that bicarbonate secretion is impaired because inadequate luminal Cl$^-$ is available for exchange with intracellular HCO$_3^-$. The blunted bicarbonate secretion contributes

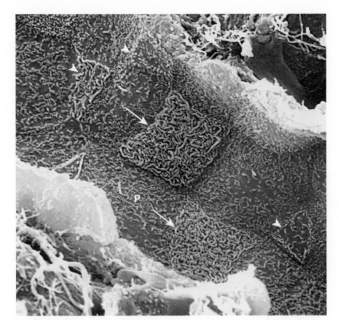

FIGURE 44-5 Scanning electron micrograph of rat cortical collecting duct viewed from the tubule lumen. Three cell types are evident. The principal cells *(P)* are large, with a single central cilium and few apical surface microprojections. The type A (acid-secreting) intercalated cells *(arrows)* have a large apical surface covered with extensive membrane folds (microplicae). The type B (bicarbonate-secreting) intercalated cells *(arrowheads)* have a small apical surface area covered with sparse microprojections. (Magnification × 4000.)

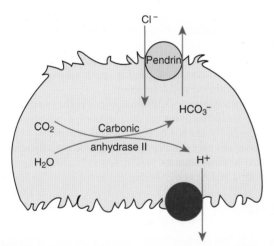

FIGURE 44-6 Schematic illustration of the mechanism of HCO_3^- secretion (H^+ reabsorption) in the type B intercalated cell of the cortical collecting duct. These cells contain H^+-ATPase in the basolateral plasma membrane and are rich in cytoplasmic carbonic anhydrase. The Cl^-/HCO_3^- exchanger, pendrin, is present in the apical plasma membrane and mediates bicarbonate secretion.

to the development and maintenance of metabolic alkalosis during Cl^- depletion, a condition commonly seen in patients after continuous gastric suction, gastrointestinal obstruction, diuretic treatment, and certain forms of diarrhea.

Little is known about the comparative physiology of renal control of acid-base balance in domestic animals, although the renal tubules are similar in all mammals examined to date, and intercalated cells have been observed at least in cat, dog, pig, and horse collecting ducts. However, it is likely that considerable anatomical and functional differences exist among species, particularly between carnivores, which usually excrete acid urine, and ruminants, which usually excrete neutral or alkaline urine.

CLINICAL CORRELATIONS

RESPIRATORY ACIDOSIS WITH RENAL COMPENSATION

History. A 6-year-old male German shepherd is brought to you with complaints of weakness, exercise intolerance, and poor appetite that have progressively worsened over the past 6 weeks.

Clinical Examination. The dog is recumbent and anxious. The heart rate is rapid, but pulses are strong and regular. Respiration is labored, and crackles are heard over all lung fields. Thoracic radiographs reveal a diffuse, severe pulmonary interstitial and alveolar infiltrate with enlargement of the hilar lymph nodes. You obtain samples of blood and urine for a complete blood cell count (CBC), serum chemistry panel, urinalysis, and arterial blood gas (ABG) measurement. The urine pH is 5.0, and the ABG results are as follows: pH, 7.37 (normal, 7.45); Po_2 (oxygen tension), 58 mm Hg (normal, 80 to 100 mm Hg); Pco_2 (carbon dioxide tension), 70 mm Hg (normal, 31 to 35 mm Hg); and HCO_3^-, 37 mEq/L (normal, 18 to 24 mEq/L).

Comment. The dog has *chronic respiratory acidosis* caused by severe pulmonary infiltrates. The lung is unable to ventilate adequately, and the blood level of CO_2 rises. The elevated CO_2 favors the production of carbonic acid, which releases H^+ and lowers the blood pH. Although the increased CO_2 level contributes to an increase in blood HCO_3^- levels, the marked increase in the blood HCO_3^- levels in this case results from enhanced renal retention of HCO_3^- and secretion of H^+. Respiratory acidosis activates the acid-secreting intercalated cells in the collecting duct, where HCO_3^- is reabsorbed and H^+ is secreted. The blood HCO_3^- concentration rises and helps return the blood pH toward normal. Despite the increased blood HCO_3^-, expression of the apical Cl^-/HCO_3^- exchanger, pendrin, is suppressed by respiratory acidosis and thus bicarbonate secretion is likely impaired. A steep H^+ gradient is established in the collecting ducts, and acid urine is excreted. (Although metabolic acidosis enhances ammoniagenesis in the proximal tubule, thereby enhancing the generation of new bicarbonate and acid excretion in the form of ammonium ion, this does not occur in respiratory acidosis, at least in rats.)

Treatment. Diagnose and correct the pulmonary disease, if possible. Bicarbonate therapy is not indicated, because the blood bicarbonate level is already high, and the blood pH is partially corrected. Oxygen therapy may improve the Pao_2 and help support the animal until specific treatment is instituted.

METABOLIC ALKALOSIS WITH PARADOXICAL ACIDURIA

History. You examine a 3-year-old Holstein-Friesian cow that has had a poor appetite for 2 to 3 days. The cow recently calved and freshened normally, but milk production has dropped in the last 2 days, and the feces are loose.

Clinical Examination. Physical examination reveals dehydration and an elevated heart rate. Percussion of the abdomen detects an area of high-pitched resonance on the right side. A distended abomasum is palpable on rectal examination. You diagnose a right displaced abomasum and suspect abomasal torsion. Attempts to correct the displacement by rolling the cow fail. The cow is transported to your clinic for surgery, and samples are obtained for a CBC, serum chemistry profile, and urinalysis. The serum K^+ level is 2.7 mEq/L (normal, 4.0 to 5.1 mEq/L), serum Cl^- level is 77 mEq/L (normal, 85 to 103 mEq/L), and total CO_2 concentration (approximately the same as serum HCO_3^- concentration) is 35 mEq/L (normal, 24 to 27 mEq/L). The urine pH is 6.0.

Comment. The cow has *hypokalemic, hypochloremic, metabolic alkalosis* secondary to abomasal displacement. The alkalosis was initiated by continued secretion of HCl by the abomasum, sequestration of the secreted HCl in the abomasal lumen, and blunted HCO_3^- secretion by the intestine after the gastrointestinal obstruction. The hypokalemia is a result largely of intracellular movement of K^+ secondary to alkalosis and may not reflect a decrease in total body K^+ levels, although in chronic chloride-depletion metabolic alkalosis, significant renal potassium losses may occur and cause K^+ depletion.

The kidney normally responds to alkalosis by excreting alkaline urine. However, in this case the volume contraction and hypochloremia prevent the formation of alkaline urine, and the result is *paradoxical aciduria.* The proximal tubule reabsorbs filtered HCO_3^-, regardless of the plasma pH or serum HCO_3^- concentration. The volume depletion enhances Na^+ reabsorption in the collecting duct and Cl^- and H_2O reabsorption are enhanced secondary to the increased Na^+ uptake.

Renal secretion of HCO_3^- occurs by apical exchange of Cl^- in the tubule fluid for intracellular HCO_3^- in type B and type C (non A, non B) intercalated cells in the collecting duct and connecting segment. Because NaCl is avidly reabsorbed to combat volume depletion, little Cl^- remains for exchange with HCO_3^-, and net HCO_3^- secretion does not occur. Acid secretion in the collecting duct increases in response to aldosterone and may be enhanced in this volume-depleted animal. In rodents, hypokalemia activates the acid-secreting intercalated cells in the collecting duct, increases apical proton pump activity, and increases ammonia excretion via principal cell and intercalated cell ammonia transporters; these events may also occur in cattle and may contribute to the excretion of acid urine and maintenance of the metabolic alkalosis in this case.

Treatment. Treatment involves vigorous volume replacement with intravenous normal saline, with KCl added, and surgical correction of the abomasal displacement.

PRACTICE QUESTIONS

1. In carnivores, the usual role of the kidney in maintaining acid-base homeostasis is to:
   a. Secrete excess bicarbonate.
   b. Secrete excess ammonia.
   c. Secrete excess acid.
   d. Secrete excess carbon dioxide.
   e. Secrete excess phosphate buffer.

2. The bulk of acid secretion (bicarbonate reabsorption) is accomplished by which renal tubule segment?
   a. Proximal tubule
   b. Thin limbs of Henle's loop
   c. Thick ascending limb of Henle's loop
   d. Distal convoluted tubule
   e. Collecting duct

3. Which of the following factors does *not* contribute to efficient acid excretion (bicarbonate reabsorption) by the renal tubules?
   a. Primary active transport of bicarbonate
   b. Intraluminal buffering by bicarbonate
   c. Intraluminal buffering by ammonia and phosphate
   d. Intracellular and membrane-associated carbonic anhydrase
   e. Transmembrane proton transport by the Na^+/H^+ exchanger, H^+-ATPase pump, and H^+,K^+-ATPase pump

4. Which of the following statements regarding mechanisms of acid-base regulation by the collecting duct is *false*?
   a. The cortical collecting duct responds to acidosis by increasing the net rate of acid secretion.
   b. The cortical collecting duct responds to alkalosis with net bicarbonate secretion.
   c. Proton and bicarbonate transport in the collecting duct are only slightly altered in response to systemic acid-base disturbances.
   d. The collecting duct determines the ultimate pH of the urine.
   e. The intercalated cells are largely responsible for acid secretion by the collecting duct.

5. What is the role of renal ammonia metabolism in the renal response to acidosis, at least in dogs and rodents?
   a. Acidosis increases ammoniagenesis in the proximal tubule, which increases the generation of new bicarbonate ions.
   b. Acidosis increases collecting duct ammonia secretion, which enhances acid secretion.
   c. Acidosis stimulates ammoniagenesis in the proximal tubule and inhibits collecting duct ammonia secretion, which increases ammonia buffering of the plasma.
   d. Renal ammonia metabolism does not contribute to renal acid-base regulation.
   e. Both a and b.

BIBLIOGRAPHY

Alpern RJ, Hebert SC: *Seldin and Giebisch's the kidney: physiology and pathophysiology,* ed 4, Philadelphia, 2007, Academic Press.

Wagner CA, Devuyst O, Bourgeois S, Mohebbi N: Regulated acid-base transport in the collecting duct, *Pflugers Arch* 458(1):137–156, 2009.

Wall SM: Recent advances in our understanding of intercalated cells, *Curr Opin Nephrol Hypertens* 14(5):480–484, 2005.

Wall SM, Pech V: The interaction of pendrin and the epithelial sodium channel in blood pressure regulation, *Curr Opin Nephrol Hypertens* 17(1):18–24, 2008.

Weiner ID, Verlander JW: Renal acidification mechanisms. In Taal MW, Chertow GM, Marsden PA, et al, editors: *Brenner & Rector's the kidney,* ed 9, Philadelphia, 2012, Saunders.

Weiner ID, Verlander JW: Role of NH_3 and NH_4^+ transporters in renal acid-base transport, *Am J Physiol Renal Physiol* 300(1):F11–F23, 2011.

CHAPTER 45

Overview of Respiratory Function: Ventilation of the Lung

KEY POINTS

Respiratory function

1. The respiratory system's primary function is the transport of oxygen and carbon dioxide between the environment and the tissues.

Ventilation

1. Ventilation is the movement of gas into and out of the lung.
2. Ventilation requires muscular energy.
3. The respiratory muscles generate work to stretch the lung and overcome the frictional resistance to airflow provided by the airways (airway resistance).
4. Lung elasticity results from tissue and surface tension forces.

5. The lung is mechanically connected to the thoracic cage by the pleural liquid.
6. Airflow is opposed by frictional resistance in the airways.
7. Smooth muscle contraction affects the diameters of the trachea, bronchi, and bronchioles.
8. Dynamic compression can narrow the airways and limit airflow.
9. The distribution of air depends on the local mechanical properties of the lung.
10. In some species, air travels between adjacent regions of lung through collateral pathways.

RESPIRATORY FUNCTION

The Respiratory System's Primary Function Is the Transport of Oxygen and Carbon Dioxide Between the Environment and the Tissues

The respiratory system provides oxygen (O_2) to support tissue metabolism and removes carbon dioxide (CO_2). *Oxygen consumption* and *carbon dioxide production* vary with the metabolic rate, which is dependent on the animal's level of activity. *Basal metabolism,* the metabolism of the resting animal, is a function of metabolic body weight ($M^{0.75}$). The consequence of this relationship is that smaller species consume more oxygen per kilogram of body weight than do larger species. For example, the 20-gram mouse consumes six times more oxygen per unit body mass than does a 70-kg pig. This difference is largely due to the metabolic requirements necessary to maintain constant body temperature. Because smaller species have a greater surface area to body weight ratio, they have a greater surface for heat loss and less heat storage capacity so they need higher basal metabolism to generate more heat.

When animals exercise, their muscles need more oxygen, which leads to an increase in oxygen consumption. *Maximal oxygen consumption* ($\dot{V}O_{2max}$) is directly related to the total mass of mitochondria within the skeletal muscles. Athletic species such as the horse and dog have greater mitochondrial density and therefore greater $\dot{V}O_{2max}$ than do less athletic species of similar body size such as the cow and goat.

Gas exchange requirements vary with metabolism and may increase up to 30 times during strenuous exercise (Figure 45-1). Surprisingly, these variations are normally accomplished with only a small energy cost. In animals with respiratory disease, the energy cost of breathing can increase. This results in less energy available for exercise or weight gain, and the owner notices the animal's poor performance. The respiratory system also is involved in communication by sound and pheromones and is important in thermoregulation; metabolism of endogenous and exogenous substances; and protection of the animal against inhaled dusts, toxic gases, and infectious agents. Additionally, the increase in abdominal pressure that facilitates urination, defecation, and parturition requires active participation of the respiratory muscles.

Figure 45-2 shows the processes involved in gas exchange, including *ventilation; distribution* of gas within the lung; *diffusion* at the alveolocapillary membrane; *transport* of O_2 in the blood from the lungs to the tissue capillaries and of CO_2 in the reverse direction; and diffusion of gases between blood and tissues.

VENTILATION

Ventilation Is the Movement of Gas Into and Out of the Lung

The oxygen needs of metabolism require that an animal take a certain volume of air into its lungs, especially its alveoli, each minute. The total volume of air breathed per minute, also known as *minute ventilation* ($\dot{V}E$), is determined by the volume of each breath, known as the *tidal volume* (VT), and the number of breaths per minute, known as *respiratory frequency* (f), as clarified next from the following equation:

$$\dot{V}E = VT \times f$$

The increase in $\dot{V}E$, which must occur when an increase in metabolic rate demands more oxygen, can be brought about through an increase in VT, f, or both.

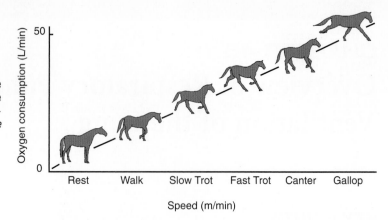

FIGURE 45-1 Effect of exercise on oxygen consumption in the horse. Oxygen consumption increases in a linear manner as the horse increases speed; the total increase is approximately thirtyfold. (Modified from Hörnicke H, Meixner R, Pollman U: *Equine exercise physiology,* Cambridge, UK, 1983, Granta Editions.)

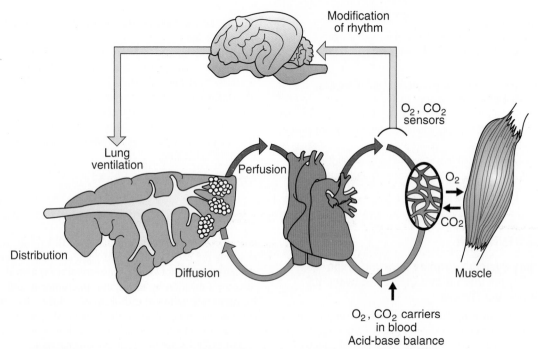

FIGURE 45-2 Diagrammatic representation of the processes involved in gas exchange. The lung is shown on the left, the heart in the center, and tissues on the right. The brain is shown at the top.

Air flows into the alveoli through the nares, nasal cavity, pharynx, larynx, trachea, bronchi, and bronchioles. These structures constitute the *conducting airways.* Because gas exchange does not occur in these pathways, they are also known as the *anatomic dead-space* (Figure 45-3). Dead-space can also occur within the alveoli. This *alveolar dead-space* is caused by alveoli that are poorly perfused with blood, so that gas exchange cannot occur optimally (see Chapter 47). *Physiologic dead-space* is the sum of the anatomic and the alveolar dead-space. Let us define the portion of each VT that enters the alveoli as VA and the part that enters the dead-space as VD. Then:

$$VT = VA + VD$$

If each side of this equation is multiplied by respiratory frequency (f) as follows:

$$VT \times f = (\dot{V}A \times f) + (VD \times f)$$

The result is:

$$\dot{V}E = \dot{V}A + \dot{V}D$$

Therefore, minute ventilation ($\dot{V}E$) is the sum of *alveolar ventilation* ($\dot{V}A$), which is essential for gas exchange, and *dead-space ventilation* ($\dot{V}d$), which is wasted ventilation.

Alveolar ventilation is regulated by control mechanisms to match the O_2 uptake and CO_2 elimination necessitated by metabolism. Thus, when an animal exercises, its alveolar ventilation increases to take in more O_2 and eliminate more CO_2.

The fraction of each breath ventilating the dead-space is known as the *dead-space/tidal volume ratio* (VD/VT). The VD/VT varies considerably among species. In smaller species, such as dogs, it approximates 33%, whereas in some larger species, such as cattle and horses, it approximates 50% to 75%. Because the volume of the anatomic dead-space is relatively constant, changes in VT, f, or both can alter the relative amounts of air that ventilate the alveoli and the dead-space. These changes in VT and f occur in animals during exercise and thermoregulation.

The anatomic dead-space is important in thermoregulation. Air entering the respiratory system is usually cooler than body temperature and not saturated with water vapor. As air passes through the dead-space into the lung, it is warmed by transfer of

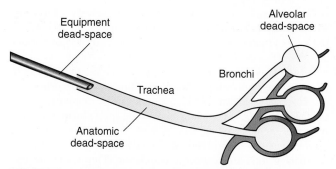

FIGURE 45-3 Respiratory dead-space includes the ventilated parts of the respiratory system where gas exchange does not occur. Three schematic alveoli are shown attached to the conducting airways and perfused by differing amounts of blood. The volume of the trachea and bronchi constitutes the anatomic dead-space; the part of the endotracheal tube extending beyond the respiratory system constitutes equipment dead-space; and the volume of air ventilating poorly perfused alveoli is alveolar dead-space. *Top,* an unperfused alveolus is dead-space because there is no blood flow to allow gas exchange; *bottom,* an ideally perfused alveolus contributes no dead-space because all of the air participates in gas exchange; *middle,* when an alveolus has less-than-sufficient perfusion for the amount of ventilation received [high ventilation/perfusion ($\dot{V}A/\dot{Q}$) ratio)], some of the air entering that alveolus is not involved in gas exchange and contributes to dead-space.

heat from respiratory mucosal capillaries and humidified by evaporation of water from the dead-space mucosal surface. When the animal exhales, heat is lost because the warmed and humidified air leaves the body. When some species such as the dog are heat stressed, they pant. The small VT and high f characteristic of panting in dogs cause more air to ventilate the dead-space in order to increase water evaporation and heat loss. Cattle, pigs, and mules subjected to heat stress also increase respiratory rate and dead-space ventilation when trying to lose heat. In contrast to the effects of heat stress, cold-stressed animals have a higher metabolic rate, which is necessary to maintain body temperature in cold conditions. This leads to an increase in both O_2 consumption and CO_2 production, making it necessary for the animal to increase alveolar ventilation and decrease dead-space ventilation. Reducing the f and increasing VT accomplishes the latter adaptations.

The veterinarian needs to ensure that equipment used for anesthesia or respiratory therapy does not increase the dead-space. Excessively long endotracheal tubes or overly large face masks create a large amount of equipment dead-space. The consequence of this is that the animal must take in a large VT to obtain adequate alveolar ventilation.

Ventilation Requires Muscular Energy

Inhalation occurs when the respiratory muscles contract to expand the thorax, stretch the lung, and create the subatmospheric alveolar pressure that causes air to enter the respiratory system. During *exhalation,* the elastic energy stored in the stretched lung and thorax causes them to decrease in volume, leading to an increase in alveolar pressure that drives air out of the respiratory system. Therefore, in most resting mammals, exhalation does not require muscular effort. Horses are an exception because they have an active phase to exhalation even at rest. During exercise or in the presence of respiratory disease by contrast, exhalation is assisted by muscle contraction in most mammals.

The most important inspiratory muscle is the *diaphragm,* which is a domed musculotendinous sheet separating the abdomen from the thorax and innervated by the *phrenic nerve.* The diaphragm consists of a costal portion, arising from the xiphoid process and the costochondral junctions of the eighth to twelfth ribs (eighth to fourteenth ribs in Equidae), and a crural portion, arising from the ventral surface of the first three to four lumbar vertebrae and extending toward the tendinous center of the diaphragm. The apex of the dome of the diaphragm extends rostrally to the seventh or eighth intercostal space at the level of the base of the heart. During contraction of the diaphragm the dome is pulled caudally and thereby enlarges the thoracic cavity. The tendinous center pushes against the abdominal contents, elevating intra-abdominal pressure, which displaces the abdominal wall and caudal ribs outward, thus also tending to enlarge the thorax. It is the enlargement of the thorax that creates the negative (subatmospheric) pressure necessary to make air flow into the lungs during inhalation.

The *external intercostal* muscles also are active during inhalation. The fibers of these muscles are directed caudoventrally, from the caudal border of one rib to the cranial border of the next, so that muscle contraction moves the ribs rostrally and outward. The relative contributions of diaphragmatic and costal movement to ventilation under different metabolic demands are not well defined in animals. Because the cranial ribs support the forelimbs in quadrupeds, they participate less in ventilation than do the more caudal ribs. Other inspiratory muscles, including those connecting the sternum to the head, contract during strenuous breathing and move the sternum rostrally and assist in thoracic enlargement.

The subatmospheric pressure generated within the respiratory tract during inhalation tends to collapse the external nares, pharynx, and larynx. Contraction of *abductor muscles* attached to these structures is essential for preventing collapse. Abductor muscle contraction during inhalation can be observed as dilation of the external nares. *Laryngeal hemiplegia* (also known as *recurrent laryngeal neuropathy*) in horses is a condition in which the muscles on the left side of the larynx undergo atrophy as a consequence of an axonopathy of the left recurrent laryngeal nerve. The left dorsal cricoarytenoid muscle, which is the most important laryngeal abductor, fails to contract during inhalation. Consequently, during exercise, the left vocal fold is not abducted and creates an abnormal breathing sound that is sometimes called *roaring.*

The principal expiratory muscles are the *abdominal and internal intercostal muscles.* Contraction of the abdominal muscles increases abdominal pressure, which forces the relaxed diaphragm forward and reduces the size of the thorax. The fibers of the internal intercostal muscles are directed cranioventrally, from the cranial border of one rib to the caudal border of the next cranial rib, so that their contraction decreases the size of the thorax by moving the ribs caudally and ventrally. As the thorax becomes smaller, the intrathoracic pressure increases and forces air out of the lungs.

During exercise, respiratory muscle activity increases in order to generate the increase in $\dot{V}E$. In cursorial (running) mammals, ventilation is synchronized with gait in the canter and gallop, but not in the walk or trot (Figure 45-4). Inhalation occurs as the forelimbs are extended and the hind limbs are accelerating the animal forward. Exhalation occurs when the forelimbs are in contact with the ground. In the galloping horse and perhaps in other galloping quadrupeds, much of the increase in size of the thorax during inhalation is a consequence of elongation of the trunk as the spine extends rather than an increase in the diameter of the thorax.

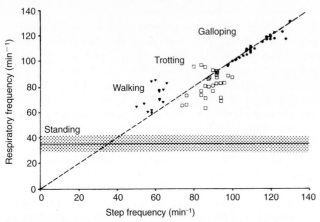

FIGURE 45-4 Relationship between gait and respiration in the horse. In the walk and trot, step and respiratory frequency are not correlated. At the gallop (and canter), respiratory and step frequency bear a 1:1 relationship. (Modified from Hörnicke H, Meixner R, Pollman U: *Equine exercise physiology,* Cambridge, UK, 1983, Granta Editions.)

The Respiratory Muscles Generate Work to Stretch the Lung and Overcome the Frictional Resistance to Airflow Provided by the Airways (Airway Resistance)

At the end of a normal exhalation, some air (~45 mL/kg) remains in the lung. This air volume is known as *functional residual capacity* (FRC). At FRC, the *pressure in the pleural cavity* (Ppl) that surrounds the lung is approximately 5 cm H_2O below atmospheric pressure (−5 cm H_2O). During inhalation, as the inspiratory muscles contract, the thorax enlarges and Ppl decreases. This decrease in Ppl stretches the elastic lung and enlarges its volume, which decreases pressure within the alveoli (Palv). The decrease in Palv causes air to flow into the lung through the tracheobronchial tree (Figure 45-5). *Lung compliance* is a measure of the elastic properties of the lungs, and *airway resistance* is a measure of the frictional resistance of the airways. The magnitude of the change in pleural pressure (ΔPpl) during each breath is determined by the tidal volume (VT), by lung compliance (C), by airflow rate ($\dot{V}$), and by airway resistance (R), as follows:

$$\Delta Ppl = (VT/C) + R\dot{V}$$

Resting animals take relatively few breaths per minute and have low airflow rates. In this situation the primary work of the respiratory muscles is against the compliance of the lung. During exercise, respiratory rate and VT increase which necessitates increased airflow. Respiratory muscles must therefore work harder to provide the necessary increase in ΔPpl to generate the greater VT and airflow. Lung diseases decrease compliance or increase airway resistance or both. As a consequence, animals with lung disease must do more work with their respiratory muscles to maintain a normal VT.

Lung Elasticity Results from Tissue and Surface Tension Forces

At FRC, the slightly subatmospheric pressure in the pleural cavity keeps the lung inflated. If the thorax is opened and the lungs are exposed to atmospheric pressure, the lungs collapse to their *minimal volume*. At this volume, some air remains trapped within the alveoli behind closed bronchioles. This trapped gas causes

collapsed normal lungs to float in water. The collapse of the lung when the thorax is opened and during exhalation is a result of the lung's inherent elasticity, which is generated by elastin tissue and by surface tension forces.

Elastin fibers form a woven mesh that extends along the length of the airways and within the interstitium of the alveolar septa. The distensible nature of this network can be demonstrated by the fact that a 10-kg dog's lung containing approximately 100 mL of air at *residual volume* can expand to 450 mL at *functional residual capacity* and to 1100 mL at *total lung capacity*. As the lung approaches total lung capacity, its inflation is limited by the collagen network of the pleural surface and also by the rib cage.

The *surface tension forces* contributing to the lung's elastic recoil arise from the air-liquid interface within the terminal airspaces (alveoli, alveolar sacs, and respiratory bronchioles). The importance of surface tension is demonstrated by the experimental observation that it takes less pressure to keep excised lungs inflated when they are filled with saline than when filled with air (Figure 45-6). Filling the lungs with saline abolishes surface tension because there is no longer an air-liquid interface. Comparison of the air and saline pressure-volume curves (see Figure 45-6) also shows that surface forces are responsible for a considerable part of the elastic recoil of the air-filled lung. These surface tension forces continually try to collapse the alveoli.

If the air spaces were simply lined with water, the surface tension would be so great that the alveoli would collapse at the inflation pressures generated during breathing. Alveolar stability is a consequence of the presence of a *pulmonary surfactant* that reduces the surface tension of the alveolar lining. Pulmonary surfactant is a mixture of lipids and proteins. The most plentiful lipid component, *dipalmitoyl phosphatidylcholine,* is responsible for the surface tension reduction. Surfactant is produced in *type II alveolar cells,* and its hydrophilic and hydrophobic portions cause it to seek the surface of the alveolar lining (Figure 45-7). As lung volume decreases and the alveolar surface area shrinks, surfactant molecules become concentrated on the alveolar surface, reducing surface tension and promoting alveolar stability.

There are four important *surfactant proteins*. Surfactant proteins B and C are hydrophobic and intimately associated with the lipid film. They regulate absorption of lipid to the surface, reversible sequestration of lipid into a surfactant reservoir in the hypophase of the alveolar liquid lining as the surface contracts and expands with breathing, and recruitment of lipids from the reservoir to spread over the expanding lung surface, for example during a sigh. Surfactant proteins A and D are hydrophilic and play important roles in innate antimicrobial defense.

Pulmonary surfactant is released into the alveolar spaces and tracheal fluid late in gestation (85% of the length of gestation in the sheep). Its appearance correlates with the rise in fetal plasma cortisol levels. Animals born prematurely have difficulty inflating their lungs because of inadequate surfactant. Synthetic surfactants can be used to treat premature newborns who lack adequate surfactant.

Postnatally and throughout life, release of surfactant from type II alveolar cells is aided by sighing, which also redistributes surfactant over the alveolar surface from stores in the hypophase. Anesthetized animals and those with pain in the chest may not sigh and consequently some of the alveoli collapse, that is, they develop *atelectasis*. Provision of deep breaths with a ventilator or bag valve mask (Ambu bag) helps to maintain surfactant activity, prevent lung collapse, and maintain normal lung compliance.

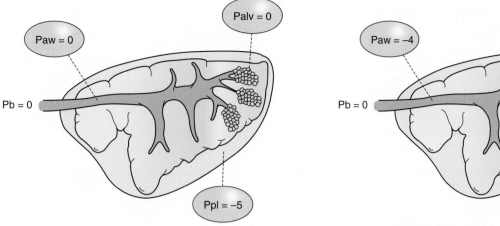

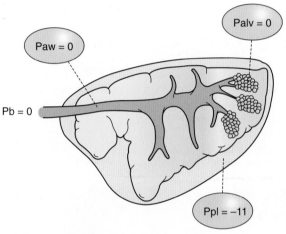

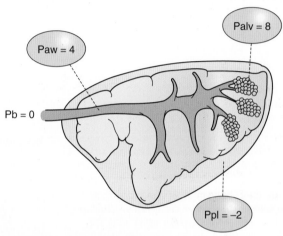

FIGURE 45-5 Examples of pressure changes that might be expected in the respiratory system during quiet breathing. *Palv*, Alveolar pressure; *Pb*, barometric pressure; *Ppl*, pleural pressure; *Paw*, pressure within the airway; *VT*, tidal volume. Numbers represent the pressure difference (cm H_2O) from atmospheric pressure (Pb). The gradient Palv − Ppl is the elastic pressure gradient necessary to keep the lung inflated. Pb − Palv is the pressure gradient that drives airflow through the airways. Pb − Ppl is the pressure gradient that inflates the lung. **A,** Before the start of inhalation, when the respiratory system is resting at functional residual capacity (FRC), there is no airflow into the lungs because Pb − Palv = 0 cm H_2O and the negative pleural pressure is keeping the lung partially inflated (Pb − Ppl = 5 cm H_2O). **B,** During inhalation, Pb − Ppl = 16 cm H_2O in order to enlarge the lung (Palv − Ppl = 8 cm H_2O) and make air flow through the airways (Pb − Palv = 8 cm H_2O). About halfway along the airways, pressure within the lumen (Paw) is −4 cm H_2O. **C,** At the end of a tidal inhalation, flow ceases because Pb − Palv = 0 cm H_2O, but the lung contains more air (Palv − Ppl = 11 cm H_2O). **D,** During exhalation, airflow reverses direction: Pb − Palv = −8 cm H_2O, the lung volume is still greater than FRC (Palv − Ppl = 10 cm H_2O), and the total pressure gradient remains slightly positive (Pb − Ppl = 2 cm H_2O). About halfway along the airways, pressure within the lumen (Paw) is 4 cm H_2O. It is important to remember that these pressure gradients change continually throughout a breath and with changes in tidal volume, respiratory frequency, lung compliance, and airway resistance.

Lung compliance is the slope of the lung-pressure volume curve (see Figure 45-6). Because the pressure-volume curve is not linear, compliance obviously varies with the state of lung inflation. It is usually measured over the range of VT and, when adjusted for differences in lung size, does not vary greatly among adult mammals. Consequently, most mammals generate similar changes in pleural pressure during breathing. Anesthesiologists frequently refer to lung compliance when trying to artificially ventilate an animal. A *compliant lung* is easy to inflate. A *lung with low compliance,* as occurs in some diseases, is difficult to inflate.

The Lung Is Mechanically Connected to the Thoracic Cage by the Pleural Liquid

The lung is covered by the *visceral pleura,* and the thorax is lined by the *parietal pleura.* These two pleural surfaces are maintained in close apposition by a thin layer of pleural fluid. The two pleural surfaces don't touch because of repulsive forces between adjacent surfaces exerted by like charges on phospholipids adhered to the mesothelial surfaces. As a consequence of this mechanical linkage of the lungs to the thorax provided by the pleural fluid, the respiratory system behaves as a single unit. When the thorax expands

FIGURE 45-6 Pressure-volume curve of the lung during inflation with saline and with air. The pressure gradient across the lung (transpulmonary pressure) is shown on the abscissa and lung volume on the ordinate. Notice that (1) a high pressure is required initially to inflate the lung with air from the gas-free state; (2) the lung reaches its elastic limits *(total lung capacity)* at PL of approximately 30 cm H$_2$0; (3) the lung's elastic properties differ during inflation and deflation; less pressure is necessary to maintain a given volume during deflation than during inflation (a phenomenon known as *pressure-volume hysteresis*); (4) when saline is used instead of air to inflate the lung, less pressure is required for inflation, and the pressure-volume hysteresis is abolished. Pressure-volume hysteresis is a result of changing surface tension forces. High surface tension is also responsible for the high pressure required initially to inflate the lung. When the lung is inflated with saline, the air-liquid interface is abolished and so is pressure-volume hysteresis; the lung becomes easier to inflate. *PL,* Transpulmonary pressure.

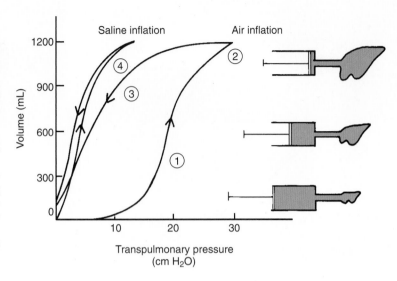

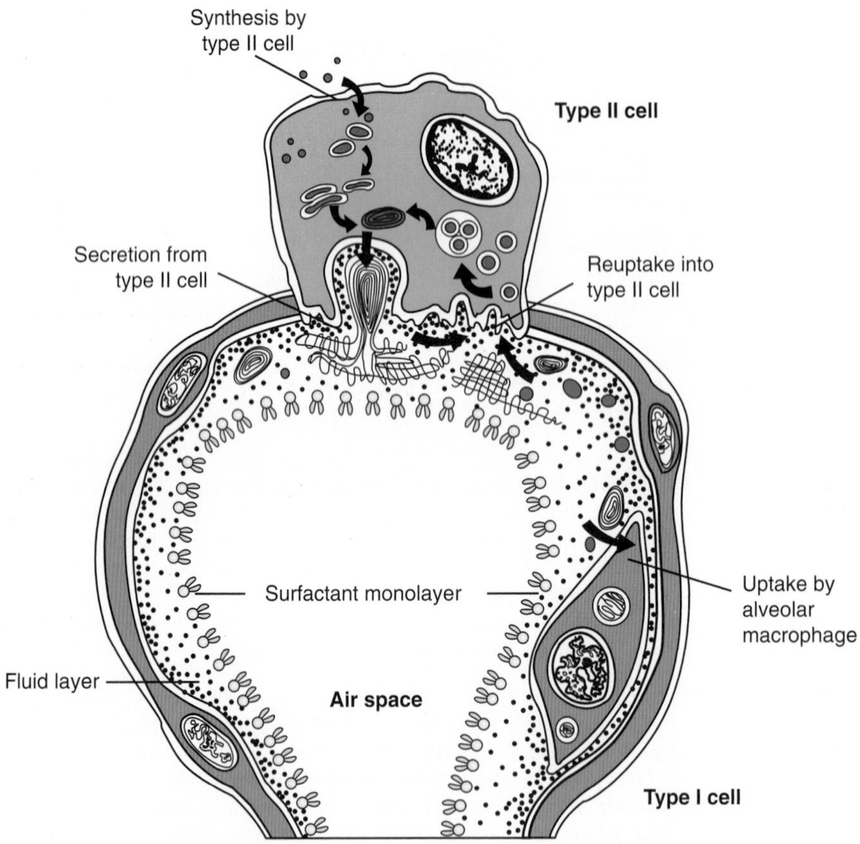

FIGURE 45-7 Diagram of an alveolus to show the movement of surfactant components through the type II cell and the alveolar liquid. Note the stores of surfactant in the hypophase (*swirls* and *concentric circles* below the surfactant monolayer).

during inhalation, for example, the lungs must expand as well. Similarly, when an animal exhales below FRC, the stiff thorax increasingly resists deformation, so that residual volume, the volume of air in the lung at the end of a maximal exhalation, is determined by the limits to which the rib cage can be compressed.

The thorax is generally stiffer—that is, it is less compliant—in large animals than small animals; the stiff chest wall of the horse and cow is in contrast to the very compliant chest wall of small rodents. Neonates need to have a compliant chest to pass through the birth canal. Lung collapse, also known as *atelectasis,* is more likely to occur in species with compliant thoraces because the

thorax cannot adequately support the lung to prevent its collapse. This is one reason that atelectasis is more common in newborn animals than in adults.

Airflow Is Opposed by Frictional Resistance in the Airways

During breathing, air flows through the tubes of the *upper airway* (i.e., nose, pharynx, and larynx) and the *tracheobronchial tree,* which present *frictional resistance* to air movement. In the resting animal the nasal cavity, pharynx, and larynx, which warm and humidify the air, provide approximately 60% of the airway resistance (Figure 45-8). Nasal resistance can be decreased (e.g.,

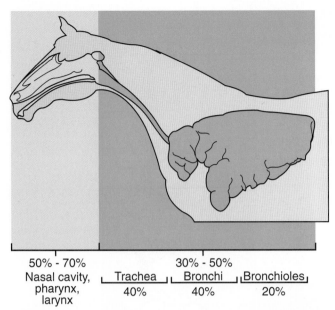

50% - 70% | 30% - 50%
Nasal cavity, | Trachea | Bronchi | Bronchioles
pharynx, | 40% | 40% | 20%
larynx

FIGURE 45-8 Distribution of airway resistance in a horse. The airways of the nose and throat comprise the majority of resistance. Within the tracheobronchial tree, the bronchioles contribute the least fraction of resistance.

during exercise) by dilation of the external nares and by vasoconstriction of the extensive vascular tissue in the nose. Vasoconstriction reduces the volume of blood in the vascular sinuses within the nasal mucosa and, as a consequence, the mucosal thickness decreases and the space available for air within the nose increases. When airflow rates increase during exercise, or when the nasal cavity is obstructed, some species, such as the cow and dog, breathe through the mouth to bypass the high-resistance nasal cavity. Other species, such as the horse, are obligate nose breathers and are solely dependent on a decrease in nasal resistance to keep the work of breathing at a reasonable level. The horse accomplishes this by flaring its nostrils and by constricting blood vessels to shrink the nasal mucosa.

The tracheobronchial tree is a branching system that delivers air to the alveoli. The number of branches depends on the animal's size. Humans have 24 branches, mice about 10, and horses 40 or more. The tracheobronchial tree is lined by a secretory, ciliated epithelium. The larger airways—*trachea* and *bronchi*—are supported by *cartilage* and supplied with *bronchial glands* and goblet cells, the secretions of which contribute to the mucous lining of the airways. The smaller airways, known as *bronchioles*, lack cartilage, glands, and goblet cells; the liquid lining over the epithelial surface originates in Clara cells. With the exception of the trachea and the cranial part of the mainstem bronchi, the airways are intrapulmonary. Alveolar septa attach to the outer layers of the airways so that the tension within the alveolar septa pulls the airways open and helps to maintain their patency.

The lungs of most species have a total of six lobes, each supplied by a *lobar bronchus*, which gives rise to daughter bronchi. Even in species such as the horse that lack lobation, the same pattern of six lobar bronchi persists. At each division of a parent bronchus, the diameters of the daughter airways are not equal; one is much narrower than the parent, whereas the diameter of the other is similar to that of the parent. This *monopodial* system of branching continues through at least the first six generations

of bronchi. At the level of the bronchioles, the diameters of parent and daughter bronchioles are similar. As a result of this branching pattern, the total *cross-sectional area* of the tracheobronchial tree through which air flows increases only slightly between the trachea and the first four generations of bronchi, but it doubles at each division of the peripheral airways. Because the total cross-sectional area increases dramatically toward the periphery of the lung, the *velocity of airflow* diminishes progressively from the trachea toward the bronchioles. The high-velocity *turbulent airflow* in the trachea and bronchi produces the *lung sounds* heard through a stethoscope in a normal animal. *Laminar airflow* (low-velocity flow) in the bronchioles produces no sound. Also as a result of the branching pattern of the tracheobronchial tree, airways larger than 2 to 5 mm in diameter contribute up to 80% of the frictional resistance to breathing in the tracheobronchial tree; bronchioles contribute as little as 20%.

Resistance to airflow is determined by the radius and length of the airways. Airway length changes minimally, but radius can be altered by several passive and active forces. As the lung inflates, airways dilate passively and airway resistance decreases. This occurs because the alveolar septa are attached to the airways, and as the alveoli inflate, tension increases in their septa, causing the attached airways to dilate (Figure 45-9). Contraction of bronchial smooth muscle is the other major factor determining airway caliber.

Smooth Muscle Contraction Affects the Diameters of the Trachea, Bronchi, and Bronchioles

There is *smooth muscle* in the walls of the airways from the trachea to the alveolar ducts. In the trachea, it forms the *trachealis muscle,* which connects the ends of tracheal cartilages. In the bronchi and the bronchioles, smooth muscle encircles the airways. Smooth muscle actively regulates airway diameter in response to neural and other stimuli. The *parasympathetic nervous system* supplies airway smooth muscle through the vagus nerve, with parasympathetic ganglia located in the walls of the airways (Figure 45-10). Activation of this system causes the release of *acetylcholine* from postganglionic fibers. The acetylcholine binds to *muscarinic receptors* on airway smooth muscle, leading to muscle contraction. This narrows the trachea, bronchi, and bronchioles, a phenomenon known as *bronchoconstriction* or *bronchospasm.* Parasympathetically mediated bronchospasm is one of the lung's protective mechanisms. Inhalation of irritating materials such as dusts can activate tracheobronchial sensory receptors that are connected to vagal afferent nerves. This, in turn, leads to activation of the parasympathetic system, resulting in bronchoconstriction.

Airway smooth muscle also contracts in response to many of the *inflammatory mediators,* particularly *histamine* and some *leukotrienes,* that are released from mast cells during an allergic reaction. Some inflammatory mediators act directly on the smooth muscle; others act in a reflexive manner involving *nonmyelinated afferent nerves* and the parasympathetic system. They are most likely responsible for the airway obstruction that occurs in diseases such as heaves in horses and asthma in cats.

Relaxation of smooth muscle, and therefore dilation of the airways, occurs during activation of *β₂-adrenergic receptors* by circulating *epinephrine* released from the adrenal medulla. *Norepinephrine* released from the *sympathetic nervous system* also causes airway dilation through β₂-adrenergic receptors, but to a lesser extent. Another bronchodilator system, the *nonadrenergic noncholinergic inhibitory nervous system,* exists in some species.

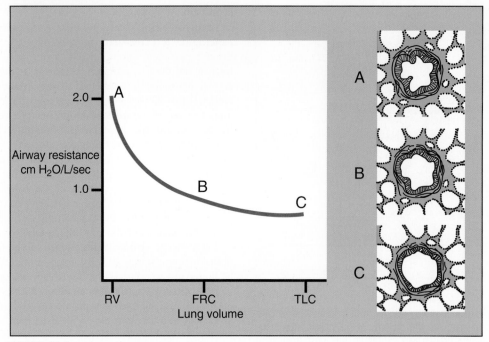

FIGURE 45-9 Effect of change in lung volume on airway resistance. The airway is represented in the diagrams on the right side of the figure by the *large circle,* to which are attached alveoli, the septa of which link the airway wall to the pleural surface. As lung volume increases, the alveolar septa become stretched, apply tension to the airway walls, and thus dilate the airway and reduce resistance. *FRC,* Functional residual capacity; *RV,* residual volume; *TLC,* total lung capacity.

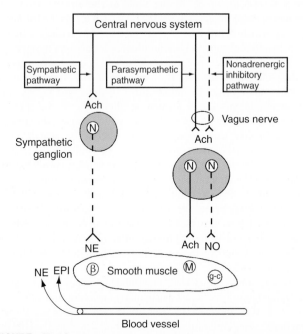

FIGURE 45-10 Diagrammatic representation of efferent autonomic innervation of tracheobronchial tree. Muscarinic receptors *(M)* are activated by acetylcholine *(Ach)* released from postganglionic parasympathetic nerve terminals. Smooth muscle β_2-adrenergic receptors (β) are activated by circulating catecholamines such as epinephrine *(EPI)* or, in a few species, by release of norepinephrine *(NE)* from sympathetic nerves. The nonadrenergic inhibitory nervous system that travels in the vagus nerve releases nitric oxide *(NO)* that activates guanylyl cyclase *(g-c)* in the smooth muscle. *N,* Neuron. (From Nadel JA, Barnes PJ, Holtzman MJ: Autonomic factors in hyperreactivity of airway smooth muscle. In Fishman AP, Macklem PT, Mead J, et al, editors: *Handbook of physiology,* section 3, vol 3, part 2, Bethesda, Md, 1985, American Physiology Society.)

The efferent fibers are in the vagus nerve, and neurotransmission involves *nitric oxide.*

Dynamic Compression Can Narrow the Airways and Limit Airflow

The walls of the airway are not rigid, and therefore the airways can be compressed or expanded by the pressure gradient across their walls. Understanding when *dynamic compression* is most likely to occur in different parts of the airways can provide diagnostic clues to the location of an airway obstruction. In the nasal cavity, pharynx, and larynx, dynamic compression of the airway occurs during inhalation. These extrathoracic airways are surrounded by atmospheric pressure, whereas the pressure within the airways is subatmospheric during inhalation. The resulting negative *transmural pressure* therefore tends to make the airways collapse. Because of its bony support, the nasal cavity is not prone to compression, but the less well-supported nares, pharynx, and larynx are prone to compression. Normally, contraction of the abductor muscles of the nares, pharynx, and larynx during inhalation prevents collapse of these regions.

Laryngeal hemiplegia provides an excellent example of dynamic collapse of the extrathoracic airway during inhalation. In this disease the intrinsic muscles on the left side of the larynx lose their nerve supply and undergo atrophy. As previously mentioned, when the abductor muscles of the larynx fail to contract during inhalation, the left vocal fold is sucked into the lumen of the airway, producing the inspiratory noise known as "roaring." In addition, the vocal fold provides an obstruction to airflow that leads to poor performance when affected horses perform strenuous exercise. Dynamic collapse of the extrathoracic airways does not occur during exhalation because the pressure within the airways is greater than atmospheric pressure, and the resulting positive transmural pressure keeps the airway open.

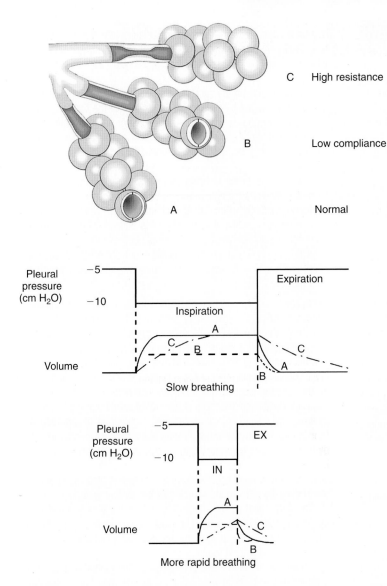

FIGURE 45-11 Effects of mechanical properties of the lung on alveolar filling. Alveolus *A* is normal, alveolus *B* has low compliance, and the airway supplying alveolus *C* has high resistance as a result of a partial obstruction. Step changes in pleural pressure are applied to these three schematic alveoli, and the changes in volume are shown during slow breathing and during more rapid breathing. During slow breathing alveoli *A* and *C* fill to equal degrees because their compliance is the same but alveolus *C* fills more slowly because its airway is partially obstructed; alveolus *B* with low lung compliance fills less. During rapid breathing, alveolus *C* does not have time to fill, it receives less ventilation than *A* and as a consequence ventilation becomes more unevenly distributed.

In the intrathoracic airways, dynamic collapse occurs during forced exhalation because intrapleural pressure exceeds pressures within the intrathoracic airway lumen. *Cough* is a *forced exhalation* during which dynamic collapse narrows the airways. The high air velocity through the narrowed portion of the airway facilitates removal of foreign material. Toy breeds of dogs have a high incidence of *collapsing trachea*. In this disease the weakened intrathoracic trachea is dynamically collapsed during the forceful ventilation of exercise. Affected dogs make a "honking" expiratory noise as air is forced past the collapsed intrathoracic portion of the trachea.

The Distribution of Air Depends on the Local Mechanical Properties of the Lung

Optimal gas exchange requires bringing together air and blood at the alveolus, that is, the *matching of ventilation and blood flow.* Obviously, gas exchange cannot occur if an alveolus receives blood but no ventilation, or vice versa. Ideally, each region of lung should receive approximately equal amounts of ventilation, but this rarely if ever occurs. Distribution of ventilation is always uneven to some degree and becomes more so in disease. Uneven distribution of ventilation can be caused by local decreases in lung compliance (e.g., in pneumonia) or local airway obstructions (e.g., by mucus or bronchospasm) (Figure 45-11).

The distribution of ventilation is very uneven in *recumbent large animals,* especially in the supine and laterally recumbent positions. This is because the lowermost regions of the lung are compressed to such an extent that they receive little or no ventilation. This can cause severe derangements of gas exchange, especially in anesthetized horses.

In Some Species, Air Travels Between Adjacent Regions of Lung Through Collateral Pathways

The lungs of mammalian species differ in the degree to which they are subdivided by connective tissue into *secondary lobules.* In the lungs of pigs and cattle, there is complete separation of lobules, and in dogs and cats there is no separation. In horses and sheep there is partial separation. The connective tissue septa prevent *collateral ventilation* (i.e., movement of air between adjacent lobules) in cattle and pigs. Collateral ventilation is extensive in dogs and intermediate in horses. Collateral ventilation provides air to alveoli when their main parent bronchus is obstructed. The differences in collateral ventilation mean that gas exchange abnormalities that follow airway obstruction are more serious in pigs and cattle than in dogs.

CLINICAL CORRELATIONS

LUNG FIBROSIS IN THE DOG

History. A 3-year-old English setter in respiratory distress is presented at a teaching hospital. The owner first noticed reluctance of the dog to exercise 3 weeks ago. Since then, the animal has had progressive difficulty in breathing. It appears hungry but cannot eat because it "gets out of breath."

Clinical Examination. Inspection reveals a thin dog breathing through its mouth. The respiratory rate is elevated, but the dog seems to be moving little air despite strong inspiratory efforts during which the intercostal spaces sink. Exhalation presents no difficulty; the ribs collapse rapidly and there is no accentuated abdominal effort.

Examination reveals slightly blue-colored mucous membranes. Lung sounds are not remarkable. All other systems are normal.

Radiographs of the thorax show diffuse miliary density (whiteness) over the parts of the lung that are normally air-filled. The bronchi are normal. An elevated change in pleural pressure during breathing, normal airway resistance, and decreased static lung compliance are the key findings on lung function testing. Tidal volume (VT) is greatly reduced.

Comment. The history and clinical signs indicate a respiratory problem. The elevated change in pleural pressure during breathing confirms the increased effort necessary to breathe. This could be caused by (1) increased air movement resulting from an increased metabolic rate, (2) airway obstruction, or (3) a decrease in lung compliance (stiffening of the lung). The increased density in the normally air-filled elastic part of the lungs, coupled with the normal air passages, suggests a decrease in lung compliance rather than airway obstruction. This was confirmed when measurements of lung function revealed a normal airway resistance and decreased lung compliance.

The retraction of intercostal spaces indicates that the stiff lung is resisting expansion. Exhalation is not a problem because the lung has an increased tendency to collapse, and the airways are normal.

This dog has a diffuse disease of the exchange area of the lung, which, by decreasing compliance, increases the work of breathing. The blue tinge to the mucous membranes indicates desaturation of hemoglobin as a result of impaired oxygen exchange in the diseased lung. A biopsy reveals diffuse fibrosis around mineral particles in the walls of the alveoli. The prognosis for the dog is poor.

CHRONIC AIRWAY DISEASE IN THE HORSE

History. A 10-year-old horse is presented with a 2-year history of coughing and a progressive loss of exercise tolerance. Recently, the horse's problem has become so severe that it has difficulty breathing while resting in its stall. The cough is frequent and is usually worse when the horse is kept inside. The horse has a normal appetite; however, it is losing weight even though the teeth are normal and it is on a good parasite control program.

Clinical Examination. Inspection reveals a thin horse with flared nostrils and an anxious expression. The respiratory rate is elevated, and respiratory movements are accentuated. During inhalation the intercostal spaces are pulled in between the ribs. The initial part of exhalation is characterized by a rapid relaxation of the rib cage. This is followed by a prolonged contraction of the abdominal muscles, which is terminated immediately before the next inhalation. During the prolonged contraction of the abdominal muscles, wheezes can be heard when you place your ear close to the nostrils.

The horse has an elevated pulse rate. The mucous membranes of the gums have a bluish tinge. Auscultation of the thorax reveals increased breath sounds over all the lung fields and musical wheezes audible at end exhalation. Excessive mucus pooled in the airway can be seen through an endoscope advanced into the trachea.

Because the horse is being examined at a teaching hospital, there are facilities for measurement of lung function. The change in pleural pressure (ΔPpl) during each breath is 25 cm H_2O (normal, 5 to 10 cm H_2O), and airway resistance is 3 cm H_2O/L/sec (normal, 1 cm H_2O/L/sec). Administration of atropine intravenously decreases ΔPpl to 7 cm H_2O and airway resistance to 1.5 cm H_2O/L/sec. The horse looks less distressed, and wheezes are reduced after atropine therapy.

Comment. The respiratory distress, cough, and lack of exercise tolerance indicate a respiratory problem. The increased effort of breathing documented by the elevated ΔPpl could be caused by airway obstruction, a decrease in lung compliance, or increased breathing resulting from increased metabolic rate. The latter cause is eliminated because the horse is resting in the clinic. The mucus in the airway and elevated airway resistance confirm airway obstruction. Musical wheezes at the end of exhalation typify airway disease and result from increased air turbulence or vibration of mucus and the airway walls. Airway obstruction is caused in part by bronchospasm resulting from parasympathetic activity, because it is reversed by atropine, a parasympathetic antagonist. Atropine does not return resistance to normal, so there is also considerable obstruction by mucus and swelling of the airway wall.

The flared nostrils are an effort to reduce the airway resistance by dilating the upper airway. The blue-tinged mucous membranes indicate desaturation of hemoglobin because of impaired oxygen uptake in the diseased lungs.

Retraction of the intercostal muscles during inhalation indicates a major decrease in pleural pressure as the respiratory muscles work to inflate the lung and pull air through the obstructed airways. The prolonged contraction of abdominal muscles, or heaving, represents an effort by the horse to force air out through obstructed airways. Weight loss is probably a result of the increased work of breathing. Coughing is an effort by the horse to expel the excessive mucus.

Treatment. This horse has *heaves* (also known as *recurrent airway obstruction* [RAO]), a problem exacerbated by stabling in a dusty barn and eating poorly cured, moldy hay. Heaves is the result of inhaling particles, antigens, and endotoxin in the hay and barn dust. The best treatment for the horse is to keep it out at pasture and supplement its diet with pelleted feed rather than hay. In many cases, including this horse, additional treatments are needed when the horse endures a crisis. Treatment is aimed at dilating the airways (bronchodilator such as clenbuterol) and reducing inflammation (inhaled or systemic corticosteroids). Oxygen therapy is rarely necessary. With good management control that involves reduction of exposure to hay dust, some horses do not need constant treatment. In advanced stages and when treating some performance horses, however, ongoing treatment with bronchodilators and inhaled steroids may be necessary.

PRACTICE QUESTIONS

1. Which of the following is true?
   a. Oxygen consumption per kilogram body weight is greater in a 50-g mammal than in a 50-kg mammal.
   b. Maximal oxygen consumption in mammals is directly related to the volume of mitochondria in the skeletal muscles.
   c. Oxygen consumption increases when metabolic rate increases.
   d. Oxygen consumption can increase up to thirtyfold during intense exercise.
   e. All of the above are true.

2. Functional residual capacity is:
   a. The volume of air remaining in the lung at the end of a maximal forced exhalation.
   b. The mechanical equilibrium of the respiratory system.
   c. Less than residual volume.
   d. Greater than total lung capacity.
   e. Determined by metabolic rate.

3. Which of the following lists includes only structures that compose the anatomic dead-space?
   a. Respiratory bronchioles, alveoli, trachea, nasal cavity
   b. Pharynx, bronchi, alveolar ducts, larynx
   c. Capillaries, respiratory bronchioles, trachea, bronchi
   d. Pharynx, nasal cavity, trachea, bronchi
   e. Capillaries, respiratory bronchioles, alveolar ducts, alveoli

4. A horse has a tidal volume (VT) of 5 L, respiratory rate of 12 breaths/min, and VD/VT ratio of 0.5. Calculate minute ventilation ($\dot{V}E$) and alveolar ventilation ($\dot{V}A$).
   a. $\dot{V}E$ = 60 L/min; $\dot{V}A$ = 2.5 L/min
   b. $\dot{V}E$ = 30 L/min; $\dot{V}A$ = 30 L/min
   c. $\dot{V}E$ = 60 L/min; $\dot{V}A$ = 30 L/min
   d. $\dot{V}E$ = 2.5 L/min; $\dot{V}A$ = 1.25 L/min
   e. $\dot{V}E$ = 5.0 L/min; $\dot{V}A$ = 2.5 L/min

5. Which of the following occur during inhalation?
   a. Diaphragm contracts, pleural pressure increases, alveolar pressure decreases.
   b. Diaphragm relaxes, external intercostal muscles contract, pleural pressure increases.
   c. Diaphragm relaxes, pleural pressure decreases, internal intercostal muscles relax.
   d. External and internal intercostal muscles contract, pleural and alveolar pressures increase.
   e. Diaphragm and external intercostal muscles contract, pleural and alveolar pressures decrease.

6. Lung compliance:
   a. Has the units of pressure per volume (cm H_2O/L).
   b. Is greater at functional residual capacity (FRC) than at total lung capacity (TLC).
   c. Is less when the lung is inflated with saline than when the lung is inflated with air.
   d. Is greater in small mammals than in large mammals, even when adjusted for differences in lung size.
   e. Is the only determinant of the change in pleural pressure during breathing.

7. Pulmonary surfactant:
   a. Can be deficient in premature newborns.
   b. Is produced in type II alveolar cells.
   c. Is in part composed of dipalmitoyl phosphatidylcholine.
   d. Decreases surface tension of the fluid lining the alveoli.
   e. All the above.

8. Which of the following *increases* the frictional resistance to breathing?
   a. Intravenous administration of a β_2-adrenergic agonist
   b. Contraction of the abductor muscles of the larynx
   c. A decrease in lung volume from FRC to residual volume
   d. Relaxation of the trachealis muscle
   e. Inhibition of the release of histamine from mast cells

9. The distribution of ventilation within the lung is influenced by:
   a. Regional variations in lung inflation
   b. Regional variations in airway resistance
   c. Regional variations in lung compliance
   d. Collateral ventilation
   e. All the above

BIBLIOGRAPHY

Boron WF: Mechanics of respiration. In Boron WF, Boulpaep EL: *Medical physiology: a cellular and molecular approach*, ed 2, Philadelphia, 2009, Saunders.

Hlastala MP, Berger AJ: *Physiology of respiration*, ed 2, New York, 2001, Oxford University Press.

Leff AR, Schumacker PT: *Respiratory physiology: basics and applications*, Philadelphia, 1993, Saunders.

Lekeux P, Art T: The respiratory system: anatomy, physiology and adaptations to exercise and training. In Hodgson DR, Rose RJ, editors: *The athletic horse: principles and practice of equine sports medicine*, Philadelphia, 1994, Saunders.

Orgeig S, Hiemstra PS, Veldhuizen EJ, et al: Recent advances in alveolar biology: evolution and function of alveolar proteins, *Respir Physiol Neurobiol* 173S:S43–S54, 2010.

Robinson NE: Some functional consequences of species differences in lung anatomy, *Adv Vet Sci Comp Med* 26:1–33, 1982.

Weibel ER, Bacigalupe LD, Schmitt B, et al: Allometric scaling of maximal metabolic rate in mammals: muscle aerobic capacity as determinant factor, *Respir Physiol Neurobiol* 140(2):115–132, 2004.

West JB: *Respiratory physiology: the essentials*, ed 8, Baltimore, 2008, Lippincott, Williams & Wilkins.

CHAPTER 46
Pulmonary Blood Flow

KEY POINTS

Pulmonary circulation
1. The structure of the small pulmonary arteries varies among species.
2. Functionally, pulmonary blood vessels can be classified as alveolar and extra-alveolar vessels.
3. The pulmonary blood vessels offer a low resistance to flow.
4. The distribution of pulmonary blood flow within the lung is influenced by several factors.
5. Passive changes in vascular resistance result from changes in vascular transmural pressure.

6. Neural and humoral factors cause contraction of the muscular pulmonary arteries.
7. Alveolar hypoxia is a potent constrictor of small pulmonary arteries.
8. During exercise the pulmonary circulation must accommodate a large increase in blood flow.

Bronchial circulation
1. The bronchial circulation provides a blood supply to airways, large vessels, and, in some species, the visceral pleura.

The lung receives blood flow from two circulatory systems: the pulmonary circulation and the bronchial circulation. The *pulmonary circulation* receives the total output of the *right ventricle,* perfuses the *alveolar capillaries,* and participates in gas exchange. The *bronchial circulation,* a branch of the systemic circulation, provides a nutritional blood supply to airways and other structures within the lung.

PULMONARY CIRCULATION

The pulmonary circulation differs from the systemic circulation in that all the blood passes through only one organ: the lung. When cardiac output increases, as occurs during exercise, the pulmonary circulation must be able to accommodate this increase in blood flow without a large increase in the work of the right ventricle. In addition, control mechanisms must exist to regulate the distribution of blood within the lung so that blood preferentially perfuses the well-oxygenated regions of the lung. The ability to regulate blood flow depends on the presence of smooth muscle in the walls of small pulmonary arteries. The quantity of smooth muscle varies among species.

The Structure of the Small Pulmonary Arteries Varies Among Species

The main pulmonary arteries that accompany the bronchi are elastic, but the smaller arteries adjacent to the bronchioles and the alveolar ducts are muscular. The adult pig and the cow have a thick muscle layer in the smaller pulmonary arteries; the horse has less muscle; and the sheep and dog have only a thin muscle layer. The amount of smooth muscle in the wall of small pulmonary arteries determines the *reactivity* of the vasculature to alveolar hypoxia and other neural and humoral stimuli (see later discussion).

The small pulmonary arteries lead into pulmonary capillaries, which form an extensive branching network of vessels within the

alveolar septum, almost covering the alveolar surface. Not all capillaries are perfused in the resting animal. As a result, vessels that are unperfused in the resting animal can be recruited when pulmonary blood flow increases (e.g., during exercise). *Pulmonary veins* with thin walls conduct blood from capillaries to the *left atrium* and also form a reservoir of blood for the *left ventricle.* The reservoir of blood in the pulmonary veins is available for sudden increases in cardiac output (e.g., at the start of a sudden burst of exercise).

Functionally, Pulmonary Blood Vessels Can Be Classified as Alveolar and Extra-Alveolar Vessels

Alveolar vessels are the thin-walled capillaries that perfuse the alveolar septum (Figure 46-1). They are exposed almost directly to the pressure changes that occur in the alveoli during breathing. *Extra-alveolar vessels* include the pulmonary arteries, and veins, which occur together with bronchi in a loose connective tissue sheath called the *bronchovascular bundle.* This bundle is bounded by a limiting membrane to which alveolar septa are attached (Figure 46-2). The behavior of extra-alveolar vessels is determined by pressure changes within the connective tissue space of the bronchovascular bundle, which approximate pleural pressure, rather than by changes in alveolar pressure. The bronchovascular bundle is also the initial site of accumulation of edema fluid when animals develop pulmonary edema.

The Pulmonary Blood Vessels Offer a Low Resistance to Flow

Pulmonary vascular pressures can be measured by advancing a catheter through the jugular vein into the right ventricle and pulmonary artery. Even though the pulmonary circulation receives the total output of the right ventricle, pulmonary arterial pressures are much less than systemic pressures. Pulmonary arterial systolic, diastolic, and mean pressures average approximately 25, 10, and 15 mm Hg, respectively, in mammals at sea level but these pressures are somewhat greater in larger than in smaller mammals. If the catheter is advanced until it becomes wedged in a pulmonary artery, the occluded vessel becomes an extension of the catheter, allowing estimation of *pulmonary venous pressure*, also known as *pulmonary wedge pressure*. Pulmonary wedge pressure (average, 5 mm Hg) is only slightly greater than left atrial pressure (average, 3 to 4 mm Hg). The small difference in pressure between the mean pulmonary artery (15 mm Hg) and left atrial (4 mm Hg) pressures indicates that the pulmonary circulation offers little vascular resistance to blood flow. *Pulmonary vascular resistance* (PVR) is calculated as follows:

$$PVR = (Ppa - Pla)/\dot{Q}$$

where *Ppa* is mean pulmonary arterial pressure, *Pla* is left atrial pressure, and $\dot{Q}$ is cardiac output.

Although PVR is low in the normal resting animal, it decreases even further when pulmonary blood flow and pulmonary vascular pressures increase, as occurs during exercise. This is because an increase in pressure recruits previously unperfused vessels and serves to distend all vessels. More importantly, pulmonary vascular smooth muscle relaxes during exercise so that small arteries and veins dilate.

Micropuncture studies have shown that approximately half the vascular resistance in the pulmonary circulation is precapillary, and that the capillaries themselves provide a considerable portion of resistance to blood flow (Figure 46-3). Unlike the arterioles in the systemic circulation, the small arteries in the pulmonary circulation neither provide large resistance nor dampen the arterial pulsations; consequently, pulmonary capillary blood flow is *pulsatile*. The pulmonary veins provide little resistance to blood flow.

The Distribution of Pulmonary Blood Flow Within the Lung Is Influenced by Several Factors

The understanding of the distribution of blood flow within the lung was based for many years on experiments performed in humans or on dog lungs postured vertically to mimic the position of lungs in humans. Such experiments indicated that there is a *vertical gradient of perfusion*, with blood flow per unit lung volume increasing from the top to the bottom of the lung. Elegant models that considered pulmonary arterial, pulmonary venous, and alveolar pressures were proposed to explain gravity-dependent distribution of blood flow.

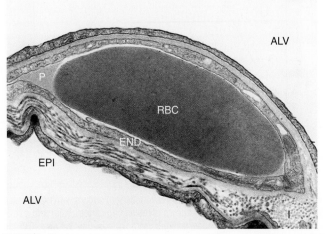

FIGURE 46-1 Transmission electron micrograph of capillary in the alveolar septum of a horse lung. A red blood cell *(RBC)* is shown bathed by plasma *(P)* in a capillary surrounded by endothelium *(END)*. Alveoli *(ALV)* are on both sides of the septum and separated from the capillary by the epithelium *(EPI)* and a layer of interstitium *(I)*. The interstitium is much thicker on one side of the capillary than on the other. Fluid exchange between the capillary and the interstitium occurs primarily on the thicker side. (Courtesy WS Tyler, Department of Anatomy, University of California–Davis.)

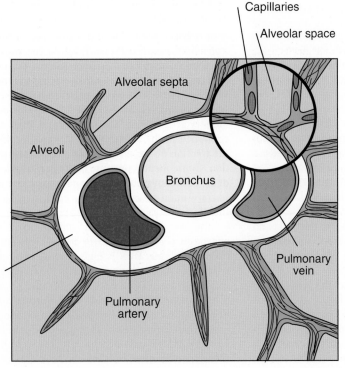

FIGURE 46-2 Diagrammatic representation of the extra-alveolar vessels (pulmonary artery and vein) in the bronchovascular bundle and *(inset)* an enlargement of the alveolar vessels (capillaries) in the alveolar septum. Notice that the alveolar septa are attached to the bronchovascular bundle so that they exert a radial traction on the bundle.

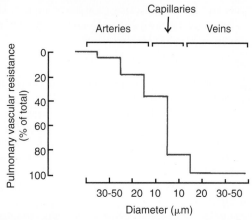

FIGURE 46-3 Distribution of vascular resistance in the pulmonary circulation, as determined by micropuncture studies. Unlike the resistance in the systemic circulation, a major portion of the resistance to blood flow in the pulmonary circulation is in the capillary bed. (From Bhattacharya J, Staub NC: Direct measurement of microvascular pressures in the isolated perfused dog lung, *Science* 210(4467):327–328, 1980. Copyright © 1980 by the American Association for the Advancement of Science.)

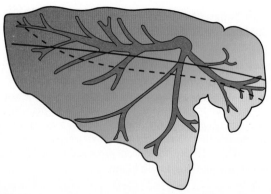

FIGURE 46-4 Graphic representation of the distribution of pulmonary blood flow in the horse's lung. Relative blood flow is indicated by the intensity of the red shading. Blood flow distribution in a dorsal-caudal direction at rest and during exercise is shown by the solid and broken lines, respectively. (Compiled from data in Hlastala MP, Bernard SL, Erikson HH, et al: Pulmonary blood flow distribution in standing horses is not dominated by gravity, *J Appl Physiol* 81(3):1051–1061, 1996.)

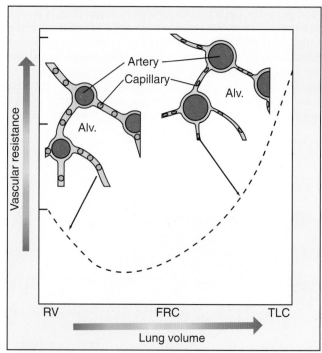

FIGURE 46-5 Change in vascular resistance that occurs with an increase in lung volume. The diagram shows alveolar capillaries *(blue)* and extra-alveolar vessels, in this case arteries *(red)*. At residual volume *(RV)* the arteries are narrowed, but the capillaries are distended. At total lung capacity *(TLC)*, the arteries are distended, but the capillaries are flattened because of the tension in the alveolar septum. Vascular resistance, which is the sum of the resistance provided by extra-alveolar vessels and capillaries, is minimal just below functional residual capacity *(FRC)*. *Alv,* Alveolus.

This description of gravitational zones provides a good theoretical basis for understanding the effects of pressures on pulmonary blood flow of bipeds. In comparison with quadrupeds, a large fraction of the human lung lies both below and above the level of the pulmonary artery so that gravity acting on the vertical height of the lung results in relative over-perfusion of the basal region and under-perfusion of the uppermost regions. In quadrupeds by contrast, the bulk of the lung is dorsal to the heart and the resting mean pulmonary perfusion pressure is sufficient to perfuse the whole lung height so gravity plays only a minor role in determining distribution of blood flow.

Blood flow is preferentially distributed to the *dorsocaudal region of the lung* of standing quadrupeds (Figure 46-4). This distribution is accentuated by exercise and may even persist when posture changes during anesthesia. The branching pattern of pulmonary arteries and arterioles and the relative resistances of each vessel are the major determinants of blood flow distribution.

Passive Changes in Vascular Resistance Result from Changes in Vascular Transmural Pressure

The diameter of blood vessels is a function of the pressure difference between the inside and the outside of the vessel, called the *transmural pressure*. Pressure within the vessels increases when the blood volume therein increases as occurs during exercise. This leads to an increase in *transmural pressure*, which causes the vessels to dilate. Transmural pressure can also increase if the pressure surrounding the vessel decreases. This occurs in large pulmonary arteries and veins as the lung inflates. These vessels are contained in the bronchovascular bundle, which is enlarged by the traction of the surrounding alveolar septa during lung inflation. Consequently, pressure in the perivascular connective tissue of the bronchovascular bundle decreases. This leads to an increase in transmural pressure, and the extra-alveolar arteries and veins therefore dilate.

The overall effects of lung volume on PVR reflect opposing effects on alveolar and extra-alveolar vessels (Figure 46-5). At residual volume, PVR is high because extra-alveolar vessels are narrowed. As the lung inflates to functional residual capacity, resistance decreases, primarily because of dilation of extra-alveolar vessels (arteries and veins). Further inflation above functional residual capacity increases PVR, primarily because alveolar capillaries are flattened by the high tension in the stretched alveolar septa. Capillaries become progressively more elliptical and therefore offer more resistance to flow.

Neural and Humoral Factors Cause Contraction of the Muscular Pulmonary Arteries

A variety of neural and humoral factors can contract or relax pulmonary vascular smooth muscle and thereby alter the resistance to blood flow. The magnitude of the response of vessels to these stimuli is largely determined by the amount of smooth muscle in the small pulmonary arteries, which varies with species (Figure 46-6). The increase in pulmonary vascular pressure in

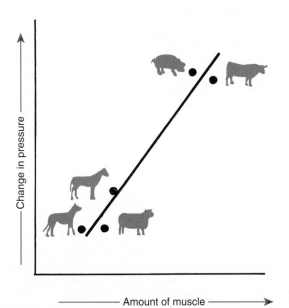

FIGURE 46-6 Relationship between the amount of muscle in the media of small pulmonary arteries and the change in pulmonary arterial pressure when animals are exposed to a hypoxic environment. Animals with thicker muscle layers, such as the cow and pig, have a greater vascular response to hypoxia than do animals with a small amount of muscle in the small pulmonary arteries, such as the dog and sheep. The horse has an intermediate response.

response to alveolar hypoxia and other stimuli is greater in calves than in sheep because of the greater amount of smooth muscle in calf pulmonary arteries.

The pulmonary arteries receive both *sympathetic* and *parasympathetic* innervation but the density of *autonomic innervation* varies among species. Although the pulmonary circulation has both alpha- and beta-adrenergic receptors, the net effect of sympathetic activation is vasoconstriction. Acetylcholine released from parasympathetic nerves activating muscarinic receptors can cause vasodilation through release of *nitric oxide* (NO) from the *endothelium* and vasoconstriction by direct effects on smooth muscle. Overall, the effect of parasympathetic activation is vasodilation.

Figure 46-7 shows the important vasoactive agents and receptors involved in regulation of pulmonary vascular resistance. Responses to receptor activation may vary among species, with the initial degree of vascular smooth muscle tone, and change between rest and exercise. Some mediators, such as acetylcholine and bradykinin, relax smooth muscle and cause vasodilation by releasing NO from the endothelium. Release of NO also occurs in response to the increased shear stress across the endothelium when blood flow increases. The increased NO release is partly responsible for the dilation of the pulmonary circulation during exercise. Catecholamines, bradykinin, and prostaglandins are metabolized by the vascular endothelium, so their effects may be modified by endothelial damage.

Alveolar Hypoxia Is a Potent Constrictor of Small Pulmonary Arteries

The air in poorly ventilated alveoli has a low partial pressure of oxygen, and it is of limited benefit to the animal to keep sending blood to such alveoli. To correct this problem, *alveolar hypoxia* results in vasoconstriction of pulmonary arteries. This *hypoxic vasoconstriction* reduces blood flow to poorly ventilated alveoli and redistributes pulmonary blood flow toward better-ventilated regions of lung. Although the vasoconstrictor response to hypoxia is present in all species, the magnitude of the response varies

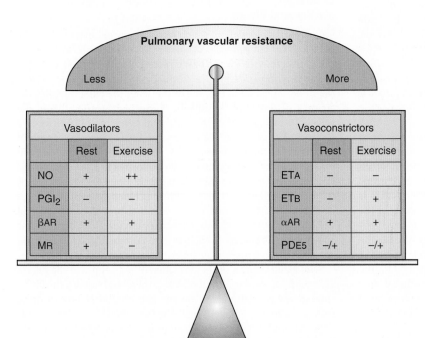

FIGURE 46-7 Important vasoactive agents and receptors regulating pulmonary vascular resistance at rest and during exercise. Vasodilators tip the scale toward less pulmonary vascular resistance and vasoconstrictors tip it toward more resistance. The small + and − signs, or their combination, represent the weight of the effect that the agent or receptor produces on its side of the scale. −, No effect; *NO*, nitric oxide; *PGI₂*, prostacyclin; *βAR*, beta-adrenergic receptor; *MR*, muscarinic receptor; *ETA*, endothelin A receptor; *ETB*, endothelin B receptor; *αAR*, alpha-adrenergic receptor; *PDE5*, phosphodiesterase-5. (Drawn with information from Merkus D, de Beer VJ, Houweling B, et al: Control of pulmonary vascular tone during exercise in health and pulmonary hypertension, *Pharmacol Therap* 119(3):242–263, 2008.)

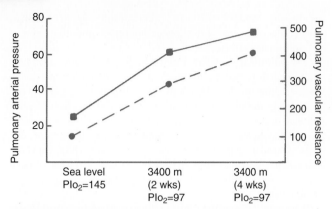

FIGURE 46-8 Change in mean pulmonary arterial pressure *(squares, solid line)* and pulmonary vascular resistance *(circles, broken line)* in calves transported from sea level to 3400 m for a 4-week sojourn. Both vascular resistance and arterial pressure increase when the calves are exposed to the hypoxia of altitude. Pressure and resistance continue to increase while at this altitude because of the proliferation of smooth muscle in the small pulmonary arteries. Pressure units are in millimeters of mercury (mm Hg); resistance units in dyne-sec/cm[5]; inspired oxygen tension (PIo$_2$) units in mm Hg. (From data in Ruiz AV, Bisgard GE, Will JA: Hemodynamic response to hypoxia and hyperoxia in calves at sea level and altitude, *Pflugers Arch* 344(4):275–286, 1973.)

greatly. Among domestic mammals, the response is most vigorous in cattle and pigs, less vigorous in horses, and trivial in sheep and dogs (see Figure 46-6).

The ability of local alveolar hypoxia to cause a local reduction in blood flow has been clearly demonstrated in several species. Under conditions of *atelectasis*, when there is no ventilation to the collapsed region of lung, local blood flow is greatly reduced by a combination of vessel closure as the lung collapses and vasoconstriction in response to the local hypoxia.

Hypoxic vasoconstriction is beneficial when there is localized alveolar hypoxia, but when hypoxia is generalized, as occurs when animals live at high altitude or have diffuse lung disease, the vasoconstriction can have serious consequences. In cattle grazing at high altitude, the hypoxia of altitude causes vigorous, generalized pulmonary hypoxic vasoconstriction (Figure 46-8). This leads to an increase in pulmonary arterial pressure, which increases the work of the right ventricle and leads to *right-sided heart failure*. The clinical syndrome is known as *brisket disease* because edematous fluid accumulates in the brisket. Because the magnitude of the response to hypoxia is genetically determined, measurements of pulmonary artery pressure in cattle grazing at high altitude has allowed selection of breeding stock that are less susceptible to brisket disease. In species such as cattle, in which the acute hypoxic constrictor response is most vigorous, chronic hypoxia results in sustained pulmonary hypertension. This is caused by an increase in the quantity of smooth muscle in the media of the small pulmonary arteries. When animals have generalized hypoxic vasoconstriction as a result of lung disease, the resultant right-sided heart failure is known as *cor pulmonale*.

Some species such as the sheep and llama, can tolerate the hypoxic conditions at high altitude because of endothelial production of the vasodilator NO. By contrast species such as cattle produce little NO to counteract the constriction induced by hypoxia.

Hypoxic vasoconstriction can be demonstrated in isolated, perfused lungs and therefore does not require intact innervation.

Under normoxic conditions, pulmonary arterial smooth muscle is relaxed because dilator factors (mitochondrial-derived hydrogen peroxide and others) keep voltage-gated potassium channels open so that muscle is hyperpolarized and does not contract. In the presence of hypoxia, these dilator factors are reduced, potassium channels close, and positivity within the cell promotes depolarization leading to an influx of calcium and smooth muscle contraction.

During Exercise the Pulmonary Circulation Must Accommodate a Large Increase in Blood Flow

To transport the extra oxygen required for muscular effort, cardiac output increases six- to eight-fold during strenuous exercise. This increase in blood flow must pass through the pulmonary circulation, where it collects oxygen. To accommodate the increase in blood flow, the pulmonary blood vessels dilate; that is, PVR decreases. This dilation is in part passive as a result of the increase in intravascular pressure, which is a result of the increased blood flow. In addition, flow-induced release of NO from the endothelium also causes relaxation of smooth muscle and vessel dilation.

In most species, pulmonary arterial pressure during strenuous exercise is about 35 mm Hg, but in the horse it increases to more than 90 mm Hg. The latter increase is attributable in large part to a very high left atrial pressure (50 mm Hg or more), which is probably necessary for rapid left ventricular filling when the heart rate exceeds 200 beats/min. When left atrial pressure is high, pulmonary arterial and capillary pressures must necessarily be even greater in order to maintain flow through the lung. These high exercise-associated intravascular pressures cause leakage of erythrocytes from the pulmonary capillaries when horses exercise strenuously, a phenomenon known as *exercise-induced pulmonary hemorrhage*.

BRONCHIAL CIRCULATION

The Bronchial Circulation Provides a Blood Supply to Airways, Large Vessels, and, in Some Species, the Visceral Pleura

The *bronchial circulation*, which receives approximately 2% of the output of the left ventricle, originates from two sources: the *bronchoesophageal artery* and a branch of the bicarotid trunk, the right apical *bronchial artery*. The former supplies the airways and the interlobular septa of most of the lung; the latter supplies the airways of the right apical lobe. Bronchial arteries follow the tracheobronchial tree to the terminal bronchioles and form a *peribronchial plexus* in the connective tissue along the length of the airways. Branches from this plexus penetrate the smooth muscle layer of the bronchial wall and form a *subepithelial vascular plexus* that serves to warm inhaled air. Branches are also given off to form the *vasa vasorum* (nutrient blood vessels) of pulmonary vessels. At the level of the terminal bronchiole, bronchial vessels *anastomose* with the pulmonary circulation. There are few anastomoses between bronchial and pulmonary arteries; most anastomoses are present at the capillary or venular level.

The extensiveness of the bronchial blood supply to the pleura varies among species. In cattle, sheep, pigs, and horses, the bronchial artery provides blood flow to the *visceral pleura;* in dogs, cats, and monkeys, it does not. The bronchial blood flow to the large extrapulmonary airways drains into the azygos vein; venous drainage of the intrapulmonary bronchial circulation enters the pulmonary circulation.

Although the bronchial circulation provides *nutrient blood flow* to many lung structures, the lung does not die if the bronchial circulation is obstructed. The extensive anastomoses between bronchial and pulmonary vessels provide pulmonary blood flow to bronchial vessels. Similarly, when parts of the pulmonary circulation are obstructed, the bronchial circulation proliferates and maintains blood flow to the affected part of the lung. The bronchial circulation also proliferates when the airways are inflamed.

Inflow pressure to the bronchial circulation is systemic arterial pressure, but outflow pressure varies, depending on whether venous drainage is through the azygos vein or pulmonary circulation. Changes in pressure in both the systemic and the pulmonary vascular bed affect the magnitude of bronchial blood flow. Increasing systemic pressure increases flow, but increasing pulmonary vascular pressures (downstream pressure) reduces and may even reverse flow. Under hypoxic conditions, bronchial arteries dilate; in contrast, pulmonary arteries constrict under these conditions.

CLINICAL CORRELATIONS

BRISKET DISEASE IN A HEIFER

History. A 2-year-old Hereford heifer was kept during the winter on a farm in the foothills of the Rocky Mountains outside Denver. In the late spring the heifer was transported to Climax, Colo. (altitude, 3400 m), for summer grazing. After 6 weeks the owners noticed that the animal was having some difficulty breathing, was reluctant to move around the pasture, and had developed an enlarged pendulous brisket and some swelling between the jaws.

Clinical Examination. Inspection of the heifer reveals a lethargic animal in poor condition. The respiratory and heart rates are elevated, and air seems to be moving well through the nostrils. The most noticeable observation is an enlarged and pendulous brisket. The swelling extends up the neck, and there is a pendulous area between the jaws. The jugular veins are distended.

Palpation of the swollen brisket reveals that it is heavy; when it is squeezed, the imprints of the fingers remain for some time. The swelling between the mandibles behaves in a similar manner when palpated. The mucous membranes of the heifer are a normal color, and the lung sounds are unremarkable.

Comment. The swelling in the brisket and between the mandibles, which pits on palpation, is evidence of accumulation of interstitial edema in the dependent areas of the heifer, in which there is loose connective tissue. Accumulation of edema in these regions is an indication of the increase in systemic venous pressure, which is also causing jugular distention. Both are caused by *right-sided heart failure.*

The most likely cause of right-sided heart failure in a heifer grazing at high altitude is diffuse vasoconstriction of the pulmonary circulation as a result of chronic hypoxia (inspired oxygen tension at 3400-m elevation is 97 mm Hg, compared with 150 mm Hg at sea level). The smooth muscle in the pulmonary arteries contracts in response to hypoxia; if this response is maintained for several weeks, the amount of smooth muscle in the pulmonary arteries increases. Furthermore, the animal produces extra erythrocytes in an attempt to transport more oxygen. These extra erythrocytes increase the hematocrit and make the blood more viscous and difficult to pump through the lung. Maintenance of cardiac output in the presence of the elevated pulmonary vascular resistance and increased blood viscosity requires an increase in pulmonary arterial and right ventricular pressure. Persistently working against the increased pressure causes right-sided heart failure.

Treatment. If this animal is returned to lowland pasture, it will recover. The vasospasm in the pulmonary circulation and the hematocrit diminish once the hypoxic stimulus is removed. For immediate treatment, this animal should be moved to an area of lower altitude and could be given oxygen to relieve the hypoxic stimulus. This would cause a reduction in pulmonary arterial pressure, which would cause some relief. However, pulmonary arterial pressure would not decrease to normal levels, because of the increased amount of smooth muscle now present in the pulmonary arteries. In early disease, this process may be reversible. When cardiac signs develop, however, the prognosis is guarded. Additional treatments include digoxin and diuretics, if desired.

STALLION WITH BILATERAL EPISTAXIS POST-RACING

History. A 2-year-old Thoroughbred stallion has been in training at the track. It has performed well at the beginning of the races, but has been fading towards the end of the races. The last time the horse raced, the trainer noted blood coming out of both nostrils at the end of the race. The horse has not had any other problems thus far.

Clinical Examination. Physical exam parameters are normal. On re-breathing exam, to detect subtle changes in the lungs, there are no abnormalities. Endoscopic exam performed at rest is normal, except for a very minimal amount of dark blood present in the distal trachea. Endoscopic exam, performed while the horse is exercising on a treadmill, demonstrates blood present in the trachea at the hilus (bifurcation to the right and left sides of the lungs). Cytology of the sample reveals predominantly erythrocytes with a small percentage of neutrophils. Culture for bacteria is negative.

Comment. This horse likely has exercise-induced pulmonary hemorrhage (EIPH). Although 65% or more of racehorses leak blood into their air passages during intense exercise, bleeding from the nostrils occurs in less than 0.5%. EIPH is a consequence of the normal physiology of the horse.

The exercising horse has a very high oxygen consumption which necessitates a high cardiac output to transport oxygen from the lungs to the muscles. The heart beats more than 200 times per minute (more than 3 times/second) and delivers about 1.5 liters per beat. For left ventricular filling to occur in the short time available, right atrial pressure and consequently pulmonary venous pressure must be very high. Maintenance of blood flow requires that pulmonary arterial pressure exceed pulmonary venous pressure so pressures throughout the pulmonary circulation are all elevated. In fact, pulmonary capillary pressure can be as high as 100 mm Hg. The high pulmonary capillary pressures create a large pressure difference between the alveoli and the pulmonary capillary bed, leading to a breakdown of the epithelial and endothelial tight junctions, resulting in bleeding into the alveoli and airways. Recently, narrowing of small pulmonary veins due to wall thickening has also been identified in horses with EIPH. By obstructing venous outflow, this would further contribute to high capillary pressure.

Treatment. Rest is not curative because EIPH is a consequence of the normal physiology of exercise. Furosemide (a diuretic) decreases bleeding severity. By increasing urination, furosemide decreases blood volume, which decreases pulmonary capillary pressure. This drug can be legally used on race day in the United States and some other countries.

PRACTICE QUESTIONS

1. Which of the following statements accurately describes the pulmonary circulation?
   a. It receives the total output of the right ventricle, except under conditions of alveolar hypoxia, when vasoconstriction reduces pulmonary blood flow.
   b. The medial layer of the main pulmonary arteries is composed of a thick layer of smooth muscle.
   c. The pulmonary veins return blood to the right atrium.
   d. Unlike systemic capillaries, the pulmonary capillaries provide a large percentage of the total resistance to blood flow.
   e. All the above.

2. During exercise, cardiac output can increase fivefold, but pulmonary arterial pressure may not even double. This occurs because:
   a. Pulmonary vascular resistance decreases during exercise.
   b. Unperfused capillaries are recruited during exercise.
   c. Previously perfused vessels are distended during exercise.
   d. Factors that dilate the pulmonary arteries are released by the endothelium during exercise.
   e. All the above

3. Which of the following will cause the greatest increase in pulmonary arterial pressure?
   a. Exposure of a cow to the hypoxia of high altitude
   b. A twofold increase in pulmonary blood flow
   c. Stimulation of the vagus nerve (parasympathetic system) in a sheep
   d. Inhalation of a tidal volume in a horse
   e. None of the above

4. The bronchial circulation:
   a. Receives the total output of the right ventricle.
   b. Drains into the pulmonary circulation and azygos vein.
   c. Vasoconstricts in response to hypoxia.
   d. Supplies nutrient blood flow only to bronchi and no other structures.
   e. Has a bronchial arterial pressure of the same magnitude as pulmonary arterial pressure.

5. In quadrupeds, pulmonary blood flow is distributed:
   a. Within the lung, as would be predicted by the action of gravity.
   b. Primarily to the ventral part of the lung during exercise.
   c. So that the dorsal-caudal regions of the lung receive the most blood flow.
   d. Uniformly among the alveoli.
   e. Uniformly when the animal is anesthetized.

BIBLIOGRAPHY

Boron WF: Ventilation and perfusion of the lungs. In Boron WF, Boulpaep EL, editors: *Medical physiology: a cellular and molecular approach*, ed 2, Philadelphia, 2009, Saunders.

Deffebach ME, Charan NB, Lakshminarayan S, et al: State of art. The bronchial circulation. Small, but a vital attribute of the lung, *Am Rev Respir Dis* 135(2):463–481, 1987.

Hinchcliff KW: Exercise-induced pulmonary hemorrhage. In McGorum BC, Dixon PM, Robinson NE, Schumacher J, editors: *Equine respiratory medicine and surgery*, St Louis, 2007, Elsevier.

Hlastala MP, Berger AJ: *Physiology of respiration*, ed 2, New York, 2001, Oxford University Press.

Leff AR, Schumacker PT: *Respiratory physiology: basics and applications*, Philadelphia, 1993, Saunders.

Lekeux P, Art T: The respiratory system: anatomy, physiology and adaptations to exercise and training. In Hodgson DR, Rose RJ, editors: *The athletic horse: principles and practice of equine sports medicine*, Philadelphia, 1994, Saunders.

Merkus D, de Beer VJ, Houweling B, et al: Control of pulmonary vascular tone during exercise in health and pulmonary hypertension, *Pharmacol Ther* 119(3):242–263, 2008.

Robinson NE: Some functional consequences of species differences in lung anatomy, *Adv Vet Sci Comp Med* 26:1–33, 1982.

West JB: *Respiratory physiology: the essentials*, ed 8, Baltimore, 2008, Lippincott Williams & Wilkins.

Williams KJ, Derksen FJ, de Feijter-Rupp H, et al: Regional pulmonary veno-occlusion: a newly identified lesion of equine exercise-induced pulmonary hemorrhage, *Vet Pathol* 45(3):316–326, 2008.

Wolin MS, Gupte SA, Mingone, CJ, et al: Redox regulation of responses to hypoxia and NO-cGMP signaling in pulmonary vascular pathophysiology, *Ann N Y Acad Sci* 1203:126–132, 2010.

CHAPTER 47
Gas Exchange

KEY POINTS

1. The composition of a gas mixture can be described by the fractional composition or partial pressure.
2. Alveolar gas composition is determined by alveolar ventilation and the exchange of oxygen and carbon dioxide.
3. Exchange of oxygen and carbon dioxide between the alveolus and pulmonary capillary blood occurs by diffusion.
4. The exchange of gases between the tissues and blood also occurs by diffusion.
5. The amount of alveolar ventilation in relation to pulmonary capillary blood flow—the $\dot{V}_A/\dot{Q}$ ratio—determines the adequacy of pulmonary gas exchange.

6. The composition of the systemic arterial blood is determined by the composition of the capillary blood that drains each alveolus.
7. Right-to-left vascular shunts allow blood to bypass ventilated lung.
8. Part of each breath ventilates dead-space and does not participate in gas exchange.
9. Arterial oxygen (Pa_{O_2}) and carbon dioxide (Pa_{CO_2}) tensions are measured to evaluate gas exchange.

The Composition of a Gas Mixture Can Be Described by the Fractional Composition or Partial Pressure

Understanding gas exchange requires an understanding of the measurement of gas composition and the forces causing gas movement within the lungs, blood, and tissues. For convenience, physiologists use many abbreviations when describing gas exchange (Table 47-1). Air contains 21% oxygen (the *fraction of oxygen in inspired air*, Fi_{O_2}, is 0.21). High in the Andes Mountains, the air still contains 21% oxygen, but visitors to those altitudes notice the lack of oxygen. Clearly, therefore, it is not only the fraction of oxygen that is important for gas exchange; the hypoxia at high altitude is a result of the low oxygen *partial pressure* that is a consequence of the low barometric pressure. At this lower barometric pressure, the oxygen molecules are less densely packed, and therefore the partial pressure of oxygen (P_{O_2}) in the air is decreased. It is this partial pressure (also called *tension*) that is important in gas transfer.

The partial pressure of oxygen (P_{O_2}) in a dry gas mixture is determined by *barometric pressure* (PB) and the *fraction of oxygen* (F_{O_2}) in the gas mixture, as follows:

$$P_{O_2} = PB \times F_{O_2}$$

In the atmosphere, Fi_{O_2} is 0.21, so P_{O_2} in dry air at sea level when PB = 760 mm Hg is approximately 160 mm Hg:

$$P_{O_2} = 760 \times 0.21 = 160 \text{ mm Hg}$$

P_{O_2} decreases at higher altitudes because barometric pressure decreases.

During inhalation, air is warmed to body temperature and humidified in the larger air passages. The concentration of oxygen and other gases is reduced by the presence of water vapor molecules; therefore, P_{O_2} is less in humidified than dry air. The P_{O_2} of humidified gas is calculated as follows:

$$P_{O_2} = (PB - PH_2O) \times Fi_{O_2}$$

where PH_2O is the *partial pressure of water vapor* at body temperature. The PH_2O is determined by the temperature and percentage saturation of the air with water. In a mammal with a body temperature of 38.2° C, PH_2O in saturated air equals 50 mm Hg; therefore, at sea level (PB = 760 mm Hg), the P_{O_2} of warmed, completely humidified gas in the conducting airways is approximately 149 mm Hg:

$$P_{O_2} = (760 - 50) \times 0.21 = 149 \text{ mm Hg}$$

Alveolar Gas Composition Is Determined by Alveolar Ventilation and the Exchange of Oxygen and Carbon Dioxide

Because there is only a negligible amount in the inspired air, the main source of carbon dioxide comes to the lungs in the blood returning from the tissues. For this reason, the PA_{CO_2} (*alveolar partial pressure of carbon dioxide*) is determined by the rate of carbon dioxide production ($\dot{V}_{CO_2}$) in relation to the amount of *alveolar ventilation* ($\dot{V}_A$):

$$PA_{CO_2} = K \times \dot{V}_{CO_2}/\dot{V}_A$$

where $K = PB - PH_2O$.

It is obvious from this equation that if $\dot{V}_{CO_2}$ increases, as occurs during exercise, $\dot{V}_A$ must also increase if PA_{CO_2} is to remain constant. If $\dot{V}_A$ does not increase sufficiently, PA_{CO_2} rises. Similarly, if $\dot{V}_{CO_2}$ remains constant and $\dot{V}_A$ halves, PA_{CO_2} doubles.

Alveolar oxygen tension (PA_{O_2}) is lower than that in inspired air because oxygen and carbon dioxide exchange occurs continuously. During breathing, PA_{O_2} fluctuates around an average value, increasing during inhalation and decreasing during exhalation.

The average oxygen tension in the alveoli of the lung can be calculated from the *alveolar gas equation,* a simplified version of which follows:

$$PAO_2 = [(PB - PH_2O) \times FiO_2] - PACO_2/R$$

where R, the *respiratory exchange ratio,* is the ratio of the rate of carbon dioxide production to that of oxygen consumption. The respiratory exchange ratio is determined by the substrates being

TABLE 47-1 Common Abbreviations Used in Gas Exchange

Abbreviation	Definition
$AaDO_2$	Alveolar-to-arterial oxygen tension difference
FiO_2	Fraction of oxygen in inspired air
FO_2	Fraction of oxygen in the gas mixture
$PaCO_2$	Arterial carbon dioxide tension
$PACO_2$	Alveolar carbon dioxide tension
PaO_2	Arterial oxygen tension
PAO_2	Alveolar oxygen tension
PB	Barometric pressure
$PcapCO_2$	Capillary carbon dioxide tension
$PcapO_2$	Capillary oxygen tension
PCO_2	Carbon dioxide tension
PH_2O	Partial pressure of water vapor
PiO_2	Inspired oxygen tension
PO_2	Oxygen tension
$PvCO_2$	Carbon dioxide tension of venous blood
PvO_2	Oxygen tension of venous blood
$\bar{v}$	Mixed venous blood
$\dot{Q}$	Perfusion
R	Respiratory exchange ratio
$\dot{V}$	Ventilation
$\dot{V}A$	Amount of alveolar ventilation
$\dot{V}CO_2$	Rate of carbon dioxide production
$\dot{V}O_2$	Rate of oxygen movement between alveolus and blood
$\dot{V}A/\dot{Q}$	Ratio of alveolar ventilation to blood flow

metabolized by the animal. This equation demonstrates that alveolar oxygen tension is determined by the inspired oxygen tension and the exchange of oxygen for carbon dioxide. Assuming an average R of 0.8 and a $PACO_2$ of 40 mm Hg, PAO_2 averages approximately 100 mm Hg at sea level, where PB is 760 mm Hg. The alveolar gas equation also shows that whenever $PACO_2$ increases, PAO_2 decreases, and vice versa.

Alveolar hypoventilation, a decrease in alveolar ventilation in relation to carbon dioxide production, elevates $PACO_2$ and decreases PAO_2. Figure 47-1 shows the causes of alveolar hypoventilation. It occurs when (1) the central nervous system is depressed by drugs or injury, (2) there is injury to the phrenic nerve that supplies the diaphragm, (3) there is damage to the thorax and respiratory muscles, (4) there is severe airway obstruction (e.g., in exercising horses with laryngeal hemiplegia), or (5) there is lung disease that severely decreases lung compliance.

The converse of alveolar hypoventilation, *alveolar hyperventilation,* causes a decrease in $PACO_2$ because ventilation is increased in relation to carbon dioxide production. Therefore, according to the alveolar gas equation, as $PACO_2$ decreases, PAO_2 increases. Hyperventilation occurs when the need to ventilate is increased by stimuli such as hypoxia, acidosis, or an increase in body temperature.

A modified form of the alveolar gas equation can be used to determine PAO_2 for clinical purposes, as follows:

$$PAO_2 = [(PB - PH_2O) \times FiO_2] - PaCO_2/R$$

In this equation, arterial carbon dioxide tension ($PaCO_2$) is substituted for alveolar carbon dioxide tension ($PACO_2$).

Exchange of Oxygen and Carbon Dioxide Between the Alveolus and Pulmonary Capillary Blood Occurs by Diffusion

Diffusion is the passive movement of gases down a concentration (partial pressure) gradient. The rate of gas movement between the alveolus and the blood ($\dot{V}O_2$) is determined by the physical properties of the gas (D), the surface area available for diffusion (A), the thickness of the air-blood barrier (x), and the driving pressure gradient of the gas between the alveolus and capillary blood ($PAO_2 - PcapO_2$), as follows:

$$\dot{V}O_2 = D \times A \times (PAO_2 - PcapO_2)/x$$

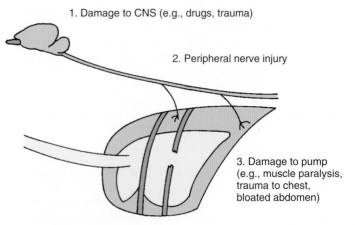

1. Damage to CNS (e.g., drugs, trauma)

2. Peripheral nerve injury

3. Damage to pump (e.g., muscle paralysis, trauma to chest, bloated abdomen)

4. Lung resisting inflation (e.g., airway obstruction, decreased lung compliance)

FIGURE 47-1 Diagrammatic representation of the brain, peripheral nerves, thorax, airways, and lung to show the causes of alveolar hypoventilation. *CNS,* Central nervous system.

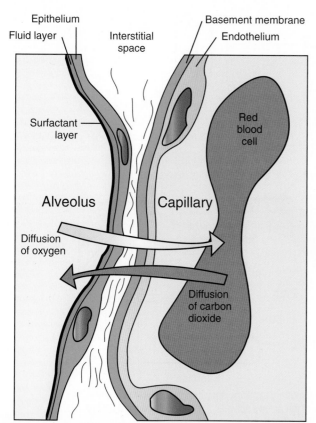

FIGURE 47-2 Diagrammatic representation of the air-blood barrier within the lung, showing the pathway for diffusion of oxygen and carbon dioxide between the alveolus and the erythrocyte within the pulmonary capillary.

D is determined by several factors, including the molecular weight and solubility of the gas. The alveolar surface area (A) available for diffusion is that occupied by perfused pulmonary capillaries. During exercise, more capillaries become perfused by blood, and thus the surface area available for diffusion increases.

In the lung the barrier separating air and blood (x) is less than 1 μm thick (Figure 47-2). However, although thin, this barrier includes a layer of liquid and surfactant lining the alveolar surface; an epithelial layer, usually formed by type I epithelial cells; a basement membrane; variable-thickness interstitium; and a layer of endothelium. In addition to moving gases through this air-blood barrier, diffusion also moves gases within the plasma, allowing oxygen to gain access to erythrocytes and hemoglobin.

Blood entering the alveolar capillary from the small pulmonary arteries is known as *mixed venous blood* because it has returned to the right side of the heart in veins from all parts of the systemic circulation. The *driving pressure* for gas diffusion is the difference in oxygen tension between the alveolus (PA_{O_2}) and the capillary blood. PA_{O_2} averages 100 mm Hg; in a resting animal, blood entering the alveolar capillary—that is, mixed venous blood—has an oxygen tension ($P\overline{v}_{O_2}$) of approximately 40 mm Hg. The driving pressure gradient of 60 mm Hg (100–40) causes rapid diffusion of oxygen into the capillary, where it combines with hemoglobin. Hemoglobin takes up oxygen from the plasma and helps maintain the gradient for oxygen diffusion.

Normally, in the resting animal, equilibration between alveolar and capillary oxygen tensions occurs within 0.25 second, approximately one third of the time the blood is in the capillary

(Figure 47-3). During strenuous exercise, muscles extract a large amount of oxygen from the blood, so the mixed venous blood returning to the lung contains little oxygen. In addition, during exercise the cardiac output is high, and the *velocity of blood flow* through the capillaries is rapid. More oxygen must therefore be transferred in less time than in the resting animal. Under these strenuous conditions, diffusion equilibrium may not occur, and the oxygen tension of blood leaving the lung and entering the systemic arteries (Pa_{O_2}) may decrease during intense exercise. This exercise-associated hypoxemia is observed in racing Thoroughbred horses.

In a diseased lung, diffusion of oxygen may be impeded as a result of inflammation and edema, which may thicken the air-blood barrier or reduce the surface area available for gas exchange. In these situations the therapeutic administration of oxygen can increase PA_{O_2} and thereby provide a greater driving pressure to deliver oxygen into the blood.

The carbon dioxide tension of venous blood returning to the lungs averages 46 mm Hg, and alveolar carbon dioxide tension (PA_{CO_2}) is 40 mm Hg. Thus the driving pressure for diffusion of carbon dioxide is only 6 mm Hg. Despite this small driving pressure, the amount of carbon dioxide that diffuses per minute between the capillaries and the alveoli is similar to the amount of oxygen. The 20-fold greater solubility of carbon dioxide compared with oxygen compensates for the small driving pressure gradient. For the same reason, carbon dioxide diffusion between the blood and the alveoli is rarely affected by lung disease.

The Exchange of Gases Between the Tissues and Blood Also Occurs by Diffusion

The Pa_{O_2} of blood entering the tissue capillaries from the systemic arteries is 85 to 100 mm Hg, and the Pa_{CO_2} is 40 mm Hg. As blood passes through the capillaries, it is exposed to the tissues that are consuming oxygen and producing carbon dioxide. *Tissue oxygen tension* is determined by the rate of delivery of oxygen in relation to its rate of consumption, but it averages 40 mm Hg. Similarly, tissue carbon dioxide tension is determined by the rate of tissue production in relation to the rate of removal by the blood, but it averages 46 mm Hg. As a result of the partial pressure differences between the tissues and capillaries, oxygen diffuses into the tissues and carbon dioxide diffuses into the blood until the partial pressures of blood and tissue are equal. Tissues with a high oxygen demand have more capillaries per gram of tissue. This provides a larger surface for diffusion and also means that the maximal distance between the tissue and the nearest capillary is less than in the poorly vascularized tissues.

During exercise, muscle blood flow increases in part as a result of recruitment of capillaries that are not perfused in the resting animal. *Capillary recruitment* brings blood closer to the metabolizing tissues and slows the rate of blood flow, which allows more time for diffusion equilibrium. In addition, the increased oxygen utilization and carbon dioxide production by muscle during exercise lowers the P_{O_2} and increases the P_{CO_2} of the muscle, which increases the driving pressure gradients for diffusion.

The Amount of Alveolar Ventilation in Relation to Pulmonary Capillary Blood Flow—the $\dot{V}A/\dot{Q}$ Ratio—Determines the Adequacy of Pulmonary Gas Exchange

In the alveoli, gas exchange is accomplished by the close approximation of air and blood. Ideally, each of the millions of alveoli should receive air and blood in amounts that are optimal for gas

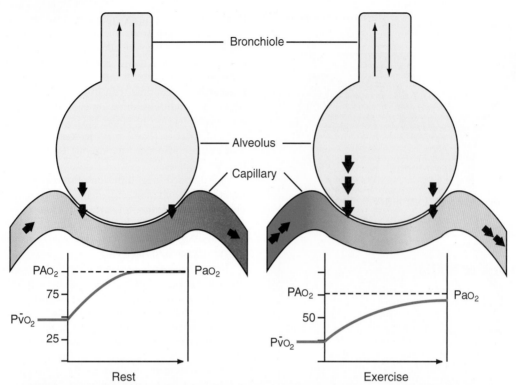

FIGURE 47-3 Schematic representation of alveolus and pulmonary capillary, showing the increase in P_{O_2} that occurs as blood passes through the capillaries. The number of the *arrows* between the alveolus and the capillary represents the magnitude of the oxygen fluxes. In the resting animal, mixed venous oxygen tension ($P\bar{v}_{O_2}$) is approximately 40 mm Hg, and blood and air equilibrate rapidly. In the exercising animal, mixed venous oxygen tension is low, and even though oxygen fluxes are high, the blood has not equilibrated with the alveolar oxygen tension before it leaves the alveolus. *PA_{O_2}*, Alveolar oxygen tension; *Pa_{O_2}*, arterial oxygen tension.

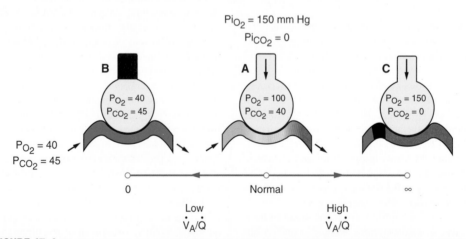

FIGURE 47-4 Diagrammatic representation of three alveoli and their capillaries, showing the effect of differing ventilation/perfusion ($\dot{V}_A/\dot{Q}$) ratios on oxygen and carbon dioxide tensions (P_{O_2} and P_{CO_2}, respectively). See text for explanation and Table 47-1 for abbreviation definitions. (Adapted from West JB: *Respiratory physiology: the essentials,* ed 8, Baltimore, 2008, Lippincott Williams & Wilkins, Figure 5-6, page 53.)

exchange; that is, ventilation ($\dot{V}_A$) and perfusion ($\dot{Q}$) should be matched. In reality, this never occurs. Even in the young healthy animal, there is some $\dot{V}_A/\dot{Q}$ mismatching, most likely resulting from branching patterns of bronchi and blood vessels and to some extent from gravitational forces. In disease, this $\dot{V}_A/\dot{Q}$ mismatching becomes more extreme and leads to *hypoxemia*, a low Pa_{O_2}.

Figure 47-4 shows schematic alveoli and capillaries with three $\dot{V}_A/\dot{Q}$ ratios. The alveolus in the center is ideal (Normal): it receives ventilation and blood flow with a $\dot{V}_A/\dot{Q}$ ratio of about 1.0. Mixed venous blood arrives at each alveolus with a P_{O_2} of 40 and a P_{CO_2} of 46 mm Hg, equilibrates with alveolar gas tensions, and leaves the normal alveolus with an end-capillary P_{O_2} and P_{CO_2} of 100 and 40 mm Hg, respectively. The alveolus on the left

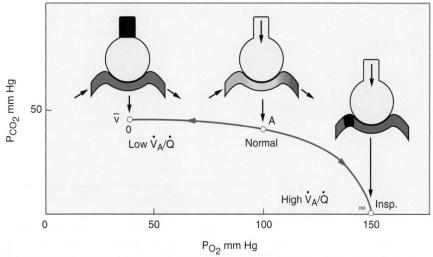

FIGURE 47-5 Effect of ventilation/perfusion ($\dot{V}A/\dot{Q}$) ratios on alveolar oxygen and carbon dioxide tensions (shown as P_{O_2} and P_{CO_2}, respectively). See text for explanation. Three alveoli are shown but $\dot{V}A/\dot{Q}$ ratios can range from zero to infinity. $\bar{v}$, Mixed venous blood composition; *Insp.,* inspired air composition. When an alveolus receives no ventilation $\dot{V}A/\dot{Q} = 0$, left), alveolar gas equilibrates with mixed venous blood and there is no gas exchange. When an alveolus receives no blood flow but ventilation continues ($\dot{V}A/\dot{Q} = \infty$, *right*), alveolar gas composition approaches that of inspired air. All alveoli between these two $\dot{V}A/\dot{Q}$ extremes have some gas exchange and their gas composition is shown by the *red line.* A normal (ideal) alveolus *(center)* with a $\dot{V}A/\dot{Q} = 0.8$ has P_{O_2} and P_{CO_2} of 100 and 40 mm Hg, respectively. (Adapted from West JB: *Respiratory physiology: the essentials,* ed 8, Baltimore, 2008, Lippincott Williams & Wilkins, Figure 5-7, page 64.)

is served by an obstructed bronchiole so receives no ventilation. Its $\dot{V}A/\dot{Q}$ ratio is therefore zero and blood passes through without participating in gas exchange. By contrast, the alveolus on the right receives no blood flow but continues to ventilate; its $\dot{V}A/\dot{Q}$ ratio is infinity. In this alveolus, the composition of the alveolar gas approaches that of inspired air but because there is no blood flow, the alveolus makes no contribution to gas exchange. It is dead space.

The millions of gas exchange units in the lung can have $\dot{V}A/\dot{Q}$ ratios ranging from zero to infinity. Any alveoli with low $\dot{V}A/\dot{Q}$ ratios are relatively overperfused and underventilated. Examination of Figure 47-5 shows that the P_{O_2} of blood leaving these low $\dot{V}A/\dot{Q}$ units is decreased substantially, but the P_{CO_2} is only slightly elevated. Low $\dot{V}A/\dot{Q}$ units occur frequently in lung disease because ventilation is reduced by airway obstruction or by localized stiffening of the lung by inflammatory processes. The alveoli to the right of the normal unit in Figure 47-5 have high $\dot{V}A/\dot{Q}$ ratios; ventilation is high in relation to blood flow. This can occur when pulmonary blood flow to part of the lung is reduced by vascular obstruction or by pulmonary hypotension. The blood leaving such units has an elevated P_{O_2} and decreased P_{CO_2}.

Extending the concepts demonstrated in Figure 47-5 to the whole lung with its multitude of alveoli requires computer simulation and the investigation of the frequency distribution of $\dot{V}A/\dot{Q}$ ratios within the lung. In the healthy animal the majority of alveoli have $\dot{V}A/\dot{Q}$ ratios close to 1, and the range of ratios is small (Figure 47-6).

The Composition of the Systemic Arterial Blood Is Determined by the Composition of the Capillary Blood That Drains Each Alveolus

Blood that returns from the lungs to the left ventricle for distribution to the tissues comes from capillaries associated with millions of alveoli, each of which may have a slightly different $\dot{V}A/\dot{Q}$ ratio. The content of oxygen and carbon dioxide in blood that leaves each alveolus varies because of these differing $\dot{V}A/\dot{Q}$ ratios (see Figure 47-5). Thus the composition of arterial blood is determined by distribution of $\dot{V}A/\dot{Q}$ ratios in the lung.

Lung disease accentuates $\dot{V}A/\dot{Q}$ mismatching because of obstruction of airways, flooding of alveoli with exudates, and local obstructions to blood flow. This mismatching has a major effect on oxygen exchange but little effect on the exchange of carbon dioxide. In the case of oxygen, overventilation of some alveoli does not compensate for underventilation of others. Because of the shape of the *oxyhemoglobin dissociation curve* (see Chapter 48) the overventilated (high $\dot{V}A/\dot{Q}$) alveoli with a high PA_{O_2} cannot add enough oxygen to the blood to compensate for the deficiency that arises from the underventilated (low $\dot{V}A/\dot{Q}$) alveoli with a low PA_{O_2}. Therefore, hypoxemia occurs to varying degrees in most lung diseases. However, in contrast to oxygen, carbon dioxide is very soluble, and because its dissociation curve (see Chapter 48) is almost linear, the overventilated alveoli can compensate for those that are underventilated. For this reason, *hypercarbia,* also called *hypercapnia* (increased Pa_{CO_2}), rarely occurs in the presence of lung disease.

As the degree of $\dot{V}A/\dot{Q}$ mismatching increases and oxygen exchange becomes less efficient, the difference between the average PA_{O_2} and Pa_{O_2} increases. Normally, this *alveolar-to-arterial oxygen tension difference* (AaD$_{O_2}$) averages 5 to 10 mm Hg, because there is a degree of $\dot{V}A/\dot{Q}$ inequality even in normal lungs, and because venous blood draining the bronchial and coronary circulations mixes with the oxygenated blood draining the alveoli. The AaD$_{O_2}$ increases when animals are anesthetized or when they have lung disease, because many poorly ventilated regions of the lung continue to receive blood flow; that is, the number of units with low $\dot{V}A/\dot{Q}$ increases (see Figure 47-5).

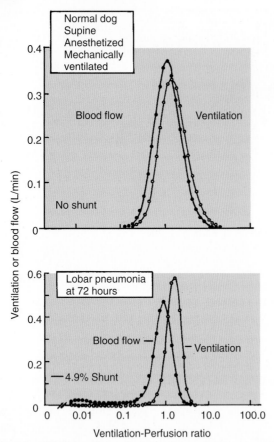

FIGURE 47-6 Distribution of ventilation and blood flow as a function of the ventilation/perfusion ($\dot{V}A/\dot{Q}$) ratio. *Top,* In the normal dog, most of the blood flow and ventilation are received by gas exchange units with a $\dot{V}A/\dot{Q}$ ratio close to 1.0. No blood flow and no ventilation are received by units with extremely high or extremely low $\dot{V}A/\dot{Q}$ ratios. *Bottom,* In the dog with pneumonia, a considerable portion of the blood flow is received by units with low $\dot{V}A/\dot{Q}$ ratios, that is, units with little ventilation. The amount of blood passing through right-to-left shunts is also increased in pneumonia. (From Wagner PD, Laravuso RB, Goldzimmer E, et al: Distributions of ventilation-perfusion ratios in dogs with normal and abnormal lungs, *J Appl Physiol* 38(6):1099–1109, 1975.)

Right-to-Left Vascular Shunts Allow Blood to Bypass Ventilated Lung

In a *right-to-left shunt,* blood from the right ventricle bypasses ventilated lung and returns to the left atrium. An example is provided in Figure 47-7 where some of the blood flow to the lung is passing through a region of severe bronchopneumonia. This shunt blood does not pick up oxygen and, when it leaves the diseased alveoli, has the same composition as the venous blood that entered the lung. When this blood mixes with that which has perfused the healthy lung, it dilutes the oxygen content so that the blood going to systemic arteries has a lower Pao_2 than normal. Right-to-left shunts have a $\dot{V}A/\dot{Q}$ ratio of zero and are formed when alveoli are collapsed *(atelectasis),* are unventilated because of complete *airway obstruction,* or are filled with exudates, as in *acute pneumonia.* Right-to-left shunts can also result from complex congenital cardiac defects, such as *tetralogy of Fallot,* which allow blood to flow directly from the right to the left chambers of the heart, bypassing the lungs. Such large right-to-left shunts cause a major impairment of oxygen exchange. In healthy animals the venous blood (low Po_2) from the bronchial and coronary veins enters the oxygenated blood leaving the lungs. This is equivalent to a right-to-left shunt and constitutes up to 5% of cardiac output.

Part of Each Breath Ventilates Dead-Space and Does Not Participate in Gas Exchange

Dead-space ventilation consists of the gas that does not participate in gas exchange. This includes both anatomic dead-space (see Chapter 45) and alveolar dead-space. The latter consists of alveoli that receive ventilation but no blood flow; that is, they have a $\dot{V}A/\dot{Q}$ ratio of infinity (see Figure 47-5, *right*). *Alveolar dead-space* can form when the pulmonary arterial pressure is so low that many capillaries are unperfused, or when the vessels are obstructed by thrombi, as in dogs with heartworm disease.

Arterial Oxygen (Pao_2) and Carbon Dioxide ($Paco_2$) Tensions Are Measured to Evaluate Gas Exchange

A systemic arterial blood sample is essential to evaluate pulmonary gas exchange because this blood has just passed through the

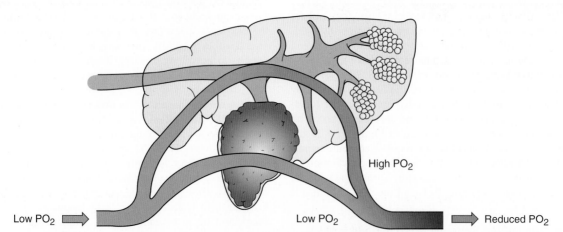

FIGURE 47-7 Diagrammatic representation of a region of pneumonia *(dark red)* in an otherwise healthy lung. The pneumonic region receives no ventilation so blood flow through that region does not pick up any oxygen (i.e., it forms a right-to-left shunt). When this poorly oxygenated blood mixes with well-oxygenated blood coming from the healthy lung, the result is a lower oxygen tension than normal in blood returning to systemic arteries for delivery to the tissues.

lung. A venous blood sample is inadequate because its composition varies depending on the blood flow/metabolism ratio of the tissue of origin. Arterial blood gas tensions are the end result of the individual processes involved in gas exchange and thus are affected by the composition of inspired air, alveolar ventilation, alveolocapillary diffusion, and ventilation/perfusion matching. All these factors must be considered when evaluating a blood gas result.

Inspired air usually contains 21% oxygen ($FiO_2 = 0.21$), but during anesthesia or oxygen therapy, the administration of oxygen increases FiO_2, which causes an increase in inspired oxygen tension (PiO_2). Although the daily fluctuations in PB cause only trivial changes in PiO_2, the decrease in PB that occurs at higher altitudes results in a major decrease in PiO_2. As a result, there is a decrease in PAO_2 and thus a decrease in PaO_2 as animals ascend in altitude. In the appropriate geographic locations, altitude-induced changes in PaO_2 must always be considered when blood gas tensions are evaluated.

Adequacy of alveolar ventilation is assessed by examination of $PaCO_2$. It is elevated above the normal value of 40 mm Hg when animals hypoventilate and is decreased during hyperventilation. At the same time, hypoventilation decreases PAO_2 and PaO_2, and hyperventilation increases these tensions.

Diffusion abnormalities and $\dot{V}A/\dot{Q}$ mismatching impair the transfer of oxygen from the alveolus to arterial blood, increase the $AaDO_2$, and reduce PaO_2. $PaCO_2$ is rarely elevated by these problems for two reasons. First, the high solubility of carbon dioxide allows easy diffusion across the remaining healthy lung. Second, the hypoxemia caused by lung disease stimulates ventilation. The resultant increase in alveolar ventilation keeps $PaCO_2$ normal or even reduces it below normal.

In animals with normal lungs, administering oxygen (increasing FiO_2) elevates PaO_2. As $\dot{V}A/\dot{Q}$ mismatching becomes more extreme, oxygen administration increases PaO_2 only modestly, especially in the presence of right-to-left shunts. Concurrently, the alveolar-arterial oxygen difference widens. The PaO_2 response to oxygen is a good way to evaluate the severity of lung disease.

PaO_2 tends to be lower in newborn animals than in adults. This is because there is greater mismatching of ventilation and blood flow in the immature lungs.

CLINICAL CORRELATIONS

HYPOVENTILATION IN A BULLDOG

History. A 5-year-old bulldog is presented to you because it refuses to exercise. Normally the dog is willing to go for short, slow walks. Over the past 6 months, the dog has been making an increasing amount of noise when it breathes. When it is awake, it makes a rattling sound during inhalation; when it sleeps, it snores loudly and wakes frequently, standing up, turning around, and then lying down again. On one occasion the owner tried to get the dog to run, but the dog collapsed, making a loud noise in its throat as it struggled to inhale.

Clinical Examination. The bulldog is in good condition, but even as you walk into the room, you notice the loud rattling noises being made by the dog during breathing. You also observe that the mucous membranes of the pendulous lips have a bluish tinge. The dog is standing when you walk into the room, but while you are talking to the owner, the dog lies down and apparently goes to sleep. This causes the breathing noises to become much louder.

Examination of the dog reveals no abnormalities in the heart or the digestive tract, but examination of the respiratory tract reveals multiple abnormalities. The external nares of the dog are extremely small, and it is difficult to introduce a speculum to examine the nasal cavity. When the dog's mouth is opened, an excessive amount of loosely folded tissue is observed in the pharynx, and it is impossible to move this aside to examine the larynx. Listening to the lungs is not helpful because all the sounds being generated by the loose, vibrating tissue in the upper airway are transmitted to the lungs. Radiographs, however, reveal no abnormalities in the lungs, but the trachea is quite narrow. An arterial blood sample is taken for measurement of oxygen and carbon dioxide tensions. PaO_2 is 50 mm Hg (normal, 95-100), and $PaCO_2$ is 75 mm Hg (normal, 40).

Comment. This bulldog's condition represents an extreme form of the brachycephalic syndrome, which is seen in short-nosed dogs, particularly bulldogs. The syndrome usually includes stenosis (narrowing) of the external nares and obstruction of the pharynx by pendulous folds of excessive soft tissue. In some of these dogs, the trachea is also very narrow. These dogs have difficulty breathing, particularly during inhalation, when the subatmospheric pressure within the upper airway sucks the loose folds of tissue into the airway lumen. This can result in total obstruction to ventilation. In general, these dogs make a lot of noise during inhalation as the loose folds of tissue vibrate. Exhalation presents less difficulty because the higher-than-atmospheric pressure in the pharynx tends to push back the loose tissue and open the airway. Over time the chronic, excessively subatmospheric pressure during inhalation can cause deformity of the larynx.

The upper airway obstruction in this bulldog is limiting ventilation so severely that the dog is suffering from alveolar hypoventilation. The elevated $PaCO_2$ indicates this. An elevation in $PaCO_2$ occurs when alveolar ventilation is not sufficient to remove the carbon dioxide being produced by the body. The accumulating carbon dioxide in the alveolus and the lack of ventilation also depress the PAO_2, which leads to a decrease in PaO_2, as in this dog. The hypoxemia then leads to hemoglobin desaturation, which accounts for the bluish color (cyanosis) of the mucous membranes of the dog.

Treatment. The treatment for this dog is surgical removal of some of the excessive tissues of the upper airway and enlargement of the external nares. This will alleviate some of the obstruction and may improve ventilation. However, with the narrowing of the trachea observed in this dog, it is unlikely that the dog will ever be able to exercise to a significant degree, although its condition may be improved sufficiently that it can make a suitable pet.

HYPOXEMIA IN AN ANESTHETIZED CLYDESDALE HORSE

History. A 2-year-old, 750-kg Clydesdale horse is presented for removal of a testicle that has been retained in the abdomen, a procedure that requires anesthesia. You know that anesthesia of heavy draft horses can lead to gas exchange problems, and therefore you have an anesthesia machine available to provide ventilation and to supplement the horse with extra oxygen. The horse is anesthetized with a short-acting intravenous anesthetic and an endotracheal tube is inserted. The horse is connected to the anesthesia machine and allowed to breathe oxygen containing isoflurane for anesthesia. Ventilation is not assisted.

Thirty minutes after the induction of anesthesia, the veterinary technician takes an arterial blood sample to monitor the horse's gas exchange. Pao_2 is 70 mm Hg, and $Paco_2$ is 65 mm Hg. Are you satisfied with the results of the blood gas analysis? If not, what can be done to improve gas exchange?

Comment. The elevation of $Paco_2$ from the normal value of 40 mm Hg to 65 mm Hg shows that the horse is suffering from alveolar hypoventilation; that is, the ventilation received by the alveoli is insufficient to remove the carbon dioxide being produced by the horse. This is probably a result of depression of the central nervous system by the anesthetic gases, so that the drive to breathe is reduced. In addition, the positioning of the horse on its back for removal of the retained testicle causes the heavy viscera to push on the diaphragm, making it difficult for the horse to ventilate. Alveolar hypoventilation in an anesthetized animal can be corrected by the use of positive-pressure ventilation. You have a ventilator as part of the anesthesia machine and choose to ventilate the horse to return the $Paco_2$ to acceptable levels.

The Pao_2 of 70 mm Hg shows that the horse has considerable problems in exchanging oxygen. Although a Pao_2 of 70 mm Hg is sufficient almost to saturate hemoglobin and would not be considered particularly low in an animal breathing air, it is very low in an animal breathing 100% oxygen. When animals breathe oxygen, PAo_2 is greater than 600 mm Hg:

$$PAo_2 = (PB - PH_2O) \times Fio_2 - Paco_2$$
$$= (760 - 50) \times 1.0 - 65$$
$$= 645 \text{ mm Hg}$$

If the lung is functioning ideally, arterial oxygen should also be close to 600 mm Hg. In this horse, Pao_2 is only 75 mm Hg, so $AaDo_2$ is 645–75, that is 570 mm Hg.

This huge $AaDo_2$ is not unusual in large, anesthetized mammals. The positioning of the horse on its back with the consequent weight of the viscera pushing forward on the diaphragm and compressing the lungs can lead to severe $\dot{V}A/\dot{Q}$ inequalities. Parts of the dependent lung are unable to ventilate, although they continue to receive blood flow and therefore become right-to-left shunts. These right-to-left shunts result in severe arterial hypoxemia. As long as the Pao_2 is sufficient to saturate hemoglobin, the horse is in no danger. The dangerous point is during recovery from anesthesia. The horse must be supplemented with oxygen until it is sufficiently conscious to be able to rest on its sternum unaided and eventually to stand. Returning to these postures eliminates right-to-left shunts, restores the $\dot{V}A/\dot{Q}$ distribution to normal, and improves gas exchange.

PRACTICE QUESTIONS

1. Calculate the alveolar oxygen tension (PAo_2) of an anesthetized cow when the barometric pressure is 750 mm Hg, PH_2O at body temperature = 50 mm Hg, and $Paco_2$ = 80 mm Hg. The cow is breathing a mixture of 50% oxygen and 50% nitrogen. Assume the respiratory exchange ratio is 1.
   a. 270 mm Hg
   b. 620 mm Hg
   c. 275 mm Hg
   d. 195 mm Hg
   e. 670 mm Hg

2. Which of the following will decrease the rate of oxygen transfer between the alveolar air and the pulmonary capillary blood?
   a. Increasing PAo_2 from 100 to 500 mm Hg
   b. Perfusing previously unperfused pulmonary capillaries
   c. Decreasing the mixed venous oxygen tension from 40 to 10 mm Hg
   d. Destruction of alveolar septa and pulmonary capillaries by a disease known as *alveolar emphysema*
   e. None of the above

3. During exercise, recruitment of muscle capillaries that are unperfused in the resting animal results in all the following except:
   a. An increase in the velocity of capillary blood flow.
   b. An increase in the surface area for gas diffusion between tissues and blood.
   c. A decrease in distance between tissue capillaries.
   d. Maintenance of tissue Po_2 in the presence of increased demand for oxygen.
   e. A shorter distance for gas diffusion.

4. Which of the following could potentially result in more low $\dot{V}A/\dot{Q}$ regions within the lung?
   a. Atelectasis of one lobe of a dog lung
   b. Obstruction of both pulmonary arteries
   c. Doubling the ventilation to the right cranial lobe while its blood flow remains constant
   d. Vasoconstriction of the pulmonary arteries of the left lung in a cow
   e. None of the above

5. Which of the following statements is correct?
   a. Right-to-left shunts represent an extremely high $\dot{V}A/\dot{Q}$ ratio.
   b. Right-to-left shunts are not a cause of elevated alveolar-arterial oxygen difference.
   c. An increase in the alveolar dead-space can result from an increase in the number of high $\dot{V}A/\dot{Q}$ units in the lung.
   d. The shape of the oxyhemoglobin dissociation curve means that low $\dot{V}A/\dot{Q}$ units in the lung are not a cause of hypoxemia (low Pao_2).
   e. Totally occluding the right pulmonary artery increases the right-to-left shunt fraction by 50%.

6. A horse has difficulty inhaling, especially during exercise. Arterial blood gas tensions at rest are $Pao_2 = 55$ mm Hg and $Paco_2 = 70$ mm Hg. After you give the horse oxygen to breathe, Pao_2 increases to 550 mm Hg, and $Paco_2$ remains unchanged. The cause of these gas tensions is:
   a. Right-to-left shunt through a complex cardiac defect.
   b. Alveolar hyperventilation.
   c. A large number of alveoli with high $\dot{V}A/\dot{Q}$ ratios.
   d. Alveolar hypoventilation.
   e. None of the above.

BIBLIOGRAPHY

Boron WF: Gas exchange in the lungs. In Boron WF, Boulpaep EL, editors: *Medical physiology: a cellular and molecular approach*, ed 2, Philadelphia, 2009, Saunders.

Boron WF: Ventilation and perfusion of the lungs. In Boron WF, Boulpaep EL, editors: *Medical physiology: a cellular and molecular approach*, second ed 2, Philadelphia, 2009, Saunders.

Hlastala MP, Berger AJ: *Physiology of respiration*, ed 2, New York, 2001, Oxford University Press.

Leff AR, Schumacker PT: *Respiratory physiology: basics and applications*, Philadelphia, 1993, Saunders.

Lekeux P, Art T: The respiratory system: anatomy, physiology and adaptations to exercise and training. In Hodgson DR, Rose RJ, editors: *The athletic horse: principles and practice of equine sports medicine*, Philadelphia, 1994, Saunders.

West JB: *Respiratory physiology: the essentials*, ed 8, Baltimore, 2008, Lippincott, Williams & Wilkins.

CHAPTER 48

Gas Transport in the Blood

KEY POINTS

Oxygen transport

1. A small amount of oxygen is transported in solution in plasma, but most is in combination with hemoglobin.
2. A molecule of hemoglobin can reversibly combine with four molecules of oxygen.
3. The binding of oxygen and hemoglobin is determined by oxygen tension.
4. The oxyhemoglobin dissociation curve can be displayed with percent saturation of hemoglobin as a function of oxygen tension.
5. The affinity of hemoglobin for oxygen varies with blood temperature, pH, carbon dioxide tension, and the intracellular concentration of certain organic phosphates.

6. As hemoglobin is depleted of oxygen, its color changes from bright red to bluish red.
7. Carbon monoxide has 200 times the affinity of oxygen for hemoglobin.
8. Methemoglobinemia occurs in certain toxic states, notably nitrite poisoning.

Carbon dioxide transport

1. Carbon dioxide is transported in the blood both in solution in plasma and in chemical combination.

Gas transport during exercise

1. Oxygen demands of exercise are met by increases in blood flow, in hemoglobin levels, and in oxygen extraction from blood.

OXYGEN TRANSPORT

A Small Amount of Oxygen Is Transported in Solution in Plasma, but Most Is in Combination with Hemoglobin

Oxygen is poorly soluble in water and therefore in plasma. Because of this low solubility, most animals need an oxygen-carrying pigment to transport sufficient oxygen to the tissues. The only animals that can exist without hemoglobin live deep in the ocean in the cold parts of the world. The depth at which they live results in a high ambient pressure and thus a high oxygen tension (P_{O_2}). In addition, the cold environment results in a low metabolic rate and therefore little need for oxygen. The high P_{O_2} and low oxygen demand enable them to exist without an oxygen-carrying pigment. All land-dwelling animals seen by veterinarians have such a pigment, and in mammals and birds, that pigment is *hemoglobin*.

When blood in the pulmonary capillaries flows past the alveoli, oxygen diffuses from the alveoli into the blood until the partial pressures (tensions) equilibrate: that is, there is no further driving pressure difference. Because oxygen is poorly soluble in water, only a very small amount dissolves in the plasma, and hemoglobin is necessary for delivery of sufficient oxygen to the tissues. Without hemoglobin, which transports the majority of the oxygen, the cardiac output would have to be inordinately high to maintain the oxygen supply to the body organs.

Even though the amount of oxygen dissolved in plasma is small, it increases directly as the partial pressure of oxygen increases; 0.003 mL of oxygen dissolves in each 100 mL (1 dL) of plasma at an oxygen tension (P_{O_2}) of 1 mm Hg (Figure 48-1). The pulmonary capillary blood equilibrates with the alveolar oxygen tension ($P_{A_{O_2}}$) of 100 mm Hg; therefore, 0.3 mL of oxygen dissolves in each deciliter of blood. If an animal breathes pure

oxygen its $P_{A_{O_2}}$ increases to at least 600 mm Hg and 1.8 mL of oxygen (600×0.003) dissolves in each deciliter of plasma.

A Molecule of Hemoglobin Can Reversibly Combine with Four Molecules of Oxygen

Mammalian hemoglobin consists of four units, each containing one heme and its associated protein (globin). *Globin* is a polypeptide composed of 140 to 150 amino acids. *Heme* is a protoporphyrin consisting of four pyrroles with a ferrous iron at the center. Each ferrous iron can combine reversibly with a single molecule of oxygen. The complete hemoglobin molecule has four hemes each with its associated globin and thus can combine reversibly with up to four molecules of oxygen (Figure 48-2). The type and sequence of amino acids that compose globin are critical to oxygen binding. Without the presence of globin, oxygen would irreversibly oxidize the ferrous iron to ferric iron. The amino acids in globin cradle the heme and limit access of oxygen to the ferrous iron. This prevents oxidation and allows uptake and release of oxygen in response to local P_{O_2}. The type and sequence of amino acids that compose globin define the different types of mammalian hemoglobin. Adult hemoglobin contains two alpha (α) and two beta (β) *amino acid chains;* fetal hemoglobin contains two α and two gamma (γ) chains. Closely related species, such as humans and anthropoid apes, have similar amino acid sequences on the side chains, whereas more divergent species have more differences in amino acid sequences.

Each hemoglobin molecule can reversibly bind up to four molecules of oxygen, one with each heme. The reversible combination of oxygen with hemoglobin is shown in the *oxyhemoglobin dissociation curve* (Figure 48-3). The binding of oxygen is a four-step process, and the oxygen affinity of a particular heme is influenced by the oxygenation of the others. This means that when the first heme unit is oxygenated, oxygen affinity of the second heme unit is increased, and so on. These *heme-heme* interactions are responsible for the sigmoid shape of the oxyhemoglobin dissociation curve.

The Binding of Oxygen and Hemoglobin Is Determined by Oxygen Tension

Figure 48-3 shows that the *oxygen content* of blood—that is, the amount of oxygen combined with hemoglobin—is determined by Po_2. At a Po_2 of more than approximately 70 mm Hg, the oxyhemoglobin dissociation curve is virtually flat, which indicates that further increases in Po_2 add little oxygen to hemoglobin. At this point, the hemoglobin is saturated with oxygen because each iron atom is associated with an oxygen molecule. The fact that hemoglobin becomes virtually saturated with oxygen at a Po_2 of more than 70 mm Hg has important clinical consequences. Many animals live at altitudes considerably above sea level, where the lower barometric pressure results in a low PIo_2 (inspired oxygen tension). Although these animals have a lower Pao_2 (arterial oxygen tension) than their sea-level–dwelling counterparts, they are still able to transport sufficient oxygen to their tissues because their hemoglobin is well saturated with oxygen. Clearly, at extreme altitudes, hemoglobin begins to desaturate.

One gram of saturated hemoglobin can hold 1.36 to 1.39 mL of oxygen; therefore, average mammalian blood with 10 to 15 g of hemoglobin per deciliter has an *oxygen capacity* of 13.6 to 21 mL of oxygen per deciliter (volume percentage [vol%]) when hemoglobin is saturated with oxygen. The oxygen capacity of the blood is the maximal amount of oxygen that can be carried in the blood at any given time. *Anemia,* a reduction in the number of circulating erythrocytes (red blood cells) with a consequent reduction in the amount of hemoglobin in the blood, decreases oxygen capacity. When the hemoglobin content of blood increases, oxygen capacity increases as well. The latter occurs during exercise; contraction of the spleen forces more erythrocytes into the circulation. More erythrocytes than normal in the blood is known as *polycythemia,* and these red blood cells increase the oxygen capacity of the blood.

When the Po_2 is less than 60 mm Hg, the oxyhemoglobin dissociation curve has a steep slope. This is in the range of tissue Po_2

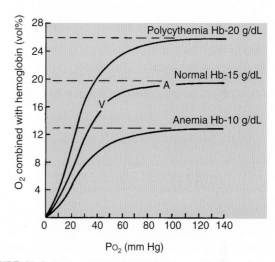

FIGURE 48-3 Oxyhemoglobin dissociation curve of *normal* (hemoglobin [Hb] = 15 g/dL), *anemic* (Hb = 10 g/dL), and *polycythemic* (Hb = 20 g/dL) blood. The amount of oxygen combined with hemoglobin (i.e., the oxygen content) is plotted as a function of oxygen tension (Po_2). *A,* Arterial; *V,* venous.

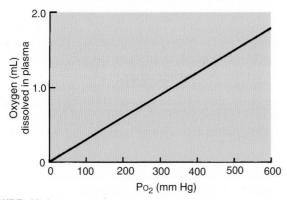

FIGURE 48-1 Amount of oxygen (in ml/dl) dissolved in plasma as a function of oxygen tension (Po_2).

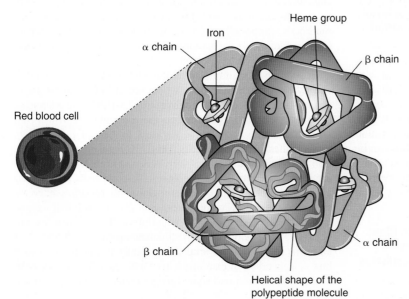

FIGURE 48-2 Structure of the hemoglobin molecule showing the two pairs of polypeptide chains. Within each chain is a heme, four in all. The ferrous iron in the center of each heme provides the binding site for molecular oxygen. (From Mader SS: *Inquiry into life,* ed 8, New York, 1997, McGraw-Hill.)

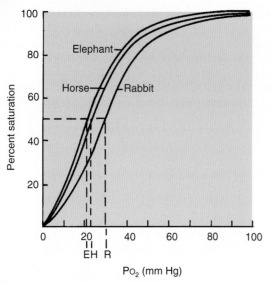

FIGURE 48-4 Oxyhemoglobin dissociation curve of three species of mammal. Percent saturation of hemoglobin is plotted as a function of oxygen tension (P_{O_2}). Although the curves have similar shapes in all mammals, they are not superimposed. The differences between the curves can be expressed by the partial pressure (tension) at which hemoglobin is 50% saturated with oxygen (P_{50}). P_{50} for each species is indicated as *E* (elephant), *H* (horse), and *R* (rabbit).

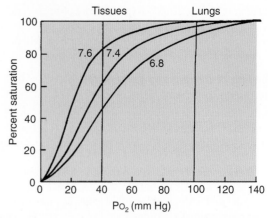

FIGURE 48-5 Effect of pH on the oxyhemoglobin dissociation curve. A decrease in pH shifts the dissociation curve to the right and therefore assists in unloading oxygen at the tissues. The shift in the dissociation curve has much less effect on the percent saturation of hemoglobin when oxygen is being loaded into the blood in the lungs (i.e., $P_{O_2} = 100$ mm Hg) than when oxygen is being unloaded in the tissues (i.e., $P_{O_2} = 40$ mm Hg).

at which oxygen is unloaded from the blood. Tissue P_{O_2} varies in accordance with the blood flow/metabolism ratio, but average tissue P_{O_2} is 40 mm Hg. Blood exposed to such a P_{O_2} loses 25% of its oxygen to the tissues. In rapidly metabolizing tissues in which tissue P_{O_2} is lower, more oxygen is unloaded from the blood. The oxygen remaining in combination with hemoglobin forms a reserve that can be tapped in emergencies.

Oxygen content is a term that describes the amount of oxygen in the blood, most bound to hemoglobin. When hemoglobin is saturated with oxygen, oxygen content and oxygen capacity are equal. When oxygen leaves the blood in the tissues, oxygen content decreases, but the oxygen capacity remains the same.

The Oxyhemoglobin Dissociation Curve Can Be Displayed with Percent Saturation of Hemoglobin as a Function of Oxygen Tension

Percent saturation of hemoglobin is the ratio of oxygen content to oxygen capacity. Hemoglobin is more than 95% saturated with oxygen when it leaves the lungs of an animal at sea level. Percent saturation of mixed venous blood averages 75%; venous oxygen tension ($P\bar{v}_{O_2}$) averages 40 mm Hg. Although all mammals have similarly shaped oxyhemoglobin dissociation curves, the position of the curve with regard to P_{O_2} varies (Figure 48-4). This can be described by measurement of P_{50}, the partial pressure at which hemoglobin is 50% saturated with oxygen. A higher P_{50} is generally found in small mammals and allows unloading of oxygen at a high P_{O_2} to satisfy their higher metabolic demands.

The Affinity of Hemoglobin for Oxygen Varies with Blood Temperature, pH, Carbon Dioxide Tension, and the Intracellular Concentration of Certain Organic Phosphates

An increase in tissue metabolism produces heat, which elevates blood temperature and shifts the oxyhemoglobin dissociation

curve to the right (increases P_{50}). Such a shift facilitates dissociation of oxygen from hemoglobin and releases oxygen to the tissues; hemoglobin is then said to have "less affinity" for oxygen. Conversely, excessive cooling of the blood, as occurs in hypothermia, shifts the dissociation curve to the left. Because of this increased affinity of hemoglobin for oxygen, tissue P_{O_2} must be lower than usual to release oxygen from hemoglobin.

Changes in carbon dioxide tension (P_{CO_2}) and pH also affect the affinity of hemoglobin for oxygen. The shift in the oxyhemoglobin dissociation curve resulting from a change in P_{CO_2} is called the *Bohr shift*. This shift results in part from the combination of carbon dioxide with hemoglobin, but mostly from the production of hydrogen ions, which decrease the pH. A change in pH alters the oxygen binding by changing the structure of hemoglobin. As a result, a higher, more alkaline pH shifts the oxyhemoglobin dissociation curve to the left, and a lower, more acidic pH shifts the curve to the right (Figure 48-5). The Bohr effect is not constant among species; a given change in pH produces a greater shift in the dissociation curve for small mammals than for large mammals, supposedly ensuring the delivery of oxygen during high rates of metabolic activity, when carbon dioxide production is greatest.

A solution of mammalian hemoglobin generally has a higher affinity for oxygen than does whole blood until organic phosphates, such as 2,3-diphosphoglycerate (2,3-DPG) and adenosine triphosphate (ATP), are added to the solution. In erythrocytes, DPG has a molar content equivalent to that of hemoglobin, much higher than in other cells. This DPG regulates the combination of oxygen with hemoglobin. When concentrations of DPG are high, as occurs under the anaerobic conditions imposed by altitude or anemia, the oxyhemoglobin dissociation curve is shifted to the right (P_{50} increases), and the unloading of oxygen is facilitated. In contrast, a reduction in DPG levels, as can occur in stored blood, shifts the dissociation curve to the left. Not all forms of hemoglobin bind DPG equally. Ruminant hemoglobin in general is unresponsive to DPG; elephant hemoglobin binds DPG weakly; and some forms of fetal hemoglobin do not bind DPG.

As Hemoglobin Is Depleted of Oxygen, Its Color Changes from Bright Red to Bluish Red

The change in the color of hemoglobin from bright red to the bluish red is known as *cyanosis*. It is observed in the mucous membranes of animals when the blood in the underlying capillaries is hypoxic. Cyanosis can result from deficient oxygen uptake in the lungs, but it can also result from reduced blood flow to the peripheral tissues. The latter can occur when animals are in cardiovascular failure.

The color change that occurs as hemoglobin loses its oxygen is the basis of *oximetry*. Oximeters use differences in light absorption to distinguish oxygenated and deoxygenated hemoglobin. A pulse oximeter is a clinical tool that can be attached to an ear or the lips of anesthetized animals to measure the hemoglobin saturation of arterial blood.

Carbon Monoxide Has 200 Times the Affinity of Oxygen for Hemoglobin

Carbon monoxide (CO) and oxygen bind to the same sites on hemoglobin, but CO is bound much more avidly. As a result of the high affinity of CO for hemoglobin, exposure to CO levels of less than 1% in air can eventually saturate hemoglobin and displace oxygen, leading to death. Fortunately, such low levels of CO must be breathed for some time to deliver sufficient CO to saturate all the blood hemoglobin, so toxic effects are not immediate. CO not only reduces the oxygen content of the blood, but also displaces the oxyhemoglobin dissociation curve to the left. This shift indicates that with the onset of CO poisoning, hemoglobin has a higher affinity for the remaining bound oxygen; thus the release of oxygen into the tissues occurs at a tissue Po_2 much lower than normal. Treatment of CO poisoning requires removal of the CO source and administration of oxygen to displace the carbon monoxide from hemoglobin.

Methemoglobinemia Occurs in Certain Toxic States, Notably Nitrite Poisoning

When the normal ferrous iron of hemoglobin is oxidized by *nitrites* and other toxins to ferric iron, brown-colored *methemoglobin* is formed. Methemoglobin does not bind oxygen; thus the oxygen capacity of the blood is reduced. Nitrite can be ingested directly from spoiled feeds, but ruminants more often form nitrite in the rumen after ingestion of nitrate-rich feeds such as Sudan grass and mangel tops. An enzyme, methemoglobin reductase, which is present in erythrocytes to reduce the normally small amounts of methemoglobin back to hemoglobin, is inadequate in the presence of excessive oxidation, so therapy must be provided.

Veterinarians Frequently Manage Oxygen Transport

Use of inhalant anesthesia and managing anemia, polycythemia, lung disease, and carbon monoxide poisoning all require an understanding of oxygen transport and the oxyhemoglobin dissociation curve. In the healthy animal (blood hemoglobin 15 g/dL) breathing air containing 21% oxygen (fraction of inspired oxygen [Fio_2] = 0.21), the hemoglobin is virtually saturated with oxygen at the normal Pao_2 of 85 to 95 mm Hg (Table 48-1). Anesthetizing such an animal with a gas mixture containing almost 100% oxygen (Fio_2 = 1.0) raises the Pao_2 to over 600 mm Hg but this has no effect on oxygen capacity (no more hemoglobin has been added to the blood) and only raises content slightly; no more oxygen can be added to hemoglobin but a little more is in solution in plasma. By contrast, breathing less than 21% oxygen decreases Pao_2 (for example, when Fio_2 is 0.15) and reduces oxygen content and percent saturation. The same situation arises when Pao_2 decreases because of lung disease or ascent to altitude.

Anemic animals lack hemoglobin and therefore have reduced oxygen capacity. Unless they also have lung disease, their PaO_2 is normal. Their oxygen content is decreased because of the low capacity but because Pao_2 is normal, all the hemoglobin is saturated so percent saturation is normal. Polycythemia is simply the converse situation.

It takes only a very small fraction of carbon monoxide in air to cause poisoning and this is not sufficient to measurably reduce the Fio_2, consequently Pao_2 is not decreased. Carbon monoxide does not reduce the amount of hemoglobin but by binding to it so avidly, it reduces the amount of hemoglobin available for oxygen binding. Therefore, oxygen content is decreased and so is percent saturation of hemoglobin by oxygen. However, hemoglobin is saturated with a mixture of carbon monoxide and oxygen.

CARBON DIOXIDE TRANSPORT

Carbon Dioxide Is Transported in the Blood Both in Solution in Plasma and in Chemical Combination

Unlike oxygen, which is bound only to hemoglobin, carbon dioxide (CO_2) is transported in several forms (Figure 48-6). Carbon dioxide is produced in the tissue; therefore tissue Pco_2 is higher than the Pco_2 of the blood arriving in the capillaries. CO_2 diffuses down a concentration gradient from the tissues into the blood. When the blood leaves the tissues, Pco_2 has risen from 40

TABLE 48-1 Effect of Some Common Situations on Arterial Oxygen Tension (Pao_2), Oxygen Content and Capacity, and Percent Saturation of Hemoglobin

	Pao_2	O_2 Capacity	O_2 Content	Percent Saturation of Hb
Breathing air (21% O_2)	Normal (85–95 mm Hg)	Normal (21 vol %)	Normal (20–21 vol %)	About 98%
Breathing 100% O_2	Increased ($\approx$ 600 mm Hg) Less with lung disease	Normal (21 vol %)	Slightly increased (22.5 vol %)	100%
Breathing 15% O_2	Reduced (55 mm Hg)	Normal (21 vol %)	Reduced (about 18 vol %)	Reduced (about 86%)
Anemia	Normal (85–95 mm Hg)	Reduced	Reduced	Normal
Polycythemia	Normal (85–95 mm Hg)	Increased	Increased	Normal
CO poisoning	Normal (85–95 mm Hg)	Normal	Reduced	Reduced*

*Reduced only if oximeter used for measurement separates oxyhemoglobin from carboxyhemoglobin. If not, percent saturation will be 100%.

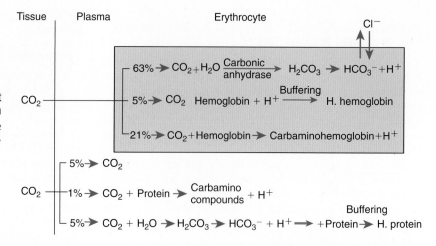

FIGURE 48-6 Forms of carbon dioxide (CO_2) transport in the blood. All reactions displayed in this diagram can be reversed when the blood reaches the lung and CO_2 diffuses into the alveolus. H_2CO_3, Carbonic acid; HCO_3^-, bicarbonate.

to approximately 46 mm Hg, with exact values depending on the ratio of blood flow to metabolism.

Approximately 5% of the CO_2 entering the blood is transported in solution. The majority of CO_2 diffuses into the erythrocyte, where it undergoes one of two chemical reactions. Most of the CO_2 combines with water and forms *carbonic acid* (H_2CO_3), which then dissociates into *bicarbonate* (HCO_3^-) and *hydrogen ion* (H^+), as follows:

$$H_2O + CO_2 \leftrightarrow H_2CO_3 \leftrightarrow H^+ + HCO_3^-$$

This reaction also occurs in plasma, but in the erythrocyte, the presence of *carbonic anhydrase* accelerates the hydration of CO_2 several hundredfold. Ionization of H_2CO_3 occurs rapidly, and H^+ and HCO_3^- accumulate within the erythrocyte. The reversible reaction is kept moving to the right because H^+ is *buffered* by hemoglobin. Most of the HCO_3^- that is produced in the erythrocyte diffuses out along a concentration gradient into the plasma. Chloride ion (Cl^-) diffuses into the erythrocyte to maintain the electrochemical neutrality.

The addition of CO_2 to capillary blood is facilitated by the deoxygenation of hemoglobin occurring in the tissues. *Deoxyhemoglobin* is a weaker acid than oxyhemoglobin and therefore a better buffer. Thus it combines more readily with H^+ and facilitates the formation of HCO_3^- from CO_2.

The *carbamino compounds* are the second form in which CO_2 is transported in the blood. Carbamino compounds are formed by coupling of CO_2 to the –NH groups of proteins, particularly hemoglobin. Although carbamino compounds account for only 15% to 20% of the total CO_2 content of the blood, they are responsible for 20% to 30% of the CO_2 exchange between the tissues and the lungs.

When venous blood reaches the lungs, CO_2 diffuses into the alveoli from plasma and erythrocytes, thus causing the reactions shown in Figure 48-6 to move to the left. Simultaneously, the oxygenation of hemoglobin releases H^+ ions, which combine with HCO_3^- to form H_2CO_3 and thus CO_2.

The blood *content of carbon dioxide* as a function of P_{CO_2} is depicted in the CO_2 equilibrium curves shown in Figure 48-7. Curves are shown for oxygenated blood ($P_{O_2} = 100$ mm Hg), for partially deoxygenated blood ($P_{O_2} = 50$), and for deoxygenated blood ($P_{O_2} = 0$). The curves are almost linear and have no plateau in the physiological range; CO_2 can be added to the blood as long as the buffering capacity is available. The higher CO_2 content of deoxygenated blood resulting from the higher buffering capacity of deoxyhemoglobin is clearly visible.

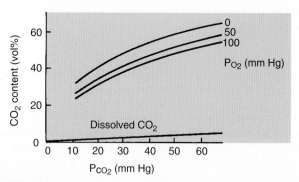

FIGURE 48-7 Carbon dioxide equilibration curves showing the amount of CO_2 contained in the blood (CO_2 content) as a function of CO_2 tension (P_{CO_2}). *Curves* are shown for dissolved CO_2 and for total CO_2 content at various oxygen tensions (P_{O_2}).

GAS TRANSPORT DURING EXERCISE

Oxygen Demands of Exercise Are Met by Increases in Blood Flow, in Hemoglobin Levels, and in Oxygen Extraction from Blood

The demands for gas transport in the blood are not constant but vary with metabolism. Strenuous exercise represents the most extreme demand placed on the gas transport mechanisms. In the galloping horse, oxygen consumption can increase to 30 times resting levels. Figure 48-8 shows how this extra demand for oxygen is met. Part of the demand is provided by an increase in *cardiac output,* which causes the amount of blood flowing through the lungs per minute to increase. This allows an increased uptake of oxygen from the lungs. The cardiac output also is redistributed, with an increased fraction of output going to the exercising muscles. The increase in cardiac output and redistribution increases muscle blood flow by twentyfold.

The horse also meets the increased oxygen demand with an increase in the number of circulating erythrocytes, and therefore an increased amount of hemoglobin. Contraction of the spleen forces stored erythrocytes into the circulation and can increase the hematocrit from 35% to 50%. This provides almost 50% more binding sites for oxygen, which raises the oxygen capacity of the blood. The usefulness of an increase in hematocrit is limited because it increases blood viscosity, which tends to slow the flow of blood through the capillaries and increase the

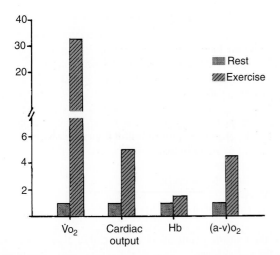

FIGURE 48-8 Oxygen consumption ($\dot{V}o_2$), cardiac output, hemoglobin level (Hb), and arteriovenous oxygen difference [(a-v)o_2] in a horse at rest and during strenuous exercise at a gallop. The thirtyfold increase in $\dot{V}o_2$ is accomplished by a fivefold increase in cardiac output, a 50% increase in Hb, and a fourfold increase in (a-v)o_2.

work of the heart. The increase in muscle blood flow and hematocrit together increase the delivery of oxygen to the muscle. An exercising muscle extracts a larger percentage of the oxygen from the blood than does a muscle at rest. This is accomplished as follows: (1) the diffusion gradient for oxygen is increased by the decrease in muscle Po_2, which results from the increase in metabolic rate, and (2) the affinity of hemoglobin for oxygen is decreased by the higher temperature of the exercising muscle and by the lower pH that results from release of carbon dioxide and hydrogen ions from the muscle. As a result of the increased extraction of oxygen, the arteriovenous oxygen content difference is increased.

Muscle itself contains an oxygen-binding pigment, *myoglobin*, which provides a small store of oxygen. However, myoglobin's main function is the transfer of oxygen within the muscle cell. Myoglobin, like hemoglobin, is an iron-containing pigment, but unlike hemoglobin, it contains only one heme group. As a result, the dissociation curve is not sigmoid but is a rectangular hyperbola. The affinity of myoglobin for oxygen is high, with 75% saturation at a Po_2 of 20 mm Hg, and the steepest slope of the dissociation curve at Po_2 equaling 5 mm Hg. As a result of these dissociation characteristics, myoglobin releases oxygen only when intracellular Po_2 is low. Myoglobin is more plentiful in slow-twitch aerobic muscle fibers, which are capable of sustained aerobic work, than in fast-twitch fibers, which are generally used for short bursts of anaerobic activity. The amount of myoglobin is increased by exercise training.

Thus, in exercise the increased demand for oxygen is met by increases in blood flow, hematocrit, oxygen extraction from blood, and to a small degree by oxygen release from myoglobin. These mechanisms are available whenever unusual demands for gas exchange arise. In anemia, for example, oxygen capacity is reduced, but oxygen delivery to the tissues can be preserved somewhat by an increase in cardiac output and increased extraction of oxygen from the hemoglobin.

The respiratory system's role in acid-base balance is discussed in Chapter 52.

CLINICAL CORRELATIONS

FLEA INFESTATION IN A CAT

History. A cat is presented to you because the owner notices that the cat seems extremely weak and recently has been staggering when it walks around the house. The cat's appetite is good, and besides the weakness, the owner thinks the cat is normal.

Clinical Examination. Inspection of the animal, which is resting quietly on the examination table, shows that it is in reasonably good condition. The respiratory rate does not appear to be elevated, and from a distance the cat shows no obvious signs of disease. When you place your hands on the cat's back, you immediately notice a gritty material in the fur. Further examination of the skin shows accumulations of this red-brown material deep within the coat, and you notice many fleas scurrying around when the coat is parted. When you moisten some of the gritty material, it produces a red liquid. The cat's mucous membranes are almost white, and the examination of the mucous membranes produces sufficient struggling that the cat begins to breathe rapidly. The cat's pulse rate is extremely elevated, but the lung sounds are normal. On physical examination, all the body systems appear to be normal. You take a blood sample; the packed cell volume (hematocrit) is 10% (normal, 30% to 45%).

Comment. This cat has a severe infestation of fleas. The gritty material in the fur is flea feces, which contains blood products that become red when wet. The infestation is further confirmed by the observation of many fleas in the coat. By their blood-sucking method of feeding, fleas can produce anemia when they are present in large numbers, as with this cat. If the flea infestation develops gradually, the anemia is slow in onset, and the host animal may show few clinical signs until the infestation and anemia become severe. The anemia is confirmed in this case by the paleness of the mucous membranes and by the low hematocrit. The rapid heart rate of the cat is a response to the anemia. To deliver sufficient oxygen to the tissues, the cardiac output needed to be increased by increasing the heart rate. When the cat is stressed by your examination, it shows signs of respiratory distress because there is inadequate oxygen delivery to the tissues; this causes production of lactic acid as a result of anaerobic metabolism. The resultant decrease in pH stimulates the chemoreceptors, causing the signs of respiratory distress.

Treatment. Your treatment approach to this cat is twofold. First, you administer blood to increase the cat's hematocrit and provide it with sufficient oxygen-carrying capacity until it can generate new erythrocytes. Second, you treat the flea infestation and instruct the owner on how to remove the fleas from the house.

Several weeks later the owner returns with the cat and notes that she has had no further problems. Occasionally she notes a flea on the cat's coat and treats the cat immediately with flea medication. She is also diligent about regular vacuuming to remove fleas from the house.

ATRIAL FIBRILLATION IN A HORSE

History. The owner of a 3-year-old Standardbred gelding is concerned because the horse is no longer able to complete its training program. Up until a week ago, the horse had been running well during its daily bouts of training. In the past 2 days, the horse has been extremely reluctant to exercise and, if pushed to do so, begins to stagger and appears weak in the rear legs.

Clinical Examination. Inspection of the horse reveals a normal appearing Standardbred in excellent condition. It is standing in its box stall, eating, and looks alert when you enter the stall. Clinical examination reveals normal-colored mucous membranes, no abnormality of lung sounds, and no abnormalities in the gastrointestinal, urinary, or nervous system. When you take the pulse, you note that it is irregular in both amplitude and rate. Several pulses follow one another rapidly, and then there are prolonged pauses, with no consistent pattern to the irregularity. Auscultation of the heart reveals a similar irregularity in the heart sounds.

You take a blood sample for measurement of the hematocrit, which is normal. You also obtain an electrocardiogram (ECG), which reveals a continuous irregular pattern of multiple P waves with occasional and irregularly occurring QRS complexes.

Comment. The history, heart rhythm, and ECG findings in this horse are typical of atrial fibrillation. The multiple P waves observed on the ECG are a result of circuitous depolarization of the atria. In atrial fibrillation the atria contract and relax in an uncoordinated manner. The atrioventricular node is activated at intervals that vary considerably from cycle to cycle; thus there is no constant interval between ventricular contractions. The variable time between ventricular contractions allows for variable degrees of ventricular filling and therefore results in uneven stroke volume; consequently, the pulse varies in amplitude as well as frequency.

The irregular ventricular rhythm may be sufficient to maintain cardiac output in the resting animal, but during exercise the cardiac output cannot be maintained. As a result, oxygen delivery to the muscles is inadequate to sustain exercise. This is an example of a failure of oxygen delivery resulting from inadequate blood flow.

Treatment. Treatment for atrial fibrillation in the horse is the administration of quinidine sulfate, which has a negative inotropic effect on the myocardium and slows atrioventricular conduction time. This allows the reestablishment of normal atrial and ventricular rhythm. The horse's heart rate will likely return to normal with treatment if there is no underlying cardiac disease. The horse is rested for at least a week, at which time training is reinstituted. Several months later the owner reports that the horse is still doing well.

This horse is a young adult, with no evidence of cardiac disease (e.g., murmur, signs of heart failure). Treating a horse with underlying cardiac disease has associated risks, and the horse may not return to normal heart rhythm. Therefore, in most cases, an echocardiogram is recommended before treatment to determine that the horse has no underlying cardiac disease. If present, any disease should be addressed first. In some horses the underlying disease is more significant, and treatment of fibrillation will not be attempted.

PRACTICE QUESTIONS

1. If 1 g of hemoglobin has an oxygen capacity of 1.36 mL of oxygen, what is the oxygen content of blood containing 10 g of hemoglobin when the blood Po_2 is 70 mm Hg?
   a. 13.6 mL/dL (vol%)
   b. 9.5 mL/dL (vol%)
   c. 6.8 mL/dL (vol%)
   d. 21 mL/dL (vol%)
   e. Cannot be calculated from the information provided.

2. An increase in pH of blood will:
   a. Shift the oxyhemoglobin dissociation curve to the right.
   b. Decrease P_{50}.
   c. Decrease the affinity of hemoglobin for oxygen.
   d. Decrease the oxygen capacity of the blood.
   e. Do all the above.

3. Which of the following decreases oxygen content but does not alter Pao_2 or percentage saturation of hemoglobin?
   a. Ascent to an altitude of 3500 m
   b. Polycythemia
   c. Breathing 50% oxygen
   d. Anemia
   e. Development of a large right-to-left shunt

4. All the following shift the oxyhemoglobin dissociation curve to the right except:
   a. An increase in pH.
   b. An increase in Pco_2.
   c. An increase in 2,3-DPG.
   d. An increase in temperature.

5. Quantitatively, the most important form of carbon dioxide (CO_2) in blood is:
   a. HCO_3^- produced in plasma.
   b. CO_2 dissolved in plasma.
   c. HCO_3^- produced in the erythrocyte.
   d. CO_2 dissolved in the erythrocyte.
   e. CO_2 combined with plasma proteins.

6. Oxygenation of hemoglobin in the lungs assists with the release of CO_2 from the blood because:
   a. Oxygen combines with the $-NH$ groups on hemoglobin and displaces CO_2 from carbamino compounds.
   b. Oxygen combines with HCO_3^- and produces CO_2.
   c. Oxygen facilitates the movement of chloride ions out of the erythrocyte.
   d. Oxygen combines with hemoglobin, making it a better buffer, which retains H^+.
   e. None of the above.

BIBLIOGRAPHY

Bartels H: Comparative physiology of oxygen transport in mammals, *Lancet* 2(7360):601–604, 1964.

Boron WF: Transport of oxygen and carbon dioxide in the blood. In Boron WF, Boulpaep EL, editors: *Medical physiology: a cellular and molecular approach*, ed 2, Philadelphia, 2009, Saunders.

Hlastala MP, Berger AJ: *Physiology of respiration*, ed 2, New York, 2001, Oxford University Press.

Kitchen H, Brett I: Embryonic and fetal hemoglobin in animals, *Ann N Y Acad Sci* 241(0):653–671, 1974.

Leff AR, Schumacker PT: *Respiratory physiology: basics and applications*, Philadelphia, 1993, Saunders.

Lekeux P, Art T: The respiratory system: anatomy, physiology and adaptations to exercise and training. In Hodgson DR, Rose RJ, editors: *The athletic horse: principles and practice of equine sports medicine*, Philadelphia, 1994, Saunders.

Prosser CL: Respiratory functions of blood. In Prosser CL, editor: *Comparative animal physiology*, ed 3, Philadelphia, 1973, Saunders.

CHAPTER 49
Control of Ventilation

KEY POINTS

1. Respiration is regulated to meet the metabolic demands for delivery of oxygen and removal of carbon dioxide.

Central control of respiration
1. Respiratory rhythmicity originates in the brainstem with inputs from higher centers.

Pulmonary and airway receptors
1. Pulmonary stretch receptors, irritant receptors, and juxtacapillary receptors can influence the rhythm of breathing.
2. Muscle spindle stretch receptors monitor the effort exerted by respiratory muscles.

Chemoreceptors
1. Hypoxia, acidosis, and hypercapnia are all potent stimuli for ventilation.

2. Peripheral chemoreceptors are the only receptors monitoring blood oxygen levels but also respond to changes in carbon dioxide and hydrogen ion concentrations.
3. The ventilatory response to carbon dioxide is mediated by central chemoreceptors.
4. Integrated breathing involves the central pattern generator, and inputs from chemoreceptors and vagal pulmonary afferents.
5. Ascent to high altitude is accompanied by a decrease in inspired oxygen tension and consequently by hypoxemia, which leads to an increase in ventilation.
6. During exercise, ventilation must increase because the tissues demand more oxygen and produce more carbon dioxide.

Respiration Is Regulated to Meet the Metabolic Demands for Delivery of Oxygen and Removal of Carbon Dioxide

During its daily activities, an animal varies its level of activity and can breathe air of varying composition and purity. To allow the respiratory system to respond to these different challenges, control mechanisms monitor (1) the chemical composition of the blood, (2) the effort being exerted by the respiratory muscles on the lungs, and (3) the presence of foreign materials in the respiratory tract. This information is integrated with the other nonrespiratory activities, such as thermoregulation, vocalization, parturition, and eructation, to produce a pattern of breathing that maintains gas exchange.

Figure 49-1 provides a diagram of feedback control for the respiratory system. The *central controller* generates the signals that regulate the activity of the respiratory muscles, which by contracting give rise to alveolar ventilation. Changes in alveolar ventilation affect blood gas tensions and pH, which are monitored by the *chemoreceptors*. These receptors send signals back to the central controller so that necessary adjustments can be made to ventilation. *Mechanoreceptors* in various parts of the respiratory system monitor the degree of stretch of the lungs and changes in the airways and vasculature. Stretch receptors *(proprioceptors)* in respiratory muscles monitor the effort of breathing.

CENTRAL CONTROL OF RESPIRATION

Respiratory Rhythmicity Originates in the Brainstem with Inputs from Higher Centers

Early attempts to understand the brain's role in the regulation of breathing indicated that rhythmic respiration originates in the medulla and pons of the brainstem but is also affected by other afferent information from the lungs, chemoreceptors, and elsewhere. After many years of investigation it is becoming clear that the apparently simple, in and out nature of breathing is the result of a complex neural network known as a *central pattern generator* (CPG) located in the brainstem. This CPG may actually involve rhythmic and nonrhythmic subnetworks that are modulated by inputs from peripheral and central chemoreceptors, pulmonary stretch receptors, and others (Figure 49-2). The status of these subnetworks is affected by sleep, wakefulness, and changes during early development. The CPG includes neurons in the *pontine respiratory group* (lateral parabrachial and Kolliker-Fuse areas) and several medullary areas especially the *Bötzinger* and *pre-Bötzinger complexes*, the retrotrapezoid nucleus (RTN), and the rostral ventral and caudal ventral respiratory groups (rVRG and cVRG, respectively) (Figure 49-3). A *dorsal respiratory group* of neurons located in the nucleus tractus solitarius relays information to the CPG from peripheral chemoreceptors, pulmonary stretch receptors, bronchial irritant receptors, and other visceral information.

The origin of rhythmic breathing is currently unknown. Pacemaker neurons have been identified in the pre-Bötzinger complex, but their role in normal breathing is unclear. Normal respiration *(eupnea)* seems to result from reciprocal inhibition of neuron groups in the CPG. During inhalation there is an increase in activity in the inspiratory neurons of the pre-Bötzinger group and rVRG that is associated with diaphragm and external intercostal contraction. This increased activity is further amplified by an increase in the chemical respiratory drive, such as hypoxia or hypercapnia. Termination of inspiration can be a result of vagal inputs from *pulmonary stretch receptors* or from a central pontine *off switch*. After vagotomy, the pontine off switch terminates

FIGURE 49-1 Feedback control diagram for the regulation of ventilation. The controller, which includes centers in the cerebrum and brainstem, drives the respiratory muscles that bring about ventilation. Changes in ventilation can cause changes in blood gas tensions (Pao_2, $Paco_2$) and pH that are monitored by central and peripheral chemoreceptors. Receptors in the lung detect the stretch in the lung tissues and the presence of materials in the lungs and airways. Proprioceptors in the respiratory muscles monitor the amount of effort being applied by the muscles. Pao_2, Arterial oxygen tension; $Paco_2$, arterial carbon dioxide tension.

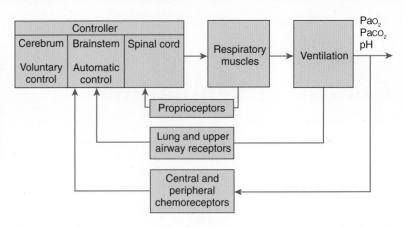

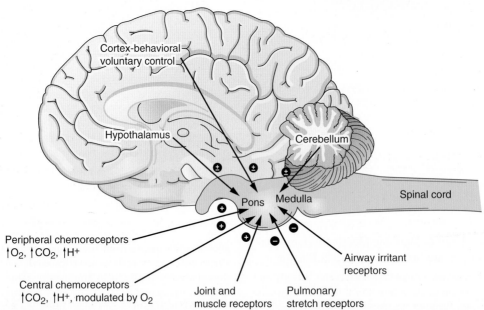

FIGURE 49-2 Overview of ventilatory control mechanisms. Respiratory rhythmicity originating in the medulla and pons is modulated by multiple inputs. Symbols: +, stimulatory; −, inhibitory; ±, stimulatory or inhibitory. Motor output to diaphragm, intercostal, and upper airway muscles not shown. (After Carroll JL, Agarwal A: Development of ventilatory control in infants, *Paediatr Respir Rev* 11(4):199–207, 2010.)

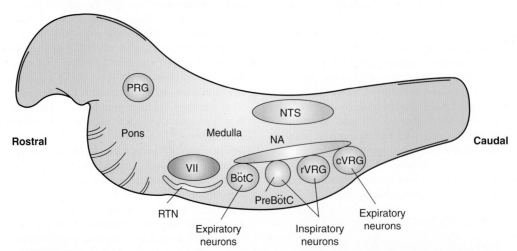

FIGURE 49-3 Diagram of the brainstem showing structures in the medulla and pons involved in the control of breathing. *BotC*, Bötzinger complex; *preBotC*, pre-Bötzinger complex; *cVRG*, caudal ventral respiratory group; *rVRG*, rostral ventral respiratory group; *NA*, nucleus ambiguus; *NTS*, nucleus tractus solitarius; *RTN*, retrotrapezoid nucleus/parafacial respiratory group; *PRG*, pontine respiratory group. VII, facial nucleus is shown for anatomical reference.

inhalation after a fixed time for inhalation, which is independent of chemical drive. When the vagus is intact, and thus signals from pulmonary stretch receptors are relayed to the brain, there is a complex interaction between the time for inhalation and the tidal volume. This interaction leads to a larger tidal volume and more rapid respiratory frequency when the chemical drive to breathe is increased.

When inhalation is terminated, inspiratory neurons are inhibited, and thus exhalation occurs passively as a result of the elastic recoil of the lung and chest wall. Activity in some inspiratory neurons (Bötzinger complex) early in exhalation leads to inspiratory muscle activity, which provides a "brake" on exhalation and regulates the rate of expiratory airflow. Later in exhalation, the braking is removed. During this latter part of exhalation, expiratory neurons may be activated (Bötzinger complex and cVRG) leading to expiratory (abdominal and internal intercostal) muscle contraction. When respiratory drive is low, this second phase of exhalation is initiated later than when drive is increased.

The rhythmic breathing just described is frequently overridden by demands from higher brain centers. Vocalization, parturition, swallowing, defecation, and many other activities require the active participation of the respiratory system.

PULMONARY AND AIRWAY RECEPTORS

Pulmonary Stretch Receptors, Irritant Receptors, and Juxtacapillary Receptors Can Influence the Rhythm of Breathing

The vagus nerve includes both myelinated and nonmyelinated afferent axons conveying sensory information from the lung. Myelinated axons originate from slowly adapting stretch receptors and *irritant receptors.* Slowly adapting stretch receptors are nerve endings associated with smooth muscle in the trachea and main bronchi, but to a lesser degree in the smaller intrapulmonary airways. They are stimulated by deformation of the wall of larger airways, as when intrathoracic airways are stretched during lung inflation. Because firing rates from these receptors increase progressively as the lung inflates, they are thought to be responsible for the inhibition of breathing caused by lung inflation *(Hering-Breuer reflex).* Termination of input from these receptors by vagotomy leads to a slowing of respiration and an increase in tidal volume. Slowly adapting stretch receptors may be responsible in part for adjustments in the rate and depth of respiration to minimize the work of the respiratory muscles.

Irritant receptors, or *rapidly adapting stretch receptors,* are thought to be myelinated nerve endings branching among epithelial cells in the larynx, trachea, large bronchi, and intrapulmonary airways. They are stimulated by mechanical deformation of the airways, such as the deformation that occurs during mechanical irritation of the airway surface. Irritant gases, dusts, mucus accumulations, histamine release, and a variety of other stimuli can also cause these receptors to respond. Stimulation of rapidly adapting irritant receptors leads to cough, bronchoconstriction, mucus secretion, and rapid, shallow breathing *(hyperpnea),* all of which are protective responses to clear irritant materials from the respiratory system. These receptors may initiate the sighs that are thought to redistribute pulmonary surfactant over the alveolar surface.

C fibers are located in the pulmonary interstitium close to pulmonary capillaries *(juxtacapillary receptors),* where they may monitor blood composition or the degree of distention of the interstitium. Similar fibers also occur in the walls of the airways.

C-fiber activation may be responsible for the increase in respiratory rate *(tachypnea)* that accompanies allergic, infectious, or vascular diseases.

In addition to intrapulmonary receptors, there are receptors located in the upper airway. Stimulation of receptors in the nasal cavity causes sniffing and sneezing, whereas stimulation of laryngeal and pharyngeal receptors may cause cough, apnea, or bronchoconstriction. Temperature receptors in the pharynx that are cooled by airflow alert the animal if there is insufficient airflow so that appropriate adjustments can be made by the inspiratory muscles to increase flow.

Muscle Spindle Stretch Receptors Monitor the Effort Exerted by Respiratory Muscles

The density of *muscle spindle stretch receptors* varies greatly in different respiratory muscles, and the effects of stimulating these receptors can vary with the anatomical location of the muscle group. The diaphragm has few muscle receptors, but intercostal muscles are well supplied with *tendon organs* and muscle spindles. In a reflexive manner, muscle receptors control the strength of respiratory muscle contraction and adjust the strength of contraction when ventilation is impeded, such as by airway obstruction.

CHEMORECEPTORS

Hypoxia, Acidosis, and Hypercapnia Are All Potent Stimuli for Ventilation

Chemoreceptors monitor oxygen, carbon dioxide, and hydrogen ion concentration (pH) at several sites in the body and provide some tonic drive to respiration during normal breathing. As blood composition departs from normal, changes in arterial carbon dioxide ($Paco_2$) and oxygen (Pao_2) tensions and pH produce major changes in ventilation.

Peripheral Chemoreceptors Are the Only Receptors Monitoring Blood Oxygen Levels but Also Respond to Changes in Carbon Dioxide and Hydrogen Ion Concentrations

Peripheral chemoreceptors include the carotid and aortic bodies, and their removal eliminates the respiratory response to hypoxia. The response to CO_2 and pH persists because these are also detected by *central chemoreceptors.*

The *carotid bodies* (Figure 49-4, *A*) are located close to the bifurcation of the internal and external carotid arteries, and the aortic bodies are located around the aortic arch. The latter appear to be most active in the fetus and of little importance in the adult. The *aortic bodies* are supplied by the vagus nerve, and the carotid bodies are supplied by a branch of the glossopharyngeal nerve. Fibers within the nerves supplying the peripheral chemoreceptors are primarily brainstem afferents, with a few parasympathetic and sympathetic efferent fibers to blood vessels.

The carotid bodies are small, nodular structures with extremely high blood flow per gram. This high blood flow to metabolism ratio allows the carotid bodies to obtain their oxygen needs from dissolved oxygen. Consequently, there is only a small arteriovenous difference in oxygen tension (Po_2) across the carotid bodies and no difference in hemoglobin saturation.

Carotid bodies contain several cell types. Type I cells, or *glomus cells,* synapse with afferent axons that transmit information back to the brain (see Figure 49-4, *B*). These glomus cells contain a variety of neurotransmitters, including catecholamines,

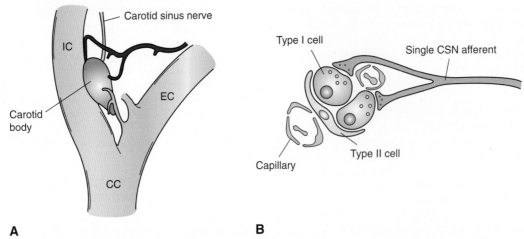

FIGURE 49-4 A, Cartoon of the carotid body located at the bifurcation of the common carotid artery *(CC)* into its external *(EC)* and internal *(IC)* branches. **B,** Cartoon of the basic cellular arrangement within the carotid body. Chemosensory CNS afferent fibers are in synaptic contact with transmitter-filled type I (glomus) cells. Clusters of type I cells are encapsulated by type II (sustentacular) cells, and the organ receives a rich capillary blood supply. (From Peers C, Wyatt CN, Evans AM: Mechanisms for acute oxygen sensing in the carotid body, *Respir Physiol Neurobiol* 174(3):292–298, 2010.)

especially *dopamine.* Glomus cells are most likely responsible for the *chemosensitivity* of the carotid bodies because they depolarize when Po_2 decreases. Alternatively, they may modify the chemosensitivity of the afferent nerve terminals. Type II cells, or *sustentacular cells,* support the axons and blood vessels that ramify within the carotid body.

When the carotid bodies are perfused with blood that has a low Po_2, high carbon dioxide tension (Pco_2), or low pH, firing rates in the carotid sinus nerve afferent fibers increase. As Pco_2 increases and pH decreases, there is an almost linear increase in ventilation. The response to Po_2 is nonlinear. Modest increases in firing rate and ventilation occur as Po_2 decreases from nonphysiological levels of 500 mm Hg down to 70 mm Hg. Further decreases cause a greater increase in ventilation, particularly at a Po_2 of less than 60 mm Hg, which is the Po_2 level at which hemoglobin begins to desaturate. Ventilation does not increase in response to either modest anemia or carbon monoxide (CO) poisoning, conditions that decrease the oxygen content of blood but not Pao_2. This is because Po_2 is more important than oxygen content as a stimulus to the carotid bodies.

Figure 49-5 shows possible mechanisms of chemosensitivity of the carotid bodies. Glomus cells are depolarized by hypoxemia. Depolarization involves potassium (K^+) channels and leads to an increase in intracellular calcium (Ca_i^{2+}). The latter causes release of neurotransmitters, primarily dopamine and acetylcholine, which activate the afferent nerve terminals. Hypercapnia (elevated Pco_2) and changes in blood pH also may release neurotransmitters by decreasing the pH in the glomus cells.

The Ventilatory Response to Carbon Dioxide Is Mediated by Central Chemoreceptors

The partial pressure of carbon dioxide in arterial blood ($Paco_2$) is tightly regulated and carbon dioxide is a potent stimulus to breathing. Increases in alveolar or brain Pco_2 of 2 mm Hg or less result in a 50% increase in ventilation while even greater increases in Pco_2 further stimulate ventilation but also cause a sensation of severe respiratory distress. Changes in $Paco_2$ and pH are detected by the peripheral chemoreceptors but it is also now well accepted

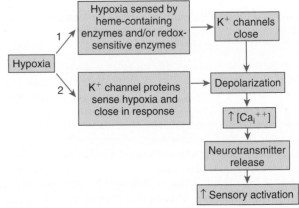

FIGURE 49-5 Hypothesized mechanisms of chemosensitivity in the carotid body. *1,* Hypoxia is sensed by enzymes in the glomus cell, leading to closure of potassium (K^+) channels, depolarization, and neurotransmitter release. *2,* Hypoxia is sensed directly by potassium channels, causing their closure. (Modified from Prabhaker NR: Oxygen sensing by the carotid body chemoreceptors, *J Appl Physiol* 88(6):2287–2295, 2000.)

that carbon dioxide, which is readily diffusible across the *blood-brain barrier,* exerts its main effects on breathing via increasing hydrogen ion concentration in the brain interstitial fluid. The decrease in brain pH activates chemosensitive neurons and perhaps even glial cells. Metabolic acidosis, by decreasing brain pH, has similar effects.

The precise location of the central chemoreceptors that affect breathing is unclear. Increases in ventilation can be provoked by local acid probing of several parts of the brain but this stimulus exerts a particularly strong effect on the ventral surface of the medulla, especially in the region of the retrotrapezoid nucleus (RTN). This is a small group of medullary glutaminergic neurons located under the facial motor nucleus and just rostral to the structures involved in the CPG. The RTN may be most critical for detecting the small carbon dioxide–induced changes in brain

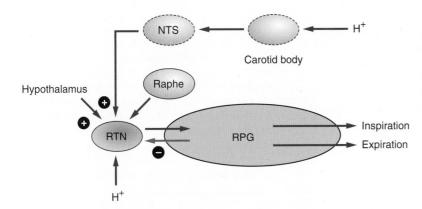

FIGURE 49-6 The possible role of chemosensitive neurons of the retrotrapezoid nucleus *(RTN)* in the regulation of breathing. RTN neurons regulate breathing according to the surrounding pH but also based on the strength of inputs received from the carotid bodies, other chemoreceptors in the hypothalamus, medullary raphe, and nucleus tractus solitarius *(NTS)*. RTN neurons provide a primary drive to the respiratory pattern generator *(RPG)* in the medulla, which can also exert negative feedback on the RTN. *Green,* Excitation; *red,* inhibition. (Modified from Guyenet PG, Stornetta RL, Bayliss DA: Central respiratory chemoreception, *J Comp Neurol* 518(19):3883–3906, 2010.)

interstitial fluid pH that regulate ventilation minute-by-minute, but other regions may be invoked when carbon dioxide becomes a noxious stimulus (Figure 49-6). This hypothesis is strongly supported by evidence from children and mice with a mutation in the transcription factor PhoxB2. The children develop central hypoventilation syndrome and the mice, in which there is loss of specific RTN neurons, lose respiratory sensitivity to carbon dioxide, have disordered breathing, and die early. The cells of the RTN are highly sensitive to acid and also vigorously activated by inputs from the carotid body. Under conditions of low respiratory drive, for example during sleep, the RTN may be the primary chemosensitive region, but it is also an integrating region for inputs from other chemosensitive tissues in the brain and especially the carotid body, and from higher brain centers, particularly the hypothalamus. The current hypothesis is that the RTN is a major driver of the CPG. During sleep, the RTN provides the major chemosensory drive but during wakefulness its function is more as a relay station for information from higher centers and other chemoreceptors.

Integrated Breathing Involves the Central Pattern Generator, and Inputs from Chemoreceptors and Vagal Pulmonary Afferents

The minute-by-minute pattern of breathing that veterinarians recognize as either normal or abnormal involves the integrated action of the CPG, chemoreceptors, the RTN, pulmonary vagal afferents, chest wall stretch receptors, and higher brain centers (see Figures 49-2, 49-3, and 49-6). The complexity of overall integrated control is illustrated by the following examples. (1) Normally, the peripheral chemoreceptors are responsible for 40% to 50% of tonic drive to ventilate. Because of this, administration of oxygen suppresses ventilation in healthy animals. (2) The changes in brain pH provide the fine control on breathing but this is greatly affected by information from the peripheral chemoreceptors, by sleeping and waking, and by body temperature. (3) *Metabolic acidosis,* which is a consequence of increased production of hydrogen ions without a change in Pa_{CO_2}, increases ventilation by activation of both central and peripheral chemoreceptors. (4) Pa_{CO_2} remains constant during aerobic exercise, in part because of an anticipatory increase in ventilation that begins at the start of exercise before CO_2 production has increased. (5) The sensation of difficult breathing and the altered respiratory frequency that accompany lung inflammation are consequences of increased input from pulmonary and airway C fibers, from carotid bodies, and from pulmonary and respiratory muscle stretch receptors.

Ascent to High Altitude Is Accompanied by a Decrease in Inspired Oxygen Tension and Consequently by Hypoxemia, Which Leads to an Increase in Ventilation

The fraction of oxygen in air is constant worldwide ($FiO_2 = 0.21$) but barometric pressure decreases with altitude. Consequently, the partial pressure of oxygen in air decreases. The ventilatory response to this hypoxia of altitude varies, depending on whether it lasts for less than an hour or for several days. The acute hypoxia experienced on first ascending to high altitude causes hyperventilation mediated through activation of the peripheral chemoreceptors. This decreases Pa_{CO_2} and increases pH, which dampens the response to hypoxia. After several hours to days, ventilation increases further and even remains somewhat elevated for hours to days after the hypoxic stimulus is removed.

This short-term *altitude acclimatization* involves three mechanisms. First, it can partly be explained by readjustments in blood pH back toward normal as the kidneys compensate by eliminating HCO_3^-. A second possible mechanism is readjustment of CSF pH toward normal. Third, the chemosensitivty of the glomus cells to hypoxia increases.

Longer-term adjustment to hypoxia involves (1) production of more erythrocytes (increased hematocrit) under the influence of erythropoietin, (2) decreased affinity of hemoglobin for oxygen because of increased concentrations of 2,3-diphosphoglycerate (2,3-DPG), (3) an increase in the pulmonary surface area available for diffusion, and (4) increased capillary density in muscle. These adjustments are sufficient to restore maximal oxygen consumption to normal at moderate (< 2000 meters) but not extreme altitudes.

During Exercise, Ventilation Must Increase Because the Tissues Demand More Oxygen and Produce More Carbon Dioxide

The increase in ventilation after the onset of exercise is initially rapid, then progresses more slowly, and, provided the workload remains constant, reaches a steady state after about 4 minutes. Although the *ventilatory response to exercise* has been well described, the reasons for the increase in ventilation are still not well understood.

The primary chemical stimuli for ventilation—Pa_{O_2}, Pa_{CO_2}, and pH—do not change in most animals during moderate aerobic exercise. This observation shows that the increase in ventilation is well matched to the needs of the tissues, and that other factors besides chemical drive increase ventilation during exercise. These factors are (1) reflexes originating from motion of the exercising limbs, (2) factors related to the increase in cardiac output, (3) thermoregulatory factors, and (4) psychogenic factors that anticipate the onset of exercise. Current exercise control theory favors *central command neurons* that are coupled through the RTN to the CPG neurons that regulate breathing. These command neurons control the responses of the respiratory and cardiovascular systems that are necessary to maintain oxygen delivery and carbon dioxide removal during exercise.

When the *anaerobic threshold* is exceeded, the production of lactic acid decreases blood pH. The latter stimulates an increase in ventilation, which leads to a decrease in $Paco_2$. In the horse, the increase in ventilation that can occur during exercise may be limited by respiratory rate being linked, one breath per stride, with stride frequency. During strenuous anaerobic exercise, the horse's arterial pH decreases progressively, although ventilation remains constant. When exercise ceases, ventilation increases further, presumably because the restrictions imposed by locomotion are removed.

CLINICAL CORRELATIONS

HYPOXEMIA WITH HYPERVENTILATION IN A SAMOYED PUPPY

History. An 8-month-old Samoyed is brought to you because it is reluctant to exercise. Ever since the owner obtained the puppy, she has noticed that its behavior is not "puppy-like"; it tires easily and prefers to sleep rather than play.

Clinical Examination. The puppy is not well grown. Even though the owner thinks it has been growing, for a Samoyed of 8 months of age the dog is rather small. When standing quietly in the examination room, the dog breathes normally, but when you call and it runs toward you, its respiratory rate increases and the dog begins to pant. At this point, you notice that the dog's tongue and gums have a distinct bluish tinge.

Before examining the dog further, you are already suspicious of a congenital cardiac anomaly. You suspect this because of the dog's age and history, and because it became cyanotic with minimal exercise.

Palpation of the dog shows that even though it is small, it is not thin. The major abnormalities are the cyanosis of the mucous membranes, an extremely elevated heart rate, and loud, abnormal cardiac sounds. A murmur is audible over the tricuspid valve area during systole. The murmur (grade 4/5) is tubulent enough to produce a palpable vibration on the chest wall. You explain your suspicions of a cardiac defect to the owner, and together you decide to request some studies to determine the nature of the defect.

An echocardiogram, which is performed to determine the type of cardiac anomaly, demonstrates a large opening between the left and right atria, caused by a patent foramen ovale. Before angiographic studies, an arterial blood gas sample is taken to determine the suitability of the dog for anesthesia; Pao_2 is 61 mm Hg and $Paco_2$ is 23 mm Hg.

Angiography is performed successfully. A catheter is floated into the right atrium of the dog, and dye is injected at this site. Some of the dye passes into the right ventricle, but a large portion passes from the right atrium into the left atrium and out into the systemic circulation.

Comment. The blood gas results are fairly typical for an animal with a major oxygen-exchange problem; this dog has a right-to-left

vascular shunt through a cardiac defect. A large amount of the mixed venous blood returning to the heart is bypassing the lungs, resulting in the low Pao_2. The Pao_2 is low enough to cause a major increase in ventilation by stimulating the peripheral chemoreceptors. This increase in ventilation causes excessive elimination of carbon dioxide, resulting in the reduced $Paco_2$. Perhaps ventilation could have increased further, but the low $Paco_2$ acting on the central chemoreceptor slows down the increase.

The echocardiogram and angiographic studies are indicative of a patent foramen ovale. Normally this would not result in right-to-left shunting of blood because the pressure in the left atrium is usually higher than that in the right atrium. However, this dog probably also has abnormalities of the tricuspid valve that cause a partial obstruction. This is sufficient to increase the pressure in the right atrium and cause blood to flow from right to left through the foramen ovale.

Treatment. The cardiac defect will need to be corrected surgically if the dog is to have any chance of life. Echocardiography is generally performed before angiography because it can better determine the extent of the abnormalities and is safer. An angiogram could then be performed, if necessary. With some limited cardiac anomalies, a transcatheter device can accomplish closure of the foramen ovale. However, if there are other tricuspid valve abnormalities, the method of repair may be altered.

HYPOVENTILATION IN AN ANESTHETIZED SAINT BERNARD

History. A 2-year-old Saint Bernard is brought to you for treatment of a fractured femur. You elect to place an intramedullary pin in the femur, and the dog will require anesthesia. The dog is anesthetized with a barbiturate, an endotracheal tube is placed, and the dog is allowed to breathe oxygen containing 2% halothane. It is not ventilated but is allowed to breathe the anesthetic mixture spontaneously. The veterinary technician observing the dog notices that the gas reservoir bag on the anesthesia machine is not moving much when the dog breathes. Therefore, she draws an arterial blood sample for measurement of blood gases. Measurement reveals a Pao_2 of 480 mm Hg and $Paco_2$ of 90 mm Hg (normal, 40 mm Hg).

Comment. This is an example of alveolar hypoventilation. Carbon dioxide is being eliminated by the lungs less quickly than it is produced by the tissues, so the $Paco_2$ is elevated above the normal value of 40 mm Hg. The lung's ability to exchange oxygen is not impaired; the measured Pao_2 is acceptable for a dog breathing oxygen. Hypoventilation is a common occurrence in anesthetized animals, particularly when anesthesia is induced with a barbiturate drug. Barbiturates depress the respiratory control centers and are prone to cause apnea. Also, the dog may have been slightly overdosed with barbiturate, resulting in the severe hypoventilation observed in this case. Hypoventilation occurs because the ventilatory response to CO_2 is depressed by anesthesia, and therefore a larger increase in $Paco_2$ than usual is required to trigger an increase in ventilation.

Treatment. The dog needs more alveolar ventilation to decrease $Paco_2$ and prevent respiratory acidosis. The additional ventilation can be supplied by squeezing the rebreathing bag on the anesthetic machine. When the dog recovers from anesthesia, its own respiratory control mechanisms will regulate alveolar ventilation and return $Paco_2$ to normal.

PRACTICE QUESTIONS

1. The rhythmicity of breathing is thought to originate in:
   a. The carotid body.
   b. The central pattern generator.
   c. The central chemoreceptor.
   d. Rapidly adapting pulmonary stretch receptors.
   e. None of the above.

2. Which of the following receptors have afferent nerve fibers in the glossopharyngeal nerve?
   a. Carotid bodies
   b. Slowly adapting pulmonary stretch receptors
   c. Aortic bodies
   d. Intercostal stretch receptors
   e. Rapidly adapting pulmonary stretch receptors

3. Which of the following statements correctly describes the carotid bodies?
   a. Carotid bodies can increase ventilation in response to low Pa_{O_2}, but not in response to an increase in Pa_{CO_2}.
   b. Carotid bodies have a low blood flow/metabolism ratio.
   c. Chemoreception is thought to occur in the sustentacular cells.
   d. Carotid bodies are located near the bifurcation of the internal and external carotid arteries.
   e. All the above.

4. The retrotrapezoidal neurons:
   a. Are highly sensitive to increases in hydrogen ion concentration.
   b. Receive inputs from the carotid body via the nucleus tractus solitarius.
   c. Provide input to the central pattern generator.
   d. Receive inputs from higher centers such as the hypothalamus.
   e. Are described by all of the above.

5. Which of the following is correct concerning the role of Pa_{CO_2} in breathing?
   a. Pa_{CO_2} exerts its effects on ventilation by changing the pH of brain interstitial fluid.
   b. Pa_{CO_2} has no effect on the carotid body.
   c. Pa_{CO_2} remains constant when hypoxia increases ventilation during the ascent to altitude.
   d. Pa_{CO_2} is much less important than Pa_{O_2} in regulation of breathing.
   e. None of the above.

6. Which of the following receptors are thought to initiate a cough in response to mechanical deformation of the airway?
   a. Juxtacapillary receptors
   b. Rapidly adapting stretch receptors
   c. Slowly adapting stretch receptors
   d. Intercostal tendon organs
   e. None of the above

BIBLIOGRAPHY

Burki NK, Lee LY: Mechanisms of dyspnea, *Chest* 138(5):1196–1201, 2010.
Carroll JL, Agarwal A: Development of ventilatory control in infants, *Paediatr Respir Rev* 11(4):199–207, 2010.
Guyenet PG, Stornetta RL, Bayliss DA: Central respiratory chemoreception, *J Comp Neurol* 518(19):3883–3906, 2010.
Hlastala MP, Berger AJ: *Physiology of respiration*, ed 2, New York, 2001, Oxford University Press.
Leff AR, Schumacker PT: *Respiratory physiology: basics and applications*, Philadelphia, 1993, Saunders.
Richerson GB, Boron WF: Control of ventilation. In Boron WF, Boulpaep EL, editors: *Medical physiology: a cellular and molecular approach*, ed 2, Philadelphia, 2009, Saunders.

CHAPTER 50

Nonrespiratory Functions of the Lung

KEY POINTS

Defense mechanisms of the respiratory system

1. The extensive, delicate gas exchange surface of an animal's lung is protected by a variety of specific and nonspecific defense mechanisms.
2. Particle deposition onto the mucociliary system depends on particle size and occurs by impaction, sedimentation, and diffusion.
3. The respiratory tract is lined by a mucociliary blanket consisting of a ciliated epithelium overlaid with a layer of mucus.
4. Alveolar macrophages scavenge particles deposited on the alveolar surface.
5. Cytokines and chemokines coordinate the defense mechanisms of the lung.

Pulmonary fluid exchange

1. The lung continuously produces lymph as a result of the net fluid movement from the pulmonary microvasculature into the pulmonary interstitium.
2. Pleural fluid originates by filtration from capillaries in the parietal pleura and is reabsorbed through stomata that connect to lymphatics.

Metabolic functions of the lung

1. The lung removes many hormones and toxins from the blood and inactivates many others.

DEFENSE MECHANISMS OF THE RESPIRATORY SYSTEM

The Extensive, Delicate Gas Exchange Surface of an Animal's Lung Is Protected by a Variety of Specific and Nonspecific Defense Mechanisms

When an animal is grazing in a rural environment, the air contains few potentially harmful particles and few pollutant gases. If the animal is intensively housed or is being transported, however, the air may be rife with organic dust that can contain particles of plant and animal origin, infectious agents such as bacteria and viruses, allergens such as spores and pollen, and other agents such as endotoxin. In addition, there may be pollutant gases such as ammonia, diesel fumes, oxides of nitrogen, and ozone. The respiratory system has a variety of defense mechanisms to protect it against these potentially injurious substances.

Nonspecific defenses (also referred to as *innate immunity*) immediately protect against many inhaled substances. Nonspecific defenses include the *mucociliary system, cough,* and the resident phagocytic cells in the alveoli. In addition, *toll-like receptors* on the surface of many types of cells recognize molecules that are common to many bacteria and fungi. When activated, these receptors immediately initiate mechanisms that lead to expression of proinflammatory cytokines.

Specific defenses involve the immune system and are directed against specific injurious agents, such as a bacterium. Specific defenses need several days to become activated and also have an immune memory that protects against future attacks by the same organism. Respiratory defense mechanisms, which may provide adequate protection to an animal in its pastoral environment, are frequently overwhelmed by the stresses of intensive housing and transportation. When these stresses are severe, for example, the stress produced by transportation, the animal can acquire an acute infectious disease such as pneumonia or pleuritis.

Noninfectious stresses that are less severe but more prolonged can lead to chronic airway diseases, such as heaves in horses.

Particle Deposition onto the Mucociliary System Depends on Particle Size and Occurs by Impaction, Sedimentation, and Diffusion

Harmful material is inhaled as aerosols suspended in air or as toxic gases. The term *aerosol* refers to collections of *particles* or *liquid droplets* that are small enough to remain suspended in air for a period of time. For epidemiological purposes, particles are generally described as inhalable or respirable. *Inhalable particulates* have a mass median diameter of 10 microns (micrometers, μm) or less (referred to as PM10). *Respirable particulates* have a diameter of 2.5 μm or less (PM2.5). Ample evidence now indicates that increases in the atmospheric concentrations of PM10 or PM2.5 are associated with worsening of respiratory disease and increased hospital admissions for cardiopulmonary disease in people. Intensively housed animals can be exposed to PM10 and PM2.5 concentrations as great as those known to cause respiratory disease in humans.

Particles and aerosols are removed from the air when they contact the moist epithelial surface of the tracheobronchial tree (Figure 50-1). The distance that particles and aerosols travel into the tracheobronchial tree depends on particle size. Larger particles, greater than 5 μm in diameter, contact the airway wall by inertial impaction. Inertial impaction occurs at the bends in the large airways because large particles traveling at high velocity have so much momentum that they fail to negotiate the turns. At sites of inertial impaction there are accumulations of lymphoid tissue, such as tonsils and bronchus-associated lymphoid tissue, presumably to orchestrate an immune response to the material landing on the airway surface. As airflow rates diminish deeper in the lung, particles 1 to 5 μm in diameter settle onto the walls

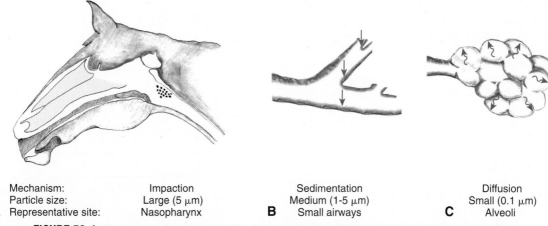

Mechanism: Impaction   Sedimentation   Diffusion
Particle size: Large (5 μm)   Medium (1-5 μm)   Small (0.1 μm)
A Representative site: Nasopharynx   **B** Small airways   **C** Alveoli

FIGURE 50-1 Mechanisms of particle deposition in the tracheobronchial tree. **A,** Large particles are deposited by impaction in the bends in the larger airways. **B,** Medium-sized particles are deposited in the smaller airways by sedimentation. **C,** Small particles contact the walls of the alveoli by diffusion.

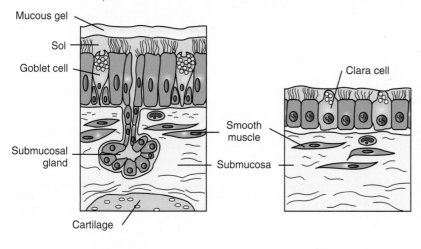

Mucous gel

Sol

Goblet cell

Clara cell

Smooth muscle

Submucosal gland

Submucosa

Cartilage

Bronchus   Bronchiole

FIGURE 50-2 Diagram of the epithelium and submucosa of a bronchus and bronchiole. In the bronchus the epithelium is pseudostratified columnar and includes goblet cells, ciliated cells, and basal cells that do not reach the surface of the epithelium. A bronchial gland is shown in the submucosa with its duct passing through the smooth muscle. Cartilage underlies the mucosal layer. The cilia beat within a sol layer over which is a layer of gel-type mucus. In the bronchiole the epithelium is cuboidal and is a mixture of ciliated cells and secretory Clara cells. Smooth muscle is shown in the submucosa. Bronchioles normally do not have submucosal glands or goblet cells, and there is no cartilage in their walls.

of the airways by sedimentation. The smallest particles reach the peripheral airways and alveoli, where they either contact the epithelial surface by diffusion or are exhaled again. Inhaled drugs must be delivered in a form with a particle size of 1 to 5 μm to be deposited onto the airway wall and remain in the lungs.

The deposition of particles within the respiratory tract is influenced by the pattern of breathing. Slow, deep breathing transports particles deep into the lung, whereas rapid, shallow breathing enhances inertial deposition in the larger airways. Bronchoconstriction enhances deposition of particles in more central airways, whereas bronchodilation favors more peripheral distribution.

The deposition of *toxic gases* depends on their solubility and concentration. Highly soluble gases, such as sulfur dioxide (SO_2), in low concentrations are removed by the nose, but in higher concentrations they can penetrate deeper into the lung. Less soluble gases can gain access to the alveoli. Toxic gases stimulate a variety of protective mechanisms, such as bronchospasm, mucus hypersecretion, coughing, and sneezing.

The Respiratory Tract Is Lined by a Mucociliary Blanket Consisting of a Ciliated Epithelium Overlaid with a Layer of Mucus

Particles deposited on the epithelial surface of the respiratory tract are transported on the *mucociliary escalator* to the pharynx, where they are then swallowed. The mucociliary system consists of sol and gel mucus layers overlying epithelial cells (Figure 50-2). The low-viscosity sol layer, in which the cilia beat, bathes the surface of the epithelial cells. On its forward stroke, the extended cilium catches the overlying viscous gel layer, in which inhaled particles are entrapped, and propels it up the tracheobronchial system or through the nasal cavity. Because the total surface area of the peripheral airways is so much greater than that of the trachea, differential rates of mucus transport are necessary in small and larger airways to prevent the accumulation of mucus in the trachea. Clearance rates and the beating frequency of cilia are slower in bronchioles than in bronchi and trachea. In large mammals, gravity also plays an important role in speeding mucociliary clearance. If a horse is prevented from lowering its head, the rate of mucociliary clearance is reduced. As a consequence, the number of bacteria in the trachea increases and this can lead to pneumonia. Inability of horses to lower their heads in a horse trailer may explain why transportation over long distances is the greatest risk factor for development of pneumonia in horses.

Respiratory tract mucus originates from several sites (see Figure 50-2). In respiratory bronchioles the conciliated *Clara cells* are a source of the fluid that lines the airways. In the larger airways, *goblet cells* produce mucous secretions. In the bronchi, submucosal *bronchial glands* produce both serous and mucous secretions. Secretion is under autonomic regulation. Throughout the respiratory tract, transepithelial movement of water and ions can change the composition of the mucus layer. Ion and fluid exchange is assisted by microvilli on the surface of epithelial cells.

Changes in the amount, composition, and viscosity of mucus occur in response to many stimuli and can be the cause or the result of respiratory disease. Normal airway epithelia regulate the rates of Na^+ absorption and Cl^- secretion to regulate the depth of the mucous layer for optimal ciliary function. A change in the depth or viscosity of the sol layer impairs ciliary function, and changes in the viscoelastic properties of the gel layer alter clearance rates. Increased viscoelasticity and decreased clearance can be caused by an increased amount of deoxyribonucleic acid (DNA) in mucus. Decreased clearance occurs during bacterial infections of the lung when both bacterial DNA and neutrophil DNA are present in mucus.

Coughing is part of the clearance mechanism of the respiratory tract and is initiated by stimulation of *subepithelial irritant receptors,* which are most numerous in the larger bronchi. Receptors can be stimulated by the mechanical deformation that results from foreign bodies or excessive amounts of material such as mucus on the epithelial surface. The cough reflex becomes hyperresponsive when the air passages are inflamed and respiratory tract epithelium is injured (e.g., by viral infections). Cough is effective in clearing mucoid secretions from the intrathoracic trachea and large bronchi, but it does not assist in removing mucus from the more peripheral bronchi and bronchioles.

Alveolar Macrophages Scavenge Particles Deposited on the Alveolar Surface

Macrophages, which constitute the majority of cells in the alveolar lining fluids, are the principal resident phagocytes in the normal lung. Macrophages originate in bone marrow as monocytes and differentiate during their passage from the blood into the alveolus, where their turnover time is in days. Surfactant proteins, complement, opsonins, and lysozymes in respiratory tract secretions assist macrophages in the killing and removal of viable particulates, such as bacteria. When phagocytized, particles are destroyed or transported out of the lung by the macrophage. Some macrophages enter the mucociliary system directly from the alveolus; others traverse the alveolar wall and enter the lymphoid tissues associated with the airways. In the lymphoid tissue, macrophages are antigen-presenting cells (APCs) and thus play a critical role in orchestrating the lung's immune responses.

Macrophages have adapted to the high oxygen levels of the alveolus, and their role as phagocytes is depressed by hypoxia. Macrophage function is also suppressed by endogenous glucocorticoids that are released from the adrenal glands at times of stress and by synthetic corticosteroids that are used to relieve inflammation (e.g., in arthritis). Stress-induced suppression of macrophage function contributes to respiratory disease in animals transported for long distances. In addition, excessive administration of synthetic corticosteroids can make animals more susceptible to bacterial infections of the lung. Viral infections also suppress macrophage function; this occurs approximately 7 days after virus inoculation (Figure 50-3) and contributes to the secondary bacterial infections that usually follow viral respiratory disease.

Alveolar macrophages are a first line of defense. When large numbers of particles are inhaled, other phagocytes from the blood, particularly *polymorphonuclear neutrophils* (PMNs), assist the macrophage. Toxic *oxygen radicals* and *proteolytic enzymes* are

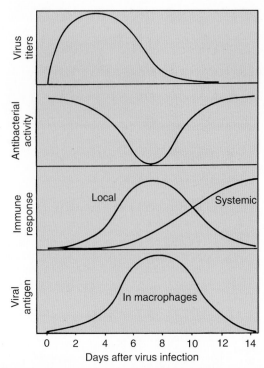

FIGURE 50-3 Effects of viral infection on antibacterial activity of alveolar macrophages. Antibacterial activity is depressed 7 days after experimental viral infection. At this time, the viral antigen is located in the macrophages, which are damaged by the local immune response to the virus. (From Jakab GT: Viral-bacterial interactions in respiratory tract infections: a review of the mechanisms of virus-induced suppression of pulmonary anti-bacterial defenses. In Loan RW, editor: *Bovine respiratory disease: a symposium,* College Station, Tex, 1984, Texas A&M University Press.)

released by phagocytic cells to break down invading bacteria, but they may also damage the lung tissue in the process. Protease inhibitors (e.g., α_1-antitrypsin) and antioxidants (e.g., glutathione peroxidase, ascorbic acid) protect the lung from its own defense mechanisms.

Cytokines and Chemokines Coordinate the Defense Mechanisms of the Lung

When the lung is injured by infectious agents, an allergic response, or inhalation of toxic particles or gases, an inflammatory process is elicited. *Cytokines* and *chemokines* are two similar groups of proteins that are produced and released by macrophages, lymphocytes, epithelial and endothelial cells, and various other cells involved in the inflammatory process. The roles of cytokines and chemokines are to attract inflammatory cells to the site of injury and to provide a means for communication between the cells involved in the inflammatory process. They also are involved in the orchestration of tissue remodeling to promote healing.

For example, physical injury to the lung epithelium or the presence of bacteria in the lung causes the release of cytokines *tumor necrosis factor* (TNF) and *interleukin-1* (IL-1) from macrophages. These cytokines act to draw neutrophils into the injured area of the lung. In addition, TNF and IL-1 initiate mechanisms that cause epithelial cells (e.g., alveolar type II) and endothelial cells to produce the chemokine *interleukin-8* (IL-8), which prolongs the inflammatory response and is also a potent chemoattractant of inflammatory cells. Injured bronchial epithelial cells are also capable of producing IL-1, IL-6, granulocyte-macrophage colony-stimulating factor (GM-CSF), and IL-8, all of which have roles in the cascade of inflammation. Other cytokines (IL-4, IL-5, IL-9, IL-13) are involved in allergic inflammation.

PULMONARY FLUID EXCHANGE

The Lung Continuously Produces Lymph as a Result of the Net Fluid Movement from the Pulmonary Microvasculature into the Pulmonary Interstitium

In the lung, as in other organs, there is continual movement of water and solutes from the capillary bed into the lung interstitium. The hydrostatic and osmotic forces governing fluid movement are the same as those in other organs, but because the lung vasculature operates at low pressure, the magnitude of the forces is different. About 60% of fluid filtration takes place from alveolar capillaries, 15% from extra-alveolar small arteries, and 20% from extra-alveolar veins.

Figure 50-4 represents a capillary in the alveolar septum. Fluid filtration normally occurs between the capillary and the interstitial tissue on the thick side of the alveolar septum, where a layer of interstitium is interposed between the endothelium and the epithelial basement membrane. Fluid filtering from pulmonary capillaries does not accumulate in this interstitium because the latter has a low compliance as a result of *proteoglycan* links between structures. On the thin side of the septum, interstitial tissue is absent because the capillary endothelium shares a basement membrane with the alveolar epithelium. Fluid movement out of the capillary is thought to occur between endothelial cells, but these gaps are too small to allow passage of *macromolecules*. The latter probably pass through endothelial cells in vesicles, which may fuse to form *transendothelial channels*. Another possibility is that these large molecules pass through gaps between cells that appear when the endothelia contract and become more permeable under the influence of mediators such as histamine. The alveolar epithelium is less permeable than the capillary endothelium, and therefore fluid does not leak into the alveoli unless the epithelium is damaged or unless there is considerable fluid accumulation in the interstitium, which occurs rapidly once proteoglycan bridges disrupt.

Forces described in *Starling's equation* govern the movement of fluid across the endothelium:

$$Qf = Kf \times [(Pcap - Pif) - \sigma(\pi cap - \pi if)]$$

Where Qf is the amount of fluid flowing per minute; Kf is the capillary filtration coefficient; $Pcap$ is capillary hydrostatic pressure; Pif is interstitial fluid hydrostatic pressure; πcap and πif are capillary and interstitial colloid osmotic (oncotic) pressures, respectively; and σ is the colloid *reflection coefficient* (see Chapter 23). Figure 50-4 shows average values for vascular and interstitial pressures.

When values shown in Figure 50-4 are inserted into Starling's equation, the net force is positive and favors fluid filtration from the capillaries to the interstitium of the lung. The fluid that is continuously filtered from capillaries does not accumulate in the low compliance interstitium of the alveolar septum but moves toward the perivascular and peribronchial tissues, where *lymphatic vessels* are located. Fluid transport out of the lung along lymphatic vessels, which is aided by lymphatic vasomotion and valves, maintains a low interstitial fluid pressure in the perivascular/peribronchial space.

Fluid filtration from the pulmonary capillaries varies with changes in vascular permeability and with hydrostatic and oncotic pressures. Increases in capillary hydrostatic pressure occur during exercise and in animals with left-sided heart failure. These elevated pressures result in an increased fluid flux into the interstitium. During exercise, the lymphatic vessels remove this filtered fluid so rapidly that there is no net fluid accumulation. This is particularly amazing in the intensely exercising horse in which pulmonary capillary pressure exceeds 60 mm Hg and fluid flux from the pulmonary capillaries has been reported to reach 8 liters/min. Similarly, in heart failure, lymphatics accommodate large increases in fluid flux. As fluid transfer across capillaries increases even further, excess fluid accumulates around the bronchi and large blood vessels in the compliant peribronchial and perivascular spaces. Clinically evident *pulmonary edema* occurs once lymphatic capacity is exceeded and the proteoglycan bridges in the alveolar septum break. The latter greatly increases the compliance of this region and allows even greater fluid fluxes. The fluid probably enters the air spaces across the alveolar epithelial cells or at the level of the bronchioles. The foaming fluid typical of clinical pulmonary edema results from the mixing of air, edema fluid, and surfactant within the airways.

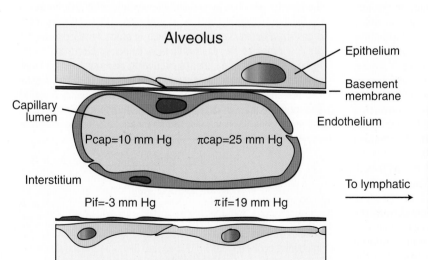

FIGURE 50-4 Diagrammatic representation of a capillary in the alveolar septum. *Top,* on the "thin" side of the septum, capillary endothelium and alveolar epithelium share a basement membrane. *Bottom,* on the "thick" side of the septum, endothelium and epithelium are separated by a layer of interstitial tissue. Values for capillary and interstitial fluid hydrostatic pressures (Pcap and Pif) and oncotic pressures (πcap and πif) are shown.

Increased fluid filtration and pulmonary edema can also result from a decrease in plasma oncotic pressure, which is a result of *hypoproteinemia*. Hypoproteinemia can be caused either by starvation or by the overvigorous administration of intravenous fluids that dilute the plasma proteins. Increased vascular permeability occurs in many inflammatory lung diseases, such as pneumonia. This results from the effects of neutrophil products, probably oxygen radicals, on the endothelium. Protein-rich fluid leaks into the interstitium, elevating interstitial fluid oncotic pressure and causing osmotic attraction of water into the interstitium from the vasculature.

Pleural Fluid Originates by Filtration from Capillaries in the Parietal Pleura and Is Reabsorbed Through Stomata That Connect to Lymphatics

The *pleural space* contains a small volume of fluid that turns over about every hour. The continual uptake of *pleural fluid* by lymphatics helps to keep the visceral and parietal surfaces in close apposition. The protein content of pleural fluid is normally low (1.5 g/dL), but the net Starling forces favor filtration of fluid into the pleural space. Under normal conditions, fluid enters the pleural space by filtration from capillaries in the parietal pleura and is removed by lymphatics that communicate directly with the pleural space through holes (stomata) in the surface of the parietal pleura. The density of *stomata* is particularly high on the tendinous part of the diaphragm and the mediastinal side of the pleural cavity. Fluid accumulates in the pleural cavity when capillary pressures increase or when *vascular permeability* is increased by inflammation of the pleura (pleuritis). If fibrin accumulates in the pleural space, lymphatic vessels may be obstructed, and drainage of the pleural space may be impaired. As a result, large volumes of fluid can accumulate between the lungs and chest wall, impeding ventilation and necessitating drainage by the use of tubes.

METABOLIC FUNCTIONS OF THE LUNG

The Lung Removes Many Hormones and Toxins from the Blood and Inactivates Many Others

Because it receives the total cardiac output, the pulmonary capillary bed with its vast endothelial surface is ideally placed to cleanse the blood of substances produced in other parts of the body. The endothelial cell surface, which is enlarged by projections and by depressions known as *caveolae,* is the site of many enzymes involved in the uptake and metabolism of vasoactive substances. *Serotonin* is almost totally removed by uptake into endothelial cells, where it is degraded by monoamine oxidase. *Norepinephrine* is also removed to some degree, but *acetylcholine, epinephrine,* and *histamine* are not removed. The peptides *bradykinin* and angiotensin are metabolized by angiotensin-converting enzyme (ACE) located on the endothelial surface. Bradykinin is inactivated, whereas angiotensin I is converted into angiotensin II. The lung degrades the majority of *prostaglandin* E_2 and prostaglandin F_2, but prostacyclin (prostaglandin I_2) is unaffected. *Leukotrienes* are broken down by neutrophils, which are numerous in the pulmonary circulation.

Many exogenous toxic substances are also removed from the blood by the pulmonary endothelium. This process at times can cause severe lung injury. For example, the toxins from *Crotalaria* species of plants can cause smooth muscle hypertrophy in the pulmonary arterioles, which leads to pulmonary hypertension.

CLINICAL CORRELATIONS

PLEURITIS IN A THOROUGHBRED HORSE

History. At your practice in California, you are asked to examine a 3-year-old Thoroughbred stallion, which arrived the previous day by truck from a racetrack in New York. On arrival the horse appeared depressed. This morning the stallion refused to eat or drink and was breathing rapidly. The owner reports that in New York the horse was at a racetrack where there was much through-traffic of young horses, many of which were coughing.

Clinical Examination. On arrival at the farm, you meet the anxious owner, who leads you to a stall where the Thoroughbred is standing with its elbows slightly abducted, its head lowered, its nostrils flared, and an anxious look in its eye. The grain and hay from the morning's feed are untouched. The horse has a respiratory rate of 65 (normal, 12 to 20). On further questioning, the owner reports that the horse looked much as it does now when it arrived from New York, but he thought it was just tired from the truck ride. The trucker reported that the horse drank little when it was offered water on its 3-day trip across country and had only nibbled at its hay. It was in the truck with four other younger horses. The condition of these horses is unknown.

You examine the horse and find that it is febrile, and its pulse rate as well as its respiratory rate is greatly elevated. The horse becomes anxious when approached and particularly when hands are laid and pressed on the thoracic cage. The horse's mucous membranes are a dull red. Auscultation of the abdomen reveals minimal gastrointestinal sounds, and there is no evidence of feces in the stall. You listen to the respiratory system and note louder, harsher sounds than normal in the trachea and in the dorsal part of the lung bilaterally. However, the ventral part of the lung is notably silent bilaterally.

You elect to take thoracic radiographs and notice that there is fluid accumulation in the ventral half of the thorax, obscuring the cardiac shadow and much of the lung. In the dorsal part of the thorax, the lung tissue has a number of radiographic densities that have a fluffy appearance, suggesting they are in the alveolar spaces. With the assistance of ultrasound, a teat cannula is placed in the right pleural cavity to drain the pleural fluid, which is foul smelling and purulent; 10 L are removed. This is repeated on the left side, with similar results. Repeat radiographs then reveal that the alveolar densities extend into the ventral part of the thorax.

Bacterial cultures of the pleural fluid grow an anaerobic organism *(Bacteroides fragilis),* which is probably responsible for the foul smell of the pleural fluid. A complete blood cell count reveals a decreased number of circulating neutrophils and a large number of immature forms of neutrophils (bands). This is an indication that the neutrophil resources of the body are being depleted and the bone marrow is putting out immature forms. Presumably, the neutrophils are being sequestered within the lung and pleural cavity.

Comment. The history and clinical findings in this horse are fairly typical of a case of pleuropneumonia. In New York the horse was exposed to other animals that were coughing, probably as a result of a viral infection, such as equine influenza or equine rhinopneumonitis. Respiratory viruses generally impair the defense mechanisms of the lung in two ways. First, they denude the tracheobronchial epithelium of cilia and therefore reduce mucociliary clearance of the airways. Second, they impair macrophage function. This combination of events results in the deposition of bacteria in the lung and failure of the lung to remove them by either the ciliary system or the macrophages. As a result, the bacteria multiply. The stress of shipping makes the situation even worse. Stress probably resulted in the release of corticosteroids from the adrenal gland, and this further suppressed the defense mechanisms of the lung. Failure to drink leads to dehydration, which can make mucus more difficult to clear. Keeping the horse's head elevated during transport also impairs mucociliary function. As a result of these events, the horse acquired a bacterial infection of the lung, which resulted in the migration of large numbers of neutrophils into the alveoli. This resulted in the fluffy densities on the radiograph.

When the infection spread to the pleural cavity, neutrophils migrated to this region as well. The release of neutrophil products designed to kill bacteria caused extensive damage to the membranes of the alveolar epithelium, pulmonary capillaries, and pleural capillaries. The protein that leaked into the alveolar spaces, interstitium of the lung, and pleural cavity raised the osmotic pressure within these regions. This resulted in the movement of fluid from the vascular space into the alveolar spaces, interstitium, and pleural cavity. Within the pleural cavity, the fluid accumulates ventrally because of gravity, and it is probably this accumulation of fluid that results in the absence of lung sounds in the ventral part of the thorax.

Treatment. Chest tubes are placed in the pleural cavity bilaterally so that the fluid can be drained repeatedly. The horse is given high levels of antibiotics and a prostaglandin synthetase inhibitor, flunixin meglumine, which should reduce the inflammation and make the horse more comfortable. However, in view of the degree of alveolar involvement, the presence of an anaerobic organism, and the large amount of fluid in the pleural cavity, the prognosis for this horse is not good.

MITRAL INSUFFICIENCY IN A DOG

History. A 12-year-old cocker spaniel is brought to a veterinary hospital because of a recent deterioration in its condition. The dog has been a faithful pet and has always enjoyed exercising with its owner, but over the past few months the owner has noticed an increasing reluctance to exercise. The dog has also coughed, especially when it gets up from resting. In the past few days the dog has refused to leave the house and has eaten little. The owner has noticed that the cough is much more frequent than previously and seems to be moist.

Clinical Examination. You have examined this dog on many occasions, and it has always been friendly, but when you walk into the examination room, the dog greets you with only a modest tail wag. It stands with its head down and its tongue hanging out; it is panting. It walks reluctantly toward you when you call it. The dog was formerly fat but is now in about normal flesh, so over the past few months it has lost some weight.

You lift the dog onto the examination table and begin by looking at the mucous membranes, which appear normal in color. The dog's temperature is normal. The dog is panting, which makes auscultation of the chest difficult, but on the occasions when the dog breathes without panting, you notice some increased sounds in the trachea and in all the lung fields, which sound like fluid bubbling within the air spaces of the lungs. The heart rate is

dramatically increased, and a loud murmur is audible over the mitral area during systole. You tell the owner that you suspect that the dog has a heart problem, which is leading to the accumulation of fluid in the lungs.

You take chest radiographs and an arterial blood sample for measurement of blood gas tensions. The chest radiograph shows an enlarged heart, particularly the left ventricle. The lungs are diffusely more dense than normal, and the densities have a fluffy appearance, which suggests that they are in the alveoli. There is also increased density along the walls of the major airways. Arterial oxygen tension (Pao_2) is 70 mm Hg, and arterial carbon dioxide tension ($Paco_2$) is 30 mm Hg (normal Pao_2 = 85 to 95 mm Hg, $Paco_2$ = 35 to 45 mm Hg). The radiographs confirm your suspicion of a heart problem. The left side of the heart is enlarged, which suggests left-sided heart failure.

An echocardiogram is performed to assess further the mitral valve regurgitation. The echocardiogram demonstrates thickening of the septal leaflet as well as the lateral leaflet. There is a flail of the mitral valve into the atria during ventricular systole. The left ventricle appears dilated, and left ventricular contractility is decreased.

Comment. Left-sided heart failure is accompanied by mitral valve insufficiency, and thus blood leaking back into the left atrium during systole creates a murmur. The elevation in left atrial pressure as a result of mitral regurgitation is leading to increased pressure in the pulmonary veins and capillaries. The increased pulmonary capillary hydrostatic pressure causes fluid filtration into the interstitium and now into the alveolar air spaces. This condition has likely been progressing for some time, and only when it became severe enough for fluid to accumulate in the air spaces of the lung did the owner notice the deterioration in the dog's condition.

The hypoxemia is a result of ventilation/perfusion mismatching because of accumulation of fluids within the alveolar spaces. These fluid-filled spaces are still perfused, but the blood passing through this region does not pick up a sufficient amount of oxygen. This results in hypoxemia. The hypoxemia stimulates ventilation, and the increase in total ventilation to the lung is sufficient to eliminate more carbon dioxide than normal, so $Paco_2$ is 30 mm Hg rather than the normal level of 40 mm Hg.

Treatment. The dog is treated with a diuretic and a digitalis glycoside. The diuretic causes fluid elimination by the kidneys, which reduces vascular volume and intravascular pressures and therefore reduces the amount of fluid being filtered into the lung. Over time this leads to resolution of the edema. The digitalis glycoside increases the contractility of the heart and thus the dog's cardiac output, which improves its ability to exercise.

PRACTICE QUESTIONS

1. Particles greater than 5 μm in diameter are deposited in the respiratory tract by:
   a. Inertial deposition in small airways.
   b. Sedimentation in airways.
   c. Diffusion in the alveoli.
   d. Inertial deposition in large airways.
   e. Sedimentation in the alveoli.

2. The mucociliary system:
    a. Consists of a gel layer in which cilia beat, overlaid by a sol layer that entraps particles.
    b. Is restricted to the nasal cavity and trachea and does not extend into the bronchi.
    c. Consists in part of mucus produced by goblet cells in the respiratory bronchioles and by Clara cells in the trachea.
    d. Has a more rapid transport rate in the trachea than in the bronchioles.
    e. Lacks ciliated cells in the bronchioles, so mucus must be pulled into the larger airways by viscous drag.

3. Phagocytosis of inhaled particles:
    a. Is generally by type II alveolar cells.
    b. Can always be accomplished by alveolar macrophages.
    c. Sometimes requires both macrophages and neutrophils.
    d. Is accentuated by alveolar hypoxia.
    e. None of the above.

4. Movement of fluid between the pulmonary capillaries and lung lymphatic vessels:
    a. Does not occur in a normal animal.
    b. Is accentuated by an increase in capillary hydrostatic pressure.
    c. Is accentuated by an increase in capillary oncotic pressure.
    d. Occurs by way of the alveolar surface.
    e. Is facilitated by a positive pressure in the peribronchial spaces of the bronchovascular bundle.

5. Which of the following occurs as a result of enzymes localized on the pulmonary endothelium?
    a. Conversion of angiotensin I to angiotensin II
    b. Conversion of angiotensinogen to angiotensin I
    c. Release of renin
    d. Conversion of renin to angiotensin II
    e. None of the above

BIBLIOGRAPHY

Chambers LA, Rollins BM, Tarran R: Liquid movement across the surface epithelium of large airways. *Respir Physiol Neurobiol* 159(3):256–270, 2007.

Leff AR, Schumacker PT: *Respiratory physiology: basics and applications*, Philadelphia, 1993, Saunders.

Lekeux P, Art T: The respiratory system: anatomy, physiology and adaptations to exercise and training. In Hodgson DR, Rose RJ, editors: *The athletic horse: principles and practice of equine sports medicine*, Philadelphia, 1994, Saunders.

Miserocchi G: Mechanisms controlling the volume of pleural fluid and extravascular lung water, *Eur Respir Rev* 18(114):244–252, 2009.

CHAPTER 51

Fetal and Neonatal Oxygen Transport

KEY POINTS

1. The fetus depends on the placenta for the exchange of gas, nutrients, and metabolic byproducts.
2. The efficiency of gas exchange at the placenta depends on the species-variable arrangement of fetal and maternal blood vessels.
3. The fetal circulation mixes oxygenated and deoxygenated blood at several points, so the fetus exists in a state of hypoxemia.
4. Fetal oxygen transport is assisted by fetal hemoglobin, which has a high affinity for oxygen.
5. The lung develops in three stages, and pulmonary surfactant must be present at birth.
6. At or shortly after birth, umbilical vessels rupture, pulmonary vascular resistance decreases, and the foramen ovale and ductus arteriosus close.

The Fetus Depends on the Placenta for the Exchange of Gas, Nutrients, and Metabolic Byproducts

From conception until birth, the *embryo* and *fetus* depend on the mother for a supply of oxygen and nutrients and for removal of carbon dioxide and other metabolic byproducts. The embryo exchanges these substances by diffusion through the uterine fluids. As the *conceptus* increases in size, the specialized exchange organ, known as the *placenta,* becomes essential. The placenta brings maternal and fetal blood into close apposition over a large surface area that is provided by a network of capillaries.

The gross appearance of the placenta of different species varies widely. In horses and pigs the placenta is *diffuse* and covers most of the uterine epithelium. In ruminants the placenta has rows of discrete circular-to-oval *cotyledons* that are attached to approximately 100 highly vascularized *caruncles* in the uterine epithelium. In dogs the placenta is *zonary,* forming a circular band around the *allantochorion* of the puppy. Table 51-1 lists types of placentation for different species.

In addition to differing in the amount of uterine surface to which they are attached, placentas also differ in the number of layers of cells that separate the maternal and fetal blood (see Table 51-1). In horses, pigs, sheep, and cows the fetal *chorion* is applied to the maternal uterine epithelium (*epitheliochorial* placentation), whereas in cats and dogs the chorion is applied to the endothelium of maternal vessels (*endotheliochorial* placentation); in rodents and most primates the chorion invades the uterine mucosa and erodes the maternal capillaries, so it becomes bathed by maternal blood (*hemochorial* placentation).

The Efficiency of Gas Exchange at the Placenta Depends on the Species-Variable Arrangement of Fetal and Maternal Blood Vessels

The exchange of gases and other substances across the placenta is determined by several factors, including the amount of surface apposition between fetal and maternal tissues and the number of layers of cells separating fetal and maternal blood. However, a major factor determining exchange is the arrangement of fetal and maternal blood vessels within the small, interdigitating villi of the placenta (Figure 51-1). *Countercurrent* flow of maternal and fetal blood provides the most efficient exchange and allows equilibration of fetal and maternal arterial gas tensions. *Concurrent* flow of fetal and maternal blood allows fetal vessels to equilibrate with the maternal venous gas tensions. In *crosscurrent* and *pool* types of equilibrators, fetal capillaries loop down to maternal vessels or into a pool of maternal blood. No simple model easily describes these types of exchangers. It is likely that several different arrangements of vessels are found in the placentas of all species, but some seem to have more of the characteristics of countercurrent exchangers, and others have those of venous equilibrators.

Figure 51-2 shows the arrangement of vessels in the *microcotyledon* of the horse, a species in which fetal and maternal blood flow is primarily countercurrent. The cotyledonary placenta of sheep functions as a venous equilibrator, whereas the hemochorial placenta of the rabbit seems to be a countercurrent exchanger.

Placental gas exchange has been best studied in the sheep (Figure 51-3). Maternal blood enters the uterus through the uterine artery with an oxygen tension (Po_2) of 80 mm Hg and leaves through the uterine vein with a Po_2 of 50 mm Hg. Some of the blood entering the uterus supplies the myometrium and endometrium, but most participates in gas exchange in the cotyledon. Fetal arterial blood reaches the placenta through the umbilical artery and enters the cotyledon with a Po_2 of 24 mm Hg. Placental gas exchange occurs, and the blood leaving the placenta in the umbilical veins has a Po_2 of only 32 mm Hg. This is because the sheep placenta is a venous equilibrator, so the maximal possible Po_2 would be 50 mm Hg. However, this maximum is not reached because venous blood, which has provided nutrient blood flow to the chorion, dilutes the better-oxygenated blood draining from the cotyledon. The countercurrent exchanger of the horse is apparently more efficient because umbilical venous Po_2 averages 48 mm Hg.

TABLE 51-1 Placentation in Domestic Mammals

Species	Classification	
	Gross	Histological
Horse	Diffuse	Epitheliochorial
Pig	Diffuse	Epitheliochorial
Cow	Cotyledonary	Epitheliochorial
Sheep	Cotyledonary	Epitheliochorial
Goat	Cotyledonary	Epitheliochorial
Dog	Zonary	Endotheliochorial
Cat	Zonary	Endotheliochorial
Rabbit	Discoid	Hemochorial
Guinea pig	Discoid	Hemochorial

The amount of placenta available for exchange partly determines the ultimate size of the fetus. If uterine caruncles are surgically removed from sheep so that there are fewer sites for formation of fetal cotyledons, the full-term weight of lambs is reduced. The diffuse placenta of the horse apparently can support only one full-size fetus. One foal in a set of twins usually dies in utero or is very small. It is rare for horse twins to survive to term and be of equal size.

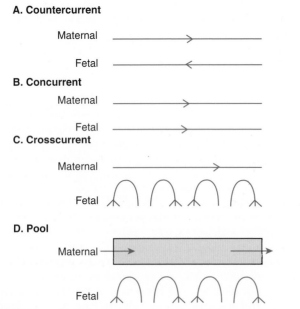

FIGURE 51-1 Schematic representation of possible arrangements of fetal and maternal blood vessels. (From Dawes GS: *Foetal and neonatal physiology: a comparative study of the changes at birth*, Chicago, 1968, Year Book Medical.)

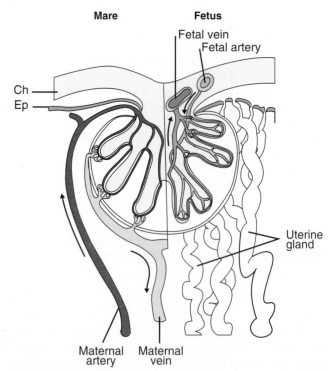

FIGURE 51-2 Diagram showing the arrangement of maternal and fetal blood vessels in the microcotyledons of the equine placenta. *Arrows* demonstrate the postulated countercurrent directions of maternal and fetal blood flow. *Ch*, Chorioallantois; *Ep*, uterine epithelium. (Based on data in Tsutsumi T: *J Agriculture Hokkaide Imperial Univ* 52:372, 1962; from Comline KS, Cross GS, Dawes GS, et al, editors: *Foetal and neonatal physiology: proceedings of the Sir Joseph Barcroft Centenary Symposium*, Cambridge, UK, 1973, Cambridge University Press.)

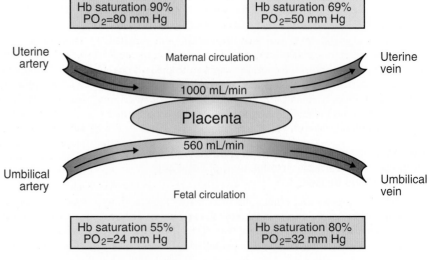

FIGURE 51-3 Placental blood flow, oxygen tension *(Po₂)*, and hemoglobin *(Hb)* saturation in the uterine and umbilical circulation of the sheep. (From Battaglia FC, Meschia G: *An introduction to fetal physiology*, Orlando, Fla, 1986, Academic Press.)

The Fetal Circulation Mixes Oxygenated and Deoxygenated Blood at Several Points, So the Fetus Exists in a State of Hypoxemia

In the adult the cardiac output of the right and left ventricles is separate and perfuses the pulmonary and systemic circulations, respectively. In the fetus the output of the two sides of the heart mixes at several points, so it is convenient to use the term *cardiac output* to refer to the combined output of the right and left ventricles. The combined cardiac output averages 500 mL/min/kg in fetal sheep; the output of the right ventricle exceeds that of the left (Figure 51-4). Because the right and left ventricles of the fetus pump into a common circulation, the two are of equal size and wall thickness.

The placenta, which has a low vascular resistance, receives 45% of the cardiac output through the *umbilical arteries*. The *umbilical veins* drain the placenta toward the liver. In species such as the sheep, most of the umbilical venous blood passes through the liver via a low-resistance channel known as the *ductus venosus;* in other species, such as the pig and horse, the ductus venosus disappears early in gestation, and umbilical venous blood flows

through the liver capillaries. Within the liver, the oxygenated blood from the placenta is mixed with a small amount of more poorly oxygenated blood draining the liver sinusoids. The hepatic venous blood enters the posterior vena cava, where it mixes with poorly oxygenated blood, draining the hind end of the fetus, so the blood returning to the right atrium has a P_{O_2} of 25 mm Hg.

A low-resistance pathway, the *foramen ovale,* connects the right and left atria, and a structure known as the *crista dividens* directs the better-oxygenated blood from the posterior vena cava through the foramen ovale to the left atrium. The poorly oxygenated blood returning to the right atrium in the cranial vena cava is directed into the right atrium and right ventricle. Most of the output of the right ventricle does not go through the lungs, however, because fetal lungs have a high vascular resistance. Another low-resistance channel, the *ductus arteriosus,* connects the *pulmonary artery* with the *aorta* and allows blood to bypass the lungs. It is important to note that the arrangement of the fetal circulation allows the better-oxygenated blood to enter the left ventricle, from which it reaches the brachycephalic vessels and the front of the animal. The less well oxygenated blood from the ductus arteriosus enters the aorta downstream from the

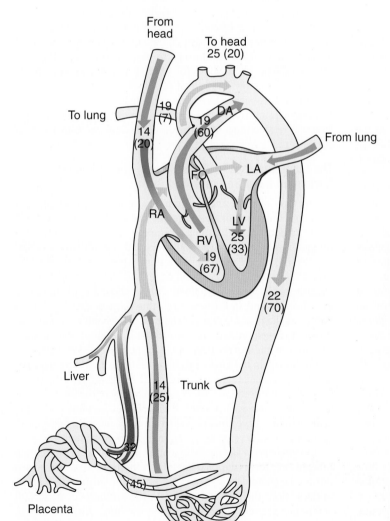

FIGURE 51-4 Diagrammatic representation of the fetal circulation showing oxygen tension (P_{O_2}) in millimeters of mercury (mm Hg) and percentage of cardiac output (in parentheses) in different parts of the circulation. *DA,* Ductus arteriosus; *FO,* foramen ovale; *LA,* left atrium; *LV,* left ventricle; *RA,* right atrium; *RV,* right ventricle.

brachycephalic vessels. The tissues of the hind end of the animal and the placenta receive blood with a Po_2 of approximately 22 mm Hg.

Flow of blood from the right atrium to the left atrium through the foramen ovale and from the pulmonary artery to the aorta through the ductus arteriosus requires that the pressure in the right side of the fetal circulation be greater than that in the left side. This pressure difference occurs because the left side of the circulation provides most of its output to the *low-resistance* placenta, whereas the right side of the fetal circulation is opposed by the *high-resistance* pulmonary circulation. At term, systemic arterial pressure in the lamb is about 42 mm Hg.

The fetal circulation is not a passive system and is capable of considerable regulation, particularly as the fetus matures. Fetal hypoxia can stimulate vasodilation in the heart and brain and vasoconstriction in the gut, kidneys, and skeletal tissues. The fetal pulmonary circulation constricts vigorously when the fetus is hypoxic. This constriction diverts more blood through the ductus arteriosus to the systemic tissues.

Fetal Oxygen Transport Is Assisted by Fetal Hemoglobin, Which Has a High Affinity for Oxygen

Fetal arterial blood has a low Po_2 because the placenta is not a highly efficient gas exchanger and because oxygenated blood and venous blood mix at several points in the fetal circulation. The fetus is adapted to this state of chronic hypoxia in two ways. First, it has a high cardiac output that delivers a large volume of blood per minute to the tissues. Second, the fetus produces erythrocytes containing hemoglobin with a *high affinity* for oxygen.

The production of erythrocytes initially occurs in the *yolk sac* and in other tissues such as endothelium. These embryonic erythrocytes are nucleated and contain embryonic hemoglobin, the oxygen affinity of which has not been clearly defined. At the termination of the embryonic period, erythrocyte production shifts to the liver and spleen and then progressively to the spleen and bone marrow. By the latter third of gestation erythrocyte production is solely by the marrow and erythrocytes lose their nuclei. Depending on the species, fetal erythrocytes contain either *fetal* or *adult hemoglobin* (see later discussion). Also, there are changes in glycolytic enzymes to provide the fetal concentrations of *2,3-diphosphoglycerate* (2,3-DPG), which regulates the combination of oxygen with hemoglobin (see Chapter 48 for discussion of role of 2,3-DPG). Fetal erythrocytes have a higher affinity for oxygen (lower partial pressure [tension] at which hemoglobin is 50% saturated with oxygen [P_{50}]) than do maternal erythrocytes; that is, the fetal blood oxyhemoglobin dissociation curve lies to the left of the adult curve (Figure 51-5). In some species, such as the cat, the difference in the P_{50} between fetus and adult is small, whereas in ruminants the difference is 10 to 20 mm Hg.

Three mechanisms account for the high affinity of *fetal hemoglobin* for oxygen. In ruminants, the higher oxygen affinity results from the synthesis of fetal hemoglobin with a high intrinsic oxygen affinity. Fetal hemoglobin of these species is unresponsive to 2,3-DPG. After birth there is gradual replacement of fetal hemoglobin by adult hemoglobin. In primates, there is little intrinsic difference in the oxygen affinity of fetal and maternal hemoglobin, but fetal hemoglobin has a decreased interaction with 2,3-DPG. In horses and pigs there is no fetal hemoglobin; embryonic hemoglobin is replaced immediately by adult hemoglobin. In these species, a low concentration of 2,3-DPG in the fetal erythrocytes is the cause of the high oxygen affinity and after

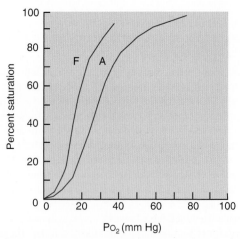

FIGURE 51-5 Oxyhemoglobin dissociation curves of fetal *(F)* and adult *(A)* sheep. Po_2, Oxygen tension. Note that the dissociation curve of the fetus is displaced to the left of the adult so that at a given Po_2, the fetal hemoglobin has a higher percent saturation than does the adult.

birth, an increase in the concentration of 2,3-DPG gives the hemoglobin its adult dissociation curve.

The high affinity of fetal hemoglobin for oxygen allows the hemoglobin in the umbilical veins, with a Po_2 of 30 mm Hg, to be 80% saturated with oxygen and allows the hemoglobin in the aorta, with a Po_2 of 22 mm Hg, to be 56% saturated. The high affinity of fetal hemoglobin for oxygen not only allows oxygen transport at the low Po_2 in fetal arteries, but also makes it necessary for fetal tissues to have an extremely low Po_2. The low tissue Po_2 provides an oxygen concentration gradient to unload oxygen from the fetal hemoglobin. Therefore the fetus exists in a state of tissue hypoxia compared with the adult.

The Lung Develops in Three Stages, and Pulmonary Surfactant Must Be Present at Birth

By the time of birth, the lung must be ready to assume the gas-exchange functions of the placenta. The lung develops in three stages of equivalent duration. Beginning as an outgrowth of the foregut, the lung bud invades the *mesenchyme* of the thorax and divides into all the major airways during the first third of gestation. Concurrently, major blood vessel branches develop. Because the primordial airways are lined with a cuboidal epithelium and look like a gland in cross section, this stage of development is known as the *pseudoglandular* stage. In the second or *canalicular* stage of development, the bronchioles develop, the airways develop lumens and the developing bronchiolar region is invaded by capillaries. In the final stage, or *alveolar sac* stage, alveolar sacs, and in some species alveoli, develop. The stage of maturity of the lung at birth in general matches the maturity of the fetus. Lambs and piglets have well-developed alveoli, but humans and especially rodents have thicker-walled alveolar sacs. In these latter species, alveoli develop as the animal grows postnatally.

Pulmonary surfactant is essential if the lung is to remain inflated after birth (see Chapter 45). Synthesis of surfactant begins during the glandular stage of development but beginning at about midgestation, there is an increase in the synthesis of surfactant components, such as lecithin, within the lung. This increase in lecithin synthesis coincides with the appearance of *type II alveolar cells* (the source of surfactant) and with an increase in pulmonary blood flow. Some of this lecithin is secreted into the alveolar lumens and appears in the amniotic fluid, where it can be measured as an indicator of the state of lung maturity. Lung maturity coincides with an increase in the serum glucocorticoid (cortisol) level in the fetus. Indeed, glucocorticoids (two thirds fetal and one third maternal in origin) play an essential role in lung maturation.

Until the time of birth, the vascular resistance of the fetal pulmonary circulation is high, for several reasons. The fetal lung is not inflated; therefore the large vessels are not pulled open by the surrounding alveolar septa. In addition, the hypoxia of the fetus maintains the pulmonary vascular smooth muscle in a state of contraction that narrows the arteries. The first few breaths alleviate both these conditions.

The fetal lung continuously secretes fluid until about 2 days before birth. This fluid, which is rich in chloride and low in bicarbonate and protein, travels up the trachea and through the fetus's mouth into the amniotic cavity. The fluid in the alveolar spaces and airways is in part squeezed out of the lung as the thorax is compressed during birth. The majority is reabsorbed into lymphatic and blood vessels shortly after birth.

Beginning at about one third of gestation, the fetus makes *breathing movements*, although it moves little of the viscous fluid to and fro in the airways. These movements apparently prepare the respiratory muscles for their postnatal function.

At or Shortly After Birth, Umbilical Vessels Rupture, Pulmonary Vascular Resistance Decreases, and the Foramen Ovale and Ductus Arteriosus Close

At term, the fetus is dependent on the placenta and the mother for exchange with the environment, but the lung and other organs must be ready to assume their postnatal functions. During a normal birth, the newborn emerges from the birth canal at about the time the placenta is detaching from the uterine wall. Placental gas exchange probably continues well into third-stage labor. If labor is prolonged, the placenta may detach before the newborn is delivered. This is a medical emergency.

Normally, the newborn takes the *first breath* immediately after delivery. The stimuli for this include (1) hypoxia and hypercarbia, which result from the loss of the placental gas exchanger; (2) cooling of the fetus as the fetal fluids evaporate from the skin; and (3) a generalized increase in sensory input to the fetus as it is licked and nuzzled by its dam. To expand the lungs initially, the respiratory muscles must create an intrathoracic pressure that is 60 cm H_2O less than atmospheric pressure. This is vastly lower than the 5 cm H_2O generated by adults breathing tidal volume. The large effort during the first breath is necessary to move viscous fluids down the airways before air can enter the alveoli and to open the fluid-filled alveoli. Not all alveoli may inflate during the first breath, but subsequent inhalations inflate the entire lung and distribute surfactant over the alveolar surface. This surfactant makes the alveoli stable and prevents their collapse so that a stable end-expiratory lung volume, known as *functional residual capacity*, can be established. After the first few breaths, arterial oxygen tension (PaO_2) is much higher than it was before birth, yet breathing continues.

Even though the fetus exists in a state of hypoxia compared to the adult, the carotid bodies do not stimulate breathing movements in utero. Rather, hypoxia inhibits breathing movements and reduces metabolic rate to reduce oxygen demand. At birth, the carotid bodies are relatively insensitive to hypoxia, but, in the presence of oxygen concentrations found in air, develop the adult sensitivity to oxygen deficits within a few weeks.

Inflation and oxygenation of the lung at birth reduces the pulmonary vascular resistance, which leads to a decreased pressure in the pulmonary artery, right ventricle, and right atrium. At about the same time, the umbilical vessels rupture because the animal struggles to stand or the umbilical cord is torn by the mother. Umbilical blood flow is arrested by local vasoconstriction in the umbilical vessels. The loss of the low-resistance placental circulation increases systemic vascular resistance, which results in an increased pressure in the aorta, left ventricle, and left atrium. As a result of these changes, aortic pressure exceeds pulmonary arterial pressure, and left atrial pressure exceeds right atrial pressure. Therefore, blood flow through the ductus arteriosus and foramen ovale reverses. Flow reversal in the foramen ovale causes a flap valve to close and occlude the foramen. Over succeeding days to weeks, this valve becomes adherent to the wall of the atrium, thus permanently closing the foramen.

Reversal of flow in the ductus arteriosus exposes the ductus wall to well-oxygenated blood. This causes constriction of smooth muscle in the wall of the ductus, thus arresting blood flow. Ductus closure involves a decrease in the concentration of *vasodilator prostaglandins*. Administration of drugs, such as indomethacin, that inhibit prostaglandin synthesis constricts the ductus in fetal sheep, and administration of prostaglandin E_2 dilates it. When the ductus has constricted and flow has been arrested, the ductus is gradually converted into a fibrous band of scar tissue.

The changes just described convert the fetal circulation into the adult circulation, which is able to support the gas-exchange function of the lung. Remarkably, these changes occur routinely and without medical assistance in almost all animal births.

CLINICAL CORRELATIONS

PATENT DUCTUS ARTERIOSUS IN A POMERANIAN

History. A 7-week-old female Pomeranian puppy is presented to you because it is not growing as fast as its littermates. The breeder says it is lethargic and prefers to sleep, whereas the other puppies play.

Clinical Examination. Clinical examination reveals a small puppy with a rapid heart rate. The mucous membranes of its gums are pink, and its temperature is normal. While holding the puppy around the thorax, you notice a vibration in the region of the heart. When you listen with a stethoscope, you hear a loud murmur that is almost continuous through systole and diastole, and you recall that this is called a *machinery murmur*. It is difficult to listen to the breath sounds because the murmur is audible all over the thorax.

A radiograph reveals a slightly enlarged heart, but the lungs appear normal, although minimally compressed by the heart. An echocardiogram is performed, which better characterizes the suspected patent ductus arteriosus (PDA). The velocity of blood flow through the ductus and its mean diameter indicate that the dog is a candidate for surgical correction of the PDA.

Comment. The clinical and radiographic findings in a puppy of this age are characteristic of PDA. In some animals the ductus fails to close after birth, and blood continues to flow through it, usually from the aorta to the pulmonary artery. This presents the animal with two problems. First, the left ventricle must increase its output to supply the systemic tissues because so much blood is passing through the ductus. Second, the pulmonary circulation has a volume overload that increases the pressure against which the right ventricle must work. Depending on the magnitude of the PDA, these extra loads result in dilation of the ventricles and sometimes in hypertrophy of the myocardium, which is seen on radiographs as an enlarged heart. The puppy is not growing and is listless because the tissues are not receiving a normal blood flow. Although surgical correction of the PDA allows the puppy to live a normal life, it would be unwise to breed this animal in the future because the condition is inherited.

Treatment. The patent ductus is closed by surgical ligation, and the puppy is expected to have a normal life.

Recently, use of a transarterial coil occlusion procedure has been successful in the treatment of animals with PDA. The treatment choice is somewhat dictated by the size of the shunt as well as the presence or absence of heart failure.

PRACTICE QUESTIONS

1. The vascular channel that allows fetal blood to pass from the pulmonary artery to the aorta is known as the:
   a. Foramen ovale.
   b. Ductus arteriosus.
   c. Ductus venosus.
   d. Fetal cotyledon.
   e. Allantois.

2. Which of the following is the correct sequence of events that follow birth?
   a. Closure of foramen ovale, first breath, rupture of umbilical vessels
   b. Decrease in right atrial pressure, first breath, closure of the ductus arteriosus
   c. First breath, closure of the ductus arteriosus, decrease in pulmonary arterial pressure
   d. First breath, decrease in pulmonary arterial pressure, closure of the foramen ovale
   e. Closure of the foramen ovale, closure of the ductus arteriosus, first breath

3. Which of the following fetal blood structures contains blood with the highest Po_2?
   a. Aorta
   b. Ductus arteriosus
   c. Pulmonary artery
   d. Left ventricle
   e. Umbilical artery

4. Which of the following statements about the fetal circulation is true?
   a. Right atrial pressure is higher than left atrial pressure.
   b. Pulmonary vascular resistance is high.
   c. The placenta receives about 45% of the combined output of both ventricles.
   d. The output of the right ventricle is greater than that of the left ventricle.
   e. All the above.

5. Which of the following does not correctly describe the lung in utero?
   a. Type II cells, which produce surfactant, are present within the first few days of gestation in sheep.
   b. Chloride-rich fluid is secreted into the airways and flows into the amniotic cavity.
   c. Components of surfactant can be detected in the amniotic fluid when the lung approaches maturity.
   d. All the major branches of the tracheobronchial tree are present at birth, but alveoli continue to multiply after birth in some species.
   e. Breathing movements occur in utero, but the volume of fluid moved in and out of the lungs is small.

6. Fetal oxygen transport is assisted by:
   a. Fetal hemoglobin, which has a lower oxygen capacity than adult hemoglobin.
   b. Fetal hemoglobin, which has a lower P_{50} than adult hemoglobin.
   c. A cardiac output that is less per kilogram of body weight than in the adult.
   d. A cardiac output that preferentially delivers the blood with the highest Po_2 to the placenta.
   e. A fetal lung, which is an efficient gas exchanger.

7. Which of the following domestic mammals has a diffuse, epitheliochorial placenta in which fetal and maternal blood flow is countercurrent in the microcotyledons?
   a. Dog
   b. Cow
   c. Horse
   d. Rabbit
   e. Sheep

BIBLIOGRAPHY

Battaglia FC, Meschia G: *An introduction to fetal physiology*, Orlando, Fla, 1986, Academic Press.

Campbell FE, Thomas WP, Miller SJ, et al: Immediate and late outcomes of transarterial coil occlusion of patent ductus arteriosus in dogs, *J Vet Intern Med* 20(1):83–96, 2006.

Carroll JL, Agarwal A: Development of ventilatory control in infants, *Paediatr Respir Rev* 11(4):199–207, 2010.

Dawes GS: *Foetal and neonatal physiology: a comparative study of the changes at birth*, Chicago, 1968, Year Book Medical.

Faber JJ, Thornburg KL: *Placental physiology: structure and function of fetomaternal exchange*, New York, 1983, Raven Press.

Jones EE: Fetal and neonatal physiology. In Boron WF, Boulpaep EL, editors: *Medical physiology: a cellular and molecular approach*, ed 2, Philadelphia, 2009, Saunders.

Leff AR, Schumacker PT: *Respiratory physiology: basics and applications*, Philadelphia, 1993, Saunders.

Silver M, Steven DH, Comline KS: Placental exchange and morphology in ruminants and the mare. In Comline KS, Cross KW, Dawes GS, et al, editors: *Foetal and neonatal physiology: proceedings of the Sir Joseph Barcroft Centenary Symposium*, Cambridge, UK, 1973, Cambridge University Press.

Smith LJ, McKay KO, van Asperen PP, et al: Normal development of the lung and premature birth, *Paediatr Respir Rev* 11(3):135–142, 2010.

CHAPTER 52
Acid-Base Homeostasis

KEY POINTS

Acid-Base Regulation

1. Relative constancy of the body's pH is essential because metabolism requires enzymes that operate at an optimal pH.
2. Hydrogen ion concentration is measured as pH.
3. An acid can donate a hydrogen ion, and a base can accept a hydrogen ion.
4. Buffers are combinations of salts and weak acids that prevent major changes in pH.
5. Hemoglobin and bicarbonate are the most important blood buffers.
6. The first defense against a change in blood pH is provided by the blood buffers, but the lungs and kidneys must ultimately correct the hydrogen ion load.
7. Changes in ventilation can rapidly change carbon dioxide tension and therefore alter pH.
8. Metabolic production of fixed acids requires that the kidneys eliminate hydrogen ions and conserve bicarbonate.
9. Intracellular pH is regulated by buffers and ion pumps.

Acid-Base Disturbances

1. Acid-base abnormalities accompany many diseases, and the restoration of normal blood pH should be a consideration in the treatment of any disease.

2. Respiratory acidosis is caused by the accumulation of carbon dioxide, which decreases blood pH.
3. Respiratory alkalosis is caused by the loss of carbon dioxide, which increases blood pH.
4. Metabolic acidosis is caused by the accumulation of fixed acids or the loss of buffer base, which decreases blood pH.
5. Metabolic alkalosis is caused by the excessive elimination of hydrogen ions or by the intake of base, such as bicarbonate, which increases blood pH.
6. Respiratory compensations for acid-base abnormalities occur rapidly; renal compensations occur over several hours.
7. Hydrogen and potassium ions are interrelated in acid-base homeostasis.
8. The diagnosis of acid-base disturbances depends on interpretation of measurements of arterial blood pH and carbon dioxide tension, from which bicarbonate concentration and total buffer base are calculated.
9. Over the years, many terms have been used to explain acid-base balance.

ACID-BASE REGULATION

Relative Constancy of the Body's pH Is Essential Because Metabolism Requires Enzymes That Operate at an Optimal pH

For optimal functioning of the cells, the ionic composition of body fluids is maintained within fairly narrow limits. Hydrogen ion (H^+, *proton*) concentration is extremely important because it determines the *acidity* or *alkalinity,* or *pH,* of the body fluids. Serious deviations of pH outside the normal range disrupt cell metabolism and therefore body function. For example, the activity of the sodium-potassium (Na^+-K^+) pump decreases by half when pH falls by one unit, and the activity of phosphofructokinase (a key regulatory enzyme in the glycolytic pathway) decreases by 90% when pH decreases by only 0.1.

When veterinarians use the terms *acidosis* and *alkalosis,* they are comparing the pH of arterial blood with the normal value of 7.4. A pH above and below 7.4 are referred to as alkalosis and acidosis, respectively. The range of pH compatible with life is 6.85 to 7.8, but such changes are rare because buffers, the lungs, and the kidneys work in concert to regulate pH.

In a 70-kg animal, 15,000 mmole of H^+ are produced daily when carbon dioxide (CO_2) is added to the blood for transport from the tissues to the lungs. If the lungs eliminate CO_2 as fast as

it is produced in the tissues, there is no net H^+ gain by the body. However, the balance between CO_2 production and CO_2 elimination may be disturbed during exercise or in respiratory disease, thus threatening the acid-base homeostasis of the body.

Forty mmole/day of H^+ are produced during protein metabolism (sulfuric and phosphoric acids), fat metabolism (keto-acids), and the incomplete oxidation of glucose (lactic acid) and another 30 mmole/day are absorbed from the intestine. Although H^+ from these sources are few compared with those produced in CO_2 transport, the kidneys must eliminate them continually. In a disease state the H^+ load imposed on the body is frequently increased because of an increase in tissue breakdown (catabolism) or because the kidneys fail to eliminate H^+. In less common situations, such as vomiting, H^+ are lost from the body.

To understand how the body regulates pH and how acid-base disorders are diagnosed, it is necessary to first review acids, bases, and buffering.

Hydrogen Ion Concentration Is Measured as pH

The *chemical potential* of H^+ is known as the acidity and is expressed in pH units. pH is the *negative logarithm* of H^+ concentration ($[H^+]$). Water with 1×10^{-7} mol/L $[H^+]$ and an equal concentration of hydroxyl ions has a pH of 7.0, that is, a neutral pH.

An increase in [H$^+$] (acidity) decreases pH. For example, a tenfold increase in [H$^+$] decreases pH by 1.0 unit, whereas doubling [H$^+$] decreases pH by 0.3 unit.

The normal range of blood pH, 6.85 to 7.80, represents [H$^+$] of 1.4×10^{-7} to 1.6×10^{-8} Eq/L. Thus, although the [H$^+$] is regulated, changes up to tenfold in magnitude can occur, much greater than the fluctuations observed in the concentration of other ions, such as sodium or potassium.

An Acid Can Donate a Hydrogen Ion, and a Base Can Accept a Hydrogen Ion

Hydrochloric acid (HCl) is a *strong acid* because it dissociates completely in water into H$^+$ and Cl$^-$. Chloride ion is a base because it has the potential to accept an H$^+$, but it is a *weak base* because HCl dissociates so completely in water. Carbonic acid (H$_2$CO$_3$), in contrast, is a *weak acid* because it dissociates incompletely in solution into hydrogen and bicarbonate ions. Bicarbonate (HCO$_3^-$), however, is a relatively *strong base* that can accept an H$^+$ and form undissociated carbonic acid. The latter reaction removes H$^+$ from solution, and the [H$^+$] decreases, causing the pH to rise. Bases do not have to be ions; for example, ammonia (NH$_3$) is a base because it can accept a proton and become ammonium ion (NH$_4^+$). This reaction is of little importance in the blood, but it is important in the renal collecting duct. In addition, proteins also act as buffers by virtue of the terminal carboxyl and amino groups, which can donate (R-COOH → R-COO$^-$ + H$^+$) or accept (R-NH$_2$ + H$^+$ → R-NH$_3^+$) protons, respectively.

Buffers Are Combinations of Salts and Weak Acids That Prevent Major Changes in pH

Buffers "soak up" free H$^+$ and prevent their accumulation in body fluids. By so doing, buffers prevent drastic changes in pH. Buffers are mixtures of weak acids and their salts. For example, sodium bicarbonate dissociates completely into sodium and bicarbonate ions; carbonic acid dissociates incompletely into hydrogen and bicarbonate ions. Thus, in a solution containing sodium bicarbonate and carbonic acid, there are sodium, hydrogen, and bicarbonate ions and undissociated carbonic acid. If a strong acid such as hydrochloric acid is added to the solution, the added H$^+$ upsets the dissociation equilibrium of carbonic acid. Hydrogen ions combine with bicarbonate ion to form carbonic acid, thus reducing the [H$^+$], that is, preventing a major change in pH.

If, in contrast, sodium hydroxide is added to the solution, the hydroxyl ions, formed by dissociation of sodium hydroxide, combine with H$^+$ to form water. The decrease in H$^+$ causes dissociation of more carbonic acid and liberation of H$^+$, again preventing a large change in pH.

The dissociation of a weak acid, and therefore the [H$^+$], base, and undissociated acid, is determined by the *dissociation constant*

(K$_a$) and can be described by the *law of mass action*. For carbonic acid:

$$K_a = [H^+][HCO_3^-]/[H_2CO_3].$$

Taking logarithms of both sides of this equation results in:

$$\log K_a = \log[H^+] + \log[HCO_3^-]/[H_2CO_3].$$

Rearrangement of this equation yields:

$$-\log[H^+] = -\log K_a + \log[HCO_3^-]/[H_2CO_3].$$

However, $-\log[H^+]$ is pH and $-\log K_a$ is called pK$_a$; therefore:

$$pH = pK_a + \log[HCO_3^-]/[H_2CO_3].$$

This is the *Henderson-Hasselbalch equation* written for the bicarbonate–carbonic acid system. It can be written for any buffering system in the generic form:

$$pH = pK_a + \log[base]/[acid].$$

This equation shows that the pH of a solution is determined by the ratio of the concentration of base (the H$^+$ acceptor) to that of undissociated acid (the H$^+$ donor) and by the pK$_a$ of the buffering system.

Figure 52-1 shows the change in pH that results when acid is added to a phosphate buffer with a pK$_a$ of 6.8. This is a graphic presentation of the Henderson-Hasselbalch equation. Initially, as acid is added, there is a large decrease in pH. As considerably more acid is added to the solution, the pH changes little. H$^+$ ions combine with HPO$_4^{2-}$ and form H$_2$PO$_4^-$. Finally, the pH decreases considerably. The zone over which the pH changes little as acid is added (i.e., where buffering capacity is optimal) is within ±1 pH unit of the pK$_a$. Note that when the pH equals the pKa, 50% of the buffer has been consumed. From this buffer curve, it is obvious that an effective buffer must have a pKa within ±1 pH unit of the solution in which it operates. Thus the optimal blood buffers should have a pK$_a$ between 6.4 and 8.4. In addition, buffers must be sufficiently plentiful to be effective.

Hemoglobin and Bicarbonate Are the Most Important Blood Buffers

Hemoglobin is an important blood buffer because it is plentiful and because the imidazole residues of globin *histidine* have a pK$_a$ close to the blood pH. In actuality, the pK$_a$ of hemoglobin changes with the degree of oxygenation. Because deoxyhemoglobin has a pK$_a$ (7.93) closer to blood pH than does oxyhemoglobin (pK$_a$ = 6.68), deoxyhemoglobin provides more buffering capacity. When arterial blood enters the tissue capillaries, oxygen leaves hemoglobin, so the resulting deoxyhemoglobin is an excellent buffer for the H$^+$ produced when CO$_2$ is added to the blood.

The other blood buffer with an optimal pK$_a$ is the HPO$_4^{2-}$/ H$_2$PO$_4^-$ system, with a pK$_a$ of 6.8 (see Figure 52-1). The normally

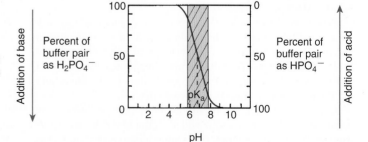

FIGURE 52-1 Titration curve for the phosphate buffer system. The pK$_a$ is 6.8. The *shaded area* represents the range of pH over which this buffer is effective.

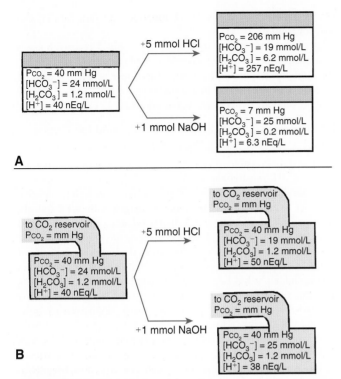

FIGURE 52-2 Buffer function of the carbonic acid–bicarbonate system under closed and open conditions. **A,** Under closed conditions, the total quantity of the buffer (acid plus base components) remains constant. **B,** Under open conditions, the carbon dioxide tension (P_{CO_2}) of the system, and thus the concentration of carbonic acid (H_2CO_3), is maintained at a fixed level by continuous equilibration of the liquid phase with a gas reservoir of constant P_{CO_2}. The term *[H_2CO_3]* denotes the combined concentration of carbonic acid and dissolved carbon dioxide. (From Madias NE, Cohen JJ: Acid-base chemistry and buffering. In Cohen JJ, Kassirer JP, editors: *Acid-base,* Boston 1982, Little, Brown.)

low phosphate concentration in the blood makes this buffering system quantitatively unimportant; however, it is important in the renal tubules, where phosphate becomes concentrated. *Plasma proteins* also provide a small amount of blood buffering.

Although a pK_a of 6.1 seems to make the HCO_3^-/H_2CO_3 buffer unimportant for blood buffering, this is not so for two reasons. First, there is a large amount (24 mEq/L) of HCO_3^- in the blood, making it readily available for buffering. Second, the kidneys can regulate the concentration of HCO_3^-, and the lungs can regulate the concentration of H_2CO_3. Because the base and acid concentration can be regulated, the HCO_3^-/H_2CO_3 system is said to be an *open system*.

Figure 52-2 shows the value of this open system in maintaining body pH. It should be noted that the concentration of H_2CO_3 ([H_2CO_3]) in solution is directly proportional to the carbon dioxide tension (P_{CO_2}); 1 molecule of H_2CO_3 is in equilibrium with 340 molecules of CO_2. Therefore, [H_2CO_3] can be calculated as $0.03 \times P_{CO_2}$. In Figure 52-2, A and B, *top panels,* 5 mmol of hydrochloric acid is added to plasma. Figure 52-2, *A,* shows what happens if the P_{CO_2} and thus [H_2CO_3] is held constant. In such a closed system, the 5 mmol of HCl reacts with 5 mmol of HCO_3^- to form 5 mmol of H_2CO_3. As a consequence of this reaction, [HCO_3^-] decreases from 24 to 19 mmol/L, [H_2CO_3] increases from 1.2 to 6.2 mmol/L, and P_{CO_2} increases from 40 to 206 mm Hg. Using the law of mass action, one can calculate that [H^+]

increases from 40 to 257 nEq/L or, stated in other terms, pH decreases from 7.4 to 6.5. If the system is open, however (as it is in the *top panel* of Figure 52-2, *B*) carbon dioxide evolves to the environment as fast as it is produced so that P_{CO_2} and therefore [H_2CO_3] remain constant, then [H^+] increases to only 50 nEq/L and the pH decreases only to 7.3. The *lower panel* in Figure 52-2, *B*, shows similar advantages to the open system when a strong base is added to the buffer system. Under most conditions, the body functions as an open system with regard to the HCO_3^-/H_2CO_3 system so that pH changes are minimized. When tissues are ischemic, however, they have no connection to the lungs, so CO_2 cannot be eliminated. The ischemic tissue then functions as a closed system, and pH changes within the tissue can therefore be drastic.

The HCO_3^-/H_2CO_3 buffering system is of great value to clinicians because its components can be readily measured in the clinical laboratory and thereby used to diagnose acid-base disturbances. It is not necessary to measure the components of every buffering system to diagnose acid-base disturbances. If one system is known, changes in other systems can be predicted. It is standard to measure pH and P_{CO_2} and to use the Henderson-Hasselbalch equation to derive [HCO_3^-]. In actual practice, these calculations are now done for the clinician by computers in the blood gas machine.

For clinical use, the Henderson-Hasselbalch equation for the HCO_3^-/H_2CO_3 system is written as follows:

$$pH = pK_a + \log[HCO_3^-]/[0.03 \times P_{CO_2}]$$

Under normal conditions, the pH of arterial blood is 7.4, [HCO_3^-] is 24 mEq/L, and the arterial carbon dioxide tension (Pa_{CO_2}) is 40 mm Hg:

$$7.4 = 6.1 + (\log 24)/(0.03 \times 40) = 6.1 + \log 20.$$

This equation demonstrates that a normal blood pH requires an [HCO_3^-]/[$0.03 \times P_{CO_2}$] ratio of 20:1. An increase or decrease in this ratio increases or decreases pH, respectively.

The First Defense Against a Change in Blood pH Is Provided by the Blood Buffers, but the Lungs and Kidneys Must Ultimately Correct the Hydrogen Ion Load

When body pH is threatened by a change in the production or elimination of H^+, the blood and tissue buffers provide the first line of defense. However, buffers only prevent drastic changes in pH; they cannot correct the problem by increasing or decreasing the elimination of H^+ or by replacing lost buffering capacity. Ultimately, pH must be corrected by adjustments in ventilation or by changes in renal function. Because the lungs can alter Pa_{CO_2} and the kidneys can regulate the concentration of HCO_3^-, the Henderson-Hasselbalch equation has been written as follows:

$$pH = pK_a + \log(\text{renal function/ventilation})$$

Changes in Ventilation Can Rapidly Change Carbon Dioxide Tension and Therefore Alter pH

As blood flows through the tissues, CO_2 diffuses into the plasma and the erythrocytes (red blood cells), where carbonic acid forms and then dissociates into hydrogen and bicarbonate ions:

$$H_2O + CO_2 \rightarrow H_2CO_3 \rightarrow H^+ + HCO_3^-$$

Because the initial [HCO_3^-] in the blood is greater than [H_2CO_3], the relative increase in [H_2CO_3] is greater than the increase in [HCO_3^-], and thus the [HCO_3^-]/[H_2CO_3] ratio (i.e.,

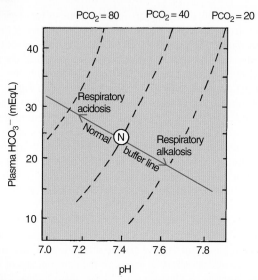

FIGURE 52-3 A pH-bicarbonate diagram showing the effect of increasing and decreasing carbon dioxide tension (Pco_2) on pH and bicarbonate (HCO_3^-) concentration. As Pco_2 increases or decreases, the changes in pH and bicarbonate concentration are predicted by the normal buffer line. *N*, Normal arterial blood composition.

$[HCO_3^-/0.03 \cdot PCO_2])$ decreases; consequently, pH decreases. In the lungs, CO_2 leaves the blood, and the pH increases again. For these reasons, venous blood is more acidic than arterial blood. Normally, the lungs eliminate CO_2 as fast as the tissues produce it, so the $Paco_2$ and pH of arterial blood remain relatively constant.

The lungs can cause rapid changes in blood pH by increasing or decreasing the elimination of CO_2. When ventilation increases in relation to CO_2 production (*hyperventilation*), $Paco_2$ decreases, the $[HCO_3^-/0.03 \times Paco_2]$ ratio increases, and pH increases. Conversely, when ventilation decreases in relation to CO_2 production (*hypoventilation*), $Paco_2$ increases, $[HCO_3^-/0.03 \times Paco_2]$ decreases, and pH decreases. Figure 52-3 shows how $[HCO_3^-]$ and pH change as the Pco_2 of the blood increases or decreases.

Metabolic Production of Fixed Acids Requires That the Kidneys Eliminate Hydrogen Ions and Conserve Bicarbonate

When fixed acids are added to the blood, for example, sulfuric acid from protein metabolism, the H^+ are buffered in part by HCO_3^-. Buffering results in the conversion of HCO_3^- to H_2CO_3 and CO_2, which is eliminated from the lungs. Fixed acids are produced continuously and would consume the body's HCO_3^- if the kidneys were not continually regenerating HCO_3^-.

The role of the kidneys in acid-base balance is described in Chapter 44. Large amounts of HCO_3^- are filtered daily through the glomerulus and subsequently reabsorbed in the renal tubule. The amount of HCO_3^- reabsorbed depends on the amount filtered, which is determined by the plasma concentration of HCO_3^-, the *glomerular filtration rate*, and the rate of H^+ secretion by renal tubular cells. This last rate is controlled in part by the acid-base status of the body.

When Pco_2 is high, the reaction:

$$H_2O + CO_2 \rightarrow H_2CO_3 \rightarrow H^+ + HCO_3^-$$

within the *renal tubules* is driven to the right, producing more H^+ for secretion into the *tubular lumen* and HCO_3^- for return to the blood. When Pco_2 is low, H^+ elimination and therefore HCO_3^- reabsorption decrease.

Ammonia, an important buffer in the distal renal tubule, is produced by the action of *glutaminase* on *glutamine*. In acidosis, the activity of glutaminase increases, resulting in increased ammonia production, an increased buffering capacity of the renal tubular fluid and, therefore, increased ability to eliminate H^+.

Intracellular pH Is Regulated by Buffers and Ion Pumps

Whereas the hemoglobin and bicarbonate provide the most immediately available source of buffers to prevent drastic changes in blood pH, *intracellular buffers* within the body tissues, other than blood, provide another large reserve of buffering capacity. In order to enter cells, H^+ must be exchanged with other cations, such as sodium or potassium. When inside the cell, H^+ is buffered by *amino acids, peptides, proteins,* and *organic phosphates*. These buffers provide approximately five times the buffering capacity of the extracellular fluid. As a general rule, intracellular pH follows extracellular pH but because of the large intracellular buffering capacity, the pH changes are less dramatic in the cytosol.

Two *ion exchangers* play a major role in regulation of intracellular pH. The Na^+/H^+ exchanger uses the energy derived from the extracellular to intracellular Na^+ gradient to move H^+ out of the cell and the Cl^-/HCO_3^- exchanger uses a similar mechanism to move HCO_3^- out of the cell. When H^+ concentration within the cell increases, the activity of the Na^+-H^+ pump increases so that more H^+ is extruded. At the same time, the activity of the Cl^--HCO_3^- pump is inhibited so that HCO_3^- accumulates within the cell. These two mechanisms can restore intracellular pH to normal as long as extracellular pH also is normal. If, however, extracellular pH is low, it is more difficult for the Na^+-H^+ pump to extrude H^+, and thus intracellular pH tends also to be acidic. If the cytosol becomes alkaline, the activity of the Cl^--HCO_3^- pump is facilitated, and the Na^+-H^+ pump is inhibited to restore pH. This corrective action is inhibited if extracellular pH also is alkaline.

ACID-BASE DISTURBANCES

Acid-Base Abnormalities Accompany Many Diseases, and Restoration of Normal Blood pH Should Be a Consideration in the Treatment of Any Disease

In most diseases the buffering systems, lungs, and kidneys keep pH within tolerable limits, but in severe disease these homeostatic mechanisms may be inadequate, and life-threatening changes in pH can occur. In the diagnosis and treatment of acid-base abnormalities, it is important to realize that a primary abnormality causes the change in blood pH, which is followed by compensatory changes. Because of the body's attempt to correct the abnormality, the clinician often must disentangle the data to differentiate the primary cause of the problem from the compensatory changes. The primary problems are excessive accumulation or elimination of carbon dioxide (respiratory abnormalities) or the excessive accumulation or elimination of fixed acids (metabolic abnormalities).

Respiratory Acidosis Is Caused by the Accumulation of Carbon Dioxide, Which Decreases Blood pH

Respiratory acidosis is caused by *alveolar hypoventilation*, which can result from damage to or depression of the respiratory control centers, injury to the respiratory pump (e.g., fractured ribs, bloated abdomen), or severe respiratory disease that either obstructs the airways or excessively stiffens the lungs. When alveolar hypoventilation occurs, P_{CO_2} increases because carbon dioxide is incompletely eliminated by the lungs. The reaction:

$$H_2O + CO_2 \rightarrow H_2CO_3 \rightarrow H^+ + HCO_3^-$$

is driven to the right by the accumulating CO_2; H^+ accumulates, and pH decreases. Bicarbonate accumulates simultaneously, but the amount is too small to keep the $[HCO_3^-/0.03 \times P_{CO_2}]$ ratio at a normal value of $20:1$.

In the blood, other nonbicarbonate buffers not only take up H^+ produced by the accumulation of CO_2 but also assist in the accumulation of HCO_3^-, as follows:

$$H_2O + CO_2 \rightarrow H_2CO_3 \rightarrow H^+ + HCO_3^-$$
$$\downarrow$$
$$H^+ + Hb^- \rightarrow HHb$$

By buffering H^+, hemoglobin (Hb^-) pulls the first reaction to the right and produces HCO_3^-. This accumulation of bicarbonate, shown on the *normal buffer line* in the pH-HCO_3^- diagram (see Figure 52-3), is still insufficient to maintain a normal $[HCO_3^-/0.03 \times P_{CO_2}]$ ratio, and therefore the pH decreases. As a result of these various reactions, the characteristic findings in acute respiratory acidosis are an elevated Pa_{CO_2}, a decreased pH, and a minor increase in $[HCO_3^-]$.

To facilitate the clinical interpretation of acid-base status, clinicians use the terms total buffer base, base excess, and base deficit. *Total buffer* base is the sum of the concentrations of available blood buffers. *Base excess* and *base deficit* refer to an increase or decrease, respectively, in total buffer base. In acute respiratory acidosis, total buffer base does not change because the accumulation of HCO_3^- is accompanied by an equivalent decrease in the concentration of other buffers, such as Hb^-. Therefore, there is no base excess or base deficit.

The ideal way for the clinician to correct respiratory acidosis is to restore alveolar ventilation. However, because disease processes that impede ventilation cause the respiratory acidosis, this option is not available to the untreated animal, and other means to correct pH, primarily renal mechanisms, must be used. The elevated P_{CO_2} and decreased pH increase H^+ and NH_3 production in the kidney. This increases the elimination of H^+ in the urine and generates new HCO_3^-, and as the plasma $[HCO_3^-]$ increases, the $[HCO_3^-/0.03 \times P_{CO_2}]$ ratio and pH are adjusted toward normal. The newly generated HCO_3^- adds to the total buffer base and therefore causes a base excess. Figure 52-4 shows how this accumulating HCO_3^- adjusts the pH toward normal during respiratory acidosis, even though P_{CO_2} remains constant.

Respiratory Alkalosis Is Caused by the Loss of Carbon Dioxide, Which Increases Blood pH

Respiratory alkalosis is caused by *alveolar hyperventilation*, which results from stimulation of the chemoreceptors by hypoxia or from stimulation of intrapulmonary receptors by lung injury or inflammation. Overly vigorous use of a ventilator also can cause hyperventilation in an anesthetized animal. Carbon dioxide is eliminated faster than the tissues produce it, and so blood P_{CO_2} decreases. The changes in blood chemistry are the inverse of those in respiratory acidosis:

$$H_2O + CO_2 \leftarrow H_2CO_3 \leftarrow H^+ + HCO_3^-$$
$$\uparrow$$
$$H^+ + Hb^- \leftarrow HHb$$

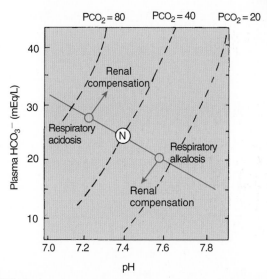

FIGURE 52-4 A pH-bicarbonate diagram showing the effects of respiratory acidosis and alkalosis on pH, bicarbonate (HCO_3^-) concentration, and carbon dioxide tension (P_{CO_2}) of arterial blood. In acute respiratory acidosis, as P_{CO_2} increases, the changes in pH and bicarbonate concentration are predicted by the normal buffer line. Renal compensation leads to an accumulation of HCO_3^-, which increases the pH, whereas P_{CO_2} remains constant. In respiratory alkalosis, Pa_{CO_2} and HCO_3^- decrease and pH increases. The kidneys compensate by increasing HCO_3^- resorption, which decreases pH. *N*, Normal arterial blood composition.

As CO_2 is eliminated, H_2CO_3 is formed from H^+ and HCO_3^-, and thus the pH increases and $[HCO_3^-]$ decreases. Hydrogen ion is supplied by release from nonbicarbonate buffers, such as hemoglobin. The net result of these processes is that Pa_{CO_2} decreases, the pH increases, and $[HCO_3^-]$ decreases and is replaced by other buffers. There is no change in total buffer base. The increase in the $[HCO_3^-/0.03 \times P_{CO_2}]$ ratio increases pH.

Figure 52-4 shows the increase in pH and decrease in $[HCO3^-]$ as P_{CO_2} decreases. To adjust the pH toward normal, hyperventilation must be stopped, or the kidneys must eliminate HCO_3^-. The latter occurs because the low P_{CO_2} and alkalosis reduce H^+ and NH_3 production by the kidney. When H^+ is not produced in sufficient amounts to capture all the filtered HCO_3^-, the latter spills into the urine and is lost from the body.

Metabolic Acidosis Is Caused by the Accumulation of Fixed Acids or the Loss of Buffer Base, Which Decreases Blood pH

Metabolic acidosis is the most common acid-base abnormality. During metabolism, there is a continuous production of fixed acids. An increase in their production or a failure of H^+ elimination by the kidneys is the cause of metabolic acidosis. Increased production of fixed acids results from protein catabolism or ketone production during starvation or from anaerobic metabolism that leads to lactic acidosis. Diarrhea can also cause metabolic acidosis because excessive amounts of HCO_3^- (buffer) are lost in the feces. In ruminants, excessive feeding of carbohydrates can lead to increased H^+ production in the rumen (*rumen acidosis*). The H^+ ions that are absorbed cause metabolic acidosis.

The accumulating H^+ in the blood combines with HCO_3^- and other buffers, which causes a base deficit. The CO_2 resulting from the combination of H^+ and HCO_3^- is eliminated by ventilation.

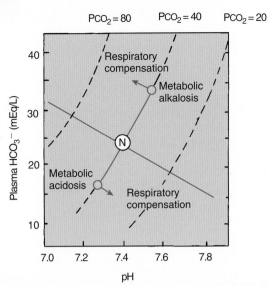

FIGURE 52-5 A pH-bicarbonate diagram showing the effects of metabolic acidosis and alkalosis on pH, bicarbonate (HCO_3^-) concentration, and carbon dioxide tension (PCO_2) of arterial blood. In uncompensated metabolic acidosis, there is a decrease in the bicarbonate concentration, which leads to a decrease in pH, whereas PCO_2 remains constant. Respiratory compensation results in a decrease in PCO_2, with a subsequent increase in pH and movement of data points parallel to the normal buffer line. In metabolic alkalosis, HCO_3^- increases and causes an increase in pH. Respiratory compensation is by alveolar hypoventilation, which leads to an increase in $PaCO_2$ and a return of pH toward normal. *N*, Normal arterial blood composition.

The HCO_3^- depletion decreases the $[HCO_3^-/0.03 \times PCO_2]$ ratio; therefore the pH decreases (Figure 52-5).

The decrease in pH accompanying metabolic acidosis stimulates ventilation. This increase in alveolar ventilation has a compensatory effect on metabolic acidosis by eliminating CO_2, leading to a decreased PCO_2, which ultimately adjusts the $[HCO_3^-/0.03 \times PCO_2]$ ratio and pH toward normal. This sequence is shown in Figure 52-5. As the PCO_2 decreases, $[HCO_3^-]$ decreases along a line that parallels the normal buffer line. This decrease in $[HCO_3^-]$ is accompanied by a decrease in pH. Complete restoration of normal acid-base balance requires the restoration of the depleted base by the kidney or by therapy with intravenous fluid that contains buffers, such as bicarbonate or lactate.

Metabolic Alkalosis Is Caused by the Excessive Elimination of Hydrogen Ions or by the Intake of Base, such as Bicarbonate, Which Increases Blood pH

The most common cause of *metabolic alkalosis* is *vomiting,* during which H^+-rich gastric contents are lost from the body. In ruminants, torsion and dilation of the abomasum cause metabolic alkalosis because H^+ ions are trapped in the *abomasum.* Metabolic alkalosis can also result from potassium (K^+) depletion because low concentrations of K^+ in the blood (hypokalemia) result in increased H^+ excretion by the kidney (see later discussion).

The loss of H^+ from the body frees buffer, and thus the plasma $[HCO_3^-]$ and total buffer base increase. The $[HCO_3^-/0.03 \cdot PCO_2]$ ratio, pH, and base excess all increase (see Figure 52-5). The increase in pH reduces the drive to ventilate; alveolar ventilation

decreases, and so PCO_2 increases. This adjusts the $[HCO_3^-/0.03 \times PCO_2]$ ratio toward normal, and thus the pH decreases toward normal (see Figure 52-5).

Respiratory Compensations for Acid-Base Abnormalities Occur Rapidly; Renal Compensations Occur Over Several Hours

This discussion of acid-base disturbances shows that the lungs compensate for metabolic problems, and the kidneys compensate for respiratory problems. Because the *chemoreceptors* respond almost immediately to changes in blood pH, and because changes in ventilation rapidly change PCO_2, respiratory compensation for metabolic acid-base problems occurs almost immediately. For this reason, it is rare to observe "pure" metabolic acidosis or alkalosis without a respiratory compensation. The response of the kidneys to a respiratory acid-base disturbance is less rapid, and changes in NH_3 and HCO_3^- production occur over about 24 hours.

As compensatory mechanisms adjust the pH toward normal, there is less "error signal" to drive the compensation; thus these mechanisms alone rarely return the pH to normal. In metabolic acidosis, for example, the low pH drives ventilation to decrease PCO_2. As the pH returns to normal, however, the respiratory drive to compensate is reduced; therefore, restoration of normal pH is rarely complete. Restoration of normal acid-base balance requires correction of the initiating cause of the acidosis or alkalosis.

Hydrogen and Potassium Ions Are Interrelated in Acid-Base Homeostasis

Acid-base disturbances affect the distribution of potassium within the body. A decrease in blood pH leads to an increase in the plasma K^+ concentration $[K^+]$ (hyperkalemia), whereas a blood alkalosis leads to a decrease in plasma $[K^+]$ (hypokalemia). The *hyperkalemia* accompanying blood acidosis is a consequence of reduced activity of the Na^+-K^+ pump and the $Na^+/K^+/Cl^-$ co-transporter, both of which normally transport K^+ back into the cell. In addition, intracellular acidosis liberates K^+ from nondiffusible intracellular anions so that more K^+ is free to diffuse out of the cell. In the case of blood alkalosis, high $[HCO_3^-]$ can stimulate K^+ uptake into cells.

Just as changes in blood pH affect $[K^+]$, the converse also is true. *Hypokalemia* is frequently associated with metabolic alkalosis, and hyperkalemia with metabolic acidosis. These changes are a consequence of the actions of K^+ on the renal tubule. Depletion of K^+ increases H^+ elimination by (1) increasing tubular Na^+/H^+ exchange and basolateral Na^+/ HCO_3^- co-transport; (2) increasing NH_3 synthesis and NH_4^+ excretion; and (3) stimulating K^+/H^+ exchange in the collecting tubules. Increases in K^+ cause metabolic acidosis by inhibition of NH_3 synthesis and NH_4^+ excretion.

The Diagnosis of Acid-Base Disturbances Depends on Interpretation of Measurements of Arterial Blood pH and Carbon Dioxide Tension, from Which Bicarbonate Concentration and Total Buffer Base Are Calculated

Arterial samples must be used to determine the respiratory component of an acid-base abnormality, and samples must be obtained

TABLE 52-1 Examples of Blood Gas Abnormalities

pH	Paco$_2$	HCO$_3^-$	Base Excess	Base Deficit	Diagnosis
7.4	40	24	0	0	Normal
7.26	60	27	0	0	Uncompensated respiratory acidosis
7.38	60	36	9	0	Partially compensated respiratory acidosis
7.2	40	15	0	12	Uncompensated metabolic acidosis
7.35	22	11	0	12	Partially compensated metabolic acidosis
7.45	20	13	0	11	Partially compensated respiratory alkalosis
7.55	40	34	11	0	Uncompensated metabolic alkalosis
7.2	50	19	0	9	Combined metabolic and respiratory acidosis
7.6	20	20	0	0	Uncompensated respiratory alkalosis
7.3	20	9	0	15	Partially compensated metabolic acidosis

Paco$_2$, Arterial carbon dioxide tension (mm Hg); *HCO$_3^-$*, bicarbonate (mEq/L).

anaerobically to prevent the loss of CO_2 from the blood. The Paco$_2$ and pH are measured with specific electrodes in an arterial blood gas (ABG) analyzer. The plasma [HCO$_3^-$] and total buffer base are determined from nomograms or frequently from a built-in program in the ABG analyzer.

When ABG data are analyzed, it is useful to ask the following questions:

1. Is the sample acidotic (pH <7.4) or alkalotic (pH >7.4)?
2. What is the respiratory component (is Paco$_2$ high, low, or normal), and will it explain the pH?
3. What is the metabolic component (is there a base excess or deficit), and will it explain the pH?
4. How can the first three questions be combined to explain the data, in view of the fact that compensations rarely return the pH toward normal?

Examples are provided in Table 52-1.

Over the Years, Many Terms Have Been Used to Explain Acid-Base Balance

The terms used to explain acid-base balance include the following:

- *Anion gap.* In the blood the total cation concentration (concentration of $Na^+ + K^+ + Mg^{2+} + Ca^{2+}$) should approximately equal the total anion concentration (concentration of $HCO_3^- + Cl^-$). Usually, the total cations exceed the total anions; the difference is called the *anion gap*. This gap results from the presence of unaccounted-for anions from fixed acids, such as lactate. In metabolic acidosis the anion gap increases because of increased production of fixed acids.
- *Standard bicarbonate.* The plasma [HCO$_3^-$] when Pco$_2$ = 40 mm Hg is known as *standard* bicarbonate. The plasma [HCO$_3^-$] can change as a result of respiratory and metabolic disturbances. An increase or decrease in [HCO$_3^-$], measured when Pco$_2$ is normal (i.e., 40 mm Hg), results only from metabolic disturbances.
- *Total carbon dioxide* (TCO$_2$). Carbon dioxide is present in the blood in solution and as carbamino compounds, but largely as HCO_3^-. TCO$_2$ can be measured by adding an acid to the blood and collecting the evolved CO_2, which comes primarily from HCO_3^-. Changes in TCO$_2$ should be interpreted as changes in plasma [HCO$_3^-$].

CLINICAL CORRELATIONS

UPPER AIRWAY OBSTRUCTION IN A BOSTON TERRIER

History. A Boston terrier exhibits signs of severe respiratory distress. It has difficulty inhaling and makes a snoring sound during inhalation. The effort of walking magnifies the distress. An arterial blood gas (ABG) sample reveals that Paco$_2$ is 80 mm Hg (normal, 40 mm Hg), pH is 7.3, [HCO$_3^-$] is 39 mEq/L, and base excess is 10 mEq/L (Figure 52-6).

Clinical Examination. Examination reveals excessively narrowed (stenotic) nares and excessive folds of tissue in the soft palate, the latter occluding the glottis. The larynx and trachea appear normal.

Treatment. Reconstructive surgery is performed on the dog to enlarge the nares and remove the excessive tissues from the palate. Two weeks after surgery, respiratory distress is greatly reduced. ABG analysis reveals that Paco$_2$ is 45 mm Hg, pH is 7.39, [HCO$_3^-$] is 27 mEq/L, and base excess is 2 mEq/L.

Comment. Before surgery the animal is acidotic with an elevated Paco$_2$ and base excess. Only the high Paco$_2$ explains the acidosis; therefore the dog has respiratory acidosis. The increase in [HCO$_3^-$] (normal, 24 mEq/L) is caused primarily by creation of new HCO_3^- (a base excess) by the kidneys and indicates the condition is of at least several days' duration. Respiratory acidosis is caused by alveolar hypoventilation resulting from the upper airway obstruction. Surgery corrects the obstruction and alleviates the hypoventilation. This returns the pH to a more normal value. Two weeks after surgery the base excess has been virtually eliminated.

TORSION OF THE ABOMASUM IN A COW

History. A Holstein cow gave birth 2 weeks ago and became inappetent 2 days ago. Over the past 12 hours she has become lethargic, and her right flank is distended. Examination shows she is depressed and dehydrated. Her extremities are cold. Rectal examination as well as percussion reveals a large, fluid-filled organ between the rumen and the right abdominal wall. A fluid sample obtained percutaneously from the distended organ is chloride rich and very acidic. An ABG sample shows that $Paco_2$ is 50 mm Hg, pH is 7.6, $[HCO_3^-]$ is 50 mEq/L, and base excess is 24 mEq/L (see Figure 52-6).

Comment. The history and physical findings are typical of a dilation or torsion of the abomasum. This condition occasionally occurs shortly after parturition in dairy cows fed high levels of concentrates and chopped feeds. The abomasum distends and may rotate, and thus its inlet and outlet are obstructed. Fluid rich in chloride and H^+ continues to be secreted into and is trapped within the abomasum. The loss of H^+ from the blood results in a base excess and causes the metabolic alkalosis. The alkalosis depresses ventilation, which elevates $Paco_2$. This is a compensation to restore pH toward normal.

Treatment. The torsion of the abomasum must be surgically corrected. However, the metabolic alkalosis and any fluid deficits should be treated concurrently to provide the best chance of recovery. The alkalosis is enhanced by loss of Cl^- into the abomasum along with H^+. Repletion of Cl^- allows the kidneys to eliminate the excess bicarbonate and restores normal pH. In practical terms, this is accomplished by treating the cow intravenously with large volumes of 0.9% NaCl solution.

NEONATAL DIARRHEA IN A FOAL

History. A 2-week-old foal has profuse diarrhea. It is lethargic and cold to the touch, its eyes are sunken and dull, and it lies in a pool of feces. The foal's hematocrit is 65 mL/dL (normal, 45), pH

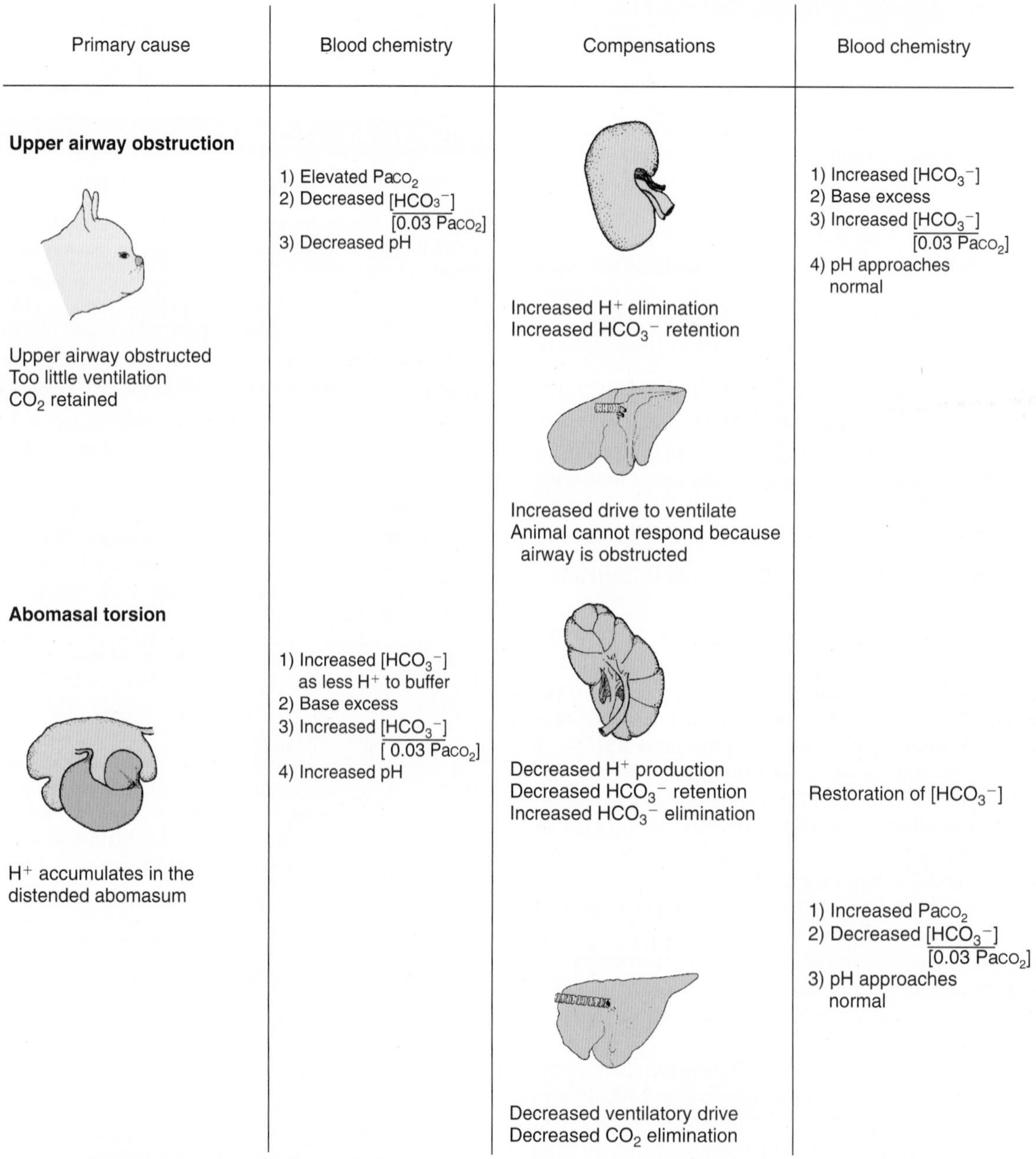

Primary cause	Blood chemistry	Compensations	Blood chemistry
Upper airway obstruction Upper airway obstructed Too little ventilation CO_2 retained	1) Elevated $Paco_2$ 2) Decreased $\dfrac{[HCO_3^-]}{[0.03\,Paco_2]}$ 3) Decreased pH	Increased H^+ elimination Increased HCO_3^- retention Increased drive to ventilate Animal cannot respond because airway is obstructed	1) Increased $[HCO_3^-]$ 2) Base excess 3) Increased $\dfrac{[HCO_3^-]}{[0.03\,Paco_2]}$ 4) pH approaches normal
Abomasal torsion H^+ accumulates in the distended abomasum	1) Increased $[HCO_3^-]$ as less H^+ to buffer 2) Base excess 3) Increased $\dfrac{[HCO_3^-]}{[0.03\,Paco_2]}$ 4) Increased pH	Decreased H^+ production Decreased HCO_3^- retention Increased HCO_3^- elimination Decreased ventilatory drive Decreased CO_2 elimination	Restoration of $[HCO_3^-]$ 1) Increased $Paco_2$ 2) Decreased $\dfrac{[HCO_3^-]}{[0.03\,Paco_2]}$ 3) pH approaches normal

FIGURE 52-6 Diagrammatic representation of the acid-base changes initiated by upper airway obstruction, abomasal torsion, and neonatal foal diarrhea.

Continued

Primary cause	Blood chemistry	Compensations	Blood chemistry
Neonatal diarrhea Fluid and electrolyte, including HCO_3^- loss in feces	1) Decreased $[HCO_3^-]$ 2) Base deficit 3) Increased $\dfrac{[HCO_3^-]}{[\alpha P_{CO_2}]}$ 4) Decreased pH	Increased H^+ elimination Complete $[HCO_3^-]$ reabsorption Increased HCO_3^- production	Restoration of $[HCO_3^-]$
		Increased ventilatory drive Increased CO_2 elimination	1) Decreased P_{CO_2} 2) Increased $\dfrac{[HCO_3^-]}{[\alpha P_{CO_2}]}$ 3) pH approaches normal

FIGURE 52-6, cont'd.

is 7.2 (normal, 7.4), P_{aCO_2} is 30 mm Hg (normal, 40), $[HCO_3^-]$ is 12 mEq/L (normal, 24), and base deficit is 15 mEq/L (see Figure 52-6).

Comment. The foal shows typical clinical signs of severe dehydration as a result of excessive fluid loss in the feces. Fluid loss from the intravascular compartment reduces blood volume and cardiac output. To maintain blood pressure, vasoconstriction occurs in the extremities, which therefore have less blood flow and become cold. The loss of fluid from the interstitial space causes the dryness of the eyes and muzzle, the sunken appearance of the eyes, and inelastic skin. The increased hematocrit of 65 mL/dL (normal, 45) confirms the dehydration.

Feces contain HCO_3^-, and its excessive loss causes a base deficit and a decrease in pH. In addition, poor tissue perfusion results in lactic acidosis. The acidosis results from loss of buffer base and accumulation of lactic acid; it is a metabolic acidosis. The acidosis stimulates ventilation, which reduces P_{aCO_2} in an attempt to correct pH. The foal has a metabolic acidosis that is partially corrected by the reduction in P_{aCO_2}.

Treatment. This foal needs fluid replacement to increase plasma volume, raise cardiac output, and restore circulatory perfusion. The fluid should contain electrolytes, to replace those lost in diarrhea, and a source of buffer, such as lactate or bicarbonate. A good choice would be lactated Ringer's solution supplemented with additional bicarbonate. If the foal's respiratory and acid-base homeostasis can be maintained until the diarrhea ceases, the foal has a moderate chance of recovery. A serious concern is that this 2-week-old foal could have an infectious cause of diarrhea. The foal could become septic from the infection, or the foal could have an initial septicemia, which is now manifested as diarrhea. In either situation, antibiotics are also warranted in most cases to treat the infection.

PRACTICE QUESTIONS

1. Elevated P_{aCO_2}, low pH, and no base excess or deficit are characteristic of:
   a. Acute respiratory acidosis.
   b. Acute respiratory alkalosis.
   c. Metabolic acidosis.
   d. Metabolic alkalosis.
   e. None of the above.

2. Elevated P_{aCO_2}, alkaline pH, and base excess are characteristic of:
   a. Chronic respiratory acidosis.
   b. Chronic respiratory alkalosis.
   c. Metabolic acidosis.
   d. Metabolic alkalosis.
   e. None of the above.

3. Low P_{aCO_2}, acid pH, and base deficit are characteristic of:
   a. Chronic respiratory acidosis.
   b. Acute respiratory alkalosis.
   c. Metabolic acidosis.
   d. Metabolic alkalosis.
   e. None of the above.

4. The most likely acid-base disturbance to be found in a dog at the top of Mount McKinley (Denali) in Alaska (height, 20,320 ft [6353 m]) is:
   a. Respiratory acidosis.
   b. Respiratory alkalosis.
   c. Metabolic acidosis.
   d. Metabolic alkalosis.
   e. None of the above.

5. The distal tubule of the kidney affects acid-base balance by:
   a. Altering the pK_a of the HCO_3^-/H_2CO_3 buffer.
   b. Concentrating CO_2 in the renal tubular cell.
   c. Generating new HCO_3^-.
   d. Using ammonia to buffer H^+.
   e. Both c and d.

6. Which of the following buffers will be most effective in blood (pH = 7.4)?
   a. HX/X^-, $pK_a = 4.2$, plentiful
   b. HY/Y^-, $pK_a = 7.2$, scarce
   c. HZ/Z^-, $pK_a = 9.6$, scarce
   d. HW/W^-, $pK_a = 7.6$, plentiful
   e. HA/A^-, $pK_a = 10.2$, plentiful

BIBLIOGRAPHY

Boron WF: Acid-base physiology. In Boron WF, Boulpaep EL: *Medical physiology: a cellular and molecular approach*, ed 2, Philadelphia, 2009, Saunders.

Cohen JP, Kassirer JJ, editors: *Acid-base*, Boston, 1982, Little, Brown.

Davenport HW: *The ABC of acid-base chemistry*, ed 6, Chicago, 1974, University of Chicago Press.

DiBartola SP: Introduction to acid-base disorders. In DiBartola SP, editor: *Fluid, electrolyte, and acid-base disorders in small animal practice*, ed 3, St Louis, 2006, Saunders.

Gamble JL: *Acid-base physiology: a direct approach*, Baltimore, 1982, Johns Hopkins University Press.

Hlastala MP, Berger AJ: *Physiology of respiration*, ed 2, New York, 2001, Oxford University Press.

CHAPTER 53
Thermoregulation

KEY POINTS

1. Temperature is a major factor affecting tissue function.
2. Homeotherms and poikilotherms use different strategies to regulate body temperature.
3. Body temperature depends on the balance between heat input and heat output.

Heat Production
1. Heat is a byproduct of all metabolic processes.
2. Shivering produces heat by muscle contraction.
3. Nonshivering thermogenesis is an increase in basal metabolic rate, caused especially by the oxidation of brown fat, to produce heat.

Heat Transfer in the Body
1. Because tissues are poor conductors, heat is most effectively transferred in the blood.
2. Countercurrent heat exchange mechanisms are used both to conserve and to lose heat.

Heat Exchange with the Environment
1. Heat loss by convection occurs when the body warms air or water.
2. Heat loss by conduction occurs when the body is in contact with a cooler surface.
3. Heat loss by radiation occurs when infrared radiation emitted by the body is absorbed by cooler objects.
4. Heat loss by evaporation occurs when the water in sweat, saliva, and respiratory secretions is converted into water vapor.

Temperature Regulation
1. Mammals and birds regulate the input and output of heat to maintain body temperature within a narrow limit.
2. Temperature-sensitive receptors are located in the central nervous system, the skin, and some internal organs.
3. Information from central and peripheral heat-sensitive neurons is integrated in the hypothalamus to regulate heat-losing or heat-conserving mechanisms.

Integrated Responses
1. The responses to heat stress are peripheral vasodilation and increased evaporative cooling.
2. The responses to cold stress are peripheral vasoconstriction, piloerection, and increased metabolic heat production by shivering and nonshivering thermogenesis.
3. Fever is an elevation of body temperature that results from an increase in the thermoregulatory set point.

Heat Stroke, Hypothermia, and Frostbite
1. Heat stroke occurs when heat production or input exceeds heat output, so body temperature rises to dangerous levels.
2. Hypothermia occurs when heat output exceeds heat production, so body temperature decreases to dangerous levels.
3. Frostbite occurs when ice crystals form in the tissues of the extremities.

Temperature Is a Major Factor Affecting Tissue Function

Because body function is the result of chemical and physical processes that are sensitive to changes in temperature, animals use a variety of strategies to regulate the temperature of their tissues. If *body temperature* is allowed to decrease too much below its normal value of about 38° C (~100° F), metabolic processes are slowed to such an extent that body functions are severely impaired. Below 34° C (93.2° F), animals become unable to regulate their own temperature, and at 27° to 29° C (80.6° to 84.2° F), cardiac fibrillation and death occur. At the other extreme, an increase in temperature to 45° C (113° F) can cause fatal brain lesions.

Homeotherms and Poikilotherms Use Different Strategies to Regulate Body Temperature

Fish, reptiles, and amphibians are called *cold-blooded animals,* or *poikilotherms*, because their body temperature varies with the temperature of the environment. However, this does not mean that these animals have no control over their body temperature. They use behavioral methods to prevent major changes in their temperature. For example, the lizard basks on a sun-baked rock to increase its temperature early in the morning and hides beneath the rock later in the day to prevent overheating. Veterinarians are sometimes asked to advise on the management of captive poikilotherms; it is important to remind owners to provide supplemental heat if they want their animals to be active at the cooler times of the year.

Mammals and birds are *homeotherms;* they maintain a constant body temperature in the presence of considerable changes in environmental temperature. Although the maintenance of a constant temperature allows mammals to live in a wide variety of environments and to remain active during the cold times of the year, it is not without cost. Homeotherms must maintain a high metabolic rate just to provide the heat necessary to maintain body temperature. This requires a high energy intake and therefore almost constant foraging for food. Poikilotherms require much less energy and are better able to survive times of food shortage. Because most veterinarians are primarily concerned with mammals and birds, this chapter focuses on the maintenance of a normal body temperature by homeotherms.

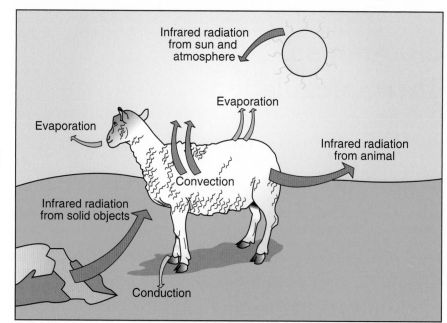

FIGURE 53-1 Representation of the heat input and heat output between a mammal and the environment.

Body Temperature Depends on the Balance Between Heat Input and Heat Output

Heat inputs to the body are from metabolism and from external sources (Figure 53-1). When food energy is ingested, heat is produced at all stages of the metabolic process. Eventually, all food energy is converted into heat, which is dissipated into the environment and radiated into space. Heat production by the body is related to metabolic rate. A basal metabolic rate is necessary to maintain the function of cells. During exercise, metabolic heat production can increase more than tenfold. If this heat is not dissipated to the environment, body temperature can increase to dangerous levels. Furthermore, this increase in body temperature increases metabolic rate, which further increases heat production.

Animals gain heat from the environment when ambient temperature exceeds body temperature and when they are exposed to *radiant heat* sources. The latter occurs when an animal is exposed to sunlight or is placed close to solid objects that are warmer than its body temperature.

Heat is lost to the environment by *radiation* from the body surface to a cooler object; by convection as the surrounding air or water is warmed by the body; by *evaporation* of respiratory secretions, sweat, or saliva; and by *conduction* to cooler surfaces with which the animal is in contact. A small amount of heat is also lost with urine and feces.

Many of the metabolic heat sources, such as the liver, heart, and limb muscles, are remote from the skin, which is the site of heat loss. Therefore, it is necessary to transfer heat among these sites. Body tissues are poor conductors, so heat is transferred mainly by convection in the circulation.

HEAT PRODUCTION

Heat Is a Byproduct of All Metabolic Processes

Table 53-1 shows the amount of heat produced by the metabolism of carbohydrates, fats, and proteins. The *basal metabolic rate* (BMR) is the rate of energy metabolism measured under minimal stress while the animal is fasting. BMR is greater in homeotherms

TABLE 53-1 Amount of Heat Produced by Metabolism of Major Food Types

Food Type	Heat Production (kcal/g)		
	Per Gram of Food	Per Liter of O_2 Consumed	Per Liter of CO_2 Produced
Carbohydrates	4.1	5.05	5.05
Fat	9.6	4.75	6.67
Proteins (to urea)	4.2	4.46	5.57

than in poikilotherms because homeotherms need to generate heat to maintain body temperature. The BMR per kilogram of body weight is greater in smaller than in larger mammals (Figure 53-2). This is necessitated partly by the greater surface/volume ratio of smaller animals. The relatively greater surface area per kilogram body weight of small animals provides a larger area for heat loss.

Shivering Produces Heat by Muscle Contraction

Shivering is one method of increasing the metabolic production of heat. Antagonistic groups of limb muscles are activated so that they produce no useful work. The chemical energy used in shivering is transferred to the body core as heat. If necessary, shivering can go on for many hours and can double heat production. Short bursts of shivering can even increase heat production up to fourfold.

Nonshivering Thermogenesis Is an Increase in Basal Metabolic Rate, Caused Especially by the Oxidation of Brown Fat, to Produce Heat

When animals are chronically exposed to cold, they develop the ability to increase metabolic heat production without shivering (*nonshivering thermogenesis*). This increase in metabolism is

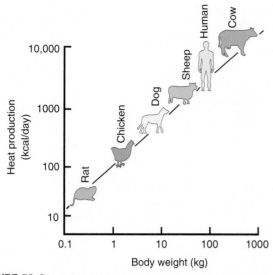

FIGURE 53-2 Relationship between body weight and heat production.

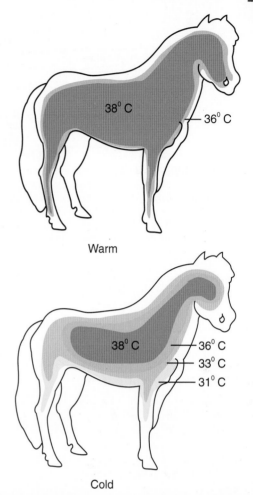

Warm

Cold

FIGURE 53-3 Representation of the distribution of temperatures in a pony under warm and cold environmental conditions. Under warm conditions, the core body temperature extends into the limbs and close to the skin surface of the animal. Under cold conditions, vasoconstriction in the peripheral blood vessels results in a gradient of temperatures between the core and the extremities. The core temperature is maintained only in the abdomen, thorax, and brain of the animal. The more peripheral tissues are allowed to cool considerably.

mediated through an increase in secretion of thyroid hormones and the calorigenic effects of catecholamines on lipids. Table 53-1 shows that fat metabolism is an effective way to produce heat. *Brown fat* is a specialized vascular, mitochondria-rich fat that is used to generate heat. It is widely distributed within the body of all mammals but is especially prevalent in small mammals where, combined with white fat it forms both subcutaneous and trunk depots. Cold stress–induced neural release of norepinephrine from the primarily adrenergic nerve supply activates β_3-adrenergic receptors on adipocytes which increases fat metabolism to produce heat that is distributed around the body through the bloodstream. Furthermore, under cold stress white adipocytes can be converted to the brown adipocytes necessary for heat generation.

HEAT TRANSFER IN THE BODY

Because Tissues Are Poor Conductors, Heat Is Most Effectively Transferred in the Blood

Because heat is produced primarily in muscles of the limbs and in the liver and is eliminated through the skin and the respiratory tract, it is necessary to transfer heat around the body. Tissues have poor *thermal conductivity;* therefore, conduction is not an efficient means of heat redistribution.

The blood perfusing a metabolically active organ collects heat and transfers it to cooler parts of the body by *circulatory convection.* Redistribution of blood flow can deliver heat preferentially to certain body regions, or it can allow regions to cool when the maintenance of the temperature of the brain and major viscera *(core temperature)* is threatened.

Under conditions of heat stress, circulatory transfer of heat to the skin can be increased dramatically by two mechanisms. First, the *arterioles* of skin vascular beds dilate, which results in increased capillary blood flow. Second, *arteriovenous anastomoses* open in the limbs, ears, and muzzle. These two actions greatly increase the total blood flow to the periphery, and the increased heat delivery increases the temperature of the skin, which facilitates heat loss. Conversely, under cold stress, skin vascular beds vasoconstrict, and arteriovenous anastomoses close; thus skin and limb temperatures decrease. This results in reduced heat loss

from the skin and in a gradient of temperatures along the limb (Figure 53-3). Under severe cold stress, the skin temperature of the extremities can approach ambient temperature. Interestingly, the lipids in the limb extremities have a lower melting point than those in the core, so fats do not solidify in extreme cold stress.

Countercurrent Heat Exchange Mechanisms Are Used Both to Conserve and to Lose Heat

When the environmental temperature is high, the blood perfusing the skin vascular beds returns to the body core through superficial veins from which heat is lost to the skin and air. Under cold conditions, limb blood flow returns to the core through deep veins that accompany arteries (Figure 53-4). Heat is transferred by *countercurrent exchange* from the warm arterial blood to the cooler venous blood and thereby returned to the core of the body.

A similar countercurrent exchange of heat occurs in a *carotid rete* in sheep and some other ungulates. In this system the carotid artery forms a rete bathed in a sinus of venous blood that has drained the nasal cavity. The colder venous blood from the nose

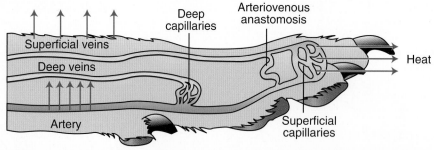

FIGURE 53-4 Representation of a limb showing the arterial supply and venous drainage by deep and superficial veins. Under warm conditions, blood perfuses the more superficial capillary beds, and heat is lost to the environment through the skin. Blood returns from these superficial vascular beds through the superficial veins, and this provides an additional source of heat loss. Under cold conditions, peripheral vasoconstriction occurs, and the blood flow to the limb is directed to the deeper vascular beds and returns to the trunk through the deep veins. Countercurrent heat exchange between the arteries and veins conserves body heat.

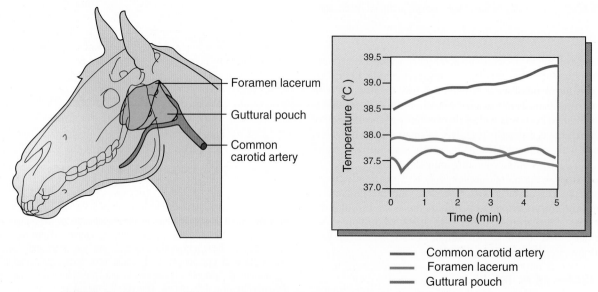

FIGURE 53-5 Guttural pouches cool the blood passing through the internal carotid artery on its way to the brain. *Left,* Anatomic arrangement of the guttural pouches and carotid arteries in the skull. The location of the temperature probes used to measure blood temperature is indicated. *Right,* Graph of blood and guttural pouch temperatures during a period of cantering. Note that even though the temperature of blood entering the guttural pouch in the common carotid artery increases with the duration of exercise, temperature at the foramen lacerum (where the internal carotid artery enters the cranium) decreases slightly.

cools the arterial blood supplying the brain and protects the temperature of the brain. This mechanism becomes important during exercise, when the increase in ventilation aids in cooling the blood that drains from the nose. As a result, the arterial blood carrying heat from the exercising muscles is cooled before it enters the brain.

Some mammals, including humans and horses, do not possess a carotid rete and must rely on other thermoregulatory mechanisms to cool their brains during exercise. In the horse the *guttural pouches* may serve as such a mechanism. The guttural pouches contain air that is cooler than the arterial blood carried in the internal carotid artery. Because anatomically these guttural pouches surround the internal carotid arteries, heat is transferred from the blood to the air in the guttural pouches, thus protecting the brain from hyperthermia (Figure 53-5). In addition, the *intracranial cavernous venous sinuses* may assist in cooling the horse's

brain during exercise. This mechanism is thought to function in the same manner as the carotid rete, but less efficiently.

HEAT EXCHANGE WITH THE ENVIRONMENT

Heat Loss by Convection Occurs When the Body Warms Air or Water

When the air or water in contact with the skin is heated, it flows away, thereby exposing the skin to cooler fluids. Because it takes more heat to warm water than it does to warm an equivalent mass of air, water-dwelling animals lose more heat by convection than do terrestrial mammals. The amount of heat lost by convection depends on the *thermal gradient* (temperature difference) between the skin of the animal and the fluid overlying the skin; a greater thermal gradient results in more heat loss. In *natural convection* the warmed air or water rises from the surface of the animal because it is less dense than the cooler fluid. In *forced convection,* cooler fluid is moved over the skin surface by a breeze or current or simply because the limbs and animal are moving. Forced convection is more effective than natural convection as a mode of heat loss because the thermal gradient is maintained by the constant renewal of the cooler air or water that blankets the surface of the skin. Young or small animals left in a cool draft can quickly lose much body heat by convection and should be protected from such situations.

The thermal gradient for heat loss can be altered by changes in skin blood flow and the amount of *insulation* separating the animal from the environment. Increasing blood flow to the skin raises skin temperature and therefore heat loss, whereas a reduction in skin blood flow reduces heat loss. Hair traps air and impairs convection. The thickness of the layer of hair can be altered by *piloerection* (making the hair stand up) and by growing a thicker hair coat in preparation for winter. The thick layer of blubber in sea mammals also provides a layer of insulation. Reducing the area of the exposed body surface also reduces convective heat loss. Animals accomplish this by curling up in a ball or by huddling with littermates.

Heat Loss by Conduction Occurs When the Body Is in Contact with a Cooler Surface

Because animals usually do not lie on cool surfaces for long periods, conduction is not usually a major form of heat loss. In some situations, however, conductive heat loss can lead to hypothermia. A cold, stainless steel surgery table can form a heat sink for a small, anesthetized bird or mammal. Insulation or a heat source should be provided for such animals. Similarly, newborn piglets can lose much heat by lying on a cold concrete floor. Adult pigs cool themselves by conduction when they wallow in cool mud puddles.

Heat Loss by Radiation Occurs When Infrared Radiation Emitted by the Body Is Absorbed by Cooler Objects

All solid objects emit invisible *electromagnetic radiation* in the *infrared* range. Warm objects emit on a shorter wavelength and emit more emissions per unit time than do cool objects. When these emissions strike another object, some are absorbed and thus transfer heat. Although all objects emit radiant heat, the net heat transfer is from warm to cool objects. It is important to realize that radiant heat loss can occur even when a thermally neutral or warm environment surrounds the animal. Heat can be lost from an animal to the uninsulated walls of a building even though the intervening air is warm.

Heat Loss by Evaporation Occurs When the Water in Sweat, Saliva, and Respiratory Secretions Is Converted into Water Vapor

The evaporation of 1 L of water into water vapor requires 580 kilocalories (kcal). If the body provides this heat, evaporation can be a major form of heat loss. Some *evaporative heat loss* occurs continuously by the diffusion of water through the skin and by loss of water vapor from the respiratory tract. This water loss is obligatory, but under thermal stress, evaporative cooling can be increased greatly either because *sweat glands* are activated, the animal begins to *pant,* or the animal smears itself with saliva. Evaporative heat loss becomes increasingly important as the ambient temperature approaches body temperature; it is the only form of heat loss available when ambient temperature exceeds body temperature. The effectiveness of evaporation is reduced as

the *relative humidity* increases, that is, as the air becomes more saturated with water vapor.

Sweating occurs from two types of coiled, tubular sweat glands located in the dermis. *Apocrine glands* produce a protein-containing secretion, whereas *eccrine glands* produce an aqueous secretion. All placental mammals except rodents and lagomorphs have sweat glands, but in the dog and pig these glands are poorly developed and of little use in thermoregulation. Apocrine glands produce the thermoregulatory sweat of hoofed animals, whereas in primates, sweat is produced by the eccrine glands. Secreted sweat has an ionic composition similar to that of plasma. As it passes to the skin surface along the duct, its composition is altered by the reabsorption of ions. If secretion rates are low, almost all the sodium and chloride, along with water, is absorbed. Therefore the sweat reaching the skin is a concentrated solution of urea, lactic acid, potassium ions, and, in the case of hoofed mammals, protein. When secretion rates are high, less sodium and chloride are absorbed, more water is lost, and the other constituents are consequently diluted. In hot environments, acclimatization increases the sweating rates, and because of increased secretion of *aldosterone,* most of the sodium and chloride is reabsorbed before the sweat reaches the skin. In most species, sweating is under the control of sympathetic cholinergic nerve fibers, but in the horse, control is through β_2 adrenoceptors activated by catecholamines originating from sympathetic nerves or the adrenal medulla.

Panting is one mode of increasing evaporation from the respiratory tract. Small tidal volumes are moved at rapid frequency (200 breaths/min) over the respiratory dead-space. The rate of panting is close to the resonant frequency of the respiratory system, and thus the work of breathing is minimized and does not add to the heat load. In the panting animal, two mechanisms act to elevate heat loss through evaporation: (1) vascular engorgement of the respiratory and oral mucosa and (2) increased salivation. By ventilating primarily dead-space, severe hyperventilation and respiratory alkalosis are avoided. In birds, *gular flutter* is another method of increasing airflow over the respiratory dead-space. Even in mammals that do not pant, such as the horse, evaporative heat loss from the respiratory tract probably increases during prolonged exercise because dead-space ventilation increases.

Mammals vary in the relative importance of different modes of evaporative heat loss. In horses and cattle, sweating is the major form of evaporative heat loss. Sheep sweat, but panting is also of considerable importance. The dog relies almost totally on panting. Even small rodents, which neither pant nor sweat, increase evaporative heat loss by smearing saliva or water on their fur.

TEMPERATURE REGULATION

Mammals and Birds Regulate the Input and Output of Heat to Maintain Body Temperature Within a Narrow Limit

It is customary to measure body temperature as a first part of the clinical examination of mammals. This is because body temperature is maintained within fairly narrow limits despite large variations in ambient conditions. In diseased animals the ability to regulate temperature can be impaired, for example, by dehydration. In addition, infectious and other agents produce pyrogens that can cause an increase in body temperature. Table 53-2 lists the normal ranges of rectal temperatures in some common domestic mammals. The *rectal temperature* is somewhat lower than the core temperature of the animal, and changes in rectal temperature lag behind changes in *core temperature*. However, rectal temperature is a convenient measure in domestic mammals and provides a useful indication of core temperature.

In well-hydrated animals living in temperate climates, the range of normal temperature is quite narrow. Mammals living in hot, arid climates tolerate a wider range of temperature, allowing body temperature to decrease during the cool nights so that more heat can be absorbed during the ensuing hot day.

To maintain temperature within narrow limits, the animal must regulate its heat inputs and outputs. The inputs and outputs clearly cannot be equal at all times. During exercise, for example, heat production exceeds heat loss. Heat is stored in the body and then dissipates when exercise ceases. The *specific heat* of body tissues is similar to that of water; therefore, large amounts of heat can be stored without a potentially lethal increase in temperature.

Temperature-Sensitive Receptors Are Located in the Central Nervous System, the Skin, and Some Internal Organs

To regulate body temperature, the animal needs a variety of *temperature sensors* at various locations within the body. These sensors relay information to the brain, which then initiates mechanisms either to increase or to decrease heat loss or production.

TABLE 53-2 Rectal Temperature (in Degrees C) of Domestic Mammals

Species	Average	Range
Cat	38.6	38.1-39.2
Cattle (beef)	38.3	36.7-39.1
Cattle (dairy)	38.6	38.0-39.3
Dog	38.9	37.9-39.9
Donkey	37.4	36.4-38.4
Goat	39.1	38.5-39.7
Horse	37.7	37.2-38.2
Pig	39.2	38.7-39.8
Sheep	39.1	38.5-39.9

Numerous heat-sensitive neurons are located in the preoptic area of the hypothalamus. These neurons increase their firing rate in response to minor increases in local temperature. In addition, experimentally warming this area immediately initiates heat-losing mechanisms, such as peripheral vasodilation and sweating. These observations suggest that this region of the brain may be the main center for temperature regulation. Other hypothalamic and midbrain neurons decrease their firing in response to heat, and still others increase firing in response to cold. All these temperature-sensitive neurons are monitoring brain or core temperature.

When an animal is exposed to a change in temperature, considerable heat loss or heat gain can occur before a change in core temperature occurs. Therefore, it is advantageous to have temperature-sensitive neurons located in the skin so that environmental temperature changes are detected before they threaten core temperature. The most numerous temperature-sensitive neurons in the skin respond to cold. If these receptors are activated, the body can initiate mechanisms for heat conservation and heat production before the core temperature decreases. *Skin cold receptors* are particularly sensitive to the rate of decrease in temperature. For this reason, shivering can occur after exercise as the skin is rapidly cooled by sweat evaporation, despite that the core temperature may be normal or slightly elevated. Skin receptors sensitive to heat also exist and can initiate heat loss when the skin temperature rises.

Temperature-sensitive neurons are also present at various locations in the viscera. Drinking large volumes of cold fluids may stimulate cold receptors in the gastrointestinal system, initiating body heat–conserving mechanisms.

Information from Central and Peripheral Heat-Sensitive Neurons Is Integrated in the Hypothalamus to Regulate Heat-Losing or Heat-Conserving Mechanisms

Figure 53-6 shows the *feedback control mechanisms* for the regulation of body temperature. Central integration of the information from various receptors occurs in the anterior hypothalamus. Information from central temperature receptors seems to predominate over information from skin and visceral receptors. For this reason, a rise in core temperature of only 0.5° C causes a sevenfold increase in the amount of skin blood flow; similarly, a

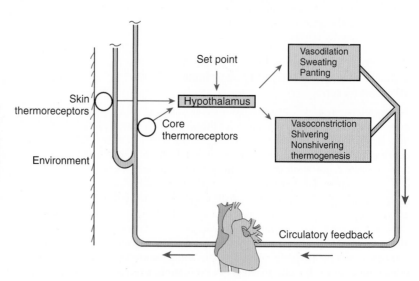

FIGURE 53-6 Feedback control mechanisms for the regulation of body temperature. Temperature receptors in the skin and the core relay information to the hypothalamus, which adjusts the responses either to conserve and produce or to lose heat. The results of these responses are relayed to the receptors through the circulatory feedback.

modest decrease in core temperature initiates vasoconstriction and shivering. The effect of central receptors is about twentyfold greater than the effect of peripheral receptors.

In the regulation of body temperature, the hypothalamus behaves as if it has a normal *set point*. When the core temperature rises above the set point, heat-losing mechanisms are initiated; when temperature decreases, heat conservation or production begins. Information from peripheral receptors modifies the set point, and thus shivering begins at a higher core temperature when the skin is cool than when it is warm. Similarly, sweating is initiated at a higher core temperature when the skin is cool than when it is warm.

INTEGRATED RESPONSES

The Responses to Heat Stress Are Peripheral Vasodilation and Increased Evaporative Cooling

For all mammals and birds, an environmental temperature exists at which body temperature can be maintained in a normal range, primarily by vasomotor mechanisms (Figure 53-7). This *thermoneutral zone* varies with the metabolic rate and the amount of insulation. The pig, which lacks fur, clearly has a higher thermoneutral temperature than does the sheep, which has thick wool. Dairy cattle that have high milk production produce so much metabolic heat that their thermoneutral zone is surprisingly low: 4° to 15° C (39° to 59° F). In the thermoneutral zone, body temperature can be regulated by vasomotor mechanisms that increase or decrease skin blood flow and therefore change the amount of heat loss by convection and radiation.

When a homeotherm is exposed to heat stress, the initial response is vasodilation, which increases skin and limb blood flow. The resulting increase in skin temperature and the extension of core temperature down the limbs increase the temperature gradient between the skin and the environment, resulting in more heat loss by radiation and convection (see Figure 53-3).

If vasodilation alone is ineffective in maintaining a normal temperature, evaporative cooling is increased by sweating, panting, or both. Evaporative cooling is the only method of heat loss available when the environmental temperature exceeds the skin temperature and is most effective when relative humidity is low. Figure 53-8 shows that at −10° C (14° F), cows lose about 10% of their heat by evaporation, but as the ambient temperature rises to about 32° C (90° F), they lose 80% by evaporation. As relative humidity rises, animals have increasing difficulty losing heat; therefore, exercise in hot, humid conditions is likely to cause heat exhaustion. This was a major concern for horses competing in the 1996 (Atlanta) and 2008 (Hong Kong) Olympics, where high temperatures were combined with high humidity.

Animals also use behavioral methods to resist heat stress. These methods, which include seeking shade, standing in water, and wallowing in mud, are not available to intensively managed livestock. The producer must assume increased responsibility for the animals' comfort and survival. Because high-producing dairy cattle have such a low thermoneutral temperature, their primary requirement is shade in hot climates, which is a greater concern than a source of heat or insulation in cold climates.

The Responses to Cold Stress Are Peripheral Vasoconstriction, Piloerection, and Increased Metabolic Heat Production by Shivering and Nonshivering Thermogenesis

As the ambient temperature decreases, homeotherms initially conserve heat by peripheral vasoconstriction. This sets up a temperature gradient along the limbs and reduces skin temperature, so there is only a narrow temperature gradient for radiation and convective heat loss (see Figure 53-3). Piloerection provides insulation and also decreases heat loss. Further cold stress initiates increases in metabolic heat production by shivering or nonshivering thermogenesis. All adult mammals can shiver, and neonates born in an advanced state of development, such as lambs and foals, can also shiver. Puppies and other less-developed neonates cannot shiver; they rely on the warmth of mother and the nest to protect them from cooling. Brown fat, which is present in some of the latter neonates and in other small mammals, provides a source of nonshivering thermogenesis.

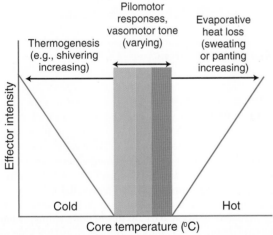

FIGURE 53-7 Relationship between the intensity of thermoregulatory responses and core temperature. The set point for temperature regulation is indicated by the pink bar zone. On either side of this set point is a zone where temperature can be maintained by vasomotor responses (*blue* and *red zones*). As the core temperature deviates more dramatically from the set point, there is a need either to increase thermogenesis during cold stress or to increase evaporative heat loss during heat stress. (Modified from Bligh J: Temperature regulation in environmental physiology of animals. In Bligh J, Cloudsley-Thompson JL, MacDonald AG, editors: *Environmental physiology of animals*, Oxford, UK, 1976, Blackwell Scientific.)

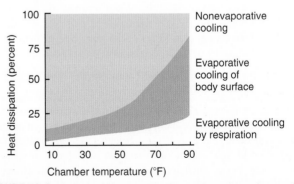

FIGURE 53-8 Methods of heat loss used by a cow as the environmental temperature increases. At low temperatures, most heat loss is by nonevaporative cooling (*pale blue shading*), but as the environmental temperature increases, the cow becomes increasingly dependent on evaporation (*darker blue shading*).

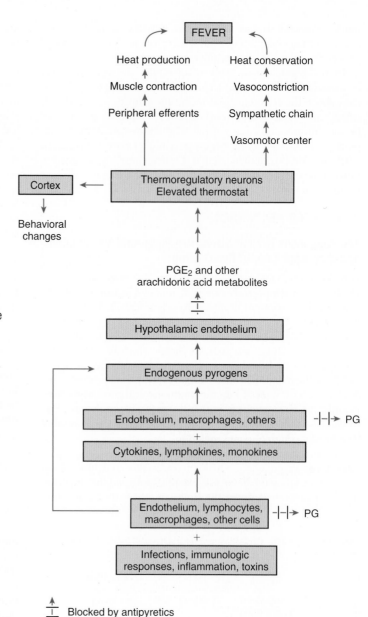

FIGURE 53-9 Peripheral and central mechanisms involved in the pathogenesis of fever. *PGE₂,* Prostaglandin E₂; *PG,* prostaglandins.

Chronic exposure of animals to cold results in increased secretion of *thyroxine* and an increase in basal metabolism, which increases basal heat production. When animals are housed in conditions where they receive natural light, the thickness of the hair coat increases at cold times of the year. Hair growth is the result of decreasing daylight as cold weather approaches.

Fever Is an Elevation of Body Temperature That Results from an Increase in the Thermoregulatory Set Point

Fever, also known as *pyrexia,* occurs in response to the elevation of an animal's thermoregulatory set point and most often accompanies infectious diseases. Fever is believed to be an evolutionary adaptation to fight off infection and can be induced in some of the ancient species, such as reptiles and amphibians. Studies indicate that during infection, an increase in body temperature enhances leukocyte activity. This results in a decrease in animal morbidity and mortality from infections.

The induction of fever begins with production by many cell types of small polypeptides known as *pyrogens* (Figures 53-9 and

54-6). This occurs when infectious agents, toxins, or the lipopolysaccharide complexes in gram-negative bacteria invade the body. Pyrogens include interleukin-1 (IL-1; considered to be the most important), tumor necrosis factor (TNF), interleukin-6 (IL-6), interferon (IFN), and macrophage inflammatory protein (MIP). In addition, prostaglandins (PGs), products of the arachidonic acid cascade that are produced by endothelial cells, are major participants in the pathogenesis of fever. When released into the blood, pyrogens reach a part of the hypothalamus called the *organa vasculosum of the lamina terminalis* (OVLT). This region of the hypothalamus is highly vascularized, and the blood-brain barrier here is almost nonexistent, so endogenous pyrogens and PGs enter the brain easily from the bloodstream. In the hypothalamus, the endogenous pyrogens act on the endothelial cells to produce additional *prostaglandin E₂* (PGE₂) and other arachidonic acid metabolites. These PGs cause the set point to rise.

When the set point increases, the animal initiates responses to conserve and produce heat until the body temperature reaches

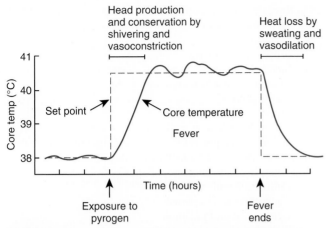

Head production and conservation by shivering and vasoconstriction

Heat loss by sweating and vasodilation

Set point

Core temperature

Fever

Exposure to pyrogen

Fever ends

Time (hours)

FIGURE 53-10 Events involved in fever. Exposure to a pyrogen increases the set point for the temperature-regulating system. This results in heat production and conservation to elevate body temperature, which in turn results in fever. When the fever ends, the set point decreases, and heat must be lost from the body through sweating and vasodilation.

the new set point (Figure 53-10). Shivering, peripheral vasoconstriction, piloerection, and huddling behavior are all characteristic of the onset of fever. When the new set point is reached, the animal maintains its body at the new temperature until the pyrogen is metabolized and production ceases. When this occurs, the set point decreases back to normal, and the animal initiates heat-losing mechanisms such as vasodilation and sweating to decrease body temperature. Because the local production of PGE$_2$ in the hypothalamus is involved in increasing the set point, nonsteroidal antiinflammatory drugs (NSAIDs; e.g., aspirin, flunixin, ibuprofen) are used to treat fever. These antipyretic drugs block the enzyme cyclooxygenase, an integral enzyme in the arachidonic acid cascade, thus blocking prostaglandin production (see Figure 53-9).

HEAT STROKE, HYPOTHERMIA, AND FROSTBITE

Heat Stroke Occurs When Heat Production or Input Exceeds Heat Output, So Body Temperature Rises to Dangerous Levels

In hot, humid weather it is difficult for animals to lose heat because evaporative cooling cannot occur effectively. Strenuous exercise under these conditions can lead to a dangerous increase in body temperature. Similarly, when dogs are closed in cars in the sun, their panting saturates the air with water vapor, so further heat loss is impossible. As the body temperature rises, the metabolic rate increases, and more heat is produced. In addition, panting or sweating (or both) lead to dehydration and can lead to circulatory collapse, which makes it more difficult to transfer heat to the skin. When the body temperature exceeds 41.5° to 42.5° C (~107° to 109° F), cellular function is seriously impaired and consciousness is lost.

Hypothermia Occurs When Heat Output Exceeds Heat Production, So Body Temperature Decreases to Dangerous Levels

Small or sick animals exposed to a cold environment may lose more heat than they can generate, and body temperature may decrease to a point at which heat-regulating mechanisms no

longer work. The ability of the hypothalamus to regulate body temperature is greatly impaired below a temperature of 29° C (84° F). Cardiac arrest occurs at around 20° C (68° F). Neonates seem to be able to withstand cooling more than adults, and apparently comatose lambs, piglets, and puppies can be revived through warming.

Frostbite Occurs When Ice Crystals Form in the Tissues of the Extremities

In extremely cold conditions, when the extremities are vasoconstricted to conserve heat, the tissues may cool below the freezing point of tissue water. Ice crystals disrupt the tissue integrity, and gangrene can result. Normally, frostbite is prevented because vascular smooth muscle dilates in extreme cold, causing an inflow of warm blood. This mechanism apparently works adequately in animals that winter outdoors in northern climates.

CLINICAL CORRELATIONS
INFLUENZA IN PIGS

History. You are called to examine a group of 3-month-old pigs in an intensively managed fattening house. The group of 20 pigs is in a pen, and there are multiple similar pens within the barn. In the last 2 days in this particular pen of pigs, the animals have been reluctant to eat and have started huddling together. The owner has observed that the outer pigs in the huddle continually try to burrow toward the center of the pile of pigs and that they appear to be trembling. At this time the remaining pigs in the barn are not affected. When you enter the barn and the pigs are disturbed, they begin sneezing and coughing, and some are reluctant to move.

Clinical Examination. Three pigs are caught, and the rectal temperature is found to be 41° C (normal, 39.2° C). There is a nasal discharge, and the conjunctiva and nasal mucosa are congested. You treat the pigs with antibiotics, and over several days, the pigs recover; however, the disease spreads progressively through the remaining pens in the fattening house. All pigs show the same clinical signs, and no pigs die from the disease. Blood samples are taken for virus neutralization tests from the acutely affected pigs 2 weeks after they have recovered.

The diagnosis from the viral neutralization test is swine influenza, which has a high morbidity rate but a low mortality rate.

Comment. The clinical signs produced by this disease are caused largely by the development of fever. The pigs that were examined had an elevated body temperature because the infection had raised the set point of their thermoregulatory centers to a high value. To raise body temperature to this new value, the pigs huddled together, and the pigs on the outside shivered to generate metabolic body heat. When the infection is overcome and pyrogens are metabolized, the behavior of the pigs changes; they need to lose heat, so they separate and move around the pens more freely.

HEAT STROKE IN A BOSTON TERRIER

History. At 3 pm on a 95° F (35° C) day in August, you receive a frantic phone call from a client. The client went to a shopping mall and left her car parked in the lot. She had her Boston terrier with her, but because she thought she would only be a few minutes, she left the dog in the car. While in the mall, she was delayed by an uncooperative clerk when her debit card was rejected. When she returned to the car, her dog was prostrate with its tongue hanging out of its mouth and was unresponsive. You instruct the owner to bring the dog to your practice immediately and to drive with the windows open for the half-mile trip.

Clinical Examination. On arrival at the clinic, the dog is laid on the examining table, where it fails to respond to its name. Its mouth is open, its tongue is distended, and its mucous membranes are dry. Body temperature is 42.2° C (normal, 38.5° C).

From the history, the animal's body temperature, and its lack of response, you diagnose heat stroke. The dog is placed in a bath of cool water, and fluids are administered intravenously. Within 5 to 10 minutes, the dog begins to look around and recognizes its owner. The water bath treatments are continued for 2 hours, at which time the body temperature is close to normal. The dog remains in the hospital overnight and is then discharged to the relieved owner the next day.

Comment. The temperature inside a car parked in the hot sun rises rapidly to above body temperature. At this time, the only mechanism available for losing heat is evaporation of water from the respiratory tract, which the dog attempts by panting and salivating. For a short time this is an effective means of losing heat, but water vapor is transferred to the air in the car and progressively saturates the atmosphere with water. As the percentage saturation of the air increases, the animal has more and more difficulty achieving evaporation and therefore heat loss. Eventually the animal cannot lose heat, and the body temperature begins to rise. When the body temperature exceeds 41.5° to 42.5° C, the animal loses consciousness. In addition, the panting results in dehydration and reduces the dog's ability to deliver heat from the core of the body to the extremities. Brachycephalic dogs, such as Boston terriers, have an added disadvantage in temperature regulation: the short nose and convolutions in the wall of the pharynx increase the work of breathing, especially when the dogs pant. This increased work is an additional source of body heat, and the anatomy of the upper airway probably makes evaporative cooling less effective.

Therapy for this condition is to reduce body temperature and to restore circulatory function as rapidly as possible. For this reason, the dog is placed in a cool water bath to reduce body temperature and also receives intravenous fluids to rehydrate it by expanding its circulatory volume and restoring the ability of the circulation to redistribute heat within the body.

PRACTICE QUESTIONS

1. Sweating is an effective cooling mechanism because:
   a. Sweat secretion produces heat, which is carried to the skin surface in the sweat.
   b. Conversion of sweat into water vapor requires heat, which is supplied to the skin by blood flow.
   c. Sweat dripping from the body carries away large amounts of heat.
   d. The ions in sweat carry large amounts of heat from the body.

2. In the cold, animals both conserve and produce heat. Which of the following is a method of heat conservation?
   a. Shivering
   b. Brown fat metabolism
   c. Increased thyroxine secretion
   d. Countercurrent heat exchange in the limbs
   e. All the above

3. Which of the following methods of heat loss can occur in an animal (body temperature = 38° C) standing in a room (temperature = 40° C) with relative humidity of zero? The walls of the room have a temperature of 30° C.
   a. Convection and evaporation
   b. Convection and radiation
   c. Evaporation and radiation
   d. Radiation alone
   e. Convection, evaporation, and radiation

4. Which of the following describes thermoregulation?
   a. Temperature receptors in both the brain and the skin can initiate thermoregulatory responses.
   b. The brain temperature receptors have a greater influence on thermoregulation than do skin receptors.
   c. The core temperature at which shivering begins is higher if the skin is cold than if it is warm.
   d. Skin cooling can initiate shivering even if core temperature is normal.
   e. All the above

5. Which of the following correctly describes fever?
   a. It results when the set point for body temperature decreases.
   b. It is accompanied by sweating to lose heat as body temperature rises.
   c. It is accompanied by shivering to gain heat as body temperature decreases when pyrogens are metabolized.
   d. It can be initiated by pyrogens from bacteria or leukocytes.
   e. All the above

BIBLIOGRAPHY

Cinti S: Between brown and white: novel aspects of adipocyte differentiation, *Ann Med* 43(2):104–115, 2011.

Eckert R, Randall D: *Animal physiology: mechanisms and adaptations,* ed 2, New York, 1983, Freeman.

Hales JR: The partition of respiratory ventilation of the panting ox, *J Physiol* 188(2):45P–46P, 1967.

Maughan RJ, Lindinger MI: Preparing for and competing in the heat: the human perspective, *Equine Vet J Suppl* 20:8–15, 1995.

Schmidt-Nielsen K: *Animal physiology: adaptation and environment,* ed 5, Cambridge, UK, 1997, Cambridge University Press.

Stitt J: Regulation of body temperature. In Boron WF, Boulpaep EL, editors: *Medical physiology: a cellular and molecular approach,* ed 2, Philadelphia, 2009, Saunders.

CHAPTER 54

Antigens and Innate Immunity

KEY POINTS

Antigens

1. Antigens (or immunogens) stimulate immune cells to induce an immune response.
2. The degree of immune response depends on several characteristics of the antigen.

Body's Defense Against Invading Antigens

1. Both nonimmune and immune mechanisms defend against invading antigens.

2. A first line of defense includes physical and chemical barriers such as the skin and internal body fluids.
3. A second line of defense consists of phagocytic cells of the myeloid and macrophage-monocyte lineages.
4. Macrophage-derived cytokines can induce a variety of physiological processes to help combat infectious antigens.

The immune system performs two vital functions that are critical for the maintenance of homeostasis and survival: (1) inducing an effective and safe response against foreign antigens (infectious and noninfectious) and (2) avoiding a response to components of "self" antigens by enforcing stringent regulatory controls over dangerous self-reactive cells that are capable of mounting devastating immune attacks on "self" tissues. Because the induction of immune responses depends on antigens, this chapter first discusses the nature and characteristics of antigens.

ANTIGENS

Antigens (or Immunogens) Stimulate Immune Cells to Induce an Immune Response

An *antigen,* or *immunogen,* is defined as any substance that is capable of stimulating immune cells (T and B cells) to induce an immune response. Antigens can be broadly divided into two large categories: (1) infectious (microbial) and (2) noninfectious (Figure 54-1). *Infectious antigens* include components that are derived from bacteria, viruses, protozoa, and helminths. *Noninfectious antigens* include those derived from "self" (autoantigens), food, plants, dust, or insect and animal venoms, as well as synthetic and cell surface proteins.

An antigen is composed of many molecular units to which an antibody binds. These small units on an antigen are called antigenic *epitopes,* or *antigenic determinants.* Thus a single antigen may be composed of many antigenic epitopes. In the strictest sense, antibodies bind to an antigenic epitope of an antigen. Some of these antigenic epitopes are shared among different bacteria (e.g., epitopes on *Brucella* and *Yersinia*) or between a bacteria and host cells (e.g., *Mycobacterium* heat shock proteins and synovial tissue; *Mycoplasma* and lung tissue). These types of antigenic epitopes are called *cross-reactive epitopes.*

Figure 54-2 shows the following antigenic structures of bacteria:

- *Bacterial cell wall.* Cell walls of gram-positive bacteria differ from those of gram-negative bacteria. Gram-positive bacteria are composed of a thick layer of short chains of amino acids or peptides and carbohydrates *(peptidoglycans).* The cell wall of gram-negative bacteria has a thin layer of peptidoglycan and is largely composed of *lipopolysaccharides,* which are potent endotoxins.
- *Capsule.* Certain bacteria produce a protective outer covering called a capsule, which is composed of polysaccharides.
- *Pili.* These small, hairlike protein structures on some bacteria enable the bacteria to adhere to target host cells and transfer genetic information from one bacterium to another.
- *Flagella.* Some bacteria possess flagella for mobility. Flagella contain a protein called *flagellin,* which can be antigenic.
- *Nucleic acids.* Nucleic acids, such as bacterial deoxyribonucleic acid (DNA), tend to be antigenic because of differences in methylation compared with mammalian DNA. The antibodies against bacterial DNA tend to cross-react with the host's DNA.

Viruses have nucleic acids (ribonucleic acid [RNA] or DNA), surrounded by a protein coat called a capsid. Some viruses have an *envelope,* a lipid membrane–like structure covering the capsid. On the envelope are glycoprotein projections that the viruses use to attach to the host target cells. All these components may be antigenic.

External structures of protozoa and helminths tend to be antigenic. Similarly, fungal spores are antigenic. Pollens, glycoproteins of certain foods, the unique biochemical structure of synthetic chemicals, insect saliva, and venoms are all good antigens. It is beyond the scope of this chapter to discuss each of these antigens in detail.

The immune system is exposed to and tolerates "self" antigens found on all of its own tissues. These antigens can be cell surface antigens (e.g., thyroglobulin, myelin peptides) or internal

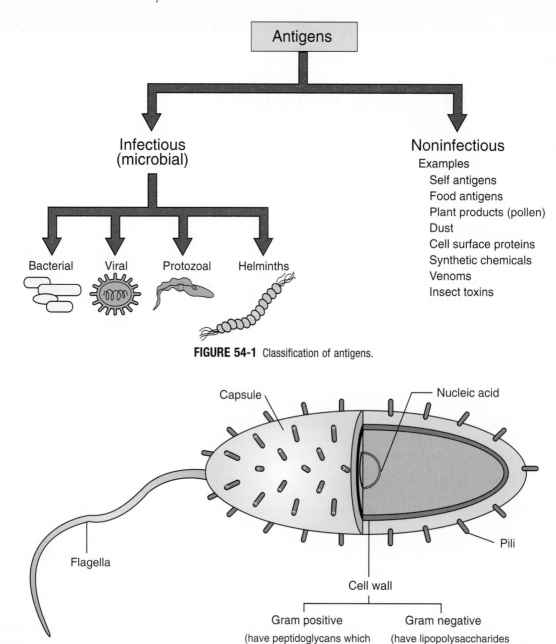

FIGURE 54-1 Classification of antigens.

FIGURE 54-2 Antigenic structures of bacteria (not all bacteria have all these structures).

antigens (e.g., cardiolipin, nucleic acids, histones). In certain individuals who are allergic, antigens derived from food (e.g., peanuts, strawberries, fish) or plants (e.g., pollen, spores) induce an immediate and potent immune reaction. Many synthetic chemicals and drugs are minute in size and tend to be adsorbed onto cell surface antigens to create a new antigenic epitope. With ever-increasing synthesis of chemicals (pesticides, agricultural chemicals, drugs, and consumer products, to name a few), it is likely that synthetic chemicals may become an important class of antigens in the future.

The Degree of Immune Response Depends on Several Characteristics of the Antigen

The degree of immune response induced by an antigen is called *antigenicity* or *immunogenicity*. Understanding the characteristics

of antigens that provoke a strong or weak immune response provides important insight into the body's ability to combat invading antigens successfully. Furthermore, this understanding is useful in designing a vaccine preparation with potent antigenicity. Characteristics that contribute to potent antigenicity include the following:

- *Foreign versus self antigens.* Antigens that are considered to be foreign to the host tend to be highly antigenic. For example, if a horse is injected separately with antigens that are derived from a dog or from its own tissues, the horse will mount a strong immune response to the dog antigens, but not to its own (self) tissues.
- *Size.* The size of an antigen also influences the level of immune response. Large antigens enable better processing by antigen-presenting cells (e.g., macrophages, dendritic cells) and

subsequent presentation of antigenic peptides to lymphocytes for induction of an immune response. Examples of large antigens include bacterial and insect toxins, viral capsids, surface proteins on protozoa and helminths, and venoms. At the other extreme, very small antigens (e.g., small synthetic antigens, endogenous hormones, pesticides) tend to be ineffective in provoking an immune response. Very small antigens are inherently incapable of inducing immune responses; however, when bound to a larger protein, they can be potent antigens. Such small compounds are referred to as *haptens*. A good example of a hapten is a poison ivy–derived chemical, urishiol, which readily combines with many proteins (e.g., skin proteins) to induce a vigorous immune response.

- *Biochemical structure and complexity.* In general, proteins tend to be more antigenic than lipids or carbohydrates. Large size alone is insufficient to provoke a good immune response. For example, many sugars and lipids, even though large in size, are ineffective in inducing an immune response because they consist of simple repeating units (e.g., repeating sugars in starch), which lack complexity. Complex carbohydrates and lipids, on the other hand, as found in many microbes, are strong immunogens. Carbohydrates and lipids, when combined with protein to form glycoproteins and lipoproteins, respectively, have increased complexity and thus are good antigens.

- *Stability and degradability.* For immune cells to respond, stability of an antigen is an important feature. Flexible antigens, such as flagellin in a bacterium, are poor immunogens. However, when stabilized and rendered less flexible, as done in vaccine preparations, flagellin tends to be a potent immunogen. For an immune response to be initiated, the antigen ingested by phagocytic cells (e.g., macrophages) must be degraded and broken down into small peptides. Lymphocytes (T cells) will only respond to the peptides and not to large, native molecules. Antigens such as steel pins or plastic heart valves, even though large and complex, are inert and not degradable and thus are not good antigens.

Large, complex proteins (or lipoproteins or glycoproteins) that can be degraded and processed therefore tend to be excellent antigens. Other parameters that influence an individual's ability to respond to antigens include genetics (e.g., major histocompatibility complex genes), endogenous biomolecules that regulate and modulate immune responses (e.g., hormones, neuropeptides), and the level and route of exposure of antigens.

An antibody that is induced in response to an antigen will specifically bind to the antigen. Any minor alteration of the antigen will negatively impact the antibody's ability to bind to an antigen. Therefore, invading microbes often alter their antigens to prevent the binding of induced antibodies, thus avoiding immune attack.

BODY'S DEFENSE AGAINST INVADING ANTIGENS

Both Nonimmune and Immune Mechanisms Defend Against Invading Antigens

The body is confronted with literally billions of antigens. Consequently, a unique challenge presented to the immune system is to respond effectively only to foreign antigens while refraining from response to "self" antigens. The induction of immune responses requires energy and protein, and antigens require extensive cellular division (and hence utilization of protein reserves); the body cannot mount immune responses to each of the innumerable antigens it encounters constantly. Instead, the body is well equipped to handle antigens effectively before resorting to a specific immune response.

Initially, most antigens are effectively handled by nonspecific defense mechanisms, such as impervious and formidable physical barriers (e.g., skin and other body surfaces) and antimicrobial body fluids (e.g., lysozymes in tears, saliva, gastric juices). These are considered the first line of defense and are discussed next. Should the antigen survive this "body armor," phagocytic cells (e.g., neutrophils, macrophages-monocytes) and natural killer (NK, NK-T) cells can effectively eliminate the invading antigens. These cells ingest and destroy a wide range of antigens and thus are non–antigen-specific. These cellular defenses constitute a second line of the body's defense. The body's initial defense (physical, chemical, and phagocytic antigen-presenting cells; natural killer cells) constitute the *innate immune system*. The antigen-presenting cells closely interact with specific T and B cells to induce a specific immune response. Thus, specific immune responses by the "adaptive" immune system tend to be the last line of the body's defense (see Chapter 55). Collectively, both nonimmune and immune mechanisms effectively counter invading microbes.

A First Line of Defense Includes Physical and Chemical Barriers such as the Skin and Internal Body Fluids

The physical nonimmune defense barriers include external body surfaces such as skin and internal body surfaces such as the gastrointestinal (GI), reproductive, respiratory, and the urogenital tracts. The skin plays a major role in preventing the entry of organisms through a variety of nonimmunological means, including the secretion of sebum from sebaceous glands, which maintains a low pH, and secretion of enzymes that are not conducive for the invading pathogens. Periodic natural desquamation of the skin also results in sloughing off any invading pathogens. Nonpathogenic bacteria also occupy skin surfaces, thereby preventing the adherence of pathogenic organisms to their target cells, which is prerequisite for entry into the body. Any changes in the skin, such as cuts, burns, and dry or very humid skin, will result in the entry of microbes. In addition to the nonimmunological mechanisms, skin is also rich in dendritic cells (Langerhans cells) and γ-δ T cells that contribute to warding off invading pathogens. The natural flushing action of urine and milk assist in elimination of infectious antigens, as evidenced by the infectious conditions that result from stasis of urine or milk.

Many body fluids are inhospitable to invading pathogens. For example, mucus in the mucosal tissues (respiratory, urogenital, and GI tracts), saliva, tears, gastric juices, and urine are rich in enzymes (e.g., lysozymes) and are low in pH. As with the skin, the GI tract is covered with nonpathogenic bacteria, which prevent the adhesion of pathogenic bacteria to their target cells. Furthermore, resident normal bacterial florae in gastric tissues secrete butyric or lactic acids, which not only maintain a low pH in gastric fluids, but also are bacteriostatic to other microbes. Vaginal epithelium is rich in glycogen and promotes the growth of *Lactobacillus,* which secretes lactic acids. In the respiratory tract the antigen load is decreased by a variety of mechanisms, including the turbulence created when air is inhaled due to the anatomical construction of the lower respiratory tract, which narrows and branches. Microorganisms in inhaled air are carried by this turbulence and are forced onto the walls of the respiratory tract, which are rich in sticky mucus and bactericidal lysozymes. The ciliary action of the respiratory tract also eliminates antigens effectively.

A Second Line of Defense Consists of Phagocytic Cells of the Myeloid and Macrophage-Monocyte Lineages

Should an antigen survive the first line of the body's defense (i.e., body surfaces) and penetrate into blood vessels and tissues, the body's defense relies on cellular response. Key cells involved in cellular defense are phagocytic cells, which are an integral part of *innate immunity*. These cells, based on their cellular origin, are broadly divided into myeloid and macrophage-monocyte lineages. Included in the myeloid lineage are neutrophils, eosinophils, and basophils. The macrophage-monocyte series includes monocytes and macrophages. *Neutrophils* constitute the largest percentage of white blood cells in most species (60% to 65%), except in ruminants (20% to 25%). Neutrophils have a short life span in the blood (half-life, ~12 hours), but in tissues their longevity increases to several days. Neutrophils are approximately 12 µm in diameter, with multilobulated nuclei and a cytoplasm rich in granules. The population of granules is composed of both primary and secondary granules. The primary granules contain important bactericidal enzymes such as myeloperoxidase, lysozymes, acid hydrolases (e.g., β-glucuronidase, cathepsin), and neutral proteases against elastase hydrolases. Neutrophils also have *defensins*, small proteins that are inserted between the lipid bilayers and disrupt the interactions emanating from lipid membranes. The secondary granules include lysozymes, lactoferrin, and collagenases.

Neutrophils are considered the first responder cells to combat invading antigens. The primary function of neutrophils is to capture and destroy antigens. Neutrophils, unlike monocytes or macrophages, respond rapidly to invading antigens and readily phagocytose antigens. However, neutrophils lack the capacity to present antigens to lymphocytes. Neutrophils destroy antigens by two different but complementary mechanisms: (1) phagocytosis and (2) respiratory burst. Phagocytosis in turn is divided into four arbitrary stages: (a) chemotaxis, (b) adherence or attachment, (c) phagocytosis, and (d) destruction (Figure 54-3).

Neutrophils are attracted to the site of infection in tissues by chemokines and chemical messengers that are released when tissues are damaged. In response to chemical signals and chemokines, vascular endothelial cells induce the expression of adhesion molecules. Neutrophils bind to these cellular adhesion molecules (CAMs) through specific receptors and are triggered to leave the circulation by crossing capillary walls (diapedesis) into tissues. When neutrophils move out of the circulation, they move toward the antigen. The contact between neutrophils and antigen is greatly facilitated when antigens are coated or bound by a host's proteins, such as complement or antibodies. These proteins that enhance contact and phagocytosis by neutrophils or other phagocytes are called *opsonins*. The contact of neutrophils with antigens triggers infolding of the cell membrane (by the action of actin and myosin), and the antigen is trapped in a vacuole called a *phagosome*. The primary granules move toward the phagosome and fuse their membrane to become *phagolysosomes,* and in the process the granules release deleterious bacteriostatic and bactericidal biomolecules. Thus, in the contained environment of phagolysosomes, the antigen is destroyed.

A concurrent mechanism by which neutrophils kill invading microbial antigens involves *respiratory burst* (see Figure 54-3). On contact of neutrophils with an antigen, consumption of oxygen is immediately increased, seventy- to 100-fold. This results in activation of an enzyme, NADPH *oxidase,* which forms an electron transport chain with cytosolic NADPH as an electron donor of oxygen. A molecule of oxygen accepts two donated electrons to result in a superoxide anion (O_2^-). This O_2^-, under the influence of the enzyme superoxide dismutase and in the presence of water, will chemically react to yield hydrogen peroxide (H_2O_2), which is toxic to microbes. This H_2O_2, under the influence of myeloperoxidase and utilizing chloride ions (Cl^-), catalyzes oxidative reactions to form H_2O_2 and halide ions. All these products are highly toxic to the antigens. Neutrophils are also known to release hydroxyl radical singlet oxygen, which is toxic to bacteria.

Neutrophils have limited energy and a relatively short life. Elastases and collagenases released from these dying neutrophils serve as a powerful chemoattractant for another group of phagocytes called *macrophages,* and therefore neutrophils are sometimes referred to as "martyrs of the immune system." Macrophages are attracted by bacterial products as well but also through the chemotactic factors released from damaged tissues. Macrophages differ from neutrophils in several important aspects. Macrophages, even though not rapid-responder cells, have extensive ability to phagocytose antigens repeatedly. These long-lived cells secrete large quantities of cytokines and chemokines that play a key role in regulating immune responses. Some of these cells even have the ability to present antigens to the immune system. Macrophages are present throughout body tissues where entry of antigens is likely.

Macrophages are round or elongated cells and express many surface receptors that include major histocompatibility complex antigens I and II (MHC class I and II). MHC classes I and II play a major role in antigen recognition and presentation (see Chapter 55). Macrophages differ in their morphology based on tissues and thus are called by different names. For example, in the lymphoid organs, these cells are macrophages, whereas in the liver they are known as *Kupffer's cells* (Figure 54-4). Macrophages are derived from the bone marrow hematopoietic cells and are initially called *monoblasts*, which mature and move into circulation and are known as *monocytes*. When monocytes move into the tissues, they are called *macrophages*. Macrophages are larger than neutrophils and are rich in rough endoplasmic reticulum and Golgi bodies, indicating their extensive ability to produce and secrete immunoregulatory proteins.

Innate immune cells, predominantly macrophages, express Toll Like Receptors (TLRs) that recognize specific sequences/molecules on microbes called pathogen-associated molecular patterns (PAMPs). These receptors serve as pattern recognition receptors that trigger an innate immune response to pathogens or other antigenic stimuli. Thus far, thirteen TLRs have been identified in mammals. TLR1, 2, 4, 5, and 6 are located on the cell surface membrane, whereas TLR3, 7, 8, and 9 are found intracellularly. The combination of TLR1 with TLR2 recognizes a wide variety of fungal and protozoal products, including peptidoglycans and lipopolysaccharide (LPS). TLR2 alone, in addition to recognizing endogenous ligands such as Heat Shock Protein 70 (Hsp70), can recognize bacterial diacylated lipopeptides when the receptor is combined with TLR6. TLR4 is activated by LPS on gram-negative bacteria. TLR5 is expressed on the basolateral surface of intestinal epithelial cells and is activated by bacterial flagellin. Intracellular TLRs recognize intracellular pathogens such as viruses. With respect to activation of TLRs, activating TLR4 can result in initiation of two distinct signaling mechanisms, one of which is a Myeloid Differentiation factor 88 (MyD88)-dependent pathway. Genes induced by this pathway are mostly those coding for proinflammatory molecules (e.g., interleukins 1α, 1β, 6, 12; cyclooxygenase 2; tumor necrosis factor α).

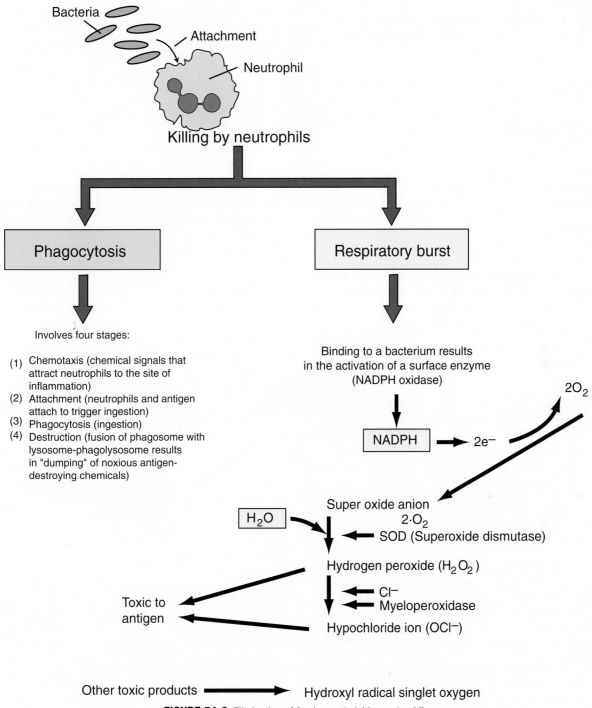

FIGURE 54-3 Elimination of foreign material by neutrophils.

Ingestion of antigen will activate the metabolic machinery of macrophages, including increasing lysosomal and bactericidal activity and upregulating the *inducible nitric oxide synthase* gene (iNOS) that encodes for iNOS protein, which in turn is responsible for enhanced release of potent antimicrobial nitric oxide. Macrophages also release several oxygen free radicals that are also antimicrobial. Thus, macrophages aid in killing of antigens by phagocytosis and by respiratory burst (oxygen and nitrogen free radicals) (see Figure 54-3). Macrophages can potentially secrete more than 100 proteins. Some of these proteins, such as interleukin-1 (IL-1), interleukin-12 (IL-12), tumor necrosis factor alpha (TNF-α), interleukin-18 (IL-18), and interleukin-27 (IL-27), play a central role in activating lymphocytes, especially naïve T lymphocytes (Figure 54-5). After an effective immune response is initiated, macrophages also secrete cytokines such as interleukin-10 (IL-10) and transforming growth factor beta (TGF-β), which downregulate the immune response.

When the antigen is cleared by macrophages, these cells also play an important role in repairing the damaged tissues. Macrophages secrete angiogenic factors to enhance the blood supply. For example, IL-1 secreted by macrophages stimulates fibroblasts to secrete collagen to rebuild tissues.

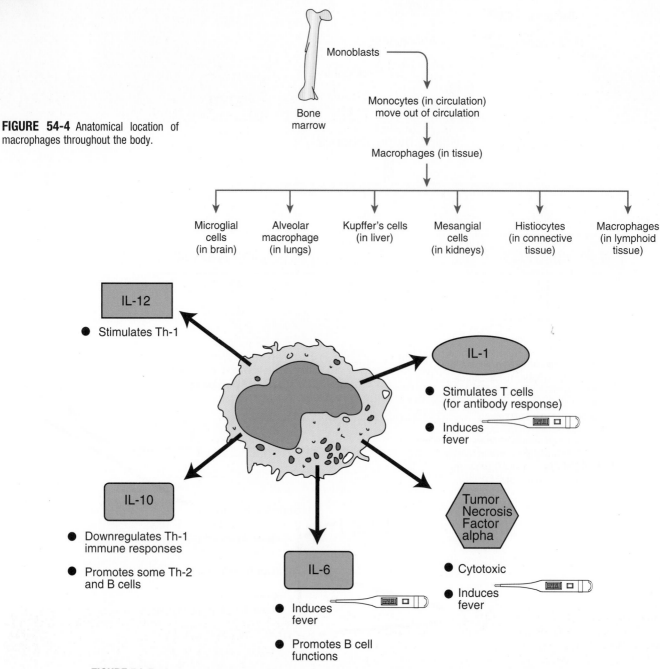

FIGURE 54-4 Anatomical location of macrophages throughout the body.

FIGURE 54-5 Macrophage-derived cytokines. *IL,* Interleukin; *Th-1,* T-helper cells type 1; *Th-2,* T-helper cells type 2.

Macrophage-Derived Cytokines Can Induce a Variety of Physiological Processes to Help Combat Infectious Antigens

Physiologically, a key component of combating infectious antigens is the induction of *fever,* which is mediated by the release of pyrogenic cytokines such as IL-1, IL-6, and TNF-α by macrophages (Figure 54-6). These cytokines act on multiple tissues to mount a coordinated effort aimed at eliminating the invading microbes. For example, they act on thermoregulatory regions in the hypothalamus to induce fever, which is an integral part of this process. Fever accelerates the mobility of neutrophils, enhances their phagocytic ability, and activates lymphocytes and complement proteins while impeding the growth of bacteria. These

cytokines also act on the liver to stimulate acute phase proteins that function as opsonins to promote phagocytosis. Further, these cytokines act on the sleep-associated regions in the hypothalamus to promote sleep in an effort to conserve energy and redirect energy toward the infectious challenge. Because major immunoprotective elements (e.g., antibodies, cytokines, complement) are all proteins, these cytokines increase the amino acid pool by acting on muscles and inducing mild proteolysis and release of amino acids, which are essential for synthesis of various immunoprotective elements.

Another important feature of some macrophages is their ability to present antigens to stimulate T cells in order to start the specific adaptive immune response. Other cells are part of the

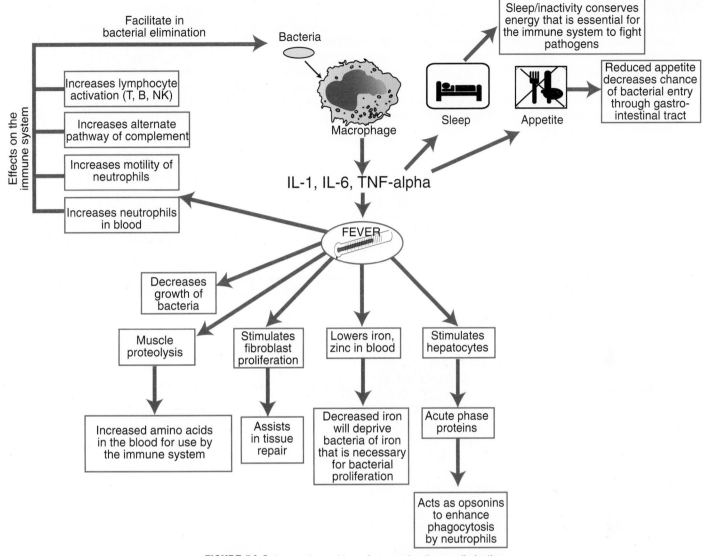

FIGURE 54-6 Pyrogenic cytokines, fever, and pathogen elimination.

innate immune system and also serve as *antigen-presenting cells* (APCs); these include dendritic cells and B cells. *Dendritic cells* are considered the most potent cells in presenting antigens. These cells have long dendrites that physically allow them to interact simultaneously with many antigens. Dendritic cells are abundant in lymphoid organs, skin, and other tissues that frequently encounter antigens. The role of APCs in the adaptive immune response is discussed in Chapter 55.

CLINICAL CORRELATIONS

SWOLLEN LYMPH NODES IN A COLT

History. A 2-year-old colt that just returned from training has shown marked bilateral nasal discharge for at least 2 days. The colt has not been eating for the last day and appears depressed. The colt also seems to have considerable swelling under the jaw and in the throatlatch area.

Clinical Examination. On physical examination the colt has a temperature of 39.2° C (102.7° F) but a normal heart rate of 36

beats/min and normal respiratory rate of 12 breaths/min. The horse has bilateral mucopurulent nasal discharge. The lymph nodes underneath the jaw and in the throat area are both greatly swollen. No other abnormalities are present.

Comment. This colt was vaccinated for Eastern and Western encephalitis as well as rhinopneumonitis, influenza, rabies, tetanus, and West Nile virus. However, the colt was not vaccinated against *Streptococcus equi (S. equi)*, the causative agent of strangles. Young horses not vaccinated against *S. equi* that have been traveling are at increased risk for disease. Based on the clinical signs of fever, bilateral mucopurulent discharge, and normal lung sounds and respiratory rate, this disease is likely an upper respiratory infection. The vaccination history and clinical signs indicate *S. equi* is the most likely pathogen.

Horses are exposed to *S. equi* through inhalation, ingestion, or exposure to conjunctival surfaces; association with other infected horses; or a contaminated environment. The bacteria enter the cells of the tonsillar crypts and ventral surface of the soft palate and migrate throughout the upper respiratory tract, infecting the lymph nodes as well and replicating there extracellularly. Most cases resolve over a prolonged period. In other horses, however, the guttural pouches can become infected, or the animal can become systemically infected and develop abscesses in other parts of the body (e.g., lymph nodes). In the latter situation the syndrome is known as "bastard strangles."

The immune response associated with infection begins with the mucosal innate response. Horses will have increased levels of neutrophils in their blood (neutrophilia). The number of lymphocytes in the blood may vary, but there is a marked reaction in the local lymph nodes to the infection. These horses have severe lymphadenopathy of the regional nodes from increased numbers of neutrophils and lymphocytes. A combination of both the innate and the acquired immune response is capable of controlling the infection, and eventually the horse eliminates the pathogen. Again, however, in a small percentage of the infected horses, *S. equi* migrates to the systemic lymph nodes to cause bastard strangles at some later time point in life.

A diagnosis can be made based on history, clinical signs, and combined diagnostic testing. Traditionally, these horses have neutrophilia in their peripheral blood. Definitive diagnosis is based on culturing the agent, often from the regional lymph nodes using an aspirate. In many cases, there is concern about an outbreak within a particular barn because the agent is highly infectious, and infected horses and barns must be quarantined to prevent further spread of the disease. Another test for a definitive diagnosis is polymerase chain reaction (PCR).

Treatment. The treatment of *S. equi* infection varies based on clinical signs and the population at risk. In the early stages of infection, with clinical signs of fever, depression, anorexia, and bilateral mucopurulent nasal discharge, but no or limited lymphadenopathy, these horses can often be treated systemically with antibiotics, and the disease will usually resolve. However, when the lymph nodes begin to become enlarged or abscessed, antibiotic treatment will often prevent further spread of infection but will not aid in clearance. When antibiotics are discontinued, the disease continues to progress. Some horses become greatly depressed, with marked lymphadenopathy that can affect breathing. In these animals the lymph nodes are often drained. Sometimes a tracheostomy is needed, in which case horses are treated with systemic antibiotics to prevent secondary infections. Disinfecting the environment is critical to the control of strangles within populations.

HEIFER CALF WITH RECURRENT INFECTION

History. An 8-week-old dairy heifer calf presents for coughing. She appeared to be fine at birth, but in the past 6 to 7 weeks, she has started to lose weight. None of the other calves of similar ages housed in pens are affected.

Clinical Examination. She has an increased temperature, and increased heart rate (tachycardic), respiratory rate (tachypnic), and effort. She has increased lung sounds consistent with pneumonia. Her feces are also a little looser than normal. Blood is collected for a complete blood count (CBC) as well as zinc sulfate turbidity test to examine immunoglobulin G (IgG) antibody levels. The CBC reveals very high neutrophil counts. The IgG levels are normal.

Comment. Bovine leukocyte adhesion deficiency (BLAD) is suspected in this calf. This is an autosomal recessive disease. There is impaired expression of the CD11/CD18 family (β2 integrins) of leukocyte adhesion molecules, and this prevents neutrophils from

emigrating into tissues. Therefore, the calves are likely to develop infection(s). Animals can be detected by polymerase chain reaction (PCR) DNA testing. Cells can also be stained with antibodies and examined by flow cytometry for expression of CD18. Affected animals often have infections of the gastrointestinal (GI) and respiratory systems as well as synovial structures (joints).

Treatment. Treatment is limited to supportive care, including antibiotics and fluid therapy, depending on the specific infection. Affected animals will succumb to infection. Euthanasia of a known affected BLAD animal should be considered as it is autosomal recessive and can be passed to future generations.

Acknowledgment
The authors would like to thank Deena Khan for her contribution in the editing of the chapters in this section.

PRACTICE QUESTIONS

1. Which of the following statements is correct in regard to macrophages?
   a. They are the first type of cells to appear in circulation and can repeatedly phagocytose in response to invasion by microbial antigens.
   b. They secrete anti-inflammatory cytokines that prevent fever.
   c. They have class I major histocompatibility complex (MHC) antigens, and selected macrophages also have class II MHC antigens and thus can serve as antigen-presenting cells.
   d. They have no ability to secrete proteins.
   e. They are actually lymphocytes.

2. Which of the following is correct about neutrophils?
   a. They can rapidly destroy antigen by phagocytosis and respiratory burst.
   b. They are lymphocytes that are the first cells to destroy antigens.
   c. They are major producers of IL-1.
   d. They are efficient antigen-processing cells.
   e. All the above.

3. Antigen-presenting cells (APCs) include which of the following?
   a. Dendritic cells
   b. Selected macrophages
   c. B cells
   d. T cells
   e. Answers a, b, and c

4. Which of the following is correct with regard to antigen?
   a. Highly degradable proteins and large, inert substances are not good antigens (i.e., not able to induce a strong immune response).
   b. Large molecules are good antigens, and therefore large molecules such as polysaccharides, with simple repeating sugars, are good antigens.
   c. Large complex proteins (especially foreign antigens) are good at inducing immune responses.
   d. Antigens do not drive an immune response.
   e. Lipids, but not lipoproteins, are excellent antigens.

BIBLIOGRAPHY

Abbas AK, Lichtman AH, Pillai S: *Cellular and molecular immunology*, ed 7, Philadelphia, 2012, Saunders.

Barrington GM, Johnson JJ: Immunologic disorders. In Smith BP, editor: *Large animal internal medicine*, ed 4, St Louis, 2009, Mosby Elsevier.

Delves PJ, Martin SJ, Burton DR, Roitt IM: *Essential immunology*, ed 12, Malden, Mass, 2011, Blackwell.

Janeway C: *Immunobiology: the immune system in health and disease*, ed 8, New York, 2011, Garland Science.

Kumar H, Kawai T, Akira S: Pathogen recognition by the innate immune system, *Int Rev Immunol* 30(1):16–34, 2011.

Nagahata H: Bovine leukocyte adhesion deficiency (BLAD): a review, *J Vet Med Sci* 66(12):1475–1482, 2004.

Parham P: *The immune system*, ed 3, New York, 2009, Garland Science.

Rao CV: *Immunology: a textbook*, Harrow, UK, 2005, Alpha Science.

Tizzard IR: *Veterinary immunology: an introduction*, ed 8, Philadelphia, 2008, Saunders.

CHAPTER 55

The Specific Immune Response: Acquired Immunity

KEY POINTS

T Cells (T Lymphocytes)

1. Mature T cells develop from lymphoid stem cells that have migrated to the thymus.
2. T cells are a heterogeneous population of cytotoxic T cells and T-helper cells.

Interactions of Antigen-Presenting Cells and T Cells

1. Major histocompatibility complex proteins are considered the central regulators of the immune system.
2. MHC class I antigens of infected nucleated cells play a major role in activating cytotoxic T cells.
3. MHC class II antigens on antigen-presenting cells play a major role in selective activation of T-helper cells.

Antibodies

1. Initial exposure to foreign antigen induces slow onset of antibody appearance, whereas subsequent exposure induces faster, longer-lasting antibody appearance.

2. Antibodies, or immunoglobulins, are glycoprotein molecules that can be divided into five isotypes, or classes.
3. The B-cell population produces antibodies to millions of different antigens, yet the antibody-antigen interaction is specific.
4. Expansion of an antigen-specific B–memory cell population on initial antigen exposure results in a faster, more pervasive, secondary immune response.

Regulation of Immune Responses

1. The actions, secretions, and surface molecule expression of immune cells play an important role in regulation of the body's immune response.

As discussed in Chapter 54, innate immunity offers effective defense against a wide range of pathogens. Key features of innate immunity include (1) rapid response against invading pathogens; (2) nonspecificity; and (3) physical, chemical, and cellular (phagocytic cells, NK cells) barriers. The response of the innate immune system, however, is not long-lasting and does not induce immunological memory (i.e., ability to recall previous exposure to antigens and respond to these effectively and specifically). For long-lasting immunity, another arm of the immune system must be activated. This is referred to as *acquired immunity,* which involves activation of T and B lymphocytes. *Antigen-presenting cells* (APCs), a part of the innate immune system, play a central role in activating lymphocytes. Activated *T lymphocytes* (T cells) secrete cytokines that are essential for defense against intracellular pathogens, activation of other cells, and coordination of immune responses. *B lymphocytes* (B cells) have two main functions: (1) secreting antibodies that bind specifically to the antigen that induced the antibody response and (2) acting as APCs.

Before discussing how antigens are presented to specific lymphocytes, it is important to understand the different types of immune cells (Figure 55-1). All cells of the immune system are derived from multipotent stem cells that are located primarily in the marrow of long bones. These multipotent stem cells subsequently give rise to primordial stem cells, such as lymphoid stem cells or myeloid stem cells. Myeloid stem cells give rise to

monocytes, which mature in tissues to become macrophages or dendritic cells. Lymphoid stem cells give rise to T, B, natural killer (NK), and lymphoid dendritic cells. Mature cells are found circulating throughout the body but concentrate in the peripheral lymphoid organs (e.g., lymph nodes, spleen) and gut-associated lymphoid tissues, where most of the complex interactions with antigens take place.

Birds, unlike mammals, have a unique lymphoid organ called the *bursa of Fabricius* where B cells develop. This round, sac-shaped organ is located above the cloaca. Analogous to the thymus, the bursa consists of lymphocytes embedded in epithelial tissues. Mammals have no precise lymphoid organ that is equivalent to this bursa. Bone marrow and ileal Peyer's patches are thought to be the principal mammalian organs where B cells develop.

T CELLS (T LYMPHOCYTES)

Mature T Cells Develop from Lymphoid Stem Cells That Have Migrated to the Thymus

Lymphoid stem cells that are destined to become T cells migrate to the thymus and are referred to as *thymocytes.* (The thymus extends approximately from the base of the trachea to the front of the heart.) The most recent immigrants from bone marrow arrive at the cortex of the thymus and lack important cell surface markers, such as T-cell receptors (TCRs), CD4, and CD8 markers,

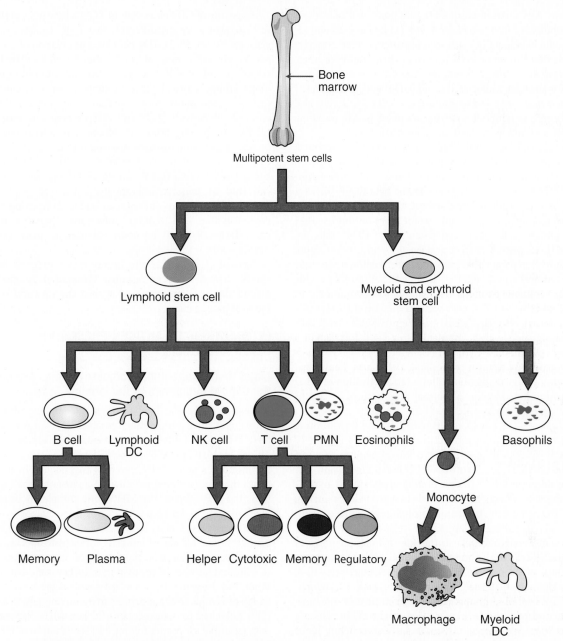

FIGURE 55-1 Lymphopoiesis: development of various types of lymphocytes. *DC,* Dendritic cell; *NK,* natural killer; *PMN,* polymorphonuclear neutrophil leukocytes.

which are essential for T-cell activation. These immature thymocytes undergo a highly complex and tightly regulated development and maturation process into mature T cells. During development the cells begin to acquire both CD4 and CD8 surface markers (double positive) and TCRs. As the cells further mature, they lose either CD4 or CD8 markers. CD4⁺/CD8⁺ cells that lose the CD8 marker become CD4⁺/CD8⁻ cells and are known as T-helper cells, whereas those double-positive cells that lose the CD4 marker become CD4⁻/CD8⁺ cells, or cytotoxic T cells.

The selection for survival of T cells during this developmental process is extremely stringent and discriminating. During development the thymocytes learn two important lessons: (1) T cells respond only to foreign antigens (positive selection), and (2) the cells will not respond to "self" antigens (negative selection). Learning these two critical lessons is essential for the survival of

the organism. Therefore, any developing thymocytes that deviate from learning these two key lessons are terminated by apoptosis (negative selection). Consequently, greater than 90% of developing thymocytes die within the thymus. Cells that are marked for intrathymic death include those cells that are defective (i.e., cannot bind to antigens or have truncated receptors) or autoreactive (bind strongly to "self" peptides). Thus, only competent, positively selected T cells (CD4⁺ or CD8⁺) are allowed to emigrate out of the thymus as T cells.

T Cells Are A Heterogeneous Population of Cytotoxic T Cells and T-Helper Cells

All T cells express a T-cell antigen receptor (TCR), CD28 and related molecules, and either CD4 (helper cells) or CD8 (cytotoxic cells). TCR specifically binds to antigenic peptides that are presented by APCs. Based on discrete functions of T cells, these cells are subdivided into two major types: (1) helper cells and (2) cytotoxic cells. T-helper (Th) cells secrete proteins called *cytokines* that act on other immune cells to provide help and coordinate immune responses. The cells express the CD4 receptor. These cells express the CD8 molecule (but not CD4) and have granules that are rich in serine esterase granzymes. Cytotoxic T cells also have perforins and lymphotoxins that are important in initiating cytotoxicity and killing infected and abnormal cells.

T-helper cells, based on the predominant cytokines secreted, are further divided into three major types: Th-1, Th-2, and Th-17. Th-1 cells predominantly secrete interleukin-2 (IL-2), interferon-gamma (IFN-γ), and tumor necrosis factor beta (TNF-β). Th-1 immunity is critical for defense against intracellular pathogens (viral, bacterial, or protozoal) and certain types of tumors. Th-1 cells are preferentially generated when naïve CD4$^+$ cells are exposed to IL-12, a cytokine from antigen-presenting cells (Figure 55-2). Failure to generate Th-1 cells creates susceptibility to these infections. Abnormal activation of Th-1 cells can result in a wide variety of inflammatory conditions, including autoimmune states.

Activation of naïve CD4$^+$ cells with interleukin-4 (IL-4) leads to differentiation into Th-2 cells (see Figure 55-2). Th-2 cells predominantly secrete IL-4, interleukin-6 (IL-6), interleukin-5 (IL-5), and interleukin-10 (IL-10). Generation of Th-2 cells is essential for defense against extracellular pathogens, neutralization of toxins and viruses in body fluids, and activation of other cells of the immune system. Abnormal regulation of Th-2 cells leads to allergies.

Activation of CD4 T-helper cells with IL-6 and transforming growth factor beta (TGFβ) induces the differentiation of Th-17 cells, which secrete a powerful pro-inflammatory cytokine, interleukin-17 (IL-17; see Figure 55-2). This cytokine is now recognized as an important mediator of inflammatory and autoimmune diseases. IL-17 acts on target cells to activate key signaling molecules to promote inflammation through several mechanisms including: (1) recruiting inflammatory cells (e.g., neutrophils, monocytes, and macrophages) to the site of inflammation; (2) acting on target cells (e.g., fibroblasts, epithelial cells) to stimulate a broad range of strong pro-inflammatory molecules (e.g., IL-6, monocyte chemotactic protein 1, nitric oxide); and (3) synergizing with TLR ligands. Although IL-17 is protective in infection, overproduction of IL-17 is known to aggravate certain disease conditions (e.g., autoimmune diseases such as systemic lupus erythematosus and multiple sclerosis).

Exposure of CD4 naïve cells to TGFβ alone (e.g., in the absence of IL-6) will drive the differentiation to T regulatory cells (Treg cells; see Figure 55-2). Treg cells are a population of T cells which act as powerful suppressors of the T cell-mediated immune response and of self-reactive T cells in autoimmune diseases. Tregs utilize a broad range of suppressive mechanisms which include release of immunosuppressive cytokines TGFβ and IL-10, and cell-cell contact. IL-10 and TGFβ secreted by Tregs are critical for dampening immune responses in allergy, burns, pregnancy, cancer, viral diseases, and autoimmune diseases. Treg cells can inhibit and downregulate all three (Th-1, Th-2, and Th-17) subsets of CD4 cells (see Figure 55-2). Dysregulation of Treg cells can lead to massive inflammatory diseases, while excessive numbers or functions of Tregs can lead to dampening of immune responses that lead to severe infections. Therefore, physiologically, Treg cells must be finely balanced to maintain immune health status.

Thus it is clear that the immune system must initiate the correct type of immune response to maintain homeostasis and defend the host appropriately against the invasion of different types of pathogens.

INTERACTIONS OF ANTIGEN-PRESENTING CELLS AND T CELLS

Major Histocompatibility Complex Proteins Are Considered the Central Regulators of the Immune System

Activation of specific T cells is highly dependent on interactions with major histocompatibility complex (MHC) proteins, which have a unique ability to bind to processed antigenic peptides. Therefore, MHC proteins are considered the central regulators of the immune system. MHC proteins are encoded by a number of genes that are clustered together on a chromosome and referred to as the *MHC locus*. The MHC gene complex is inherited as a block of genes and is known to encode three categories of proteins or antigens: class I, class II, and class III antigens. The number of genes that encode class I antigens varies from species to species, with a large number in humans (> 30) at one end of the spectrum to a limited number of genes in pigs, turkeys, and cheetahs at the other end. In general, all nucleated cells express class I antigen, which is a single α-chain peptide of approximately 45 kilodaltons (kD) linked to β2-microglobulin (a non-MHC protein thought to be essential for proper folding and stabilization of the α chain). Class I antigens can bind to peptides (e.g., viral peptides) and serve as receptors for CD8 molecules on cytotoxic T cells. Class I antigens have a high rate of mutation, but no recombination. These mutations allow class I antigens to alter their ability to bind to endogenous, processed antigenic peptides.

MHC Class I Antigens of Infected Nucleated Cells Play A Major Role in Activating Cytotoxic T Cells

Cytotoxic killing of intracellularly infected, cancer, or autoreactive cells is an essential step in survival by containing infected cells or the spread of deleterious cells. For example, a viral infection of any cell in the body yields to viral replication within the cell, and some of these viral peptides will physically bind to intracellular MHC class I antigens (Figure 55-3). This viral peptide–MHC class I complex is carried to the surface and displayed as an altered MHC class I molecule. TCR molecules of effector CD8$^+$ cytotoxic T cells will recognize the class I molecule–peptide complex to initiate cytotoxicity by at least four different, but complementary, mechanisms. First, contact of a cytotoxic CD8$^+$

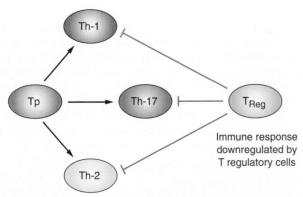

FIGURE 55-2 T precursor cells (Tp) differentiate into Th-1, Th-2, or Th-17 cells based on the cytokine signals. Generation of T regulatory (Treg) cells will inhibit all three types of cells to downregulate immune responses.

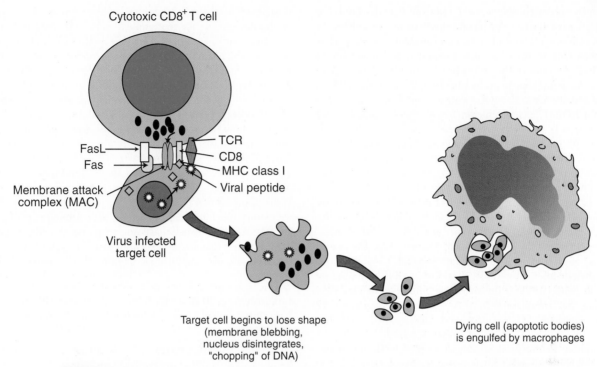

FIGURE 55-3 Mechanism of CD8-mediated cytotoxicity. *FasL,* Fas ligand; *MHC,* major histocompatibility complex; *TCR,* T-cell receptor.

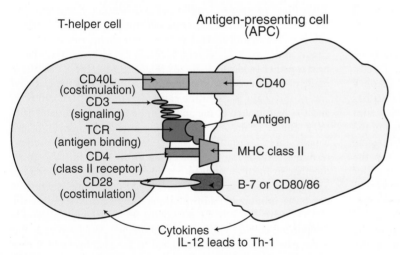

FIGURE 55-4 Interacting molecules of T-helper cells and antigen-presenting cells. *IL,* Interleukin; *MHC,* major histocompatibility complex; *TCR,* T-cell receptor; *Th-1,* T-helper cell type 1; *Th-2,* T-helper cell type 2.

cell with an infected cell that is displaying a MHC class I–peptide complex will immediately result in cytoplasmic reorganization within the CD8⁺ cell. This includes the alignment of granules and Golgi apparatus at the site of contact. Perforins in the cytotoxic cells polymerize to form tiny injectable tubes referred to as membrane attack complexes (MACs) that "drill" holes into the target cells. Granzymes are passed from the cytotoxic cells into the target cells through these perforin tubes to initiate apoptosis.

The other three mechanisms by which CD8⁺ cells induce apoptosis of target cells are (1) the secretion of lymphotoxin α (tumor necrosis factor alpha, TNF-α), which binds to its specific receptor on the target cells to initiate apoptosis; (2) the interactions of CD95 ligand on T cells with the CD95 "death" receptor on target cells; and (3) secretion of granulysin, an antibacterial peptide found in granules that activates lipid-degrading enzymes

(sphingomyelinases). This in turn results in an increase in saponins, including ceramide, which increase apoptosis. Granulysin kills not only infected target cells, but also bacteria, thus containing the infection.

MHC Class II Antigens on Antigen-Presenting Cells Play A Major Role in Selective Activation of T-Helper Cells

The expression of cell surface MHC class II antigens is highly restricted. They are only present on select types of cells including dendritic cells, select macrophages, B cells, and keratinocytes. The presence of class II antigens on their surfaces endows these cells with a unique ability to present antigens to CD4⁺ Th cells (Figure 55-4). Therefore these cells are called professional APCs. Class II antigens are two-chain molecules composed of a glycoprotein, 33-kD α chain and a shorter, 27-kD β chain that form a groove onto which processed (exogenous) antigenic peptides bind. For example, when a macrophage phagocytoses an antigen and breaks it down into peptides within a vacuole, intracellular MHC class II antigens bind to these processed peptides, and this complex moves to the surface of the cell to be presented to CD4+ T cells. The processed antigenic peptide specifically binds to the TCR on T cells, and the class II MHC proteins (on APCs) specifically interact with the CD4 molecule on T cells. These interactions are the first steps in activation of Th cells. Activation of T cells is highly regulated because their inadvertent activation has profound and widespread consequences; the cytokines secreted by activated Th cells can affect a wide range of both lymphoid and nonlymphoid cells.

Activation of CD4+ T cells requires at least two signals for activation. The primary activation signal determines the specificity through interactions of antigenic peptides and MHC molecules on APCs with the TCR/CD3 complex on T cells. The second signal is referred to as a *co-stimulatory signal*. Co-stimulatory signals include interaction of CD28 and/or CD40L, both residing on T cells, with CD80/86 and/or CD40, both residing on APCs. Cytokines that are released from APCs, such as interleukin-12 (IL-12), interleukin-18 (IL-18), and interleukin-27 (IL-27), promote the generation of a Th-1 subset of cells.

Activation of T cells is strictly controlled, with two major restrictions. First, T cells cannot recognize free antigens; rather, they recognize short peptides that are a product of processed antigens by the APCs. Second, the processed antigen must be physically associated with the MHC molecules. This results in molecular interactions of antigenic peptide bond to MHC class I or class II molecules on cells or APCs, with the TCR and CD8, or TCR and CD4 on T cells, respectively.

As mentioned, T cells will specifically interact with antigenic peptides through specific recognition by the TCR on T cells, analogous to the B-cell receptor (BCR) on B cells. The TCR on T cells belongs to the immunoglobulin superfamily and thus has variable and constant regions along with transmembrane and cytosolic domains. Similar to B cells, the variable portion of the TCR chain determines the specific binding to the antigenic peptide. Because more antigens exist in the universe than the actual number of T cells, these cells have adapted a variety of molecular mechanisms to interact specifically with an innumerable number of antigens. These mechanisms include recombination of TCR genes (similar to the BCR), unequal sister-chromatid exchange, and nucleotide insertion at various locations of the variable gene segments. An important difference between the TCR and BCR is that the TCR does not undergo somatic mutation. If the TCR could undergo somatic mutation, there would be an increased chance of inadvertently generating a TCR reactive against "self" antigens, resulting in devastating autoimmune conditions. This attribute is critical for survival because T cells, unlike B cells, can affect a large number of diverse lymphoid and nonlymphoid cells through secretion of cytokines.

ANTIBODIES

Initial Exposure to Foreign Antigen Induces Slow Onset of Antibody Appearance, Whereas Subsequent Exposure Induces Faster, Longer-Lasting Antibody Appearance

The exposure of an animal to a foreign antigen usually elicits a specific immune response. This response may involve the production of (1) specifically reactive T cells or (2) antibodies able to bind specifically with the foreign antigen. Typically, if an animal is exposed to a particular foreign antigen for the first time, no antibodies specific for that antigen will be detected in blood or secretions for several days. This "lag" period can last for up to 1 week, at which time antibodies capable of binding to the antigen appear in circulation and start increasing in quantity for the next 2 or 3 weeks. After that time, antibody quantities plateau and eventually decrease until they essentially disappear. The amount of antibodies produced and the duration of the response depend greatly on the nature of the antigen, quantity and route of exposure, and whether the antigen is given in combination with immune enhancers (adjuvants).

The type of response obtained after a first exposure to a specific antigen is called the primary immune response (Figure 55-5). If the animal is reexposed to the antigen, the lag period is very short, much higher levels of specific antibodies are obtained, and the response usually lasts for a significantly longer period. This response to a second exposure to an antigen is called a secondary immune response or anamnestic (memory) immune response.

Antibodies, or Immunoglobulins, Are Glycoprotein Molecules That Can Be Divided into Five Isotypes, or Classes

Antibodies are glycoprotein molecules that are the products of B lymphocytes. Antibodies, also called immunoglobulins, are basically made of four glycoprotein molecules. They are found on the surface of B cells, where they serve as antigen receptors (BCRs), or free in blood and secretions after being secreted by B cells. These free, or soluble, antibodies can neutralize antigens and assist in their removal. The basic structure of an antibody molecule has two identical short glycoprotein chains called light (L) chains and two identical longer chains called heavy (H) chains held together by disulfide bonds (Figure 55-6). The L chains are made of two halves, or domains; the half located at the carboxyl end of the chain is called the constant part of the L chain (C_L), and the half located at the amino end is called the variable part (V_L). The H chain is made of one variable domain (V_H) and usually three constant domains (CH_1, CH_2, CH_3). The amino terminal ends of the L chain (V_L) and the H chain (V_H) come together to form an antigen-binding or combining site (Figure 55-7). Therefore, two identical antigen-combining sites exist per basic immunoglobulin molecule. The carboxyl end of the two H chains form the Fc portion of the molecules; this end is the portion able to bind to Fc receptors on specialized cells and is the part of the molecule attached to the membrane of B cells when the immunoglobulin serves as the antigen receptor (BCR) for the cell.

Depending on molecular weight and other characteristics, immunoglobulins can be divided into classes, or isotypes. Basically, there are five isotypes: IgM, IgG, IgA, IgE, and IgD. Soluble immunoglobulin M (IgM) consists of five basic antibody molecules that bind together by disulfide bonds and an additional short protein chain to form a pentamer. Therefore, one IgM molecule has 10 identical antigen-combining sites. Its molecular weight is about 900 kD. In primary immune responses, IgM is the predominant immunoglobulin. Because of its large size, IgM is rarely found in body fluids other than blood. The BCR form of IgM is a monomer of 180 kD.

Immunoglobulin G (IgG) has the structure of the basic antibody molecule (monomer) previously described, and its molecular weight is 180 kD. IgG has two antigen-combining sites and is the predominant immunoglobulin detected in the secondary

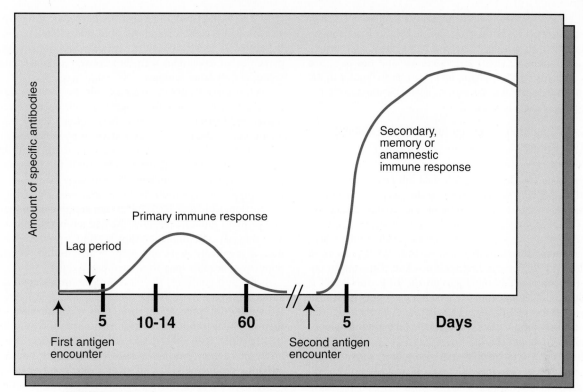

FIGURE 55-5 General dynamics and characteristics of the primary and secondary antibody responses.

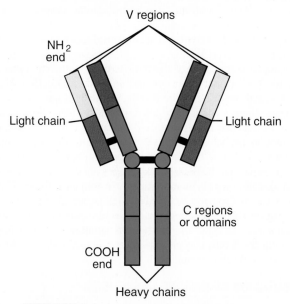

FIGURE 55-6 Basic structure of an antibody molecule.

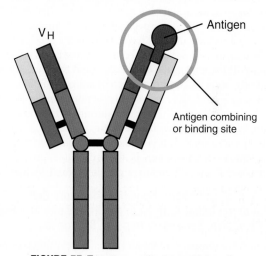

FIGURE 55-7 Antigen-antibody combining site.

immune response. It is able to move out of the circulatory system and appears in body fluids and also in secretions.

Immunoglobulin A (IgA) is found in small amounts in circulation as a monomer and in much larger amounts in secretions, where it is found as the predominant immunoglobulin and primarily as a dimer. It is produced by plasma cells (mature B cells) located under body surfaces such as skin, mammary glands, and the intestinal, respiratory, genital, and urinary tracts. IgA is found in secretions and has an attached secretory molecule that protects

IgA from intestinal proteases. Secretory IgA is the main immunoglobulin found on mucosal surfaces and has four antigen-combining sites in its dimeric structure. Its main role is to prevent antigen from attaching to these surfaces. Thus, IgA blocks penetration of antigen into the body. IgA responses are mainly elicited if antigen exposure is through contact with mucosal surfaces, such as the upper respiratory and intestinal tracts. IgM and IgG responses are elicited through parenteral contact with antigen (intradermal, subcutaneous, intramuscular, and systemic routes).

Immunoglobulin E (IgE) is a monomer, and its H chain contains four constant domains in addition to the variable domain. It is found in very low levels systemically, and most IgE is bound to basophils and mast cells (inflammatory and allergic reaction mediators) through its Fc portion. IgE is able to bind antigen while attached to these cells, thereby eliciting allergic reactions.

Immunoglobulin D (IgD) is a monomer and has only two constant domains on its H chain. IgD is primarily bound to the membrane of B cells and is secreted in negligible amounts in the serum. Negligible IgD is secreted.

The B-Cell Population Produces Antibodies to Millions of Different Antigens, Yet the Antibody-Antigen Interaction Is Specific

Antibodies bind to antigen through their antigen-binding sites. Each antigen-binding site is formed by the steric interaction of the V_L and V_H domains, which come in close contact because of the three-dimensional folding of the glycoprotein chains on which they reside. This steric interaction essentially forms a cleft, and any antigenic structure that fits into this cleft is recognized and binds to the antigen-binding site. Therefore, if an antigen can bind to the antigen-combining site on the BCR, the B cell is eventually (after a complex set of signal interactions) triggered to replicate (clonally expand), giving rise to many "identical" B cells, which eventually produce and secrete the soluble immunoglobulin specific for that antigen.

It is important to stress that antibody-antigen responses are specific. Antibodies produced after exposure to an antigen will only bind to that antigen or to other antigens structurally similar to the original antigen (cross-reaction). The question is, "how does the immune system manage to respond to literally several million different foreign antigens in a specific way?" Three facts are crucial to understand this situation. First, the BCR is an immunoglobulin, and the specificity of the immunoglobulin secreted by a particular B cell is the same as the specificity of its BCR. Second, an individual B cell can only have BCRs of identical specificity. Third, essentially each B cell (and there are millions) in the body has a BCR with a different antigen-combining site, because B cells undergo random genetic mutations in the genes coding for their V_L and V_H domains during their early development (ontogeny). Because these domains make up the antigen-combining site, a single amino acid change in either of the regions changes the steric interaction of these domains, giving rise to different "clefts" with different antigen-combining abilities.

Expansion of an Antigen-Specific B–Memory Cell Population on Initial Antigen Exposure Results in a Faster, More Pervasive, Secondary Immune Response

As the host is exposed to a foreign antigen, all existing B cells that have a BCR capable of binding the foreign antigen are able to react to such an antigen. Initially, among the millions of different B cells, the BCR of a few will bind to the antigen. This binding allows those matching B cells to multiply, creating many more B cells with the same BCR. This rather rapid expansion of antigen-specific B cells is often referred to as specific clonal expansion. The newly generated B cells start producing specific antibodies and secreting them. Specific antibodies begin appearing in circulation, and as clonal expansion increases, the quantity of specific antibodies in circulation increases. All B cells start their specific antibody production by producing IgM isotypes. Given the right milieu (e.g., appropriate sequence of signals), B cells stop producing IgM and switch production to IgG or another isotype (IgA or IgE). For example, IL-4 secreted by Th-2 cells will induce the switch from IgM to IgE. On the other hand, T regulatory cells (Treg) can block the production of cytokines from Th-1 and Th-2

cells, which could lead to the decrease of specific antibody isotype switching in B cells. It is important to understand, however, that the antigenic specificity of the antibody does not change. These dynamics are consistent with those observed in a primary and secondary immune response.

As the host encounters an antigen for the first time, few of the existing B cells are able to recognize it, but once the antigen is recognized by those few B cells, they undergo clonal expansion. Therefore, antibody production starts increasing, shows up in circulation, and IgM predominates during the primary immune response. The long "lag" period represents the time needed to process significant numbers of antibody-producing B cells through clonal expansion. Some B cells start switching to IgG production, which is why some IgG appears during the later parts of a primary immune response. As antigen is neutralized by the antibodies, B-cell stimulation stops, antibody production declines until it eventually stops, and many B cells within the expanded population become long-lived memory B cells.

If the host confronts the same antigen for a second time, the antigen is recognized by the vastly expanded, antigen-specific B–memory cell population, many cells of which have switched their antibody production capability to an isotype other than IgM, mainly IgG. This expanded cell population starts antibody production quickly because of the larger population of antibody-producing cells and greater likelihood of being in an IgG-producing state. The lag period is therefore very short, and a large amount of IgG is produced, typical of a secondary immune response. Eventually, as in a primary immune response, clonal expansion stops, and antibody production decreases and eventually stops. Future confrontations with the same antigen will lead to secondary immune responses, which are characterized by short "lag periods" and high sustained production of IgG or other isotypes (IgA or IgE).

Antigen stimulation of the BCR is not a sufficient signal to initiate B-cell clonal expansion and antibody production. Many other signals must reach the B cell after its BCR has recognized antigen. These signals, often represented by interleukins, come from Th cells that have recognized the antigen through complex interaction mechanisms with APCs (see earlier discussion). Interestingly, B cells that have bound antigen through their BCR and have internalized the BCR-bound antigen are also able to interact with Th cells, helping them to recognize antigen. A B cell–T cell interaction is also necessary for B cells to switch their production from IgM to other isotypes. The B cells must interact with interleukins from Th cells. The timing and nature of the interleukins reaching the B cells play an important role in deciding to which isotype the B cell is switching.

REGULATION OF IMMUNE RESPONSES

The Actions, Secretions, and Surface Molecule Expression of Immune Cells Play an Important Role in Regulation of the Body's Immune Response

When the antigen is cleared by antibodies or T cells, it is imperative that the immune response return to its normal state to maintain homeostasis. Failure to downregulate the heightened immune reactivity will likely result in a number of pathological conditions, including autoimmunity, lymphoid tumors, allergies, amyloidosis, and abortion. The body has multiple mechanisms to downregulate the immune system. Immune cells themselves secrete various biomolecules that downregulate immune activity. These include prostaglandin E_1 (PGE_1), which increases cyclic adenosine monophosphate (cAMP) to suppress physiological activity of cells. As previously noted, immune cells also secrete cytokines, such as TGF-β and IL-10, which downregulate immune responses. The importance of these cytokines in downregulating immune responses is evident in the immune-mediated inflammation that results in mice with a deleted TGF-β gene. Antibodies themselves can downregulate their immune responses by binding to Fc receptors on B cells. This cross-ligation of Fc receptors results in delivery of inhibitory signals. Immune responses are antigen driven, so clearing of antigen by immune mechanisms leads to a decrease in antigenic load and thus diminishes the antigen-induced activation of lymphocytes.

As mentioned earlier, activation of T cells requires at least two signals. The second signal is altered by the increased secretion of molecules or the T cells that deliver a negative signal to dampen T-cell activation. Important in this regard are the aforementioned, recently discovered Treg cells, a small percentage of T cells (< 5%) that are CD4$^+$/CD25$^+$/FoxP3$^+$ and that have powerful downregulatory effects. The importance of these cells in downregulation of immune responses is evident because defects in these cells lead to widespread autoimmune diseases in many experimental models. Conversely, administration of Treg cells leads to prevention of inflammatory attacks. These cells hold promise in understanding the biology of immunoregulation and in therapy of various inflammatory diseases. There is a growing body of knowledge on these subsets of T cells in domestic animals.

CLINICAL CORRELATIONS

UNTHRIFTY FOAL

History. You are presented with a 4-week-old Arabian filly for depression, coughing, and nasal discharge. The foal was born with no apparent problems. Immunoglobulin levels were checked and were normal. However, the foal has been unhealthy and seems to be repeatedly sick with skin and respiratory infections.

Clinical Examination. The foal has a temperature of 38.8° C (102° F) (elevated), heart rate of 60 beats/min (elevated), and a respiratory rate of 48 breaths/min (elevated). On auscultation the foal has both crackles and wheezes (abnormal lung sounds). The capillary refill time (CRT) is prolonged, and the mucous membranes are darker pink than normal. The foal also has some abrasions and cellulitis in these areas on the skin.

Comment. With the increased temperature, abnormal lung sounds, poor perfusion (prolonged CRT, darker-than-normal mucous membranes), and increased respiratory rate, this foal probably has a respiratory infection, most likely bacterial in origin. Additionally, based on the skin abrasions, the filly probably has a skin infection, which is uncommon in normal, healthy foals. Based on the age, breed, and recurrent infections, this foal likely has combined immunodeficiency (CID), a genetic autosomal recessive disorder. Foals with CID have a defect in a DNA-dependent protein kinase. This results in inability to produce mature B and T cells. As a result, the foal's immune responses are limited. A normally functioning innate response is present, composed of neutrophils, macrophages, dendritic cells, and NK cells, but a normal adaptive immune response is lacking. The B cells do not make antibodies, and insufficient T cells are present to produce cytokines to help with the immune response and control infection. This foal

has evidence of recurrent infections based on the history and appears to have concurrent skin and respiratory infections on presentation.

Foals with this type of history, including those with low lymphocyte counts and low immunoglobulin levels, are suspect candidates for CID. However, a definitive diagnosis is based on genetic testing and necropsy. Typically, foals with CID have rudimentary thymuses and lymph nodes because of the lack of lymphocytes and germinal centers. The spleen is usually reduced in size as well.

Treatment. Because CID is a genetic disorder that the filly cannot overcome, the prognosis is poor. In many cases, until a definitive diagnosis is made, these foals are treated with antibiotics for the infection. When a definitive diagnosis is made based on genetic testing, however, the foals are usually euthanized because of the poor long-term prognosis for life.

PRACTICE QUESTIONS

1. On their surface, T cells have:
   a. T-cell antigen receptor.
   b. CD3 molecules.
   c. CD4 or CD8.
   d. CD28 molecules.
   e. All the above.
   f. Both a and b.

2. Which of the following statements is correct with regard to CD4$^+$ T cells?
   a. They are regarded as a suppressor/cytotoxic type of T cell.
   b. CD4 molecule on T cells is a receptor for class I molecules on antigen-presenting cells.
   c. They provide help to T, B, and NK cells and to macrophages by secreting critical cytokines such as IL-2.
   d. CD4 molecules recognize CD8.
   e. CD4 molecules bind to class I MHC.

3. Which of the following is correct concerning cytotoxic cells?
   a. Viral-infected target cells undergo necrotic cell death by cytotoxic cells.
   b. Cytotoxic cells release granzymes (through holes "drilled" by perforin) into target cells.
   c. Cytotoxic cells express CD4 molecules but lack TCR.
   d. Cytotoxic cells do not secrete interferon-γ and are not T cells.

4. Cytotoxic T cells can kill their target cells through:
   a. Perforins and granzymes.
   b. Phagocytosis.
   c. Respiratory burst.
   d. All of the above.
   e. None of the above.

5. A simple antibody molecule consists of:
   a. One heavy chain and one light chain.
   b. Two heavy chains and two light chains bound by peptide bonds.
   c. Two heavy chains and two light chains bound by dipeptide bonds.
   d. Two heavy chains and two light chains bound by disulfide bonds.

6. Which of the following is correct regarding primary and secondary antibody response?
   a. Primary response has a short lag phase, rapid exponential phase, short steady/peak phase, and slow decline.
   b. Secondary response has a long lag phase, slow exponential phase, short steady/peak phase, and slow decline.
   c. Primary response has a long lag phase, slow exponential phase, short steady/peak phase, and rapid decline.
   d. Secondary response has a short lag phase, slow exponential phase, long steady phase, and slow decline.

BIBLIOGRAPHY

Abbas AK, Lichtman AH: *Cellular and molecular immunology*, ed 7, Philadelphia, 2012, Saunders.

Delves PJ, Martin SJ, Burton DR, Roitt IM: *Essential immunology*, ed 12, Malden, Mass, 2011, Blackwell.

Janeway C: *Immunobiology: the immune system in health and disease*, ed 8, New York, 2011, Garland Science.

Jonuleit H, Tuettenberg A, Steinbrink K: Research in practice: regulatory T cells—targets for therapeutic approaches? *J Dtsch Dermatol Ges* 9(1):8–11, 2011.

LeRoith T, Ahmed S: Regulatory T cells and viral disease. In Khatami M, editor: *Open access book project; inflammatory diseases/book 1*, Rijeka, Croatia, 2011, INTECH Open Access Publisher.

Parham P: *The immune system*, ed 3, New York, 2009, Garland Science.

Rao CV: *Immunology: a textbook*, Harrow, UK, 2005, Alpha Science.

Sakaguchi S: Regulatory T cells: history and perspective, *Methods Mol Biol* 707:3–17, 2011.

Tizzard IR: *Veterinary immunology: an introduction*, ed 8, Philadelphia, 2008, Saunders.

Chapter 1	1 b	2 c	3 d	4 b	5 d	
Chapter 2	1 d	2 b	3 b	4 e	5 c	

Chapter 3	1 d	2 a	3 c	4 d		
Chapter 4	1 e	2 c	3 a	4 b	5 a	
Chapter 5	1 b	2 d	3 c	4 b	5 a	
Chapter 6	1 d	2 a	3 d	4 c	5 d	6 b
Chapter 7	1 c	2 c	3 a	4 c	5 d	
Chapter 8	1 a	2 c	3 b	4 d		
Chapter 9	1 c	2 a	3 c	4 a	5 e	6 e
Chapter 10	1 c	2 e	3 b	4 c	5 e	6 a
Chapter 11	1 c	2 b,e	3 c	4 a	5 c,e	
Chapter 12	1 c	2 b	3 e	4 b	5 a	
Chapter 13	1 d	2 b	3 a	4 e	5 a	
Chapter 14	1 b	2 a	3 c	4 d	5 c	
Chapter 15	1 a	2 c	3 a	4 e	5 a,e	
Chapter 16	1 c	2 d	3 c	4 a	5 a	
Chapter 17	1 d	2 c,e	3 b	4 c	5 a	

Chapter 18	1 c	2 e	3 a	4 a	5 e	6 e
	7 b					
Chapter 19	1 e	2 a	3 c	4 b	5 d	6 c
	7 b					
Chapter 20	1 b	2 b	3 e	4 d	5 a	
Chapter 21	1 b	2 d	3 e	4 e	5 a	
Chapter 22	1 d	2 b	3 e	4 c	5 a	6 a
Chapter 23	1 d	2 a	3 a	4 c	5 b	
Chapter 24	1 d	2 b	3 c	4 a	5 b	6 d
Chapter 25	1 a	2 e	3 b	4 c	5 a	
Chapter 26	1 b	2 d	3 c	4 e	5 e	

Chapter 27	1 b	2 c	3 c	4 a	5 d	6 d
	7 b	8 c	9 d			
Chapter 28	1 d	2 d	3 b	4 c	5 e	6 d
	7 d	8 a	9 c	10 b	11 d	
Chapter 29	1 d	2 a	3 b	4 a	5 c	
Chapter 30	1 b	2 c	3 e	4 b	5 a	6 c
Chapter 31	1 d	2 c	3 a	4 c	5 d	
Chapter 32	1 c	2 d	3 e	4 b	5 a	

Chapter 33	1 c	2 c	3 c	4 e	5 b	
Chapter 34	1 a	2 c	3 b	4 d	5 d	

Chapter 35	1 d	2 d	3 d	4 c	5 c	
Chapter 36	1 b	2 b	3 a	4 e	5 c	
Chapter 37	1 e	2 e	3 c	4 e	5 f	6 f
Chapter 38	1 a,c,d,e,f	2 b	3 c	4 e	5 f	
Chapter 39	1 d	2 d	3 b	4 c	5 c	
Chapter 40	1 c	2 b	3 d	4 d	5 e	

Chapter 41	1 c	2 d	3 a	4 d	5 e	
Chapter 42	1 a	2 d	3 d	4 e	5 a,b	
Chapter 43	1 a	2 e	3 c	4 d	5 e	
Chapter 44	1 c	2 a	3 a	4 c	5 e	

Chapter 45	1 e	2 b	3 d	4 c	5 e	6 b
	7 e	8 c	9 e			
Chapter 46	1 d	2 e	3 a	4 b	5 c	
Chapter 47	1 a	2 d	3 a	4 a	5 c	6 d
Chapter 48	1 e	2 b	3 d	4 a	5 c	6 e
Chapter 49	1 b	2 a	3 d	4 a	5 a	6 b
Chapter 50	1 d	2 d	3 c	4 b	5 a	

Chapter 51	1 b	2 d	3 d	4 e	5 a	6 b
	7 c					
Chapter 52	1 a	2 d	3 c	4 b	5 e	6 d
Chapter 53	1 b	2 d	3 c	4 e	5 d	

Chapter 54	1 c	2 a	3 e	4 c		
Chapter 55	1 e	2 c	3 c	4 a	5 d	6 c

INDEX

Page numbers followed by "f" indicate figures, "t" indicate tables, and "b" indicate boxes.